Multiple Sclerosis as a Neuronal Disease

Multiple Sclerosis as a Neuronal Disease

Edited by

Stephen G. Waxman, M.D., Ph.D.

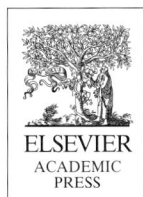

ELSEVIER
ACADEMIC
PRESS

Amsterdam • Boston • Heidelberg • London • New York • Oxford • Paris • San Diego
San Francisco • Singapore • Sydney • Tokyo

Elsevier Academic Press
300 Corporate Drive, Suite 400, Burlington, MA 01803, USA
525 B Street, Suite 1900, San Diego, California 92101-4495, USA
84 Theobald's Road, London WC1X 8RR, UK

This book is printed on acid-free paper. ∞

Library of Congress Cataloging-in-Publication Data

Multiple sclerosis as a neuronal disease / edited by Stephen G. Waxman.
    p. ; cm.
  Includes bibliographical references and index.
  ISBN 0-12-738761-7 (alk. paper)
  1. Multiple sclerosis–Pathophysiology. 2. Neurons.
  [DNLM: 1. Multiple Sclerosis–physiopathology. 2. Neurons–pathology.
WL 360 M956373 2005] I. Waxman, Stephen G.
  RC377.M8445 2005
  616.8′34–dc22
                                      2004030224

British Library Cataloguing in Publication Data
A catalogue record for this book is available from the British Library

ISBN: 0-12-738761-7

For all information on all Academic Press publications
visit our Web site at www.academicpress.com

Printed in China
05 06 07 08 09   9 8 7 6 5 4 3 2 1

Contents

VI Other Aspects of Neuronal Injury in Multiple Sclerosis

VII Lessons from the Peripheral Nervous System

VIII Prognosis, Reparative Mechanisms, and Therapeutic Approaches

Preface

Although multiple sclerosis is a very frequent cause of neurologic disability in young adults, and despite the introduction of disease-modifying medications over the past decade, the etiology, pathogenesis, and pathophysiology of MS remain incompletely understood. We now know that MS is more than a demyelinating disorder, that neurons are injured in MS, and that MS affects more than white matter. But perhaps because it has been eclipsed by rapid advances in immunopathogenesis that have led to disease-modifying therapies, the neuron has been neglected as a player in MS.

This volume focuses on MS as a disease affecting neurons. It does not attempt to cover all aspects of MS, but rather emphasizes one particular perspective—that is, the *neuro*biology of multiple sclerosis—by examining what happens to neurons in MS. The propelling force for this sharp focus is simple: an understanding of the neuron as a target of the disease process, and the development of therapeutic strategies that can limit or prevent neuronal injury, is of critical importance not only in terms of pathogenesis and pathophysiology, but also in terms of therapy. If neurons are injured or die in multiple sclerosis, it is not necessarily bad news. We know a lot about neuronal injury and degeneration and, by interceding in the molecular cascades that lead to the dysfunction or death of neurons, it may be possible to slow or halt the development of disability in MS.

The concept that neurons are injured in MS is not new. It was recognized about a century ago by Charcot, Jakob, and Marburg; and Doinikow devoted an entire monograph to it in 1915. What *is* new is recognition that axonal degeneration occurs frequently in MS, that it occurs early in the course of the disease, and that it produces non-remitting deficits, thereby leading to disability. Also new is the beginning of an understanding of *how axons die* in multiple sclerosis; specific molecules and pathways have been indicted, providing hints about potential therapeutic strategies and about well-defined molecular targets. In parallel, magnetic resonance imaging and spectroscopy are providing new methods for the non-invasive assessment of the integrity of axons and neurons, so that biomarkers may soon be available for human trials of potential neuroprotective agents.

Axonal degeneration is not the sole response of neurons to the assaults that occur in MS. Neuronal apoptosis may occur, and requires study. Importantly, demyelinated axons can rebuild their membranes, in some cases via changes in ion channel organization that support restoration of impulse conduction after demyelination. But this is not the only change in ion channel expression that occurs: in addition, maladaptive changes in channel organization occur in models of MS and in MS, and these can contribute to conduction failure, to axonal degeneration, and to mis-tuning of neurons, which distorts their ability to reliably transmit information. This book examines all of these processes.

The title of the book, *Multiple Sclerosis as a Neuronal Disease*, is not meant to imply that MS is a *primary* neuronal disease (i.e., that neuronal injury precedes or triggers demyelination or glial cell injury). We do not yet know for sure whether neuronal injury is a primary or a secondary event. When we answer this question we will be in a better position to prevent loss of neurons, and loss of myelin, in MS. The emphasis, in this book, on the neurobiology of MS, moreover, is not intended to devalue immunobiological approaches. In fact, it is likely that neuroprotective strategies that directly target neurons may complement immunomodulatory interventions that act on immune cells and molecules, so that the two therapeutic approaches can be used in combination.

One overall goal of this book is to stimulate research on neuronal injury in MS. A second goal is to discuss the ways in which neuronal dysfunction and injury in MS might be forestalled or halted. A third goal is to attract additional neuroscientists to the battle against MS. This is, after all, a battle that will be won. By understanding the roles of neurons in MS, we will hopefully quicken the pace of progress.

ACKNOWLEDGMENTS

A small army of supporters is helping to propel research on multiple sclerosis. The research of each author in this volume has been supported by individuals, agencies, and organizations who share the goal of understanding, and then curing, MS. On behalf of all the contributors to this volume, I extend deep thanks to these partners. My own research program has been helped immeasurably by support from many agencies, organizations, and individuals, including the Department of Veterans Affairs, the National Multiple Sclerosis Society, the National Institutes of Health, the Paralyzed Veterans of America, the United Spinal Association, the Allen Charitable Trust, the Nancy Davis Foundation, Destination Cure, Dundas Flaherty, and Sandra Kulli.

This book could not have been written without the efforts of its authors, and to them I am deeply appreciative.

The editing of this book was made much easier by the expert support of Sheila MacMillan at Yale and Karen Dempsey at Elsevier, and I express deep thanks to both. Finally, I thank Jasna Markovac of Elsevier for encouragement throughout the writing of this volume.

Stephen G. Waxman, M.D., Ph.D.
New Haven, CT

Contributors

Mathias Bähr
Zentrum Neurologische Medizin Neurologie Georg-August-Universität Göttingen

Mark D. Baker
Department of Biology, University College, London

Narendra L. Banik
Department of Neurology, Medical University of South Carolina

Christopher T. Bever
Department of Neurology, University of Maryland Hospital

Scott Thomas Brady
Department of Anatomy/Cell Biology, University of Illinois at Chicago

Shing-Yan Chiu
Department of Physiology, University of Wisconsin Medical School

Theodore R. Cummins
Stark Neuroscience Research Institute, Indiana University School of Medicine

Gabriele C. DeLuca
Department of Clinical Neurology, University of Oxford

Ricarda Diem
Neurologische Universitätsklinik, University Hospital, Göttingen

Margaret M. Esiri
Departments of Neuropathology and Clinical Neurology Radcliffe Infirmary, University of Oxford

Massimo Filippi
Neuroimaging Research Unit, Department of Neuroscience, Scientific Institute and University Ospedale, San Raffaele

Elizabeth Fisher
Department of Biomedical Engineering, Lerner Research Institute, The Cleveland Clinic Foundation

Robert M. Gould
Department of Anatomy/Cell Biology, University of Illinois at Chicago

John W. Griffin
Department of Neurology; Departments of Neuroscience and Pathology, Johns Hopkins University, School of Medicine

Mary Kelly Guyton
Department of Microbiology and Immunology, Department of Neurology, Medical University of South Carolina

Claes Hildebrand
Department of Biomedicine and Surgery, Division of Cell Biology, Faculty of Health Science, University of Linkoping

Ahmet Hoke
Department of Neurology and Neuroscience; Neuromuscular Pathology Laboratory, Johns Hopkins University, School of Medicine

Charles L. Howe
Department of Neurology, Divison of Neuroimmunology, Mayo Clinic

Steve Jones
Department of Clinical Neurophysiology, National Hospital for Neurology and Neurosurgery

Katia Kazarinova-Noyes
Department of Community and Preventive Medicine, University of Rochester Medical Center

Grahame J. Kidd
Department of Neurosciences / NC30, Lerner Research Institute, The Cleveland Clinic Foundation

Jeffery D. Kocsis
Rehabilitation Research and Development, Veteran's Affairs, Connecticut Healthcare Systems, Inc.

Hans Lassmann
Institute of Brain Research, Division of
Neuroimmunology, Medical University of Vienna

Albert C. Lo
Neuroscience Research (127A), Veteran's Affairs,
Connecticut Healthcare Systems, Inc.

Paul M. Matthews
Oxford Centre for Functional Magnetic Resonance
Imaging of the Brain, John Radcliffe Hospital

Isabelle M. Medana
Nuffield Department of Clinical and Laboratory
Sciences, University of Oxford

David H. Miller
Department of Neuroinflammation, NMR Research
Unit, Institute of Neurology

Klaus-Armin Nave
Department of Neurogenetics, Max-Planck-Institute for
Experimental Medicine

Elior Peles
Department of Molecular Cell Biology, The Weizmann
Institute of Science

V. Hugh Perry
School of Biological Sciences, CNS Inflammation
Group, University of Southampton

John W. Peterson
Department of Neurosciences / NC30, Lerner Research
Institute, The Cleveland Clinic Foundation

Matthew Rasband
Neuroscience Department, University of Connecticut
Health Center

Swapan K. Ray
Department of Neurology, Medical University of South
Carolina

Maria A. Rocca
Neuroimaging Research Unit, Department of
Neuroscience, Scientific Institute and University
Ospedale, San Raffaele

Moses Rodriguez
Department of Neurology, Divison of
Neuroimmunology, Mayo Clinic

Richard A. Rudick
Mellen Center for Multiple Sclerosis Treatment and
Research, Department of Neurology, The Cleveland
Clinic Foundation

Masanori Sasaki
Rehabilitation Research and Development, Veteran's
Affairs, Connecticut Healthcare Systems, Inc.

Kazim A. Sheikh
Department of Neurology, Johns Hopkins University,
School of Medicine

Peter Shrager
Department of Neurobiology and Anatomy, University
of Rochester Medical Center

Mohseni Simin
Department of Biomedicine and Surgery, Division of
Cell Biology Faculty of Health Science, University of
Linkoping

William Simon
Department of Biochemistry and Biophysics, University
of Rochester Medical Center

Kenneth J. Smith
Division of Clinical Neurosciences, Department of
Neuroimmunology, Guy's, Kings' and St. Thomas'
Medical School, Guy's Campus

Eric A. Sribnick
Department of Neurology, Medical University
of South Carolina

Peter K. Stys
Division of Neuroscience, Ottawa Health Research
Institute

Bruce D. Trapp
Department of Neurosciences / NC30 , Lerner Research
Institute, The Cleveland Clinic Foundation

Stephen G. Waxman
Department of Neurology, Yale University School
of Medicine

Hauke Werner
Department of Neurogenetics, Max-Planck-Institute for
Experimental Medicine

J. M. Wingrave
Department of Neurology, Medical University of South
Carolina

1

The Structure of Myelinated Axons in the CNS

Claes Hildebrand, Ph.D.
Simin Mohseni, Ph.D.

I. Introduction

The myelinated nerve fiber is one of the most beautiful examples of how structure and function go hand-in-hand in biology. The axon, a slender living process from a single neuron, possesses the molecular apparatus for generating and propagating nerve impulses, one of the important information units that the nervous system uses to promote our survival. The myelin sheath, a living compacted membrane duplicature from a glial cell, helps to control the developmental, anatomical, and molecular differentiation of the axon into nodal, paranodal, juxtaparanodal, and undifferentiated internodal segments and isolates some segments of the axon electrically so that saltatory conduction becomes possible. The myelinated nerve fiber is designed by evolution to provide the body with a rapid and efficient transfer of

information from peripheral receptors to the central nervous system (CNS), from the CNS to peripheral effectors, and between different centers within the CNS. The two former functions are provided by peripheral nervous system (PNS)-type myelinated nerve fibers, and the latter function is mediated by CNS-type myelinated axons. The structure of PNS-type axons is relatively well understood today. However, the structure of myelinated axons in the CNS is less well appreciated. That type of knowledge is, of course, vital for an analysis of the function of CNS-type myelinated axons as well as for an understanding of the various diseases that affect CNS-type myelinated nerve fibers, such as multiple sclerosis (MS). Hence, the purpose of the present chapter is to provide the reader with an up-to-date survey of the structure of myelinated axons in the CNS.

II. The Myelinated Axon

The ability of the nervous system to generate and propagate repetitive nerve impulses at a high speed depends on the myelinated axon—a highly complex biological structure, which has been characterized as ". . . the most unique cytological feature in the animal kingdom . . ." (Fig. 1) (Schnapp and Mugnaini, 1978). A large myelinated axon represents an

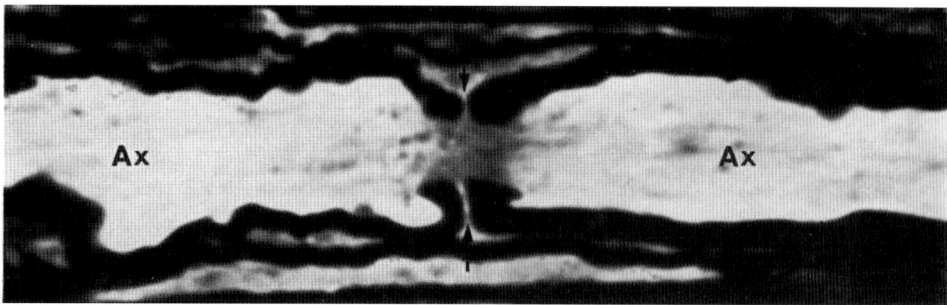

Figure 1 Light micrograph from a longitudinal section from adult cat spinal cord white matter showing a node-paranode-juxtaparanode region of a large fiber. The axon (Ax) is constricted at the node and the paranodes. Note the density of the nodal-paranodal axoplasm. The juxtaparanodal myelin sheaths turn in toward the axon and delimit a narrow and deep node gap (*arrows*) (×2,000). (With permission from Hildebrand, 1971.)

extraordinary union between cellular components with remarkable dimensions. A human S1 α-motoneuron with a diameter of 50 μm has a soma volume of about 65,400 μm³. The volume of the dendritic tree may amount to three to four times the soma volume (Ulfhake and Cullheim, 1988). If the axon has a diameter of 12.5 μm and a length of 1.3 meter (distance from the S1 segment to a plantar muscle), and disregarding the terminal branching of the axon, its volume is about 160 million μm³, 2,400 times the soma volume. If this axon has an average nodal spacing of 1,300 μm, there are altogether 1,000 mainly PNS-type myelin sheaths along its course. Assuming that the average myelin sheath has 119 lamellae, each outrolled sheath measures 1.3 × 5.5 = 7.1 mm². If we add all the myelin in the 1,000 internodes we get a strip of myelin that measures 1.3 × 5,500 mm. During the myelination period, oligodendrocytes synthesize myelin at a fast rate. It has been estimated that one oligodendrocyte produces 5,000 μm² of myelin membrane per day and 10^5 myelin protein molecules per minute (Pfeiffer et al., 1993). According to other calculations, a rat brain oligodendrocyte produces twice its own weight of myelin membrane per day at the peak of myelination (Norton and Poduslo, 1973; Norton and Cammer, 1984).

A. The Axon

PNS and CNS axons have a similar structure. Indeed, many axons (motor axons, preganglionic autonomic axons, primary sensory axons) course uninterrupted from the CNS to the PNS or vice versa. The axon membrane (the axolemma), which is about 8 nm thick, contains key molecules responsible for maintaining the resting potential and for action potential generation and propagation (voltage gated ionic channels, ion pumps, enzymes, cell adhesion molecules). Examination of the axolemma by freeze fracture electron microscopy (EM) shows that the outside of the inner leaflet (the P-face) displays numerous particles assumed to represent macromolecules. In unmyelinated axons, the inside of the outer leaflet (the E-face) presents

few particles. However, at initial axon segments and at nodes of Ranvier in myelinated axons, the E-face exhibits clusters of 10 nm particles, which may be related to sodium channels (Fig. 13; Rosenbluth, 1976, see further later). Subjacent to the axolemma there is a cytoskeletal cortex (Ichimura and Ellisman, 1991).

The axolemma encloses cytosol, axoplasmic organelles and inclusions. Axonal mitochondria are prominent among the organelles (Fig. 2). A typical axonal mitochondrion is 0.1 to 0.3 μm thick and 0.5 to more than 10 μm long, and the cristae are longitudinally oriented. In transverse sections the mitochondrial concentration varies from 2/μm² axoplasm in unmyelinated axons to 0.1/μm² axoplasm in myelinated axons. The axoplasmic reticulum, a system of membranous tubules (20 to 60 nm) and flattened sacs (<100 nm), extends from the axon hillock to the axon terminals (Fig. 2). It may be involved in slow anterograde transport and it acts as a reservoir for calcium ions (see Berthold and Rydmark, 1995).

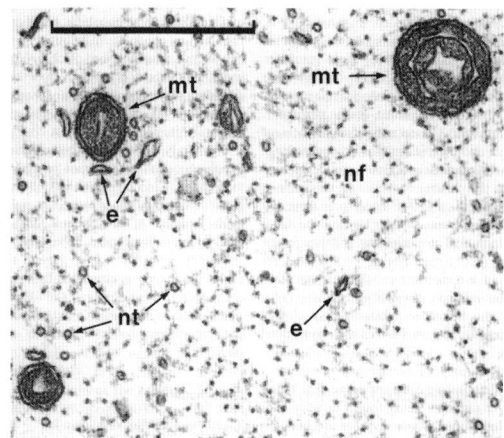

Figure 2 Electron micrograph showing axoplasm of a transversely sectioned large mammalian myelinated axon (nf = neurofilaments; nt = neurotubules; mt = mitochondria; e = axoplasmic reticulum). Scale bar = 0.5 μm. (With permission from Landon, 1981.)

The cytoskeleton includes microtubules, neurofilaments, and the microtrabecular matrix (Figs. 2 and 3). Axonal microtubules resemble microtubules elsewhere, that is, 25-nm, thick, unbranched discontinuous tubes. Thin axons have 100 microtubules/μm^2 cross-sectional area, and thick axons 10/μm^2. The average microtubule length seems to be relatively limited (Tsukita and Ishikawa, 1981: 370–760 μm; Bray and Bunge, 1981: 108 μm). They have a light core surrounded by a 6-nm thick wall composed of 13 protofilaments (Figs. 2 and 3). The filaments consist of tubulin subunits, each of which is a heterodimer of two globular proteins (α-tubulin and β-tubulin) bound together. The end of a microtubule pointing away from the cell body (the plus end, β subunits exposed) is where new monomers are added for growth. The other end (the minus end, α subunits exposed) is where monomers are removed for shortening. A major function of microtubules is to provide tracks for fast anterograde transport, mediated by kinesin, and fast retrograde transport mediated by dynein (see Berthold and Rydmark, 1995; Alberts et al., 2002).

Neurofilaments, 10-nm unbranched stable fibers of unknown length, belong to the family of intermediate filaments (Figs. 2 and 3). There are 150 to 300 neurofilaments/μm^2 axoplasm, independent of axon size (Hirano and Dembitzer, 1978). Three types of neurofilament protein (NF-L, 68 kD; NF-M, 150 kD; NF-H, 200 kD) coassemble *in vivo* to heteropolymers with NF-L plus one of the others. The neurofilaments are linked together by protein cross-bridges believed to contribute to the tensile strength of the axon and accounting for the regular interfilament spacing (Fig. 3)

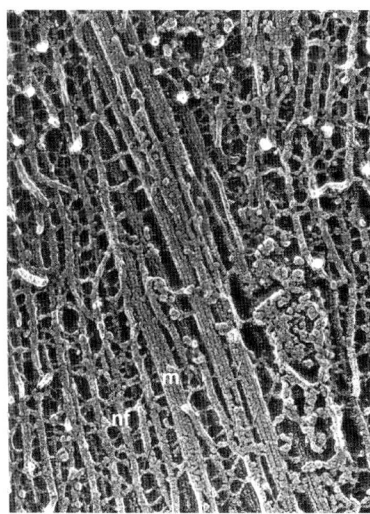

Figure 3 Electron micrograph showing part of an axon in a quick-frozen and deep-etched frog spinal nerve treated with saponin. Microtubules (m) and neurofilaments (nf) are shown. The microtubules, which were stabilized with taxol, run across the central part of the field in a bundle. The protofilaments are clearly visible. Some cross-bridges join adjacent microtubules. The neurofilaments are also linked by cross-bridges ($\times 200,000$). (With permission from Peters et al., 1991.)

(Alberts et al., 2002). There is ample evidence that axon diameter increases with increasing neurofilament number and with the degree of neurofilament phosphorylation. When neurofilament transport or assembly is prevented, axonal radial growth is much reduced. Phosphorylation induces neurofilaments to extend side arms that increase the filament spacing. Myelination promotes axon radial growth by causing an accumulation of neurofilaments and by induction of neurofilament phosphorylation (Starr et al., 1996; Yin et al., 1998; Jessen and Mirsky, 1999). In that respect, there is evidence that oligodendrocytes control the axonal phenotype in the same way as Schwann cells (Sanchez et al., 1996).

The microtrabecular matrix, which can be visualized with special techniques, is a network cross-linking neurofilaments, microtubules and membranous organelles (Fig. 3; Hirokawa, 1982; Schnapp and Reese, 1982; Hirokawa et al., 1984; Langford et al., 1987; Ichimura and Ellisman, 1991). Vesiculotubular membranous profiles act as transport vectors for newly synthesized protein and lipid and tend to accumulate proximal to a transport blockage (Ellisman et al., 1984). Finally the axon contains a few lamellated bodies and multivesicular bodies and various electron dense granules (Berthold and Rydmark, 1995).

B. The Myelin Sheath

1. Myelin Geometry

Most myelinated CNS axons are very thin. The critical diameter for myelination in the mammalian CNS is about 0.2 μm, whereas PNS axons myelinate at a diameter of approximately 1 μm (Waxman and Bennett, 1972). Both the radial and longitudinal dimensions of CNS myelin sheaths are coupled to axon diameter. The number of myelin lamellae is related to axon diameter according to a curvilinear function that varies among species (Fig. 4) (Hildebrand and Hahn, 1978). A mature CNS sheath may have up to 160 compacted lamellae. Conduction velocity is maximized when the g ratio (ratio axon diameter/fiber diameter [d/D]) is approximately 0.6, and this ratio is found in most myelinated mammalian CNS fibers (Waxman and Bennett, 1972). Since a single oligodendrocyte may produce sheaths with different numbers of myelin lamellae, the thickness of a myelin sheath seems to be regulated locally by the axon (Friedrich and Mugnaini, 1983; Waxman and Sims, 1984). One and the same oligodendrocyte can myelinate fibers in different tracts (Sternberger et al., 1978), and one cell can produce myelin sheaths spiralling in different directions (Remahl and Hildebrand, 1990; Waxman and Sims, 1984).

As in the PNS, the internodal length (L) of myelinated CNS axons increases with D, but CNS axons show a shorter and more variable L than PNS axons (Fig. 5). Older data from various species have been reviewed elsewhere (Blakemore, 1981; Hildebrand et al., 1993). Murray and

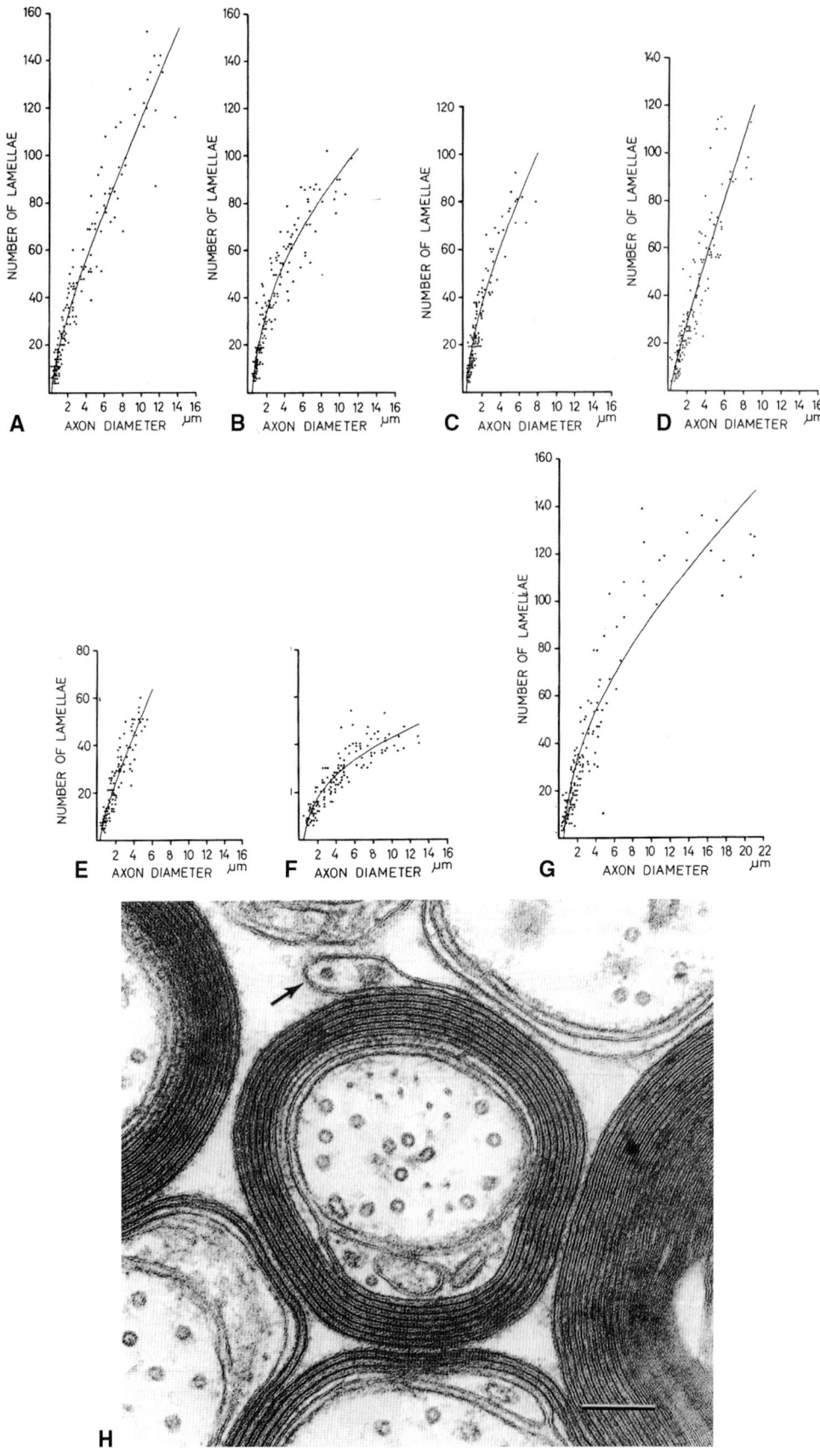

Figure 4 The relation between axon diameter and number of myelin lamellae in spinal cord white matter of various species; (**A**) cat, (**B**) rabbit, (**C**) rat, (**D**) guinea pig, (**E**) mouse, (**F**) frog, and (**G**) perch. (From Hildebrand and Hahn, 1978.) Electron micrograph showing a transversely sectioned thin myelinated axon with eight myelin lamellae in the canine spinal cord (**H**). The outer loop (*arrow*), the inner loop, the spiral nature of the myelin sheath, the alternating major and minor dense lines and the axonal cytoskeleton are apparent. Scale bar = 0.1 μm. (With permission from Raine, 1984a.)

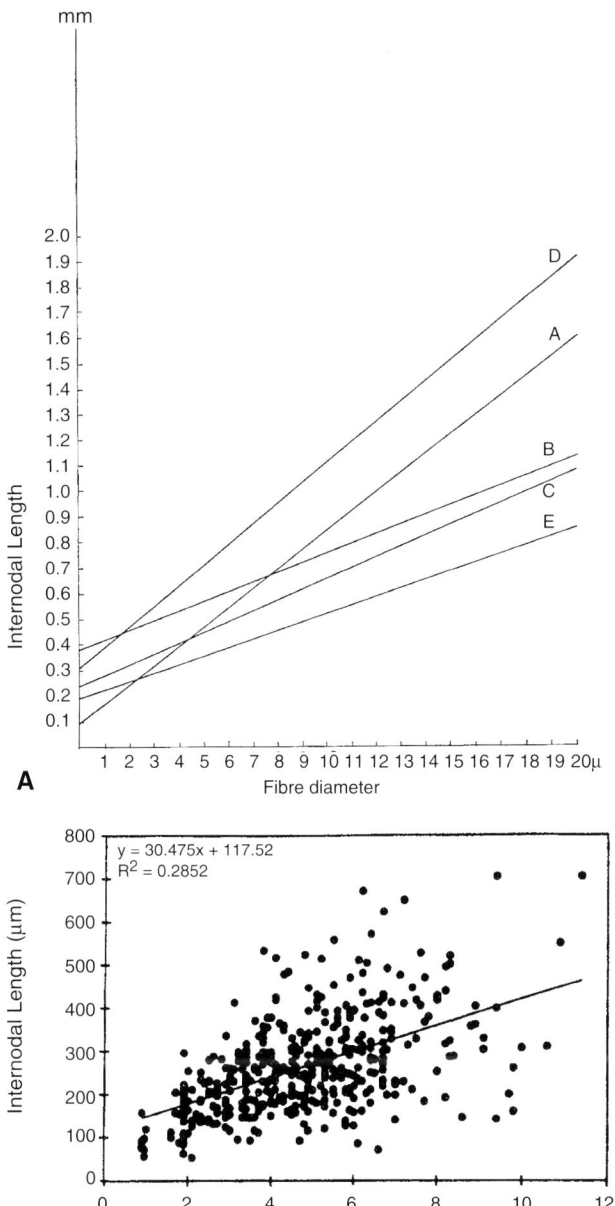

Figure 5 Regression lines describing the relation between internodal length (L) and fiber diameter (D) in teased preparations of cat spinal cord white matter, as described by different investigators (**A**). The line indicated by A refers to measurements of distances between intact nodes. The line indicated by D shows the observed relation when internodes bordered by broken nodes (heminodes) were also measured. The latter approach allowed observation of longer large-diameter internodes. (Modified from Murray and Blakemore, 1980, with permission.) (**B**) Scatterplot illustrating the relation L/D observed in myelinated axons in whole-mounts of the rat anterior medullary velum. Note that this regression line has a smaller slope than those shown in the top graph. (With permission from Ibrahim. et al. 1995.)

Blakemore (1980) noted that cat spinal cord fibers with a diameter of 3 μm have 300 μm long sheaths (range 100–600 μm), while fibers with a diameter of 20 μm possess 1,500 μm long internodes (range 1,100–2,000 μm; Fig. 5A). After dye injection of oligodendrocytes in the optic nerve of young rats, Butt and Ransom (1989) found 150 to 200 μm long myelin segments. In the anterior medullary velum (AMV) of the adult rat L is poorly correlated to D compared to spinal cord fibers. In the AMV the total range of D is 0.4 to 12 μm and L ranges between 50 and 750 μm. For thin fibers (D <1 μm) L varies around approximately 100 μm. For thick fibers (D = 9-10 μm) L varies around approximately 300 μm (Fig. 5B). The different relation L/D in the AMV compared to the spinal cord may be due to a different developmental length growth after myelination (Ibrahim et al., 1995; Butt et al., 1998a).

2. Myelin Fine Structure

Like PNS myelin, CNS myelin exhibits compact and cytoplasmic domains. In EM, the compact domains show alternating electron-dense and electron-lucent layers (Figs. 4H, 6A, B). The major dense line, or period line, forms where the cytoplasmic surfaces of the plasma membrane of the spiralling oligodendroglial process appose. The fused outer leaflets facing the extracellular space form the intraperiod line, or minor dense line, which sometimes is split (Figs. 4H, 6D; Hirano and Dembitzer, 1978). One major PNS/CNS difference is that the myelin repeating period (i.e., the distance between the midpoints of two successive major dense lines) is about 16 nm in fresh CNS myelin, but 18 nm in fresh PNS myelin (see Kirschner and Blaurock, 1992). In addition, the average CNS myelin period, but not the PNS counterpart, shrinks differentially during preparation for EM, so that it is 9 nm in thick sheaths, but 11 nm in thin sheaths (Hildebrand, 1972; Hildebrand and Muller, 1974) (Fig. 6D, E). This difference seems to reflect different effects of lipid solvents on thick and thin sheaths during dehydration and embedding. Another PNS/CNS dissimilarity is that myelinated CNS fibers lack a delimiting basal lamina. Since the outer surfaces of adjoining sheaths may appose each other directly, a minor dense line may sometimes form (Figs. 4H, 6B) (Peters et al., 1991).

In cross-sections the string-shaped cytoplasmic domains of a CNS myelin sheath show up as inner and outer loops (Fig. 4H). In thin myelinated CNS fibers, both loops are very small; but in large CNS fibers, and in all PNS fibers (see Peters et al., 1991), the outer loop may include the myelinating glial cell soma (Hildebrand, 1971). The other cytoplasmic domains in CNS sheaths—lateral or paranodal loops and incisures of Schmidt and Lanterman—are best seen in longitudinal sections. The paranodal loops represent expansions of the major dense line at the nodal end of each myelin lamella, which attach to the paranodal axon (Fig. 7B, C). Expansions of the major dense line in internodal parts of the myelin sheath stacked in sequence on top of each other form incisures of Schmidt and Lanterman. Although it has been stated that incisures are lacking in the CNS, many investigators (see Blakemore, 1969; Hildebrand et al., 1993) have noted Schmidt-Lanterman incisures in thick spinal cord fibers. All the cytoplasmic

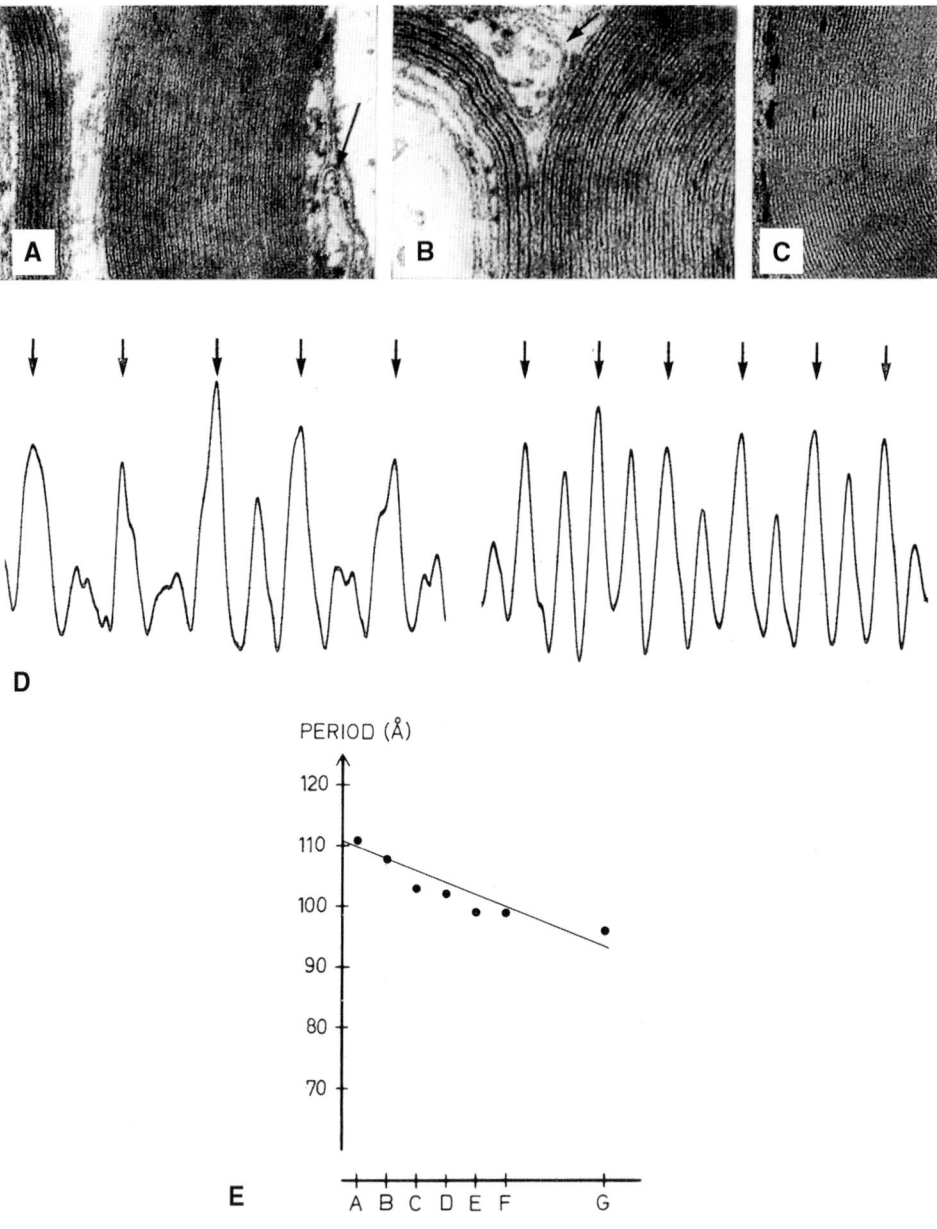

Figure 6 (**A, B**) Electron micrographs showing details of thin (*left*) and thick (*right*) myelin sheaths in cat white matter. Note the difference in period. (**C**) Aberrant uniform lamellar pattern that can be found in myelinoid bodies. (×113,000 [**A**] and ×124,000 [**B, C**]). (With permission from Hildebrand, 1971.) (**D**) Densitometric graphs made from high-magnification EM plates showing myelinated cat CNS fibers. The left graph shows the lamellar pattern in a thin sheath, and the right graph shows the pattern in a thick sheath. Arrows indicate deflections corresponding to major dense lines. (**E**) Mean myelin period in myelin sheaths with 0–10 (A), 11–20 (B), 21–30 (C), 31–40 (D), 41–50 (E), 51–60 (F), and >60 lamellae (G). (With permission from Hildebrand, 1972.)

strings contain microtubules. Longitudinally oriented tight junctions anchor the inner and outer loops to the myelin and seal the intramyelinic space. Paranodal and incisural junctions follow a transverse course (Raine, 1984a; Rosenbluth, 1984). In cross-cut myelinated CNS axons, the outer and inner loops tend to be located in the same quadrant. In the sector between the outer and inner loops CNS myelin may show a "radial component" (i.e., longitudinally oriented

junction strands at the extracellular apposition—an intramyelinic tight junction) (Fig. 7A; Peters, 1964; Dermietzel, 1974; Dermietzel et al., 1980; Shinowara et al., 1980; Kosaras and Kirschner, 1990).

The unrolled myelin sheath has a trapezoidal shape (Fig. 8). Compact myelin forms most of the trapezoid. The outer, inner, and paranodal loops form a continuous cytoplasmic string along the edge of the compact myelin plate.

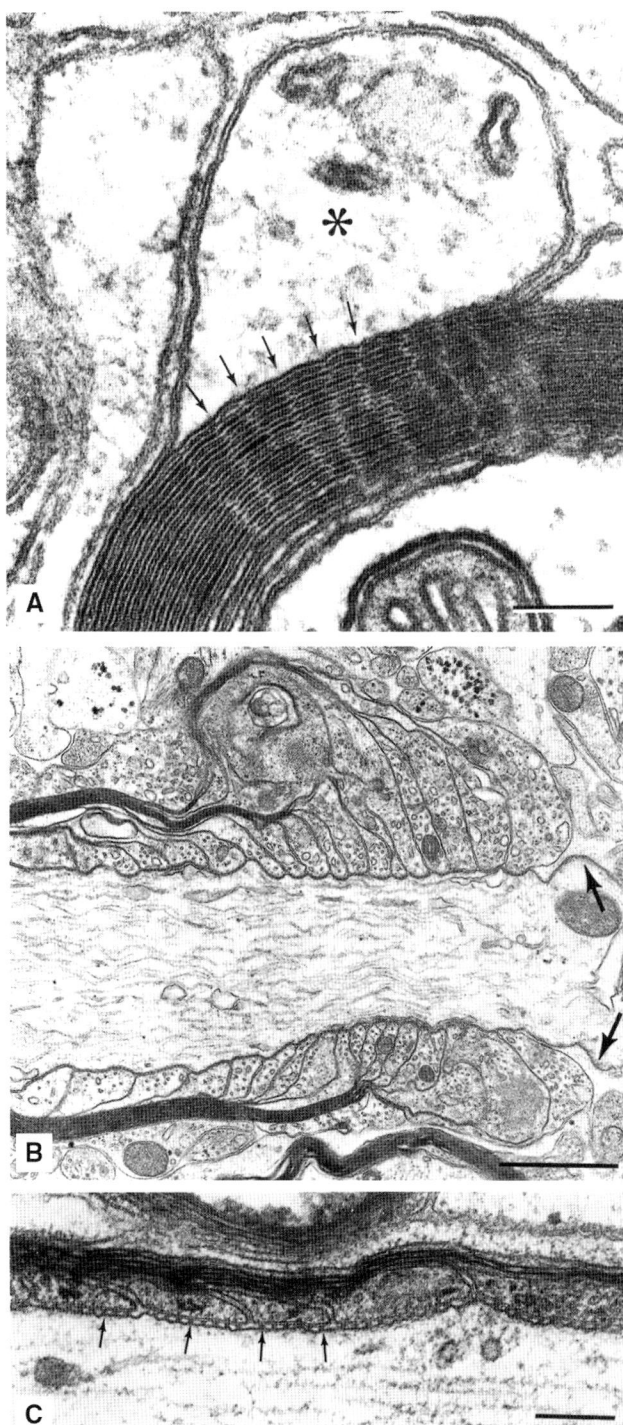

Figure 7 Electron micrographs showing details from myelinated CNS fibers. (**A**) Mouse white matter. Note radial component (*arrows*) below outer tongue (*). The radial component is composed of radially arranged tight junctions seen here as light zones where the minor dense line is narrowed. Scale bar = 0.1 µm. (With permission from Nagara and Suzuki, 1982.) (**B**) Node-paranode region of myelinated fiber in kitten spinal cord. Each myelin lamella terminates as a lateral loop apposing the axolemma. Arrows indicate nodal axolemma. Scale bar = 1 µm. (**C**) Paranode in mature small myelinated CNS fiber. Note the presence of regularly spaced densities (*arrows*), the so-called transverse bands, between the lateral loops and the axolemma. Scale bar = 0.2 µm. (With permission from Raine, 1984a.)

In large myelinated CNS fibers, the compact myelin plate is subdivided into subplates by cytoplasmic strings forming the incisures in the rolled sheath.

3. The Myelin-Oligodendrocyte Unit

When Del Rio Hortega studied oligodendrocytes in the early 1900s he recognized four subtypes (Types I-IV) without sharp boundaries, different types being associated to fibers of different diameters (Fig. 9) (reviewed by Bunge, 1968; Friedrich et al., 1980; Wood and Bunge, 1984; Hildebrand et al., 1993; Szuchet, 1995). This view was confirmed by Penfield (1932) and has been supplemented by EM data from the toad (Stensaas and Stensaas, 1968), the cat (Remahl and Hildebrand, 1990), and the rat (Bjartmar et al., 1994a), as well as by light microscopic observations on dye-injected rat oligodendrocytes (Butt et al., 1994a, 1998a, 1998b; Berry et al., 1995; Weruaga-Prieto et al., 1996). The Type I oligodendrocyte emits many thin radially directed processes, and Type II has fewer and thicker processes. Direct observations on stained myelin-oligodendrocyte units show that rodent optic nerve oligodendrocytes are Type I or II (Butt et al., 1994a). Rat and mouse optic nerve oligodendrocytes are linked to 15 to 20 internodes via 15- to 30-µm long processes (Fig. 10; Butt and Ransom, 1989, 1993; Butt et al., 1994a, 1994c). In the kitten corpus callosum Remahl and Hildebrand (1990) observed Type I/II cells connected to 4 to 11 myelin sheaths. The rat AMV contains thin myelinated axons linked to Type I/II cells as well as thick myelinated trochlear fibers (d = 4-15 µm), supplied by Type III or Type IV oligodendrocytes. In the AMV Type I/II, oligodendrocytes extend thin branching processes long distances (up to over 100 µm) to 5 to 18 fibers with a mean diameter of 1.25 µm. Type III cells are bipolar or tripolar and send processes to two to five fibers with a mean diameter of 3.5 µm (Fig. 11A). The Type IV unit has a Schwann cell-like anatomy, being associated with a single large myelinated fiber with a mean diameter of 6.2 µm (Fig. 11B; see Berry et al., 1995; Butt et al., 1998a, 1998b).

Whether immature oligodendrocytes are intrinsically committed to develop into a particular subtype or induced to develop into a specific phenotype by the axon or other external factors is unknown. Oligodendrocytes exhibit an axon-independent differentiation *in vitro*, ending up in process elaboration and production of myelin-like sheets (see Szuchet, 1995). Since oligodendrocytes from immature rat spinal cord and cerebrum, respectively, develop different process morphologies *in vitro*, in the absence of neurons, it was concluded that they follow dissimilar intrinsic programs (Bjartmar, 1998). On the other hand, Fanarraga and co-workers (1998) concluded from transplantation experiments that oligodendrocytes develop a Type I-IV anatomy depending on which axon they contact.

The amount of myelin produced by an oligodendrocyte varies strongly, depending on its subtype. Blakemore (1981) calculated that a single large CNS internode contains 400

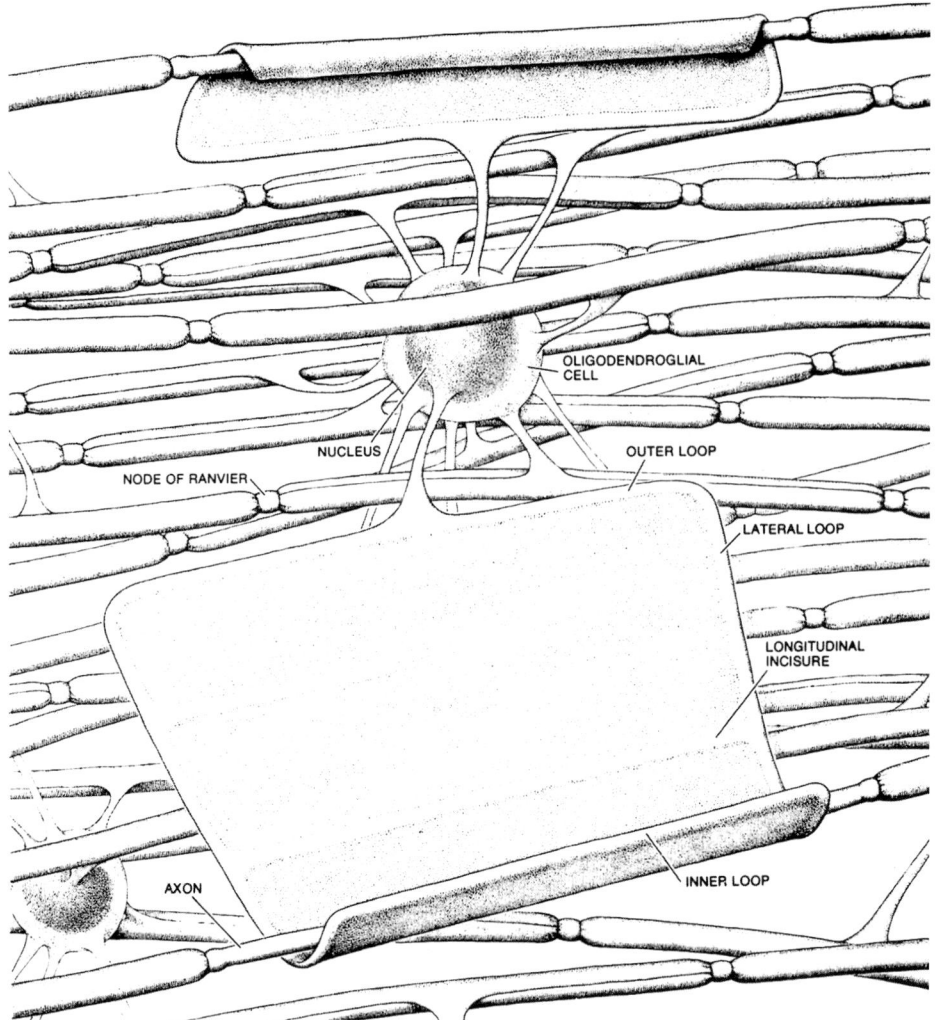

Figure 8 Type I/II oligodendroglial cell body (*top center*) attached to 14 myelin sheaths, two of which have been unrolled to varying degrees to show the arrangement of the cytoplasmic strings in the sheet of myelin. (With permission from Morell and Norton, 1980.)

times as much myelin as a single small internode. He also found that the volume of myelin supported by an oligodendrocyte providing one 11.4-μm thick axon with a 1,250-μm long myelin sheath is 10 times greater than the volume supported by a cell providing 39 thin (d = 1.5 μm) axons with 200-μm long sheaths. According to Butt et al. (1998a), the mean myelin volume amounts to 600 μm^3 in Type I/II units and 30,000 μm^3 in Type III/IV units in the AMV. If so, a Type III/IV cell maintains 50 times more myelin than a Type I/II cell. A third calculation (Anderson, 2003) indicates that a Type IV oligodendrocyte providing a 16-μm thick axon with a single thick long sheath maintains 100 times more myelin than a Type I cell with 50 thin short sheaths along 0.5-μm thick axons. These calculations show that Type IV cells produce and maintain a greater volume of myelin than Type I cells.

In addition to the occurrence of anatomical subtypes, adult oligodendroglial cells show a molecular heterogeneity. The chemical composition of bovine white matter areas con-

taining thick and thin myelinated fibers differs from the composition of areas with thin fibers only (Amaducci et al., 1962), and the chemical composition of spinal cord myelin differs from the composition of brain myelin (Norton and Camner, 1984). Further, myelin in rat white matter areas with both thin and thick fibers is more strongly myelin basic protein (MBP) immunoreactive than myelin in areas with thin fibers only. The reverse is valid for proteolipid protein (PLP) immunoreactivity (Hartman et al., 1982). More recently, Butt et al. (1995) showed that carbonic anhydrase II is present in Type I-II rat AMV oligodendrocytes, but not in Type III-IV oligodendrocytes. Moreover, the large isoform of myelin associated glycoprotein is present in all oligodendrocytes, but the small isoform is only present in Type III-IV cells (Butt et al., 1998b). Since various demyelinating toxic agents cause greater demyelination where carbonic anhydrase II is low than where it is high, presence or absence of this enzyme may be a key factor in the pathology of white matter (see Butt et al., 1995). Further, it seems pos-

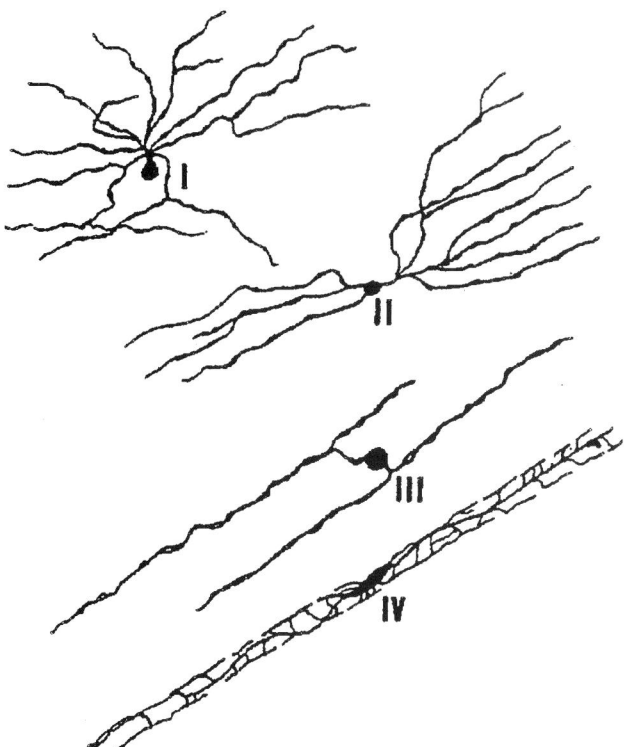

Figure 9 As described by Del Rio Hortega (1928), the oligodendroglial population includes four varieties, Types I–IV, in terms of number of processes and branching pattern. (With permission from Wood and Bunge, 1984.)

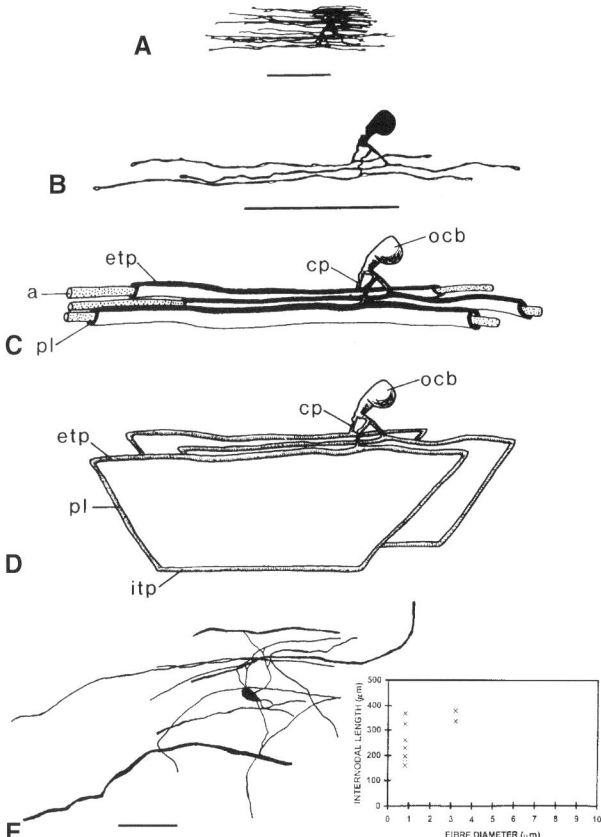

Figure 10 Camera lucida drawings showing an HRP-filled Type I oligodendrocyte in young rat optic nerve. (**A**) The whole cell. Scale bar = 100 µm. (**B**) Drawing at a higher magnification (×1,250) showing the cell body and three selected longitudinal processes. Scale bar = 100 µm. (**C**) Schematic interpretation of the parts of this cell seen in (**B**). (**D**) The picture shown in (**C**) would look like this if the myelin sheaths could be unwrapped. Each sheath has been transformed into a trapezoidal sheet bordered by strings of cytoplasm corresponding to the outer, the inner, and the lateral loop (a = axon, etp = outer loop, pl = lateral loop, itp = inner loop, ocb = oligodendroglial cell body, cp = connecting process). (Modified from Butt and Ransom, 1989, with permission.) (**E**) Camera lucida drawing showing a Type II oligodendrocyte in the adult rat medullary velum visualized by application of the antibody Rip to a velum whole mount. Diagram on the right side shows the relation L/D for the fibers in this unit. Scale bar = 50 µm. (With permission from Butt et al., 1998a.)

sible that a molecular heterogeneity of the type described might underlie the fact that tracts myelinating late (Type I/II cells) and early (Type III/IV cells), respectively, are differentially affected by some inborn errors of myelin metabolism, such as Krabbe's disease (Suzuki and Suzuki, 1983).

The cytoplasmic strings of the myelin sheath are used for distribution of myelin molecules. MBP and PLP are major components of CNS myelin. It turns out that MBP is synthesized near its site of assembly in the myelin sheath. This is accomplished by a trafficking of MBP mRNA along the string-related microtubules from the nucleus to the myelin compartment (Barbarese et al., 1999). Indeed, EM examination of oligodendrocytes *in vitro* and *in situ* reveals the presence of ribosome clusters in distal oligodendroglial processes (Waxman and Sims, 1984; Barry et al., 1996). As to the biological value of this RNA trafficking, various hypotheses have been discussed (see Barbarese et al., 1999). PLP, on the other hand, is synthesized on endoplasmic reticulum-bound ribosomes in the oligodendroglial cell body, shifted to the Golgi system via microtubules, and transferred to the myelin via transport vesicles budding off from transitional ER elements. In the mutant *taiep* rat, a microtubular defect causes a deficient incorporation of PLP into myelin through a blockage of membrane movement from the ER to the Golgi system, which causes abnormal myelination and progressive demyelination of CNS axons (Couve et al.,

1997). The microtubule defect is present in all oligodendrocytes, but the myelination problem affects mainly thin axons (Lunn et al., 1997; Song et al., 2001). Hence, the logistic functions mediated by the microtubular system might be more important in oligodendrocytes myelinating several thin axons than in cells with few myelin sheaths or a single one.

C. The Compound Myelinated Nerve Fiber

From a longitudinal point of view, the compound myelinated axon is organized into segments: the node, paranode, juxtaparanode and the unspecialized internodal segment. Each of these domains has a unique structure and carries unique molecules. A detailed account of the molecular

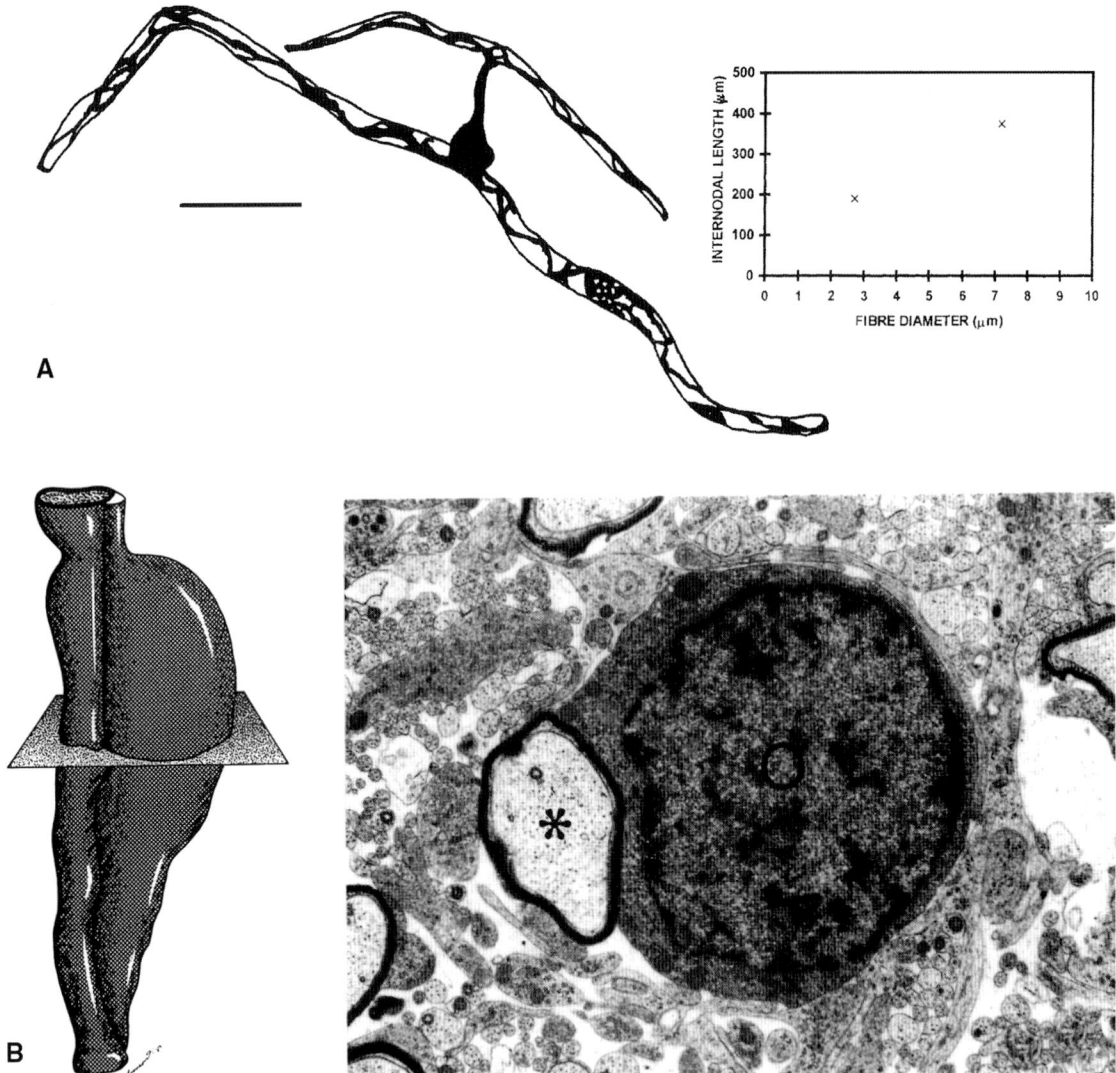

Figure 11 (**A**) Camera lucida drawing showing a Type III oligodendrocyte in the adult rat medullary velum. The oligodendrocyte was visualized by application of the antibody Rip to a velum whole mount. The diagram on the right side shows the relation L/D for the fibers in this unit. Scale bar = 50 μm. (With permission from Butt et al., 1998a.) (**B**) Type IV oligodendrocyte in fetal day 47 cat spinal cord white matter. The drawing to the left was made from an EM reconstruction based on serial thin sections. It shows a myelinating oligodendrocyte associated with a single axon. Note the close relation between the oligodendroglial perikaryon and the myelin sheath. Electron micrograph on the right side shows a transverse section through this unit at the level indicated in the drawing. Asterisk indicates axon. (×12,400). (With permission from Remahl and Hildebrand, 1990.)

anatomy of the oligodendrocyte-axon interface is presented elsewhere in this book.

1. Nodal Features

a. The Nodal Axon   Successive myelin sheaths are separated by short gaps, the nodes of Ranvier, where the axolemma is exposed to the extracellular space over a length of about 1 μm (Hildebrand, 1971; Hildebrand and Waxman, 1984; Peters et al., 1991), as in the PNS (Berthold and Rydmark, 1995). Longer nodes have been observed in preterminal-terminal CNS axon domains (see Peters et al., 1991). As at PNS nodes (Reles and Friede, 1991; Berthold and Rydmark, 1995) the cross-cut CNS nodal axon usually has a circular outline and is barrel-shaped in longitudinal

sections. The diameter of the nodal axon is less than the internodal diameter, particularly in the largest fibers, where the ratio between the nodal and the internodal diameter may be 1/3 (Fig. 12; Hildebrand, 1971).

A few spherical invaginations (75-85 nm) regularly occur in the nodal axolemma. In the nodal axoplasm microtubules and neurofilaments are relatively tightly packed, together with mitochondria, empty vesicles, some lamellated bodies, and small irregular membranous profiles (Fig. 12) (Hildebrand, 1971). In EM the nodal axolemma is very distinct because of the presence of a dense granular undercoating, which is 25 to 35 nm thick and separated from the axolemma by a 10-nm light zone (Fig. 12) (Hildebrand, 1971; Reles and Friede, 1991). The undercoating seems to

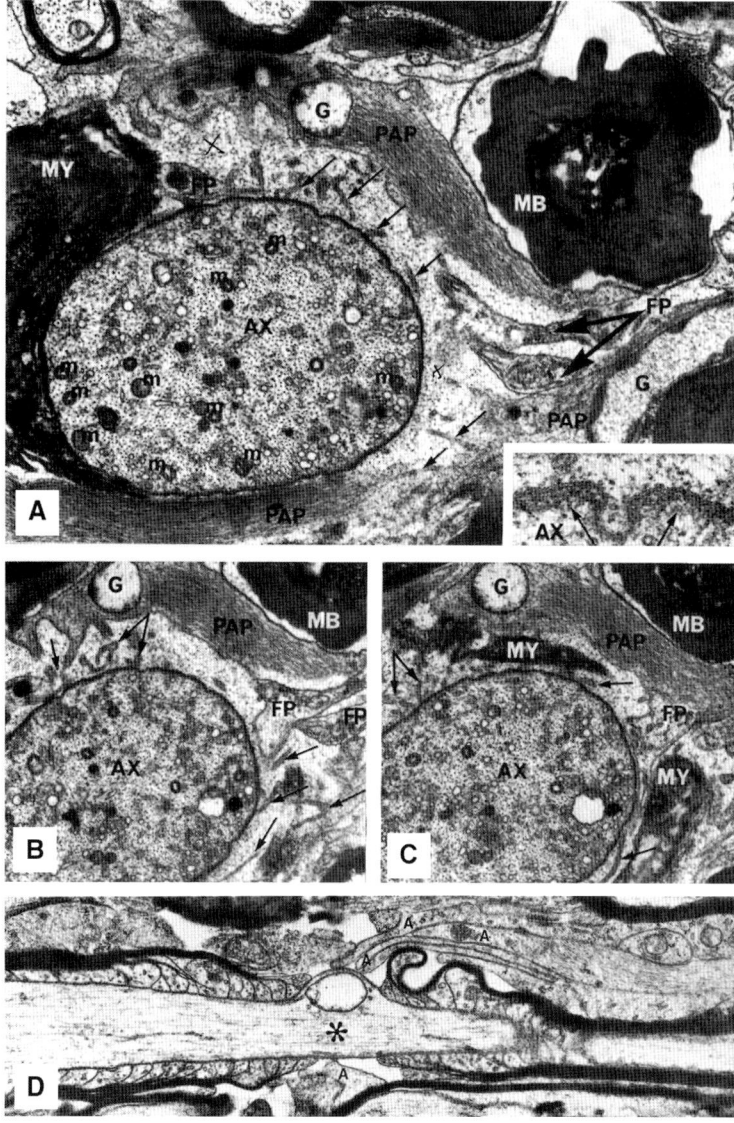

Figure 12 Electron micrographs from thin sections through nodes of Ranvier. (**A**) Transverse section through large node in cat spinal cord white matter. The nodal axon (AX) contains many vesicles and mitochondria (m) in addition to various other bodies. Note the close packing of microtubules and neurofilaments. The nodal axon membrane has a dense appearance. The axon is apposed by terminating myelin (MY) on the left side. The uncovered right side of the axon is surrounded by an extracellular material that separates the axon from perinodal astrocytic processes (PAP) containing filaments and gliosomes (G). The perinodal astrocytic processes emit microvilli-like processes (*small arrows*) and other processes (FP), which approach the nodal axolemma. Note presence of a myelinoid body (MB) in the upper right corner. (×17,400). Inset shows nodal axon membrane at a higher magnification (AX = axon). Arrows indicate a dense undercoating on the axoplasmic side of the axon membrane. (**B, C**) Later in the series of sections. (×13,800). (With permission from Hildebrand, 1971.) (**D**) Longitudinal section from node in a thin axon in a 30-day-old rat optic nerve. Asterisk indicates nodal axon. Note that the nodal axon is contacted by astrocytic processes (A). (×16,700). (With permission from Hildebrand and Waxman, 1984.)

represent a cytoskeletal anchoring for protein molecules in the nodal axolemma (Ellisman, 1979; Bray et al., 1981; Koenig and Repasky, 1986). Freeze-fracture EM studies show a high density (1,000-1,500 per μm^2) of large (>10 nm) particles in the E-face of the nodal axolemma, whereas the internodal axolemma (25-150 per μm^2) and the axolemma of unmyelinated axons (25-250 per μm^2) have a low density of such particles (Fig. 13) (Schnapp and Mugnaini, 1978; Rosenbluth, 1983; Waxman, 1984; Black et al., 1990; Waxman and Ritchie, 1993).

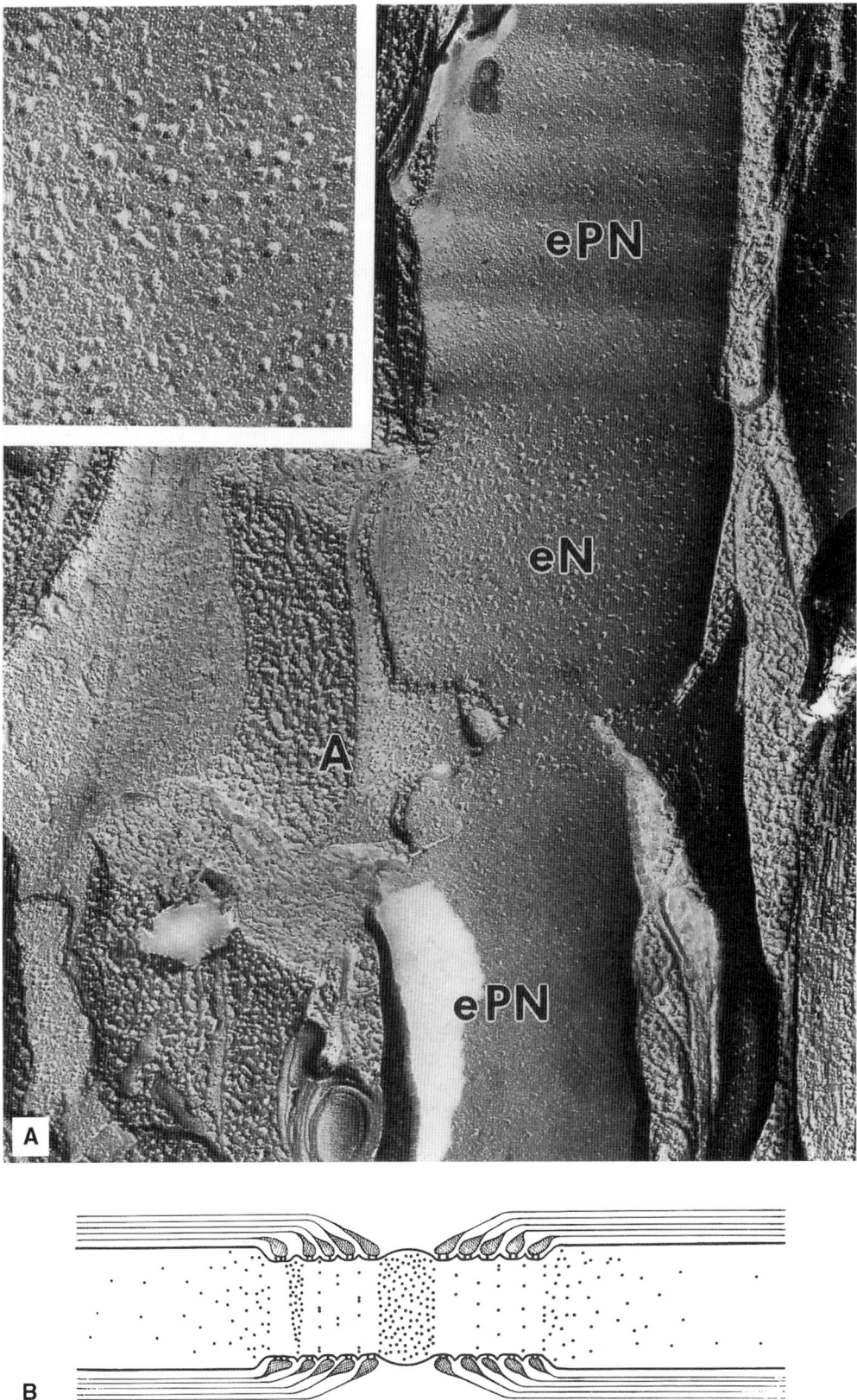

Figure 13 Freeze-fracture electron micrographs showing a node of Ranvier in the adult rat optic nerve. The fracture has exposed the E-face of the axon membrane, which exhibits numerous large particles at the node (eN), but not at the flanking paranodes (ePN). (**A**) Perinodal astrocytic process. (×70,000). Inset shows the E-face of the nodal axon membrane at a higher magnification. (×175,000). (With permission from Waxman and Black, 1995.) (**B**) Distribution of large intramembranous E-face particles (*black dots*) in the nodal-paranodal-juxtaparanodal region of a myelinated CNS axon. Note that such particles are enriched at the node. They also form linear strings in the paranodal region and occur in the juxtaparanode adjacent to the paranode. (Modified from Rosenbluth, 1989, with permission.)

Since the nodal axolemma exhibits a distinct Na$^+$ channel immunoreactivity and a high binding of the Na$^+$ channel probe saxitoxin (see Rosenbluth, 1983; Waxman and Ritchie 1993), it has been suggested that these particles may represent sodium channels (Rosenbluth, 1976, 1984; Kristol et al., 1978).

b. Nodal Adnexa   The perinodal astrocyte: When the diameter of a large CNS axon decreases as the node is approached, the emerging perinodal space becomes filled by fibrous astrocytic processes. Nodes of small myelinated CNS fibers decrease less in diameter and are less well shielded. EM analysis of CNS nodes shows that fingerlike or sheetlike astrocytic extensions course from the perinodal shield down to within 10 nm from the nodal axolemma (Fig. 12) (Hildebrand, 1971; Hildebrand and Waxman, 1984). There are gap junctions between perinodal astrocytic processes and nodal oligodendrocytic components (Massa and Mugnaini, 1982; Waxman and Black, 1984; Waxman, 1986). Large nodes have more nodal processes than small nodes, but the system of nodal astrocytic processes always remains less impressive than the elaborate collar of Schwann cell processes seen at medium-size and large PNS nodes (Bjartmar et al., 1994b). The perinodal astrocytic extensions, from which the nodal extensions emerge, contain filament bundles and occasional gliosomes (Fig. 12). A single astrocyte may send processes to more than one node, and a single node may receive processes from more than one astrocyte. Similar observations have been made on CNS nodes in the cat (Hildebrand, 1971), the rat (Hildebrand and Waxman, 1984; Butt et al., 1994b), the guinea pig (Raine, 1984b), the chicken (Anderson et al., 2000), reptiles and amphibia (Bodega et al., 1987, Sims et al., 1991), and in fish (Maggs and Scholes, 1990). For a comprehensive discussion of the molecular anatomy of the nodal glial processes see Black et al. (1990, 1995). It has been suggested that the nodal astrocytic processes produce and maintain the node gap substance (see later) and/or influence the ionic composition of the node gap. It has also been speculated that node-contacting glial cells might transfer glial Na$^+$ channels to the nodal axon membrane (Bevan et al., 1985; Gray and Ritchie, 1985). However, more recent evidence indicates that the clustering of sodium channels in the nodal axolemma is due to oligodendroglial signals (Kaplan et al., 1997).

The nodal NG2 immunoreactive cell: Rat CNS nodes of Ranvier are contacted by processes from fibrous astrocytes and glial cells expressing the NG2 (neuron-glial antigen 2) integral membrane chondroitin sulfate proteoglycan (Fig. 14) (Butt et al., 1999, 2002). The NG2 molecule has a large extracellular domain and interacts with other membrane molecules and extracellular matrix molecules. The NG2 cells are not astrocytes since they are devoid of GFAP (glial fibrillary acidic protein). Their expression of PDGFα

(platelet-derived growth factor α) receptors and the O4 antigen indicates that they may be related to immature oligodendrocytes (Fig. 15). Thus, NG2 cells are distinct from neurons, astrocytes, microglia, and mature oligodendrocytes, and they are at least as common as other glial types (Nishiyama et al., 1999; Nishiyama, 2001).

The CNS node of Ranvier is a meeting place for four different cell types: the neuron, the myelinating oligodendrocyte, the perinodal astrocyte, and the nodal NG2 cell. It has been suggested that nodal NG2 cells might participate in sodium channel clustering at nodes of Ranvier (Butt et al., 1999, 2002). After rat brain injury, NG2 cells proliferate and their NG2 expression increases (Levine, 1994). NG2 cells occur in MS lesions, and these cells proliferate and differentiate into myelinating cells in experimentally demyelinated areas. NG2 cells undergo reactive changes in inflammatory CNS conditions and occur in oligodendrogliomas (Nishiyama et al., 1999). Finally, NG2 cells in the hippocampus receive a glutamatergic synaptic input from CA3 pyramidal cells (Bergles et al., 2000; Nishiyama, 2001). The function of this neuronal-glial synapse remains an enigma (LoTurco, 2000).

The node gap substance: In EM images from CNS nodes of Ranvier, a granular extracellular material is present in the node gap (Figs. 12A-C) (Hildebrand, 1971; Hildebrand and Waxman, 1984; Raine, 1984b; Remahl and Hildebrand, 1985). Staining of sections from cat white matter according to a histochemical method for demonstration of polyanions (Langley and Landon, 1969) results in a reaction product at the nodes with a pattern that is very similar to that seen at rat PNS nodes (Fig. 16) (Langley and Landon, 1969; Hildebrand and Skoglund, 1971). A similar pattern is seen in adult rat white matter nodes of Ranvier after application of antibodies against chondroitin sulfate or J1 glycoprotein molecules (Bjartmar et al., 1994b). These antibodies seem to label the node gap substance. According to Langley (1969) and Zagoren (1984), the node gap substance at PNS nodes acts as a cationic exchange resin, being strategically present where ion exchange takes place during impulse propagation. Since the PNS and CNS node gap substance can be visualized with the same reagents, they may be chemically similar and might play analogous roles. One function of this component of the CNS node could be to control the nodal ionic milieu (Hildebrand and Skoglund, 1971). It may also counteract sprouting from the nodal axon (Faissner and Schachner, 1995) and/or anchor nodal glial processes to the node (Davis et al., 1996).

2. Paranodal Features

Each node is flanked by two paranodes, where the myelin lamellae attach to the paranodal axolemma. Some previous investigators, including Ranvier himself, used the term *paranode* to describe a longer part of the myelin sheath, including both the paranodal myelin attachment

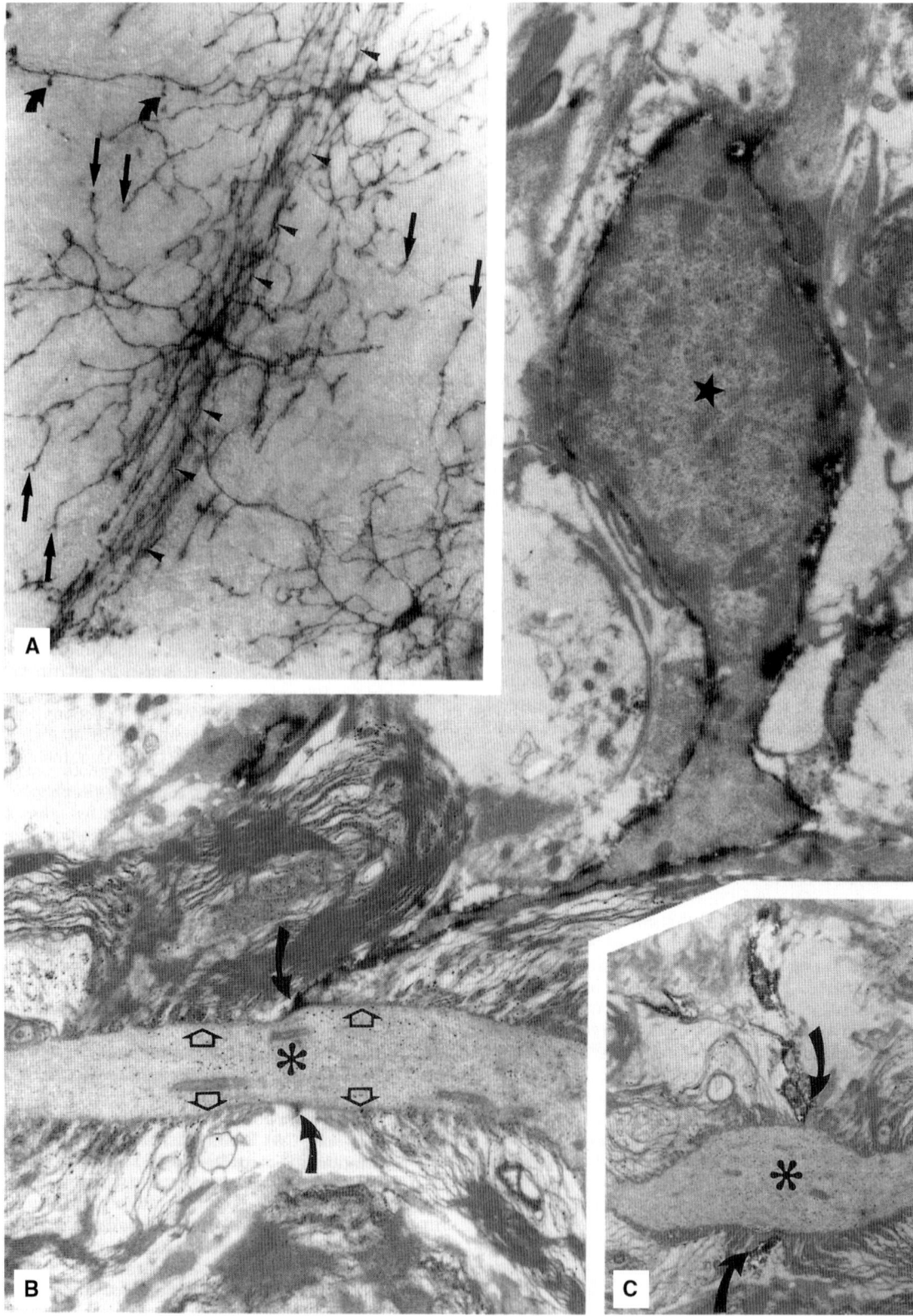

Figure 14 NG2[+] glial cells visualized light microscopically by immunoperoxidase staining of a whole mount of the rat anterior medullary velum (**A**) and by preembedding EM immunocytochemistry (**B, C**). (**A**) Two NG2[+] cells with a small soma and multiple branching primary processes, which either ramify along axon bundles (*arrowheads*) or terminate on individual axons (*arrows*). Some processes have spines that terminate on axons (*curved arrows*). (**B**) Electron micrograph showing an NG2[+] cell (star = nucleus). Note the immunoreactive membrane. This cell sends a process (*curved arrows*) to a node of Ranvier nearby (*asterisk, open arrows* indicate paranodes). (**C**) Node of Ranvier (*asterisk*) contacted by NG2[+] processes (*curved arrows*). ×330, ×10,600, and ×7,600, respectively, for **A**, **B,** and **C**. (With permission from Butt et al., 1999.)

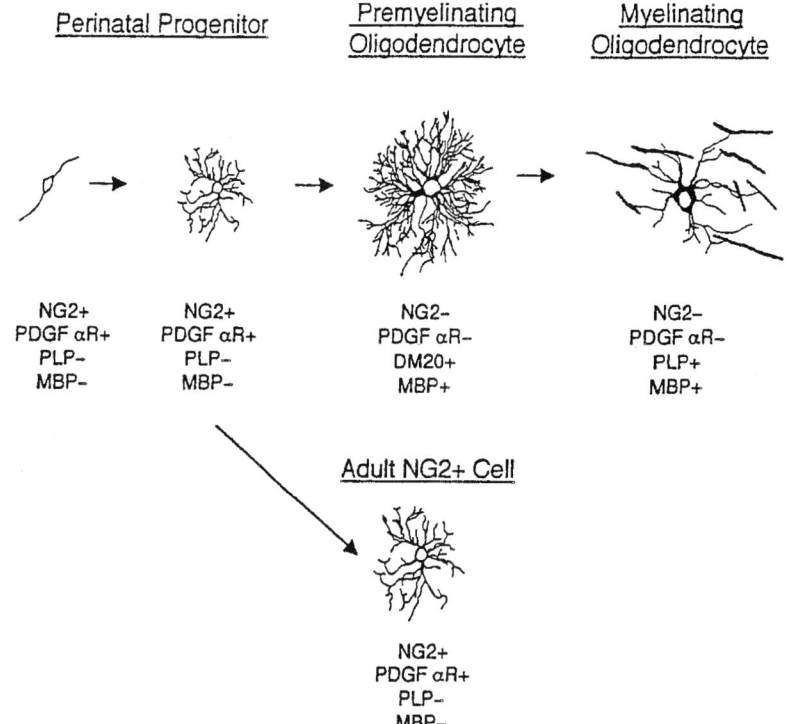

Perinatal Progenitor

NG2+
PDGF αR+
PLP–
MBP–

NG2+
PDGF αR+
PLP–
MBP–

Premyelinating
Oligodendrocyte

NG2–
PDGF αR–
DM20+
MBP+

Myelinating
Oligodendrocyte

NG2–
PDGF αR–
PLP+
MBP+

Adult NG2+ Cell

NG2+
PDGF αR+
PLP–
MBP–

Figure 15 Possible differentiation route for oligodendrocyte lineage cells. The neonatal and adult CNS contains numerous NG2$^+$ cells with PDGF α receptors, but those present in the adult do not proliferate as rapidly as the perinatal counterpart and do not readily differentiate into oligodendrocytes. They appear to be arrested at the NG2$^+$/PDGF αR stage and persist in the adult CNS. (With permission from Nishiyama et al., 1999.)

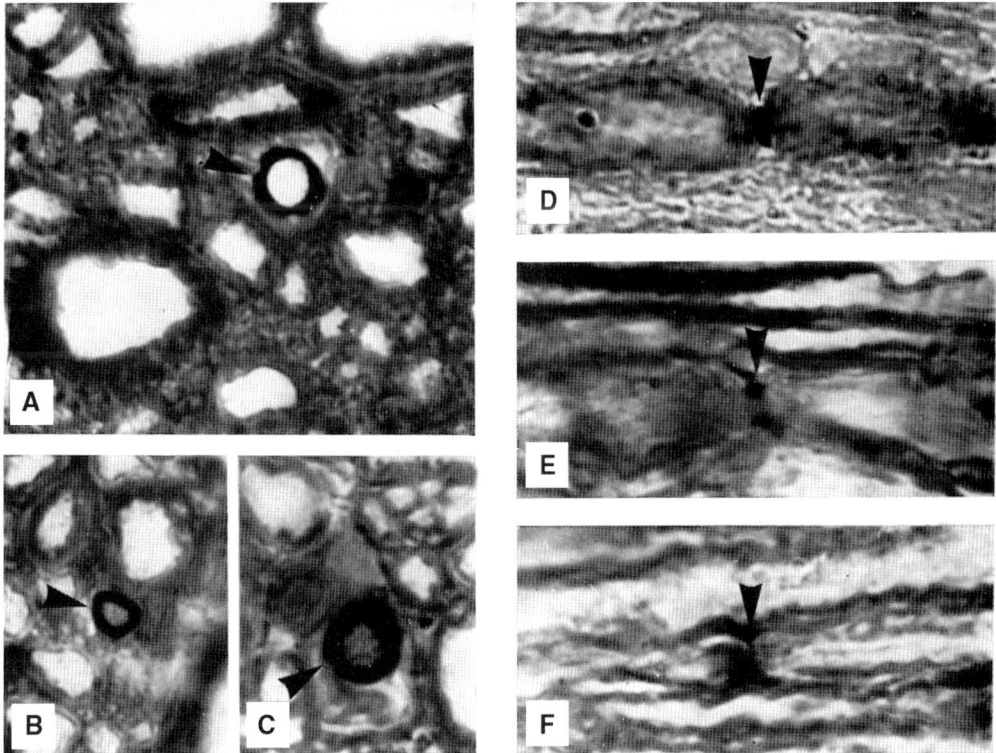

Figure 16 Transverse (**A, B, C**) and longitudinal (**D, E, F**) sections through nodes of Ranvier in glutaraldehyde-fixed and paraffin-embedded spinal cord white matter of the adult cat. The tissue was processed according to the procedure described by Langley and Landon (1969) for demonstration of the extracellular node gap substance in PNS nodes. Note distinct presence of reaction product in relation to nodes of Ranvier (*arrowheads*). (×1,500). (With permission from Hildebrand and Skoglund, 1971.)

zone and the juxtaparanode (Thomas et al., 1993). As seen in longitudinal sections, each myelin lamella terminates as a lateral loop (Figs. 7B and 13B). Here, the major dense line splits and forms a membrane-bounded drop-shaped cytoplasmic compartment containing a few microtubules, an occasional vesicle and varying amounts of electron-dense particles. In cat CNS fibers of all sizes, the lateral loops appose the paranodal part of the axon, on each side of the node, over a length of about 4 μm (Hildebrand, 1971). Since each loop occupies a specific length, the paranodal axon allows direct apposition of a limited number of loops. When the number of myelin lamellae exceeds that number, some loops pile up on top of each other forming the "spiny bracelets of Nageotte" (Hess and Young, 1952; Hildebrand, 1971). Adjacent loops are linked to one another through tight junctions, which separate the extracellular compartment inside myelin from the general extracellular space (Kosaras and Kirschner, 1990).

Relative to the unspecialized internodal part of the axon, the paranodal part is slightly constricted in thin fibers, and markedly so in thick fibers. In the thickest fibers the paranodal axon diameter is one-third the internodal diameter (Fig. 1) (Hildebrand, 1971). The lateral loops indent the paranodal axolemma forming scallops. Here the gap between the axolemma and the lateral loops is only 2.5 to 3 nm (Dermietzel, 1974; Schnapp and Mugnaini, 1978; Rosenbluth, 1983, 1984). The loops in direct contact with the axolemma form a junction, the features of which vary with the method of preparation. Hence, the exact structure of this region is disputed (see Schnapp and Mugnaini, 1978; Peters et al., 1991). In EM images from longitudinal sections of aldehyde- and osmium-fixed material, the paranodal axoglial gap is interrupted by thickenings protruding from the axolemma toward the plasma membrane of the terminal loops, the transverse bands (Fig. 7C) (Dermietzel, 1974).

The transverse bands form segments of a circumaxonal helix, which is interrupted between the lateral loops. As seen by freeze-fracture EM, the bands comprise rows of regularly spaced particles in glial and axonal membranes, which are associated with cytoskeletal filaments and which appear to tighten the paranodal axoglial junction (Fig. 17) (Ichimura and Ellisman, 1991). This junction is reminiscent of a septate junction, an invertebrate equivalent to the tight junction (Schnapp and Mugnaini, 1978). The complex membrane anatomy of this region as seen by freeze-fracture EM has been described in detail elsewhere and will not be further commented on here (see Wiley and Ellisman, 1980; Rosenbluth, 1983, 1984, 1995; Waxman 1997). The paranodal junction is not tight in the conventional sense since small tracer molecules, but not larger ones, can reach the periaxonal space from the node gap (Hirano and Dembitzer, 1969; see Peters et al., 1991). The node gap and the periaxonal space seem to be connected

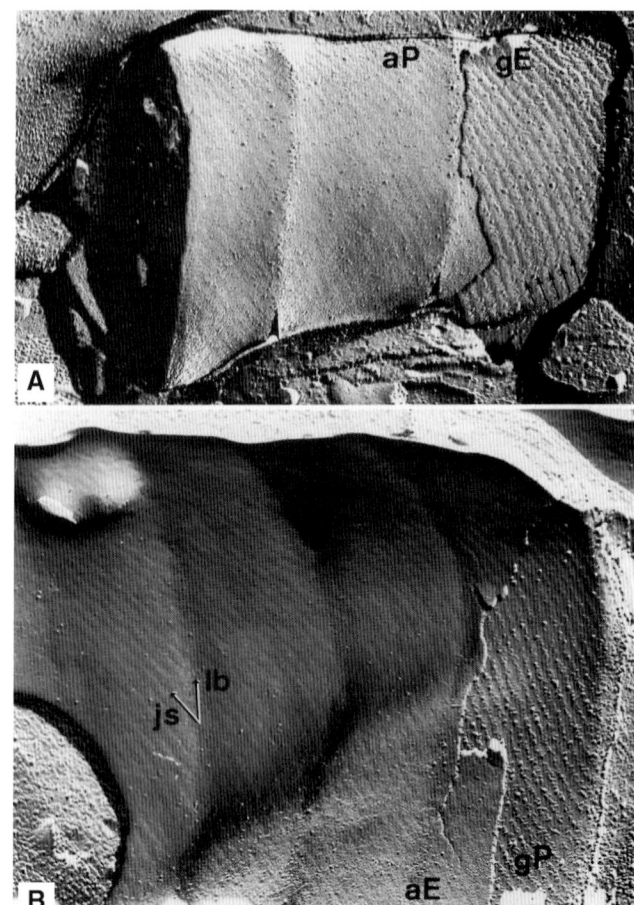

Figure 17 Turtle optic nerve. Freeze-fracture electron micrographs illustrating the four fracture faces associated with the paranodal axo-glial junction. (**A**) The glial E-face (gE) and the axonal P-face (aP) are seen. Note that the junctional pattern is more obvious in the glial than in the axonal membrane. The glial membrane is undulated and exhibits parallel chains of particles in register with shallow grooves (*arrows*). Arrowheads indicate strips of axolemma that face the intervals between the paranodal loops. This nonjunctional band of the axolemma contains randomly distributed particles. Compare with Fig. 13B. (×63,750.) (**B**) The axonal E-face (aE) appears above the glial P-face (gP). The undulations in the axolemma are more obvious in this figure. Their coincidence with the undulations in the glial membrane are clearly discernible. The chains of particles in the glial P-face are located on narrow ridges. In the middle left part of the picture the long axis of the paranodal lateral loop (lb) and of the junctional specialization (js) are indicated. The angle between them is about 30 degrees. (×57,700.) (With permission from Schnapp and Mugnaini, 1978.)

by a narrow helical channel. The paranodal axoglial junction has been attributed a variety of functions: to anchor lateral loops to the axon, to form a partial diffusion barrier from the node gap into the periaxonal space, to demarcate axonal domains by limiting lateral diffusion of membrane components, to be a site for signaling between axons and myelinating glial cells, and/or to play an active role in the ion exchange underlying saltatory conduction (Schnapp and Mugnaini, 1978; Wiley and Ellisman, 1980; Peles and Salzer, 2000).

3. Juxtaparanodal Features

a. The Juxtaparanodal Segment of the Myelinated Axon The juxtaparanode is markedly different in PNS and CNS axons. In a thick myelinated PNS axon, this region extends some 35 μm in an abnodal direction from the paranode. In the juxtaparanodes of a large myelinated PNS axon, the axon and the Schwann cell form a complex structural relation, the axon-Schwann cell network, which is composed of axonal and Schwann cell processes containing lysosomes and residual bodies. In each juxtaparanode-paranode-node-paranode-juxtaparanode region, the network tends to be most prominent in the distal juxtaparanode. It has been suggested that the network takes care of (potentially injurious) material taken up by peripheral terminals and transported in a retrograde fashion toward the CNS. The transported material interacts with primary lysosomes so that secondary lysosomes form. Large myelinated CNS axons exhibit few axoglial networks and secondary lysosomes. Although such formations are prominent in the ventral root part of motor axons, they are lacking or weakly developed in the CNS segments of the same axons. Similarly, dorsal root ganglion axons show more robust network formations in their dorsal root part than in their dorsal column part (Gatzinsky and Berthold, 1990; Gatzinsky et al., 1997).

There is another major juxtaparanodal PNS/CNS difference. In large myelinated PNS axons the juxtaparanodal myelin sheath exhibits three to five longitudinal crests, with intervening furrows, which extend to a distance of about 40 μm from the node. Hence, the juxtaparanodal segment of the axon has a markedly noncircular shape. The axon-Schwann cell network resides on the axonal side of the crests. The furrows on the outside of the juxtaparanodal myelin sheath are filled with mitochondrion- and glycogen-loaded Schwann cell cytoplasm. These "mitochondrion bags" are continuous with the nodal Schwann cell processes (Berthold and Rydmark, 1995). Large myelinated CNS axons are devoid of any direct counterpart to the juxtaparanodal myelin crests and mitochondrion bags (Hildebrand, 1971).

As revealed by freeze-fracture EM, the juxtaparanodal region of CNS axons shows accumulations of large E-face particles, possibly representing K$^+$ channels (Fig. 13B) (Arroyo and Scherer, 2000; Peles and Salzer, 2000). These accumulations show a sharp boundary toward the paranode and a gradually decreasing concentration in the direction of the unspecialized internodal segment. Such juxtaparanodal particle accumulations do not occur in PNS axons (Rosenbluth, 1983; Tao-Cheng and Rosenbluth, 1984). A detailed consideration of the molecular anatomy of the juxtaparanodal region is presented elsewhere (see Arroyo and Scherer, 2000; Peles and Salzer, 2000, and elsewhere in this volume).

b. The Myelinoid Bodies Marchi's histochemical method stains degenerating PNS and CNS myelin fragments and associated lipid droplets brown or black, while normal myelin remains unstained (Adams, 1965). Marchi-positive bodies are also ubiquitous in normal white matter, where they occur in rows or clusters along juxtaparanodes of large myelinated fibers (Fig. 18A-D) (Hildebrand and Skoglund, 1971; Hildebrand, 1977). Since the Marchi-positive bodies were found to correspond to myelin-like lamellated bodies in the EM (Fig. 18E-G) they were named *myelinoid bodies* (Hildebrand and Skoglund, 1971). The lamellar pattern either shows alternating minor and major dense lines, like myelin, or uniform dense lines, unlike myelin (Figs. 18F,G). The two patterns probably reflect different stages in the life history of these bodies. Myelinoid bodies have a size range of <1 μm to >25 μm, and a peak frequency at 3 μm. They occur in spinal cord white matter of various vertebrate species, including humans, being particularly prominent in areas with large myelinated fibers (Hildebrand, 1977; Corneliuson et al., 1989). In the lateral funiculus of the cat, the incidence and size of Marchi-positive myelinoid bodies increase with development (Remahl et al., 1977). While some myelinoid bodies are linked to oligodendroglial/myelin units, others reside within astrocytes or in microglial cells (Fig. 18E, H) (Hildebrand and Aldskogius, 1976; Hildebrand, 1977). Juxtaparanodal Marchi-positive myelinoid bodies occur also in the PNS (Berthold, 1973, 1974), but they are much less frequent than in white matter. This difference may be due to the greater speed with which degenerating myelin fragments are removed in the PNS compared to the CNS (Franson and Ronnevi, 1984).

Since myelinoid bodies resemble degenerating myelin fragments formed during wallerian degeneration (Fig. 18E) (Hildebrand and Aldskogius, 1976; Hildebrand, 1977), and since myelinoid bodies inside astrocytes and within microglia are surrounded by acid phosphatase activity (Fig. 18H) (Hildebrand and Skoglund, 1971; Hildebrand, 1982), these bodies seem to reflect the catabolic side of myelin turnover. This view has gained support from biochemical studies. Ultracentrifugation of a rabbit CNS homogenate in a 0.32 /0.85 M sucrose gradient gives a myelin fraction at the interface, and a small floating fraction (FF) on top of the light sucrose. The FF is highly enriched in Marchi-negative and Marchi-positive myelinoid bodies. Similar fractions from pathological CNS tissue have been interpreted as partially degraded myelin (Persson and Corneliuson, 1989; Persson, 1991). The protein composition of the FF is myelin-like, except for partly degraded myelin proteins and some nonmyelin proteins (Persson and Corneliuson, 1989; Persson, 1991; Persson et al., 1992). In addition, calpains, which participate in the degradation of myelin proteins during degeneration, are present in the FF (Persson and Karlsson, 1991). These biochemical analyses

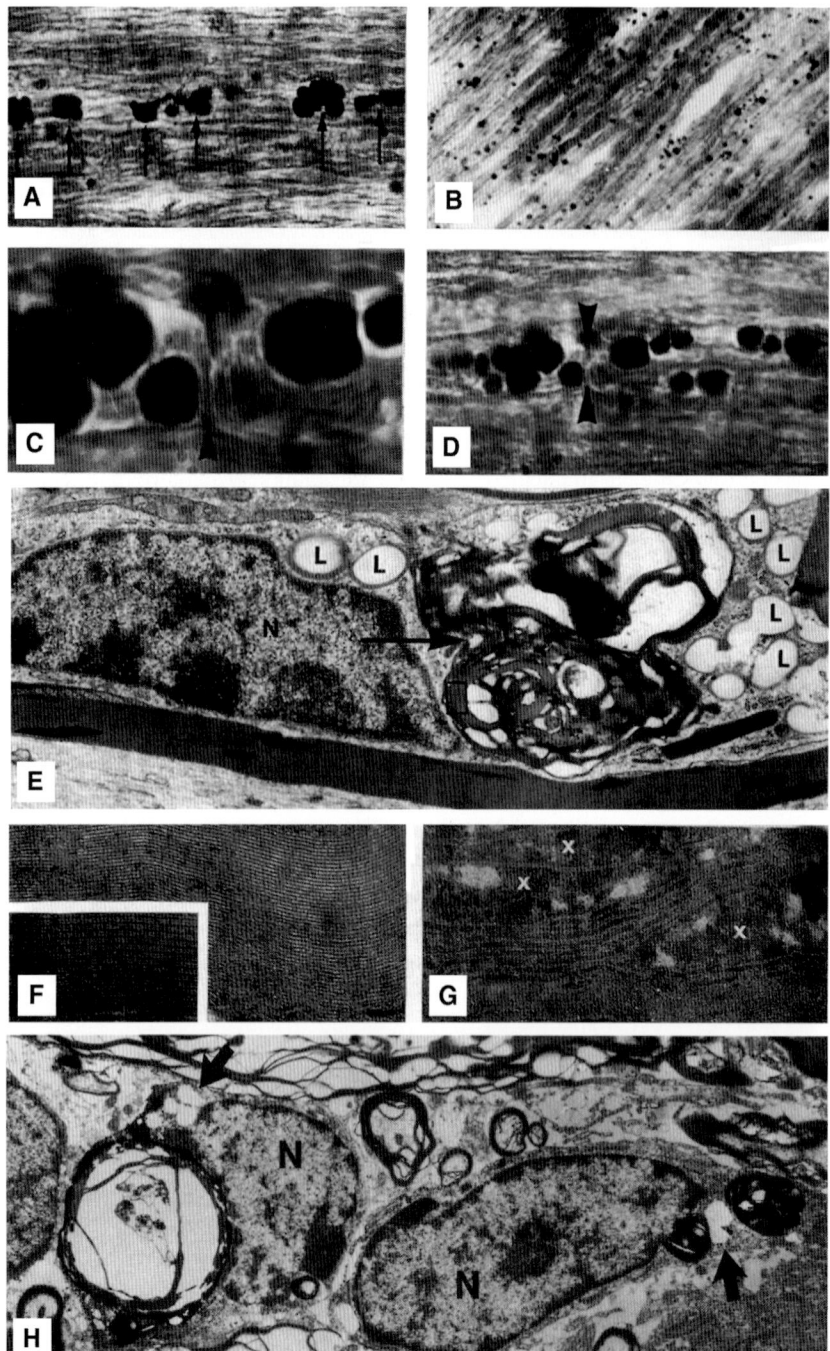

Figure 18 Marchi-positive myelinoid bodies in longitudinal slices from cat spinal cord white matter. (**A**) Row of Marchi-positive myelinoid bodies (*arrows*); (**B**) Survey illustrating the high general incidence of such bodies; (**C, D**) Paranode-juxtaparanode region with Marchi-positive myelinoid bodies at different magnifications. Arrowheads indicate node gap. (**A**) (×1,000) (**B**) (×200) (**C**) (×1,500) (**D**) (×640). (With permission from Hildebrand and Skoglund, 1971.) (**E**) Microglial cell (N = nucleus) in cat white matter. Note that this cell contains a myelinoid body (*arrow*) and lipid droplets (L). (**F, G**) Examples of the lamellar pattern in the outer compact part (**F**) and in the inner less compact part (**G**) of a myelinoid body (see also Fig. 6C). Inset in (**F**) shows lamellar pattern in normal myelin. X in (**G**) indicates a dense flocculent nonlamellar material possibly cytoplasmic remnants. (**E**) (×11,300) (**F**) (×113,000) (**G**) (×63,400) (With permission from Hildebrand, 1971.) (**H**) Electron micrograph from slice of adult guinea pig white matter incubated for the demonstration of acid phosphatase activity. The picture shows two microglial cells (N = nucleus). The left cell contains a hollow myelinoid body surrounded by a dense precipitate indicating acid phosphatase activity. The right cell exhibits two massive lamellated bodies containing reaction product. In both cells lipid droplets can be seen (*arrows*). (×6,500.) (With permission from Hildebrand, 1982.)

18

of purified subcellular fractions agree with the view that myelin turnover in large myelinated CNS fibers includes a degradation step via formation of myelinoid bodies in the juxtaparanodal region (Fig. 19).

4. The Unspecialized Internodal Segment

The segment of a myelinated axon extending between the juxtaparanodes (Fig. 4B) has been called the internode by some workers. However, it is more appropriate to use this term for the entire myelin sheath, as we do when we talk about internodal length. Here the segment extending between the juxtaparanodes is called the unspecialized internodal segment. In this segment the CNS myelin sheath is separated from the axolemma by a space of at least 12 nm. As in myelinated PNS axons, the inner aspect includes a thin cytoplasmic lamella terminating in a small inner loop that is part of the inner mesaxon (Fig. 4B). With respect to thin myelinated axons the oligodendroglial cytoplasm associated with the outer aspect of the internodal segment of a CNS myelin sheath is limited to a small outer tongue and the outer mesaxon (Fig. 4B; see Hirano and Llena, 1995). However, in large myelinated axons associated with Type IV oligodendrocytes, the glial perikaryon may be directly apposed to the internodal sheath in a Schwann cell-like manner (Fig. 11B; Hildebrand, 1971; Remahl and Hildebrand, 1990; Anderson et al., 2000). Otherwise the internodal anatomy of CNS fibers is devoid of specific features. The molecular anatomy of this region is considered elsewhere (Arroyo and Scherer, 2000; Peles and Salzer, 2000; Arroyo et al., 2001).

III. Some Special Regions

A. The CNS/PNS Transitional Zone

Dorsal and ventral spinal roots and cranial nerves III-XII are attached to the CNS by thin rootlets. At this attachment afferent axons shift from PNS to CNS features, and efferent axons shift from CNS to PNS characteristics. The rootlet segment containing both CNS and PNS tissue is the transitional zone (TZ). In the TZ, CNS tissue is separated from PNS tissue by the glia limitans and its basal lamina.

With respect to the structure of the TZ, there is a considerable variation between different nerves and between individual rootlets of a given nerve (Fig. 20A; see Fraher, 1992). The CNS-PNS borderline may be convex with projection of CNS tissue into the PNS, flat, or concave with projection of PNS tissue into the CNS. At the CNS-PNS transition of some nerves, PNS tissue forms isolated islands within the CNS. Similarly, isolated islands of CNS tissue may be located within the PNS part of a rootlet (Fig. 20A; see Fraher 1992). As a rule, CNS tissue extends into the rootlets, forming a central tissue projection (see Berthold and Carlstedt, 1977a; Berthold et al., 1984; Fraher, 1992).

On the CNS side of the glia limitans, the nerve fibers coursing between the CNS and the PNS are surrounded mainly by astrocytic processes emerging from perikarya in the glia limitans. Oligodendrocytes and a few microglial cells are also present. On the PNS side of the glia limitans, the nerve fibers are surrounded by endoneurial connective

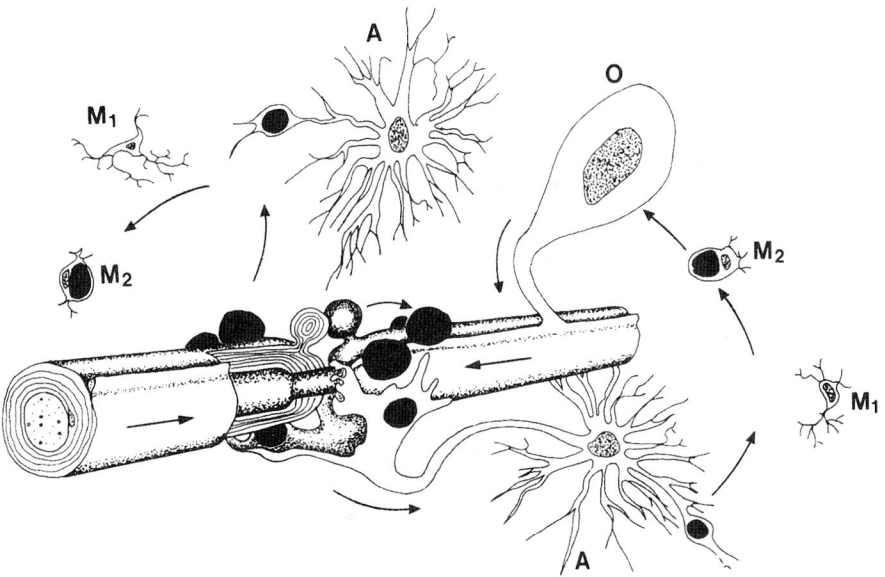

Figure 19 Hypothetical scheme illustrating the theory of myelin turnover discussed in Section II. Nodal-paranodal-juxtaparanodal region of a large CNS fiber with associated Marchi-negative (*stippled*) and Marchi-positive (*black*) myelinoid bodies. The latter are detached from the fiber, taken up by perinodal astrocytic processes (A = astrocyte) and transferred to microglial cells (M). The latter digest the engulfed myelinoid bodies and the breakdown products are reutilized by oligodendroglia (O). (With permission from Hildebrand et al., 1993.)

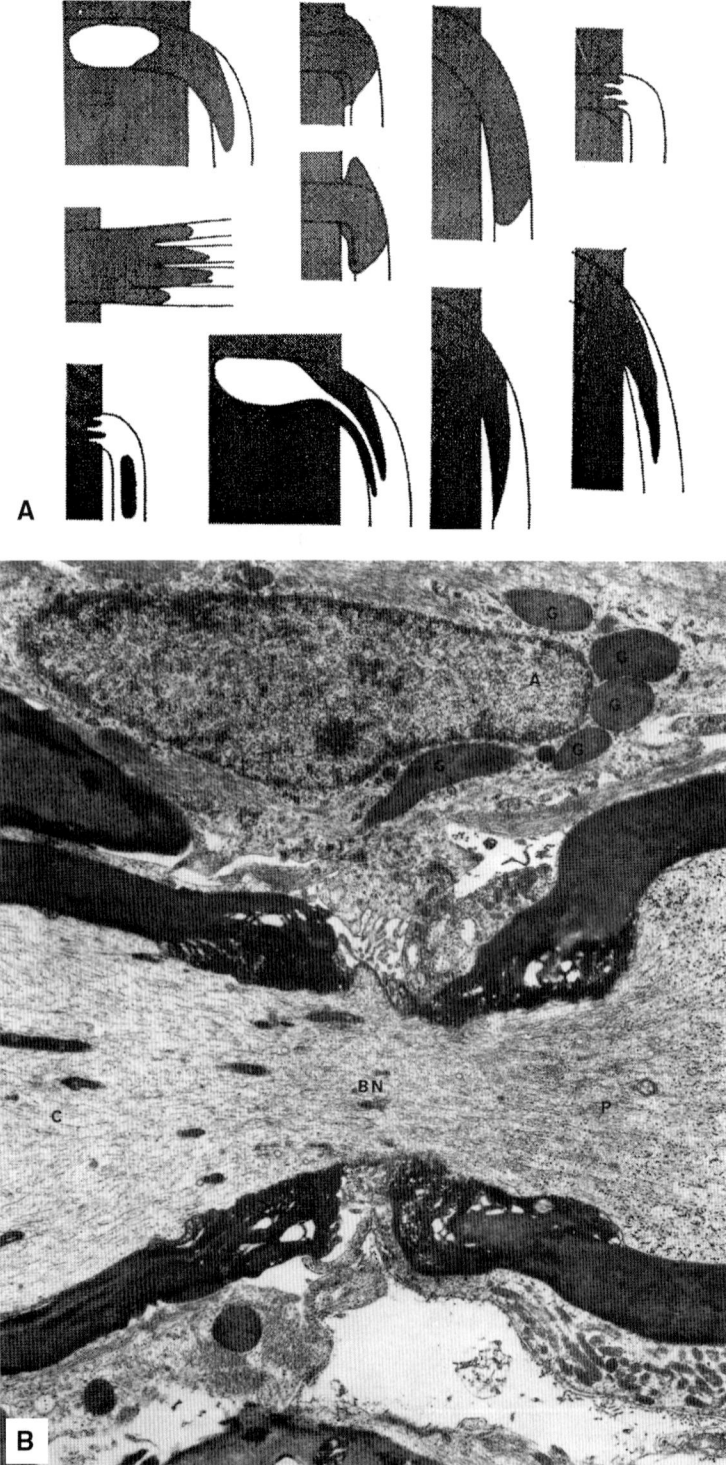

Figure 20 (**A**) Principal types of anatomy at the TZ. Black indicates CNS tissue; white indicates PNS tissue. (With permission from Fraher, 1992.) (**B**) Transitional node of Ranvier (BN) in a S1 dorsal rootlet in an adult cat. The PNS part is located to the right (P) and the central part is located to the left (C). Note that the node gap contains both astrocytic processes and Schwann cell extensions. A perinodal astrocyte containing some gliosomes is located close to the node. (×7,700.) (With permission from Berthold and Carlstedt, 1977b.)

tissue, including Schwann cells, fibroblasts, pericytes, and collagen (Berthold and Carlstedt, 1977a). Schwann cells enveloping the most proximal PNS axon segment lie in an invagination of the glia limitans (see Fraher, 1992). At the site of CNS-PNS transition the basal lamina of the Schwann cell is continuous with the basal lamina of the glia limitans, and both unmyelinated and myelinated axons are surrounded by astrocytic process as they traverse the TZ (Fraher, 1992). Most unmyelinated PNS axons continue as unmyelinated axons into the CNS compartment. Where a bundle of unmyelinated axons is about to cross the CNS-PNS borderline, the Schwann cell cytoplasm surrounding the PNS axons attenuates and terminates (Carlstedt, 1977). At the point of transition, some axons may be covered partly by Schwann cell cytoplasm and partly by astrocytic cytoplasm. Other axons lose their Schwann cell sheaths a few micromillimeters distal to the CNS-PNS borderline and are covered only by a basal lamina. Unmyelinated PNS axons with diameters of 0.6 to 0.8 μm or more become myelinated as they enter the CNS (Carlstedt, 1977). Myelinated fibers have a transitional node at the CNS-PNS interface. Such nodes are bordered by a CNS and a PNS myelin sheath and exhibit a mixture of CNS and PNS features (Fig. 20B). Node density is very high in the TZ. In the TZ of rat, lumbar ventral rootlets the node density is 7 times that in the ventral root and more than twice that in the intramedullary rootlet (Fraher and Bristol, 1990). In addition, Marchi-positive myelinoid bodies are clearly more frequent here than in white matter in general and much more frequent than on the PNS side of the TZ (Corneliuson et al., 1989).

After a crush lesion of a dorsal root in an adult rat the axons regenerate toward the spinal cord, but they stop at the TZ (Fraher and Dockery, 2002). Embryonic human dorsal root ganglion (DRG) neurons, which have been implanted into adult rat DRGs, emit axons into the dorsal rootlets. These axons can enter the CNS, but axon density decreases abruptly when the TZ is approached. This suggests that adult as well as embryonic neurons are sensitive to some growth inhibitory factor(s) emanating from the TZ (Kozlova et al., 1997). These and other similar experiments may eventually promote a more complete understanding of the biology of the PNS-CNS interface, so that we will be able to treat traumatic dorsal root avulsions in the future. With respect to ventral root avulsions, some progress has been made in recent years. Experiments in the cat show that replantation of a divided ventral root into the spinal cord is followed by growth of axons from motoneurons in the ventral horn into the denervated root. Trials in patients show that motor axons can enter implanted ventral roots and grow from the cervical spinal cord into peripheral nerves of the arm, with a resultant useful recovery of motor function (Carlstedt et al., 1995; Fraher, 2000; Carlstedt, 2002). For a more comprehensive discussion of injury-induced changes in the TZ and of regeneration of sensory axons across the

CNS-PNS interface see Cafferty and Ramer (2002) and Fraher and Dockery (2002).

B. The Nerve Fiber Layer of the Retina

The nerve fiber layer (NFL) of the rat retina is composed of unmyelinated ganglion cell axons en route to the optic nerve. These axons, which become myelinated after entering the optic nerve, range in size from 0.12 to 0.8 μm, with a few reaching 2.0 μm. The peak frequency is 0.3 to 0.4 μm (Hildebrand and Waxman, 1983). In the EM rat, NFL axons show membrane patches with a 12- to 20-nm thick undercoating, as seen in thin sections (Figs. 21A-D), and clusters of large E-face particles, as seen in freeze-fracture preparations (Fig. 21E). The undercoating always occupies a limited part of the axon circumference and it extends 0.5-5.0 μm along the axon. Clouds of a granular material may project from the undercoating into the axoplasm. Müller cell processes are always present outside undercoated patches (Fig. 21) (Hildebrand and Waxman, 1983; Black et al., 1984). Undercoated patches and glial adnexa are not usually seen along unmyelinated CNS axons. Whether this specialization of NFL axons results in a nonuniform but continuous or a saltatory-like type of conduction is unknown. Similar patches have been observed in pathological unmyelinated axons or chronically demyelinated white matter (Blakemore and Smith, 1983; Black et al., 1985a, 1991). Thus, some unmyelinated, demyelinated, dysmyelinated, and glial cell-deprived axons exhibit focal regions of node-like membrane despite absence of myelination (see Black et al., 1991).

C. The Retina-Optic Nerve Junction

The first part of the optic nerve is a site of transition where unmyelinated retinal axons become myelinated and enter the optic nerve proper (Fig. 22A; see Hildebrand and Waxman, 1983, 1984). The first 300 μm of the retina optic nerve junction (ROJ), which passes through the sclera, is composed of unmyelinated axons and fibrous astrocytic processes. Oligodendrocytes are absent. At places, the axons in this part of the optic nerve head present patches of an axolemmal undercoating with external astrocytic processes. As seen with freeze-fracture EM such axolemmal areas show a high density of large E-face particles (Hildebrand et al., 1985; Black et al., 1985b). Behind this segment follows a 250-μm long transition part, where an increasing proportion of the axons achieve myelin sheaths with increasing distance from the eye.

In the transition part of the ROJ, oligodendroglial processes appose some unmyelinated axons along part of their circumferences and form paranodal-like junction patches. Other axons are ensheathed by short cytoplasmic glial sheaths, or by 1- to 120-μm long myelin sheaths (Fig. 22B-E). Sheath

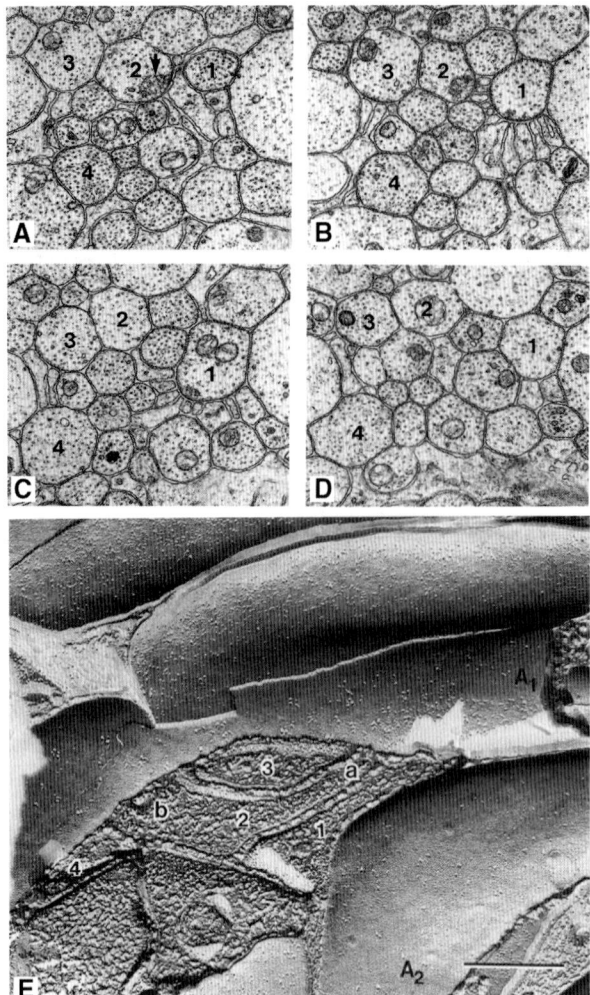

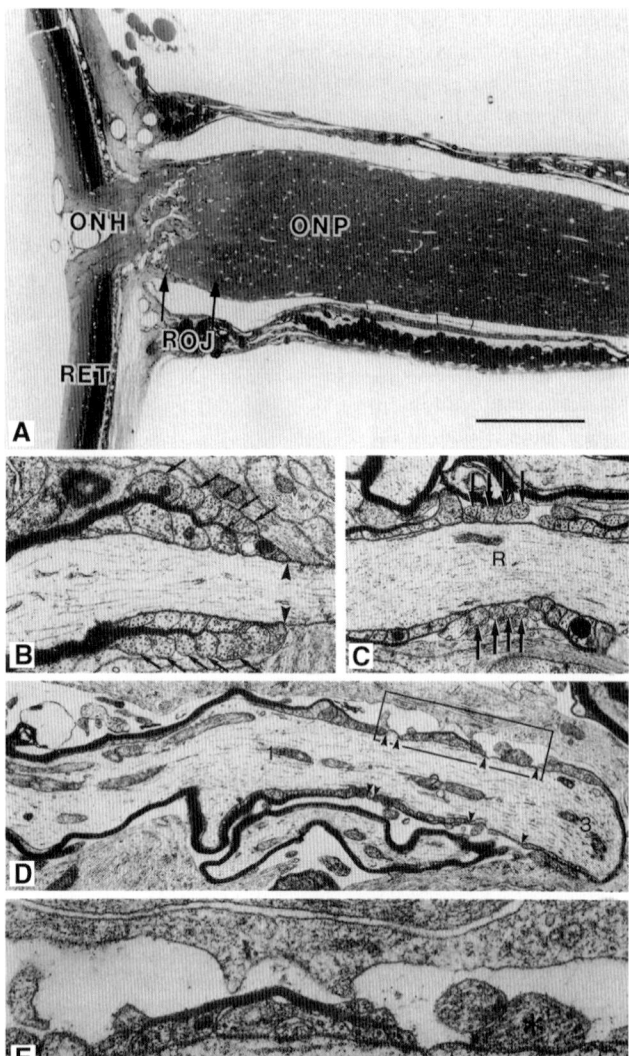

Figure 21 Electron micrographs from a series of transverse sections through the nerve fiber layer of the adult rat retina. At each level, the same four axons are indicated by numbers 1–4. (**A**) Axon 1 shows no unusual features. Axon 2 has an undercoating, an axoplasmic cloud of electron dense material (*arrow*) and associated glial processes. Axons 3 and 4 are also apposed by glial processes and there may be a feeble undercoating at these sites. (**B**) Seven sections later (section thickness 65 nm) a distinct undercoating has appeared in the lower left half of axon 1 and several glial processes are associated to this area. The undercoating and the glial processes in relation to axon 2 persist. An undercoating is clearly present in the lower half of axon 3 but axon 4 does not show any specialization. (**C**) Eight sections later undercoated patches and glial profiles are seen in relation to the lower part of axons 1 and 3 but not in axons 2 and 4. Note the cloud of dense material in axon 1. (**D**) Another 27 sections later axon 3, but not axons 1, 2, and 4, retains an undercoated patch with associated glial adnexa. (×18,400.) (With permission from Hildebrand and Waxman, 1983.) (**E**) Freeze-fracture electron micrograph from adult rat retinal nerve fiber layer. Glial processes 1 through 4 abut the the axon A1 and the E-face of this axolemmal area is visible. Note that the E-face exhibits a higher occurrence of large intramembranous particles than does the E-face of the adjacent axon A2. Scale bar = 0.5 μm. (With permission from Black et al., 1984.)

Figure 22 (**A**) Light micrograph from longitudinal section through the retina (RET), the optic nerve head (ONH), the retina-optic nerve junction (ROJ) and the optic nerve proper (ONP) in the rat. In the retina and the ONH, all axons are unmyelinated; in the ROJ the axons gradually become myelinated; in the ONP nearly all axons are myelinated. (×28.) Scale bar = 500 μm. (With permission from Black et al., 1985b.) (**B-E**) Electron micrographs from longitudinal sections through the ROJ of the adult rat. (**B**) In this paranode about half the lateral loops face outward instead of apposing the axolemma (*arrows*). Arrowheads indicate nodal-paranodal border. (×26,100.) (**C**) Node of Ranvier (R = nodal axon). Note that isolated loop-like profiles without obvious continuity with the myelin cover the nodal axolemma (*arrows*). (×11,500.) (**D**) This ROJ axon shows three successive myelin sheaths (1, 2, 3, arrowheads indicate sheath edges). The myelin sheath enclosed by the rectangular frame is 1.3 μm long only. (**E**). Sheath shown at higher magnification has four outer compacted and 2 inner uncompacted lamellae. Some of the lateral loops face outwards. In the 0.8 μm long gap between sheath 2 and 3, a small oligodendroglial profile apposes the axon (*asterisk* in E. On both sides of this profile the axolemma has an electron-dense undercoating (*arrows* in (**E**). (×17,900) **D**) and (× 37,600 **E**). (With permission from Hildebrand et al., 1985.)

length and number of myelin lamellae are not related to axon diameter. Between successive myelin sheaths are gaps of varying lengths, with or without a nodally differentiated axolemma. Freeze-fracture EM shows the presence of bands of large E-face particles in this region (Black et al., 1982; see Waxman, 1984). The optic axons have relatively small diameters where they are unmyelinated in the retina and optic nerve head, somewhat larger diameters in the ROJ, and clearly larger sizes in the optic nerve proper (Hildebrand et al., 1985). This suggests a trophic dependence of axon diameter on myelination in the rat optic system, similar to that seen in the PNS (Bray et al., 1981).

These results show that the shift from an unmyelinated to a myelinated state in the ROJ is gradual. In the transition zone, the axon-myelin relations are similar to those seen in remyelinated CNS fibers (Clifford-Jones et al., 1980; Blakemore and Murray, 1981), along myelinated dendrites (see later) and in some dysmyelinating conditions (Aguayo and Bray, 1982; Duncan et al., 1983). Similarly, freeze-fracture EM observations show the presence of axon membrane morphologies previously observed only in dysmyelinated mutants (Black et al., 1985a). Dysmyelinating conditions sometimes depend on a deficient oligodendroglial differentiation. It has been suggested that oligodendroglial differentiation in this area is inhibited through a local blood-brain barrier deficiency (Hildebrand et al., 1985).

D. Myelinated Dendrites

Myelin ensheathment is not an exclusively axonal feature. In some CNS areas, neuronal perikarya are covered by myelin (Braak et al., 1977; Cooper and Beal, 1977; Burd, 1980; Tigges and Tigges, 1980) and nerve cells in certain PNS ganglia are myelinated (Peters et al., 1991). In some mammals, mitral cell and tufted cell dendrites in the olfactory bulb are partly myelinated (Pinching, 1971; Willey, 1973; Burd, 1980; Tigges and Tigges, 1980). This is the only localization where myelinated dendrites are known to occur in the normal mammalian CNS, and it has been suggested that these dendrites may generate and propagate action potentials (Willey, 1973). If so, they would be expected to possess nodes of Ranvier.

According to studies in the cat, dendritic myelin sheaths are very thin and short (Fig. 23A-D). There are approximately eight myelin lamellae, the sheath is 5 to 20 μm long, and neither parameter is related to dendritic diameter. In contrast, the mitral cell axons present a strict relation between diameter and number of myelin lamellae (Remahl and Hildebrand, 1985). Where dendritic myelin sheaths end, the lamellae shift into terminal loops, but the terminal loops do not form paranodal-like junctions with the dendritic membrane. Instead, glial or neuronal profiles often intervene between the paranodal myelin and the dendritic mem-

brane (Fig. 23B-D). Of importance, the structural specializations typical for CNS nodes of Ranvier are not seen between successive sheaths along myelinated dendrites or in relation to the end of a single sheath (Fig. 23B-D). There is no diameter alteration of the dendrite, no undercoating of the dendritic membrane, and no "nodal" astrocytic processes and extracellular matrix. In contrast, these features are obvious in mitral cell axons (Remahl and Hildebrand, 1985). Obviously, mitral cell dendrites can attract myelinating oligodendroglial processes and support some preliminary myelination, but they do not possess the signals specifying development of mature myelin sheath characteristics and nodes.

It has been suggested that mitral cell dendrites have spike-generating foci (Yamamoto et al., 1963; Mori and Takagi, 1975). If this applies to the cat, these foci do not seem to have a distinctive thin section EM morphology. The absence of nodes along myelinated dendrites suggests that the myelin is not there to support saltatory conduction. It is possible that the presence of dendritic myelin sheaths facilitates electrotonic spread of potentials along these long dendrites (Rall and Shepherd, 1968; Pinching and Powell, 1971; Scheibel and Scheibel, 1975). Of interest, experimental deafferentation of neurons in the cerebellar cortex or the lateral geniculate nucleus is followed by partial dendritic and perikaryal myelination (Hamori et al., 1980; Hamori and Silakov, 1981). Hence, dendritic myelination may possibly serve as a "protective" response to generation of vacated synaptic sites.

IV. Final Overview

As outlined previously, the myelinated axon is a highly complex structure with impressive dimensions. Linked via specialized interfaces with three different cell types—myelinating oligodendrocytes, perinodal astrocytes, and nodal NG2 cells—it displays a remarkable morphological, as well as molecular and functional, heterogeneity along its length. In addition to reflecting a rich set of interactions between the axon and associated glial cells, this polymorphism presents multiple targets for the disease process in multiple sclerosis (MS). In view of the complex structure of the myelinated CNS fiber, and of the more-or-less symbiotic relations between the axon and the glial cells associated with it, it is not surprising that axons are subject to injury in MS, a disease classically considered as primarily affecting myelin. Continued studies of the morphological, molecular, and functional properties of normal myelinated CNS nerve fibers will bring us close to a more complete understanding of the cellular mechanisms that are deranged in MS. It is hoped that this knowledge will enable us to treat and/or prevent the disease in the not-too-distant future.

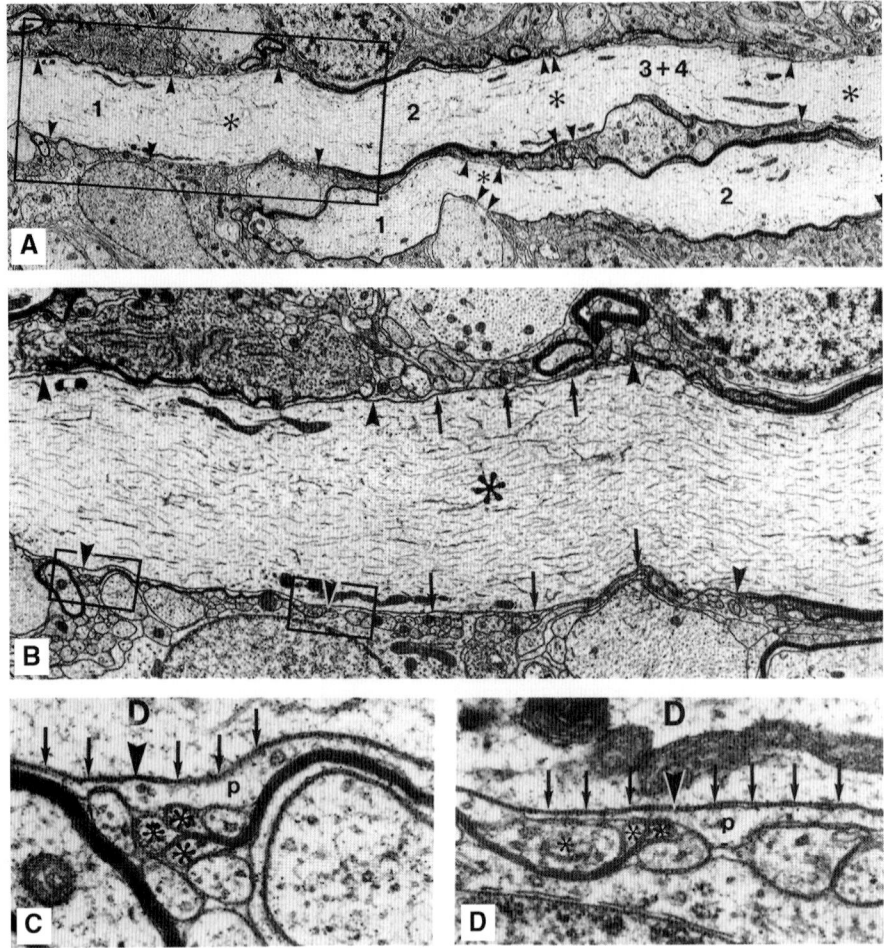

Figure 23 Longitudinally sectioned myelinated mitral cell dendrites in the adult cat olfactory bulb. (**A**) Two myelinated dendrites. The top one has four successive thin sheaths labeled 1, 2, and 3+4; the bottom one has two thin sheaths labeled 1 and 2. Arrowheads indicate myelin sheath terminations and asterisks indicate unmyelinated dendritic segments. (×3,500.) (**B**) Higher magnification of the framed area in (**A**). Arrowheads indicate myelin sheath ends and arrows point at a 7-μm long stretch of bare dendritic membrane. Note that this dendritic segment (*asterisk*) is devoid of a nodal differentiation. (×8,160.) (**C, D**) Details from framed areas in (**B**) showing lateral loops (*asterisks*) completely separated from the dendritic membrane (D = dendrite) by glial processes (p). Note that the dendritic membrane lacks specializations at as well as beyond the myelin sheath terminations (*arrows*). Arrowhead positions correspond to those in (**B**). (×53,700.) (With permission from Remahl and Hildebrand, 1985.)

Acknowledgments

The authors' studies cited in this chapter were supported by grants from the Swedish Science Council (Proj. No. 3761), from the Karolinska Institute, from the University of Linköping, and from the County Council of Östergötland.

References

Adams, C. W. M. (1965). "Neurohistochemistry." Elsevier, Amsterdam.
Alberts, B., Johnson, A., Lewis, J., Raff, M., Roberts, K., and Walter, P. (2002). "Molecular Biology of the Cell." 4th ed. Garland Science, New York.
Aguayo, A., and Bray, G. M. (1982). Developmental disorders of myelination in mouse mutants. *In* "Neuronal-Glial Cell Interrelationships" (T. A. Sears, Ed.), Dalhem Konferenzen, pp. 57-76. Springer Verlag, Berlin, Heidelberg and New York.
Amaducci, L., Pazzaglia, A., and Pessina, G. (1962). The relation of proteolipids and phosphatidopeptides to tissue elements in the bovine nervous system. *J. Neurochem.* **9**, 509–515. **32**, 1045–1053.
Anderson, E. S. (2003). Morphology of early developing oligodendrocytes in the ventrolateral chicken spinal cord. *J. Neurocytol.* **32**, 1045–1053.
Anderson, E. S., Bjartmar, C., and Hildebrand, C. (2000). Myelination of prospective large fibres in chicken ventral funiculus. *J. Neurocytol.* **29**, 755–764.
Arroyo, E. J., and Scherer, S. S. (2000). On the molecular architecture of myelinated fibers. *Histochem. Cell Biol.* **113**, 1–18.
Arroyo E. J., Xu, T., Poliak, S., Watson, M., Peles, E., and Scherer, S. S. (2001). Internodal specialization of myelinated axons in the central nervous system. *Cell Tiss. Res.* **305**, 53–66.

Barbarese, E., Brumwell, C., Kwon, S., Cui, H., and Carson, J. H. (1999). RNA on the road to myelin. *J. Neurocytol.* **28,** 263–270.

Barry, C., Pearson, C., and Barbarese, E. (1996). Morphological organization of oligodendrocyte processes during development in culture and *in vivo. Dev. Neurosci.* **18,** 233–242.

Bergles, D. E., Roberts, J. D. B., Somogyi, P., and Jahr, C. E. (2000). Glutamatergic synapses on oligodendrocyte precursor cells in the hippocampus. *Nature* **405,** 187–191.

Berry, M., Ibrahim, M., Carlile, J., Ruge, F., Duncan, A., and Butt, A. M. (1995). Axon-glial relationships in the anterior medullary velum of the adult rat. *J. Neurocytol.* **24,** 963–983.

Berthold, C.-H. (1973). Histochemistry of postnatally developing feline spinal roots. I. A study with the OTAN method. *Neurobiology* **3,** 275–290.

Berthold, C.-H. (1974). A comparative morphological study of the developing node-paranode region in lumbar spinal roots. I. Electron microscopy. *Neurobiology* **4,** 82–104.

Berthold, C.-H., and Carlstedt, T. (1977a). Observations on the morphology at the transition between the peripheral and the central nervous system in the cat. II. General organisation of the transitional region in S1 dorsal rootlets. *Acta Physiol. Scand.,* **Suppl. 446,** 23–42.

Berthold, C.-H., and Carlstedt, T. (1977b). Observations on the morphology at the transition between the peripheral and the central nervous system in the cat. III. Myelinated fibres in S1 dorsal rootlets. *Acta Physiol. Scand.,* **Suppl. 446,** 43–60.

Berthold, C.-H., Carlstedt, T., and Corneliuson, O. (1984). Anatomy of the nerve root at the central-peripheral transitional region. *In:* "Peripheral Neuropathy" (P. J. Dyck, P. K. Thomas, and E. H. Lambert, Eds.), pp. 156–170. W.B. Saunders and Co, Philadelphia.

Berthold, C.-H., and Rydmark, M. (1995). Morphology of normal peripheral axons. *In* "The Axon" (S. G. Waxman, J. D. Kocsis, and P. K. Stys, Eds.), pp. 13–48. Oxford University Press, New York and Oxford.

Bevan, S., Chiu, S. Y., Gray, P. T. A., and Ritchie, J. M. (1985). The presence of voltage gated sodium, potassium and chloride channels in rat cultured astrocytes. *Proc. Roy. Soc. Lond. B* **225,** 229–313.

Bjartmar, C. (1998). Morphological heterogeneity of cultured spinal and cerebral rat oligodendrocytes. *Neurosci. Lett.* **247,** 91–94.

Bjartmar, C., Hildebrand, C., and Loinder, K. (1994a). Morphological heterogeneity of rat oligodendrocytes: Electron microscopic studies on serial sections. *Glia* **11,** 235–244.

Bjartmar, C., Karlsson, B., and Hildebrand, C. (1994b). Cellular and extracellular components at nodes of Ranvier in rat white matter. *Brain Res.* **667,** 111–114.

Black, J. A., Waxman, S. G., and Foster, R. E. (1982). Spatial heterogeneity of the axolemma of nonmyelinated fibers in the optic disc of the adult rat. *Cell Tiss. Res.* **224,** 239–246.

Black, J. A., Waxman, S. G., and Hildebrand, C. (1984). Membrane specialization and axo-glial association in the rat retinal nerve fiber layer: Freeze-fracture observations. *J. Neurocytol.* **13,** 417–430.

Black, J. A., Sims, T. J., Waxman, S. G., and Gilmore, S. A. (1985a). Membrane ultrastructure of developing axons in glial cell deficient spinal cord. *J. Neurocytol.* **14,** 79–104.

Black, J. A., Waxman, S. G., and Hildebrand, C. (1985b). Axo-glial relations in the retina-optic nerve junction of the adult rat: freeze-fracture observations on axon membrane structure. *J. Neurocytol.* **14,** 887–907.

Black, J. A., Kocsis, J. D., and Waxman, S. G. (1990). Ion channel organization of the myelinated fiber. *Trends Neurosci.* **13,** 48–54.

Black, J. A., Felts, P., Smith, K. J., Kocsis, J. D., and Waxman, S. G. (1991). Distribution of sodium channels in chronically demyelinated spinal cord axons: Immunoultrastructural localization and electrophysiological observations. *Brain Res.* **544,** 59–70.

Black, J. A., Sontheimer, H., Oh, Y., and Waxman S. G. (1995). The oligodendrocyte, the perinodal astrocyte and the central node of Ranvier. *In* "The Axon" (S. G. Waxman, J. D. Kocsis, and P. K. Stys, Eds.), pp. 116–143. Oxford University Press, New York and Oxford.

Blakemore, W. F. (1969). Schmidt-Lanterman incisures in the central nervous system. *J. Ultrastruct. Res.* **29,** 496–498.

Blakemore, W. F. (1981). Observations on myelination and remyelination in the central nervous system. *In* "Development in the Nervous System" (D. R. Garrod and J. D. Feldman, Eds.), pp. 289–308. Cambridge University Press, Cambridge.

Blakemore W. F., and Murray, J. A. (1981). Quantitative examination of internodal lengths of remyelinated nerve fibres in the central nervous system. *J. Neurol. Sci.* **49,** 273–284.

Blakemore, W. F., and Smith, K. J. (1983). Node-like axonal specializations along demyelinated central nerve fibers. Ultrastructural observations. *Acta Neuropathol.* **60,** 291–296.

Bodega, G., Suarez, J., and Fernandez, B. (1987). Fine structural relationships between astrocytes and the node of Ranvier in the amphibian and reptilian spinal cord. *Neurosci. Lett.* **80,** 7–10.

Braak, E., Braak, H., and Strenge, H. (1977). The fine structure of myelinated nerve cell bodies in the bulbus olfactorius of man. *Cell Tiss. Res.* **182,** 221–233.

Bray, D., and Bunge, M. B. (1981). Serial analysis of microtubules in cultured rat sensory axons. *J. Neurocytol.* **10,** 589–605.

Bray, G. M., Rasminsky, M., and Aguayo, A. (1981). Interactions between axons and their sheath cells. *Annu. Rev. Neurosci.* **4,** 127–162.

Bunge, R. P. (1968). Glial cells and the central myelin sheath. *Physiol. Rev.* **48,** 197–210.

Burd, G. D. (1980). Myelinated dendrites and neuronal perikarya in the olfactory bulb of the mouse. *Brain Res.* **181,** 450–454.

Butt, A. M., and Ransom, B. R. (1989). Visualization of oligodendrocytes and astrocytes in the intact rat optic nerve by intracellular injections of Lucifer Yellow and horseradish peroxidase. *Glia* **2,** 470–475.

Butt, A. M., and Ransom, B. R. (1993). Morphology of astrocytes and oligodendrocytes during development in the intact rat optic nerve. *J. Comp. Neurol.* **338,** 141–158.

Butt, A. M., Colquhoun, K., and Berry, M. (1994a). Confocal imaging of glial cells in the intact rat optic nerve. *Glia* **10,** 315–322.

Butt, A. M., Duncan, A., and Berry, M. (1994b). Astrocyte association with nodes of Ranvier: Ultrastructural analysis of HRP-filled astrocytes in the mouse optic nerve. *J. Neurocytol.* **23,** 486–499.

Butt, A. M., Colquhoun, K., Tutton, M., and Berry, M. (1994c). Three-dimensional morphology of astrocytes and oligodendrocytes in the intact mouse optic nerve. *J. Neurocytol.* **23,** 469–485.

Butt, A. M., Ibrahim, M., Ruge, F. M., and Berry, M. (1995). Biochemical subtypes of oligodendrocytes in the anterior medullary velum of the rat, as revealed by the monoclonal antibody Rip. *Glia* **14,** 185–197.

Butt, A. M., Ibrahim, M., and Berry, M. (1998a). Axon-myelin sheath relations of oligodendrocyte unit phenotypes in the adult rat anterior medullary velum. *J. Neurocytol.* **27,** 259–269.

Butt, A. M., Ibrahim, M., Gregson, N., and Berry, M. (1998b). Differential expression of the L- and S-isoforms of myelin-associated glycoprotein (MAG) in oligodendrocyte unit phenotypes in the adult rat anterior medullary velum. *J. Neurocytol.* **27,** 271–280.

Butt, A. M., Duncan, A., Hornby, M. F., Kirvell, S. L., Hunter, A., Levine, J. M., and Berry, M. (1999). Cells expressing the NG2 antigen contact nodes of Ranvier in adult CNS white matter. *Glia* **26,** 84–91.

Butt, A.M., Kiff, J., Hubbard, P., Ibrahim M., and Berry, M. (2002). Synantocytes: New functions for novel NG2 expressing glia. *J. Neurocytol.* **31,** 551–565.

Cafferty, W. B. J., and Ramer, M. S. (2002). Promoting sensory axon regeneration across the PNS-CNS interface. *In* "Glial interfaces in the nervous system. Role in repair and plasticity" (H. Aldskogius and J. Fraher, Eds.), pp. 23–40. IOS press, Amsterdam.

Carlstedt, T. (1977). Observations on the morphology at the transition between the peripheral and the central nervous system in the cat. IV. Unmyelinated fibres in S1 dorsal rootlets. *Acta Physiol. Scand.,* **Suppl 446,** 61–71.

Carlstedt, T. (2002). Overcoming PNS-CNS boundaries: clinical approach. *In* "Glial interfaces in the nervous system. Role in repair and plasticity" (H. Aldskogius and J. Fraher, Eds.), pp. 71–75. IOS press, Amsterdam.

Carlstedt, T., Grane, P., Hallin, R. G., and Norén, G. (1995). Return of function after spinal cord implantation of avulsed spinal nerve roots. *Lancet* **346,** 1323–1325.

Clifford-Jones, R. E., Landon, D. N., and McDonald, W. I. (1980). Remyelination during optic nerve compression. *J. Neurol. Sci.* **46,** 239–243.

Cooper, M. H., and Beal, J. A. (1977). Myelinated granule cell bodies in the cerebellum of the monkey (*Saimiri sciureus*). *Anat. Rec.* **187,** 249–256.

Corneliuson, O., Berthold, C.-H., Fabricius, C., Gatzinsky, K., and Carlstedt, T. (1989). Marchi-positive myelinoid bodies at the transition between the central and the peripheral nervous system in some vertebrates. *J. Anat.* **163,** 17–31.

Couve, E., Cabello, J. F., Krsulovic, J., and Roncagliolo, M. (1997). Binding of microtubules to transitional elements in oligodendrocytes of the myelin mutant *taiep* rat. *J. Neurosci. Res.* **47,** 573–581.

Davis, J. Q., Lambert, S., and Bennett, V. (1996). Molecular composition of the node of Ranvier: identification of ankyrin-binding cell adhesion molecules neurofascin (mucin + /third FNIII domain-) and NrCAM at nodal axon segments. *J. Cell Biol.* **135,** 1355–1367.

Dermietzel, R. (1974). Junctions in the central nervous system of the cat II. A contribution to the tertiary structure of the axonal-glial junctions in the paranodal region of the node of Ranvier. *Cell Tiss. Res.* **148,** 577–586.

Dermietzel, R., Leibstein, A. G., and Schunke, D. (1980). Interlamellar tight junctions of central myelin. II. A freeze-fracture and cytochemical study on their arrangement and composition. *Cell Tiss. Res.* **213,** 95–108.

Duncan, I. D., Griffiths, I. R., and Munz, M. (1983). "Shaking pups": a disorder of central myelination in the spaniel dog. III. Quantitative aspects of glia and myelin in the spinal cord and optic nerve. *Neuropath. Appl. Neurobiol.* **9,** 355–368.

Ellisman, M. H. (1979). Molecular specializations of the axon membrane at nodes of Ranvier are not dependent upon myelination. *J. Neurocytol.* **8,** 719–735.

Ellisman, M. H., Wiley, C. A., Lindsey, J. D., and Wurtz, C. C. (1984). Structure and function of the cytoskeleton and endomembrane systems at the node of Ranvier. *In* "The Node of Ranvier" (J. C. Zagoren and S. Fedoroff, Eds.), pp. 153–181. Academic Press, Orlando.

Faissner, A., and Schachner, M. (1995). Tenascin and janusin: Glial recognition molecules involved in neural development and regeneration. *In* "Neuroglia" (H. Kettenmann and B. R. Ransom, Eds.), pp. 411–426. Oxford University Press, New York and Oxford.

Fanarraga, M. L., Griffiths, I. R., Zhao, M., and Duncan, I. D. (1998). Oligodendrocytes are not inherently programmed to myelinate a specific size of axon. *J. Comp. Neurol.* **399,** 94–100.

Fraher, J. P. (1992). The CNS-PNS transitional zone of the rat. Morphometric studies at cranial and spinal levels. *Prog. Neurobiol.* **38,** 261–316.

Fraher, J. P. (2000). The transitional zone and CNS regeneration. *J. Anat.* **196,** 137–158.

Fraher, J. P., and Bristol, D. (1990). High density of nodes of Ranvier in the CNS-PNS transitional zone. *J. Anat.* **170,** 131–137.

Fraher, J., and Dockery, P. (2002). Injury-induced changes in spinal root transitional zones: Morphometric ultrastructural studies. *In* "Glial Interfaces in the Nervous System. Role in Repair and Plasticity" (H. Aldskogius and J. Fraher, Eds.), pp. 41–59. IOS press, Amsterdam.

Franson, P., and Ronnevi, L.-O. (1984). Myelin breakdown and elimination in the posterior funiculus of the adult cat after dorsal rhizotomy: A light and electron microscopic qualitative and quantitative study. *J. Comp. Neurol.* **223,** 138–151.

Friedrich, V. L., and Mugnaini, E. (1983). Myelin sheath thickness in the CNS is regulated near the axon. *Brain Res.* **274,** 329–331.

Friedrich, V. L., Massa, P., and Mugnaini, E. (1980). Fine structure of oligodendrocytes and central myelin sheaths. *In* "Search for the Cause of Multiple sclerosis and Other Chronic Diseases of the Central Nervous System" (A. Boese, Ed.), pp. 27–49. Verlag Chemie, Weinheim.

Gatzinsky, K. P., and Berthold, C.-H. (1990). Lysosomal activity at nodes of Ranvier during retrograde axonal transport of horseradish peroxidase in alpha-motor neurons of the cat. *J. Neurocytol.* **19,** 989–1002.

Gatzinsky, K. P., Persson, H., and Berthold, C.-H. (1997). Removal of retrogradely transported material from rat lumbosacral alpha-motor axons by paranodal axon-Schwann cell networks. *Glia* **20,** 115–126.

Gray, P. T., and Ritchie, J. M. (1985). Ion channels in Schwann and glial cells. *Trends Neurosci.* **8,** 411–415.

Hamori, J., and Silakov, V. L. (1981). Myelinated perikarya and dendrites in lateral geniculate nucleus of adult cat following chronic cortical deafferentation. *J. Neurocytol.* **10,** 879–888.

Hamori, J., Lakos, I., and Mezey, E. (1980). Myelinated dendrites of Purkinje cells in deafferented cerebellar cortex. *J. Hirnforsch.* **21,** 391–407.

Hartman, B. K., Agrawal, C. H., Agrawal, D., and Kalmbach, S. (1982). Development and maturation of central nervous myelin: comparison of immunohistochemical localization of proteolipid protein and basic protein in myelin and oligodendrocytes. *Proc. Natl. Acad. Sci. U. S. A.* **79,** 4217–4220.

Hess, A., and Young, J. Z. (1952). The nodes of Ranvier. *Proc. Roy. Soc. Lond. B* **140,** 301–320.

Hildebrand, C. (1971). Ultrastructural and light microscopic studies of the nodal region in large myelinated fibres of the adult feline spinal cord white matter. *Acta Physiol. Scand.* **Suppl. 364,** 43–81.

Hildebrand, C. (1972). Evidence for a correlation between myelin period and number of myelin lamellae in fibres of the feline spinal cord white matter. *J. Neurocytol.* **1,** 223–232.

Hildebrand, C. (1977). Presence of Marchi-positive myelinoid bodies in the spinal cord white matter of some vertebrate species. *J. Morphol.* **153,** 1–22.

Hildebrand, C. (1982). Electron microscopic identification of Gomori-positive rings in normal spinal cord white matter. *Acta Neuropathol.* **56,** 29–34.

Hildebrand, C., and Aldskogius, H. (1976). Electron microscopic identification of Marchi-positive and argyrophilic bodies in the spinal cord white matter of the guinea pig. *J. Comp. Neurol.* **170,** 191–204.

Hildebrand, C., and Hahn, R. (1978). Relation between myelin sheath thickness and axon size in spinal cord white matter of some vertebrate species. *J. Neurol. Sci.* **38,** 421–434.

Hildebrand, C., and Muller, H. (1974). Low-angle X-ray diffraction studies on the period of central myelin sheaths during preparation for electron microscopy. A comparison of different anatomical areas. *Neurobiology* **4,** 71–81.

Hildebrand, C., and Skoglund, S. (1971). Histochemical studies of adult and developing feline spinal cord white matter. *Acta Physiol. Scand.* **Suppl. 364,** 145–166.

Hildebrand, C., and Waxman, S. G. (1983). Regional node-like membrane specializations in non-myelinated axons of rat retinal nerve fiber layer. *Brain Res.* **258,** 23–32.

Hildebrand, C., and Waxman, S. G. (1984). Postnatal differentiation of rat optic nerve fibers: electron microscopic observations on the development of nodes of Ranvier and axoglial relations. *J. Comp. Neurol.* **224,** 25–37.

Hildebrand, C., Remahl, S., and Waxman, S. G. (1985). Axo-glial relations in the retina-optic nerve junction of the adult rat: electron-microscopic observations. *J. Neurocytol.* **14,** 597–617.

Hildebrand, C., Remahl, S., Persson, H., and Bjartmar, C. (1993). Myelinated nerve fibers in the CNS. *Prog. Neurobiol.* **40,** 319–384.

Hirano, A., and Dembitzer, H. M. (1969). The transverse bands as a means of access to the periaxonal space of the central myelinated nerve fiber. *J. Ultrastruct. Res.* **28,** 141–149.

Hirano, A., and Dembitzer, H. M. (1978). Morphology of normal central myelinated axons. *In* "Physiology and Pathobiology of Axons" (S. G. Waxman, Ed.), pp. 65–82. Raven Press, New York.

Hirano, A., and Llena, J. F. (1995). Morphology of central nervous system axons. *In* "The Axon" (S. G. Waxman, J. D. Kocsis, and P. K. Stys, Eds.), pp. 49–67. Oxford University Press, Oxford and New York.

Hirokawa, N. (1982). Cross-linker system between neurofilaments, microtubules and membranous organelles in frog axons revealed by the quick-freeze deep-etching method. *J. Cell Biol.* **94**, 129–142.

Hirokawa, N., Glicksman, M. A., and Willard, M. B. (1984). Organization of mammalian neurofilament polypeptides within the neuronal cytoskeleton. *J. Cell Biol.* **98**, 1523–1536.

Ibrahim, M., Butt, A. M., and Berry, M. (1995). The relationship between myelin sheath diameter and internodal length in axons of the anterior medullary velum of the adult rat. *J. Neurol. Sci.* **133**, 119–127.

Ichimura, T., and Ellisman, M., H. (1991). Three-dimensional fine structure of cytoskeletal-membrane interactions at nodes of Ranvier. *J. Neurocytol.* **20**, 667–681.

Jessen, K. R., and Mirsky, R. (1999). Schwann cells and their precursors emerge as major regulators of nerve development, *Trends Neurosci.* **22**, 402–410.

Kaplan, M. R., Meyer-Franke, A., Lambert, S., Bennett, V., Duncan, I. D., Levinson, S. R., and Barres, B. A. (1997). Induction of sodium channel clustering by oligodendrocytes. *Nature* **386**, 724–728.

Kirschner, D. A., and Blaurock, A. E. (1992). Organization, phylogenetic variations and dynamic transitions of myelin. *In* "Myelin: Biology and Chemistry" (R. E. Martenson, Ed.), pp. 3–78. CRC Press, Boca Raton.

Koenig, E., and Repasky, E. (1986). A regional analysis of α-spectrin in the isolated Mauthner neuron and in isolated axons of the goldfish and rabbit. *J. Neurosci.* **5**, 705–714.

Kosaras, B., and Kirschner, D. A. (1990). Radial component of CNS myelin: Junctional subunit structure and supramolecular assembly. *J. Neurocytol.* **19**, 187–199.

Kozlova, E., Seiger, Å., and Aldskogius, H. (1997). Human dorsal root ganglion neurons from embryonic donors extend axons into the host rat spinal cord along laminin-rich peripheral surroundings of the dorsal root transitional zone. *J. Neurocytol.* **26**, 811–822.

Kristol, C., Sandri, C., and Akert, K. (1978). Intramembranous particles at the nodes of Ranvier of the cat spinal cord: a morphometric study. *Brain Res.* **142**, 391–400.

Landon, D. N. (1981). Structure of normal peripheral myelinated nerve fibres. *In* "Demyelinating Diseases: Basic and Clinical Electrophysiology" (S. G. Waxman and J. M. Ritchie, Eds.), pp. 25–49. Raven Press, New York.

Langford, G. M., Allen, R. D., and Weiss, D. G. (1987). Substructure of sidearms of squid axoplasmic vesicles and microtubules visualized by negative contrast electron microscopy. *Cell Motil. Cytoskel.* **7**, 20–30.

Langley, O. K. (1969). Ion exchange at the node of Ranvier. *Histochem. J.* **1**, 295–309.

Langley, O. K., and Landon, D. N. (1969). Copper binding at nodes of Ranvier: A new electron histochemical technique for the demonstration of polyanions. *J. Histochem. Cytochem.* **17**, 66–69.

Levine, J. M. (1994). Increased expression of the NG2 chondroitin-sulfate proteoglycan after brain injury. *J. Neurosci.* **14**, 4716–4730.

LoTurco, J. (2000). Neural circuits in the 21st century: Synaptic networks of neurons and glia. *Proc. Natl. Acad. Sci. U. S. A.* **97**, 8196–8197.

Lunn, K. F., Clayton, M. K., and Duncan, D. (1997). The temporal progression of the myelination defect in the taiep rat. *J. Neurocytol.* **26**, 267–281.

Maggs, A., and Scholes, J. (1990). Reticular astrocytes in the fish optic nerve: Macroglia with epithelial characteristics form an axially repeated lacework pattern, to which nodes of Ranvier are apposed. *J. Neurosci.* **10**, 1600–1614.

Massa, P. T., and Mugnaini, E. (1982). Cell junctions and intramembrane particles of astrocytes and oligodendrocytes. *Neuroscience* **7**, 523–538.

Morell, P., and Norton, W. T. (1980). Myelin. *Sci. Amer.* **242**, 88–90.

Mori, K., and Takagi, S. F. (1975). Spike generation in the mitral cell dendrite of the rabbit olfactory bulb. *Brain Res.* **100**, 685–689.

Murray, J. A., and Blakemore, W. F. (1980). The relationship between internodal length and fibre diameter in the spinal cord of the cat. *J. Neurol. Sci.* **45**, 29–41.

Nagara, H., and Suzuki, K. (1982). Radial component of the central myelin in neurologic mutant mice. *Lab. Invest.* **47**, 51–59.

Nishiyama, A. (2001). NG2 cells in the brain: a novel glial population. *Hum. Cell* **14**, 77–82.

Nishiyama, A., Chang, A., and Trapp, B. D. (1999). NG2+ glial cells: a novel glial cell population in the adult brain. *J. Neuropath. Exp. Neurol.* **58**, 1113–1124.

Norton, W. R., and Cammer, W. (1984). Isolation and characterization of myelin. *In* "Myelin" (P. Morell, Ed.), pp. 147–195. Plenum Press, New York.

Norton, W. R., and Poduslo, S. E. (1973). Myelination in rat brain: changes in myelin composition during brain maturation. *J. Neurochem.* **21**, 759–773.

Peles, E., and Salzer, J. L. (2000). Molecular domains of myelinated axons. *Curr. Opin. Neurobiol.* **10**, 558–565.

Penfield, W. (1932). "Cytology and Cellular Pathology of the Nervous System," Vol. 2, pp. 481–534. P. B. Hoeber, New York.

Persson, H. (1991). Degradation products of myelin-oligodendrocyte-associated proteins in a light CNS subcellular fraction. *Neurochem. Res.* **16**, 1113–1120.

Persson, H, and Corneliuson, O. (1989). Degradation products of myelin proteins in a light CNS subcellular fraction. *Neurochem. Res.* **14**, 1177–1180.

Persson, H., and Karlsson, J. O. (1991). Calpain activity in a subcellular fraction enriched in partially degraded CNS myelin fragments compared with myelin. *Neurosci. Lett.* **130**, 81–84.

Persson, H., Berthold, H., Rydmark, M., and Fabricius, C. (1992). Metabolic relationships between proteins of myelin and paranodally shedded, partially degraded myelin fragments in the rabbit CNS. *J. Neurosci. Res.* **33**, 310–318.

Peters, A. (1964). Further observations on the structure of myelin sheaths in the central nervous system. *J. Cell Biol.* **20**, 281–291.

Peters, A., Palay, S. L., and Webster, H. de F. (1991). "The Fine Structure of the Nervous System. Neurons and their Supporting Cells." 3rd ed. Oxford University Press, New York and Oxford.

Pfeiffer, S. E., Warrington, A. E., and Bansal, R. (1993). The oligodendrocyte and its many cellular processes. *Trends Cell Biol.* **3**, 191–197.

Pinching, A. J. (1971). Myelinated dendritic segments in the monkey olfactory bulb. *Brain Res.* **29**, 133–138.

Pinching, A. J., and Powell, T. P. S. (1971). The neuron types of the glomerular layer of the olfactory bulb. *J. Cell Sci.* **9**, 305–345.

Raine, C. S. (1984a). Morphology of myelin and myelination. *In* "Myelin" (P. Morell, Ed.), pp. 1–51, Plenum Press, New York.

Raine, C. S. (1984b). On the association between perinodal astrocytic processes and the node of Ranvier in the CNS. *J. Neurocytol.* **13**, 21–27.

Rall, W., and Shepherd, G. M. (1968). Theoretical reconstruction of field potentials and dendrodendritic synaptic interactions in olfactory bulb. *J. Neurophysiol.* **31**, 884–915.

Reles, A., and Friede, R. L. (1991). Axonal cytoskeleton at the nodes of Ranvier. *J. Neurocytol.* **20**, 450–458.

Remahl, S., and Hildebrand, C. (1985). Myelinated non-axonal neuronal elements in the feline olfactory bulb lack sites with a nodal structural differentiation. *Brain Res.* **325**, 1–11.

Remahl, S., and Hildebrand, C. (1990). Relation between axons and oligodendroglial cells during initial myelination. I. The glial unit. *J. Neurocytol.* **19**, 313–328.

Remahl, S., Risling, M., and Hildebrand, C. (1977). Age-related changes in occurrence of Marchi-positive myelinoid bodies in postnatally developing feline white matter. *J. Neurol. Sci.* **34**, 71–86.

Rosenbluth, J. (1976). Intramembranous particle distribution at the node of Ranvier and adjacent axolemma in myelinated axons of the frog brain. *J. Neurocytol.* **5,** 731–746.

Rosenbluth, J. (1983). Structure of the node of Ranvier. *In* "Structure and Function of Excitable Cells" (D. C. Chang, I. Tasaki, W. J. Adelman, and H. J. Leuchtag, Eds.), pp. 25–53. Plenum Press, New York.

Rosenbluth, J. (1984). Membrane specializations at the nodes of Ranvier and paranodal and juxtaparanodal regions of myelinated central and peripheral nerve fibers. *In* "The Node of Ranvier" (J. C. Zagoren and S. Fedoroff, Eds.), pp. 31–67. Academic Press, Orlando.

Rosenbluth, J. (1989). Role of Schwann cells in differentiation of the axolemma: Consequences of myelin deficiency in spinal roots of the dystrophic mouse mutant. *In* "Peripheral Nerve Development and Regeneration. Recent Advances and Clinical Applications" (E. Scarpini, M. G. Fiori, D. Pleasure, and D. Scarlato, Eds.), pp. 39–53. Livania Press, Padova.

Rosenbluth, J. (1995). Glial membranes and axonal junctions. *In* "Neuroglia" (H. Kettenmann, and B. Ransom, Eds.), pp. 613–633. Oxford University Press, New York.

Sanchez, I., Hassinger, L., Paskevich, P. A., Shine, H. D., and Nixon, R. A. (1996). Oligodendroglia regulate the regional expansion of axon caliber and local accumulation of neurofilaments during development independently of myelin formation. *J. Neurosci.* **16**, 5095–5105.

Scheibel, M. E., and Scheibel, A. B. (1975). Dendrite bundles, central programs and the olfactory bulb. *Brain Res.* **95**, 407–421.

Schnapp, B., and Mugnaini, E. (1978). Membrane architecture of myelinated fibres as seen by freeze-fracture. *In* "Physiology and Pathobiology of Axons" (S. G. Waxman, Ed.), pp. 83–123. Raven Press, New York.

Schnapp, B. J., and Reese, T. S. (1982). Cytoplasmic structure in rapid-frozen axons. *J. Cell Biol.* **94**, 667–679.

Sims, T. J., Gilmore, S. A., and Waxman, S. G. (1991). Radial glia give rise to perinodal processes. *Brain Res.* **549**, 25–35.

Shinowara, N. L., Beutel, W., and Revel, J.-P. (1980). Comparative analysis of junctions in the myelin sheath of central and peripheral axons of fish, amphibians and mammals. A freeze fracture study using complementary replicas. *J. Neurocytol.* **7**, 15–38.

Song, J., Goetz, B. D., Kirvell, S. L., Butt, A. D., and Duncan, I. D. (2001). Selective myelin defects in the anterior medullary velum of the *taiep* mutant rat. *Glia* **33**, 1–11.

Starr, R., Attema, B., De Vries, G. H., and Monteiro, M. J. (1996). Neurofilament phosphorylation is modulated by myelination. *J. Neurosci. Res.* **44**, 328–337.

Stensaas, L. J., and Stensaas, S. S. (1968). Astrocytic neuroglial cells, oligodendrocytes and microgliacytes in the spinal cord of the toad. I. Light microscopy. *Z. Zellforsch.* **84**, 473–489.

Sternberger, N. H., Itoyama, Y., Kies, M. W., and Webster, H. de F. (1978). Immunocytochemical method to identify basic protein in myelin-forming oligodendrocytes of newborn rat CNS. *J. Neurocytol.* **7**, 251–263.

Suzuki, K., and Suzuki, Y. (1983). Galactosylceramide lipoidosis: Globoid cell leukodystrophy (Krabbe's disease). *In* "The Metabolic Basis of Inherited Disease" (J. B. Wyngaarden, D. S. Fredrickson, J. L. Goldstein, and M. S. Brown, Eds.), pp. 857–880. McGraw-Hill, New York.

Szuchet, S. (1995). The morphology and ultrastructure of oligodendrocytes and their functional implications. *In* "Neuroglia" (H. Kettenmann and B. Ransom, Eds.), pp. 23–43. Oxford University Press, New York and Oxford.

Tao-Cheng J.-H., and Rosenbluth, J. (1984). Extranodal particle accumulations in the axolemma of myelinated frog optic axons. *Brain Res.* **308**, 289–300.

Thomas, P. K., Berthold, C.-H., and Ochoa, J. (1993). Microscopic anatomy of the peripheral nervous system. *In*: "Peripheral Neuropathy" 3rd edition, (P. J. Dyck, and P. K. Thomas, Eds.), pp. 28–91. W. B. Saunders, Philadelphia.

Tigges, M., and Tigges, J. (1980). Distribution and morphology of perikarya and dendrites in the olfactory bulb of primates. *J. Neurocytol.* **9**, 825–834.

Tsukita, S., and Ishikawa, H. (1981). The cytoskeleton in myelinated axons: Serial section study. *Biomed. Res.* **2**, 424–437.

Ulfhake, B., and Cullheim, S. (1988). Postnatal development of cat hind limb motoneurons. III: Changes in size of motoneurons supplying the triceps surae muscle. *J. Comp. Neurol.* **278**, 103–120.

Waxman, S. G. (1984). Nodelike membrane at extranodal sites: Comparative morphology and physiology. *In* "The Node of Ranvier" (J. C. Zagoren, and S. Fedoroff, Eds.), pp. 311–351. Academic Press, New York.

Waxman, S. G. (1986). The astrocyte as a component of the node of Ranvier. *Trends Neurosci.* **9**, 250–253.

Waxman, S. G. (1997). Axon-glia interactions: Building a smart nerve fiber. *Curr. Biol.* **7**, R406–R410.

Waxman, S. G., and Bennett, M. V. L. (1972). Relative conduction velocities of small myelinated and non-myelinated fibres in the central nervous system. *Nature* **238**, 217–219.

Waxman, S. G., and Black, J. A. (1984). Freeze-fracture ultrastructure of the perinodal astrocyte and associated glial junctions. *Brain Res.* **308**, 77–88.

Waxman, S. G., and Black, J. A. (1995). Axoglial interactions at the cellular and molecular levels in central nervous system myelinated fibers. *In* "Neuroglia" (H. Kettenmann and B. R. Ransom, Eds.), pp. 587–610. Oxford University Press, New York and Oxford.

Waxman, S. G., and Sims, T. J. (1984). Specificity in central myelination: Evidence for local regulation of myelin thickness. *Brain Res.* **292**, 179–185.

Waxman, S. G., and Ritchie, J. M. (1993). Molecular dissection of the myelinated axon. *Ann. Neurol.* **33**, 121–136.

Weruaga-Prieto, E., Eggli, P., and Celio, M. R. (1996). Topographic variation in rat brain oligodendrocyte morphology elucidated by injection of Lucifer Yellow in fixed tissue slices. *J. Neurocytol.* **25**, 19–31.

Wiley, C. A., and Ellisman, M. H. (1980). Rows of dimeric-particles within the axolemma and juxtaposed particles within the glia, incorporated into a new model for the paranodal glial-axonal junction at the node of Ranvier. *J. Cell Biol.* **84**, 261–280.

Willey, T. J. (1973). The ultrastructure of the cat olfactory bulb. *J. Comp. Neurol.* **152**, 211–232.

Wood, P., and Bunge, R. P. (1984). The biology of the oligodendrocyte. *In* "Oligodendroglia" (W. T. Norton, Ed.), pp. 1–46. Plenum Press, New York and London.

Yamamoto, C., Yamamoto, T., and Iwama, K. (1963). The inhibitory systems in the olfactory bulb studied by intracellular recording. *J. Neurophysiol.* **26**, 403–415.

Yin, X., Crawford, T. O., Griffin, J. W., Tu, P.-H., Lee, V. M.-Y., Li, C., Roder, J., and Trapp, B. D. (1998). Myelin-associated glycoprotein is a myelin signal that modulates the caliber of myelinated axons. *J. Neurosci.* **18**, 1953–1962.

Zagoren, J. C. (1984). Cation binding at the node of Ranvier. *In* "The Node of Ranvier" (J. C. Zagoren, and S. Fedoroff, Eds.), pp. 69–91. Academic Press, Orlando.

2

Dialogues: Communication Between Axons and Myelinating Glia

Robert M. Gould, Ph.D.
Scott T. Brady, Ph.D.

I. Introduction

The structure and function of the nervous system are determined by cell-cell interactions. Genes and genetic programs provide the algorithms and molecular players needed to assemble and maintain a nervous system. Successful execution of these programs is dependent on the ensemble of cellular interactions that the neuron or glial cell experiences. Both temporal and spatial coding of cell-cell interactions is important. If the timing of a contact occurs out of sequence, the intended exchange of information will likely fail because the ligand or the receptor may either be absent or not recognized. If the interaction occurs in the wrong place, then the intended partner will not be available. Regardless, when an appropriate interaction is missing, communication between cells fails to occur and, consequently, genetic algorithms fail to run or alter the outcome, and a different nervous system is the result. These principles, most dramatically in evidence during development, also apply to the adult nervous system. The profound changes seen in the nervous system when damage or disease disrupts normal cellular interactions demonstrate a need for appropriate spatial and temporal cell-cell interactions in the nervous system.

Many neuroscientists consider nervous system development and function solely in a neuronal context, viewing the nervous system primarily in terms of synaptic contacts and circuitry. However, nerve-glia interactions are more extensive than synaptic contacts, and these interactions play a critical role in the generation and maintenance of a nervous system. In this chapter, we consider the relationship between neurons and myelinating glia (MG). Specific examples exist of neurons directing differentiation of MG, as well as MG modulating the differentiation and functional architecture of neurons. Although many of the signals and pathways that compose these dialogues remain to be identified, consequences of disrupting the dialogues are well documented.

The matching of glial cells with appropriate neuronal populations is one of the earliest examples of a dialogue between neurons and glia. Only a subset of central nervous system (CNS) and PNS axons are destined to receive a myelin sheath, and selection is made from populations of axons whose members have a variety of different fates and destinations. Schwann cells (SCs) must settle on a single axon and then begin myelination. Oligodendrocytes (OLs) choose a set of axon segments more or less concurrently before initiating myelination. What are the criteria used by MG in choosing axons? What confirms that the choice is appropriate and triggers differentiation in the MG? How are competitions with nearby SCs and OLs for axon segments controlled?

Once myelination begins, neurons and axons respond to the developing myelin sheath in characteristic ways that may differ between the CNS and PNS. Multiple pathways are involved, so a neuron with a developing or thin myelin sheath differs in many respects from the mature neuron. Moreover, some of these pathways involve local actions with local consequences, whereas other pathways require transport of one or more signals from or back to the neuronal perikaryon. Transported signals may have profound effects on the transcription and translation of neuronal proteins, affecting the differentiation and maturation of the neuron. Concurrent with this effect, the MG is being transformed with both quantitative and qualitative changes in gene expression and organization.

Gaps between myelinating segments (i.e., nodes of Ranvier) represent another region in which both axons and MG create highly specialized domains through a series of interactions. These nodes have distinctive organization of ion channels, receptors, transporters, membrane cytoskeleton, cell adhesion, and cell recognition molecules. Both the structure and molecular organization of nodal and paranodal domains need to be highly stereotyped and precisely maintained for proper nerve conduction.

Finally, axonal diameters, myelin sheath thickness, and internodal lengths are remarkably consistent over the entire length of an unbranched axon. In humans, forming and maintaining an axon 1 m or more long involves hundreds to thousands of MG. In the CNS, the problem is compounded because OL independently maintain myelin sheath thickness and internode length for many different axons at the same time. Each of these parameters is dynamic, changing during development and maturation of the nervous system, as well as being altered again when an axon or sheath is damaged by disease or injury. Feedback mechanisms must exist to allow adjustment and coordination of these parameters, but we are just beginning to understand these mechanisms.

The extent to which these dialogues must be coordinated for a properly functioning nervous system is extraordinary. The deceptively simple task of picking up a cup of hot coffee and bringing it to the mouth for a sip without spilling cannot be accomplished without successful execution of these essential dialogues between neurons and MG. We are just beginning to understand the nature of these dialogues and how they may be disrupted in dysmyelinating and demyelinating diseases such as Krabbe's disease and multiple sclerosis. Identifying the molecular and cellular bases of individual steps and characterizing the relevant signaling pathways will go a long way toward understanding the causes of neuronal pathology in these diseases and developing treatment strategies.

II. Developmental Matching of Axons and Myelinating Glia

Many, but not all, axons in the CNS and PNS are myelinated. In the CNS, extensive studies have characterized the origins and stages of OL differentiation (Miller, 1996; Miller and Reynolds, 2004). Less attention has been paid to the sequence of events by which axons match up with OL precursors and induce them to initiate myelination. The signaling involved in recruiting MG to cover and myelinate axons with appropriately sized sheaths is one of the first examples of communication between neurons and MG.

OL, the myelin forming cells of the CNS, originate in neuroepithelial precursor cell populations in developing brain and spinal cord (reviewed by Bongarzone, 2002; Noble et al., 2004; and Rao, 2004). Although cells originating in multiple regions have the capacity to develop into myelinating OL (Hardy and Friedrich, 1996), the cells that actually myelinate axons come from spatially restricted cell populations (reviewed by Liu and Rao, 2003; Miller, 1996; Noble et al., 2004; Rogister et al., 1999; Rowitch et al., 2002). Formation of OL progenitors is dependent on positive local sonic hedgehog signaling and negative bone morphogenetic protein pathways (Miller, 2002; Orentas et al., 1999; Rogister et al., 1999). Other factors also play roles during OL differentiation. One example is PDGF-A, an OL mitogen (Calver et al., 1998) and an attractant that influences OL progenitor migration (Simpson and Armstrong, 1999). PDGF-A appears necessary for the spreading of OL progenitors to territories occupied by maturing axons (Rowitch et al., 2002; Woodruff et al., 2001). How these and other factors influencing developmental pathways leading to myelination are coordinated with axon maturation is poorly understood.

As is often the case during development in the CNS, proliferation in the OL precursor population overshoots the numbers of available axon segments and OL death occurs as matches are made (Barres et al., 1992; Burne et al., 1996).

Early developmental interactions with axons are required for survival and further differentiation of OL progenitors. A large and growing number of growth factors, hormones, chemokines and small molecules influence OL differentiation and myelination (reviewed by Du and Dreyfus, 2002; Miller and Reynolds, 2004; Rogister et al., 1999). Detailed descriptions of OL development are outside the scope of this chapter. Instead, we will try to place the expression of these stimulation and repression factors in the framework of the developing axon-glial cell contacts that occur throughout the various stages of myelination.

Migrating OL precursors must distribute throughout the regions destined to contain myelinated fibers in numbers and at times when axons destined to be their partners are ready. The earliest migration of OL progenitors, at least in the spinal cord, is triggered at least in part by the expression of chemorepulsive molecules (including netrin-1) in regions where they are produced (Tsai et al., 2003). The trigger for this event is uncertain, but PDGF is a known stimulant of OL-precursor migration (Simpson and Armstrong, 1999). Once OL precursors are in motion, they appear to migrate along tracks that contain guidance cues for axons (Tsai and Miller, 2002), ensuring that they will encounter axons at appropriate stages of maturation. When the migrating OL precursors encounter axon-rich fields, a signal is needed to prevent further migration. Such cues must be titrated appropriately to the number of axons that require myelination. This number may change over time, as enlarging axons are the first to be selected for myelination. Smaller axons are avoided, although they may be picked subsequently for myelination as they enlarge later in development. To accomplish appropriate pairing, the chemokine CXCL1 or a related molecule appears to be secreted by the axon and recognized by the CXCR2 receptor on the OL precursor (Tsai et al., 2002). In the absence of this signaling pathway, OL precursors migrate past the axon tracts and accumulate in the periphery. Significantly, inhibition of OL precursor migration occurs in a critical CXCL1 concentration range, with higher or lower levels having minimal effect (Tsai et al., 2002). This tight concentration dependence may ensure a distribution of OL precursors in axon tracts sufficiently dispersed to encompass all areas where the precursors are needed.

The timing for early stages of myelination is likely to be set by the first axons to reach a developmental stage where they require myelin sheaths for further differentiation. OL progenitors first appear in developing brain and spinal cord tracts around the time when a population of axons can be distinguished that are larger in caliber than neighboring axons. In animals as evolutionarily separated as mammals and cartilaginous fishes, we can identify stages before the appearance of OL, when all axons, for example, in the medial longitudinal fascicle and ventral spinal cord are small. At slightly later stages, when the first few axons are enlarged,

OLs enter the area (Gould and Gilland, unpublished observation).

After OL precursors enter a tissue region where myelination is to occur, they extend processes. Light and electron microscopy have documented the stages of development and maturation of contacts between OL processes and axons as they segregate and myelinate selected axons (Bunge, 1968; Ogawa et al., 2004; Peters et al., 1991; Trapp and Kidd, 2004). Such studies provide a basis for identifying when and where signaling molecules might be needed. These processes must recognize large caliber axons through a set of poorly understood mechanisms. At this stage, cell surface and adhesion molecules are likely to play an important role. Contact between OL precursor and axon surface appears to be key to subsequent OL differentiation and myelination.

An important player in this initial interaction is the Notch1 receptor expressed on OL precursors (Wang et al., 1998). Neurons and to some extent OL precursors express the Jagged1, an integral membrane protein and Notch1 ligand that inhibits further differentiation of the OL precursor. Expression of both Notch1 and its ligand in OL precursors may prevent differentiation of the OL in the absence of axonal contact. When an axon in contact with an OL precursor process down-regulates Jagged1 expression, myelination of the axon can proceed (Wang et al., 1998). The developmental program that causes an axon to increase in diameter presumably also reduces Jagged1 expression. Another potential axonal ligand for notch 1 is F3/contactin (Hu et al., 2003; Popko, 2003), a protein that associates in paranodal junctions of the forming node of Ranvier. If jagged-1 and F3/contactin are expressed on the surface of maturing axons, these molecules may signal OL differentiation leading to myelination. Once an appropriate axon is identified, the OL process begins to spread along the axon surface, separating the larger axon from adjacent smaller fibers (Hardy and Friedrich, 1996; Ogawa et al., 2004).

The fact that one OL can interact with multiple axons greatly increases the complexity of the signaling between these two cell populations. For myelination to occur in a timely manner, the signaling between individual OL processes and the axon segments they select to myelinate must be tightly regulated. This requirement suggests that different OL processes may be involved in different stages of myelination and receiving different signals. In such cases, different processes must act independently, although the main source of myelin proteins is a common OL soma. There must also be coordination between neighboring OL as each establishes a specific field of axon segments under its influence with a density that assures all suitable axon segments will be myelinated. Subsequent signaling between OL and axons is needed to target specific axonally transported proteins to nodes of Ranvier (sodium channels, adhesion molecules, actin cytoskeleton-linkers), adjacent paranodes (adhesion molecules) and juxtaparanodes (adhesion molecules and potassium channels).

The sequence of events that occurs during peripheral nerve development differs in some key respects, although it still involves interactions between axons and MG (SC) precursors as well as between different SC precursors. SC precursors arise in the neural crest, along with peripheral sensory neurons and a range of other cell types (Le Douarin and Dupin, 1993; Le Douarin and Dupin, 2003). Detailed information on SC development can be found in recent reviews (Jessen and Mirsky, 2004; Lobsiger et al., 2002). Here, we focus on results that illuminate the cross-talk between developing axons and SC used to attain normal functioning peripheral nerves, particularly those aspects that differ from interactions occurring during CNS development. During PNS development, SC precursors are initially concentrated at the margins of axon bundles. They enter the bundles and associate with axons in one of two ways. Precursors either separate individual axons from all their neighbors to establish a 1:1 relationship as prelude to myelin sheath formation, or they separate clusters of small caliber axons into unmyelinated fiber bundles. For a correct pairing of SC with axons, SC numbers increase through extensive proliferation in the developing nerve (Asbury, 1967; Cheng et al., 1998; Stewart et al., 1993). This proliferation requires contact with the axonal membrane (Ratner et al., 1985). Subsequently, SC that fail to develop proper interactions with axons die (Grinspan et al., 1996; Syroid et al., 1996).

Under both myelinating and nonmyelinating conditions, SCs form a basal lamina that covers each nerve fiber or fiber bundle along its length. Although a complete basal lamina was thought to be an essential prerequisite for myelination (Bunge et al., 1986), newer evidence suggests that laminins expressed by SC plus mechanical stability may be sufficient (Podratz et al., 2001). By the time the nerve reaches maturity, all SCs are associated with axons (Webster, 1971). In addition to the SCs that develop associations with axons in peripheral nerves, SCs also form associations with neurons in ganglia as satellite cells and in association with sensory and motor terminal specializations. Differentiation of these SCs is likely to be controlled by signals from the cell specializations they contact, as well as additional environmental cues.

The importance of axons in determining the SC phenotype was demonstrated in an elegant manner with nerve transplantation studies (Aguayo et al., 1976; Weinberg and Spencer, 1976) and reviewed in Bray et al., 1981. In these studies, nerve fibers containing a preponderance of large caliber axon bundles were cut and rerouted to proximal cut ends of nerve fibers that were occupied by SCs largely associated with small caliber nonmyelinated axons. The regenerating axons not only regrew into the mismatched distal stump and became large caliber axons, but they induced SCs originally associated with small caliber axons and/or their progeny to produce myelin sheaths of thick-

nesses appropriate for their caliber. Conversely, when fibers that contained small caliber axons were rerouted into a cut nerve that originally contained large caliber myelinated axons, the regenerating axons induced SC progeny from large caliber axons to take on a nonmyelinating phenotype. SC responses to changed target axons demonstrated the instructive role axons play in determining the formation of myelin by SC. Further, SCs that are originally committed to a specific size class of axons have the plasticity to adapt to either myelinating or nonmyelinating conditions depending on signals from the axons encountered.

The ability of SCs to respond to axonal signals was also shown by an elegant study in which axons in a sympathetic postganglionic nerve were manipulated experimentally (Voyvodic, 1989). Limiting the target by reducing the size of the target (submandibular salivary gland) also reduced the sizes of axons innervating the gland (mainly unmyelinated fibers). Consequently, SCs clustered a larger number of axons into each bundle. If axon input was reduced, effectively increasing target size, axons responded by increasing in caliber. These increases in axon caliber induced SCs to form myelin sheaths. Using several different experimental manipulations, investigators showed that axons control both SC population numbers and myelination. More recently, a variety of axon effectors, SC responders, and signal transduction mechanisms important for axon/SC communication have been elucidated.

The neuregulins make up one of the most important axon-to-SC signaling systems, particularly type III neuregulin-1, which contains an N-terminal cysteine-rich domain believed to intercalate into the membrane (Bao et al., 2003) and erbB2/erbB3 receptor heterodimers (Adlkofer and Lai, 2000; Falls, 2003a; Garratt et al., 2000a; Gassmann and Lemke, 1997; Topilko et al., 1996). Neuregulin/erbB interactions are essential for normal development. Although knockout mice lacking either neuregulin-1 (all subtypes) or erb-B2 receptor die of cardiac failure at E10.5 well before peripheral nerves develop, gene targeting strategies show the importance of the neuregulin-erbB receptor system in SC survival (Garratt et al., 2000b; Wolpowitz et al., 2000). Neuregulin-1 type III expression on the surface of early developing axons is required to signal SC precursors and allow them to survive. Once these differentiate into early SC, they develop an autocrine system that allows survival in the absence of axons. Significantly, these studies also reveal a dependence of neurons on SC survival. In the absence of neuregulin-1 type III, SC died and the absence of SC led to a consequent loss of both motor and sensory neurons. SC appear to provide paracrine factors that are needed for peripheral neuron survival, even in the presence of factors generated from targets (Davies, 1998). A recent study (Esper and Loeb, 2004) identified several SC-derived factors that elicit axonal release of neuregulin. Even before myelination has occurred, a mutual dependence exists between neurons and MG.

Although mutual dependence is established, many questions remain about how neuregulin-1 type III expression is controlled and the identity of other signaling pathways that help to establish this link. What signals neurons to increase expression of the neuregulins and release them from axonal domains where the signals will reach SCs? Since membrane bound neuregulin-1 type III can possibly receive information through contact with erbB receptors (Bao et al., 2003; Falls, 2003b), interactions with numerous SCs along the length of growing axon may in turn regulate neuregulin expression and transport. In addition to neuregulin, insulin-like growth factor (Syroid et al., 1999) and endothelins (Brennan et al., 2000) may participate in the signaling important for SC/axon pairing during development.

III. Local Influences of Myelin on Axon Cytoskeleton

Traditionally, changes in synthesis of cytoskeletal proteins, connection with suitable targets, patterns of activity, and availability of target-derived neurotrophic factors were thought to regulate axon diameter. From this viewpoint, the number of MTs and NFs (Friede and Samorajski, 1970) supplied by slow axonal transport (Hoffman et al., 1988, 1985, 1983; Lasek et al., 1983; Wujek et al., 1986) were believed to be the primary determinants of axon diameter. Synthesis of cytoskeletal and membrane proteins in neurons was presumably affected by contact with an appropriate target, largely by increasing the return of neurotrophins to the neuronal perikaryon by retrograde axonal transport ensuring neuronal survival and differentiation (Burek and Oppenheim, 1996; Thoenen, 2000). Neurotrophin uptake and retrograde transport by neurons could be enhanced by increased neuronal activity, enhancing neuronal plasticity (Thoenen, 2000). Glial cell influences on neuronal growth were thought to act primarily through mechanisms like glial production of neurotrophins (Althaus and Richter-Landsberg, 2000). However, release of neurotrophins in the adult nervous system by MG was thought to be modest compared to release by targets, although it could be upregulated in some cases by nerve injury (Heumann et al., 1987) or disease (Burbach et al., 2004; Heese et al., 1998).

In fact, myelination by either SC or OL has profound effects on the local axon. The absence of myelin, whether due to demyelination or failure to form myelin, leads to characteristic alterations in the organization, biochemistry, and composition of the axonal cytoskeleton. Such changes in the neuronal cytoskeleton have a dramatic impact on neuronal function. Studies with myelin mutant mouse models, Trembler and Shiverer, provided the initial evidence for this influence.

Trembler mice have a point mutation in a gene (PMP22) expressed in SC, but not OLs (Suter and Snipes, 1995; Suter et al., 1992b). As a result, Trembler mice have a phenotype that includes demyelination of large caliber axons in the PNS with no apparent effect on myelination of CNS axons (Low and McLeod, 1975). Affected PNS SC exhibit continuing cycles of myelination and demyelination that get progressively worse, eventually resulting in a high percentage of large axons with little or no compact myelin (Low, 1976a, 1976b). In Trembler, PMP22 is a dominant mutation with several alleles (Suter et al., 1992a, 1992b; Suter and Snipes, 1995). Although specific functions of PMP22 in myelination are poorly understood, a variety of human peripheral neuropathies have defects in PMP22 or in levels of its expression. For example, missense mutations lead to hypomyelinating phenotypes (Trembler, Dejerine-Sottas syndrome, and some cases of CMT1a), whereas deletions in PMP22 are implicated in hereditary neuropathy with liability to pressure palsies and PMP22 gene duplication gives rise to most cases of CMT1a in humans.

PMP22 is an SC integral membrane tetraspan protein, but most PMP22 is degraded without insertion into the plasma membrane. Interaction with an axon during myelination increases PMP22 synthesis and promotes insertion of glycosylated protein into the plasma membrane (Pareek et al., 1997). One effect of point mutations is to reduce PMP22 insertion into plasma membrane (Colby et al., 2000). The sensitivity of PNS myelin to both the presence of PMP22 and levels expressed on the myelin surface suggests that PMP22 functions in signaling to neurons. That disruption of PMP22 function or distribution leads to a neuropathy suggests a neuronal target.

Electron microscopic images of Trembler peripheral nerves in cross-section typically show many axons undergoing active demyelination or lacking myelin. Axons were smaller and thinner than normal (Ayers and Anderson, 1976). Remarkably, this reduction in axonal caliber was a local phenomenon (Aguayo et al., 1977; de Waegh and Brady, 1991; de Waegh et al., 1992). When sciatic nerve segments from Trembler mice are grafted into wild-type sciatic nerve and axons are allowed to regenerate, axon regions in the Trembler graft have a Trembler phenotype, demyelinated axons, and reduced axonal caliber in graft regions (Aguayo et al., 1977; de Waegh and Brady, 1991). In these nerves, axons proximal and distal to the graft had normal compact myelin and axon caliber. The reverse graft experiment (normal sciatic nerve segment grafted in Trembler sciatic nerve) had normal myelin and axonal caliber in the graft, but Trembler phenotype proximal and distal to the graft (Aguayo et al., 1977; de Waegh and Brady, 1991).

Axonal parameters that are altered locally included rates of slow axonal transport (de Waegh and Brady, 1990; de Waegh et al., 1992), phosphorylation of neurofilament and microtubule proteins (de Waegh et al., 1992; Kirkpatrick and Brady, 1994), and neurofilament density (de Waegh and Brady, 1991; de Waegh et al., 1992). Neurofilament phosphorylation appeared to be the primary determinant of axonal caliber in these models (de Waegh et al., 1992), and the loss of compact myelin in Trembler PNS axons led to a significant reduction in neurofilament phosphorylation and consequential increase in neurofilament densities (Fig. 1). Two hypomyelinating transgenic mice with different severity of demyelination showed that the effects on neurofilament phosphorylation and density scaled with the severity of the demyelination (Cole et al., 1994).

The influence of myelin sheaths on organization of the axonal cytoskeleton begins to explain how SC myelin can alter the functional architecture of the axon. For example, myelin sheaths formed by SCs specifically influence phosphorylation of axonal NFs (Cole et al., 1994; de Waegh et al., 1992; Hsieh et al., 1994). Neurofilament phosphorylation was sensitive to myelination levels both *in vivo* and in culture (Cole et al., 1994; Starr et al., 1996). Remarkably, short gaps in compact myelin such as those found at nodes of Ranvier were sufficient to change neurofilament density (Figure 1B) and phosphorylation (de Waegh, 1990; Hsieh et al., 1994; Mata et al., 1992). Changes in phosphorylation of axonal NFs thus appear to be responsible for the characteristic structure of larger caliber axons at PNS and CNS nodes of Ranvier (Brady, 1993; de Waegh et al., 1992), with reduced caliber and increased NF density (Berthold, 1982; Scherer et al., 2004).

CNS myelin also affects local properties of the axon, with some differences in the effects. Not only fine structure (Peters et al., 1991; Raine, 1984) but also protein and lipid composition (Morell and Quarles, 1999) differ between CNS and PNS myelin. Moreover, some functions of SC in the PNS may be split between OL and astrocytes in the CNS. Shiverer is a recessive mutation with a more severe pheno-

type than Trembler. Shiverer mutant mice lack compact myelin in the CNS and develop a severe tremor in early postnatal development (Readhead and Hood, 1990). They have a mean life span of 100 to 120 d (Chernoff, 1981). The absence of compact myelin in the CNS is due to deletion of coding regions after the first exon in the myelin basic protein (MBP) gene (Roach et al., 1985). MBP is a major structural protein of CNS myelin, but a minor component of PNS myelin (Campagnoni and Macklin, 1988). Two PNS-specific proteins, P0 and P2, appear to have functional overlap with MBP, so PNS myelination is near normal (Rosenbluth, 1980a, 1980b), albeit with some structural differences (Gould et al., 1995).

Whereas PNS axons in Trembler mice are subject to a constant cycle of myelination and demyelination, the absence of MBP in Shiverer means that CNS axons never see normal myelin. One advantage of studying Shiverer mouse as an animal model is that transgenic mice are available that express different levels of MBP (Popko et al., 1987). Studies with mouse strains having different levels of MBP expression indicate that MBP levels limit myelin sheath thickness (Shine et al., 1992) with an minimum of 50% of wild-type MBP required for normal thickness in CNS myelin sheaths. Mice homozygous for an MBP transgene expressed only 25% of wild-type MBP levels, resulting in a thin compact myelin with relatively few lamellae. However, this thin myelin sheath was sufficient to suppress tremors and increase life spans to near normal (Readhead et al., 1987). Availability of Shiverer and transgenic Shiverer mice homozygous for the MBP transgene (MBP/MBP) permitted evaluation of how myelin sheath thicknesses affect CNS axons (Brady et al., 1999).

Both CNS axons lacking myelin (Shiverer) and CNS axons with abnormally thin myelin sheaths (transgenic Shiverer: TG Shiverer) exhibit changes in local properties relative to CNS

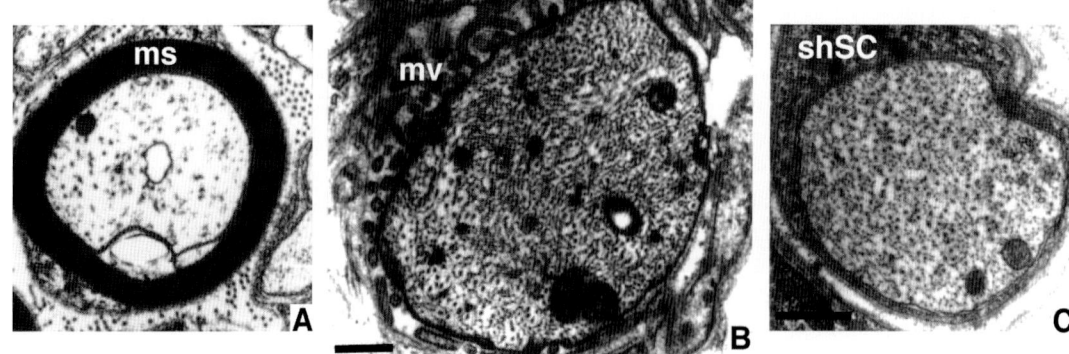

Figure 1 Local influences of myelination on the axon cytoskeleton. The use of mutant mouse strains such as Trembler show that the presence of compact myelin has a dramatic effect on the organization of axonal neurofilaments and axonal caliber. Contrast the number and density of neurofilaments in wild-type (**A**) and Trembler (**C**) axons in cross-section. The increased density of neurofilaments is accompanied by a reduction in axonal caliber and neurofilament phosphorylation (de Waegh et al., 1992). At a node of Ranvier (**B**), there is a gap in the myelin sheath that leads to a similar dephosphorylation of axonal neurofilaments and reduction in axonal caliber (ms: myelin sheath; sc: Schwann cell cytoplasm; mv: Schwann cell microvilli at node of Ranvier). (Adapted from Kirkpatrick and Brady, 1999.) (Micrographs by S. de Waegh and S. Brady.)

axons with normal myelin sheaths (wild-type). These differences are analogous in some, but not all, respects to those seen in Trembler PNS axons. Relative to wild-type, axonal diameters of optic axons were reduced in Shiverer mice; NF densities were increased in Shiverer; and NFH phosphorylation was reduced (Brady et al., 1999; Kirkpatrick et al., 2001). However, changes in these parameters were less pronounced than corresponding changes in Trembler PNS nerve (de Waegh et al., 1992). In TG Shiverer mice with 25% of normal MBP and fewer layers of compact myelin than wild-type, these same parameters were intermediate between Shiverer and wild-type (Brady et al., 1999). In adult myelinated axons, Na(v) 1.2 channels are restricted to unmyelinated zones like the axon hillock and Na(v) 1.6 channels are restricted to the nodes of Ranvier (Boiko et al., 2001). Consistent with this pattern, Na(v) 1.2 channels are abundant on nonmyelinated fibers and appear first in development, but Na(v) 1.6 channels do not appear in significant amounts until myelin forms. Targeting of sodium channel isoforms is altered in Shiverer axons (Boiko et al., 2001) with a distribution similar to that seen in nonmyelinated axons (i.e., Na(v)1.2) all along the axons and very little Na(v) 1.6 is detected.

Other local axonal parameters were the same in TG Shiverer and wild-type optic axons. For example, slow axonal transport rates were increased in Shiverer, but were indistinguishable in TG Shiverer and wild-type nerves (Brady et al., 1999). These observations indicate that OL influence local axonal parameters during development and that the full effect of myelination is not expressed until the thickness of the myelin sheath approaches wild-type levels.

Changes in other myelin-related proteins also affect local axonal parameters. For example, absence of either PMP22 or connexin 32 (another SC protein) leads to specific changes in axonal properties and architecture (Neuberg et al., 1999). Both of these knockouts allow formation of compact myelin that is subsequently removed and exhibit axonal atrophy. Notably, there are also changes in the distribution of a nodal K_v-channel in these mice (Neuberg et al., 1999). Connexin 32 mutant mice also have changes in the axonal cytoskeleton similar to those seen in Trembler along with indications of altered axonal transport (Sahenk and Chen, 1998).

Mice with a null mutation in proteolipid protein (PLP) exhibit axonal swellings and degeneration consistent with a local effect on fast axonal transport (Griffiths et al., 1998). A detailed study of axons in PLP null mice (Edgar et al., 2004) showed significant accumulations of axonal vesicles and alterations in the molecular motor protein cytoplasmic dynein. This action of PLP-deficient myelin was local because similar phenotypes were seen in axonal segments surrounded by PLP-null OL in a Shiverer background (Edgar et al., 2004).

Mice lacking myelin-associated glycoprotein (MAG) form compact myelin sheaths, but these sheaths are not closely apposed to the axonal membrane (Yin et al., 1998).

With increasing age, the axons in MAG knockout mice develop significantly smaller calibers and reduced neurofilament phosphorylation. Another indication that MAG affects neuronal properties is found in the observation that MAG is also an important modulator of neurite growth (Filbin, 1995). A similar phenotype is observed in mice that lack the ability to make complex gangliosides (Sheikh et al., 1999), raising the possibility that complex gangliosides are ligands for MAG (Vyas et al., 2002). Whether another MAG ligand, Nogo receptor (Barton et al., 2003; Liu et al., 2002), influences axonal properties is not yet known. Studies on mice lacking both MAG and the complex gangliosides (Marcus et al., 2002) suggest that these two components interact to stabilize glial-axonal interactions. Developmental studies (Yin et al., 1998) suggest that MAG-based signaling is not solely responsible for local alteration of axonal parameters, but interactions between myelin and axons mediated by MAG influence phosphorylation of axonal cytoskeletal proteins and axonal caliber (Dashiell et al., 2002).

Local axonal parameters of both CNS and PNS fibers are affected by dysmyelination or demyelination, but the changes are not identical. What they share is an increase in neurofilament density coupled to a reduction in both neurofilament phosphorylation and axonal caliber. The stability of axonal microtubules is also affected in both mouse models, but the composition of axonal microtubules is affected differentially (Kirkpatrick and Brady, 1994; Kirkpatrick et al., 2001). Slow axonal transport is also affected by lack of myelin in both CNS and PNS, but is increased over wild-type in Shiverer axons that have never seen myelin and slower in Trembler PNS axons that have been demyelinated (Brady et al., 1999; de Waegh and Brady, 1988, 1990; de Waegh et al., 1992). These effects all result from local effects of MG on axons, but equally striking are differences in neuronal properties that result from changes in gene expression in the neuron.

IV. Distal Effects of Myelination and Myelin as a Neuronal Maturation Factor

The influence of myelination is not restricted to local changes in the axon. The signaling pathways responsible for changes in the phosphorylation of cytoskeletal proteins in the axon also have other actions. Either directly or indirectly, local signals about myelination are communicated to the neuronal cell body where both translational and transcriptional changes occur. Mouse strains with altered or defective myelin provided direct evidence of this retrograde communication pathway.

A wide variety of neuronal parameters are altered in Shiverer mouse CNS tissues. These included differences in slow axonal transport, cytoskeletal composition, posttranslational modification of cytoskeletal proteins, and axon caliber. Even more striking than these local changes are alterations in the cytoskeletal composition of Shiverer neurons that reflect changes in neuronal gene transcription and translation. By a number of criteria, neurons in the Shiverer mouse exhibit characteristics similar to early postnatal neurons (i.e., before myelination occurs) and to neurons with nonmyelinated axons. Remarkably, analysis of these same parameters in the CNS of TG Shiverer mice producing 25% of normal myelin with minimal tremor and normal life spans reveals a phenotype exhibiting features in common with both wild-type and Shiverer neurons as well as some features intermediate between the two.

Quantitative analysis of cytoskeletal proteins in slow axonal transport provided the first evidence that the axonal cytoskeleton in a Shiverer nerve was very different from that seen in wild-type axons (Brady et al., 1999; Kirkpatrick et al., 2001). Specifically, the stoichiometries of neurofilament subunits indicated that protein levels for high and medium molecular weight neurofilament subunits (NFH and NFM) were significantly and selectively lower in Shiverer axons (Brady et al., 1999). In contrast, NFM levels were restored to normal in TG Shiverer axons with a thin myelin sheath, but NFH was still reduced. NFL levels were not significantly different among the three mouse strains. Analysis of NF mRNA levels showed that NFH mRNA levels were reduced in both Shiverer and TG Shiverer brains, suggesting that transcription of the NFH gene was regulated by myelination (Brady et al., 1999). Because NFM mRNA levels were comparable in all three genotypes, however, control of NFM expression by myelination was not regulated at the level of transcription, but rather during mRNA translation and protein expression.

Myelination levels in CNS axons dramatically affected axonal microtubules (Fig. 2). In both Shiverer and TG Shiverer axons, the number of microtubules per axon was twice that seen in comparable wild-type axons (Kirkpatrick

et al., 2001). This increase was accompanied by an increase in tubulin mRNA consistent with an effect of myelin on transcription. The increased ratio of microtubules to NF and reductions in NFH/NFM levels resemble ratios obtained for the cytoskeleton of nonmyelinated axons in the CNS. These findings are consistent with the idea that formation of compact myelin sheath is a requisite step for the differentiation and maturation of large-caliber axons.

The primary phase of myelination in the rodent CNS begins 1 to 2 weeks after birth and continues for several more weeks. A number of changes in the properties of CNS neurons exhibit a similar time course. For example, NFH is low at birth and increases to approach adult levels several weeks after birth in rats (Carden et al., 1987) and levels of tubulin as well as expression of different tubulin ioforms also change during this interval (Lewis et al., 1985). Slow axonal transport is high in neonates and decreases at approximately 3 weeks postnatal (McQuarrie et al., 1989; Willard and Simon, 1983). The temporal pattern of these events, along with a failure to observe comparable changes in Shiverer, indicates that formation of compact myelination triggers these neuronal changes.

Other axonal parameters are also affected by myelination in the CNS. The density and expression levels of voltage-gated sodium channels are increased in Shiverer CNS (Noebels et al., 1991). This change reflects both a change in the distribution of the Na channels and a difference in the specific Na-channel isoforms being expressed. In nonmyelinated nerves, the predominant voltage dependent Na-channel is $Na(v)$ 1.2. Although $Na(v)$ 1.2 is still present in unmyelinated regions of myelinated axons, the dominant voltage dependent Na-channel in nodes of Ranvier is $Na(v)$ 1.6 (Caldwell et al., 2000). Expression of $Na(v)$ 1.2 is elevated in Shiverer CNS (Westenbroek et al., 1992). Moreover, $Na(v)$ 1.2 is distributed all along the axon in Shiverer axons, much as in nonmyelinated fibers, and little

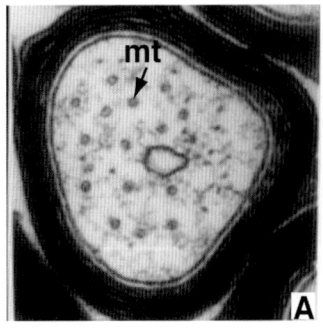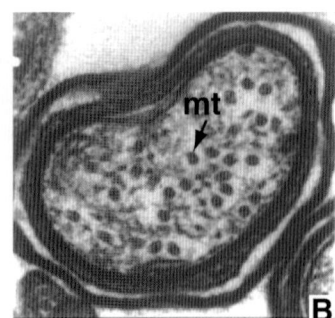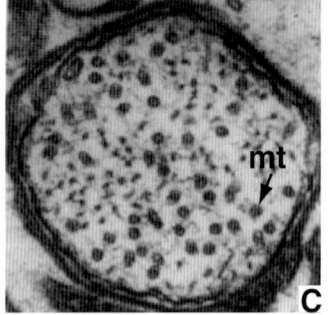

Figure 2 Distal effects of myelination on the axon cytoskeleton. Some changes in the axon reflect a change in gene transcription and protein synthesis in the neuronal cell body as a response to retrograde signals generated in the axon by myelination. Comparing the microtubule cytoskeleton of wild type axon (**A**) with normal myelin to a transgenic Shiverer mouse axon (**B**) expressing only 25% of normal myelin basic protein sufficient for a myelin sheath about 25% of wild-type; and to a Shiverer mouse axon (**C**) with no myelin. Both Shiverer and transgenic Shiverer axons have twice the normal number of microtubule seen in a comparable sized wild-type axon. Both Shiverer and the transgenic Shiverer nerves have increased tubulin mRNA levels as well (Kirkpatrick et al., 2001). Changes in other neuronal mRNAs including neurofilament subunits and ion channels are also seen in Shiverer. (Figure adapted from Kirkpatrick et al., 2001.)

or no Na(v) 1.6 is expressed (Boiko et al., 2001). Normally Na(v) 1.2 accumulates in forming nodes of Ranvier and is then replaced by Na(v) 1.6. Concurrently, voltage-gated potassium channels (K(v) 1.1 and 1.2) appear to redistribute from a broad distribution along the nerve to a restricted distribution in juxtaparanodes as myelination proceeds (Wang et al., 1995). Expression levels and localization of K-channels are also altered in Shiverer mice with a significant increase in both neuronal and glial K-channels (Wang et al., 1995).

PNS dysmyelination mutants may also exhibit altered levels of cytoskeletal and membrane proteins. For example, MAG-deficient axons have reductions in NF protein levels that become more apparent in older axons (Yin et al., 1998). In Charcot-Marie-Tooth Type 1a disease, there appears to be reduced numbers of neurofilaments (Watson et al., 1994). Similarly, the level of specific immature β-tubulin isotypes is elevated in CMT-1a nerves (Watson et al., 1994). Finally, K-channel expression is elevated in Trembler mouse PNS axons, as well as in Shiverer CNS axons (Wang et al., 1995).

In Trembler axons, levels of neurofilament and tubulin subunits were not dramatically altered (de Waegh et al., 1992; Kirkpatrick and Brady, 1994). However, there are a number of changes in the microtubule cytoskeleton of Trembler axons. The stable fraction of Trembler axonal microtubules is significantly reduced relative to that of wild-type axons (Kirkpatrick and Brady, 1994). This stable tubulin fraction normally increases in axons as they mature (Brady, 1984; Yan et al., 1985). The microtubule-associated protein composition in Trembler mice also is altered. Trembler axons are enriched in low-molecular-weight tau protein and the high-molecular-weight tau protein characteristic of mature peripheral nerve is reduced in Trembler relative to wild-type axons (Kirkpatrick and Brady, 1994). High-molecular-weight tau proteins result from alternative splicing of mRNAs from a single tau gene and correlate with increased maturation and MT stability (Oblinger et al., 1991).

Trembler axons are myelinated and then lose that myelin. Expression of all three NF subunits during regeneration is coordinate (McKerracher et al., 1993), but during development NFH gene expression lags behind NFL and NFM (Kost et al., 1992). This suggests that myelination of an axon may trigger a differentiation step that alters regulation of NF subunit expression. For example, MAG-null mice form myelin, but that myelin is never properly apposed to the axonal membrane, and the myelination signal may not be completed. This may explain why MAG-null mice show reductions in NF protein levels in PNS axons (Yin et al., 1998) and Trembler mice do not (de Waegh and Brady, 1991; de Waegh et al., 1992).

Dysmyelination affects neuronal gene expression in both CNS and PNS. As with the local effects of myelin, there are both similarities and differences between CNS and PNS effects of myelination. Some of these changes may reflect differences in the nature of the dysmyelination (e.g., demyelination/remyelination, failure to form compact myelin). Other differences may reflect differences in signaling between axons and OL or SC. For example, pathways expressed by SC may be split between OL and astrocytes in the CNS. Alternatively, the ability of PNS axons to regenerate more effectively than CNS fibers indicates that differences exist in the maturation of large neurons in the PNS and CNS. This may be relevant to the milder axonal phenotype seen in many peripheral demyelinating diseases as compared to multiple sclerosis.

V. Nodes of Ranvier

The influence of myelination on expression and distribution of Na- and K-channels (Noebels et al., 1991; Wang et al., 1995; Westenbroek et al., 1992) draws attention to another essential element of neuronal architecture that is largely defined by interactions between MG and axons. In both the CNS and PNS, the establishment and maintenance of nodes of Ranvier separated by much larger internodal myelin sheaths form the basis of saltatory conduction, an evolutionary breakthrough that led to the increasingly complex nervous systems of modern-day vertebrates. In humans and other large animals, long projection axons may have more than a thousand nodes located at precisely spaced intervals (0.5 to 3 mm) along meter-long axons. At each node, there is a highly structured organization of channels, adhesion molecules, and cytoskeletal elements that ensure high current flow and efficient saltatory conduction (Poliak and Peles, 2003; Scherer et al., 2004). The task faced by neurons in distributing and maintaining lipids and proteins components to each of these nodal, paranodal, and juxtaparanodal specializations distinct from the myriad other functional microdomains in an axon is daunting. A detailed description of nodal architecture and nodal development is outside the scope of this chapter. However, many lines of evidence support the essential roles played by MG and myelination on establishing and maintaining nodes of Ranvier. A brief overview of this evidence and consideration of pathways that may participate in the formation and maintenance of nodes are merited.

The classic description of cellular membranes as fluid mosaic structures with rapid movement of membrane proteins in the plane of the membrane is at odds with the requirements of a neuron maintaining functional axons and synapses. The size of large projection neurons and their need to maintain highly specialized functional microdomains like those present at nodes dictate that membrane proteins inserted into the plasma membrane remain in place. Indeed, axolemmal proteins, synthesized during pulse-labeling studies, were shown to maintain a constant location for months after labeling (Griffin et al., 1981).

Consistent with this line of reasoning, nodal location of channels is retained for a rather long time after demyelination, before Na channels appear widely distributed over the demyelinated axonal membrane (England et al., 1990; Foster et al., 1980; Shrager, 1989). Two lines of evidence support the conclusion that Na channels appearing in demyelinated internodal axon membranes represent newly synthesized channels delivered by fast axonal transport rather than a redistribution of the old nodal channels. First, reorganization of channels requires an increase in synthesis of new channels (England et al., 1991; Foster et al., 1980), and this increased synthesis occurs in neurons (England et al., 1996). Second, the Na channel isotype that appears in the demyelinated membrane is in many cases predominantly Na(v) 1.2 rather than the Na(v)1.6, the channel typically found in nodal regions (Craner et al., 2003). Given that mouse mutants with defective myelination also have increased synthesis of channels (Noebels et al., 1991; Wang et al., 1995; Westenbroek et al., 1992) and the channels increased are typical of nonmyelinated fibers (Boiko et al., 2001; Westenbroek et al., 1992), it is highly likely that newly synthesized and transported channels are the ones appearing in demyelinated axon membranes.

Taken together with observations that OL (Kaplan et al., 2001, 1997) and SC (Ching et al., 1999) induce clustering of Na channels, there is little doubt that MG interaction with axons plays a critical role in the targeting of proteins that form and maintain nodal architecture. A key remaining question is how MG accomplish this regulation of channel expression and organization. Considerable information about the axonal and glial cell proteins that assemble in nodes, paranodes, and juxtaparanodes is now available (Girault and Peles, 2002; Poliak and Peles, 2003; Salzer, 2003; Scherer et al., 2004). This information provides a framework for understanding nodal complex formation and maintenance, but much remains to be learned about targeting mechanisms and signaling pathways involved in assembly or maintenance.

In the PNS, SC initiate node formation by contacting an axon to be ensheathed. When ensheathment reaches more than one turn and MAG begins to be expressed (Martini and Schachner, 1986), the leading edges at either end of an SC approach leading edges of neighboring SC and Na channels are seen to cluster in these regions (Vabnick et al., 1996; Vabnick and Shrager, 1998). Similar clustering of channels in response to SC contact is seen in remyelination (Dugandzija-Novakovic et al., 1995; Novakovic et al., 1996) and can be used to study targeting of nodal proteins. Remyelinated internodes are thinner and shorter than those formed during development (Hirano, 1989).

A number of other proteins are also targeted to these developing nodal specializations. On the neuronal side, these include proteins important in attaching membrane proteins to the membrane cytoskeleton, including ankyrin

G, spectrin α II and β-IV, and protein 4.1 (Berghs et al., 2000; Denisenko-Nehrbass et al., 2003; Kordeli et al., 1990); cell adhesion molecules important for interaction with SC microvillae including NrCAM and neurofascin-186 (Davis et al., 1996); and at least two types of K-channels (Devaux et al., 2003, 2004). On the glial microvillae side, clustering of Na channels correlates with the appearance of FERM proteins (4.1, ezrin, radixin, and moesin) and FERM interacting proteins in SC microvilli suggest that these structures play a role in the signaling responsible for Na-channel clustering, possibly through the syndecans (Goutebroze et al., 2003) and possibly also tenascins (Weber et al., 1999). The axonal partner and signaling pathway responsible remains to be understood, but phosphoinositide signaling has been associated with ERM activity (Bretscher et al., 2002). In addition, a recent report suggests a role for small GTPase signaling on the SC side, because inhibition of Rho kinase activity significantly alters SC morphology and induces additional nodal specializations along myelinating fibers in SC-dorsal root ganglion co-culture (Melendez-Vasquez et al., 2004).

Clustering of Na channels is also a feature of developing CNS nodes, but there is evidence that OL can induce clustering of Na channels without direct contact, presumably through a diffusible element (Kaplan et al., 2001, 1997). The nature of this signal is unclear. Differences in nodal structure and composition between CNS and PNS nodes suggest that the signals provided by OL and SC may overlap, albeit incompletely. For example, the ERM proteins that are so prominent in SC processes associated with clustering of Na channels are not present in OL processes (Melendez-Vasquez et al., 2001; Scherer et al., 2001). CNS nodes are also less stable than PNS nodes based on the relative severity of node disruption observed in knockouts of nodal components (Poliak and Peles, 2003). Mutations that affect expression of galactolipids (Dupree et al., 1998) or paranodal proteins (Bhat et al., 2001; Boyle et al., 2001; Rios et al., 2003) disrupt CNS nodes preferentially. A possible explanation is that the role of stabilizing nodal structures is taken by SC alone in the PNS, but is split between OL and a unique type of astrocyte (Butt et al., 1999, 2002). OL directly interact to form the glial loops of paranodal domains, but have no contact with nodal membranes. Instead, cells in the astrocyte lineage stabilize nodal membranes in the CNS.

A key feature of both PNS and CNS nodes is a reduced axonal diameter (Hildebrand et al., 1993) that is more apparent as fiber size increases. As noted previously, a major determinant of reduced axonal caliber at nodes of Ranvier is reduced phosphorylation of NF proteins. This observation led to the proposal that formation of compact myelin plays a role in targeting membrane proteins like Na channels to nodes of Ranvier as well as influencing cytoskeletal organization in the axon (de Waegh et al., 1992). Consistent with this, Na channels begin to appear in internodal membrane after demyelination (Foster et al., 1980). Neuronal phosphatases and kinases typically have multiple substrates, so myelination may affect phosphorylation of multiple axonal proteins. A variety of kinase and phosphatase pathways are reported to play a role in targeting of neuronal membrane proteins to specific functional domains (Beffert et al., 2004; Donelan et al., 2002; Morfini et al., 2004, 2002, 2001; Tsai et al., 2000). Thus, observed changes in phosphorylation of axonal proteins may be a way to target vesicles containing Na channels and other nodal components to the node of Ranvier membrane (Morfini et al., 2001). For example, a pathway for activating protein phosphatase PP1 in axons inhibits kinesin-based motility through the GSK3 pathway (Morfini et al., 2004). Whether or not this is the pathway for targeting nodal proteins like Na channels to the node of Ranvier, the spatially restricted dephosphorylation of NF proteins implicates one or more kinase/phosphatase pathways in the generation of nodal structures.

VI. Axonal Diameter, Myelin Sheath Thickness, and Internode Lengths

Myelin sheath thickness and internodal length vary with axonal caliber (Fraher, 1978; Friede and Miyagishi, 1972). An important feature of myelination in both the CNS and PNS is the matching of axon diameter, myelin sheath thickness, and nodal length because this matching is required to optimize nerve conduction properties (Rushton, 1951; Waxman, 1997). The specific combination of axon diameter, myelin sheath thickness, and internodal length is established during development and maturation of a myelinated fiber. A given myelinated axon will exhibit remarkable consistency in diameter, sheath thickness, and internodal distance as long as the axon is unbranched and the type of MG responsible is unchanged. Neighboring axons with comparable diameters will have comparable sheath thicknesses and internodal lengths (Friede and Miyagishi, 1972). The specific values of these parameters are established during development and maturation of an axon population. However, when axons are denuded and subsequently remyelinated or when regenerating axons become myelinated, the values are typically reduced relative to the original ones (Blakemore, 1974).

Although the matching of axon caliber to myelin sheath thickness has long been recognized (Elder et al., 2001; Friede and Miyagishi, 1972), the molecular mechanisms that regulate the interrelationships between axon caliber, myelin sheath thickness, and internodal length are still poorly understood. Recent studies begin to dissect this pathway in the PNS. Mice lacking erbB2 receptor form unusually thin myelin sheaths (Garratt et al., 2000a, 2000b). This focused attention on the possibility of axonal expression of neuregulins, the ligands for erbB receptors (Falls,

2003a, 2003b). Subsequent studies showed that axonal expression of a specific neuregulin, (neuregulin-1 type III with an N-terminal cysteine-rich domain) plays a key role in the relationship between myelin sheath thickness and axon caliber. Neuregulin-1 type III, is expressed in myelinated axons and its receptors, erbB2 and erbB3, are expressed in SC and in myelin (Michailov et al., 2004). As with reduced erbB2 receptor (Garratt et al., 2000b), lowering levels of neuregulin-1 type III, but not other nrg-1 family members, leads to hypomyelination. To show that the effect was on the ligand and not the receptor, overexpression of ligand, but not receptor, resulted in hypermyelinated axons. Interestingly, internodal length was unaffected by altered nrg-1 or altered erbB2 receptor, suggesting that other mechanisms were involved in controlling internodal length. Such studies pave the way for future analyses of the underlying signaling mechanisms.

Signals generated through axonal neuregulins and myelin erbB receptors regulate myelination in the PNS. However, control of myelin sheath thickness by axons in the CNS is a more complex event. In the CNS, individual OL extend multiple processes that simultaneously myelinate axons with different calibers and sheaths of different thicknesses (Elder et al., 2001; Friedrich and Mugnaini, 1983; Waxman and Sims, 1984). Control of myelin sheath thickness must be locally controlled at the level of the axon-glia interface. It is not currently known whether neuregulin/erbB interactions or other yet-to-be-uncovered mechanisms are involved.

VII. Conclusion

The time when neuroscientists could treat neurons as autonomous cells defined primarily by target interactions is long past. The interdependence of neurons and glia in both the PNS and CNS is a complex and essential relationship for both partners. Neither fully differentiates in the absence of their appropriate partners. Furthermore, the relationship changes as the nervous system develops and matures. Much remains to be understood about the nature of these dialogues shared between MG and neurons. However, significantly altering either the neuronal or the glial components has profound effects on the function of the nervous system.

Acknowledgments

Preparation of this chapter was supported in part by grants from the NINDS (NS23868, NS23320, NS41170 and NS43408) to STB and from NSF (1000624) to RMG.

References

Adlkofer, K., and Lai, C. (2000). Role of neuregulins in glial cell development. *Glia* **29**, 104–111.

Aguayo, A., Attiwell, M., Trecarten, J., Perkins, S., and Bray., G. (1977). Abnormal myelination in transplanted Trembler mouse Schwann cells. *Nature* **265**, 73–74.

Aguayo, A. J., Charron, L., and Bray, G. M. (1976). Potential of Schwann cells from unmyelinated nerves to produce myelin: a quantitative ultrastructural and radiographic study. *J. Neurocytol.* **5**, 565–573.

Althaus, H. H., and Richter-Landsberg, C. (2000). Glial cells as targets and producers of neurotrophins. *Int. Rev. Cytol.* **197**, 203–277.

Asbury, A. K. (1967). Schwann cell proliferation in developing mouse sciatic nerve. A radioautographic study. *J. Cell Biol.* **34**, 735–743.

Ayers, M., and Anderson, R. (1976). Development of onion bulb neuropathy in the Trembler mouse. Morphometric study. *Acta Neuropath. (Berlin)* **36**, 137–152.

Bao, J., Wolpowitz, D., Role, L. W., and Talmage, D. A. (2003). Back signaling by the Nrg-1 intracellular domain. *J. Cell Biol.* **161**, 1133–1141.

Barres, B. A., Hart, I. K., Coles, H. S., Burne, J. F., Voyvodic, J. T., Richardson, W. D., and Raff, M. C. (1992) Cell death and control of cell survival in the oligodendrocyte lineage. *Cell*, **70**, 31–46.

Barton, W. A., Liu, B. P., Tzvetkova, D., Jeffrey, P. D., Fournier, A. E., Sah, D., Cate, R., Strittmatter, S. M., and Nikolov, D. B. (2003). Structure and axon outgrowth inhibitor binding of the Nogo-66 receptor and related proteins. *EMBO J.* **22**, 3291–3302.

Beffert, U., Weeber, E. J., Morfini, G., Ko, J., Brady, S. T., Tsai, L. H., Sweatt, J. D., and Herz, J. (2004). Reelin and cyclin-dependent kinase 5-dependent signals cooperate in regulating neuronal migration and synaptic transmission. *J. Neurosci.* **24**, 1897–1906.

Berghs, S., Aggujaro, D., Dirkx, R., Jr., Maksimova, E., Stabach, P., Hermel, J. M., Zhang, J. P., Philbrick, W., Slepnev, V., Ort, T., and Solimena, M. (2000). BetaIV spectrin, a new spectrin localized at axon initial segments and nodes of ranvier in the central and peripheral nervous system. *J. Cell Biol.* **151**, 985–1002.

Berthold, C. (1982). Some aspects of the ultrastructural organization of peripheral myelinated axons in the cat. *In* "Axoplasmic Transport" (D. Weiss, ed.), pp. 40–54. Springer-Verlag, New York.

Bhat, M. A., Rios, J. C., Lu, Y., Garcia-Fresco, G. P., Ching, W., St Martin, M., Li, J., Einheber, S., Chesler, M., Rosenbluth, J., Salzer, J. L., and Bellen, H. J. (2001). Axon-glia interactions and the domain organization of myelinated axons requires neurexin IV/Caspr/Paranodin. *Neuron* **30**, 369–383.

Blakemore, W. F. (1974). Pattern of remyelination in the CNS. *Nature* **249**, 577–578.

Boiko, T., Rasband, M. N., Levinson, S. R., Caldwell, J. H., Mandel, G., Trimmer, J. S., and Matthews, G. (2001). Compact myelin dictates the differential targeting of two sodium channel isoforms in the same axon. *Neuron* **30**, 91–104.

Bongarzone, E. R. (2002). Induction of oligodendrocyte fate during the formation of the vertebrate neural tube. *Neurochem. Res.* **27**, 1361–1369.

Boyle, M. E., Berglund, E. O., Murai, K. K., Weber, L., Peles, E., and Ranscht, B. (2001). Contactin orchestrates assembly of the septate-like junctions at the paranode in myelinated peripheral nerve. *Neuron* **30**, 385–397.

Brady, S. T. (1984). Increases in cold-insoluble tubulin during aging. *Soc. Neurosci. Abstr.*, **10**, 273.

Brady, S. T. (1993) Axonal dynamics and regeneration. *In* "Neuroregeneration" (A. Gorio, ed.), pp. 7–36. Raven Press, New York.

Brady, S. T., Witt, A. S., Kirkpatrick, L. L., de Waegh, S. M., Readhead, C., Tu, P.-H., and Lee, V. M.-Y. (1999). Formation of compact myelin is required for maturation of the axonal cytoskeleton. *J. Neurosci.* **19**, 7278–7288.

Bray, G. M., Rasminsky, M., and Aguayo, A. J. (1981). Interactions between axons and their sheath cells. *Annu. Rev. Neurosci.* **4**, 127–162.

Brennan, A., Dean, C. H., Zhang, A. L., Cass, D. T., Mirsky, R., and Jessen, K. R. (2000). Endothelins control the timing of Schwann cell generation in vitro and in vivo. *Dev. Biol.* **227**, 545–557.

Bretscher, A., Edwards, K., and Fehon, R.G. (2002). ERM proteins and merlin: Integrators at the cell cortex. *Natl. Rev. Mol. Cell Biol.* **3**, 586–599.

Bunge, R. P. (1968). Glial cells and the central myelin sheath. *Physiol. Rev.* **48**, 197–251.

Bunge, R. P., Bunge, M. B., and Eldridge, C. F. (1986). Linkage between axonal ensheathment and basal lamina production by Schwann cells. *Annu. Rev. Neurosci.* **9**, 305–328.

Burbach, G. J., Hellweg, R., Haas, C. A., Del Turco, D., Deicke, U., Abramowski, D., Jucker, M., Staufenbiel, M., and Deller, T. (2004). Induction of brain-derived neurotrophic factor in plaque-associated glial cells of aged APP23 transgenic mice. *J. Neurosci.* **24**, 2421–2430.

Burek, M. J., and Oppenheim, R. W. (1996). Programmed cell death in the developing nervous system. *Brain Pathol.* **6**, 427–446.

Burne, J. F., Staple, J. K., and Raff, M. C. (1996). Glial cells are increased proportionally in transgenic optic nerves with increased numbers of axons. *J. Neurosci.*, **16**, 2064–2073.

Butt, A. M., Duncan, A., Hornby, M. F., Kirvell, S. L., Hunter, A., Levine, J. M., and Berry, M. (1999). Cells expressing the NG2 antigen contact nodes of Ranvier in adult CNS white matter. *Glia* **26**, 84–91.

Butt, A. M., Kiff, J., Hubbard, P., and Berry, M. (2002). Synantocytes: new functions for novel NG2 expressing glia. *J. Neurocytol.* **31**, 551–565.

Caldwell, J. H., Schaller, K. L., Lasher, R. S., Peles, E., and Levinson, S. R. 2000. Sodium channel Na(V)1.6 is localized at nodes of ranvier, dendrites, and synapses. *Proc. Nat. Acad. Sci. USA* **97**, 5616–5620.

Calver, A. R., Hall, A. C., Yu, W. P., Walsh, F. S., Heath, J. K., Betsholtz, C., and Richardson, W. D. (1998). Oligodendrocyte population dynamics and the role of PDGF in vivo. *Neuron* **20**, 869–882.

Campagnoni, A. T., and Macklin, W. B. (1988). Cellular and molecular aspects of myelin protein gene expression. *Mol. Neurobiol.* **2**, 41–89.

Carden, M. J., Trojanowski, J. Q., Schlaepfer, W. W., and Lee, V. M.-Y. (1987). Two stage expression of neurofilament polypeptides during rat neurogenesis with early establishment of adult phosphorylation patterns. *J. Neurosci.* **7**, 3489–3504.

Cheng, L., Esch, F. S., Marchionni, M. A., and Mudge, A. W. (1998). Control of Schwann cell survival and proliferation: autocrine factors and neuregulins. *Mol. Cell Neurosci.* **12**, 141–156.

Chernoff, G. F. (1981). Shiverer: an autosomal recessive mutant mouse with myelin deficiency. *J. Hered.* **72**, 128.

Ching, W., Zanazzi, G., Levinson, S. R., and Salzer, J. L. (1999). Clustering of neuronal sodium channels requires contact with myelinating Schwann cells. *J. Neurocytol.* **28**, 295–301.

Colby, J., Nicholson, R., Dickson, K. M., Orfali, W., Naef, R., Suter, U., and Snipes, G. J. (2000). PMP22 carrying the trembler or trembler-J mutation is intracellularly retained in myelinating Schwann cells. *Neurobiol. Dis.* **7**, 561–573.

Cole, J. S., Messing, A., Trojanowski, J. Q., and Lee, V. M.-Y. (1994). Modulation of axon diameter and neurofilaments by hypomyelinating Schwann cells in transgenic mice. *J. Neurosci.*, **14**, 6956–6966.

Craner, M. J., Lo, A. C., Black, J. A., and Waxman, S. G. (2003). Abnormal sodium channel distribution in optic nerve axons in a model of inflammatory demyelination. *Brain* **126**, 1552–1561.

Dashiell, S. M., Tanner, S. L., Pant, H. C., and Quarles, R. H. (2002). Myelin-associated glycoprotein modulates expression and phosphorylation of neuronal cytoskeletal elements and their associated kinases. *J. Neurochem.* **81**, 1263–1272.

Davies, A. M. (1998). Neuronal survival: early dependence on Schwann cells. *Curr. Biol.* **8**, R15–18.

Davis, J. Q., Lambert, S., and Bennett, V. (1996). Molecular composition of the node of Ranvier: Identification of ankyrin-binding cell adhesion molecules neurofascin (mucin+/third FNIII domain-) and NrCAM at nodal axon segments. *J. Cell Biol.* **135**, 1355–1367.

de Waegh, S., and Brady, S. T. (1988). Altered slow axonal transport in optic nerve of shiverer mutant mice. *Soc. Neurosci. Abstr.* **14**, 118.

de Waegh, S., and Brady, S. T. (1990). Altered slow axonal transport and regeneration in a myelin deficient mutant mouse: he Trembler mouse as an in vivo model for Schwann cell-axon interactions. *J. Neurosci.*, **10**, 1855–1865.

de Waegh, S. M. (1990). The importance of Schwann cell/axon interactions in the local control of neuronal shape and function: the Trembler mouse as an *in vivo* model. *Cell Biology,* p. 202. University of Texas Southwestern Medicial Center, Dallas, TX.

de Waegh, S. M., and Brady, S. T. (1991). Local control of axonal properties: Neurofilaments and axonal transport in homologous and heterologous nerve grafts. *J. Neurosci. Res.* **30**, 201–212.

de Waegh, S. M., Lee, V. M.-Y., and Brady, S. T. (1992). Local modulation of neurofilament phosphorylation, axonal caliber, and slow axonal transport by myelinating Schwann cells. *Cell* **68**, 451–463.

Denisenko-Nehrbass, N., Oguievetskaia, K., Goutebroze, L., Galvez, T., Yamakawa, H., Ohara, O., Carnaud, M., and Girault, J. A. (2003). Protein 4.1B associates with both Caspr/paranodin and Caspr2 at paranodes and juxtaparanodes of myelinated fibres. *Eur. J. Neurosci.* **17**, 411–416.

Devaux, J., Alcaraz, G., Grinspan, J., Bennett, V., Joho, R., Crest, M., and Scherer, S. S. (2003). Kv3.1b is a novel component of CNS nodes. *J. Neurosci.* **23**, 4509–4518.

Devaux, J. J., Kleopa, K. A., Cooper, E. C., and Scherer, S. S. (2004). KCNQ2 is a nodal K+ channel. *J. Neurosci.* **24**, 1236–1244.

Donelan, M. J., Morfini, G., Julyan, R., Sommers, S., Hays, L., Kajio, H., Briaud, I., Easom, R. A., Molkentin, J. D., Brady, S. T., and Rhodes, C. J. (2002). Ca2+-dependent dephosphorylation of kinesin heavy chain on beta-granules in pancreatic beta-cells. Implications for regulated beta-granule transport and insulin exocytosis. *J. Biol. Chem.* **277**, 24232–24242.

Du, Y., and Dreyfus, C.F. (2002). Oligodendrocytes as providers of growth factors. *J. Neurosci. Res.* **68**, 647–654.

Dugandzija-Novakovic, S., Koszlowski, A. G., Levinson, S. R., and Shrager, P. (1995). Clustering of Na+ channels and node of Ranvier formation in remyelinating axons. *J. Neurosci.*, **15**, 492–503.

Dupree, J. L., Coetzee, T., Blight, A., Suzuki, K., and Popko, B. (1998). Myelin galactolipids are essential for proper node of Ranvier formation in the CNS. *J. Neurosci.* **18**, 1642–1649.

Edgar, J. M., McLaughlin, M., Yool, D., Zhang, S. C., Fowler, J. H., Montague, P., Barrie, J. A., McCulloch, M. C., Duncan, I. D., Garbern, J., Nave, K. A., and Griffiths, I. R. (2004). Oligodendroglial modulation of fast axonal transport in a mouse model of hereditary spastic paraplegia. *J. Cell Biol.* **166**, 121–131.

Elder, G. A., Friedrich, V. L., Jr., and Lazzarini, R. A. (2001). Schwann cells and oligodendrocytes read distinct signals in establishing myelin sheath thickness. *J. Neurosci. Res.* **65**, 493–499.

England, J. D., Gamboni, F., and Levinson, S. R. (1991). Increased numbers of sodium channels form along demyelinated axons. *Brain Res.* **548**, 334–337.

England, J. D., Gamboni, F., Levinson, S. R., and Finger, T. E. (1990). Changed distribution of sodium channels along demyelinated axons. *Proc. Natl. Acad. Sci. U. S. A.* **87**, 6777–6780.

England, J. D., Levinson, S. R., and Shrager, P. (1996). Immunocytochemical investigations of sodium channels along nodal and internodal portions of demyelinated axons. *Microsc. Res. Tech.* **34**, 445–451.

Esper, R. M., and Loeb, J. A. (2004). Rapid axoglial signaling mediated by neuregulin and neurotrophic factors. *J. Neurosci.* **24**, 6218–6227.

Falls, D. L. (2003a). Neuregulins and the neuromuscular system: 10 years of answers and questions. *J. Neurocytol.* **32**, 619–647.

Falls, D. L. (2003b). Neuregulins: Functions, forms, and signaling strategies. *Exp. Cell Res.* **284**, 14–30.

Filbin, M. T. (1995). Myelin-associated glycoprotein: A role in myelination and in the inhibition of axonal regeneration? *Curr. Opin. Neurobiol.* **5**, 588–595.

Foster, R. E., Whalen, C. C., and Waxman, S. G. (1980). Reorganization of the axon membrane in demyelinated peripheral nerve fibers: Morphological evidence. *Science* **210**, 661–663.

Fraher, J. P. (1978). Quantitative studies on the maturation of central and peripheral parts of individual ventral motoneuron axons: I. Myelin sheath and axon caliber. *J. Anat.* **126**, 509–533.

Friede, R. L., and Miyagishi, T. (1972). Adjustment of the myelin sheath to changes in axonal caliber. *Anat. Rec.* **17**, 1–14.

Friede, R. L., and Samorajski, T. (1970). Axon caliber related to neurofilaments and microtubules in sciatic nerve fibers of rats and mice. *Anat. Rec.* **167**, 379–388.

Friedrich, V. L., Jr., and Mugnaini, E. (1983). Myelin sheath thickness in the CNS is regulated near the axon. *Brain Res.* **274**, 329–331.

Garratt, A. N., Britsch, S., and Birchmeier, C. (2000a). Neuregulin, a factor with many functions in the life of a Schwann cell. *Bioessays* **22**, 987–996.

Garratt, A. N., Voiculescu, O., Topilko, P., Charnay, P., and Birchmeier, C. (2000b). A dual role of erbB2 in myelination and in expansion of the Schwann cell precursor pool. *J. Cell Biol.* **148**, 1035–1046.

Gassmann, M., and Lemke, G. (1997). Neuregulins and neuregulin receptors in neural development. *Curr. Opin. Neurobiol.* **7**, 87–92.

Girault, J. A., and Peles, E. (2002). Development of nodes of Ranvier. *Curr. Opin. Neurobiol.* **12**, 476–485.

Gould, R. M., Byrd, A. L., and Barbarese, E. (1995). The number of Schmidt-Lanterman incisures is more than doubled in shiverer PNS myelin sheaths. *J. Neurocytol.* **24**, 85–98.

Goutebroze, L., Carnaud, M., Denisenko, N., Boutterin, M. C., and Girault, J. A. (2003). Syndecan-3 and syndecan-4 are enriched in Schwann cell perinodal processes. *BMC Neurosci.* **4**, 29.

Griffin, J. W., Price, D. L., Drachman, D. B., and Morris, J. R. (1981). Incorporation of transported glycoproteins into axolemma during regeneration. *J. Cell Biol.* **88**, 205–214.

Griffiths, I., Klugmann, M., Anderson, T., Yool, D., Thomson, C., Schwab, M. H., Schneider, A., Zimmermann, F., McCulloch, M., Nadon, N., and Nave, K. A. (1998). Axonal swellings and degeneration in mice lacking the major proteolipid of myelin. *Science* **280**, 1610–1613.

Grinspan, J. B., Marchionni, M. A., Reeves, M., Coulaloglou, M., and Scherer, S. S. (1996). Axonal interactions regulate Schwann cell apoptosis in developing peripheral nerve: Neuregulin receptors and the role of neuregulins. *J. Neurosci.* **16**, 6107–6118.

Hardy, R. J., and Friedrich, V. L., Jr. (1996). Oligodendrocyte progenitors are generated throughout the embryonic mouse brain, but differentiate in restricted foci. *Development* **122**, 2059–2069.

Heese, K., Hock, C. and Otten, U. (1998). Inflammatory signals induce neurotrophin expression in human microglial cells. *J. Neurochem.* **70**, 699–707.

Heumann, R., Korsching, S., Bandtlow, C., and Thoenen, H. (1987). Changes in nerve growth factor synthesis in nonneuronal cells in response to sciatic nerve transsection. *J. Cell Biol.* **104**, 1623–1631.

Hildebrand, C., Remahl, S., Persson, H., and Bjartmar, C. (1993). Myelinated nerve fibres in the CNS. *Prog. Neurobiol.* **40**, 319–384.

Hirano, A. (1989). Review of the morphological aspects of remyelination. *Dev. Neurosci.* **11**, 112–117.

Hoffman, P., Koo, E., Muma, N., Griffin, J., and Price, D. (1988). Role of neurofilaments in the control of axonal caliber in myelinated nerve fibers. *In* "Intrinsic Determinants of Neuronal Forms and Functions" (R. J. Lasek, and M. M. Black (eds.)), pp. 389–402. Alan R. Liss Inc., New York.

Hoffman, P., Thompson, G., Griffin, J., and Price, D. (1985). Changes in neurofilament transport coincide temporally with alterations in the caliber of axons in regenerating motor fibers. *J. Cell Biol.* **101**, 1332–1340.

Hoffman, P. M., Lasek, R. J., Griffin, J. W., and Price, D. L. (1983). Slowing of the axonal transport of neurofilament protein during development. *J. Neurosci.* **3**, 1694–1700.

Hsieh, S.-T., Kidd, G. J., Crawford, T. O., Xu, Z., Lin, W.-M., Trapp, B. D., Cleveland, D. W., and Griffin, J. W. (1994). Regional modulation of neurofilament organization by myelination in normal axons. *J. Neurosci.* **14**, 6392–6401.

Hu, Q. D., Ang, B. T., Karsak, M., Hu, W. P., Cui, X. Y., Duka, T., Takeda, Y., Chia, W., Sankar, N., Ng, Y. K., Ling, E. A., Maciag, T., Small, D.,

Trifonova, R., Kopan, R., Okano, H., Nakafuku, M., Chiba, S., Hirai, H., Aster, J. C., Schachner, M., Pallen, C. J., Watanabe, K., and Xiao, Z. C. (2003). F3/contactin acts as a functional ligand for Notch during oligodendrocyte maturation. *Cell* **115**, 163–175.

Jessen, K. R., and Mirsky, R. (2004). Schwann cell development. *In* "Myelin Biology and Disorders" (R. A. Lazzarini, ed.), Vol. 1, pp. 329–370. Elsevier Academic Press, Amsterdam.

Kaplan, M. R., Cho, M. H., Ullian, E. M., Isom, L. L., Levinson, S. R., and Barres, B. A. (2001). Differential control of clustering of the sodium channels Na(v)1.2 and Na(v)1.6 at developing CNS nodes of Ranvier. *Neuron* **30**, 105–119.

Kaplan, M. R., Meyer-Franke, A., Lambert, S., Bennett, V., Duncan, I. D., Levinson, S. R., and Barres, B. A. (1997). Induction of sodium channel clustering by oligodendrocytes. *Nature* **386**, 724–728.

Kirkpatrick, L. L., and Brady, S. T. (1994). Modulation of the axonal microtubule cytoskeleton by myelinating Schwann cells. *J. Neurosci.* **14**, 7440–7450.

Kirkpatrick, L. L., and Brady, S. T. (1999). Cytoskeleton of neurons and glia. *In* "Basic Neurochemistry: Molecular, Cellular and Medical Aspects" (G. J. Siegel, B. W. Agranoff, R. W. Albers, S. K. Fisher, and M. D. Uhler, eds.), pp. 155–174. Lippincott-Raven, Philadelphia.

Kirkpatrick, L. L., Witt, A. S., Payne, H. R., Shine, H. D., and Brady, S. T. (2001). Changes in microtubule stability and density in myelin-deficient shiverer mouse CNS axons. *J. Neurosci.* **21**, 2288–2297.

Kordeli, E., Davis, J., Trapp, B., and Bennett, V. (1990). An isoform of ankyrin is localized at nodes of Ranvier in myelinated axons of central and peripheral nerves. *J. Cell Biol.* **110**, 1341–1352.

Kost, S. A., Chacko, K., and Oblinger, M. M. (1992). Developmental patterns of intermediate filament gene expression in the normal hamster brain. *Brain Res.* **595**, 270–280.

Lasek, R., Oblinger, M., and Drake, P. (1983). Molecular biology of neuronal geometry: Expression of neurofilament genes influences axonal diameter. *Cold Spring Harbor Symp. Quant. Biol.* **28**, 731–744.

Le Douarin, N. M., and Dupin, E. (1993). Cell lineage analysis in neural crest ontogeny. *J. Neurobiol.* **24**, 146–161.

Le Douarin, N. M., and Dupin, E. (2003). Multipotentiality of the neural crest. *Curr. Opin. Genet. Dev.* **13**, 529–536.

Lewis, S. A., Lee, M. G., and Cowan, N. J. (1985). Five mouse tubulin isotypes and their regulated expression during development. *J. Cell Biol.* **101**, 852–861.

Liu, B. P., Fournier, A., GrandPre, T., and Strittmatter, S. M. (2002). Myelin-associated glycoprotein as a functional ligand for the Nogo-66 receptor. *Science* **297**, 1190–1193.

Liu, Y., and Rao, M. (2003). Oligodendrocytes, GRPs and MNOPs. *Trends Neurosci.* **26**, 410–412.

Lobsiger, C. S., Taylor, V., and Suter, U. (2002). The early life of a Schwann cell. *Biol. Chem.* **383**, 245–253.

Low, P. A. (1976a). Hereditary hypertrophic neuropathy in the Trembler mouse. Part 1. Histological studies: light microscopy. *J. Neurol. Sci.* **30**, 327–341.

Low, P. A. (1976b). Hereditary hypertrophic neuropathy in the Trembler mouse. Part 2. Histological studies: Electron microscopy. *J. Neurol. Sci.* **30**, 343–368.

Low, P. A., and McLeod, J. G. (1975). Hereditary demyelination neuropathy in the Trembler mouse. *J. Neurol. Sci.* **26**, 565–574.

Marcus, J., Dupree, J. L., and Popko, B. (2002). Myelin-associated glycoprotein and myelin galactolipids stabilize developing axo-glial interactions. *J. Cell Biol.* **156**, 567–577.

Martini, R., and Schachner, M. (1986). Immunoelectron microscopic localization of neural cell adhesion molecules (L1, N-CAM and MAG) and their shared carbohydrate epitope and myelin basic protein in developing sciatic nerve. *J. Cell Biol.* **103**, 2439–2448.

Mata, M., Kupina, N., and Fink, D. J. (1992). Phosphorylation-dependent neurofilament epitopes are reduced at the node of Ranvier. *J. Neurocytol.* **21**, 199–210.

McKerracher, L., Essagian, C., and Aguayo, A. J. (1993). Temporal changes in b-tubulin and neurofilament mRNA levels after transection of adult rat retinal ganglion cell axons in the optic nerve. *J. Neurosci.*, **13**, 2617–2626.

McQuarrie, I. G., Brady, S. T., and Lasek, R. J. (1989). Retardation in axonal transport of cytoskeletal elements during maturation and aging. *Neurobiol. Aging* **10**, 359–365.

Melendez-Vasquez, C. V., Einheber, S., and Salzer, J. L. (2004). Rho kinase regulates Schwann cell myelination and formation of associated axonal domains. *J. Neurosci.* **24**, 3953–3963.

Melendez-Vasquez, C. V., Rios, J. C., Zanazzi, G., Lambert, S., Bretscher, A., and Salzer, J. L. (2001). Nodes of Ranvier form in association with ezrin-radixin-moesin (ERM)-positive Schwann cell processes. *Proc. Natl. Acad. Sci. U. S. A.* **98**, 1235–1240.

Michailov, G. V., Sereda, M. W., Brinkmann, B. G., Fischer, T. M., Haug, B., Birchmeier, C., Role, L., Lai, C., Schwab, M. H., and Nave, K. A. (2004). Axonal neuregulin-1 regulates myelin sheath thickness. *Science* **304**, 700–703.

Miller, R. H. (1996). Oligodendrocyte origins. *Trends Neurosci.* **19**, 92–96.

Miller, R. H. (2002). Regulation of oligodendrocyte development in the vertebrate CNS. *Prog. Neurobiol.* **67**, 451–467.

Miller, R. H., and Reynolds, R. (2004). Oligodendroglial lineage. *In* "Myelin Biology and Disorders" (R. A. Lazzarini, ed.), Vol. 1, pp. 289–310. Elsevier Academic Press, Amsterdam.

Morell, P., and Quarles, R. H. (1999). Myelin formation, structure, and biochemistry. *In* "Basic Neurochemistry. Molecular, Cellular, and Medical Aspects" (G. J. Siegal, B. W. Agranoff, R. W. Albers, S. K. Fisher, and M. D. Uhler, eds.), pp. 69–93. Lippincott-Raven Press, Philadelphia.

Morfini, G., Szebenyi, G., Brown, H., Pant, H. C., Pigino, G., DeBoer, S., Beffert, U., and Brady, S. T. (2004). A novel CDK5-dependent pathway for regulating GSK3 activity and kinesin-driven motility in neurons. *EMBO J.* **23**, 2235–2245.

Morfini, G., Szebenyi, G., Elluru, R., Ratner, N., and Brady, S. T. (2002). Glycogen synthase kinase 3 phosphorylates kinesin light chains and negatively regulates kinesin-based motility. *EMBO J.* **23**, 281–293.

Morfini, G., Szebenyi, G., Richards, B., and Brady, S. T. (2001). Regulation of kinesin: Implications for neuronal development. *Dev. Neurosci.* **23**, 364–376.

Neuberg, D. H., Sancho, S., and Suter, U. (1999). Altered molecular architecture of peripheral nerves in mice lacking the peripheral myelin protein 22 or connexin32. *J. Neurosci. Res.* **58**, 612–623.

Noble, M., Proschel, C., and Mayer-Proschel, M. (2004). Getting a GR(i)P on oligodendrocyte development. *Dev. Biol.* **265**, 33–52.

Noebels, J. L., Marcom, P. K., and Jalilian-Tehrani, M. H. (1991). Sodium channel density in hypomyelinated brain increased by myelin basic protein gene deletion. *Nature* **352**, 431–434.

Novakovic, S. D., Deerinck, T. J., Levinson, S. R., Shrager, P., and Ellisman, M. H. (1996). Clusters of axonal Na+ channels adjacent to remyelinating Schwann cells. *J. Neurocytol.*, **25**, 403–412.

Oblinger, M. M., Argasinski, A., Wong, J., and Kosik, K. S. (1991). Tau gene expression in DRG neurons during development and regeneration. *J. Neurosci.* **11**, 2453–2459.

Ogawa, T., Suzuki, M., Matoh, K., and Sasaki, K. (2004). Three-dimensional electron microscopic studies of the transitional oligodendrocyte associated with the initial stage of myelination in developing rat hippocampal fimbria. *Brain Res. Dev. Brain Res.* **148**, 207–212.

Orentas, D. M., Hayes, J. E., Dyer, K. L., and Miller, R. H. (1999). Sonic hedgehog signaling is required during the appearance of spinal cord oligodendrocyte precursors. *Development* **126**, 2419–2429.

Pareek, S., Notterpek, L., Snipes, G. J., Naef, R., Sossin, W., Laliberte, J., Iacampo, S., Suter, U., Shooter, E. M., and Murphy, R. A. (1997). Neurons promote the translocation of peripheral myelin protein 22 into myelin. *J. Neurosci.* **17**, 7754–7762.

Peters, A., Palay, S. L., and Webster, H. D. (1991). "The Fine Structure of the Nervous System: Neurons and Their Supporting Cells." Oxford University Press, New York.

Podratz, J. L., Rodriguez, E., and Windebank, A. J. (2001). Role of the extracellular matrix in myelination of peripheral nerve. *Glia* **35**, 35–40.

Poliak, S., and Peles, E. (2003). The local differentiation of myelinated axons at nodes of Ranvier. *Nat. Rev. Neurosci.* **4**, 968–980.

Popko, B. (2003). Notch signaling: A rheostat regulating oligodendrocyte differentiation? *Dev. Cell* **5**, 668–669.

Popko, B., Puckett, C., Lai, E., Shine, H. D., Readhead, C., Takahashi, N., Hunt, S. W. D., Sidman, R. L., and Hood, L. (1987). Myelin deficient mice: expression of myelin basic protein and generation of mice with varying levels of myelin. *Cell* **48**, 713–721.

Raine, C. S. (1984). The morphology of myelin and mylination. *In* "Myelin" (P. Morrell, ed.), pp. 1–41. Plenum, New York.

Rao, M. (2004). Neural cell specification during development. *In* "Myelin Biology and Disorders" (R. A. Lazzarini, ed.), Vol. 1, pp. 223–258. Elsevier Academic Press, Amsterdam.

Ratner, N., Bunge, R. P., and Glaser, L. (1985). A neuronal cell surface heparan sulfate proteoglycan is required for dorsal root ganglion neuron stimulation of Schwann cell proliferation. *J. Cell Biol.* **101**, 744–754.

Readhead, C., and Hood, L. (1990). The dysmyelinating mouse mutants shiverer (*shi*) and myelin deficient (*shi^{mld}*). *Behav. Genet.* **20**, 213–234.

Readhead, C., Popko, B., Takahashi, N., Shine, H. D., Saavedra, R. A., Sidman, R. L., and Hood, L. (1987). Expression of a myelin basic protein gene in transgenic shiverer mice: Correction of the dysmyelinating phenotype. *Cell* **48**, 703–712.

Rios, J. C., Rubin, M., St. Martin, M., Downey, R. T., Einheber, S., Rosenbluth, J., Levinson, S. R., Bhat, M., and Salzer, J. L. (2003). Paranodal interactions regulate expression of sodium channel subtypes and provide a diffusion barrier for the node of Ranvier. *J. Neurosci.* **23**, 7001–7011.

Roach, A., Takahashi, N., Pravtcheva, D., Ruddle, F. and Hood, L. (1985). Chromosomal mapping of mouse myelin basic protein gene and structure and transcription of the partially deleted gene in Shiverer mutant mice. *Cell* **42**, 149–155.

Rogister, B., Ben-Hur, T., and Dubois-Dalcq, M. (1999). From neural stem cells to myelinating oligodendrocytes. *Mol. Cell Neurosci.* **14**, 287–300.

Rosenbluth, J. (1980a). Central myelin in the mouse mutant shiverer. *J. Comp. Neurol.* **194**, 639–648.

Rosenbluth, J. (1980b). Peripheral myelin in the mouse mutant Shiverer. *J. Comp. Neurol.* **193**, 729–739.

Rowitch, D. H., Lu, Q. R., Kessaris, N., and Richardson, W. D. (2002). An "oligarchy" rules neural development. *Trends Neurosci.* **25**, 417–422.

Rushton, W. A. (1951). A theory of the effects of fibre size in medullated nerve. *J. Physiol.* **115**, 101–122.

Sahenk, Z., and Chen, L. (1998). Abnormalities in the axonal cytoskeleton induced by a connexin32 mutation in nerve xenografts. *J. Neurosci. Res.* **51**, 174–184.

Salzer, J. L. (2003). Polarized domains of myelinated axons. *Neuron* **40**, 297–318.

Scherer, S. S., Arroyo, E. J., and Peles, E. (2004). Functional organization of the nodes of Ranvier. *In* "Myelin Biology and Disorders" (R. A. Lazzarini, ed.),. Vol. 1, pp. 89–116. Elsevier Academic Press, Amsterdam.

Scherer, S. S., Xu, T., Crino, P., Arroyo, E. J., and Gutmann, D. H. (2001). Ezrin, radixin, and moesin are components of Schwann cell microvilli. *J. Neurosci. Res.* **65**, 150–164.

Sheikh, K. A., Sun, J., Liu, Y., Kawai, H., Crawford, T. O., Proia, R. L., Griffin, J. W., and Schnaar, R. L. (1999). Mice lacking complex gangliosides develop Wallerian degeneration and myelination defects. *Proc. Natl. Acad. Sci. U. S. A.* **96**, 7532–7537.

Shine, H. D., Readhead, C., Popko, B., Hood, L., and Sidman, R. L. (1992). Morphometric analysis of normal, mutant, and transgenic cns: correlation of myelin basic protein expression to myelinogenesis. *J. Neurochem.* **58**, 342–349.

Shrager, P. (1989). Sodium channels in single demyelinated mammalian axons. *Brain Res.* **483**, 149–154.

Simpson, P. B., and Armstrong, R.C. (1999). Intracellular signals and cytoskeletal elements involved in oligodendrocyte progenitor migration. *Glia* **26**, 22–35.

Starr, R., Attema, B., DeVries, G. H., and Monteiro, M. J. (1996). Neurofilament phosphorylation is modulated by myelination. *J. Neurosci. Res.* **44**, 328–337.

Stewart, H. J., Morgan, L., Jessen, K.R., and Mirsky, R. (1993). Changes in DNA synthesis rate in the Schwann cell lineage in vivo are correlated with the precursor: Schwann cell transition and myelination. *Eur. J. Neurosci.* **5**, 1136–1144.

Suter, U., Moskow, J. J., Welcher, A. A., Snipes, G. J., Sidman, R. L., Buchberg, A. M., and Shooter, E. M. (1992a). A leucine-to-proline mutation in the putative first transmembrane domain of the 22-kDa peripheral myelin protein in the trembler-J mouse. *Proc. Natl. Acad. Sci. U. S. A.* **89**, 4382–4386.

Suter, U., and Snipes, G. J. (1995). Peripheral myelin protein 22: Facts and hypotheses. *J. Neurosci. Res.* **40**, 145–151.

Suter, U., Welcher, A. A., Ozcelik, T., Snipes, G. J., Kosaras, B., Francke, U., Billings-Gagliardi, S., Sidman, R. L., and Shooter, E. M. (1992b). Trembler mouse carries a point mutation in a myelin gene. *Nature*, **356**, 241–243.

Syroid, D. E., Maycox, P. R., Burrla, P. G., Liu, N., Wen, D., Lee, K. F., Lemke, G., and Kilpatrick, T. J. (1996). Cell death in the Schwann cell lineage and its regulation by neuregulin. *Proc. Natl. Acad. Sci. U. S. A.* **93**, 9229–9234.

Syroid, D. E., Zorick, T. S., Arbet-Engels, C., Kilpatrick, T. J., Eckhart, W., and Lemke, G. (1999). A role for insulin-like growth factor-I in the regulation of Schwann cell survival. *J. Neurosci.* **19**, 2059–2068.

Thoenen, H. (2000). Neurotrophins and activity-dependent plasticity. *Prog. Brain Res.* **128**, 183–191.

Topilko, P., Murphy, P., and Charnay, P. (1996). Embryonic development of Schwann cells: Multiple roles for neuregulins along the pathway. *Mol. Cell Neurosci.* **8**, 71–75.

Trapp, B. D., and Kidd, G. J. (2004). Structure of the myelinated axon. *In* "Myelin Biology and Disorders" (R. A. Lazzarini, ed.), Vol. 1, pp. 3–27. Elsevier Academic Press, Amsterdam.

Tsai, H. H., Frost, E., To, V., Robinson, S., French-Constant, C., Geertman, R., Ransohoff, R. M., and Miller, R. H. (2002). The chemokine receptor CXCR2 controls positioning of oligodendrocyte precursors in developing spinal cord by arresting their migration. *Cell* **110**, 373–383.

Tsai, H. H., and Miller, R. H. (2002). Glial cell migration directed by axon guidance cues. *Trends Neurosci.* **25**, 173–175; discussion 175–176.

Tsai, H. H., Tessier-Lavigne, M., and Miller, R. H. (2003). Netrin 1 mediates spinal cord oligodendrocyte precursor dispersal. *Development* **130**, 2095–2105.

Tsai, M.-Y., Morfini, G., Szebenyi, G., and Brady, S. T. (2000). Modulation of kinesin-vesicle interactions by hsc70: implications for regulation of fast axonal transport. *Mol. Biol. Cell* **11**, 2161–2173.

Vabnick, I., Novakovic, S. D., Levinson, S. R., Schachner, M., and Shrager, P. (1996). The clustering of axonal sodium channels during development of the peripheral nervous system. *J. Neurosci.* **16**, 4914–4922.

Vabnick, I., and Shrager, P. (1998). Ion channel redistribution and function during development of the myelinated axon. *J. Neurobiol.* **37**, 80–96.

Voyvodic, J. T. (1989). Target size regulates calibre and myelination of sympathetic axons. *Nature* **342**, 430–433.

Vyas, A. A., Patel, H. V., Fromholt, S. E., Heffer-Lauc, M., Vyas, K. A., Dang, J., Schachner, M., and Schnaar, R. L. (2002). Gangliosides are functional nerve cell ligands for myelin-associated glycoprotein (MAG), an inhibitor of nerve regeneration. *Proc. Natl. Acad. Sci. U. S. A.* **99**, 8412–8417.

Wang, H., Allen, M. L., Grigg, J. J., Noebels, J. L., and Tempel, B. L. (1995). Hypomyelination alters K+ channel expression in mouse mutants shiverer and Trembler. *Neuron* **15**, 1337–1347.

Wang, S., Sdrulla, A. D., diSibio, G., Bush, G., Nofziger, D., Hicks, C., Weinmaster, G., and Barres, B. A. (1998). Notch receptor activation inhibits oligodendrocyte differentiation. *Neuron* **21**, 63–75.

Watson, D. F., Nachtman, F. N., Kuncl, R. W., and Griffin, J. W. (1994). Altered neurofilament phosphorylation and beta tubulin isotypes in Charcot-Marie-Tooth disease type 1. *Neurology* **44**, 2383–2387.

Waxman, S. G. (1997). Axon-glia interactions: building a smart nerve fiber. *Curr. Biol.* **7**, R406–410.

Waxman, S. G., and Sims, T. J. (1984). Specificity in central myelination: evidence for local regulation of myelin thickness. *Brain Res.* **292**, 179–185.

Weber, P., Bartsch, U., Rasband, M. N., Czaniera, R., Lang, Y., Bluethmann, H., Margolis, R. U., Levinson, S. R., Shrager, P., Montag, D., and Schachner, M. (1999). Mice deficient for tenascin-R display alterations of the extracellular matrix and decreased axonal conduction velocities in the CNS. *J. Neurosci.* **19**, 4245–4262.

Webster, H. D. (1971). The geometry of peripheral myelin sheaths during their formation and growth in rat sciatic nerves. *J. Cell Biol.* **48**, 348–367.

Weinberg, H. J., and Spencer, P. S. (1976). Studies on the control of myelinogenesis. II. Evidence for neuronal regulation of myelin production. *Brain Res.* **113**, 363–378.

Westenbroek, R. E., Noebels, J. L., and Catterall, W. A. (1992). Elevated expression of type II Na+ channels in hypomyelinated axons of shiverer mouse brain. *J. Neurosci.* **12**, 2259–2267.

Willard, M., and Simon, C. (1983). Modulations in neurofilament axonal transport during development of rabbit retinal ganglion cells. *Cell* **35**, 551–559.

Wolpowitz, D., Mason, T. B., Dietrich, P., Mendelsohn, M., Talmage, D. A., and Role, L. W. (2000). Cysteine-rich domain isoforms of the neuregulin-1 gene are required for maintenance of peripheral synapses. *Neuron* **25**, 79–91.

Woodruff, R. H., Tekki-Kessaris, N., Stiles, C. D., Rowitch, D. H., and Richardson, W. D. (2001). Oligodendrocyte development in the spinal cord and telencephalon: Common themes and new perspectives. *Int. J. Dev. Neurosci.* **19**, 379–385.

Wujek, J., Lasek, R. J., and Gambetti, P. (1986). The amount of slow axonal transport is proportional to the radial dimensions of the axon. *J. Neurocytol.* **15**, 75–83.

Yan, S. B., Hwang, S., Rustan, T. D., and Frey, W. H. (1985). Human brain tubulin purification: Decrease in soluble tubulin with age. *Neurochem. Res.* **10**, 1–18.

Yin, X., Crawford, T. O., Griffin, J. W., Tu, P. H., Lee, V. M. Y., Li, C., Roder, J., and Trapp, B. D. (1998). Myelin-associated glycoprotein is a myelin signal that modulates the caliber of myelinated axons. *J. Neurosci.* **18**, 1953–1962.

3

Molecular Specializations at the Glia-Axon Interface

Elior Peles, Ph.D.

I. Introduction

To achieve optimal conduction properties, the axonal membrane of myelinated axons is divided into distinct molecular, structural, and functional domains at and around the nodes of Ranvier. This local differentiation of the axon is highly regulated by the myelinating glial cell trough contact-dependent and -independent mechanisms. Voltage-gated Na$^+$ channels concentrated at the nodes are separated from K$^+$ channels clustered at the juxtaparanodal region by a specialized axoglial contact formed between the axon and the myelinating cell at the paranodes. The juxtaparanodal region, paranodes, and nodes contain several molecular complexes of cell adhesion molecules (CAMs) that mediate axoglial interactions and several cytoplasmic adaptor proteins, which link these CAMs to the axonal cytoskeleton. At the nodes of Ranvier, Na$^+$ channels are found together with the two immunoglobulin CAMs, neurofascin 186 (NF186) and NrCAM, all of which associate with ankyrin$_G$ and βIV-spectrin located at this site. The paranodal junction contains a complex of three CAMs: the axonal Caspr and contactin and the glial isoform of neurofascin (NF155). The Caspr-contactin complex is further linked to the axonal cytoskeleton through protein 4.1B. At the juxtaparanodal region Shaker-like K$^+$ channels are associated with Caspr2 and the contactin-related CAM, TAG-1. Recent experiments revealed that these protein complexes are crucial for the specific clustering of different ion channels to distinct locations along the axon and provided an insight into the mechanisms by which the local differentiation of myelinated axons is regulated by oligodendrocytes and myelinating Schwann cells.

The reciprocal communication between the axon and its myelinating glial cell results in the differentiation of the axonal membrane into distinct molecular, structural, and functional domains, a feature that allows them to maximize their conduction velocities. These domains include the nodes of Ranvier, the paranodal junction, the juxtaparanodes, and the internodal region (Poliak and Peles, 2003; Salzer, 2003) (Fig. 1). This chapter summarizes current

45

knowledge of the molecular mechanisms of axon-glia interactions at the nodal environ that is involved in the generation and maintenance of specialized axonal domains necessary for the physiology of myelinated nerves. Given that the mechanisms underlying the generation of nodal specialization in the CNS may share common principles with those operating in peripheral nerves, both are described.

II. The Nodes of Ranvier

A. Morphology

The nodes are short, periodical interruptions in the myelin sheath that are regularly spaced at intervals that are about 100 times the axonal diameter. At the nodes and the adjacent paranodes, the axon constricts 15% to 30% of the internodal cross-sectional area. This constriction may facilitate eliciting axon potentials and causes an accumulation of synaptic vesicles, microtubules, and mitochondria, suggesting retardation in axonal transport around the nodes (Fabricius et al., 1993). One of the main differences between the PNS and the CNS is the origin of the membrane that contacts the nodal axolemma. In peripheral nerves, the entire myelin unit is covered by a basal lamina, and the outermost layer (the outer collar) of the Schwann cell extends

microvillus processes that cover the nodes (Fig. 1B). At the proximal region of the microvilli, the membranes of two adjoining Schwann cells are connected by tight junctions (Poliak et al., 2002). However, these junctions do not seal the nodal gap, as it is permeable to horseradish peroxidase applied outside the nerve fibers (Hall and Williams, 1971). The perinodal space (i.e., between the axolemma and the basal lamina), which contains the microvilli, is also filled with a filamentous matrix (Landon and Langley, 1971). In the central nervous system (CNS), there is no basal lamina and the nodes are contacted by perinodal astrocytes (Black and Waxman, 1988; Raine, 1984).

B. Molecular Composition

The nodes are characterized by the presence of high density ($>1,200/\mu m^2$) of Na^+ channels that are essential for the generation of the action potential during saltatory conduction (Waxman and Ritchie, 1993). Several other transmembrane and cytoskeletal proteins were also identified at the nodal axolemma: the cell adhesion molecules of the immunoglobulin superfamily (Ig-CAMs) NrCAM and Neurofascin-186 (NF186) (Davis et al., 1996), the cytoskeletal adaptor ankyrin$_G$ (Kordeli et al., 1990, 1995), and the actin-binding protein spectrin βIV (Berghs et al., 2000) (Fig. 2A). Recent studies have also revealed the pres-

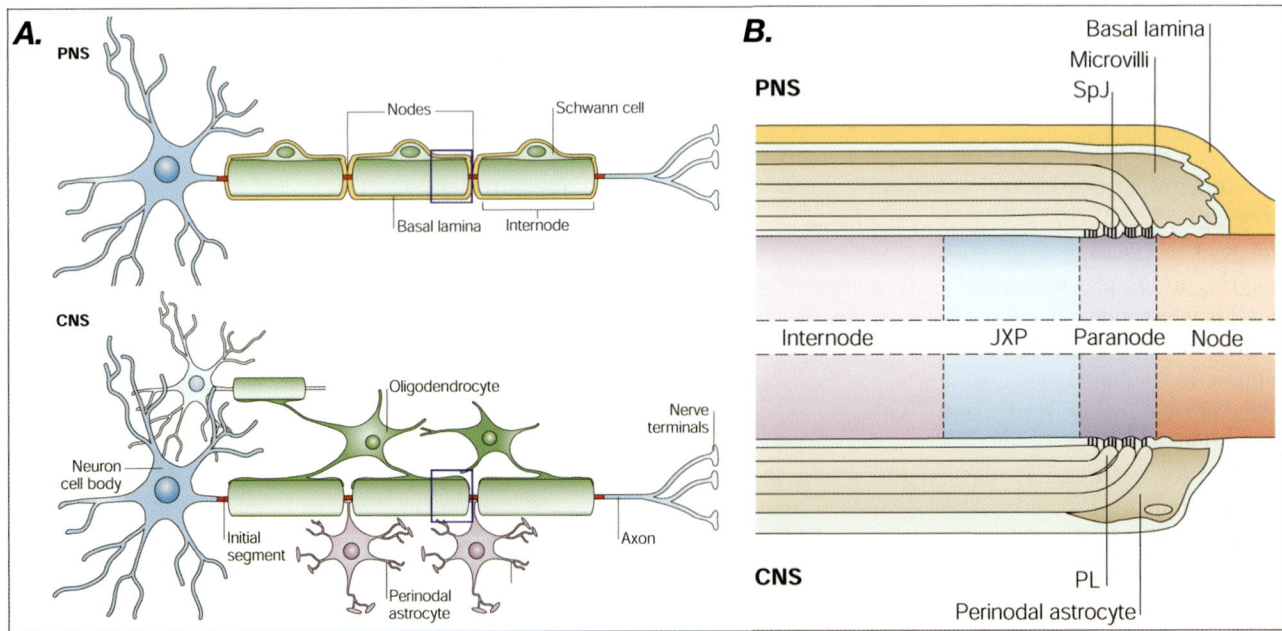

Figure 1 Schematic structure of myelinated axons. (**A**) Myelinating glial cells, oligodendrocytes in the CNS, or Schwann cells (SC) in the PNS form the myelin sheath by enwrapping their membrane multiple times around the axon. The myelin covers the axon at intervals (internodes) leaving bare gaps, the nodes of Ranvier. (**B**) Schematic longitudinal cut of a myelinated fiber around the node of Ranvier showing a heminode. The node, paranode, juxtaparanode (JXP), and internode are labeled. The node is contacted by SC microvilli in the PNS or processes from perinodal astrocytes in the CNS. Myelinated fibers in the PNS are covered by a basal lamina (BL). The paranodal loops form a septate-like junction (SpJ) with the axon. The juxtaparanodal region resides beneath the compact myelin next to the paranode. The internode extends from the juxtaparanodes and lies under the compact myelin. (Modified from Poliak and Peles, 2003.)

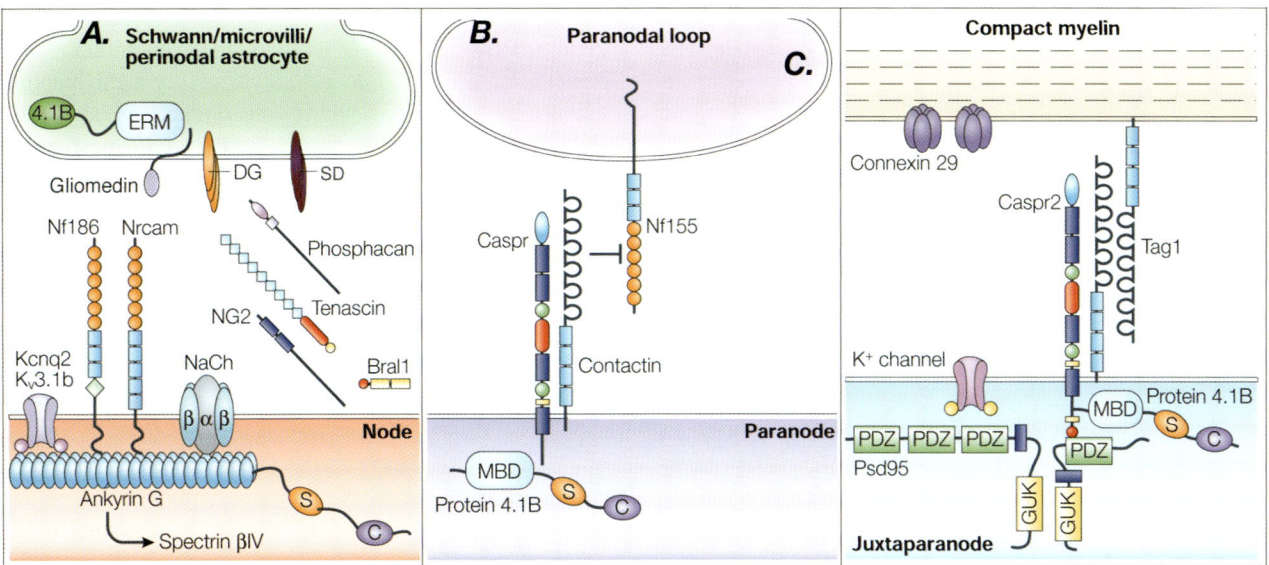

Figure 2 **Molecular composition of the nodal domains.** The specialized domains around the node of Ranvier are composed of a distinct set of molecules. (**A**) At the nodal axolemma, voltage dependent Na$^+$ channels are anchored to the cytoskeleton by ankyrin$_G$, which also binds NF186, NrCam, and Kv3.1b. Ankyrin$_G$ further connects these proteins to the axonal cytoskeleton through βIV-spectrin. In the PNS, Schwann cell microvilli express ERM proteins Dystroglycan (DG), and Syndecan, as well as Gliomedin, which binds to the axolemmal CAMs. The nodal gap also contains several ECM proteins: phosphacan, tenescin, and Bral1. (**B**) At the paranodes, Caspr-Contactin complex in the axolemma faces NF155 at the glial membrane. While Contactin alone is able to bind NF155, Caspr inhibits this interaction, suggesting that the Caspr-Contactin complex may bind an as yet unidentified ligand present at the glial loops. The cytoplasmic tail of Caspr interacts with protein 4.1B, providing a potential link with the actin cytoskeleton. (**C**) At the juxtaparanode's axolemma, voltage-gated K$^+$ channels are found in a macromolecular complex with Caspr2, 4.1B, PSD95, and TAG-1. The latter is also expressed on the glial membrane and binds the axonal Caspr2/TAG-1 complex. Connexin 29, localized at the juxtaparanodal glial membrane could form functional hemichannels. (Modified from Poliak and Peles, 2003.)

ence of two K$^+$ channels, Kv3.1 (Devaux et al., 2003) and KCNQ2 (Devaux et al., 2004) at the nodes. The nodes are enriched in ankyrin$_G$, a membrane-cytoskeleton adaptor that links integral membrane proteins to the spectrin cytoskeleton (Kordeli et al., 1990, 1995). Ankyrin$_G$ interacts with Na$^+$ channels (Srinivasan et al., 1988), both with their α (Lemaillet et al., 2003) and β (Malhotra et al., 2000) subunits, as well as with NF186, NrCAM (Garver et al., 1997), and Kv3.1b (Devaux et al., 2003). The β subunit recruits ankyrin$_G$ to the plasma membrane (Malhotra et al., 2000), and this interaction is regulated by tyrosine phosphorylation (Malhotra et al., 2002). The binding of ankyrin$_G$ to the α subunit is mediated through a sequence of nine amino acids present in all known voltage-gated Na$^+$ channels (Lemaillet et al., 2003). This nine amino acid motif is required for the accumulation of this subunit in the axon initial segment (Garrido et al., 2003), which may be considered as the first node along the axon. Ankyrin$_G$ also binds βIV spectrin, a spectrin isoform enriched at the nodes of Ranvier and axon initial segments (Berghs et al., 2000), further anchoring the nodal Na$^+$ channel and Ig-CAMs to the axonal cytoskeleton.

C. Axoglial Contact at the Nodes

Voltage-gated Na$^+$ channels are multimeric complexes that consist of a pore forming α subunit and one or more smaller β subunits (Yu and Catterall, 2003). An important feature of β subunit proteins is their ability to function as cell adhesion molecules (CAMs) (Isom, 2002). The extracellular domain of these β subunits exhibits a single immunoglobulin (Ig) domain (Isom et al., 1995), which mediates homophilic interactions (Malhotra et al., 2000), as well as binding to other nodal components. β1 and β3 subunits interact in *cis* with NF186 (Ratcliffe et al., 2001), and β1 also binds contactin (Kazarinova-Noyes et al., 2001; McEwen et al., 2004), a glycosylphosphatidylinositol-(GPI) anchored glycoprotein that is found in all paranodes (see later), but also in CNS nodes (Rios et al., 2000). The interaction with contactin enhances the expression of Na$^+$ channels on the surface of transfected cells, suggesting that this CAM may be important for the expression of Na$^+$ channels in the node of Ranvier (Kazarinova-Noyes et al., 2001; Liu et al., 2001). In agreement, the expression of these channels is markedly reduced in the optic nerve of *contactin*-null mice (Kazarinova-Noyes and Shrager, 2002). β1 and β2 subunits also interact with the extracellular matrix molecules tenascin-C and tenascin-R (Srinivasan et al., 1998; Xiao et al., 1999), as well as with the secreted form of receptor protein tyrosine β (RPTPβ), phosphacan (Ratcliffe et al., 2000).

In the PNS, the nodal gap is filled with Schwann cell microvilli emanating from the outer aspect of the cell (Fig. 1B). Three ERM proteins, ezrin, radixin, and moesin, as well as the ezrin-binding protein EBP50 and Rho-A GTPase, are localized at the microvilli (Gatto et al., 2003; Melendez-Vasquez et al., 2001; Scherer et al., 2001). These proteins may potentially link the actin-rich microvilli with integral membrane proteins such as syndecans (Goutebroze et al., 2003). In addition, several extracellular matrix proteins are present in the nodal gap under the basal lamina, including the hyaluronan-binding proteoglycan versican (Apostolski et al., 1994), tenascin C (Martini et al., 1990; Rieger et al., 1986), and the NG2 proteoglycan (Martin et al., 2001). Dystroglycan, which is abundantly expressed at the abaxonal surface of myelinating Schwann cells (Saito et al., 1999), is also located at the nodes (Saito et al., 2003). Schwann cell-specific ablation of dystroglycan results in disorganization of the microvilli, marked reduction in nodal Na^+ channels and consequently impaired nerve conduction (Saito et al., 2003). It was recently suggested that in the PNS, the two axonal CAMs, neurofascin and NrCAM bind to a specific receptor on the Schwann cell microvilli (Eshed and Peles, unpublished observation). This receptor, termed Gliomedin, was identified using an expression cloning approach as a type II transmembrane protein that contains two-collagen triple helix repeats and a single olfactomedin domain. Gliomedin is precisely localized with NrCAM, NF186, and Na^+ channels during development and may function in recruiting these proteins to the forming nodes in the PNS.

In contrast to the PNS, processes of perinodal astrocytes are contacting most of the nodes in the CNS. Here, the nodal gap has been shown to include several proteoglycans and extracellular matrix proteins that are produced by oligodendrocytes, including tenascin (Ffrench-Constant et al., 1986), and the secreted extracellular domain of RPTPβ, phosphacan (Xiao et al., 1997). The CNS nodal gap also contains the versican-binding protein Bral-1, which is produced by neurons (Oohashi et al., 2002). The function of these proteins is presently unclear, although it was suggested that due to their high content of acidic disaccharides, they could provide a strong negative environment that serves as an extracellular Na^+ reservoir in the perinodal space (Oohashi et al., 2002). Both tenascin C and tenascin R bind to Na^+ channels (Srinivasan et al., 1998) and alter their electrophysiological properties (Xiao et al., 1999). Genetic ablation of tenascin-R resulted in slower nerve conduction, but had no effect on the distribution of Na^+ channels at the nodes, indicating that this interaction may stabilize nodal complexes or regulate channel activity, but is not required for the initial clustering of these channels (Weber et al., 1999). Na^+ channels were also reported to bind the cytoplasmic tail and the extracellular domain of RPTPβ (Ratcliffe et al., 2000). The significance of these interactions for the normal physiology of myelinated nerves is not clear, as the distribution of nodal Na^+ channels, as well as conduction velocity of CNS myelinated axons, is normal in RPTPβ-deficient mice (Harroch et al., 2000). Interestingly, it was

reported that RPTPβ is induced in MS lesions and that RPTPβ-deficient mice show impaired recovery from EAE induced by myelin oligodendrocyte glycoprotein peptide, suggesting that axoglial interactions mediated by this phosphatase may regulate oligodendrocyte survival (Harroch et al., 2002). Both tenascin-R and RPTPβ also interact with contactin and NrCAM (Peles et al., 1995; Pesheva et al., 1993; Sakurai et al., 1997) present at CNS nodes, suggesting the existence of large macromolecular complexes at the perinodal space.

III. The Paranodal Junction

These junctions that are formed between the axon and the myelinating cell border the nodes of Ranvier (Fig. 1B). In this region, the compact myelin lamellae open up into a series of cytoplasmic loops that spiral around the axon. These glial loops are closely opposed to the axon; being separated by a gap of only 2.5 to 3 nm, form a series of ridges (transverse bands) that are reminiscent of invertebrate septate junctions (Rosenbluth, 1995). The axoglial junctions appear relatively late during myelination, being first generated closer to the nodes by the most outer paranodal loop, and continue gradually as additional loops are attached to the axon (Tao-Cheng and Rosenbluth, 1983). As a result, they are composed of a number of rings, each representing a turn of the myelin wrap.

A. Molecular Composition

The axonal membrane at the axoglial junction contains a complex of two cell-recognition molecules: Caspr (contactin-associated protein; also known as paranodin) (Einheber et al., 1997; Menegoz et al., 1997) and contactin (Rios et al., 2000) (Fig. 2B). Caspr is a Type I transmembrane protein that belongs to a distinct subgroup of the neurexins, a polymorphic protein family involved in cell adhesion and intercellular communication (Bellen et al., 1998; Missler and Sudhof, 1998). There are five human genes in the Caspr family (Caspr-Caspr5 [Peles et al., 1997; Poliak et al., 1999; Spiegel et al., 2002]), two in Drosophila (nrxIV and axo [Baumgartner et al., 1996; Yuan and Ganetzky, 1999]), and two in C. elegans (itx and nlr; Haklai-Topper and Peles, unpublished observations). These proteins bind several cell adhesion molecules and thus considered as CAM-associated-proteins (acronym CASPR). Their extracellular region consists of several domains implicated in mediating protein-protein interactions, including a discoidin and a fibrinogen-like domain, EGF motifs, and several regions with homology to the G domain of laminin A. Caspr, but not other members of the Caspr family, forms a complex with contactin when both are present in the same cell (i.e., in cis) (Peles et al., 1997). The interaction between Caspr and contactin is required for the efficient export of Caspr from the endoplasmic reticulum to the plasma membrane (Faivre-Sarrailh et al., 2000) and regulates the glycosylation and transport of contactin (Bonnon et al., 2003; Gollan et al., 2003). In accordance with these in vitro findings, Caspr is retained in the neuronal cell bodies and does not reach the axons in *contactin*-deficient mice (Boyle et al., 2001), while Caspr is necessary to maintain contactin at the paranodes (Bhat et al., 2001; Gollan et al., 2002, 2003).

Both Caspr and contactin are essential for the generation of the axoglial junction, and their absence results in the disappearance of septa and a widening of the space between the axon and the paranodal loops (Bhat et al., 2001; Boyle et al., 2001; Gollan et al., 2003). These results suggest that Caspr and contactin are part of a paranodal adhesion complex required for the tight attachment of the two membranes. This phenotype is similar to two other paranodal mutants: the galactolipids–deficient mice (UDP-galactose ceramide galactosyltransferase, cgt), which do not synthesize galactocerebroside (GalC) and sulfatide, and cerebroside sulfotransferase (cst) null mice, which are lacking only sulfatide (Bosio et al., 1996; Coetzee et al., 1998, 1996; Honke et al., 2002; Ishibashi et al., 2002). In all of these mice mutants, Caspr and contactin are absent from the paranodes (Bhat et al., 2001; Boyle et al., 2001; Dupree et al., 1999; Ishibashi et al., 2002; Poliak et al., 2001). The way in which the absence of GalC and sulfatide causes paranodal abnormalities is not clear, but it may result from direct binding of sulfatide to the Caspr/contactin complex, or misrouting of junctional glial components to noncompact myelin (Schafer et al., 2004).

B. Generation of Molecular Complexes at the PNJ

1. Cytoplasmic Linkage to the Axonal Cytoskeleton

The intracellular regions of Caspr and Caspr2 contain a juxtamembrane sequence that binds protein 4.1B (Denisenko-Nehrbass et al., 2003; Gollan et al., 2002; Menegoz et al., 1997; Peles et al., 1997), which is present at the paranodes and juxtaparanodes (Denisenko-Nehrbass et al., 2003; Ohara et al., 2000; Parra et al., 2000; Poliak et al., 2001). Similar to other 4.1 proteins, 4.1B contains a conserved actin-spectrin-binding domain and thus, could immobilize Caspr (and hence contactin) to the cytoskeleton (Gollan et al., 2002). Consistent with this notion, protein 4.1B is abnormally distributed along peripheral myelinated axons of mice lacking either contactin and galactolipids, both of which lack paranodal Caspr (Gollan et al., 2002; Poliak et al., 2001). In these mutants, the position of protein 4.1B is strongly correlated with those of Caspr and Caspr2, suggesting that they determine its localization. Furthermore, the cytoplasmic tail of Caspr is required for stabilizing the

Caspr/contactin complex at the paranodes, as a Caspr mutant lacking this domain is not properly maintained at the axoglial junction (Gollan et al., 2002). Thus, Caspr appears to serve as a transmembrane scaffold that stabilizes the Caspr/contactin adhesion complex at septatelike junctions by connecting it to the axonal cytoskeleton via protein 4.1B.

2. Extracellular Interactions Mediating Axoglial Contact

The intracellular regions of Caspr and the distribution of Caspr and contactin along the internodes (Arroyo et al., 1999; Poliak et al., 2001; Rios et al., 2003) (discussed later), their accumulation at the paranodes as a number of rings that represent each turn of the myelin wrap during development (Pedraza et al., 2001; Rasband et al., 1999; Rios et al., 2000), and the abnormal distribution of Caspr in multiple sclerosis tissue (Wolswijk and Balesar, 2003), as well as in several myelin mutants (Arroyo et al., 2002; Dupree et al., 1999; Ishibashi et al., 2002; Jenkins and Bennett, 2002; Poliak et al., 2001; Rasband et al., 1999), all indicate that the myelin sheath dictates their localization in the axolemma. Furthermore, the addition of a soluble RPTPβ protein that binds contactin to myelinating co-cultures perturbs the paranodal accumulation of Caspr, suggesting that the localization of the Caspr/contactin complex to this site is mediated by its interaction with a glial ligand (Rios et al., 2000). The most likely candidate to serve as a glial ligand of the Caspr/contactin complex is NF155, a glial isoform of the cell adhesion molecule neurofascin, which is located across Caspr and contactin at the axoglial junction (Tait et al., 2000) and is not localized to this site in the absence of Caspr (Bhat et al., 2001; Boyle et al., 2001; Marcus et al., 2002; Poliak et al., 2001). In agreement, it was recently reported that a soluble NF155-Fc chimera binds to cells expressing Caspr and contactin and precipitates these proteins from rat brain lysates, suggesting that NF155 indeed serves as a receptor for the Caspr/contactin complex (Charles et al., 2002). However, it was recently shown that while NF155 binds directly to contactin, Caspr inhibits this interaction, suggesting the existence of other receptors for the Caspr/contactin complex in myelinating glia (Gollan et al., 2003). This conclusion aligns with previous observations that demonstrate that NF155 appears much later than Caspr in the paranodes (Marcus et al., 2002), suggesting that other ligands for the Caspr/contactin complex exist.

3. Functional Aspects of the PNJ

The paranodal junction was proposed to attach the myelin sheath to the axon, to separate the electrical activity at the node of Ranvier from the internodal region under the compact myelin sheath, and to serve as a fence that limits the lateral diffusion of axolemmal proteins (Rosenbluth, 1976). Recent studies using four different paranodal mutant mice (i.e., *Caspr, Contactin, cgt*, and *cst*), all of which lack the characteristic septa in their axoglial junction, allowed close examination of these original ideas. In the CNS of these mutants, the paranodal loops are disorganized, with many overlapping and inverted loops that face away from the axon (Bhat et al., 2001; Dupree et al., 1998; Honke et al., 2002). In the PNS, possibly due to the presence of the basal lamina, the morphological alterations are much milder, the paranodes are well organized, but there is an increase in the space between the glial membrane and the axon. Even in the absence of septa, however, the paranodal loops are still closely attached to the axon in many sites in the PNS and CNS, suggesting the presence of yet unidentified paranodal components that mediate axoglial contact at this site. Together with ultrastructural data demonstrating that the transverse bands are generated rather late during myelination (Marcus et al., 2002; Tao-Cheng and Rosenbluth, 1983), these studies suggest a role for the septa in securing the paranodal loops to the axon at the axoglial junction. In agreement, a gradual, age-dependent detachment of the paranodal loops from the axon was observed in the CNS of *Caspr*-null mice (Rios et al., 2003).

The absence of paranodal septa in all four paranodal mutants results in a reorganization of the axonal membrane (Bhat et al., 2001; Boyle et al., 2001; Dupree et al., 1999; Ishibashi et al., 2002; Poliak et al., 2001). In these mutants, the *Shaker*-type K^+ channels normally present in the juxtaparanodal region are mislocalized to the paranodal axonal membrane (Bhat et al., 2001; Boyle et al., 2001; Dupree et al., 1999; Ishibashi et al., 2002; Poliak et al., 2001). Thus, it appears that the paranodal septate junction functions as a barrier that restricts the movement of K^+ channels from under the compact myelin, separating them from the Na^+ channels at the nodes. In contrast to the juxtaparanodal K^+ channels, disruption of the paranodal septa only minimally affects the distribution of the nodal Na^+ channels (Bhat et al., 2001; Boyle et al., 2001; Dupree et al., 1999). There is a small increase in the nodal length, accompanied by a reduction in membrane particles at the nodal axolemma detected by freeze-fracture EM, suggesting that the paranodal septate junction is not required for the generation of the nodes (Bhat et al., 2001; Rios et al., 2003; Rosenbluth et al., 2003). In the CNS, however, glial attachment at the paranodes is required to maintain Na^+ clustering at the nodal axolemma (Ishibashi et al., 2002; Rasband et al., 2003a; Rios et al., 2003; Rosenbluth et al., 2003).

IV. Juxtaparanodal Specialization

The juxtaparanode is located in a short zone just beyond the innermost paranodal junction (Fig. 1B). In freeze-fracture EM, this region exhibits randomly distributed particles, which are more concentrated near the paranodes and diffuse away toward the internodes (Rosenbluth, 1976). These particles

most likely correspond to heteromultimers of the delayed rectifier K^+ channels of the Shaker family, Kv1.1, Kv1.2, and their Kvβ2 subunit (Rhodes et al., 1997; Wang et al., 1993). At the juxtaparanodal axolemma, these channels co-localize and create a complex with Caspr2, the second member of the Caspr family (Poliak et al., 1999). Two other proteins that are found at the juxtaparanodes are TAG-1, a GPI-anchored cell adhesion molecule related to contactin (Traka et al., 2002), and connexin 29 (Cx29), which is found at the glial membrane (Altevogt et al., 2002). The association of Caspr2 with K^+ channels is mediated by their C-terminal region, most likely through a yet unidentified PDZ-containing protein. Although one such protein, PSD95, is located at the juxtaparanodes and associates with K^+ channels, it does not mediate the interaction of these channels with Caspr2 or their accumulation at this site (Baba et al., 1999; Rasband et al., 2002). Caspr2 and TAG-1 form a juxtaparanodal complex, consisting of a glial TAG-1 molecule and an axonal Caspr2/TAG-1 heterodimer (Poliak et al., 2003; Traka et al., 2003) (Fig. 2C). This complex is essential for the accumulation of K^+ channels in the juxtaparanodes, as targeted disruption of *Caspr2* or *TAG-1* genes results in a striking reduction in the accumulation of these channels in this site in both PNS and CNS axons. These results suggest that Caspr2 and TAG-1 form a scaffold that enables the positioning of ion channels at specific sites of the plasma membrane, thus resembling the mechanisms operating during synapse formation (Poliak and Peles, 2003). It should be noted that despite the dramatic abolishment in juxtaparanodal clustering of Kv1.1/Kv1.2 in *Caspr-2* and *TAG-1* nulls, there is no change in the excitability of myelinated nerves, leaving the question of what these channels are doing under the myelin sheath unresolved (Poliak et al., 2003; Traka et al., 2003).

V. Development of the Nodal Environ

A. The Role of Myelinating Glia

During the development of myelinated nerves in the PNS, the different nodal domains are formed gradually; Na^+ channels are first clustered at the nodes, followed by the generation of the paranodal junction and only then by the clustering of K^+ channels at the juxtaparanodal region (Boiko et al., 2001; Vabnick et al., 1996, 1999). In both the CNS and PNS, Na^+ channels cluster initially at sites adjacent to the edges of processes extended by oligodendrocytes (Boiko et al., 2001; Rasband et al., 1999) and myelinating Schwann cells (Ching et al., 1999; Vabnick et al., 1996). Further longitudinal growth of these processes causes displacement of the clusters until ultimately two neighboring clusters appear to fuse, thus forming a new node of Ranvier. These results indicate that these Na^+ clusters are positioned by direct glial cell contact. In agreement, Na^+ channels are diffuse along retinal ganglion cells, but are clustered at the nodes right after these axons cross the lamina cribrosa and become myelinated (Boiko et al., 2001). These channels are not clustered after ablation of oligodendrocytes (Mathis et al., 2001) or Schwann cells (Vabnick et al., 1996) and are dispersed during demyelination (Dugandzija-Novakovic et al., 1995). Nodal Na^+ channels were also found to be associated with the edges of myelinating Schwannn cells in nerves that display shorter internodes as a result of remyelination (Dugandzija-Novakovic et al., 1995), or a genetic mutation, as seen in the *Claw Paw* mutant mouse (Koszowski et al., 1998). Furthermore, it was recently found that pharmacological inhibition of Rho kinase in myelinating Schwann cells results in multiple myelin segments produced by the same cell, each flanked by paranodes and Na^+ channel-containing nodes, supporting the notion that the location of the nodes of Ranvier along the axon is determined by the overlying myelin sheath (Melendez-Vasquez et al., 2004). Studies using retinal ganglion cells, however, revealed that Na^+ clustering could be induced in vitro by soluble factors secreted by cultured oligodendrocytes (Kaplan et al., 2001, 1997). Although Schwann cells do not secrete such clustering activity (Ching et al., 1999), some clustering of Na^+ channels has been detected in the absence of myelinating Schwann cells in the dystrophic mouse (Deerinck et al., 1997). Analyses of dysmyelinating (Ishibashi et al., 2003; Ulzheimer et al., 2003) or paranodal mutants (Rasband et al., 2003b; Rios et al., 2003), as well as demyelinating models (Craner et al., 2003; Rasband et al., 2003a), revealed that the presence of intact myelinating oligodendrocytes is also required for the developmental switch of Na^+ channel isoform in the nodes. In contrast, Nav1.6 is found in the nodes of two myelin mutants that are associated with oligodendrocyte death and lack normal paranodal junctions, *md* rats and *jimpy* mutant mice, suggesting that the switch may occur in the absence of normal paranodal contact or myelin (Arroyo et al., 2002; Jenkins and Bennett, 2002). Notably, analysis of the Shiverer mutant revealed that while axoglial contact is necessary for the expression of Nav1.6 at nodes, it is not required for targeting of this subunit to the axon initial segment, suggesting the existence of multiple targeting mechanisms in myelinated axons (Boiko et al., 2003).

B. Spatial and Temporal Events during Node Formation

During development of myelinated nerves in the PNS, NrCAM and NF186 are detected at the nodes first, followed by the appearance of ankyrin$_G$ and Na^+ channels (Lambert et al., 1997). In the CNS, however, ankyrin$_G$ is detected at the nodes before the clustering of NF186 and Na^+ channels (Jenkins and Bennett, 2002). These results suggest that NrCAM, NF186, or a yet-unidentified ankyrin$_G$-binding receptor, bind ankyrin$_G$, which in turns recruits Na^+ chan-

nels. In support of this model, the addition of a soluble NrCAM to myelinating dorsal root ganglia cultures was shown to inhibit Na^+ clustering (Lustig et al., 2001). Moreover, the appearance of ankyrin$_G$ and Na^+ channels at the nodes is delayed in *NrCAM* null mice (Custer et al., 2003), indicating that this adhesion molecule participates in the clustering of these channels. The eventual formation of nodes in these animals could be explained by the presence of NF186, which contains a similar ankyrin$_G$ binding site and could thus compensate for the absence of NrCAM. The significance of the interaction between ankyrin$_G$ and these nodal components was demonstrated in mice lacking the cerebellar isoform of ankyrin$_G$, in which Na^+ channel, Ig-CAMs, and βIV spectrin are not clustered in the initial segment of Purkinje cells (Jenkins and Bennett, 2001; Zhou et al., 1998). Similarly, spontaneous mutations of βIV spectrin in the *quivering* mice (Parkinson et al., 2001) or target disruption of this gene by a gene-trap (Komada and Soriano, 2002) results in nodal abnormalities and altered ion channel distribution. However, during the early development of myelinated axons ankyrin$_G$ is also present at the paranodes, suggesting that it is not directly involved in the initial targeting of Na^+ channels to the nodes, but rather is important for their stabilization (Jenkins and Bennett, 2002; Rasband et al., 1999). Furthermore, ankyrin$_G$ normally localized at the nodes in *dystroglycan*-null mice, which display a marked reduction of nodal Na^+ channel clusters (Saito et al., 2003). After the initial clustering of nodal components in PNS fibers, NF155 and the Caspr/contactin complex accumulate in the paranodal junction (Boiko et al., 2001; Rios et al., 2000), followed by the arrival of Caspr2 and K^+ channels to the juxtaparanodal region (Poliak et al., 2001; Vabnick et al., 1999). Caspr2, K^+ channel, and TAG-1 are first detected at the paranodes, and subsequently relocate to the juxtaparanodes as the paranodal junction is forming (Poliak et al., 2001; Rasband et al., 1998; Traka et al., 2003; Vabnick et al., 1999). In the absence of this junction, K^+ channels do not move to the juxtaparanodes and remain adjacent to the nodes (Bhat et al., 2001; Boyle et al., 2001; Dupree et al., 1999; Ishibashi et al., 2002; Poliak et al., 2001). Further maintenance of K^+ channels at the juxtaparanodal region requires Caspr2 and TAG-1, as in their absence these channels are redistributed along the internodes (Poliak et al., 2003; Traka et al., 2003).

C. Mechanisms

Several mechanisms were suggested to operate during the formation of the nodal environ (Poliak and Peles, 2003; Salzer, 2003). The exclusion of Na^+ channels from the extending edges of myelinating glia during development may be mediated by a selective molecular "filter" (Rosenbluth, 1976), or "sieve" (Pedraza et al., 2001), that is found at the paranodes. It was proposed that such a sieve selectively excludes large protein complexes, including Na$^+$ channels and Ig-CAMs that are connected to ankyrin, while allowing the passage of small membrane particles, such as the ones that correspond to K$^+$ channels (Pedraza et al., 2001; Rosenbluth, 1976). This process requires axoglial contact, but is not mediated by the Caspr/contactin complex, as their absence does not prevent Na$^+$ channels from clustering at the nodes (Bhat et al., 2001; Boyle et al., 2001; Gollan et al., 2003). Hence, the generation of mature, septa-containing paranodal junction may not be required for the efficient clustering of Na$^+$ channels. This conclusion is further supported by freeze-fracture EM studies, revealing an early differentiation of the nodes before the generation of the paranodal septa (Tao-Cheng and Rosenbluth, 1983). This implies that the initial axoglial contact at the paranodes is required for node formation, independently of the generation of septa. Accordingly, the accumulation of Caspr at the paranodes, as well as nodal clustering of Na$^+$ channels, occurs before the appearance of the septa (Marcus et al., 2002). It should be noted that gradual detachment of the paranodal loops in the CNS of paranodal mutants is accompanied by the widening of the nodal gap and dispersion of nodal Na$^+$ channels, suggesting that, although the septa are not required for the initial assembly of Na$^+$ channels at the nodes, stabilized glial contact (which is depending on septa) at the paranodes is necessary to maintain these clusters (Ishibashi et al., 2002; Rios et al., 2003; Rosenbluth et al., 2003).

In contrast to the clustering of Na$^+$ channels at the nodes, the formation of a septa-containing axoglial junction is essential for the sequestering of K$^+$ channels at the juxtaparanodes (Bhat et al., 2001; Boyle et al., 2001; Dupree et al., 1999; Poliak et al., 2001). These observations suggest that, once formed, the axoglial septate junction functions as a fence that restricts the movement of these channels, as well as of other components from beneath the myelin sheath toward the nodes. The generation of this fence may be mediated by the attachment of the Caspr/contactin complex to the axonal cytoskeleton (Gollan et al., 2002), binding to a glial ligand, as well as by the assembly of specific lipid-microdomains. In addition to the paranodal junction, a membrane barrier may also exist at the nodes. Although in the absence of the paranodal junction, Caspr2/K$^+$ channel complex and TAG-1 are aberrantly located at the paranodal region, these proteins do not invade the nodes, indicating the existence of an additional membrane barrier at this site (Bhat et al., 2001; Boyle et al., 2001; Dupree et al., 1999). A nodal barrier may be similar to the diffusion barrier (or a membrane fence) found at the axonal initial segment, which could be regarded as the first node in most myelinated axons (Winckler et al., 1999). At the axon initial segment, this fence is formed by a high local concentration of transmembrane proteins that are anchored to the actin cytoskeleton, which are able to block the diffusion of membrane proteins and phospholipids (Nakada et al., 2003). Interestingly, an

intact actin cytoskeleton is also required for the clustering of Na$^+$ channels along retinal ganglion axons by a soluble factor secreted from oligodendrocytes (Kaplan et al., 2001). In the PNS, clustering of nodal Na$^+$ channels during development could also be mediated by contacting glial processes that "drag" Na$^+$ channels and Ig-CAMs toward their final position on the axolemma. This may be mediated by binding of Na$^+$ channels to the Schwann cell microvilli, either directly through their β subunits, or indirectly through NrCAM and NF186 (Lambert et al., 1997) and Gliomedin (Eshed and Peles, unpublished observations). During development, the ERM-positive Schwann cell microvilli were shown to make early contact with the nodes during their formation (Melendez-Vasquez et al., 2001). These contact sites (termed caps) contain the phosphorylated EBP50 adaptor protein and face across axonal ankyrin$_G$ (Gatto et al., 2003). Disruption of the microvilli organization in mice lacking Schwann cells dystroglycan resulted in a striking reduction in clustering of nodal Na$^+$ channel (Saito et al., 2003). Although CNS nodes are not covered by microvilli, they do contain a similar protein complexes, including ion channels, cell adhesion molecules, and cytoplasmic linkers, suggesting the basic mechanisms that operate in their formation and maintenance may be similar.

Acknowledgments

The work carried out in the author's laboratory is supported by the National Multiple Sclerosis Society, the NIH, the United States-Israel Science Foundation (BSF), Jerusalem, Israel, the Minerva Foundation, and the Israel Science Foundation. E.P. is an Incumbent of the Madeleine Haas Russell Career Development Chair.

References

Altevogt, B. M., Kleopa, K. A., Postma, F. R., Scherer, S. S., and Paul, D. L. (2002). Connexin29 is uniquely distributed within myelinating glial cells of the central and peripheral nervous systems. *J. Neurosci.* **22**, 6458–6470.

Apostolski, S., Sadiq, S. A., Hays, A., Corbo, M., Suturkova-Milosevic, L., Chaliff, P., Stefansson, K., LeBaron, R. G., Ruoslahti, E., Hays, A. P., and et al. (1994). Identification of Gal(beta 1-3)GalNAc bearing glycoproteins at the nodes of Ranvier in peripheral nerve. *J. Neurosci. Res.* **38**, 134–141.

Arroyo, E. J., Xu, T., Grinspan, J., Lambert, S., Levinson, S. R., Brophy, P. J., Peles, E., and Scherer, S. S. (2002). Genetic dysmyelination alters the molecular architecture of the nodal region. *J. Neurosci.* **22**, 1726–1737.

Arroyo, E. J., Xu, Y. T., Zhou, L., Messing, A., Peles, E., Chiu, S. Y., and Scherer, S. S. (1999). Myelinating Schwann cells determine the internodal localization of Kv1.1, Kv1.2, Kvbeta2, and Caspr. *J. Neurocytol.* **28**, 333–347.

Baba, H., Akita, H., Ishibashi, T., Inoue, Y., Nakahira, K., and Ikenaka, K. (1999). Completion of myelin compaction, but not the attachment of oligodendroglial processes triggers K(+) channel clustering. *J. Neurosci. Res.* **58**, 752–764.

Baumgartner, S., Littleton, J. T., Broadie, K., Bhat, M. A., Harbecke, R., Lengyel, J. A., Chiquet-Ehrismann, R., Prokop, A., and Bellen, H.

J. (1996). A Drosophila neurexin is required for septate junction and blood-nerve barrier formation and function. *Cell* **87**, 1059–1068.

Bellen, H. J., Lu, Y., Beckstead, R., and Bhat, M. A. (1998). Neurexin IV, caspr and paranodin: Novel members of the neurexin family: Encounters of axons and glia. *Trends Neurosci.* **21**, 444–449.

Berghs, S., Aggujaro, D., Dirkx, R., Jr., Maksimova, E., Stabach, P., Hermel, J. M., Zhang, J. P., Philbrick, W., Slepnev, V., Ort, T., and Solimena, M. (2000). BetaIV spectrin, a new spectrin localized at axon initial segments and nodes of ranvier in the central and peripheral nervous system. *J. Cell Biol.* **151**, 985–1002.

Bhat, M. A., Rios, J. C., Lu, Y., Garcia-Fresco, G. P., Ching, W., St Martin, M., Li, J., Einheber, S., Chesler, M., Rosenbluth, J., et al. (2001). Axonglia interactions and the domain organization of myelinated axons requires neurexin IV/Caspr/Paranodin. *Neuron* **30**, 369–383.

Black, J. A., and Waxman, S. G. (1988). The perinodal astrocyte. *Glia* **1**, 169–183.

Boiko, T., Rasband, M. N., Levinson, S. R., Caldwell, J. H., Mandel, G., Trimmer, J. S., and Matthews, G. (2001). Compact myelin dictates the differential targeting of two sodium channel isoforms in the same axon. *Neuron* **30**, 91–104.

Boiko, T., Van Wart, A., Caldwell, J. H., Levinson, S. R., Trimmer, J. S., and Matthews, G. (2003). Functional specialization of the axon initial segment by isoform-specific sodium channel targeting. *J. Neurosci.* **23**, 2306–2313.

Bonnon, C., Goutebroze, L., Denisenko-Nehrbass, N., Girault, J. A., and Faivre-Sarrailh, C. (2003). The paranodal complex of F3/contactin and Caspr/paranodin traffics to the cell surface via a non-conventional pathway. *J. Biol. Chem.* **278**, 48339–48347.

Bosio, A., Binczek, E., and Stoffel, W. (1996). Functional breakdown of the lipid bilayer of the myelin membrane in central and peripheral nervous system by disrupted galactocerebroside synthesis. *Proc. Natl. Acad. Sci. U. S. A.* **93**, 13280–13285.

Boyle, M. E., Berglund, E. O., Murai, K. K., Weber, L., Peles, E., and Ranscht, B. (2001). Contactin orchestrates assembly of the septate-like junctions at the paranode in myelinated peripheral nerve. *Neuron* **30**, 385–397.

Charles, P., Tait, S., Faivre-Sarrailh, C., Barbin, G., Gunn-Moore, F., Denisenko-Nehrbass, N., Guennoc, A. M., Girault, J. A., Brophy, P. J., and Lubetzki, C. (2002). Neurofascin is a glial receptor for the paranodin/Caspr-contactin axonal complex at the axoglial junction. *Curr. Biol.* **12**, 217–220.

Ching, W., Zanazzi, G., Levinson, S. R., and Salzer, J. L. (1999). Clustering of neuronal sodium channels requires contact with myelinating Schwann cells. *J. Neurocytol.* **28**, 295–301.

Coetzee, T., Dupree, J. L., and Popko, B. (1998). Demyelination and altered expression of myelin-associated glycoprotein isoforms in the central nervous system of galactolipid-deficient mice. *J. Neurosci. Res.* **54**, 613–622.

Coetzee, T., Fujita, N., Dupree, J., Shi, R., Blight, A., Suzuki, K., and Popko, B. (1996). Myelination in the absence of galactocerebroside and sulfatide: Normal structure with abnormal function and regional instability. *Cell* **86**, 209–219.

Craner, M. J., Lo, A. C., Black, J. A., and Waxman, S. G. (2003). Abnormal sodium channel distribution in optic nerve axons in a model of inflammatory demyelination. *Brain* **126**, 1552–1561.

Custer, A. W., Kazarinova-Noyes, K., Sakurai, T., Xu, X., Simon, W., Grumet, M., and Shrager, P. (2003). The role of angyrin-binding protein NrCAM in node of Ranvier formation. *J. Neurosci.* **23**, 10032–10039.

Davis, J. Q., Lambert, S., and Bennett, V. (1996). Molecular composition of the node of Ranvier: identification of ankyrin-binding cell adhesion molecules neurofascin (mucin+/third FNIII domain-) and NrCAM at nodal axon segments. *J. Cell Biol.* **135**, 1355–1367.

Deerinck, T. J., Levinson, S. R., Bennett, G. V., and Ellisman, M. H. (1997). Clustering of voltage-sensitive sodium channels on axons is independent of direct Schwann cell contact in the dystrophic mouse. *J. Neurosci.* **17**, 5080–5088.

Denisenko-Nehrbass, N., Oguievetskaia, K., Goutebroze, L., Galvez, T., Yamakawa, H., Ohara, O., Carnaud, M., and Girault, J. A. (2003). Protein 4.1B associates with both Caspr/paranodin and Caspr2 at paranodes and juxtaparanodes of myelinated fibres. *Eur. J. Neurosci.* **17**, 411–416.

Devaux, J., Alcaraz, G., Grinspan, J., Bennett, V., Joho, R., Crest, M., and Scherer, S. S. (2003). Kv3.1b is a novel component of CNS nodes. *J. Neurosci.* **23**, 4509–4518.

Devaux, J. J., Kleopa, K. A., Cooper, E. C., and Scherer, S. S. (2004). KCNQ2 is a nodal K+ channel. *J. Neurosci.* **24**, 1236–1244.

Dugandzija-Novakovic, S., Koszowski, A. G., Levinson, S. R., and Shrager, P. (1995). Clustering of Na+ channels and node of Ranvier formation in remyelinating axons. *J. Neurosci.* **15**, 492–503.

Dupree, J. L., Coetzee, T., Blight, A., Suzuki, K., and Popko, B. (1998). Myelin galactolipids are essential for proper node of Ranvier formation in the CNS. *J. Neurosci.* **18**, 1642–1649.

Dupree, J. L., Girault, J. A., and Popko, B. (1999). Axo-glial interactions regulate the localization of axonal paranodal proteins. *J. Cell Biol.* **147**, 1145–1152.

Einheber, S., Zanazzi, G., Ching, W., Scherer, S., Milner, T. A., Peles, E., and Salzer, J. L. (1997). The axonal membrane protein Caspr, a homologue of neurexin IV, is a component of the septate-like paranodal junctions that assemble during myelination. *J. Cell Biol.* **139**, 1495–1506.

Fabricius, C., Berthold, C. H., and Rydmark, M. (1993). Axoplasmic organelles at nodes of Ranvier. II. Occurrence and distribution in large myelinated spinal cord axons of the adult cat. *J. Neurocytol.* **22**, 941–954.

Faivre-Sarrailh, C., Gauthier, F., Denisenko-Nehrbass, N., Le Bivic, A., Rougon, G., and Girault, J. A. (2000). The glycosylphosphatidyl inositol-anchored adhesion molecule F3/contactin is required for surface transport of paranodin/contactin-associated protein (caspr). *J. Cell Biol.* **149**, 491–502.

Ffrench-Constant, C., Miller, R. H., Kruse, J., Schachner, M., and Raff, M. C. (1986). Molecular specialization of astrocyte processes at nodes of Ranvier in rat optic nerve. *J. Cell Biol.* **102**, 844–852.

Garrido, J. J., Giraud, P., Carlier, E., Fernandes, F., Moussif, A., Fache, M. P., Debanne, D., and Dargent, B. (2003). A targeting motif involved in sodium channel clustering at the axonal initial segment. *Science* **300**, 2091–2094.

Garver, T. D., Ren, Q., Tuvia, S., and Bennett, V. (1997). Tyrosine phosphorylation at a site highly conserved in the L1 family of cell adhesion molecules abolishes ankyrin binding and increases lateral mobility of neurofascin. *J. Cell Biol.* **137**, 703–714.

Gatto, C. L., Walker, B. J., and Lambert, S. (2003). Local ERM activation and dynamic growth cones at Schwann cell tips implicated in efficient formation of nodes of Ranvier. *J. Cell Biol.* **162**, 489–498.

Gollan, L., Sabanay, H., Poliak, S., Berglund, E. O., Ranscht, B., and Peles, E. (2002). Retention of a cell adhesion complex at the paranodal junction requires the cytoplasmic region of Caspr. *J. Cell Biol.* **157**, 1247–1256.

Gollan, L., Salomon, D., Salzer, J. L., and Peles, E. (2003). Caspr regulates the processing of contactin and inhibits its binding to neurofascin. *J. Cell Biol.* **163**, 1213–1218.

Goutebroze, L., Carnaud, M., Denisenko, N., Boutterin, M. C., and Girault, J. A. (2003). Syndecan-3 and syndecan-4 are enriched in Schwann cell perinodal processes. *BMC Neurosci.* **4**, 29.

Hall, S. M., and Williams, P. L. (1971). Studies on the "incisures" of Schmidt-Lanterman. *J. Cell Sci.* **6**, 767–795.

Harroch, S., Furtado, G. C., Brueck, W., Rosenbluth, J., Lafaille, J., Chao, M., Buxbaum, J. D., and Schlessinger, J. (2002). A critical role for the protein tyrosine phosphatase receptor type Z in functional recovery from demyelinating lesions. *Nat. Genet.* **32**, 411–414.

Harroch, S., Palmeri, M., Rosenbluth, J., Custer, A., Okigaki, M., Shrager, P., Blum, M., Buxbaum, J. D., and Schlessinger, J. (2000). No obvious abnormality in mice deficient in receptor protein tyrosine phosphatase beta. *Mol. Cell Biol.* **20**, 7706–7715.

Honke, K., Hirahara, Y., Dupree, J., Suzuki, K., Popko, B., Fukushima, K., Fukushima, J., Nagasawa, T., Yoshida, N., Wada, Y., and Taniguchi, N. (2002). Paranodal junction formation and spermatogenesis require sulfoglycolipids. *Proc. Natl. Acad. Sci. U. S. A.* **99**, 4227–4232.

Ishibashi, T., Dupree, J. L., Ikenaka, K., Hirahara, Y., Honke, K., Peles, E., Popko, B., Suzuki, K., Nishino, H., and Baba, H. (2002). A myelin galactolipid, sulfatide, is essential for maintenance of ion channels on myelinated axon but not essential for initial cluster formation. *J. Neurosci.* **22**, 6507–6514.

Ishibashi, T., Ikenaka, K., Shimizu, T., Kagawa, T., and Baba, H. (2003). Initiation of sodium channel clustering at the node of Ranvier in the mouse optic nerve. *Neurochem. Res.* **28**, 117–125.

Isom, L. L. (2002). The role of sodium channels in cell adhesion. *Front Biosci.* **7**, 12–23.

Isom, L. L., Ragsdale, D. S., De Jongh, K. S., Westenbroek, R. E., Reber, B. F., Scheuer, T., and Catterall, W. A. (1995). Structure and function of the beta 2 subunit of brain sodium channels, a transmembrane glycoprotein with a CAM motif. *Cell* **83**, 433–442.

Jenkins, S. M., and Bennett, V. (2001). Ankyrin-G coordinates assembly of the spectrin-based membrane skeleton, voltage-gated sodium channels, and L1 CAMs at Purkinje neuron initial segments. *J. Cell Biol.* **155**, 739–746.

Jenkins, S. M., and Bennett, V. (2002). Developing nodes of Ranvier are defined by ankyrin-G clustering and are independent of paranodal axoglial adhesion. *Proc. Natl. Acad. Sci. U. S. A.* **99**, 2303–2308.

Kaplan, M. R., Cho, M. H., Ullian, E. M., Isom, L. L., Levinson, S. R., and Barres, B. A. (2001). Differential control of clustering of the sodium channels Na(v)1.2 and Na(v)1.6 at developing CNS nodes of Ranvier. *Neuron* **30**, 105–119.

Kaplan, M. R., Meyer-Franke, A., Lambert, S., Bennett, V., Duncan, I. D., Levinson, S. R., and Barres, B. A. (1997). Induction of sodium channel clustering by oligodendrocytes. *Nature* **386**, 724–728.

Kazarinova-Noyes, K., Malhotra, J. D., McEwen, D. P., Mattei, L. N., Berglund, E. O., Ranscht, B., Levinson, S. R., Schachner, M., Shrager, P., Isom, L. L., and Xiao, Z. C. (2001). Contactin associates with Na+ channels and increases their functional expression. *J. Neurosci.* **21**, 7517–7525.

Kazarinova-Noyes, K., and Shrager, P. (2002). Molecular constituents of the node of Ranvier. *Mol. Neurobiol.* **26**, 167–182.

Komada, M., and Soriano, P. (2002). [Beta]IV-spectrin regulates sodium channel clustering through ankyrin-G at axon initial segments and nodes of Ranvier. *J. Cell Biol.* **156**, 337–348.

Kordeli, E., Davis, J., Trapp, B., and Bennett, V. (1990). An isoform of ankyrin is localized at nodes of Ranvier in myelinated axons of central and peripheral nerves. *J. Cell Biol.* **110**, 1341–1352.

Kordeli, E., Lambert, S., and Bennett, V. (1995). AnkyrinG. A new ankyrin gene with neural-specific isoforms localized at the axonal initial segment and node of Ranvier. *J. Biol. Chem.* **270**, 2352–2359.

Koszowski, A. G., Owens, G. C., and Levinson, S. R. (1998). The effect of the mouse mutation claw paw on myelination and nodal frequency in sciatic nerves. *J. Neurosci.* **18**, 5859–5868.

Lambert, S., Davis, J. Q., and Bennett, V. (1997). Morphogenesis of the node of Ranvier: co-clusters of ankyrin and ankyrin-binding integral proteins define early developmental intermediates. *J. Neurosci.* **17**, 7025–7036.

Landon, D. N., and Langley, O. K. (1971). The local chemical environment of nodes of Ranvier: a study of cation binding. *J. Anat.* **108**, 419–432.

Lemaillet, G., Walker, B., and Lambert, S. (2003). Identification of a conserved ankyrin-binding motif in the family of sodium channel alpha subunits. *J. Biol. Chem.* **278**, 27333–27339.

Liu, C. J., Dib-Hajj, S. D., Black, J. A., Greenwood, J., Lian, Z., and Waxman, S. G. (2001). Direct interaction with contactin targets voltage-gated sodium channel Na(v)1.9/NaN to the cell membrane. *J. Biol. Chem.* **276**, 46553–46561.

Lustig, M., Zanazzi, G., Sakurai, T., Blanco, C., Levinson, S. R., Lambert, S., Grumet, M., and Salzer, J. L. (2001). Nr-CAM and neurofascin interactions regulate ankyrin$_G$ and sodium channel clustering at the node of Ranvier. *Curr. Biol.* **11**, 1864–1869.

Malhotra, J. D., Kazen-Gillespie, K., Hortsch, M., and Isom, L. L. (2000). Sodium channel beta subunits mediate homophilic cell adhesion and recruit ankyrin to points of cell-cell contact. *J. Biol. Chem.* **275**, 11383–11388.

Malhotra, J. D., Koopmann, M. C., Kazen-Gillespie, K. A., Fettman, N., Hortsch, M., and Isom, L. L. (2002). Structural requirements for interaction of sodium channel beta 1 subunits with ankyrin. *J. Biol. Chem.* **277**, 26681–26688.

Marcus, J., Dupree, J. L., and Popko, B. (2002). Myelin-associated glycoprotein and myelin galactolipids stabilize developing axo-glial interactions. *J. Cell Biol.* **156**, 567–577.

Martin, S., Levine, A. K., Chen, Z. J., Ughrin, Y., and Levine, J. M. (2001). Deposition of the NG2 proteoglycan at nodes of Ranvier in the peripheral nervous system. *J. Neurosci.* **21**, 8119–8128.

Martini, R., Schachner, M., and Faissner, A. (1990). Enhanced expression of the extracellular matrix molecule J1/tenascin in the regenerating adult mouse sciatic nerve. *J. Neurocytol.* **19**, 601–616.

Mathis, C., Denisenko-Nehrbass, N., Girault, J. A., and Borrelli, E. (2001). Essential role of oligodendrocytes in the formation and maintenance of central nervous system nodal regions. *Development* **128**, 4881–4890.

McEwen, D. P., Meadows, L. S., Chen, C., Thyagarajan, V., and Isom, L. L. (2004). Sodium channel beta1 subunit-mediated modulation of Nav1.2 currents and cell surface density is dependent on interactions with contactin and ankyrin. *J. Biol. Chem.* **279**, 16044–16049.

Melendez-Vasquez, C. V., Einheber, S., and Salzer, J. L. (2004). Rho kinase regulates Schwann cell myelination and formation of associated axonal domains. *J. Neurosci.* **24**, 3953–3963.

Melendez-Vasquez, C. V., Rios, J. C., Zanazzi, G., Lambert, S., Bretscher, A., and Salzer, J. L. (2001). Nodes of Ranvier form in association with ezrin-radixin-moesin (ERM)-positive Schwann cell processes. *Proc. Natl. Acad. Sci. U. S. A.* **98**, 1235–1240.

Menegoz, M., Gaspar, P., Le Bert, M., Galvez, T., Burgaya, F., Palfrey, C., Ezan, P., Arnos, F., and Girault, J. A. (1997). Paranodin, a glycoprotein of neuronal paranodal membranes. *Neuron* **19**, 319–331.

Missler, M., and Sudhof, T. C. (1998). Neurexins: three genes and 1001 products. *Trends Genet.* **14**, 20–26.

Nakada, C., Ritchie, K., Oba, Y., Nakamura, M., Hotta, Y., Iino, R., Kasai, R. S., Yamaguchi, K., Fujiwara, T., and Kusumi, A. (2003). Accumulation of anchored proteins forms membrane diffusion barriers during neuronal polarization. *Nat. Cell Biol.* **5**, 626–632.

Ohara, R., Yamakawa, H., Nakayama, M., and Ohara, O. (2000). Type II brain 4.1 (4.1B/KIAA0987), a member of the protein 4.1 family, is localized to neuronal paranodes. *Mol. Brain Res.* **85**, 41–52.

Oohashi, T., Hirakawa, S., Bekku, Y., Rauch, U., Zimmermann, D. R., Su, W. D., Ohtsuka, A., Murakami, T., and Ninomiya, Y. (2002). Bral1, a brain-specific link protein, colocalizing with the versican V2 isoform at the nodes of Ranvier in developing and adult mouse central nervous systems. *Mol. Cell Neurosci.* **19**, 43–57.

Parkinson, N. J., Olsson, C. L., Hallows, J. L., McKee-Johnson, J., Keogh, B. P., Noben-Trauth, K., Kujawa, S. G., and Tempel, B. L. (2001). Mutant beta-spectrin 4 causes auditory and motor neuropathies in quivering mice. *Nat. Genet.* **29**, 61–65.

Parra, M., Gascard, P., Walensky, L. D., Gimm, J. A., Blackshaw, S., Chan, N., Takakuwa, Y., Berger, T., Lee, G., Chasis, J. A., et al. (2000). Molecular and functional characterization of protein 4.1B, a novel member of the protein 4.1 family with high level, focal expression in brain. *J. Biol. Chem.* **275**, 3247–3255.

Pedraza, L., Huang, J. K., and Colman, D. R. (2001). Organizing principles of the axoglial apparatus. *Neuron* **30**, 335–344.

Peles, E., Nativ, M., Campbell, P. L., Sakurai, T., Martinez, R., Lev, S., Clary, D. O., Schilling, J., Barnea, G., Plowman, G. D., and Schlessinger,

J. (1995). The carbonic anhydrase domain of receptor tyrosine phosphatase beta is a functional ligand for the axonal cell recognition molecule contactin. *Cell* **82**, 251–260.

Peles, E., Nativ, M., Lustig, M., Grumet, M., Schilling, J., Martinez, R., Plowman, G. D., and Schlessinger, J. (1997). Identification of a novel contactin-associated transmembrane receptor with multiple domains implicated in protein-protein interactions. *Embo J.* **16**, 978–988.

Pesheva, P., Gennarini, G., Goridis, C., and Schachner, M. (1993). The F3/11 cell adhesion molecule mediates the repulsion of neurons by the extracellular matrix glycoprotein J1-160/180. *Neuron* **10**, 69–82.

Poliak, S., Gollan, L., Martinez, R., Custer, A., Einheber, S., Salzer, J. L., Trimmer, J. S., Shrager, P., and Peles, E. (1999). Caspr2, a new member of the neurexin superfamily, is localized at the juxtaparanodes of myelinated axons and associates with K⁺ channels. *Neuron* **24**, 1037–1047.

Poliak, S., Gollan, L., Salomon, D., Berglund, E. O., Ohara, R., Ranscht, B., and Peles, E. (2001). Localization of Caspr2 in myelinated nerves depends on axon-glia interactions and the generation of barriers along the axon. *J. Neurosci.* **21**, 7568–7575.

Poliak, S., Matlis, S., Ullmer, C., Scherer, S. S., and Peles, E. (2002). Distinct claudins and associated PDZ proteins form different autotypic tight junctions in myelinating Schwann cells. *J. Cell. Biol.* **159**, 361–372.

Poliak, S., and Peles, E. (2003). The local differentiation of myelinated axons at nodes of Ranvier. *Nat. Rev. Neurosci.* **4**, 968–980.

Poliak, S., Salomon, D., Elhanany, H., Sabanay, H., Kiernan, B., Pevny, L., Stewart, C. L., Xu, X., Chiu, S.-Y., Shrager, P., et al. (2003). Juxtaparanodal clustering of Shaker-like K⁺ channels in myelinated axons depends on Caspr2 and TAG-1. *J. Cell Biol.* **162**, 1149–1160.

Raine, C. S. (1984). On the association between perinodal astrocytic processes and the node of Ranvier in the C.N.S. *J. Neurocytol.* **13**, 21–27.

Rasband, M. N., Kagawa, T., Park, E. W., Ikenaka, K., and Trimmer, J. S. (2003a). Dysregulation of axonal sodium channel isoforms after adult-onset chronic demyelination. *J. Neurosci. Res.* **73**, 465–470.

Rasband, M. N., Park, E. W., Zhen, D., Arbuckle, M. I., Poliak, S., Peles, E., Grant, S. G., and Trimmer, J. S. (2002). Clustering of neuronal potassium channels is independent of their interaction with PSD-95. *J. Cell Biol.* **159**, 663–672.

Rasband, M. N., Peles, E., Trimmer, J. S., Levinson, S. R., Lux, S. E., and Shrager, P. (1999). Dependence of nodal sodium channel clustering on paranodal axoglial contact in the developing CNS. *J. Neurosci.* **19**, 7516–7528.

Rasband, M. N., Taylor, C. M., and Bansal, R. (2003b). Paranodal transverse bands are required for maintenance but not initiation of Nav1.6 sodium channel clustering in CNS optic nerve axons. *Glia* **44**, 173–182.

Rasband, M. N., Trimmer, J. S., Schwarz, T. L., Levinson, S. R., Ellisman, M. H., Schachner, M., and Shrager, P. (1998). Potassium channel distribution, clustering, and function in remyelinating rat axons. *J. Neurosci.* **18**, 36–47.

Ratcliffe, C. F., Qu, Y., McCormick, K. A., Tibbs, V. C., Dixon, J. E., Scheuer, T., and Catterall, W. A. (2000). A sodium channel signaling complex: modulation by associated receptor protein tyrosine phosphatase beta. *Nat. Neurosci.* **3**, 437–444.

Ratcliffe, C. F., Westenbroek, R. E., Curtis, R., and Catterall, W. A. (2001). Sodium channel beta1 and beta3 subunits associate with neurofascin through their extracellular immunoglobulin-like domain. *J. Cell Biol.* **154**, 427–434.

Rhodes, K. J., Strassle, B. W., Monaghan, M. M., Bekele-Arcuri, Z., Matos, M. F., and Trimmer, J. S. (1997). Association and colocalization of the Kvbeta1 and Kvbeta2 beta-subunits with Kv1 alpha-subunits in mammalian brain K⁺ channel complexes. *J. Neurosci.* **17**, 8246–8258.

Rieger, F., Daniloff, J. K., Pincon-Raymond, M., Crossin, K. L., Grumet, M., and Edelman, G. M. (1986). Neuronal cell adhesion molecules and cytotactin are colocalized at the node of Ranvier. *J. Cell. Biol.* **103**, 379–391.

Rios, J. C., Melendez-Vasquez, C. V., Einheber, S., Lustig, M., Grumet, M., Hemperly, J., Peles, E., and Salzer, J. L. (2000). Contactin-associated protein (Caspr) and contactin form a complex that is targeted to the paranodal junctions during myelination. *J. Neurosci.* **20**, 8354–8364.

Rios, J. C., Rubin, M., St Martin, M., Downey, R. T., Einheber, S., Rosenbluth, J., Levinson, S. R., Bhat, M., and Salzer, J. L. (2003). Paranodal interactions regulate expression of sodium channel subtypes and provide a diffusion barrier for the node of Ranvier. *J. Neurosci.* **23**, 7001–7011.

Rosenbluth, J. (1976). Intramembranous particle distribution at the node of Ranvier and adjacent axolemma in myelinated axons of the frog brain. *J. Neurocytol.* **5**, 731–745.

Rosenbluth, J. (1995). Glial membranes and axoglial junctions. *In* "Neuroglia" (H. Kettenmann, and B. R. Ransom, eds.), pp. 613–633, Oxford University Press, New York.

Rosenbluth, J., Dupree, J. L., and Popko, B. (2003). Nodal sodium channel domain integrity depends on the conformation of the paranodal junction, not on the presence of transverse bands. *Glia* **41**, 318–325.

Saito, F., Masaki, T., Kamakura, K., Anderson, L. V., Fujita, S., Fukuta-Ohi, H., Sunada, Y., Shimizu, T., and Matsumura, K. (1999). Characterization of the transmembrane molecular architecture of the dystroglycan complex in schwann cells. *J. Biol. Chem.* **274**, 8240–8246.

Saito, F., Moore, S. A., Barresi, R., Henry, M. D., Messing, A., Ross-Barta, S. E., Cohn, R. D., Williamson, R. A., Sluka, K. A., Sherman, D. L., et al. (2003). Unique role of dystroglycan in peripheral nerve myelination, nodal structure, and sodium channel stabilization. *Neuron* **38**, 747–758.

Sakurai, T., Lustig, M., Nativ, M., Hemperly, J. J., Schlessinger, J., Peles, E., and Grumet, M. (1997). Induction of neurite outgrowth through contactin and Nr-CAM by extracellular regions of glial receptor tyrosine phosphatase beta. *J. Cell Biol.* **136**, 907–918.

Salzer, J. L. (2003). Polarized domains of myelinated axons. *Neuron* **40**, 297–318.

Schafer, D. P., Bansal, R., Hedstrom, K. L., Pfeiffer, S. E., and Rasband, M. N. (2004). Does paranode formation and maintenance require partitioning of neurofascin 155 into lipid rafts? *J Neurosci* **24**, 3176–3185.

Scherer, S. S., Xu, T., Crino, P., Arroyo, E. J., and Gutmann, D. H. (2001). Ezrin, radixin, and moesin are components of Schwann cell microvilli. *J. Neurosci. Res.* **65**, 150–164.

Spiegel, I., Salomon, D., Erne, B., Schaeren-Wiemers, N., and Peles, E. (2002). Caspr3 and caspr4, two novel members of the caspr family, are expressed in the nervous system and interact with PDZ domains. *Mol. Cell Neurosci.* **20**, 283–297.

Srinivasan, J., Schachner, M., and Catterall, W. A. (1998). Interaction of voltage-gated sodium channels with the extracellular matrix molecules tenascin-C and tenascin-R. *Proc. Natl. Acad. Sci. U. S. A.* **95**, 15753–15757.

Srinivasan, Y., Elmer, L., Davis, J., Bennett, V., and Angelides, K. (1988). Ankyrin and spectrin associate with voltage-dependent sodium channels in brain. *Nature* **333**, 177–180.

Tait, S., Gunn-Moore, F., Collinson, J. M., Huang, J., Lubetzki, C., Pedraza, L., Sherman, D. L., Colman, D. R., and Brophy, P. J. (2000). An oligodendrocyte cell adhesion molecule at the site of assembly of the paranodal axo-glial junction. *J. Cell Biol.* **150**, 657–666.

Tao-Cheng, J. H., and Rosenbluth, J. (1983). Axolemmal differentiation in myelinated fibers of rat peripheral nerves. *Brain Res.* **285**, 251–263.

Traka, M., Dupree, J. L., Popko, B., and Karagogeos, D. (2002). The neuronal adhesion protein TAG-1 is expressed by Schwann cells and oligodendrocytes and is localized to the juxtaparanodal region of myelinated fibers. *J. Neurosci.* **22**, 3016–3024.

Traka, M., Goutebroze, L., Denisenko, N., Bessa, M., Nifli, A., Havaki, S., Iwakura, Y., Fukamauchi, F., Watanabe, K., Soliven, B., et al. (2003). Association of TAG-1 with Caspr2 is essential for the molecular organization of juxtaparanodal regions of myelinated fibers. *J. Cell Biol.* **162**, 1161–1172.

Ulzheimer, J. C., Peles, E., Levinson, S. R., and Martini, R. (2003). Altered expression of ion channel isoforms at the node of Ranvier in P0 deficient myelin mutants. *Mol. Cell Neurosci.* **25**, 83–94.

Vabnick, I., Novakovic, S. D., Levinson, S. R., Schachner, M., and Shrager, P. (1996). The clustering of axonal sodium channels during development of the peripheral nervous system. *J. Neurosci.* **16**, 4914–4922.

Vabnick, I., Trimmer, J. S., Schwarz, T. L., Levinson, S. R., Risal, D., and Shrager, P. (1999). Dynamic potassium channel distributions during axonal development prevent aberrant firing patterns. *J. Neurosci.* **19**, 747–758.

Wang, H., Kunkel, D. D., Martin, T. M., Schwartzkroin, P. A., and Tempel, B. L. (1993). Heteromultimeric K+ channels in terminal and juxtaparanodal regions of neurons. *Nature* **365**, 75–79.

Waxman, S. G., and Ritchie, J. M. (1993). Molecular dissection of the myelinated axon. *Ann. Neurol.* **33**, 121–136.

Weber, P., Bartsch, U., Rasband, M. N., Czaniera, R., Lang, Y., Bluethmann, H., Margolis, R. U., Levinson, S. R., Shrager, P., Montag, D., and Schachner, M. (1999). Mice deficient for tenascin-R display alterations of the extracellular matrix and decreased axonal conduction velocities in the CNS. *J. Neurosci.* **19**, 4245–4262.

Winckler, B., Forscher, P., and Mellman, I. (1999). A diffusion barrier maintains distribution of membrane proteins in polarized neurons. *Nature* **397**, 698–701.

Wolswijk, G., and Balesar, R. (2003). Changes in the expression and localization of the paranodal protein Caspr on axons in chronic multiple sclerosis. *Brain* **126**, 1638–1649.

Xiao, Z. C., Bartsch, U., Margolis, R. K., Rougon, G., Montag, D., and Schachner, M. (1997). Isolation of a tenascin-R binding protein from mouse brain membranes. A phosphacan-related chondroitin sulfate proteoglycan. *J. Biol. Chem.* **272**, 32092–32101.

Xiao, Z. C., Ragsdale, D. S., Malhotra, J. D., Mattei, L. N., Braun, P. E., Schachner, M., and Isom, L. L. (1999). Tenascin-R is a functional modulator of sodium channel beta subunits. *J. Biol. Chem.* **274**, 26511–26517.

Yu, F. H., and Catterall, W. A. (2003). Overview of the voltage-gated sodium channel family. *Genome Biol.* **4**, 207.

Yuan, L. L., and Ganetzky, B. (1999). A glial-neuronal signaling pathway revealed by mutations in a neurexin-related protein. *Science* **283**, 1343–1345.

Zhou, D., Lambert, S., Malen, P. L., Carpenter, S., Boland, L. M., and Bennett, V. (1998). Ankyrin$_G$ is required for clustering of voltage-gated Na channels at axon initial segments and for normal action potential firing. *J. Cell Biol.* **143**, 1295–1304.

4

Potassium Channel Organization of Myelinated and Demyelinated Axons

Matthew N. Rasband, Ph.D.

beneath the myelin sheath adjacent to nodes of Ranvier. The unmasking of Kv1 channels is thought to be a major contributor to the altered electrical properties of demyelinated and remyelinating axons. In this chapter I discuss the kinds of channels expressed in myelinated axons with special emphasis on the Kv1 channels that are exposed as a consequence of demyelination. I discuss the cellular and molecular mechanisms responsible for Kv1 channel localization and the consequences of demyelination for Kv1 channel localization and function.

I. Introduction

Potassium (K^+) channels regulate a variety of neuronal properties, including frequency of firing, neurotransmitter release, resting membrane potential, and action potential amplitude and duration. These properties depend on both the kinds of channels expressed in the plasma membrane and their spatial localization. An assortment of K^+ channels are present in myelinated axons and are localized to distinct domains at or near nodes of Ranvier. For example, KCNQ2 channels have been found clustered at nodes of Ranvier, while Kv1 channels have been shown to be restricted

II. Potassium Channel Structure and Function

Potassium (K^+) channels regulate a variety of neuronal properties, including frequency of firing, neurotransmitter release, resting membrane potential, and action potential amplitude and duration (Hille, 2001). These properties depend on both the kinds of channels expressed in the plasma membrane and their spatial localization. One of the best examples demonstrating the heterogeneous expression and localization of different voltage-gated K^+ (Kv) channels is the myelinated nerve fiber. This chapter briefly summarizes general properties about Kv channels, describes in detail the localization and composition of Kv channel protein complexes in myelinated nerve fibers, and discusses the consequences of demyelination for Kv channel localization and function.

The K$^+$ channels form a large and diverse gene family (Fig. 1A), with many properties that are common among the proteins (Jan and Jan, 1997; Trimmer and Rhodes, 2003). For example, Kv channels share a common topology including intracellular N- and C-termini, six transmembrane domains (S1-S6) with S4 being the positively charged voltage-sensor, and a pore or P-loop between S5 and S6 responsible for ion selectivity (Fig. 1A). Based on their sequence homology and their ability to form heterotetrameric proteins, Kv channels have been divided into subfamilies Kv1-Kv10. Several of these Kv channels have been shown to be present in myelinated nerve fibers. Structural and biophysical studies have begun to elucidate the underlying mechanisms responsible for the selectivity and high rate of ion flux through K$^+$ channels (for a recent review see MacKinnon, 2003).

A. K$^+$ Channels Are Multisubunit Protein Complexes

Kv channels are multisubunit protein complexes. The main pore-forming complex consists of a tetramer of α subunits. Often, Kv channels also have accessory subunits. For example, the Kv1 channels consist of four membrane-spanning and pore-forming α subunits and up to four cytoplasmic β subunits (Isacoff et al., 1990; Rhodes et al., 1997). In heterologous cells, Kv1 α and β subunits have been shown to heteromultimerize promiscuously, resulting in channels with biophysically and pharmacologically distinct properties (Ruppersberg et al., 1990; Hopkins et al., 1994; Rettig et al., 1994; Shamotienko et al., 1997). For example, homotetrameric channels consisting of Kv1.1 or Kv1.2 encode channels that give rise to slow, noninactivating outward rectifiers (Fig. 1B). In contrast, channels consisting of only Kv1.4 α subunits encode a fast transient (A-type) channel. When these Kv1 α subunits are co-expressed, channels with

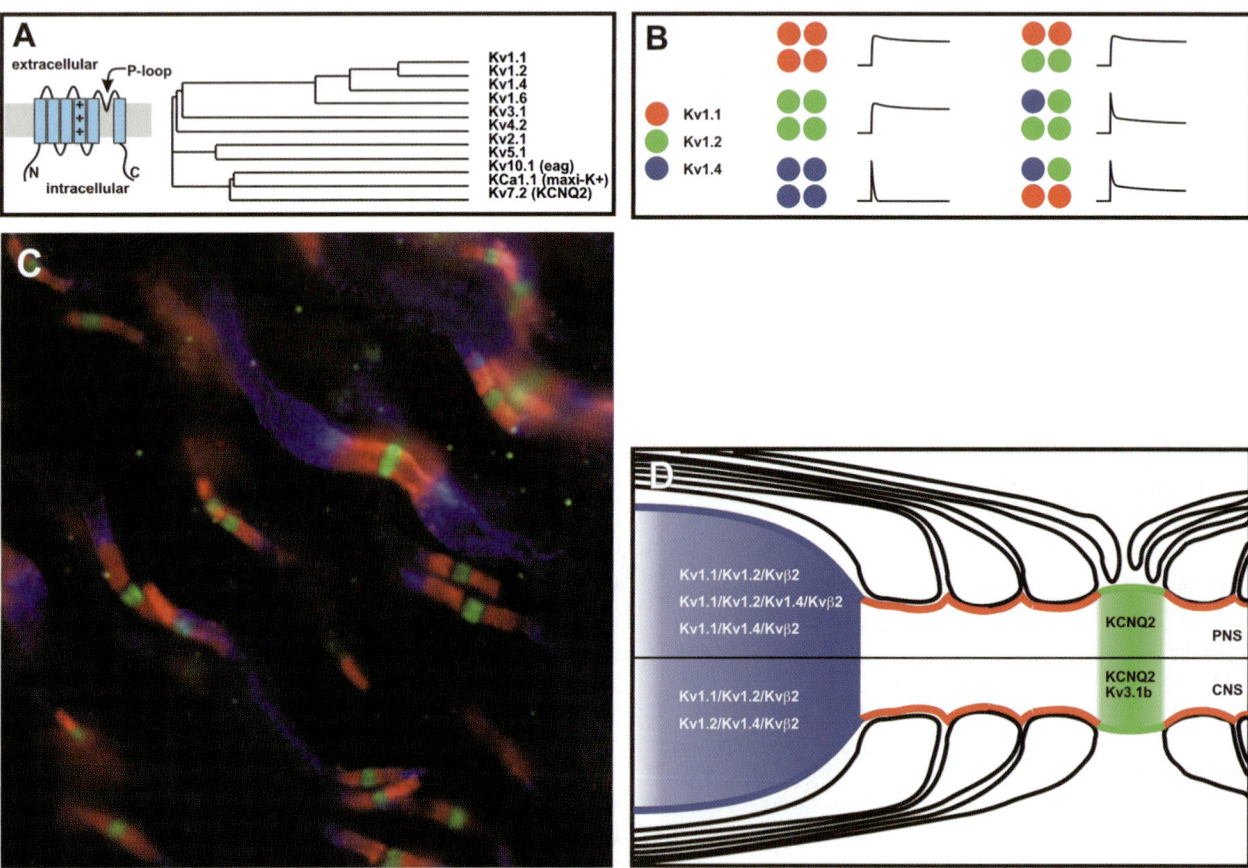

Figure 1 Voltage-dependent K$^+$ (Kv) channels are localized at and near nodes of Ranvier. (**A**) The Kv channels make up a large family of homologous proteins (dendrogram created using ClustalW). Kv channel subunits are topologically similar with intracellular N- and C-termini, a positively charged transmembrane segment, and a K$^+$ selective pore (P-loop). (**B**) Heteromultimerization of Kv1 channels results in channels with properties intermediate to those of homomultimeric channels. For example, addition of Kv1.4 into a channel containing Kv1.1 and/or Kv1.2 converts the channel from noninactivating to inactivating. (**C**) A rat optic nerve triple-labeled for Kv1.2 (*blue*), Caspr (*red*), and Nav channels (*green*), which label juxtaparanodes, paranodes, and nodes, respectively. (Reprinted with permission from Rasband and Shrager, 2000, copyright 2000 by the *Journal of Physiology*.) (**D**) Kv channels and their localization in myelinated nerve fibers.

intermediate biophysical properties result (e.g., inclusion of a Kv1.4 α subunit can convert channels with Kv1.1 or Kv1.2 subunits to inactivating channels with transient currents (Ruppersberg et al., 1990; Fig. 1B).

Kv channel subunits also heteromultimerize in vivo to form K+ channels. This conclusion is based on a variety of data including co-immunoprecipitation, co-purification via column chromatography, and co-localization (Sheng et al., 1993; Wang et al., 1993; Rhodes et al., 1995). For example, Kv4.2 and Kv4.3 subunits have been shown to form functional heteromultimers in mammalian heart (Guo et al., 2002), whereas Kv3.1 and Kv3.2 form heteromultimeric channels in neurons of the globus pallidus (Hernandez-Pineda et al., 1999). Since Kv1α subunits are expressed widely throughout the nervous system (Monaghan et al., 2001), the heteromultimerization of subunits could, in principle, result in the expression of an enormous number of Kv channels with different properties. However, co-immuno-precipitation experiments have shown that only a relatively small number of subunit combinations can be detected (Rhodes et al., 1997; Shamotienko et al., 1997).

In addition to altering the biophysical properties of channels, recent experiments have shown that the kinds of Kv1 α subunits present in a channel can dramatically influence the surface expression of the channel, and that these properties are regulated by a retention signal localized to the channel pore (Manganas and Trimmer, 2000; Manganas et al., 2001; Zhu et al., 2001, 2003). Thus, excitable cells may modulate K+ currents through regulating the kinds of subunits expressed in a channel complex, which in turn regulates both the biophysical properties of the channels and their surface expression.

III. The Repertoire and Localization of K+ Channels in Myelinated Axons

A variety of Kv currents have been described in myelinated nerve fibers (Roper and Schwarz, 1989; Safronov et al., 1993). However, the precise localization and the molecular correlates that underlie these currents have only recently been elucidated through the use of subtype specific Kv channel antibodies. This work has shown that various channel types and combinations are found clustered in discrete domains at and near nodes of Ranvier.

Nodes of Ranvier have three well-defined functional and spatial domains. These are (1) the node, (2) the paranode, and (3) the juxtaparanode. The node itself is the site where voltage-gated Na+ (Nav) channels are found clustered in high densities to support the inward Na+ currents responsible for generation and conduction of the action potential (Fig. 1C, green). The paranode is the site where the myelin sheath terminates in cytoplasm rich axoglial junctions that closely abut the axolemma (Fig. 1C, red). Although the paranode usually

does not contain Kv channels, the cellular and molecular interactions responsible for formation and maintenance of the paranode are thought to be important to restrict channels to specific regions (see later; Poliak and Peles, 2003; Salzer, 2003). Finally, the juxtaparanode is a region just inside the innermost axoglial junction, entirely covered by compact myelin, that extends into the internode (Fig. 1C, blue). Both nodal and juxtaparanodal domains have been shown to possess a unique set of Kv channels (Fig. 1D).

A. Nodal K+ Channels

The molecular identities of several nodal K+ channels were identified by Devaux et al., (2003, 2004). The first to be described was Kv3.1b, the major splice variant of Kv3.1 found in brain (Perney et al., 1992). Interestingly, Kv3.1b is expressed mainly in the central nervous system (CNS), but only in a subset of nodes. For example, in the lateral and ventral columns nearly every node of Ranvier has Kv3.1b, however, in the corticospinal tract relatively few nodes have Kv3.1b. Furthermore, the presence of Kv3.1b in nodes appears to correlate with increasing fiber diameter. The significance of these differences is unknown. Several investigators showed previously that the K+ channel blocker 4-aminopyridine (4-AP) increases the amplitude and broadens the action potential of myelinated fibers in the adult CNS, but not peripheral nervous system (PNS) (Gordon et al., 1988, 1989; Rasband et al., 1998, 1999). These results suggest the existence of a nodal 4-AP-sensitive K+ channel restricted to the CNS. Since Kv3.1 is relatively sensitive to block by 4-AP (Kirsch and Drewe, 1993) but is very rare in the PNS, it is an ideal candidate channel to explain the earlier electrophysiological results. However, recordings of compound action potentials from Kv3.1-null mice in the presence or absence of 4-AP show no difference from WT mice (Devaux et al., 2003). As a result, additional experiments are needed to determine the function of Kv3.1b in CNS nodes and whether the properties of the action potential in Kv3.1-null mice are due to some other 4-AP-sensitive nodal Kv channel (e.g., Kv3.3), either through compensatory upregulation or heterotetrameric channels that in WT animals consist of both Kv3.1b and another Kv3 subunit.

In addition to Kv3.1b, the channel subunit KCNQ2 (also known as Kv7.2) is clustered in high densities at nodes of Ranvier (Devaux et al., 2004). In contrast to Kv3.1b, however, KCNQ2 appears to be ubiquitous throughout the CNS and PNS. Furthermore, KCNQ2 is present at axon initial segments, whereas Kv3.1b cannot be detected at these sites. As for Nav channels, KCNQ2 forms high density clusters in the nodal gap, and is part of a larger macromolecular complex including ankyrin$_G$, a cytoskeletal scaffolding protein thought to link nodal membrane proteins to the actin/spectrin based cytoskeleton (Kordeli et al., 1995). This channel is particularly interesting, as mutations in KCNQ2 have been shown to cause a variety of pathological states, including neonatal epilepsy and myokymia. Application of the KCNQ2 agonist retigabine reduces axonal excitability, while the antagonist linopirdine has little effect on the action potential in adult animals (Devaux et al., 2004). However, linopirdine increased both the amplitude and duration of the action potential in immature, myelinating nerve fibers. These studies suggest that KCNQ2 forms functional channels at nodes of Ranvier and that these channels contribute to the electrical properties of the axon. However, the contribution may be more significant during periods of myelination than in normal mature myelinated nerve fibers, a fact that may prove important for demyelinated and remyelinating axons, as these states recapitulate many aspects of developmental myelination.

B. Juxtaparanodal K⁺ Channels

The first Kv channel subunits to be identified in mammalian myelinated nerves were Kv1.1 and Kv1.2. As such, they are also the channels in myelinated fibers that have been most extensively studied. The most surprising thing about these ion channels is that they are restricted to axolemma beneath the myelin sheath and flanking each node of Ranvier (Figs. 1C and 1D, blue). As a result, the function of these channels is not immediately obvious. It is clear, however, that loss of the myelin sheath exposes this large pool of channels and radically alters the active, voltage-dependent properties of the axon (see later), above and beyond the already dramatic consequences that the loss of the myelin sheath has on the passive electrical properties of the axon.

Based on co-immunoprecipitation and co-localization experiments, juxtaparanodal channels are thought to consist of both Kv1 α and β subunits. Specifically, these experiments suggest that these complexes consist of Kv1.1/1.2/Kvβ2, Kv1.1/1.4/Kvβ2, Kv1.2/Kv1.4/Kvβ2, and Kv1.1/1.2/1.4/Kvβ2 heteromultimers (Fig. 1D; Wang et al., 1993; Rasband et al., 1999, 2001). For example, immunolabeling optic nerve using Kv1 channel subunit specific antibodies shows that Kv1.1 and Kv1.2 co-localize at nearly every juxtaparanode (Fig. 2A, overlap is yellow). In contrast, relatively few juxtaparanodes have Kv1.4 that co-localizes with Kv1.2 (Fig. 2B, arrow). While it is clear that most juxtaparanodes express a combination of Kv1 channel subunits in varying amounts (Rasband et al., 1998), the significance of the different levels of subunit expression in distinct fibers is unknown. It is possible that these differences reflect unique requirements for membrane excitability and function, and the addition of Kv1.4 α subunits would be predicted to noticeably alter the K⁺ currents within a myelinated fiber. Alternatively, given the fact that subunit composition can affect the surface expression of channels, the addition of Kv1.4 would be predicted to promote surface

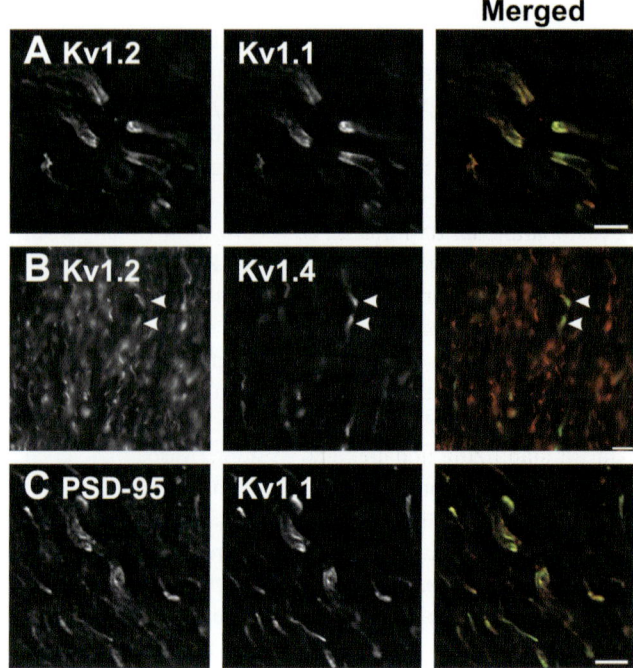

Figure 2 Heteromultimeric, juxtaparanodal Kv channels are part of a larger protein complex. (**A**) Kv1.1 (*green*) and Kv1.2 (*red*) co-localize at juxtaparanodes (*overlap is yellow*) of optic nerve axons. There is a pronounced gap in immunoreactivity corresponding to the paranodal and nodal domains. Note that immunoreactivity is most intense adjacent to the paranodal zone and decreases towards internodal regions. (**B**) In the optic nerve, Kv1.4 (*green*) co-localizes with a minority of the Kv1.2 (*red*) labeled juxtaparanodes (*arrowhead*). (**C**) PSD-95 (*red*) is present at juxtaparanodes, co-localizes with Kv1 channels (*green*), and is part of the juxtaparanodal Kv channel protein complex. Scalebars: (**A–C**) = 10 μm.

expression of heteromultimers containing this subunit (Manganas et al., 2001).

The cytoplasmic Kvβ subunits of Kv1 channels associate with α subunits during early channel biosynthesis and are thought to promote channel surface expression (Shi et al., 1996). Juxtaparanodal Kv1 channel complexes include Kvβ2 subunits, although other Kvβ subunits associate with Kv1 channels at various locations throughout the nervous system (Rhodes et al., 1997; Rasband et al., 1998). The crystal structure of the Kvβ subunit has shown that there is significant structural similarity to aldo-keto reductases, including the conservation of key catalytic and cofactor binding sites (Gulbis et al., 1999). However, mutation of the catalytic site has no effect on the intracellular trafficking of channels, suggesting that any role for the enzymatic activity of the Kvβ-subunit likely lies outside of its function in promoting the surface expression of channels (Campomanes et al., 2002). It is somewhat surprising, then, that mice lacking Kvβ2 apparently have no change in either the surface expression of Kv1 channels, or in the localization of channels to juxtaparanodes (McCormack et al., 2002). However, whether other kinds of Kvβ subunits compensate for the lack of Kvβ2 has not been addressed. Furthermore, these results are unable to account for the fact that Kvβ2-null mice have seizures, reduced life span, and cold-swim induced tremors, a phenotype that is quite similar to that observed for Kv1.1-deficient mice (Zhou et al., 1998b). Thus, additional experiments will be needed to determine the consequence of the Kvβ2 deletion and its precise role with respect to juxtaparanodal Kv1 channels.

As shown in Fig. 1C, Kv1 channels (blue) are localized to very discrete domains and do not overlap with paranodal proteins. This high degree of regulation in channel localization implies that these channels play an important role in nervous system function. However, while the role of these channels during early development suggests they are important for stabilizing nodal excitability (Vabnick et al., 1999), their function in normal adult myelinated fibers remains an enigma. An in-depth discussion of the normal function of these juxtaparanodal channels is provided by Chiu (see Chapter 5); the function of these channels subsequent to demyelination and during remyelination is discussed later.

1. Juxtaparanodal K⁺ Channels Are Part of a Larger Protein Complex

Besides Kv1 α and β subunits, other proteins have now been recognized at juxtaparanodes. Together with Kv1 channels, these form a large protein complex consisting of cell adhesion molecules, cytoskeletal, and scaffolding proteins. The first component of juxtaparanodes, besides K⁺ channel subunits, was identified by Poliak et al. (1999) and named Caspr2 based on its similarity to the paranodal axoglial junction component contactin-associated protein (Caspr; also known as paranodin or NCP1; Einheber et al., 1997; Menegoz et al., 1997; Peles et al., 1997). Caspr2 is a 180 kD cell adhesion molecule clustered at juxtaparanodes. That it interacts with the Kv1 channel was demonstrated through the reciprocal co-immunoprecipitation of Kv1 α and β subunits and Caspr2 (Poliak et al., 1999). Despite being in the same protein complex, the interaction between Kv1 channels and Caspr2 is likely indirect, because mutation of the C-terminal PDZ (*PSD-95, d*iscs-large, *z*onula occludens) binding motifs of either Kv1 channels or Caspr2 abolishes their interaction (Poliak et al., 1999). Caspr2 deficient mice have a dramatic reduction in juxtaparanodal clustering of channels, without an overall reduction in the total number of channels (Poliak et al., 2003). These results indicate that Caspr2 is required for the localization and/or maintenance of Kv1 channels at juxtaparanodes.

When Caspr2 was first identified, it was proposed to be involved in the localization of Kv1 channels to juxtaparanodes through interaction with a glial binding partner (Poliak et al., 1999). This hypothesis is based, in part, on the fact that dysmyelination, hypomyelination, and demyelination result in the loss of clustered Kv1 channels (Wang et al., 1995; Rasband et al., 1998; Baba et al., 1999). Caspr2's binding partner has now been identified as the glyco-sylphosphatidyl-inositol (GPI) anchored Transient Axonal Glycoprotein, or TAG-1. While other functions unrelated to myelinated nerve fibers have been ascribed to this molecule (Furley et al., 1990), TAG-1 is also present at juxtaparanodes and is expressed by myelinating glia (Traka et al., 2002). More recently, both Poliak et al. (2003) and Traka et al. (2003) have shown that TAG-1 and Caspr2 form a protein complex in the brain, as they can reciprocally co-immunoprecipitate one another. The molecular basis of this interaction was determined by transfecting COS-7 cells with Caspr2 or TAG-1, or co-transfecting cells with both TAG-1 and Caspr2. In these transfected cells, TAG-1 Fc fusion proteins bound only to cells transfected with TAG-1 or TAG-1 and Caspr2 (Poliak et al., 2003; Traka et al., 2003). Together, these results indicate that the interaction between axonal Caspr2 and glial TAG-1 is not direct, but requires the *cis*-interaction of Caspr2 and TAG-1 in the same membrane. Thus, axonal *cis*-interacting TAG-1 and Caspr2 bind in *trans* with glial TAG-1. The significance of this interaction for juxtaparanodal Kv1 channel localization was shown in TAG-1-null mice as these animals have a phenotype identical to the Caspr2-null mouse: reduced juxtaparanodal Kv1 channels without any reduction in Kv1 channel subunit protein levels (Poliak et al., 2003; Traka et al., 2003). Since TAG-1 is mislocalized in Caspr2-null mice, a reciprocal interaction must organize the glial juxtaparanodal domains. Together, these results suggest that neuroglial interactions regulate the reciprocal subcellular differentiation of juxtaparanodal axolemma and myelin membrane.

An important component of the juxtaparanodal protein complex not yet identified is a protein linking Kv1 channels and the Caspr2/TAG-1 complex. This protein likely consists of multiple PDZ domains, as mutation of the PDZ binding motifs in either Caspr2 or Kv1 channel subunits abolishes their interaction (Poliak et al., 1999). Multi-PDZ-domain scaffolding proteins, such as PSD-95 have been shown to cluster Kv1 channels in vitro (Kim et al., 1995). As a result, it is reasonable to postulate that this type of protein might link and cluster Kv1 channels and Caspr2. Indeed PSD-95 is present at juxtaparanodes (Fig. 2C, the co-localization of Kv1.1 and PSD-95 appears yellow) and forms a macromolecular protein complex with Kv1 channels as demonstrated by co-immunoprecipitation (Rasband et al., 2002; Menon et al., 2003). Surprisingly, however, loss of PSD-95 from juxtaparanodes disrupts neither the localization of Kv1 channels and Caspr2 nor their biochemical interaction (Rasband et al., 2002). Although PSD-95 is present at juxtaparanodes, either its function lies outside of mediating the interaction between Caspr2 and Kv1 channels or there is another multi-PDZ domain protein that can link Caspr2 and Kv1 channel subunits and fully compensate for loss of PSD-95.

Membrane proteins are often anchored to the cytoskeleton through adaptor and/or scaffolding proteins. Both Caspr and Caspr2 have an intracellular, c-terminal motif similar to the erythrocyte protein 4.1 binding motif found in gly-cophorin C (Denisenko-Nehrbass et al., 2003). Among the 4.1 proteins, type II or 4.1B has been described at both para-nodes and juxtaparanodes (Ohara et al., 2000; Poliak et al., 2001). Pull-down assays have shown that 4.1B binds the intracellular GNP (glycophorin C, Neurexin, Paranodin/ Caspr) motif of both Caspr and Caspr2 (Denisenko-Nehrbass et al., 2003). During development 4.1B is detected at both paranodes and juxtaparanodes, but is detected at these sites after Caspr and Caspr2, suggesting that the pri-mary role for 4.1B may be to anchor and maintain Kv1 channel/Caspr2 protein complexes in their respective domains rather than initiating clustering.

Besides TAG-1, the only other glial juxtaparanodal pro-tein to have been described is Connexin29 (Cx29; Altevogt et al., 2002). Cx29 is expressed in myelinating glia and co-localizes with Kv1 channels at juxtaparanodes in the PNS and in small diameter myelinated fibers in the CNS. However, no adjacent axolemmal Connexin has been found, bringing into question whether Cx29 forms functional gap junctions at these sites. Thus, the role(s) of Cx29 at juxta-paranodes is unknown, although Altevogt et al. (2002) spec-ulate that Cx29 may form functional hemichannels involved in the removal of K^+ from the periaxonal space.

Finally, one other protein has been reported to be present in the juxtaparanodal K^+ channel protein complex. Recently, Nie et al. (2003) reported that oligodendroglial Nogo-A, Caspr, and Kv1 channels reciprocally co-precipitated each other from brain membranes and transfected cells (suggest-ing that these proteins form a complex and that Caspr and Kv1 channels interact directly). It was also reported that in adult animals Nogo-A is present in paranodal domains (Nie et al., 2003). These results are surprising since Kv1 channels are normally excluded from paranodal domains. Subsequent experiments attempting to repeat these controversial results have not met with success (Rasband, 2004). Thus, while Nogo-A appears to be localized at paranodes in adult ani-mals, more experiments are needed to determine whether a macromolecular protein complex exists that includes both paranodal and juxtaparanodal components.

2. Cellular Mechanisms of Juxtaparanodal K^+ Channel Localization

As described previously, a variety of proteins (most notably cell adhesion molecules) interact with and partici-pate in the localization of juxtaparanodal Kv1 channels. This fact is clearly demonstrated in Caspr2 and TAG-1 defi-cient mice where Kv1 channels are no longer clustered in their appropriate domains (Poliak et al., 2003; Traka et al., 2003). In addition to these molecular interactions, cellular mechanisms also play important roles in organizing and restricting the localization of Kv1 channels. In particular, axoglial junctions participate in channel localization. The idea that sites of axoglial contact regulate the localization of channels was first suggested after careful analysis of myeli-

nated nerve fibers by freeze-fracture and electron micro-scopic methods. These studies showed a high density of intramembranous particles confined to regions between adjacent axoglial junctions (Rosenbluth, 1988). Later, using immunofluorescence methods, it was found that during development Kv1 channels were often present in distinct bands that were oriented parallel to the direction of axoglial junctions. Double-immunostaining using markers for para-nodal junctions showed that the Kv1 channel bands were confined between axoglial junctions (Rasband et al., 1999; Vabnick et al., 1999). A careful analysis of the internodal localization of Caspr and Kv1 channels in the PNS showed that a thin strand of Caspr runs adjacent to the inner mesaxon and is flanked on each side by a double strand of Kv1 channels (Arroyo et al., 1999). Together, these results point to a role for myelinating glial cells as primary deter-minants of channel localization.

The conclusion that axoglial junctions restrict the lateral diffusion of Kv1 channels in the axolemma and confine them to juxtaparanodal domains has been confirmed by sev-eral important studies examining mutant animals with altered paranodal junctions. For example, mice lacking para-nodal components such as Caspr (Bhat et al., 2001) or con-tactin (Boyle et al., 2001), or lacking key myelin galactolipids such as Galc and sulfatide (Dupree et al., 1998, 1999) or sulfatide alone (Ishibashi et al., 2002), do not have the transverse bands that are a hallmark of mature, well-defined axoglial junctions. These mice all have conduction deficits, tremors, reduced densities of Nav channels at nodes of Ranvier, and in many cases everted paranodal loops that point away from the axolemma. In these animals, there is a dramatic redistribution and invasion of Kv1 channels from the juxtaparanode into the paranode. Together, these results show that paranodal junctions are essential to restrict Kv1 channels to juxtaparanodes and that these junctions provide a diffusion barrier within the axonal membrane.

In contrast to the juxtaparanodal Kv1 channels, we do not yet have any information about the cellular or molecular mech-anisms of either Kv3.1b or KCNQ2 channel trafficking, tar-geting, and clustering at nodes of Ranvier. Since both Kv3.1b and KCNQ2 can co-immunoprecipitate ankyrin$_G$ (Devaux et al., 2003, 2004), and ankyrin$_G$ is thought to be a primary determinant of Nav channel clustering (Zhou et al., 1998a), the mechanisms of nodal ion channel localization and clustering may be common for KCNQ2, Kv3.1b, and Nav channels.

IV. K⁺ Channel Organization and Function in Demyelinated and Remyelinating Axons

Although the function of juxtaparanodal Kv1 channels in normal myelinated nerve fibers is not well understood, sev-eral lines of evidence suggest that disruption or loss of the myelin sheath can dramatically alter the conduction properties of an axon and reduce excitability. In some instances, this disruption appears to be almost entirely a consequence of aberrant localization and expression of Kv1 channels, as the use of Kv1 channel blockers can restore conduction (Bostock et al., 1981; Targ and Kocsis, 1985, 1986; Rasband et al., 1998; Nashmi et al., 2000). The consequences of demyelination and or myelin disruption for the localization and expression of Kv1 channels has been investigated mainly in two separate kinds of model systems: (1) experimentally demyelinated axons and (2) dysmyelinating, hypomyelinating, or demyelinating mutant mice. The evidence that Kv1 channels are important contributors to axonal dysfunction in each of these experimental paradigms is described next.

A. Kv1 Channel Localization and Function in Demyelinated and Remyelinating Axons

Kv1 channel localization after demyelination and during remyelination was described using the lysolecithin model of peripheral demyelination (Rasband et al., 1998). In these experiments, lysolecithin was injected directly into the sciatic nerve, resulting in activation of macrophages, and the disruption and eventual phagocytosis of myelin. In this model, complete, focal demyelination occurs at the site of injection within about 1 week. After demyelination, Schwann cells proliferate and are able to remyelinate the injured region. However, the structure of remyelinated axons is different than before the drug injection: there are fewer layers of myelin, and the internodal length is decreased to about one-fourth the length found in uninjured animals. As a result, new nodes of Ranvier form in regions that were formerly internodal with low densities of ion channels. Finally, it is relatively easy to isolate the sciatic nerve and record action potentials in the demyelinated/remyelinating nerve. Thus, this model provides an excellent system in which to examine the localization and relative contribution of ion channels to nervous system dysfunction after disease or injury. This model has also been used to study the mechanisms of Nav channel localization after demyelination and during remyelination (Dugandzija-Novakovic et al., 1995). An indepth discussion of Na$^+$ channel clustering during remyelination is given by Shrager et al. (see Chapter 8).

One week after injection of lysolecithin myelin is cleared from the injected site, and broad regions of denuded axons are apparent. Double-immunostaining with antibodies against Kv1.1 and Nav channels reveals former nodal sites, as these can be easily distinguished based on the presence of a focal Nav channel cluster (Fig. 3A,B, arrowheads). In constrast, Kv1 channels were not retained at juxtaparanodes, but instead were very labile in the axolemma and were able to diffuse into formerly paranodal and internodal zones. A quantitative analysis of this dispersion showed that 6 days after injection, 60% of nodal regions had some detectable Kv1 channel immunoreactivity. Just 1 day later, however,

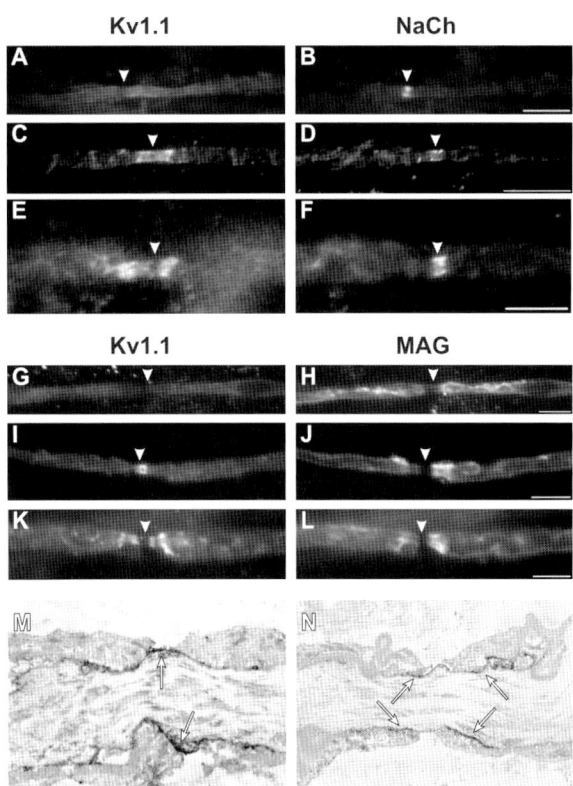

Figure 3 Kv1 channel localization in demyelinated and remyelinating rat sciatic nerve fibers. Demyelinated and remyelinating nerve fibers double-labeled for Kv1.1 (**A, C, E, G, I, K**) and Nav channels (**B, D, F**) or the myelin associated glycoprotein (MAG; **H, J, L**). 6 days postinjection (**A, B**), 9 days postinjection (**G, H**), 18 days postinjection (**C, D, I, J**), and 24 days postinjection (**E, F, K, L**). (**M, N**) Immunoelectron microscopy showing Kv1.1 in nodal (**M**) and paranodal (**N**) regions at 19 and 27 days postinjection, respectively. Scalebars: **A–H** = 25 μm; **I–L** = 12 μm. (Figure modified from Rasband et al. 1998, copyright 1998 by the Society for Neuroscience.)

immunoreactivity was reduced to only 20% of sites. These results suggest that either Kv1 channels are rapidly internalized on demyelination, or that they are able to freely diffuse in the axolemma in the absence of an overlying myelin sheath. Since Caspr2 and TAG-1 deficient mice have dramatically reduced amounts of juxtaparanodal channels, but no decrease in the total numbers of channels (Poliak et al., 2003; Traka et al., 2003), it is more likely that in the absence of myelin, the juxtaparanodal K$^+$ channel complex is unable to interact with glial TAG-1 and remain restricted to the juxtaparanode.

At the start of the second week after injection (7 to 9 days after injection) Schwann cells associate with axons, extend processes, and begin to remyelinate damaged regions. Although Nav channels can be detected at the edges of these extending Schwann cell processes (Dugandzija-Novakovic et al., 1995), Kv1 channels are undetectable and do not accumulate at these sites. For example, Figs. 3G and 3H show a remyelinating nerve fiber double-labeled for Kv1.1 (Fig. 3G) and the myelin-associated glycoprotein (MAG, a marker of early myelination; Fig. 3H). This figure shows that newly forming nodes of Ranvier (arrowhead) are devoid of any Kv1 channel immunoreactivity.

Although initially new nodes of Ranvier lack Kv1 channels, they rapidly acquire a high density as remyelination progresses. These Kv1 channels co-localize with nodal Nav channels (Figs. 3C, D, arrowheads) and are restricted to the gap between adjacent MAG-labeled, myelinating Schwann cells (Figs. 3I, J, arrowheads). By the end of the third week after injection, as many as 60% of nodal sites have Kv1 channel immunoreactivity. This result is surprising and significant, as it suggests that although remyelination may occur with appropriate Nav channel clustering, the aberrant localization of Kv1 channels may position them in a region where they can block normal conduction. Further, this result suggests that in contrast to Nav channels clustered at new nodes of Ranvier (which derive from a preexisting pool of axolemmal channels [Tzoumaka et al., 1995]), the Kv1 channels are manufactured de novo and inserted at nascent nodes of Ranvier. The nodal localization of these channels has been confirmed by immunoelectron microscopy: Fig. 3M shows a new node of Ranvier with a dense, dark precipitate at the node (arrows).

At the start of the fourth week after lysolecithin injection, the formerly nodal Kv1 channels begin to redistribute into paranodal and finally their normal, juxtaparanodal zones. Figures 3E and F show the initial stage where these Kv1 channels begin to split and become restricted beneath the myelin sheath. Interestingly, the split occurs precisely at the site where Nav channels are clustered at the highest density (Figs. 3E, F, arrowhead). Double-immunostaining with anti-MAG shows that the point where Kv1 channels begin to be removed from the node corresponds to the edges of MAG immunoreactivity (compare Figs. 3K and L, arrowhead), suggesting that

myelin sheath may actively participate in determining the localization of Kv1 channels. Immunoelectron microscopy of remyelinating sciatic nerve fibers shows the redistribution of Kv1 channels into paranodal and juxtaparanodal domains (Fig. 3N, arrows).

The results described here indicate that demyelination and the lack of glial binding partners, possibly TAG-1, results in the redistribution of Kv1 channel proteins throughout the axolemma due to the latter's intrinsic mobility within the membrane. Remyelination also initiates the clustering of Nav channels (Dugandzija-Novakovic et al., 1995) at the edges of elongating processes. As new nodes form and are defined, newly synthesized Kv1 channels are inserted at nascent nodes by mechanisms that remain unknown. At this stage of remyelination, Kv1 channels are transient in their localization to nodes of Ranvier; they soon become sequestered beneath the myelin sheath in paranodal and juxtaparanodal domains. Of importance, if remyelination is delayed by addition of the mitotic inhibitor mitomycin-C, Schwann cells do not proliferate, axons remain unmyelinated, and channels fail to cluster. Although there is an apparent increase in the amount of Kv1 channels in these demyelinated axons at 3 to 4 weeks after lysolecithin injection, the channels remain diffusely distributed throughout the axolemma. Under these conditions, remyelination eventually occurs and Kv1 channels eventually become localized first at nodal, then juxtaparanodal domains (Rasband et al., 1998).

Significantly, the localization of Kv1 channels during remyelination closely parallels the degree of pathophysiology and sensitivity to K+ channel blockers such as 4-AP. Thus, before demyelination and when Kv1 channels are sequestered beneath the myelin sheath in juxtaparanodal

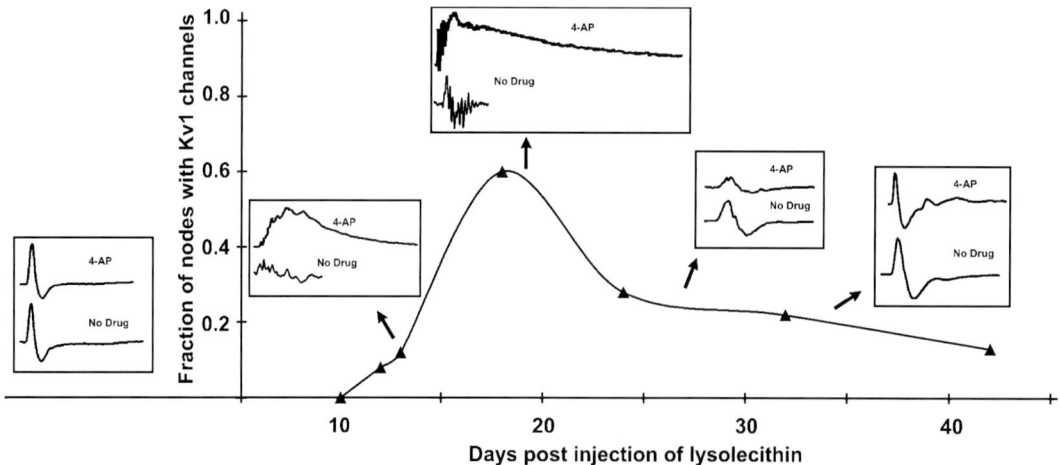

Figure 4 The sensitivity of remyelinating nerve fibers to 4-aminopyridine (4-AP) correlates closely with the fraction of nodes that have Kv1 channels. Kv1 channels are transiently detected at nodes of Ranvier with a peak at about 18 days postinjection. Boxed insets show, for the times after lysolecithin injection indicated, compound action potentials before and after exposure to 1 mM 4-AP. The boxed inset on the left shows compound action potentials from noninjected, control sciatic nerves before and after exposure to 1 mM 4-AP. (Figure modified from Rasband et al., 1998, copyright 1998 by the Society for Neuroscience.)

domains, peripheral myelinated nerve fibers are insensitive to 4-AP (Fig. 4). However, 2 weeks after demyelination these fibers become sensitive to 4-AP. The most dramatic effects of 4-AP occur when the majority of new nodes have Kv1 channels. Addition of 4-AP at these times significantly increased both the amplitude and duration of the action potential. It is important to note that at this stage of remyelination axons are well-wrapped, and there are significant densities of nodal Nav channels, suggesting that the pathophysiology is a consequence of the misplaced Kv1 channels rather than too little myelin or too few nodal Nav channels. As Kv1 channels become sequestered beneath the myelin sheath, the sensitivity to 4-AP decreased (Fig. 4A). Taken together, these results suggest that subsequent to demyelination and during remyelination, axolemmal Kv1 channels are exposed, aberrantly localized to nodes of Ranvier, and block conduction by their activity at these sites.

B. K+ Channel Localization and Function in Dysmyelinating Mutant Mice

Most studies examining Kv1 channel localization in the CNS when myelin is damaged or lost have used hypomyelinating and dysmyelinating mutant mice. Unfortunately, these studies have been confined mostly to a descriptive analysis of channel localization and expression levels rather than a description of Kv1 channel function. Nevertheless, several important insights have been gained from these studies. For example, Wang et al. (1995) showed that there was a large increase in Kv1.1 and Kv1.2 subunit expression in the hypomyelinating Shiverer mutant mouse. In this same mouse model, the localization of Kv1 channels in optic nerve is dramatically disrupted (Rasband et al., 1999), with a significant reduction in the clustering of Kv1.1 and Kv1.2 at juxtaparanodes. Together these studies have pointed to a role for myelin in regulating both the expression levels and the localization of juxtaparanodal Kv1 channels.

Although instructive, Shiverer and other dysmyelinating and hypomyelinating mutants as models for demyelination are not ideal, as the redistribution and misexpression of Kv1 channels may be a consequence of developmental defects rather than demyelination per se. In an effort to more closely approximate adult onset, chronic demyelination, as in multiple sclerosis, Baba et al. (1999) examined Kv1 channel localization and expression in a transgenic animal that has two extra copies of the proteolipid protein gene (Plp; Kagawa et al., 1994). This mouse undergoes spontaneous, adult-onset demyelination beginning at about 3 months of age, with full demyelination by 7 months of age (Inoue et al., 1996). In these animals, demyelination is not accompanied by either inflammation or axon degeneration. However, Kv1 channels are no longer restricted to juxtaparanodal domains. Further, the expression levels of these channels remained constant in both demyelinated optic nerves and spinal cord, suggesting that the loss of the myelin sheath did not result in an upregulation of channels but rather that the sheath is required for maintenance of the normal localization of the channels.

V. Conclusion

A variety of Kv channels are expressed in myelinated nerve fibers. Those present at nodes of Ranvier have only recently been described, and the consequences of demyelination for both expression and localization of these channels are unknown. In contrast, much more is known about the function and role of juxtaparanodal Kv1 channels, as these have been examined during development, in transgenic knockouts of Kv1 channel proteins, and in a variety of demyelinating models. Together, these studies all point to axonal Kv1 channels as important modulators of nervous system function after demyelination. Furthermore, it is clear that there exists a dynamic interaction between axons and myelinating glia that regulates the localization and density of channels in specific regions. Current and future therapies designed to block Kv1 channels or induce a redistribution of Kv1 channels to regions where they do not affect conduction may prove to be useful in treating demyelinating diseases.

References

Altevogt, B. M., Kleopa, K. A., Postma, F. R., Scherer, S. S., and Paul, D. L. (2002). Connexin29 is uniquely distributed within myelinating glial cells of the central and peripheral nervous systems. *J. Neurosci.* **22,** 6458–6470.

Arroyo, E. J., Xu, Y. T., Zhou, L., Messing, A., Peles, E., Chiu, S. Y., and Scherer, S. S. (1999). Myelinating Schwann cells determine the internodal localization of Kv1.1, Kv1.2, Kvbeta2, and Caspr. *J. Neurocytol.* **28,** 333–347.

Baba, H., Akita, H., Ishibashi, T., Inoue, Y., Nakahira, K., and Ikenaka, K. (1999). Completion of myelin compaction, but not the attachment of oligodendroglial processes triggers K+ channel clustering. *J. Neurosci. Res.* **58,** 752–764.

Bhat, M. A., Rios, J. C., Lu, Y., Garcia-Fresco, G. P., Ching, W., St. Martin, M., Li, J., Einheber, S., Chesler, M., Rosenbluth, J., Salzer, J. L., and Bellen, H. J. (2001). Axon-glia interactions and the domain organization of myelinated axons requires neurexin IV/Caspr/Paranodin. *Neuron* **30,** 369–383.

Bostock, H., Sears, T. A., and Sherratt, R. M. (1981). The effects of 4-aminopyridine and tetraethylammonium ions on normal and demyelinated mammalian nerve fibres. *J. Physiol.* **313,** 301–315.

Boyle, M. E., Berglund, E. O., Murai, K. K., Weber, L., Peles, E. and Ranscht, B. (2001). Contactin orchestrates assembly of the septate-like junctions at the paranode in myelinated peripheral nerve. *Neuron* **30,** 385–397.

Campomanes, C. R., Carroll, K. I., Manganas, L. N., Hershberger, M. E., Gong, B., Antonucci, D. E., Rhodes, K. J., and Trimmer J. S. (2002). Kv beta subunit oxidoreductase activity and Kv1 potassium channel trafficking. *J. Biol. Chem.* **277,** 8298–8305.

Denisenko-Nehrbass, N., Oguievetskaia, K., Goutebroze, L., Galvez, T., Yamakawa, H., Ohara, O., Carnaud, M., and Girault, J. A. (2003). Protein

4.1B associates with both Caspr/paranodin and Caspr2 at paranodes and juxtaparanodes of myelinated fibres. *Eur. J. Neurosci.* **17,** 411–416.

Devaux, J., Alcaraz, G., Grinspan, J., Bennett, V., Joho, R., Crest, M., and Scherer, S. S. (2003). Kv3.1b is a novel component of CNS nodes. *J. Neurosci.* **23,** 4509–4518.

Devaux, J. J., Kleopa, K. A., Cooper, E. C., and Scherer S. S. (2004). KCNQ2 Is a Nodal K+ Channel. *J. Neurosci.* **24,** 1236–1244.

Dugandzija-Novakovic, S., Koszowski, A. G., Levinson, S. R., and Shrager, P. (1995). Clustering of Na+ channels and node of Ranvier formation in remyelinating axons. *J. Neurosci.* **15,** 492–503.

Dupree, J. L., Girault, J.-A., and Popko, B. (1999). Axo-glial interactions regulate the localization of axonal paranodal proteins. *J. Cell Biol.* **147,** 1145–1151.

Dupree, J. L., Coetzee, T., Blight, A., Suzuki, K., and Popko, B. (1998). Myelin galactolipids are essential for proper node of Ranvier formation in the CNS. *J. Neurosci.* **18,** 1642–1649.

Einheber, S., Zanazzi, G., Ching, W., Scherer, S., Milner, T. A., Peles, E., and Salzer, J. L. (1997). The axonal membrane protein Caspr, a homologue of neurexin IV, is a component of the septate-like paranodal junctions that assemble during myelination. *J. Cell Biol.* **139,** 1495–1506.

Furley, A. J., Morton, S. B., Manalo, D., Karagogeos, D., Dodd, J., and Jessell, T. M. (1990). The axonal glycoprotein TAG-1 is an immunoglobulin superfamily member with neurite outgrowth-promoting activity. *Cell* **61,** 157–170.

Gordon, T. R., Kocsis, J. D., and Waxman S. G. (1988). Evidence for the presence of two types of potassium channels in the rat optic nerve. *Brain Res.* **447,** 1–9.

Gordon, T. R., Kocsis, J. D., and Waxman, S. G. (1989). Pharmacological sensitivities of two afterhyperpolarizations in rat optic nerve. *Brain Res.* **502,** 252–257.

Gulbis, J. M., Mann, S., and MacKinnon, R. (1999). Structure of a voltage-dependent K+ channel beta subunit. *Cell* **97,** 943–952.

Guo, W., Li, H., Aimond, F., Johns, D. C., Rhodes, K. J., Trimmer, J. S., and Nerbonne, J. M. (2002). Role of heteromultimers in the generation of myocardial transient outward K+ currents. *Circ. Res.* **90,** 586–593.

Hernandez-Pineda, R., Chow, A., Amarillo, Y., Moreno, H., Saganich, M., Vega-Saenz de Miera, E. C., Hernandez-Cruz, A., and Rudy, B. (1999). Kv3.1-Kv3.2 channels underlie a high-voltage-activating component of the delayed rectifier K+ current in projecting neurons from the globus pallidus. *J. Neurophysiol.* **82,** 1512–1528.

Hille, B. (2001). *Ionic Channels of Excitable Membranes,* ed 3. Sinauer Associates, Inc., Sunderland, MA.

Hopkins, W. F., Allen, M. L., Houamed, K. M., and Tempel, B. L. (1994). Properties of voltage-gated K+ currents expressed in Xenopus oocytes by mKv1.1, mKv1.2 and their heteromultimers as revealed by mutagenesis of the dendrotoxin-binding site in mKv1.1. *Pflugers Arch.* **428,** 382–390.

Inoue, Y., Kagawa, T., Matsumura, Y., Ikenaka, K., and Mikoshiba, K. (1996). Cell death of oligodendrocytes or demyelination induced by overexpression of proteolipid protein depending on expressed gene dosage. *Neurosci. Res.* **25,** 161–172.

Isacoff, E. Y., Jan, Y. N., and Jan, L. Y. (1990) Evidence for the formation of heteromultimeric potassium channels in Xenopus oocytes. *Nature* **345,** 530–534.

Ishibashi, T., Dupree, J. L., Ikenaka, K., Hirahara, Y., Honke, K., Peles, E., Popko, B., Suzuki, K., Nishino, H. and Baba, H. (2002). A myelin galactolipid, sulfatide, is essential for maintenance of ion channels on myelinated axon but not essential for initial cluster formation. *J. Neurosci.* **22,** 6507–6514.

Jan, L. Y., and Jan, Y. N. (1997). Cloned potassium channels from eukaryotes and prokaryotes. *Annu. Rev. Neurosci.* **20,** 91–123.

Kagawa, T., Ikenaka, K., Inoue, Y., Kuriyama, S., Tsujii, T., Nakao, J., Nakajima, K., Aruga, J., Okano, H., and Mikoshiba, K. (1994). Glial cell degeneration and hypomyelination caused by overexpression of myelin proteolipid protein gene. *Neuron* **13,** 427–442.

Kim, E., Niethammer, M., Rothschild, A., Jan, Y. N., and Sheng, M. (1995). Clustering of Shaker-type K+ channels by interaction with a family of membrane-associated guanylate kinases. *Nature* **378,** 85–88.

Kirsch, G. E., and Drewe, J. A. (1993). Gating-dependent mechanism of 4-aminopyridine block in two related potassium channels. *J. Gen. Physiol.* **102,** 797-816.

Kordeli E., Lambert S., and Bennett V. (1995). AnkyrinG. A new ankyrin gene with neural-specific isoforms localized at the axonal initial segment and node of Ranvier. *J. Biol. Chem.* **270,** 2352–2359.

MacKinnon, R. (2003). Potassium channels. *FEBS Lett.* **555,** 62–65.

Manganas, L. N., and Trimmer, J. S. (2000). Subunit composition determines Kv1 potassium channel surface expression. *J. Biol. Chem.* **275,** 29685–29693.

Manganas, L. N., Wang, Q., Scannevin, R. H., Antonucci, D. E., Rhodes, K. J., and Trimmer, J. S. (2001). Identification of a trafficking determinant localized to the Kv1 potassium channel pore. *Proc. Natl. Acad. Sci. U. S. A.* **98,** 14055–14059.

McCormack, K., Connor, J. X., Zhou, L., Ho, L. L., Ganetzky, B., Chiu, S. Y., and Messing, A. (2002). Genetic analysis of the mammalian K+ channel beta subunit Kvbeta 2 (Kcnab2). *J. Biol. Chem.* **277,** 13219–13228.

Menegoz, M., Gaspar, P., Le Bert, M., Galvez, T., Burgaya, F., Palfrey, C., Ezan, P., Arnos, F., and Girault, J. A. (1997). Paranodin, a glycoprotein of neuronal paranodal membranes. *Neuron* **19,** 319–331.

Menon, K., Rasband, M. N., Taylor, C. M., Brophy, P. J., Bansal, R., and Pfeiffer, S. E. (2003). The myelin-axolemmal complex: biochemical dissection and the role of galactosphingolipids. *J. Neurochem.* **87,** 995–1009.

Monaghan, M. M., Trimmer, J. S., and Rhodes, K. J. (2001). Experimental localization of Kv1 family voltage-gated K+ channel alpha and beta subunits in rat hippocampal formation. *J. Neurosci.* **21,** 5973–5983.

Nashmi, R., Jones, O. T., and Fehlings, M. G. (2000). Abnormal axonal physiology is associated with altered expression and distribution of Kv1.1 and Kv1.2 K+ channels after chronic spinal cord injury. *Eur. J. Neurosci.* **12,** 491–506.

Nie, D. Y., Zhou, Z. H., Ang, B. T., Teng, F. Y., Xu, G., Xiang, T., Wang, C. Y., Zeng, L., Takeda, Y., Xu, T. L., Ng, Y. K., Faivre-Sarrailh, C., Popko, B., Ling, E. A., Schachner, M., Watanabe, K., Pallen, C. J., Tang, B. L., and Xiao Z. C. (2003). Nogo-A at CNS paranodes is a ligand of Caspr: possible regulation of K(+) channel localization. *EMBO J* **22,** 5666–5678.

Ohara, R., Yamakawa, H., Nakayama, M., and Ohara, O. (2000). Type II brain 4.1 (4.1B/KIAA0987), a member of the protein 4.1 family, is localized to neuronal paranodes. *Brain Res. Mol. Brain Res.* **85,** 41–52.

Peles, E., Nativ, M., Lustig, M., Grumet, M., Schilling, J., Martinez, R., Plowman, G. D., and Schlessinger, J. (1997). Identification of a novel contactin-associated transmembrane receptor with multiple domains implicated in protein-protein interactions. *EMBO J.* **16,** 978–988.

Perney, T. M., Marshall, J., Martin, K. A., Hockfield, S., and Kaczmarek, L. K. (1992). Expression of the mRNAs for the Kv3.1 potassium channel gene in the adult and developing rat brain. *J Neurophysiol* **68,** 756–766.

Poliak, S., and Peles, E. (2003). The local differentiation of myelinated axons at nodes of Ranvier. *Nature Rev. Neurosci.* **4,** 968–980.

Poliak, S., Gollan, L., Salomon, D., Berglund, E. O., Ohara, R., Ranscht, B., and Peles, E. (2001). Localization of Caspr2 in myelinated nerves depends on axon-glia interactions and the generation of barriers along the axon. *J. Neurosci.* **21,** 7568–7575.

Poliak, S., Gollan, L., Martinez, R., Custer, A., Einheber, S., Salzer, J. L., Trimmer, J. S., Shrager, P., and Peles, E. (1999). Caspr2, a new member of the neurexin superfamily, is localized at the juxtaparanodes of myelinated axons and associates with K+ channels. *Neuron* **24,** 1037–1047.

Poliak, S., Salomon, D., Elhanany, H., Sabanay, H., Kiernan, B., Pevny, L., Stewart, C. L., Xu, X., Chiu, S. Y., Shrager, P., Furley, A. J., and Peles, E. (2003). Juxtaparanodal clustering of Shaker-like K+ channels in myelinated axons depends on Caspr2 and TAG-1. *J. Cell Biol.* **162,** 1149–1160.

Rasband, M. N. (2004). It's "juxta" potassium channel. *J. Neurosci. Ref.* **76,** 749–757.

Rasband, M. N., Park, E. W., Zhen, D., Arbuckle, M. I., Poliak, S., Peles, E., Grant, S. G. N., and Trimmer, J. S. (2002). Clustering of neuronal potassium channels is independent of their interaction with PSD-95. *J. Cell Biol.* **159,** 663–672.

Rasband, M. N., Park, E. W., Vanderah, T., Lai, J., Porreca, F., and Trimmer, J. S. (2001). Distinct K+ channels on pain sensing neurons. *Proc. Natl. Acad. Sci. U. S. A.* **98,** 13373–13378.

Rasband, M. N., and Shrager, P. (2000). Ion channel sequestration in central nervous system axons. *J. Physiol. (Lond)* **525,** 63–73.

Rasband, M. N., Trimmer, J. S., Peles, E., Levinson, S. R., and Shrager, P. (1999). K+ channel distribution and clustering in developing and hypomyelinated axons of the optic nerve. *J. Neurocytol.* **28,** 319–331.

Rasband, M. N., Trimmer, J. S., Schwarz, T. L., Levinson, S. R., Ellisman, M. H., Schachner, M., and Shrager, P. (1998). Potassium channel distribution, clustering, and function in remyelinating rat axons. *J. Neurosci.* **18,** 36–47.

Rettig, J., Heinemann, S. H., Wunder, F., Lorra, C., Parcej, D. N., Dolly, J. O., and Pongs, O. (1994). Inactivation properties of voltage-gated K+ channels altered by presence of beta-subunit. *Nature* **369,** 289–294.

Rhodes, K. J., Keilbaugh, S. A., Barrezueta, N. X., Lopez, K. L., and Trimmer, J. S. (1995). Association and colocalization of K+ channel alpha- and beta-subunit polypeptides in rat brain. *J. Neurosci.* **15,** 5360–5371.

Rhodes, K. J., Strassle, B. W., Monaghan, M. M., Bekele-Arcuri, Z., Matos, M. F., and Trimmer, J. S. (1997). Association and colocalization of the Kvbeta1 and Kvbeta2 beta-subunits with Kv1 alpha-subunits in mammalian brain K+ channel complexes. *J. Neurosci.* **17,** 8246–8258.

Roper, J., and Schwarz, J. R. (1989). Heterogeneous distribution of fast and slow potassium channels in myelinated rat nerve fibres. *J. Physiol. (Lond.)* **416,** 93–110.

Rosenbluth, J. (1988). Role of glial cells in the differentiation and function of myelinated axons. *Int. J. Dev. Neurosci.* **6,** 3–24.

Ruppersberg, J. P., Schroter, K. H., Sakmann, B., Stocker, M., Sewing, S., and Pongs, O. (1990). Heteromultimeric channels formed by rat brain potassium-channel proteins. *Nature* **345,** 535–537.

Safronov, B. V., Kampe, K., and Vogel, W. (1993). Single voltage-dependent potassium channels in rat peripheral nerve membrane. *J. Physiol.* **460,** 675–691.

Salzer, J. L. (2003). Polarized domains of myelinated axons. *Neuron* **40,** 297–318.

Shamotienko, O. G., Parcej, D. N., and Dolly, J. O. (1997). Subunit combinations defined for K+ channel Kv1 subtypes in synaptic membranes from bovine brain. *Biochemistry* **36,** 8195–8201.

Sheng, M., Liao, Y. J., Jan, Y. N., and Jan L. Y. (1993). Presynaptic A-current based on heteromultimeric K+ channels detected in vivo. *Nature* **365,** 72–75.

Shi, G., Nakahira, K., Hammond, S., Rhodes, K. J., Schechter, L. E., and Trimmer, J. S. (1996). Beta subunits promote K+ channel surface expression through effects early in biosynthesis. *Neuron* **16,** 843–852.

Targ, E. F., and Kocsis, J. D. (1985). 4-Aminopyridine leads to restoration of conduction in demyelinated rat sciatic nerve. *Brain Res.* **328,** 358–361.

Targ, E. F., and Kocsis, J. D. (1986). Action potential characteristics of demyelinated rat sciatic nerve following application of 4-aminopyridine. *Brain Res.* **363,** 1–9.

Traka, M., Dupree, J. L., Popko, B., and Karagogeos, D. (2002). The neuronal adhesion protein TAG-1 is expressed by Schwann cells and oligodendrocytes and is localized to the juxtaparanodal region of myelinated fibers. *J. Neurosci.* **22,** 3016–3024.

Traka, M., Goutebroze, L., Denisenko, N., Bessa, M., Nifli, A., Havaki, S., Iwakura, Y., Fukamauchi, F., Watanabe, K., Soliven, B., Girault, J. A., and Karagogeos, D. (2003). Association of TAG-1 with Caspr2 is essential for the molecular organization of juxtaparanodal regions of myelinated fibers. *J. Cell Biol.* **162,** 1161–1172.

Trimmer, J. S., and Rhodes, K. J. (2003). Localization of voltage-gated ion channels in mammalian brain. *Annu. Rev. Physiol.* **66,** 477–519.

Tzoumaka, E. E., Novakovic, S. D., Levinson, S. R., and Shrager, P. (1995). Na+ channel aggregation in remyelinating mouse sciatic axons following transection. *Glia* **15,** 188–194.

Vabnick, I., Trimmer, J. S., Schwarz, T. L., Levinson, S. R., Risal, D., and Shrager, P. (1999). Dynamic potassium channel distributions during axonal development prevent aberrant firing patterns. *J. Neurosci.* **19,** 747–758.

Wang, H., Kunkel, D. D., Martin, T. M., Schwartzkroin, P. A., and Tempel, B. L. (1993). Heteromultimeric K+ channels in terminal and juxtaparanodal regions of neurons. *Nature* **365,** 75–79.

Wang, H., Allen, M. L., Grigg, J. J., Noebels, J. L., and Tempel, B. L. (1995). Hypomyelination alters K+ channel expression in mouse mutants Shiverer and Trembler. *Neuron* **15,** 1337–1347.

Zhou, D., Lambert, S., Malen, P. L., Carpenter, S., Boland, L. M., and Bennett, V. (1998a). AnkyrinG is required for clustering of voltage-gated Na channels at axon initial segments and for normal action potential firing. *J. Cell Biol.* **143,** 1295–1304.

Zhou, L., Zhang, C. L., Messing, A., and Chiu, S. Y. (1998b). Temperature-sensitive neuromuscular transmission in Kv1.1 null mice: role of potassium channels under the myelin sheath in young nerves. *J. Neurosci.* **18,** 7200–7215.

Zhu, J., Watanabe, I., Gomez, B., and Thornhill, W. B. (2001). Determinants involved in Kv1 potassium channel folding in the endoplasmic reticulum, glycosylation in the Golgi, and cell surface expression. *J. Biol. Chem.* **276,** 39419–39427.

Zhu, J., Watanabe, I., Gomez, B., and Thornhill, W. B. (2003). Heteromeric Kv1 potassium channel expression: Amino acid determinants involved in processing and trafficking to the cell surface. *J. Biol. Chem.* **278,** 25558–25567.

5

The Roles of Potassium and Calcium Channels in Physiology and Pathophysiology of Axons

S.Y. Chiu, Ph.D.

I. Introduction

Voltage-gated ion channels act like field-effect transistors that gate the flow of ions across excitable membranes in a voltage-dependent fashion (Jiang et al., 2003; MacKinnon, 2003). Sodium (Na), potassium (K), and calcium (Ca) channels are three major classes of ion channels that determine the excitability of excitable membranes (Hille, 2001). Na channels are responsible for the rapid upstroke of an action potential for local excitation, for providing axial current to depolarize neighboring membrane patches for impulse propagation, and are the primary depolarizing force that activates the other two channel types. K channels contribute to the resting potential, to repolarization of an action potential, and to frequency modulation. Another channel activated by the Na-triggered membrane depolarization is Ca channel. Unlike the other two channel types, Ca channels are usually expressed at a lower density and are normally not sufficient to generate an action potential. However, Ca channels are important modulators of excitability in different ways and over different time scales. For example, Ca influx can activate cytoplasmic proteins capable of chemically modifying Na and K channels, as well as activating biochemical cascades that affect the integrity of axons.

Historically, the important role of Na and K channels was first recognized in axons through the pioneering work of Hodgkin and Huxley on the physiological properties of the squid giant axons (Hodgkin and Huxley, 1952). The physiological landscape has now been repainted with molecular strokes aided by gene cloning of ion channels, mapping of ion channel localization in the nervous system with highly specific antibodies, and recently by crystallographic determination of the three-dimensional structure of individual channel proteins (MacKinnon, 2003). From a clinical aspect, the new molecular knowledge promises, probably within the next 5 to 10 years, design of highly specific drugs that can fundamentally alter the excitability of the nervous system by targeting single residues within an ion channel protein. This chapter summarizes our current knowledge of the physiology and pathophysiology of ion channels on myelinated axons as they relate to demyelinating diseases.

II. Na Channels

A. Physiological Studies of Na Channels on Axons

The node of Ranvier is the site of excitation enriched with voltage-gated Na (Nav) channels. Gating current measurement reveals that a single large mammalian node has ~83,000 Na channels (Chiu, 1980), translating to ~1,400 channels/μm^2 when a nodal area of 60 μm^2 is assumed. Historically, nodal clustering of ion channels was first hypothesized by Rosenbluth (1976) based on observations of nodal particles in freeze fracture studies in myelinated axons. Subsequent physiological evidence for nodal segregation of Nav channels came from studies by Ritchie and Rogart (1977) on binding of ^{3}H-saxitoxin to sodium channels of intact and homogenized myelinated nerves. The critical finding is that homogenization, which exposed the internodal axon under the myelin, did not reveal extra ^{3}H-saxitoxin binding, suggesting that Nav channels are concentrated at the node with little present under the myelin sheath. This finding was later confirmed in voltage-clamp studies of single mammalian myelinated fibers, in which acute paranodal demyelination was found to add little to the nodal sodium currents (Fig. 1A) (Chiu and Ritchie, 1980).

B. Molecular Identity of Nav Channels on Axons

Gene cloning has identified up to 10 different Na channel genes in the mammals, with many expressed in neurons (Goldin, 1999; Goldin et al., 2000). These genes encode sodium channel proteins with similar structural motifs but different kinetic properties due to variation in other regions of their primary amino acid sequence. The location, density, and type of Nav isoforms expressed in myelinated axons greatly affect their physiological responses in health and diseases. The availability of isoform-specific antibodies allows cellular mapping of Nav expression in various normal and pathological axons. Nav1.2 is expressed predominantly in nonmyelinated axons, while Nav1.6 is expressed predominantly at nodes of Ranvier. Developmentally, Nav expression switches from Nav1.2 to Nav1.6 when the axon becomes myelinated (Boiko et al., 2001; Rasband and Trimmer, 2001), a switch that may reflect

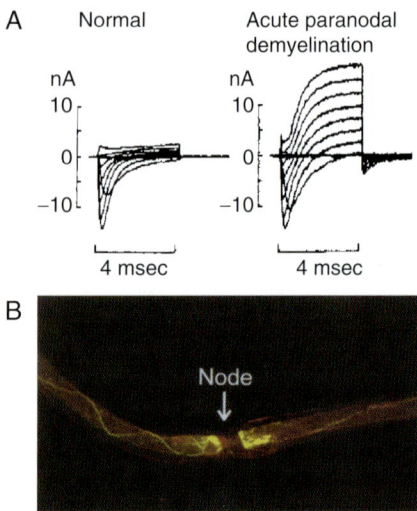

Figure 1 **Juxtaparanodal clustering of Kv1 channels in mature myelinated axons.** (**A**) Voltage clamp recordings of total ionic currents from a single mammalian node of Ranvier before (*left*) and after (*right*) acute paranodal demyelination. Note paranodal demyelination reveals a large outward K current (upward deflections) that is absent in the intact node. Note also that inward Na currents (downward deflections) remain unaffected. (**B**) Kv1.1 immunofluorescence (*green*) in a single myelinated fiber, showing juxtaparanodal localization. The fiber is also double-stained with anti-MAG (*red*). (Reproduced from Chiu, Zhou, Zhang, and Messing, 1999, with permission.)

adaptation to a change in firing pattern as axons become myelinated.

C. The Role of Nav Channels in Demyelinating Diseases

Nav channel expression undergoes two types of changes in demyelinating diseases that impact the pathophysiological properties of axons. The first type of change is Nav channel desegregation, leading to a dilution of the locally intense Na influx normally needed for saltatory conduction. The molecular mechanisms for normal clustering of Nav channels and channel desegregation in demyelination are being clarified at a rapid pace, and readers should consult Chapters 3, 7, 8, and 19 for greater details. The second type of change in demyelination is alteration in Nav gene expression. Demyelinated axons can lose certain Nav isoforms or acquire new Nav isoforms, resulting in new excitability properties in pathological axons. A notable example is the downregulation of Nav1.6 and acquisition of Nav1.2 in dysmyelinated axons and the inappropriate acquisition of Nav1.8 channels in Purkinje cells in demyelinating disorders. Readers should consult Chapter 7. We now turn to the main focus of this chapter: K and Ca channels on normal and demyelinated axons.

III. K Channels

A. Molecular Overview of K Channels

K channels have more diverse roles in axons than Na channels (Hille, 2001). Molecular cloning and structure-function studies have revealed that K channels are built on a common structure plan, composing a selectivity filter that is present in all K channels, and a voltage sensor that could be absent in some K channels (Jan and Jan, 1997). The voltage-dependent, or Kv, channels have 9 gene families (Kv1 to Kv9) in the mammalian nervous system. The voltage-insensitive K channels (having only the selectivity filter but no voltage sensor) come in two different subclasses. The first subclass is inward rectifiers (Kir) whose open pore configuration preferentially allows K ions to flow into rather than out of the cell. The other subclass of voltage-insensitive K channels is the more recently characterized 2-P domain channels (Goldstein et al., 2001), where each α subunit has 2 selectivity loops rather than a single loop in a more traditional α subunit. 2-P channels have minimal rectification in open pore configuration (i.e., allowing K ions to flow in and out of the cell with equal efficacy); are sensitive to pH, second messengers, and volatile anesthetics; and are typically referred to as background K channels. There are three major areas of research on axonal K channels: identification of Kv subtypes and mapping of axonal location (see Chapter 4 for more detail), molecular basis for K channel clustering (see Chapter 3 for more detail), and physiological roles of axonal Kv channels in health and in disease (the focus of this chapter).

B. Identification of K Channel Subtypes and Mapping of Axonal Localization

1. Juxtaparanodal Tripartite of Kv1.1/Kv1.2/Kvβ2

Fast, delayed rectifier is historically the first K channel to be studied in axons. This channel was first characterized in the squid giant axon in 1952 (Hodgkin and Huxley, 1952), then later in amphibian nodes of Ranvier. These channels are partially open at the resting potential, but are strongly activated by depolarization with fast activation kinetics. As shown by Hodgkin and Huxley, fast delayed rectifiers play an indispensable role in repolarization of an action potential. Surprisingly, subsequent voltage-clamp studies on single mammalian myelinated axons from various peripheral nerves, including human nerves, showed that the nodal membrane of these fibers lacks fast delayed rectifiers (Brismar, 1980; Chiu et al., 1979; Schwarz et al., 1995). Action potential repolarization in a mammalian node, in contrast to the nonmyelinated axons, relies only on Nav channel inactivation and passive leakage current (Chiu et al., 1979). Of interest, Chiu and Ritchie (1980) first showed in acute paranodal demyelination studies that fast delayed rec-

tifiers are normally present under the myelin sheath (Fig. 1A). Subsequent immunohistochemistry with Kv-specific antibodies shows that Kv1.1 and Kv1.2, as well as the auxiliary subunit Kvβ2, are localized to the juxtaparanodal region of both peripheral nervous system (PNS) and central nervous system (CNS) myelinated axons (Fig. 1B) (Wang et al., 1993). Genetic studies on Kv1.1 mutants have suggested that juxtaparanodal Kv1 channels act as transition zone stabilizer, as discussed in detail later.

2. Nodal Kv3.1 Channels

Even though Kv1.1 and Kv1.2 are sequestered at the juxtaparanode of mature CNS nerves, the K channel blocker 4-AP still significantly broadens the action potential in mature myelinated CNS fiber tracts such as the optic nerves. This suggests the presence of nodal Kv channels responsible for action potential repolarization. The first nodal Kv component was recently identified to be Kv3.1 (Devaux et al., 2003), present mainly in large myelinated axons of the CNS. Kv3.1 is activated at a higher threshold than most Kv channels, has fast deactivation rate (Rudy and McBain, 2001), and is uniquely suitable for high frequency signaling for certain CNS axons. However, the function of Kv3.1 in axons remains enigmatic: genetic ablation of Kv3.1 neither broadens the action potential nor eliminates the effect of 4-AP on the action potential waveform (Devaux et al., 2003).

3. Internodal Kir

Baker and colleagues (1987) defined the presence, as well as the probable function, of three types of rectifying channels (one sensitive to 4-AP, one to TEA, and the third to cesium) under intact myelin in rat spinal root myelinated axons. Of particular interest is the inferred presence of internodal Kir channels under intact myelin. The functions of these channels in normal nerves remain unclear. Since Kir conductance is increased only when the membrane is hyperpolarized, an attractive hypothesis is that Kir channels tend to limit a tetanus-induced, after-hyperpolarization (due, for example, to action of the electrogenic Na/K pumps) that if unopposed may lead to nerve conduction block.

4. 2P Leakage Channels

The stability of excitable cell is critically determined by K channels that determine the resting membrane potential. While some Kv channels such as Kv1.1 (which has a low threshold for activation and is partially open at the resting potential) may contribute to the resting potential, the 2P leakage K channels are thought to be important contributors to the resting potential in neurons. In axons, however, the role of 2-P channels and their molecular identity have not yet been addressed. TREK-1, a member of the 2P TREK family, is present in DRG neurons (Maingret et al., 2000), making its presence in axons likely.

C. Normal and Pathological Roles of K Channels in Myelinated Axons

1. Overview of K Channel Function in Axonal Tree

Between the neuronal cell soma and the nerve terminals lies a complex morphological landscape, commonly referred to as the axonal tree, that an action potential has to navigate to reach the nerve terminal (Fig. 2) (Waxman, 1972). The bulk of the journey for an action potential takes place along monotonous cables designed in a rushtonian fashion optimized geometrically for conduction velocity (Rushton, 1951). However, the axonal tree is capable of signal integration through differential routing and frequency modulation as action potentials pass through branch points and local variation in geometry collectively referred to as transition zones (Fig. 2) (Swadlow et al., 1980; Waxman, 1972). How might axonal K channels modulate nerve signaling in this complex axonal tree? Are K channels more important in transition zones than in the rest of the axons? Do specific types of axonal Kv channels subserve different functions? In this chapter, we focus on the juxtaparanodal Kv1.1, as the availability of various Kv1.1 mutants has made this axonal channel the best characterized in terms of functions in myelinated axons. As discussed in great detail later, a major conclusion of physiological analysis of Kv1 mutants is that juxtaparanodal Kv1 channels play an important role in stabilizing transition zones in an axonal tree. Before going into functional issues, we first discuss the nature of transition zones.

2. Transition Zones

Transition zones in general refer to the regions in an axonal tree where there is a local change in geometry because of certain functional requirements. Important examples are the branch points or the nerve terminal region where the myelinated segment ends and the nonmyelinated segment begins (Fig. 2). The safety factor for nerve conduction is altered at these sites as a result of impedance mismatch. Impedance *mis*-matching is normally minimized by local variation in fiber geometry. For example, the internodes shorten as the nerve terminal is approached (Fig. 2, arrow) (Quick et al., 1979), and this has been shown theoretically to facilitate invasion of the nerve terminal (Khodorov and Timin, 1975). In pathological situations, remyelination proceeds by forming short internodes preceding lesion sites, providing impedance matching that contributes to successful propagation (Waxman and Brill, 1978).

Other variations in local fiber geometry may also prove important. First, postbranching internodes are significantly smaller than the rest of the fiber (Pfeiffer and Friede, 1985). Second, in dorsal root ganglion (DRG) neurons, the first internode after the initial segment has an unusually thin myelin sheath (Spencer et al., 1973). At the branch point of DRG neurons, the caliber of the CNS-directed axon is different than the PNS-directed axon (Spencer et al., 1973).

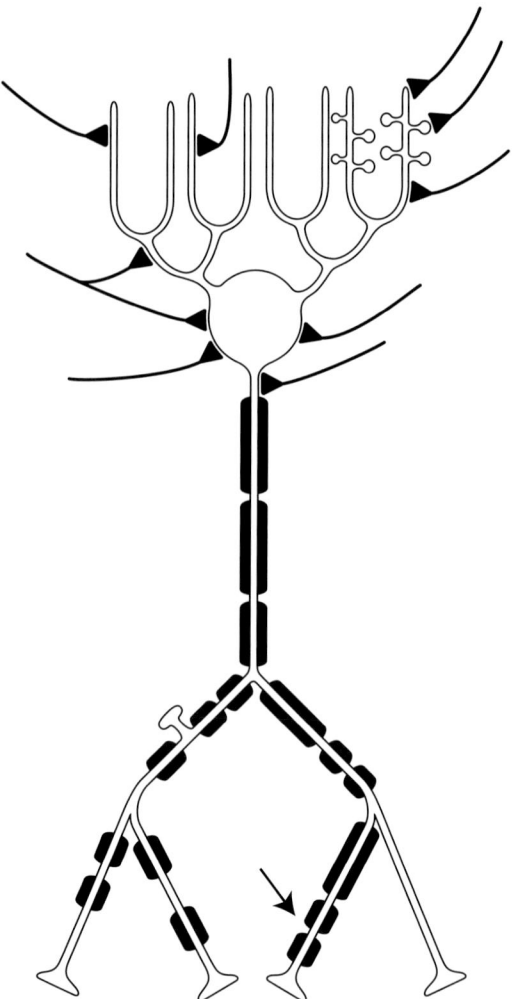

Figure 2 **Schematic drawing of an axonal tree.** Arrows show presynaptic shortening of internodes. Existing immunohistochemistry suggests that Kv1.1 is present at the juxtaparanodes, but absent from the nerve terminals (Brew et al., 2003; Zhou et al., 1998). The major function of juxtaparanodal Kv1.1 is to stabilize transition zones (branch points and presynaptic regions) in the axonal tree. (Modified after Waxman, 1972, with permission.)

Third, action potentials could fail at branch points, and frequency-dependent failures at branch points could act as safety measures to prevent an injurious level of axonal activity from permeating other regions of the axonal tree. Collectively, transition zone excitability has profound implications for signal integration in normal and pathological axonal trees. Analysis of Kv1.1 mutants suggests that juxtaparanodal Kv1.1 stabilizes transition zones at nerve terminals and branch points.

a. Stabilization of Axonal Segment before the Nerve Terminal   The internodal shortening ahead of the nerve terminal (Fig. 2, arrow), while facilitating impulse invasion of the nerve terminal (Quick et al., 1979; Waxman and Brill, 1978), also raises the local excitability by increasing the Na channel content per unit fiber length (Chiu et al., 1999). Do Kv channels function to stabilize this region, and, if so, by what mechanisms? Genetic ablation of Kv1.1 results in no detectable change in the morphology of the myelinated nerves (Chiu et al., 1999). There is only a slight change in the action potential waveform and refractory period (Smart et al., 1998). However, the most dramatic excitability change is traced to a short nerve segment of probably not more than one to two internodal lengths just before neuromuscular junction, where a single action potential in the mutant elicits multiple action potentials (Fig. 3) (Zhou et al., 1998, 1999). This occurs only when the temperature is cooled below the physiological level, contributing to an intense myokymia seen in mutant mice forced to swim in cold water (Zhou et al., 1998).

Stabilization of branch points of myelinated axons
Branch points (Fig. 2) represent another site of impedance mismatch where a propagating action potential can be rerouted, reflected backwards, blocked, or its frequency of transmission altered. Analysis of Kv1.1 mutant mice, in conjunction with computer modeling, has shed light on how Kv1.1 might modulate branch point transmission.

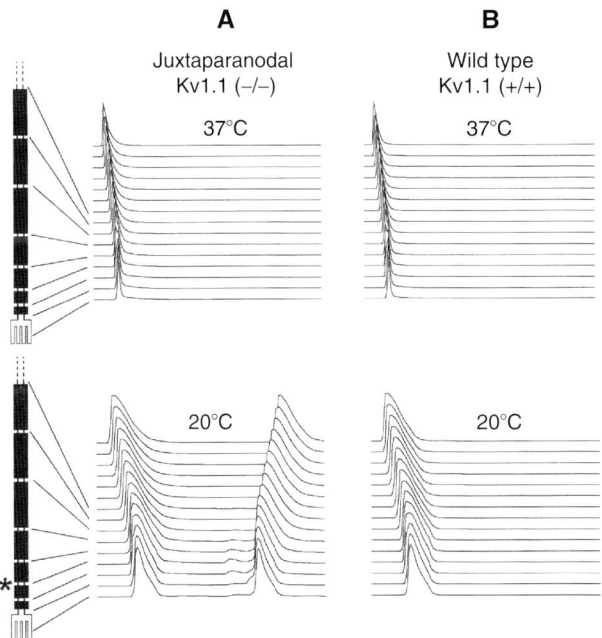

Figure 3 Ablation of juxtaparanodal Kv1.1 destabilizes the axonal segment before the nerve terminal. (**A**) Computer simulations of action potential propagation (from top to bottom) toward the nerve terminal with Kv1.1 deleted. (Top) 37°C. (Bottom) 20°C. Note that at the lower temperature, a single action potential elicits a second impulse at segment (*), causing a backfiring, as well as another forward firing. (**B**) In the wild-type, the segment before the nerve terminal is electrically stable, thus ensuring a faithful 1-to-1 transmission irrespective of temperature changes. (Modified from Zhou et al., 1999, with permission.)

The excitability of the basket cell axon plexus that innervates the Purkinje cells in the cerebellum was examined in Kv1.1 null mice (Zhang et al., 1999). Kv1.1 deletion does not affect the spontaneous firing rate of the basket cell soma, suggesting that Kv1.1 does not alter the number of action potentials emitted down the axonal tree. Yet an increase in the inhibitory postsynaptic current (IPSC) is recorded in the Kv1.1 null mice. This increase in IPSP could not be explained by an increase in the excitability of the basket cell axon terminals (such as an increase in bouton density, in the spontaneous firing rate at the nerve terminal, or in the action potential duration at the nerve terminal), because both the miniature IPSP and the amplitude of the IPSP are unaffected in the mutants. The conclusion, by a process of elimination, is that Kv1.1 deletion elevates excitability by reducing the failure rates of action potential propagation through branch points. A similar conclusion was reached using a transgenic mouse in which point mutations were engineered in the Kv1.1 gene to reproduce the human neurological disorder episodic ataxia (Herson et al., 2003). Since basket cell axons are nonmyelinated, these studies do not address whether Kv1.1 is a stabilizer of branch points in myelinated axons.

That Kv1.1 destabilizes branch points in myelinated axons is evoked to explain alterations in the excitability of the auditory system in the Kv1.1 null mice (Kopp-Scheinpflug et al., 2003). In a technically demanding study, in vivo single-unit recordings were made from bushy cells, their axonal endings, and the MNTB neurons (calyces of Held) the bushy cells innervate. Two interesting observations emerge. First, no apparent changes in the excitability were observed in cell body or the calyceal terminals of the bushy cells; the latter is consistent with the nondetectability of Kv1.1 proteins in the calyceal terminals (Brew et al., 2003). Rather, Kv1.1 deletion diminishes the ability of the bushy cell axons to follow high frequency, sound-driven stimulations. Second, the jitter of the first spike measured at the MNTB cells (innervated by the bushy cells) is significantly increased in the Kv1.1 null mice, leading to a degradation of the highly precise processing of temporal information required of the auditory system. The hypothesis is that these excitability changes in the auditory system result from *destabilization* of branch points of the bushy cell axonal tree (Kopp-Scheinpflug et al., 2003). This study provides the first empirical evidence to suggest a change in excitability of branch points in myelinated axons upon genetic ablation of Kv1.1.

b. Theoretical Considerations and Computer Simulations
Why should transition zones be particularly sensitive to Kv1.1 deletion? One reason is the existence of internodal shortening before some transition zones (Quick et al., 1979), as in PNS neuromuscular junctions and in the vicinity of some branch points. Local internodal shortening ahead of a

transition zone translates into excitability augmentation due to an increase in the Na channel content per unit length. In a normal nerve, this augmentation of excitability is counteracted by juxtaparanodal Kv1.1 and a background K conductance. The countereffect of juxtaparanodal Kv1.1 also increases on a per unit length basis as a result of internodal shortening. However, if one assumes that the background K conductance per unit length remains constant, which would be true if the background conductance is distributed uniformly along the axons, and that the internodal portion of the myelinated axon contributes significantly to the background resting conductance (Chiu, 1982; Chiu and Ritchie, 1984), then it is immediately apparent that deletion of juxtaparanodal Kv1.1 would produce a disproportionately larger loss of counteracting force at the transition zone over the rest of the nerve. This theoretical consideration, therefore, corroborates the conclusion from physiological analysis of the Kv1.1 mutants that juxtaparanodal Kv1.1 is an important modifier of transition zone excitability. However the directionality of the excitability change observed in the mutants is complex. For example, the types of transition zones appear to be important: Kv1.1 deletion elevates the excitability of transition zones ahead of the nerve terminal (Zhou et al., 1999), but depresses the excitability in transition zones at branch points (Kopp-Scheinpflug et al., 2003).

c. Computer Modeling   Because direct, empirical measurement of branch point transmission is notoriously difficult to achieve, theoretical modeling becomes an important complementary tool to address the role of juxtaparanodal Kv1 at branch points. Mathematical modeling of a single branch point for myelinated axons has been achieved in our laboratory (Zhou and Chiu, 2001), and extension to an axonal tree with multiple branch points is now under way (Chan and Chiu, unpublished observations). Computer simulations show that action potential propagation through a single branch point in a myelinated axon is very sensitive to the prebranch internodal lengths, minor changes in the paranodal junctions and potassium accumulations at vicinity of the branch point (Zhou and Chiu, 2001). Further, preliminary calculations show that deletion of juxtaparanodal Kv1 channels shifts the cut-off frequency of high-frequency trains through a branch point to a higher frequency level, effectively augmenting the excitability of the axonal tree (Chan and Chiu, unpublished observations). Further computer modeling of myelinated axonal trees with complex branch point distribution will be needed to shed light on how Kv1 affects global signaling processing in an axonal tree.

d. Mechanism of Stabilization of Transition Zones
Even though analysis of Kv1.1 mutants suggests that transition zones are stabilized by juxtaparanodal Kv1.1, it is unclear by what mechanism the stabilization is achieved.

One mechanism of stabilization is prevention of reentrant excitation of the node of Ranvier (Chiu and Ritchie, 1981) by flanking the node with a high-density band of juxtaparanodal Kv1.1 channels. In this scheme, the juxtaparanodal Kv1.1 channels only interact dynamically with nodal currents during excitation to prevent re-excitation, but the Kv1.1 channels do not contribute to the steady-state resting potential. The other mechanism of stabilization is maintaining a resting potential for the axon under the myelin (Chiu, 1982; Chiu and Ritchie, 1984). Kv1.1 is a strong candidate in this later mechanism, as its low threshold for activation (Hopkins et al., 1994) allows this channel to be partially open at the resting potential and contributes to stabilizing it. In the first mechanism (dynamic prevention of reentrant excitation), the pattern of Kv1.1 distribution (i.e., juxtaparanodal clustering) is important. In the second mechanism (maintaining a steady resting potential), the total Kv1.1 content per internode, rather than the pattern of channel distribution, is important. Recent studies of the Caspr-2 knockout mice lend credence to the second mechanism. The unique feature of Caspr-2 ablation (see Chapter 3) is that it desegregates Kv1.1 without altering the total Kv1.1 content per internode (Poliak et al., 2003). If Kv1.1 stabilizes transition zones primarily by maintaining a resting potential for the axons, then there should be no change in the excitability of transition zones in the Caspr-2 knockout mice because in these mice, Kv1.1 simply randomizes over the internode without a reduction in total channel numbers, which should not lead to any change in the steady resting potential. Transition zone analysis of this mouse has so far been restricted to the neuromuscular junction (Poliak et al., 2003), and the excitability there is normal. Other transition zones, such as branch points, have not been evaluated. Thus, the best current working hypothesis from studies of Kv1.1 (Zhou et al., 1998) and Caspr-2 mutants (Poliak et al., 2003) is that Kv1.1 stabilizes transition zones by a mechanism involving stabilization of the resting potential. Evidently, transition zones are highly vulnerable to resting potential perturbation than the rest of the axon.

D. Function of Kv1 Channels in Demyelination

What is the role of Kv1 channels in demyelinating diseases? Two key changes in demyelination are germane to this question. First is the well-known morphological change of exposure of the internodal axon. The unmasked Kv1 channels will antagonize action potential propagation across the demyelinated region already poor in Na channels. Second is the possible change in Kv1 expression after demyelination. Desegregation of Kv1 aside, any change in overall expression level in demyelination is important: a downregulation of Kv channels may be favorable to conduction, while an upregulation of Kv channels is not.

Information on the directionality of changes in Kv expression in demyelination is sparse, but new data are emerging. An early report demonstrated that in CNS fiber tracts of the dysmyelinating Shiverer mice, Kv1.1 expression is upregulated in both axons and glia as revealed by immunocytochemistry and mRNA analysis (Wang et al., 1995). If Kv1.1 is a transition zone stabilizer, then the creation of more transition zones in demyelinating axons suggests that Kv1.1 will play an important role in neuropathologic axons. In this regard, an upregulation of Kv1.1 in demyelination might confer stability to branch point transmission in pathological nerves. The role of Kv1.1 in remyelination also is of clinical interest. Computer simulations show that a short remyelinated internode ahead of a denuded axonal segment can restore nerve conduction (Waxman and Brill, 1978). Here again, an upregulation of Kv1.1 might stabilize transition zones in remyelination.

IV. Ca Channels

Traditionally, translation of electricity to biochemistry is thought to take place at the nerve terminal of a neuron, where electricity (the action potential) is translated into biochemical events occurring during calcium-mediated vesicular release of neurotransmitters. Before the nerve terminal, the axon has been regarded as a high-speed conduit whose major role is transmission of electricity via Na and K channels, rather than translation of electricity to biochemistry. This picture of axons is no longer tenable, as Ca channels (both voltage-gated and ligand-gated), which are instrumental for synaptic signal transduction, have been discovered in mammalian axons.

A. Voltage-Gated Calcium Channels

In the mammals, three subfamilies of voltage-gated calcium genes (Cav) have been cloned: Cav1, Cav2, and Cav3. Cav1 and Cav2 are also commonly referred to as HVA channels, as they require relatively high-membrane depolarizations (> −30 mV) for activation (Hille, 2001). Cav3 is also called LVA channels because they are activated by lower depolarizations (> −70 mV). The HVA Cav1 subfamily (Cav1.1-1.4) is also called L-type calcium channels, whereas the HVA Cav2 subfamily consists of P/Q (Cav2.1), N (Cav2.2) and R (Cav2.3). Which type of Cav channels are found in axons? Our focus is on recent discoveries in the mammalian axons, though we are fully cognizant that Cav channels have long been described in the squid giant axons.

Four different approaches have been used to establish the presence of Ca channels on mammalian axons. In the first approach, Ca channel contribution to the waveform of action potentials is unmasked by blocking Na and/or K channels. In the second approach, subtype-specific anti-

bodies are used in immunohistochemistry to establish the presence of certain Cav channel isoforms. In the third approach, the protective action of calcium channel blockers on ischemic axons is examined, from which the calcium channel subtypes that contribute to axonal damage are inferred (Fern et al., 1995a; Stys et al., 1995). In the fourth and final approach, Ca imaging technique is used to measure directly activity-dependent calcium influx in mammalian axons. In this last approach, which receives more attention here because of the author's current interest, the Ca dyes must be selectively introduced into axons and not the surrounding glial cells. Our laboratory has developed a technique where a tight suction pipette is used to load Ca dyes into thousands of axonal cylinders through the cut end of an optic nerve (Fig. 4A) (Verbny et al., 2002). We use a dextran-conjugated Ca dye that significantly increases its molecular size. The use of this dye has three advantages in analysis of axonal Ca signals. First, the large size of dextran excludes glial cell staining because the dye cannot pass through gap junctions. Second, it allows better retention in axons. Third, a dextran-conjugated Ca dye has low mobility, allowing a more faithful analysis of spatial Ca signals (Gabso et al., 1997) (Sabatini et al., 2001). Fig. 4B shows an image of axons stained with Ca dyes using this technique. Once axons are loaded with Ca indicators, and activity-dependent Ca influx detected, it becomes a straightforward experiment to discern various Cav channel subtypes based on the excellent availability of subtype-specific toxins.

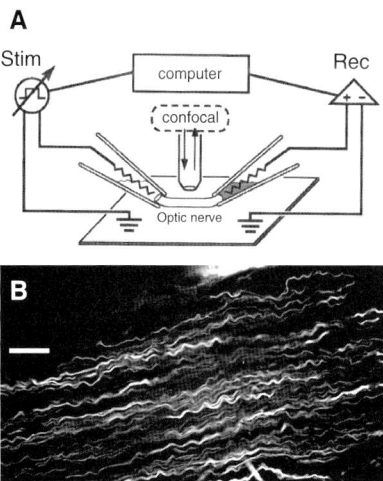

Figure 4 **Confocal imaging of calcium fluorescence in axons of mammalian optic nerves.** (**A**) Schematics of the imaging setup. An isolated piece of optic nerve is tightly drawn into a glass pipette on the right filled with calcium indicators. The calcium indicators diffuse into the axonal cylinders. The other nerve end is loosely drawn into a glass stimulation pipette. In this setup, simultaneous recordings of axonal calcium and action potentials can be achieved. (**B**) Representative images of axons stained with calcium indicators. Bar is 20 μm. (Reproduced from Zhang et al., 2004, with permission.)

Results using this approach from our laboratory on the mammalian optic nerves are summarized here.

1. N-type Ca Channels (Cav2.2)

Activity-dependent Ca transients are detected in neonatal optic nerve axons (Fig. 5A, B) (Sun and Chiu, 1999). These Ca transients are reversibly eliminated by removal of external Ca, suggesting that they arise primarily from Ca influx, and are blocked by the wide-spectrum Cav channel blockers Cd and Ni. About 58% of the Ca transients are blocked by ωconotoxin-GVIA (Fig. 5C, left), an N-type Cav-specific blocker, demonstrating the presence of axonal N-type Ca channels (Sun and Chiu, 1999). However, the identity of the remaining Ca transients remains unclear, as L-type Ca channel blockers, as well as P/Q specific toxins (Fig. 5C, right), did not affect the Ca transient. Of interest, activation of GABA$_B$ receptors by baclofen leads to a rapid downregulation

of N-type Ca transients in the neonatal optic nerves (Fig. 5A) (Sun and Chiu, 1999). Neuromodulation of axonal Ca signals might be neuroprotective in pathological axons. Fern et al. (1995b) demonstrated that GABA$_B$ receptor activation is linked to protection of white matter during metabolic insults, and it is tempting to speculate that this protection stems from inhibition of N-type Ca channels. However, it is unclear if N-type Ca channels exist in adult myelinated nerves (Brown et al., 2001). As described next, N-type Ca channels are upregulated in nerves of certain demyelinated models.

2. L-Type Calcium Channels

Ischemic studies carried out in adult mammalian white matter show that L-type Ca channel blockers are neuroprotective, suggesting that L-type Ca channels are present on axons and mediate damaging Ca influx during ischemia (Fern et al., 1995a; Brown et al., 2001; Quardouz et al.,

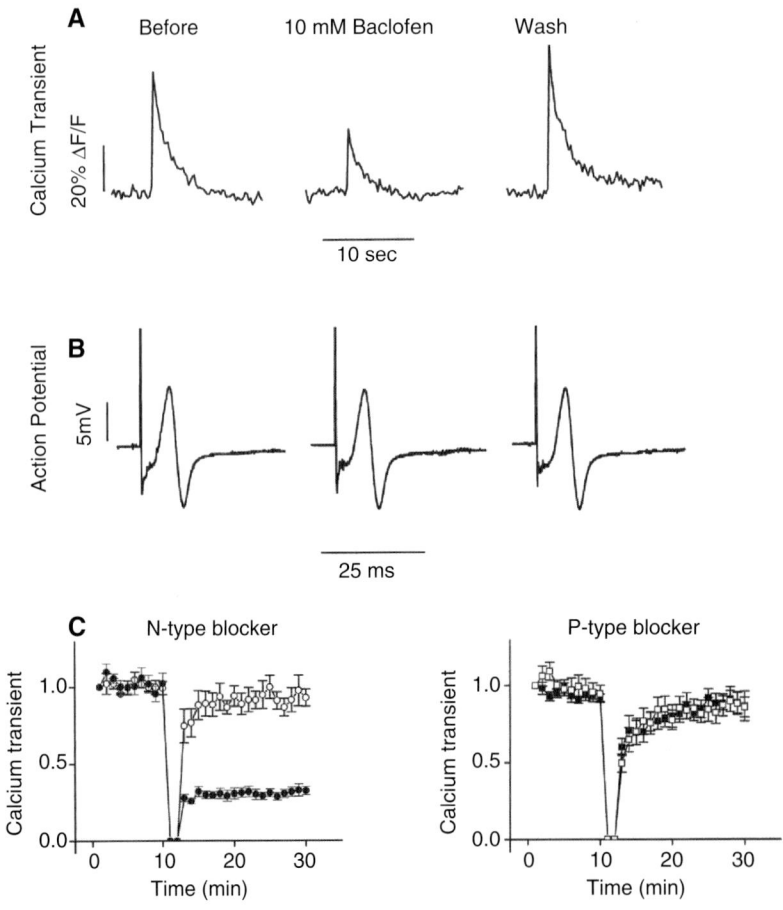

Figure 5 N-type calcium channels in neonatal rat optic nerves. (A, B) Simultaneous recordings of axonal calcium transients (**A**) and action potentials (**B**) using the setup shown in Fig. 4. Note difference in time scale between the calcium and the action potential recordings. Baclofen rapidly reduces the calcium transient (**A**) without affecting the action potentials (**B**). (**C**) Application of ωconotoxin-GVIA, an N-type calcium channel blocker, blocks the calcium transients by ~58% (left). Application of ω-Aga-IVA, a P-type channel blocker, is without effect (right). Note that the baclofen-sensitive component of the calcium transient is identical to the ωconotoxin-GVIA-sensitive component, suggesting that N-type calcium channels are coupled to GABA$_B$ receptors. (Modified from Sun and Chiu, 1999, with permission.)

2003). Immunohistochemistry suggests that L-type Ca channels, unlike Na channels, have a more diffuse distribution on the axons and are not localized at the nodes of Ranvier (Brown et al., 2001). A more recent immunohistochemical study shows that L-type Ca channels in myelinated axons form clusters with ryanodine receptors, and that these channel-receptor clusters mediate damaging elevation of intracellular Ca in ischemia (Quardouz et al., 2003). Of interest, L-type Ca channels could not be detected pharmacologically in Ca image analysis of neonatal optic nerves (Sun and Chiu, 1999), suggesting that axonal L-type Ca channels are upregulated during myelinogenesis.

3. Ligand-Gated Ca Channels

Various receptors for neurotransmitters are coupled to an ion channel that exhibits significant permeability to Ca. Ligand-gated Ca channels have been extensively characterized in synapses, notable examples being the NMDA receptor, the AMPA receptor, and the nicotinic acetylcholine receptor (nAChR). Recently, nAChR receptors have been demonstrated in mammalian optic nerve axons in Ca imaging studies (Zhang et al., 2004). In axons loaded with Ca indicators, bath application of nicotine induces a robust Ca elevation in the axons (Fig. 6). The Ca elevation is abolished on removal of bath calcium, indicating that nicotine induces Ca influx into axons. The nicotine response is blocked by various nAChR antagonists including curare, suggesting that the Ca influx is receptor mediated. Further, nicotine abruptly shunts the action potential, consistent with the opening of the cationic nAChR on axons. These observations have led Zhang and co-workers (Zhang et al., 2004) to postulate the presence of functional nAChR on axons of

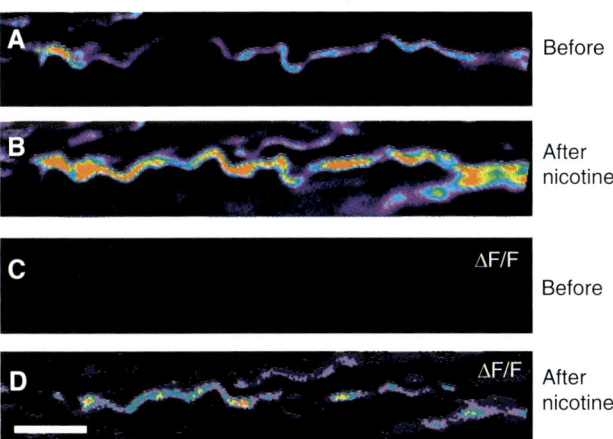

Figure 6 Calcium-permeable, nicotinic acetylcholine receptors on axons of neonatal mouse optic nerves. Axons were loaded with calcium indicators according to Fig. 4A, and pseudo-color calcium images of axons were monitored before (**A**) and after (**B**) 50 μM nicotine was bath applied. (**C**, **D**) Computed ΔF/F from images in A and B, showing the percent calcium change on a pixel-by-pixel basis. Bar is 5 μm. (Reproduced from Zhang et al., 2004, with permission.)

mouse optic nerves. Of interest, the nAChR-mediated calcium response declines as the optic nerve matures, suggesting a downregulation or masking of axonal nAChR as myelin is formed. In the neonatal nerves, repetitive stimulation causes a curare-sensitive shunting of the action potential, suggesting that acetylcholine is released during repetitive activity (Zhang et al., 2004). It is possible that part of the activity-dependent axonal Ca elevation is mediated by endogenous acetylcholine release.

B. Functions of Axonal Calcium Channels

Unlike Na and K channels, axonal Ca channels apparently are expressed at a lower density that precludes them from having a significant influence on the waveform of the action potentials. Rather, the most likely function of axonal Cav channels is a translation of nerve activity into graded axonal calcium elevation that may be relevant to axon biology. For example, Ca transients mediated by both voltage-gated and ligand-gated Ca channels might alter the dynamics of actin/cytoskeletal assembly (Bentley and O'Connor, 1994; Lankford et al., 1996) and modulate axonal elongation during development. Further, Ca ion is an important modulator of transport of axonal proteins that is crucial to structural integrity of axons (Breuer et al., 1992; Chan et al., 1980; Worth and Ochs, 1982).

C. Roles of Ca Channels in Demyelinating Diseases

Since axonal degeneration is now recognized to be a prominent feature in demyelinating diseases, Ca channels might be pathologically relevant if they predispose axons to Ca-mediated damage. There are three mechanisms by which axonal Ca influx can be modulated in demyelination: unmasking of existing Ca channels in the internode, changes in gene expression of other ion channels, and changes in gene expression of Ca channels.

1. Increased Ca Influx per Unit Length by Unmasking Ca Channels on the Internode

The diffuse staining pattern for L-type Ca channels in a mature optic nerve suggests that the channels are normally masked by the myelin (Brown et al., 2001). Demyelination will markedly increase activity-dependent Ca influx per unit axon length by unmasking these existing internodal Ca channels, potentially contributing to excitotoxity. It is possible that Ca clearance will also be compromised in demyelinated axons if they accumulate excessive Na. Na accumulation during repetitive activity has been shown to inhibit Ca clearance (Verbny et al., 2002), possibly by retardation of Ca extrusion via the Na/Ca exchanger. Figure 7A shows superimposed traces of axonal Ca elevation in a neonatal optic nerve evoked by a single and a train of 20 action potentials. Axonal Ca rises and then falls after cessation of the action

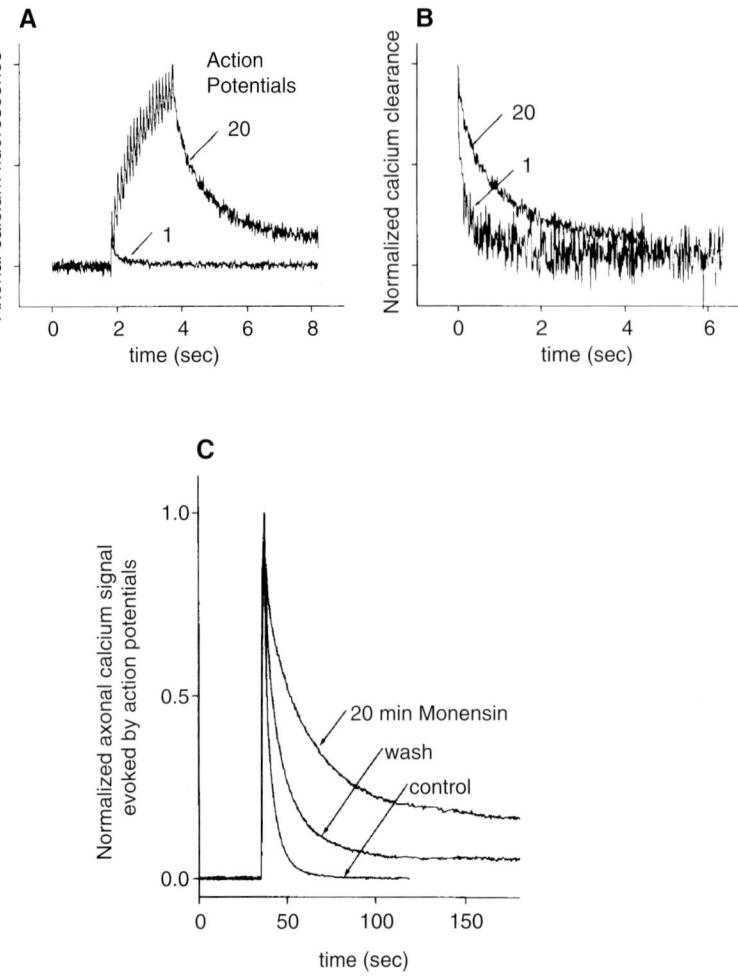

Figure 7 Coupling of calcium clearance to Na accumulation in axons of repetitively stimulated neonatal mouse optic nerves. (**A**) Axonal calcium fluorescence during a single and a train of 20 action potentials. (**B**) Normalized time course of the return of axonal calcium to the resting level following the action potentials. Note that return (i.e., calcium clearance) is slower after the 20 action potential train. (**C**) Increasing axonal Na with the Na-ionophore monensin retards the calcium clearance following action potentials. These studies suggest that activity-dependent Na accumulation in axons retards calcium clearance following repetitive action potentials. (Reproduced from Verbny et al., 2002, with permission.)

potentials. The restoration of Ca to the resting level is slower after more action potentials (Fig. 7B). This slow Ca clearance appears to be coupled to Na loading during the repetitive nerve activity, as artificially increasing axonal Na with an ionophore (monensin) also retards post-tetanus Ca clearance (Fig. 7C). Na-loading in metabolically compromised demyelinated axons will exacerbate the effect of unmasked Ca influx by retarding Ca clearance. Finally, L-type Ca channels are coupled to ryanodine receptors in clusters, and these clusters have been suggested to mediate a toxic level of Ca release from intracellular stores in ischemic axons (Quardouz et al., 2003). Whether the unmasking of L-type channels/ryanodine clusters in demyelination contributes to excitotoxcity remains to be examined.

2. Modulation of Axonal Ca Loading via Changes in Gene Expression of Other Ion Channels

Changes in gene expression of Na and K channels in demyelination could modulate Ca influx in demyelination axons. For example, upregulation of Na channels seen in some demyelinating lesions might augment Ca influx by virtue of Ca permeation through Na channels. Further, increasing Na channel expression might result in higher activity-dependent Na accumulation, thereby augmenting Ca loading via retardation of Ca extrusion (Verbny et al., 2002). Changes in K channel expression in demyelination also can indirectly regulate activity-dependent Ca influx. In general, overexpression of K channels in demyelinating diseases should be neuroprotective (by limiting activation of voltage-gated Ca channels), whereas downregulation of K channels should be pathological (by exacerbating Ca channel activation via prolonged membrane depolarization). Highly specific K channel toxins are now available to identify K channel subtypes important in modulating activity-dependent Ca influx in axons. For example, in mouse postganglionic sympathetic axon bundles, blocking Kv1.2 augments activity-dependent Ca transient (Jackson et al., 2001). Upregulation of Kv1.1/Kv1.2 in the CNS fiber tracts of the dysmyelinating mutant Shiverer mice might be neuroprotective against calcium-mediated damage (Wang et al., 1995).

3. Upregulation of Calcium Channels in Demyelination

Besides unmasking existing Ca channels, demyelination also can increase axonal Ca influx if there is an unregulation of Ca channels. Kornek and co-workers (Kornek et al., 2001) observed that N-type Ca channel immunoreactivity is nondetectable in normal adult myelinated nerves, but upregulated in multiple sclerosis and experimental autoimmune encephalomyelitis (EAE) model of demyelination. The N-type Ca channel proteins are ectopically expressed in actively demyelinating lesion sites, and the pore-forming subunit appears to be inserted onto the axolemma (Kornek et al., 2001). This article is important, because it shows for the first time that certain axonal Ca channel subtypes are upregulated in multiple sclerosis, leading to the suggestion that expression of Ca channels might contribute to axonal degeneration in inflammatory demyelinating disorders (Kornek et al., 2001). An important issue is whether the Ca channel proteins observed in the study of Kornek et al. (2001) are functional and mediate Ca influx. We have addressed this issue by measuring activity-dependent Ca transients in hypomyelinated PNS axons from the Po-over-expressor mice. Activity-dependent Ca transients are absent in normal axons, but strongly present in hypomyelinated axons, suggesting that Ca channels expressed in hypomyelinated axons are functional. Whether these Ca transients contribute to axonal degeneration in these nerves remains to be explored.

Besides voltage-gated Ca channels, ligand-gated Ca channels also might contribute to Ca-mediated axonal injury. In the mammalian optic nerves, nicotine-induced axonal Ca elevation declines as the nerve matures, suggesting a downregulation or masking of nAChR by the myelin sheath (Zhang et al., 2004). Of interest, nAChR-mediated Ca response is present in hypomyelinated axons of the Jimpy optic nerves, suggesting either an upregulation of nAChR or an unmasking of existing nAChR during demyelination. Thus, both voltage-gated and ligand-gated Ca channels are operative in demyelinated axons and potentially contribute to Ca-mediated axonal degeneration.

V. Therapeutic Treatments Targeting Ion Channels

All three axonal ion channels (Na, K, and Ca) described in this chapter are potential targets in therapeutic treatment of multiple sclerosis. Pharmacological manipulation of these three channels can produce (1) short-term neurological effects and (2) changes in glial-axon relationship that might be beneficiary for long-term functional restoration.

A. Na Channel Therapy

Na channels are needed for nerve conduction, but their overexpression in certain demyelination lesions (Westenbroek et al., 1992), while functionally compensating for conduction deficits, could produce adverse long-term Ca overload to axons (e.g., by interacting with the Na/Ca exchanger, or by Ca permeation through Na channels). In a recent study on EAE, an inflammatory model of demyelination, Nav1.6 is found to co-localize with the Na/Ca exchanger in degenerating axons labeled with β-APP (Craner et al., 2004). The idea is that Nav1.6, which has a persistent sodium current component to it (Herzog et al., 2003), interacts with the Na/Ca exchanger (driving it to run in a reverse mode to deliver Ca influx) to cause damaging Ca overload. Reducing Ca overload by Na channel blockage also blocks nerve conduction. Given that multiple Nav genes are turned on and off in neuropathy, however, it is possible that a subset of Nav gene products can be targeted to improve axonal viability with minimal negative impact on nerve conduction. For example, Na channel therapy is neuroprotective in ischemic axons. A detailed discussion of Na channel therapy in MS can be found in Chapter 7.

B. K Channel Therapy

Since K channels act as excitation brakes, blocking K channels should increase the amplitude of action potentials and promote conduction across demyelination sites. Schauf and Davis (1974) first suggested that blockage of Kv1 channels with 4-AP should increase the safety factor of conduction in demyelinated axons. This idea was later confirmed in animal models of demyelination (Bostock et al., 1981; Targ and Kocsis, 1985). This was followed by clinical trials (Stefoski et al., 1987) showing that oral dosages of 4-AP transiently improve neurological functions in multiple sclerosis patients (see Chapter 10 for more detail).

What are the mechanisms by which K channel blockage improves neurological functions? First, neurological improvement may result from restoration of nerve conduction across demyelinated regions by blocking internodal K channels. Second, besides acting on the axons, 4-AP might also improve neurological functions by modulating synaptic transmissions in multiple sclerosis. Studies have shown extensive morphological remodeling of synaptic terminals in animal models of hypomyelination. It is unclear if synaptic remodeling is accompanied by alterations in K channel expression at the nerve terminals. If K channels are upregulated at the synapse after demyelination, blocking the channels with 4-AP may facilitate neurotransmission. Another issue concerns the effect of K channel antagonists on branch points of an axonal tree. Impedance mismatch created by denuded axons at or near a branch point might be effective in blocking conduction. Computer simulations show that minor changes in local environment or morphology at a branch point have profound effects on action potential passage through the branch point. For example, a preshortening of internodes ahead of the branch point can bolster passage of high-frequency trains through the branch point (Zhou and Chiu, 2001). Blockage of Kv channels might impact nerve conduction at branch points more so than at other sites on the demyelinated nerve.

Besides acute effects on excitability, K channel blockage may lead to changes in axoglial relationship potentially resulting in long-lasting changes in nerve excitability. One reason is that glial cells express K channels, and blocking glial K channels affect glial cell mitosis and myelinogenesis (Chiu and Wilson, 1989; MacFarlane and Sontheimer, 2000a, 2000b). A novel question raised by these studies is whether normal myelinogenesis requires normal expression of glial K channels. Several provocative studies have shed light on this issue. Genetic ablation of K channels has produced hypomyelination in certain transgenic mouse models. A striking example is genetic ablation of a Kir channel (Kir4.1), which causes severe hypomyelination in the CNS axons (Neusch et al., 2001). Kir4.1 is expressed in oligodendrocytes and deleting Kir4.1 channels from oligodendrocytes results in a depolarized resting membrane potential and immature morphology in these cells (Neusch et al., 2001). Global genetic ablation of Kir2.1, the Kir species found in Schwann cells, results in early postnatal death in mice, which has prevented any study of possible perturbation on myelination (Zaritsky et al., 2000). Mutations in Kir2.1 in humans cause *Andersen's syndrome* (AS), a rare disorder characterized by periodic paralysis and cardiac arrhythmias (Andelfinger et al., 2002; Plaster et al., 2001). Whether AS patients have dysmyelination in the PNS remains unexplored. Kir2.1 channels maintain a stable resting potential that is important for cell function (Jongsma and Wilders, 2001), and it remains possible that mutation of this channel causes a deviation of the resting potential of Schwann cells to a pathological level that is compatible with normal myelination. More recently, preliminary studies in our laboratory have shown that genetically ablating Kv1.2 from the Po-overexpressor mutants improves myelination of the sciatic nerve. Since Schwann cells normally express Kv1.2 mRNA (Chiu et al., 1994), this improvement of myelination may result from forcing these cells to exit from a persistent mitotic cycle to enter myelinogenesis after Kv1.2 deletion. These various genetic studies suggest that glial K channel expression might be functionally linked to myelinogenesis, and that K channel manipulation could result in long-term changes in myelinogenesis with major impact on excitability.

C. Ca Channel Therapy

Ca channel antagonists are neuroprotective in ischemic white matter (see Chapter 29). Might Ca antagonists prove useful in multiple sclerosis, particularly in light of the upregulation of Ca channels in certain demyelination models? Early clinical trials treating MS patients with the Ca channel blocker verapamil have produced inconclusive results (Komoly et al., 1986; Gilmore et al., 1985). This issue is now being revisited in several laboratories as the Ca channel subtypes on axons are increasingly being clarified. Most of the current studies on Ca antagonists focus on nimodipine, which easily penetrates the blood-brain barrier and is known to exert both CNS and PNS effects (Bar et al., 1990). In a recent in vivo study, the effects of nimodipine on nerve regeneration and functional recovery were examined in mice after intracranial facial nerve crush. Several important results emerged (Mattsson et al., 2001). First, nimodipine accelerates the time course of functional recovery measured by analysis of vibrissae movement and induces increased numbers and sizes of remyelinated axons during the recovery. Second, nimodipine intriguingly enlarges the axons and myelin sheaths in normal, uncrushed nerves. Are Ca antagonists effective in demyelination models? Based on the upregulation of N-type Ca channels in certain demyelination models, this particular Ca channel subtype becomes the target of two recent studies. In one study, administering N-type Ca channel blockers reduces disease severity in EAE models of demyelination in mice (Smith et al., 2003). In the other study, induction of EAE in N-type Ca channel knockout mice produces less severe neurological symptoms than when EAE was induced in wild-type mice (Tokuhara et al., 2003). The conclusion from these two preliminary studies is that antagonizing a Ca channel subtype that is upregulated in demyelinating diseases is beneficial. The most important issue is a mechanistic one: How might Ca antagonists improve neurological functions in demyelinating diseases? One possibility is that it attenuates axonal degeneration by inhibiting Ca influx through voltage-gated Ca channels. The other possibility is that some of these Ca antagonists can actually improve the Ca buffering capacity of neurons. For example, various Ca-binding proteins (parvalbumin, S-100, and calbindin-D28K) are upregulated by nimodipine (Buwalda et al., 1994). The mechanism for the augmentation of Ca buffering capacity by nimodipine remains unclear, but it may be related to inhibition of Ca influx and the consequential downstream effect on gene expression of the Ca binding proteins. Treatments that block Ca channels or produce long-lasting enhancement of axonal Ca buffering capacity might be neuroprotective in multiple sclerosis.

VI. Conclusion

This chapter discusses three major classes of ion channels on axons of mammalian myelinated fibers and their roles in normal axons and pathological axons in multiple sclerosis (MS). The first class of ion channel is Na channels. These channels are clustered at a normal node of Ranvier and provide the primary trigger for a normal nerve impulse. Na channels are pathologically relevant in MS in three ways: their deficiency in the internodes contributes to conduction block, their plasticity in gene expression contributes to abnormal firing patterns in MS, and their linkage to Ca homeostasis might contribute to Ca-mediated axonal injury. Clever targeting of certain Na channel subtypes in MS could simultaneously restore normal excitability and achieve neuroprotection. The second class of ion channel is K channels. Most of the axonal K channels are sealed by myelin in a normal nerve, and the best functional analysis has been carried out for the juxtaparanodal Kv1.1 using transgenic mice. Gene knockout studies suggest that juxtaparanodal Kv1 channels stabilize action potential propagation through transition zones of an axonal tree, probably through maintaining a normal resting potential that is particularly important in transition zones than the rest of the axon. Unmasking of internodal Kv channels contributes to conduction block, and pharmacological manipulation of Kv channels can restore nerve conduction across demyelinated lesions. The third class of axonal ion channel is Ca channels. Both voltage-gated and ligand-gated Ca channels are present on myelinated and demyelinated axons. The normal physiological roles of axonal Ca channels remain unclear, but they may translate nerve activity into graded axonal Ca elevation that can drive various processes including axonal elongation and axonal transport. Axonal Ca channels are relevant in MS because augmented Ca influx through these channels, either resulting from unmasking of existing channels or upregulation of certain Ca channel subtype, might be excitotoxic. Recent preliminary results on the beneficial role of Ca antagonists in various animal models of demyelination suggest that a supplementary Ca channel therapy should be considered with other treatments.

Acknowledgments

Work in the author's laboratory was supported by grants from the National Institute of Health, the National Multiple Sclerosis Society, and a Pew Scholar Award in the Biomedical Sciences.

References

Andelfinger, G., Tapper, A. R., Welch, R. C., Vanoye, C. G., George, A. L., Jr., and Benson, D. W. (2002). KCNJ2 mutation results in Andersen syndrome with sex-specific cardiac and skeletal muscle phenotypes. *Am. J. Hum. Genet.* **71**, 663–668.

Baker, M., Bostock, H., Grafe, P., and Martius, P. (1987). Function and distribution of three types of rectifying channel in rat spinal root myelinated axons. *J. Physiol.* **383**, 45–67.

Bar, P. R., Traber, J., Schuurman, T., and Gispen, W. H. (1990). CNS and PNS effects of nimodipine. *J. Neural Transm. Suppl.* **31**, 55–71.

Bentley, D., and O'Connor, T. P. (1994). Cytoskeletal events in growth cone steering. *Curr. Opin. Neurobiol.* **4**, 43–48.

Boiko, T., Rasband, M. N., Levinson, S. R., Caldwell, J. H., Mandel, G., Trimmer, J. S., and Matthews, G. (2001). Compact myelin dictates the differential targeting of two sodium channel isoforms in the same axon. *Neuron* **30**, 91–104.

Bostock, H., Sears, T. A., and Sherratt, R. M. (1981). The effects of 4-aminopyridine and tetraethylammonium ions on normal and demyelinated mammalian nerve fibres. *J. Physiol.* **313**, 301–315.

Breuer, A. C., Bond, M., and Atkinson, M. B. (1992). Fast axonal transport is modulated by altering trans-axolemmal calcium flux. *Cell Calcium* **13**, 249–262.

Brew, H. M., Hallows, J. L., and Tempel, B. L. (2003). Hyperexcitability and reduced low threshold potassium currents in auditory neurons of mice lacking the channel subunit Kv1.1. *J. Physiol.* **548**, 1–20.

Brismar, T. (1980). Potential clamp analysis of membrane currents in rat myelinated nerve fibres. *J. Physiol.* **298**, 171–184.

Brown, A. M., Westenbroek, R. E., Catterall, W. A., and Ransom, B. R. (2001). Axonal L-type Ca2+ channels and anoxic injury in rat CNS white matter. *J. Neurophysiol.* **85**, 900–911.

Buwalda, B., Naber, R., Nyakas, C., and Luiten, P. G. (1994). Nimodipine accelerates the postnatal development of parvalbumin and S-100 beta immunoreactivity in the rat brain. *Brain Res. Dev. Brain Res.* **78**, 210–216.

Chan, S. Y., Ochs, S., and Worth, R. M. (1980). The requirement for calcium ions and the effect of other ions on axoplasmic transport in mammalian nerve. *J. Physiol.* **301**, 477–504.

Chiu, S. Y. (1980). Asymmetry currents in the mammalian myelinated nerve. *J. Physiol.* **309**, 499-519.

Chiu, S. Y. (1982). Resting potential of a frog myelinated axon: The role of the internode. *Asbtr. Soc. Neurosci.* **8**, 253.

Chiu, S. Y., and Ritchie, J. M. (1980). Potassium channels in nodal and internodal axonal membrane of mammalian myelinated fibres. *Nature* **284**, 170–171.

Chiu, S. Y., and Ritchie, J. M. (1981). Evidence for the presence of potassium channels in the paranodal region of acutely demyelinated mammalian single nerve fibres. *J. Physiol.* **313**, 415–437.

Chiu, S. Y., and Ritchie, J. M. (1984). On the physiological role of internodal potassium channels and the security of conduction in myelinated nerve fibres. *Proc. R. Soc. Lond B Biol. Sci.* **220**, 415–422.

Chiu, S. Y., Ritchie, J. M., Rogart, R. B., and Stagg, D. (1979). A quantitative description of membrane currents in rabbit myelinated nerve. *J. Physiol.* **292**, 149–166.

Chiu, S. Y., Scherer, S. S., Blonski, M., Kang, S. S., and Messing, A. (1994). Axons regulate the expression of Shaker-like potassium channel genes in Schwann cells in peripheral nerve. *Glia* **12**, 1–11.

Chiu, S. Y., and Wilson, G. F. (1989). The role of potassium channels in Schwann cell proliferation in Wallerian degeneration of explant rabbit sciatic nerves. *J. Physiol. (London)* **408**, 199–222.

Chiu, S. Y., Zhou, L., Zhang, C. L., and Messing, A. (1999). Analysis of potassium channel functions in mammalian axons by gene knockouts. *J. Neurocytol.* **28**, 349–364.

Craner, M. J., Hains, B. C., Lo, A. C., Black, J. A., and Waxman, S. G. (2004). Co-localization of sodium channel Nav1.6 and the sodium-calcium exchanger at sites of axonal injury in the spinal cord in EAE. *Brain* **127**, 294–303.

Devaux, J., Alcaraz, G., Grinspan, J., Bennett, V., Joho, R., Crest, M., and Scherer, S. S. (2003). Kv3.1b is a novel component of CNS nodes. *J. Neurosci.* **23**, 4509–4518.

Fern, R., Ransom, B. R., and Waxman, S. G. (1995a). Voltage-gated calcium channels in CNS white matter: role in anoxic injury. *J. Neurophysiol.* **74**, 369–377.

Fern, R., Waxman, S. G., and Ransom, B. R. (1995b). Endogenous GABA attenuates CNS white matter dysfunction following anoxia. *J. Neurosci.* **15**, 699–708.

Gabso, M., Neher, E., and Spira, M. E. (1997). Low mobility of the Ca2+ buffers in axons of cultured Aplysia neurons. *Neuron* **18**, 473–481.

Gilmore, R. L., Kasarskis, E. J., and McAllister, R. G. (1985). Verapamil-induced changes in central conduction in patients with multiple sclerosis. *J. Neurol. Neurosurg. Psychiatry* **48**, 1140–1146.

Goldin, A. L. (1999). Diversity of mammalian voltage-gated sodium channels. *Ann. NY Acad. Sci.* **868**, 38–50.

Goldin, A. L., Barchi, R. L., Caldwell, J. H., Hofmann, F., Howe, J. R., Hunter, J. C., Kallen, R. G., Mandel, G., Meisler, M. H., Netter, Y. B., Noda, M., Tamkun, M. M., Waxman, S. G., Wood, J. N., and Catterall, W. A. (2000). Nomenclature of voltage-gated sodium channels. *Neuron* **28**, 365–368.

Goldstein, S. A., Bockenhauer, D., O'Kelly, I., and Zilberberg, N. (2001). Potassium leak channels and the KCNK family of two-P-domain subunits. *Nat. Rev. Neurosci.* **2**, 175–184.

Herson, P. S., Virk, M., Rustay, N. R., Bond, C. T., Crabbe, J. C., Adelman, J. P., and Maylie, J. (2003). A mouse model of episodic ataxia type-1. *Nat. Neurosci.* **6**, 378–383.

Herzog, R. I., Cummins, T. R., Ghassemi, F., Dib-Hajj, S. D., and Waxman, S. G. (2003). Distinct repriming and closed-state inactivation kinetics of Nav1.6 and Nav1.7 sodium channels in mouse spinal sensory neurons. *J. Physiol.* **551**, 741–750.

Hille, B. (2001). "Ionic Channels of Excitable Membranes." Sinauer, Sunderland, MA.

Hodgkin, A. L., and Huxley, A. F. (1952). A quantitative description of membrane current and its application to conduction and excitation in nerve. *J. Physiol. (London)* **115**, 500.

Hopkins, W. F., Allen, M. L., Houamed, K. M., and Tempel, B. L. (1994). Properties of voltage-gated K+ currents expressed in Xenopus oocytes by mKv1.1, mKv1.2 and their heteromultimers as revealed by mutagenesis of the dendrotoxin-binding site in mKv1.1. *Pflugers Arch.* **428**, 382–390.

Jackson, V. M., Trout, S. J., Brain, K. L., and Cunnane, T. C. (2001). Characterization of action potential-evoked calcium transients in mouse postganglionic sympathetic axon bundles. *J. Physiol.* **537**, 3–16.

Jan, L. Y., and Jan, Y. N. (1997). Cloned potassium channels from eukaryotes and prokaryotes. *Annu. Rev. Neurosci.* **20**, 91–123.

Jiang, Y., Ruta, V., Chen, J., Lee, A., and MacKinnon, R. (2003). The principle of gating charge movement in a voltage-dependent K+ channel. *Nature* **423**, 42–48.

Jongsma, H. J., and Wilders, R. (2001). Channelopathies: Kir2.1 mutations jeopardize many cell functions. *Curr. Biol.* **11**, R747–R750.

Khodorov, B. I., and Timin, E. N. (1975). Nerve impulse propagation along nonuniform fibres. *Prog. Biophys. Mol. Biol.* **30**, 145–184.

Komoly, S., Jakab, G., and Fazekas, A. (1986). Multiple sclerosis: failure of treatment with verapamil in a pilot trial. *J. Neurol.* **233**, 59–60.

Kopp-Scheinpflug, C., Fuchs, K., Lippe, W. R., Tempel, B. L., and Rubsamen, R. (2003). Decreased temporal precision of auditory signaling in Kcna1-null mice: An electrophysiological study in vivo. *J. Neurosci.* **23**, 9199–9207.

Kornek, B., Storch, M. K., Bauer, J., Djamshidian, A., Weissert, R., Wallstroem, E., Stefferl, A., Zimprich, F., Olsson, T., Linington, C., Schmidbauer, M., and Lassmann, H. (2001). Distribution of a calcium

channel subunit in dystrophic axons in multiple sclerosis and experimental autoimmune encephalomyelitis. *Brain* **124**, 1114–1124.

Lankford, K. L., Kenney, A. M., and Kocsis, J. D. (1996). Cellular mechanisms regulating neurite initiation. *Prog. Brain Res.* **108**, 55–81.

MacFarlane, S. N., and Sontheimer, H. (2000a). Changes in ion channel expression accompany cell cycle progression of spinal cord astrocytes. *Glia* **30**, 39–48.

MacFarlane, S. N., and Sontheimer, H. (2000b). Modulation of Kv1.5 currents by Src tyrosine phosphorylation: Potential role in the differentiation of astrocytes. *J. Neurosci.* **20**, 5245–5253.

MacKinnon, R. (2003). Potassium channels. *FEBS Lett.* **555**, 62–65.

Maingret, F., Lauritzen, I., Patel, A. J., Heurteaux, C., Reyes, R., Lesage, F., Lazdunski, M., and Honore, E. (2000). TREK-1 is a heat-activated background K(+) channel. *EMBO J.* **19**, 2483–2491.

Mattson, P., Janson, A. M., Aldskogins, H., and Svensson, M. (2001). Nimodipine promotes regeneration and functional recovery after intercranial facial nerve crush. *J. Comp. Neurol.* **437**, 106–117.

Neusch, C., Rozengurt, N., Jacobs, R. E., Lester, H. A., and Kofuji, P. (2001). Kir4.1 potassium channel subunit is crucial for oligodendrocyte development and in vivo myelination. *J. Neurosci.* **21**, 5429–5438.

Pfeiffer, G., and Friede, R. L. (1985). A morphometric study of nerve fiber atrophy in rat spinal roots. *J. Neuropathol. Exp. Neurol.* **44**, 546–558.

Plaster, N. M., Tawil, R., Tristani-Firouzi, M., Canun, S., Bendahhou, S., Tsunoda, A., Donaldson, M. R., Iannaccone, S. T., Brunt, E., Barohn, R., Clark, J., Deymeer, F., George, A. L., Fish, F. A., Hahn, A., Nitu, A., Ozdemir, C., Serdaroglu, P., Subramony, S. H., Wolfe, G., Fu, Y. H., and Ptácek, L. J. (2001). Mutations in Kir2.1 cause the developmental and episodic electrical phenotypes of Andersen's syndrome. *Cell* **105**, 511–519.

Poliak, S., Salomon, D., Elhanany, H., Sabanay, H., Kiernan, B., Pevny, L., Stewart, C. L., Xu, X., Chiu, S. Y., Shrager, P., Furley, A. J., and Peles, E. (2003). Juxtaparanodal clustering of Shaker-like K+ channels in myelinated axons depends on Caspr2 and TAG-1. *J. Cell Biol.* **162**, 1149–1160.

Quardouz, M., Nikolaeva, M. A., Coderre, E., Zamponi, G. W., McRory, J. E., Trapp, B. D., Yin, X., Wang, W., Woulfe, J., and Stys, P. K. (2003). Depolarization-induced Ca2+ release in ischemic spinal cord white matter involves L-type Ca2+ channel activation of ryanodine receptors. *Neuron* **40**, 53–63.

Quick, D. C., Kennedy, W. R., and Donaldson, L. (1979). Dimensions of myelinated nerve fibers near the motor and sensory terminals in cat tenuissimus muscles. *Neuroscience* **4**, 1089–1096.

Rasband, M. N., and Trimmer, J. S. (2001). Developmental clustering of ion channels at and near the node of Ranvier [Review]. *Dev. Biol.* **236**, 5–16.

Ritchie, J. M., and Rogart, R. B. (1977). Density of sodium channels in mammalian myelinated nerve fibers and nature of the axonal membrane under the myelin sheath. *Proc. Natl. Acad. Sci. U. S. A.* **74**, 211–215.

Rosenbluth, J. (1976). Intramembranous particle distribution at the node of Ranvier and adjacent axolemma in myelinated axons of the frog brain. *J. Neurocytol.* **5**, 731–745.

Rudy, B., and McBain, C. J. (2001). Kv3 channels: voltage-gated K+ channels designed for high-frequency repetitive firing. *Trends Neurosci.* **24**, 517–526.

Rushton, W. A. H. (1951). A theory of the effects of fibre size in medullated nerve. *J. Physiol.* **115**, 101–122.

Sabatini, B. L., Maravall, M., and Svoboda, K. (2001). Ca(2+) signaling in dendritic spines. *Curr. Opin. Neurobiol.* **11**, 349–356.

Schauf, C. L., and Davis, F. A. (1974). Impulse conduction in multiple sclerosis: a theoretical basis for modification by temperature and pharmacological agents. *J. Neurol. Neurosurg. Psychiatry* **37**, 152–161.

Schwarz, J. R., Reid, G., and Bostock, H. (1995). Action potentials and membrane currents in the human node of Ranvier. *Pflugers Arch.* **430**, 283–292.

Smart, S. L., Lopantsev, V., Zhang, C. L., Robbins, C. A., Wang, H., Chiu, S. Y., Schwartzkroin, P. A., Messing, A., and Tempel, B. L. (1998).

Deletion of the Kv1.1 potassium channel causes epilepsy in mice. *Neuron* **20**, 809–819.

Smith, T., Groom, A., Rivers, L., Barden, L., Yamauchi, T., Niidome, T., Limura, Y., Nishizawa, Y., and Yamanishi, Y. (2003). The N-type calcium channel antagonists E2050 and ER-129002-02 ameliorate experimental autoimmune encephalomyelitis (EAE). *Society of Neuroscience* **214**, 7.

Spencer, P. S., Raine, C. S., and Wisniewski, H. (1973). Axon diameter and myelin thickness. Unusual relationships in dorsal root ganglia. *Anatomical Record* **176**, 225–243.

Stefoski, D., Davis, F. A., Faut, M., and Schauf, C. L. (1987). 4-Aminopyridine improves clinical signs in multiple sclerosis. *Ann. Neurol.* **21**, 71–77.

Stys, P. K., Ransom, B. R., Black, J. A., and Waxman, S. G. (1995). Anoxic/ischemic injury in axons. *In* "The Axon: Structure, Function, and Pathophysiology" (S. G. Waxman, J. D. Kocsis, and P. K. Stys, eds.) pp. 464–479. Oxford University Press, New York.

Sun, B. B., and Chiu, S. Y. (1999). N-type calcium channels and their regulation by GABA(B) receptors in axons of neonatal rat optic nerve. *J. Neurosci.* **19**, 5185–5194.

Swadlow, H. A., Kocsis, J. D., and Waxman, S. G. (1980). Modulation of impulse conduction along the axonal tree. *Annu. Rev. Biophys. Bioeng.* **9**, 143–179.

Targ, E. F., and Kocsis, J. D. (1985). 4-Aminopyridine leads to restoration of conduction in demyelinated rat sciatic nerve. *Brain Res.* **328**, 358–361.

Tokuhara, N., Yamauchi, T., Ohgoh, M., Hanada, T., Takahashi, E., Miyamoto, N., and Niidome, T. (2003). Experimental autoimmune encephalomyelitis in N-type calcium channel knockout mice. *Society for Neuroscience* **214**, 8.

Verbny, Y., Zhang, C. L., and Chiu, S. Y. (2002). Coupling of calcium homeostasis to axonal sodium in axons of mouse optic nerve. *J. Neurophysiol.* **88**, 802–816.

Wang, H., Allen, M. L., Grigg, J. J., Noebels, J. L., and Tempel, B. L. (1995). Hypomyelination alters K$^+$ channel expression in mouse mutants *Shiverer* and *Trembler*. *Neuron* **15**, 1337–1347.

Wang, H., Kunkel, D. D., Martin, T. M., Schwartzkroin, P. A., and Tempel, B. L. (1993). Heteromultimeric K$^+$ channels in terminal and juxtaparanodal regions of neurons. *Nature* **365**, 75–79.

Waxman, S. G. (1972). Regional differentiation of the axon: a review with special reference to the concept of the multiplex neuron. *Brain Res.* **47**, 269–288.

Waxman, S. G., and Brill, M. H. (1978). Conduction through demyelinated plaques in multiple sclerosis: computer simulations of facilitation by short internodes. *J. Neurol. Neurosurg. Psychiatry* **41**, 408–416.

Westenbroek, R. E., Noebels, J. L., and Catterall, W. A. (1992). Elevated expression of type II Na$^+$ channels in hypomyelinated axons of *shiverer* mouse brain. *J. Neurosci.* **12**, 2259–2267.

Worth, R. M., and Ochs, S. (1982). Dependence of batrachotoxin block of axoplasmic transport on sodium. *J. Neurobiol.* **13**, 537–549.

Zaritsky, J. J., Eckman, D. M., Wellman, G. C., Nelson, M. T., and Schwarz, T. L. (2000). Targeted disruption of Kir2.1 and Kir2.2 genes reveals the essential role of the inwardly rectifying K(+) current in K(+)-mediated vasodilation. [see comments]. *Circ. Res.* **87**, 160–166.

Zhang, C. L., Messing, A., and Chiu, S. Y. (1999). Specific alteration of spontaneous GABAergic inhibition in cerebellar Purkinje cells in mice lacking the potassium channel Kv1.1. *J. Neurosci.* **19**, 2852–2864.

Zhang, C. L., Verbny, Y., Malek, S. A., Stys, P. K., and Chiu, S. Y. (2004). Nicotinic acetylcholine receptors in mouse and rat optic nerves. *J. Neurophysiol.* **91**, 1025–1035.

Zhou, L., and Chiu, S. Y. (2001). Computer model for action potential propagation through branch point in myelinated nerves. *J. Neurophysiol.* **85**, 197–210.

Zhou, L., Messing, A., and Chiu, S. Y. (1999). Determinants of excitability at transition zones in Kv1.1-deficient myelinated nerves. *J. Neurosci.* **19**, 5768–5781.

Zhou, L., Zhang, C. L., Messing, A., and Chiu, S. Y. (1998). Temperature-sensitive neuromuscular transmission in Kv1.1 null mice: role of potassium channels under the myelin sheath in young nerves. *J. Neurosci.* **18**, 7200–7215.

6

The Conduction Properties of Demyelinated and Remyelinated Axons

Kenneth J. Smith, Ph.D.
Stephen G. Waxman, M.D., Ph.D.

I. Introduction

Although demyelination is an event that primarily affects the myelinating glial cell, the important consequences of demyelination are imposed first on the axon in the form of disturbed impulse conduction, and thence on the individual in terms of symptoms. Indeed, many of the conduction deficits resulting from demyelination can be mapped directly to the expression of different forms of neurological deficit in patients with multiple sclerosis (MS).

In broad outline, demyelination first results in reduced excitability of axons so that conduction block is the dominant electrophysiological feature. This block results in the expression of "negative" symptoms, namely loss of function result-ing in deficits such as blindness, paralysis, and numbness. During the next few weeks the axon adapts to its demyelinated state, resulting in a gradual increase in excitability and then, if conditions are favorable, conduction through the demyelination lesion may be restored. Where this occurs, it will contribute to clinical recovery and the remission of the negative symptoms, although conduction remains insecure and some residual deficits may persist. Some axons may become hyperexcitable, resulting in the expression of "positive" symptoms such as tingling sensation or pain. Repair of the axons by remyelination, when and if this occurs, results in the restoration of relatively normal conduction properties and the resolution of symptoms; however, some neurological deficit may persist if many axons degenerate. This chapter details the changing electrophysiological properties of axons as they undergo demyelination and remyelination.

Although demyelination has profound effects on axonal function, in most lesions the occurrence of demyelination has no detectable consequences for the patient because the lesions may occur in clinically "silent" areas of the brain where even the local complete destruction of nerve tissue does not produce symptoms. However, in clinically "eloquent" areas, such as the optic nerves or motor pathways, even a physically small lesion can have major consequences for the patient, causing profound neurological deficits.

Development of a lesion in such a pathway can produce a clinical relapse. The form of the relapse (e.g., whether it is sensory or motor) and the modality or body part affected are determined directly by the location of the lesion and thus by the axons affected. The occurrence of lesions with similar pathology in silent areas of the brain, even if the lesions are large, would be overlooked by both patient and physician during life, in the absence of imaging. In fact, the physical changes to the structure of the nerve fiber imposed by demyelination and remyelination are not the only events that result directly in neurological deficits in patients with MS, and factors associated with inflammation can also impair conduction. In Chapter 18, we document the consequences of exposing axons to the inflammatory mediator nitric oxide.

II. Conduction Properties of Demyelinated Axons

A. Conduction Block

Demyelination markedly impairs axonal function, and the complete loss of myelin over a single internode (segmental demyelination) is more than sufficient to block conduction completely. Indeed, even myelin thinning along the internode can be sufficient to cause conduction failure, and failure is especially likely if an equivalent quantity of myelin is lost from the paranodes, resulting in widening of the nodal gap (see later). Conduction block is often the dominant electrophysiological feature of experimental demyelinating lesions, and the block occurs specifially at the site of the lesion; the other parts of the axon appear to retain normal conduction properties (McDonald, 1963). We shall see later that demyelinated axons can regain the ability to conduct, but conduction block is favored (indeed, it appears to be mandatory) in freshly segmentally demyelinated axons. Although some computer simulations suggest that conduction can occur in newly segmentally demyelinated axons (see also Waxman et al., 1989), our experience in the laboratory suggests that such an event is rare, if it occurs at all. Certainly it is routine to find that conduction is blocked for several days following segmental demyelination (McDonald and Sears, 1970; Smith et al., 1979), a fact that probably derives from the initial paucity of sodium channels in the freshly exposed internodal axolemma (Waxman, 1977; Ritchie and Rogart, 1977).

B. Nodal Widening

Sometimes demyelination does not involve the whole internode, but only the paranodes, resulting in widening of the nodal gap. As noted previously, nodal widening is sufficient to block conduction (Gilliatt, 1982; Lu et al., 2000; Sumner et al., 1982), in agreement with predictions made by computer modeling (Koles and Rasminsky, 1972; Bostock, 1994; Chiu and Ritchie, 1981).

An increased nodal gap can block conduction because the loss of the myelin means that the local current generated by the driving node (i.e., the last intact node before the demyelinated region) is now dispersed across a much wider area of axonal membrane than normal, and, in particular, the nodal capacitance is greatly increased. Cell membranes, such as the axolemma, have a significant capacitance as they are very thin, and this capacitance has to be discharged as the axon is depolarized. The nodal capacitance is effectively determined by the area of the denuded axolemma, and so demyelination can dramatically increase nodal capacitance, thereby increasing the amount of local current required to depolarize the membrane to its firing threshold (Smith, 1994; Hille, 1992; Bostock, 1984; Waxman and Brill, 1978). The dispersal of the current and the increase in capacitance both serve to reduce the safety factor for conduction (see later).

C. Restoration of Conduction to Demyelinated Axons in the Absence of Remyelination

Although conduction is initially blocked by segmental demyelination, the block is not necessarily permanent. The loss of the myelin triggers a series of adaptive responses in the axon, including changes in the ion channel population along the demyelinated membrane (see Chapters 7 and 8). If several conditions are favorable, these changes can result in the restoration of conduction. In peripheral axons, conduction can be restored within only a week of the initiation of demyelination (Smith et al., 1982; Smith and Hall, 1980), although restoration often takes longer in central axons (e.g., 2 to 3 weeks after lesion induction) (Smith et al., 1981). The presence of conduction in demyelinated axons was first proven in elegant experiments that examined conduction along rat spinal roots experimentally demyelinated with diphtheria toxin (Bostock and Sears, 1978). A sophisticated recording technique revealed that the action potential crossed the demyelinated region by reverting from the normal saltatory mode of conduction, exhibited along the myelinated portion of the axon, to a slow, continuous (see later) mode of conduction along the demyelinated axolemma; saltatory conduction was resumed along the normal tissue on the other side of the lesion. Subsequent experiments revealed that conduction along axons demyelinated by the action of lysolecithin proceeded not in a continuous manner, but rather by adopting a microsaltatory mode of conduction (Smith et al., 1982), perhaps reflecting the organization of sodium channels into new nodelike foci, termed phi-nodes. These foci occurred along the demyelinated axolemma every 100 to 400 μm (mean, 255 μm) and were probably formed in preparation for remyelination.

That conduction could occur in central demyelinated axons was proven in a study where the conduction properties of single axons passing through demyelinated lesions were determined electrophysiologically, and then the axons were labeled so that they could be identified and reconstructed in three dimensions at the electron microscope level (Fig. 1) (Felts et al., 1997). This study established that conduction could occur along central demyelinated axons in which several internodes of myelin had been lost, and in the proven absence of any repair by remyelination (Felts et al., 1997). Furthermore, the demyelinated central axons were able to conduct even when at least 88% of their surface area

was deprived of glial contacts for several internodes; glial ensheathment, even without myelin formation, is likely to aid conduction by affecting the passive cable properties of the axons (Shrager and Rubinstein, 1990). Thus conduction may be possible even in "open" MS lesions (Barnes et al., 1991), where there is a paucity of glial processes and a greatly expanded extracellular space.

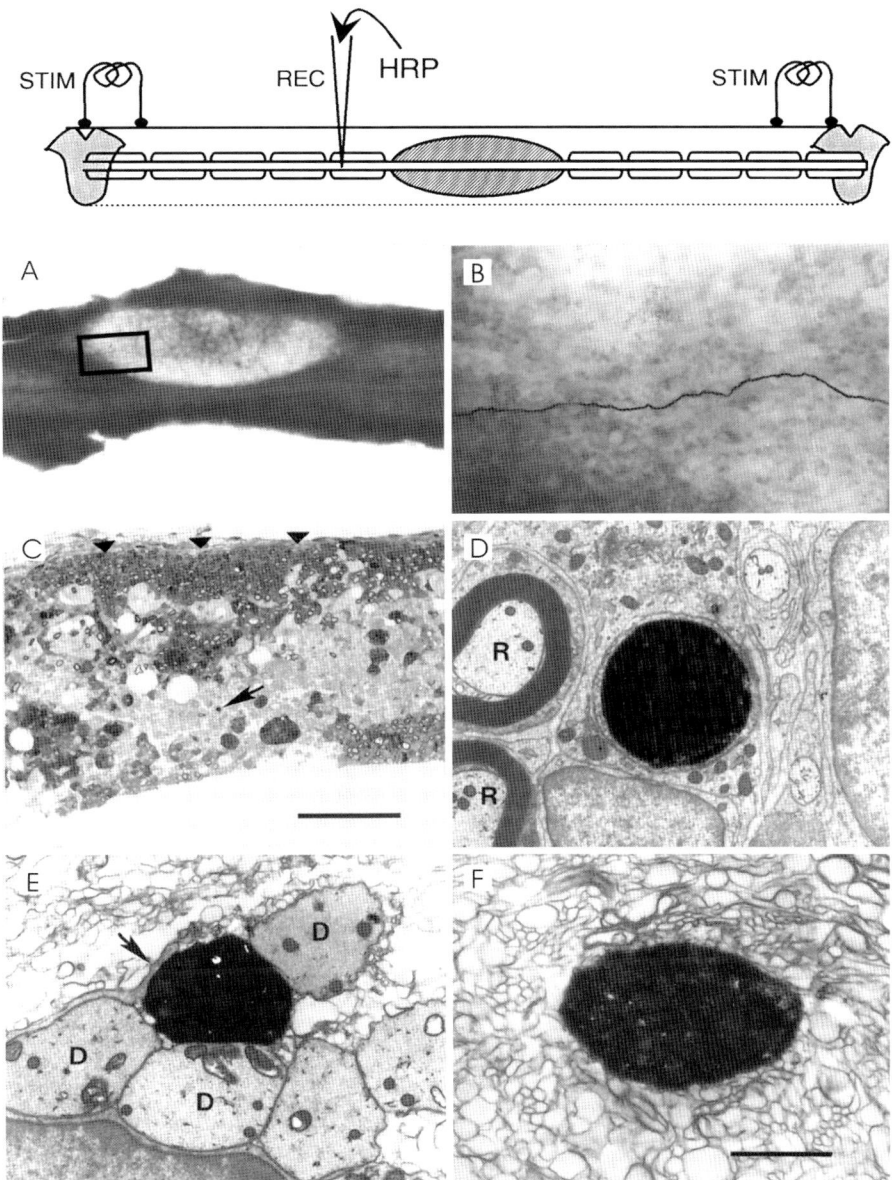

Figure 1 **Correlating the electrophysiological and ultrastructural properties of A** l The ultrastructural description of a central demyelinated axon with known conduction properties. Recordings from the axon (*diagram*) revealed that it conducted through the lesion with a slow velocity and prolonged refractory period for transmission. The axon was labeled by the iontophoresis of horseradish peroxidase (HRP) so that it could later be identified microscopically. Longitudinal sections through the lesion (**A**) allowed the identification of the labeled axon (**B**), the only axon in the tissue for which the conduction properties were known. Transverse sections through the axon (**C–F**) were studied at different locations taken over several millimeters, using light (**C**) and electron (**D–F**) microscopy. The axon passed through regions where it was demyelinated but ensheathed by a Schwann cell (**D**, two adjacent axons are remyelinated), or demyelinated and largely (**E**) or entirely (**F**) free of glial processes. The axon is embedded in vesicular myelin debris in **F.** (Reproduced modified from Felts et al., 1997.)

It seems reasonable to believe that the restoration of conduction to demyelinated axons will tend to reverse symptoms imposed by demyelination-induced conduction block, and so to believe that the restoration may make an important contribution to remissions. The presence of conduction in demyelinated axons can also explain the observation that large, but clinically "silent" (i.e., asymptomatic) demyelinating lesions can occur in patients in pathways where symptoms may have been expected (Wisniewski et al., 1976; Ghatak et al., 1974; Phadke and Best, 1983).

D. Changes in the Distribution and Expression of Ion Channels

The restoration of conduction to demyelinated axons involves substantial remodeling of the demyelinated axolemma at the molecular level. The nature of these changes is becoming clearer with the advent of suitable antibodies for immunohistochemistry, and it is now possible, for example, to view the exquisite precision with which Nav1.6 sodium channels are segregated at nodes of Ranvier (Fig. 2) (Arroyo and Scherer, 2000; Caldwell et al., 2000; Black et al., 2002). Earlier morphological evidence that sodium channel density can increase in demyelinated axons (Foster et al., 1980; England et al., 1991) reviewed in (Kazarinova-Noyes and Shrager, 2002) has been augmented by the discovery that two different isoforms of voltage-sensitive sodium channels, Nav1.2 and Nav1.6, become expressed along demyelinated axons (Craner et al., 2003)., this volume (see also Chapter 7).

E. Persistence of Conduction Block

Although conduction can be restored to demyelinated axons, conduction block remains a common feature of such axons. Whether conduction is restored in practice depends

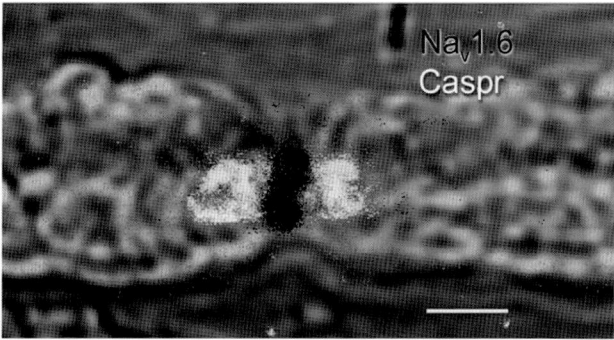

Figure 2 Clustering of Nav1.6 sodium channels at a node of Ranvier. The Nav1.6 channels (*black*) are flanked by Caspr (a constituent of the paranodal axoglial junction; *white*) without significant overlap. This flourescent image of a node after immunostaining for Nav1.6 and Caspr was merged with a differential interference image to show the myelin on either side of the node. (Modified from Black et al., 2002.)

on a number of factors. Factors favoring the persistence of conduction block include a large axon diameter (Bostock and Sears, 1978; Waxman, 1989); a long internode preceding the demyelinated region (especially if the internode is partially demyelinated) (Waxman and Brill, 1978; Shrager and Rubinstein, 1990; Bostock, 1994); a long overall length of demyelination (e.g., many internodes lost); the dysregulation of the composition of the extracellular fluid due, for example, to failure of the blood-brain barrier; the presence of factors deleterious for conduction such as nitric oxide and other factors associated with inflammation (Redford et al., 1997); the absence of any glial ensheathment (Shrager and Rubinstein, 1990); a short period of time elapsed since the occurrence of demyelination; a recent (seconds/minutes) history of sustained impulse conduction (see later); an inopportune composition of ion channels and pumps along the demyelinated axolemma, perhaps theoretically influenced by genetic background; and a warm body temperature (see later). Some of these points deserve further comment, and with regard to axon diameter, it is known that conduction can occur in demyelinated axons as large as 5.5 μm in diameter (Felts et al., 1997). As most demyelinated axons are smaller than this, especially in the central nervous system (CNS), it seems likely that most peripheral and central demyelinated axons should be capable of conduction if conditions are optimal. Also with regard to the preceding list, a long internode before the demyelinated region impedes the depolarization of the demyelinated axolemma by reducing the local current available at this site due to capacitative and resistive loss over the internode (Fig. 3). Even limited remyelination at the margin of an otherwise demyelinated lesion can therefore be expected to promote the restoration of conduction along the axon, as remyelinated internodes are short. Glial ensheathment is probably beneficial to conduction even in the absence of myelin formation as, even apart from any passive electrical benefit conferred by the apposition of glial membranes, glial contacts can be associated with morphological evidence of nodelike axolemmal specializations suggestive of increased excitability (Blakemore and Smith, 1983; Rosenbluth et al., 1985). It is likely that the efficacy of the repair process could vary over time (Black and Waxman, 1996).

Given this list of reasons why conduction may fail in demyelinated axons, it is less surprising that conduction block can persist for years in axons affected by multifocal motor neuropathy, despite the maintenance of axonal continuity (Lewis et al., 1982). Although the pathology of such axons is not yet certain, threshold tracking techniques have suggested that the axons might be hyperpolarized distal to the site of the block, perhaps linked to a depolarization within the lesion itself (Kiernan et al., 2002); such depolarization could favor conduction block. Whether similar mechanisms might contribute to persistent conduction block in MS currently remains unclear.

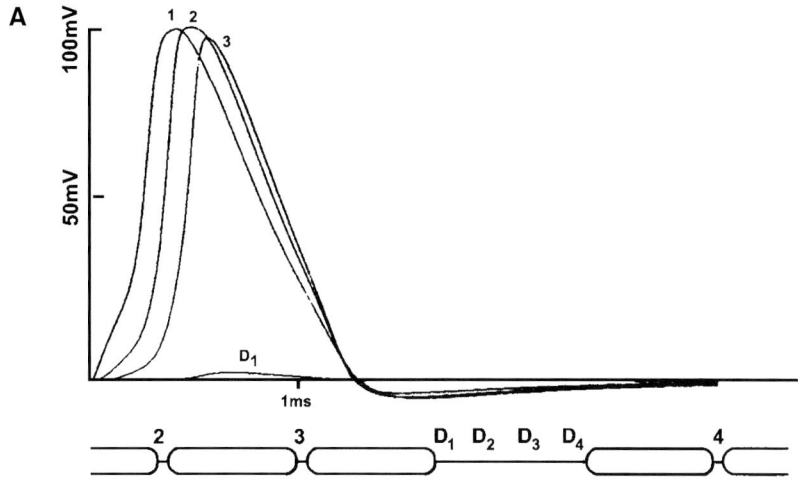

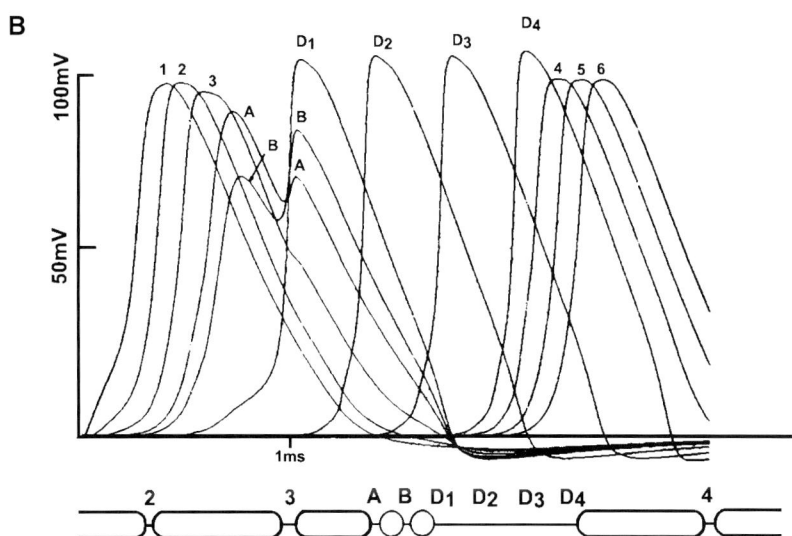

Figure 3 Computer simulations showing conduction through a focally demyelinated axon. Action potentials at nodes 1, 2, 3, the demyelinated region (D_1-D_4), and nodes 4, 5, and 6 are shown. A high density of sodium channels (similar to the density in the nodal membrane) was built into the demyelinated part of the axon (D_1-D_4). (**A**) Even in the presence of a high density of sodium channels in the demyelinated zone, conduction can fail as a result of impedance mismatch. (**B**) Interposition of two short myelinated internodes, just proximal to the demyelinated zone, provides impedance matching that facilitates conduction into, and then through, the demyelinated zone. (Reproduced from Waxman and Brill, 1978.)

F. Safety Factor for Conduction

The concept of safety factor is useful in the pathophysiology of demyelination. It can be defined as the "current available to depolarize the axolemma, divided by the current necessary to do so" (Rushton, 1937). In normal myelinated axons, the action potential at an individual node generates approximately three to seven times more current than is actually required to fire the next node along the axon (Tasaki, 1953), giving a safety factor of 3 to 7. In demyelinated axons, however, several factors conspire to reduce the safety factor

and in some axons it falls to around unity. This is a critical level, because if the safety factor is fractionally higher than 1, the axon will conduct and the patient will have few symptoms; but if the safety factor is fractionally lower, conduction will be blocked and a neurological deficit may ensue. Some patients have many axons with a safety factor near unity, and thus many axons in which function is balanced on a "knife edge." This can result in noticeable, quite sudden changes in the severity of symptoms, because the safety factor is not absolutely fixed for any particular axon and it can be modulated slightly by small changes in the environment of the axons, especially temperature. In fact, even subtle changes in temperature can have dramatic effects on the success of conduction, and thereby on the expression of symptoms, by shifting the safety factor of axons balanced on the verge of successful conduction (see Effects of Temperature).

G. Factors that may Modulate Conduction in Demyelinated Axons

The low safety factor of demyelinated axons means that conduction along the axons is not only particularly sensitive to changes in temperature but also vulnerable to chemical factors that may impair conduction. For example, conduction may be perturbed if an imbalance occurs in the normal composition of the extracellular fluid bathing axons, such as may arise from impairments in the blood-brain barrier. It is suspected that this imbalance can include the appearance of factors that directly affect axonal physiology. Historically, there has been much interest in serum-derived neuroelectric blocking factors that were found to impair different types of neurophysiological function (reviewed in Smith, 1994), but the identity of the factors remained elusive, results were inconsistent, and interest in them waned. More recently, however, interest in the topic has been revived by evidence suggesting that factors associated with inflammation may be able to produce brief exacerbations in patients with MS (Moreau et al., 1996), apparently by acutely and reversibly blocking conduction in demyelinated axons. Nitric oxide has been identified as a candidate for mediating the acute and reversible block (Redford et al., 1997; Shrager et al., 1998; Garthwaite et al., 1999) (see Chapter 18), as has a pentapeptide with the sequence QYNAD (Brinkmeier et al., 2000; Meuth et al., 2003; Weber et al., 2002). Both factors are reported to be present in MS cerebrospinal fluid, and also to impair both axonal conduction and the function of sodium channels. The findings with nitric oxide have been reproduced in different laboratories, but those relating to QYNAD have been questioned (Cummins et al., 2003; Quasthoff et al., 2003). The factors are discussed in Chapter 18 (nitric oxide) and Chapter 22 (QYNAD).

H. Conduction Properties of Conducting Demyelinated Axons

Although demyelinated axons can sometimes conduct impulses successfully, they never conduct as well as normal axons. Conduction remains much slower and less secure than normal, and it is also prone to conduction failure, especially if conducting trains of impulses at higher frequencies. These conduction deficits result in a range of functional deficits in patients.

1. Conduction Slowing

Techniques that allow the progress of the action potential to be monitored as it conducts along the demyelinated axolemma (Bostock and Sears, 1978) have clearly revealed that while conduction remains fast in the normally myelinated portions of the axolemma, it is markedly slowed along the demyelinated region (McDonald and Sears, 1970). In fact, conduction is slowed to approximately 1 m/sec (0.5 to 2.5 m/sec), and so each 1 mm of demyelination contributes approximately 1 mssec of delay. Except in particular pathways, this slowing usually has little consequence for patients (Halliday et al., 1973), but it has proven to be particularly valuable clinically, assisting in the diagnosis of demyelinating disease because of delays in the latency of the sensory or motor compound action potentials in patients with peripheral neuropathy, or in delays in the latency of the visual (Halliday et al., 1973), somatosensory, or auditory-evoked potentials in patients with MS.

2. Conduction of Pairs of Impulses

The slow conduction along demyelinated axolemma inevitably limits the ability of the axons to transmit pairs (and trains) of impulses because the second action potential of a pair, traveling close behind the first, will run into the relative and absolute refractory periods of the first impulse as this is slowed at the site of demyelination. McDonald and Sears (1970) coined the phrase the *refractory period of transmission* (RPT) to describe this deficit, defining the RPT as the maximum interval between two conducted impulses such that the second impulse fails to be conducted successfully through the lesion. In a subsequent study of central axons proven to be segmentally demyelinated, the refractory period of the normal portion of the axon was always in the range 0.5 to 1.4 m/sec, but this was prolonged to 1.0 to 6.0 m/sec if the site of demyelination was included in the conduction pathway (Fig. 4). In one axon the RPT was prolonged to 27 m/sec when the lesion was included in the pathway (Felts et al., 1997).

3. Conduction of Trains of Impulses

The problems associated with conducting pairs of impulses are magnified when considering the conduction of trains of impulses. One consideration is that the RPT of the second and later impulses is longer than that of the first (McDonald and Sears, 1970), slightly increasing with increasing numbers of impulses until a plateau is reached. This effect is due, in part, to the fact that the second impulse conducts across the demyelinated region in the relative refractory period of the first, and so conducts a little more slowly than it, and so on. The maximum frequency of transmission therefore slowly declines over time. In a classic study (Fig. 5) (McDonald and Sears, 1970) conduction through the lesion was restricted to only 410 Hz, although the normal portion of the same axon was conducted at 1,000 Hz. Even the low frequency was maintained for only three impulses before alternate impulses failed to be transmitted.

Another problem arising with repeated activation is the appearance of intermittent periods of complete conduction

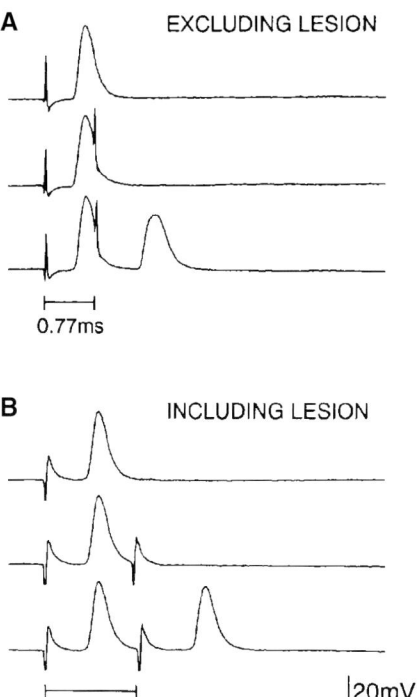

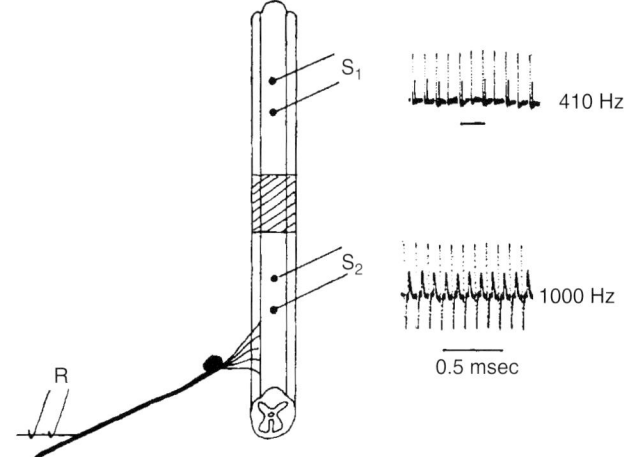

Figure 5 Single unit activity in a dorsal root filament teased from an intercostal nerve caudal to an experimental demyelinating lesion in the dorsal columns induced by the prior injection of diphtheria toxin (*hatched region*). The stimulus artifacts appear as dotted lines and the action potentials as solid lines. Whereas stimulation at S_2 excludes the lesion from the conduction pathway and the axon can conduct faithfully at 1,000 Hz, stimulation at S_1 includes the lesion and conduction sometimes fails even at 410 Hz. (Reproduced from McDonald and Sears, 1970.)

Figure 4 Recordings from a central demyelinated axon either excluding (**A**) or including (**B**) the lesioned portion in the conduction pathway. The normal portion of the axon can conduct two closely spaced impulses resulting from electrical stimuli presented 0.77 ms apart (**A**, third record), but not less than 0.77 ms apart (**A**, second record). However, the demyelinated portion of the same axon was only able to conduct impulses spaced by more than 1.32 ms (**B**). (Reproduced from Felts et al., 1995.)

block (Fig. 6) (Felts et al., 1995); a high-frequency impulse train is abruptly "chopped" into periods where impulses are transmitted faithfully at high frequency, separated by periods of conduction failure. These periods are due to membrane hyperpolarization in response to potentiated activity

of the electrogenic Na^+/K^+ ATPase (sodium pump) caused by the raised intra-axonal sodium concentration resulting from the impulse activity (Bostock and Grafe, 1985; Vagg et al., 1998). The phenomenon can appear after just 1 second of stimulation at 500 Hz (McDonald and Sears, 1970) or within 10 to 30 seconds of stimulation at 100 to 200 Hz (R. Kapoor, P. A. Felts, and K. J. Smith, unpublished observations). These latter frequencies are within the physiological range, and so the phenomenon is likely to impair normal sensation and motor function, contributing to the reduced flicker fusion frequency in some patients (Titcombe and Willison, 1961), to the "fading" or blurring of vision upon prolonged fixation of gaze (McDonald, 1998; Waxman,

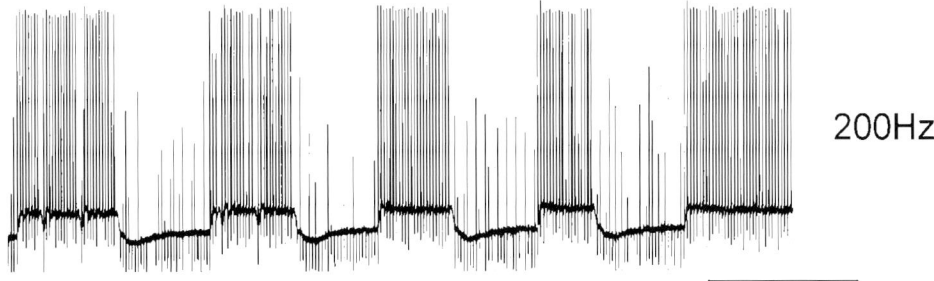

200Hz

Figure 6 Intermittent complete conduction block exhibited by a central demyelinated axon in an intra-axonal record (resting potential –60mV) obtained at or near a site of demyelination induced by the injection of ethidium bromide into the dorsal column 14 days previously. The axon was initially able faithfully to follow a stimulus applied at 200 Hz (not shown), but after about 10 seconds of such stimulation, the axon entered intermittent periods of complete conduction block. The action potentials are the tall spikes of regular amplitude. The irregular spikes during the periods of conduction block are due to stimulus artefacts occasionally captured by the analog-to-digital converter. The axon conducted trains of 20 or so action potentials separated by periods of conduction block. The periods of conduction block coincide exactly with periods of membrane hyperpolarization, indicating that the block is mediated by activity of the electrogenic sodium/potassium ATPase. Calibration bar = 0.5 sec. (Reproduced from Felts et al., 1995.)

1981), and to the progressive weakness experienced by some patients upon walking only a short distance (McDonald, 1975). Drugs that inhibit the Na^+/K^+ ATPase have been reported to improve conduction in central demyelinated axons (Kaji and Sumner, 1989) and some patients with MS (Kaji et al., 1990). Intermittent conduction block has now been demonstrated in a range of human neuropathies (e.g., Cappelen-Smith et al., 2000).

Although preceding impulse activity typically impairs function in demyelinated axons, it can happen, at least in demyelinated Xenopus axons, that successful impulse transmission is enhanced by prior activity. The enhancement occurs if the axon is conditioned by the timing of the preceding activity so that a subsequent impulse arrives at the lesion while it exhibits supernormality (Shrager, 1993).

4. Temporary Exacerbation Caused by Warming: Uhthoff's Phenomenon

The security of conduction in demyelinated axons is markedly affected by temperature, and this effect can readily be demonstrated in the laboratory in both central (Fig. 7) (Smith et al., 2000) and peripheral experimentally demyelinated axons (Bostock et al., 1981; Davis et al., 1975; Rasminsky, 1973). The effects can be sufficiently strong that even subtle changes in body temperature can have a profound effect on the expression of symptoms by patients with

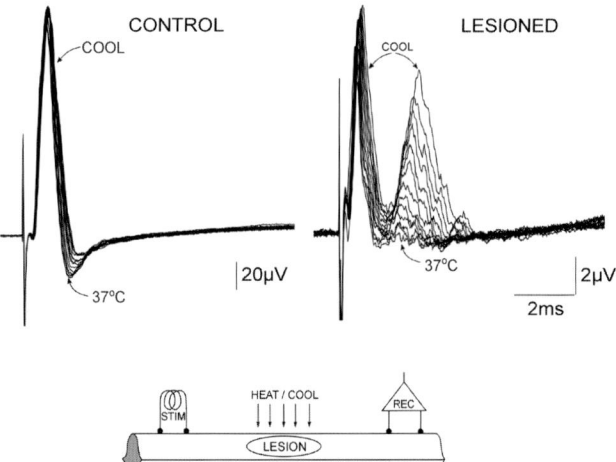

Figure 7 Two families of superimposed records obtained from excised dorsal columns examined *in vitro,* showing the effects of temperature on axonal conduction. The records on the left are from normal tissue, while those on the right include an experimental demyelinating lesion in the conduction pathway, induced 21 days previously. The records were obtained as the temperature in the central recording lane (containing the lesion, where present) was raised from 25°C to 37°C in 1°C intervals. (**A**) The temperature changes had little effect on conduction along normal axons. (**B**) In contrast, temperature changes had prominent effects on conduction in demyelinated axons, distinguished by their longer latency. At cooler temperatures many more demyelinated axons were able to conduct than at normal body temperature, when nearly all the demyelinated axons failed to conduct. (Reproduced from Smith et al., 2000.)

MS. Indeed, many patients with MS exhibit a worsening of some symptoms upon body warming, and the worsening is sufficiently robust and reproducible that at one time the phenomenon was used in the diagnosis of MS in the form of the "hot bath test" (Guthrie, 1951; Malhotra and Goren, 1981). The effect was first described in 1890 by Uhthoff, and the phenomenon now bears his name. Uhthoff-like phenomena can be provoked by a hot shower (Waxman and Geschwind, 1983), sunbathing (Berger and Sheremata, 1985; Harbison et al., 1989; Avis and Pryse-Phillips, 1995), exercise (van Diemen et al., 1992; Edmund and Fog, 1955), or even by the normal circadian change in body temperature (Fig. 8) (Scherokman et al., 1985). Just as warming can be deleterious to function, so cooling can be beneficial and can sometimes be realized after a cool bath or simply after drinking cold water. Indeed, improvement in vision has been documented after drinking iced water, and these functional improvements are accompanied by an increase in the amplitude of the visual-evoked potential (McDonald, 1986; Hopper et al., 1972).

It is generally accepted that temperature affects the success of conduction in demyelinated axons mainly by affecting the duration of the action potential (Paintal, 1966) at the driving node, the node just before the demyelinated region that is responsible for driving the current to depolarize the demyelinated axolemma to its firing threshold. The change in duration arises from the fact that the temperature coefficient for sodium inactivation is larger than that for sodium activation (Davis and Schauf, 1981). In axons balanced on the "knife edge" between conduction block and successful conduction (see Safety Factor) this change can easily be sufficient to decide whether conduction succeeds or fails. Thus although warming will increase the conduction velocity (Fig. 9) (Swadlow et al., 1981), thereby offsetting the reduction in conduction velocity produced by demyelination, the net effect of warming is typically deleterious to the patient, at least with regard to the expression of symptoms. It is worth mentioning that although the mechanism described (changes in action potential duration) may be paramount in most lesions in patients, the expression of Uhthoff's phenomenon may involve multiple mechanisms, perhaps including the modulation of nitric oxide production (see Chapter 18).

5. Therapeutic Strategies Based on Uhthoff's Phenomenon

That cooling can improve conduction in demyelinated axons has encouraged the search for pharmacological agents that might be able to achieve the same benefit, but at normal body temperature. At a time when it was believed that potassium currents curtailed action potential duration in mammalian axons, it was imaginatively surmised that blocking these currents might mimic the effects of body cooling and so restore conduction to demyelinated axons (Bostock et al., 1978; Sherratt et al., 1980; Davis and Schauf, 1981;

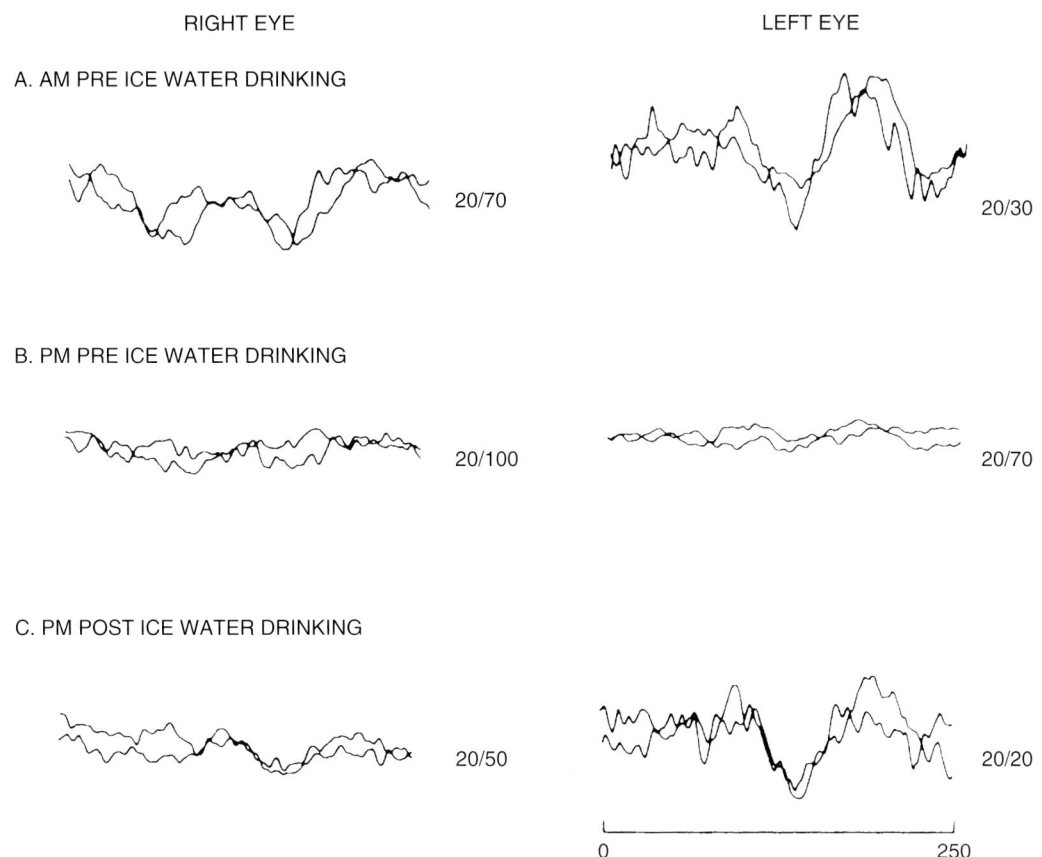

Figure 8 Visual-evoked potentials from a pilot with MS who experienced blurred vision each afternoon (visual acuity indicated). Visual acuity improved substantially in the afternoon within 3 minutes of drinking iced water, and this improvement was accompanied by an increase in the visual-evoked response. On a different day a similar improvement in acuity was accompanied by a reduction in the temperature of the tympanic membrane of 0.25°C. (Reproduced from Scherokman et al., 1985.)

McDonald and Sears, 1970). Indeed, the potassium channel blocking agent 4-aminopyridine can be effective in restoring conduction to demyelinated axons (Sears and Bostock, 1981; Targ and Kocsis, 1985; Bowe et al., 1987), and prolonging action potential duration with scorpion toxin is also effective (Bostock et al., 1978). Based on findings such as these, 4-AP is being evaluated as a possible symptomatic therapy in MS (see Chapter 10), although whether the undoubtedly beneficial effects of the drug in patients are due to effects at the lesion or on synapses (Smith et al., 2000) is currently uncertain. Laboratory studies (Smith et al., 2000) have noted that at the very low concentrations that can safely be achieved in patients (the drug is strongly proconvulsant) it has no apparent effects on demyelinated axons, but it strongly potentiates synaptic transmission.

III. Hyperexcitability

Demyelinated axons not only can develop excitability along the demyelinated portion over time but also can become hyperexcitable, such that they generate trains of ectopic impulses. Such impulses are generated at the site of demyelination, conducting away from it in both directions (Smith and McDonald, 1982; Baker and Bostock, 1992). The impulse trains are composed of either continuous (at 10 to 50 Hz) or bursting discharges (e.g., 0.1 to 5 sec bursts separated by gaps of 0.1 to 100 sec) (Fig. 10), with the discharge pattern typically being consistent for any particular axon if left undisturbed. However, different patterns of impulse activity can continue simultaneously in different axons within a single lesion. Continuous discharges can arise because of the appearance of a slow, persistent inward sodium current along the demyelinated axolemma (Kapoor et al., 1997; Rizzo et al., 1996), whereas bursting discharges can arise from an inward potassium current that can arise if potassium ions accumulate in a compartment surrounding axons (Kapoor et al., 1993; Felts et al., 1995), although a definitive link between these mechanisms and these particular patterns of hyperexcitability has not been established (see reviews by Smith et al., 1997; Mogyoros et al., 2000; Baker, 2000; and Chapter 9).

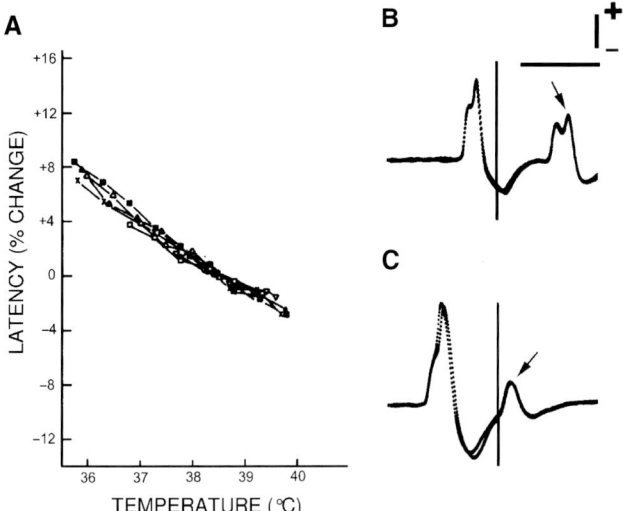

Figure 9 Axonal conduction velocity increases, but safety factor is reduced, as temperature increases. (**A**) Changes in conduction latency for callosal axons, measured in rabbits, as body temperature is altered. Note the decrease in latency, reflecting increased conduction velocity, as temperature rises. (**B, C**) Extracellular recordings of action potentials elicited in a callosal efferent neuron by stimulation of its axon in the corpus callosum, at 36.5°C (**B**) and at 38.7°C (**C**), display more rapid conduction (resulting in earlier onset of the action potential) at higher temperature. For the second action potential evoked at high frequency, the safety factor is reduced, resulting in an inflection (**arrow in B**) between the initial segment spike and somatodendritic spike at 36.5°C. At 38.7C° the action potential fails to invade the soma (arrow in **C**) because of a superimposed temperature-induced decrease in safety factor. (Reproduced from Swadlow et al., 1981.)

Ectopic activity is more common in sensory demyelinated axons than motor, probably because of their greater expression of persistent sodium currents (Mogyoros et al., 2000). In this regard, it is interesting that Nav1.6 and Nav1.2 sodium channels are both expressed along demyelinated axons (Craner et al., 2003, 2004), and both of these sodium channels are known to produce persistent sodium currents (which are larger in Nav1.6; see Chapter 7), although neither type of channel has yet been indicted as contributing to hyperexcitability of demyelinated axons. Some hyperexcitability of axons in inflammatory MS lesions might be attributable to exposure to nitric oxide, as this agent can enhance persistent sodium currents (Hammarstrom and Gage, 1999) (see Chapter 18). Hyperexcitability is also enhanced by hyperventilation (Davis et al., 1970; Burchiel, 1981), perhaps mediated by changes in the extracellular concentration of H^+ and Ca^{2+} ions (Mogyoros et al., 1997).

The more frequent occurrence of ectopic activity in sensory axons correlates with the fact that sensory manifestations of ectopic activity are much more common than their motor counterparts in patients with MS (Matthews, 1998), although manifestations such as facial myokymia and paroxysmal dystonia do occur (Andermann et al., 1961;

Kapoor et al., 1992). It is intuitively likely that the trains of ectopic activity arising in sensory axons will contribute to, if not underlie, the positive sensory symptoms commonly associated with MS, such as tingling paraesthesia and perhaps pain. Evidence to support this view has been provided by recordings made during neck movement in patients exhibiting Lhermitte's sign (Nordin et al., 1984) (see Mechanosensitivity).

Observations in patients that sodium channel blocking agents (e.g., carbamazepine, lamotrigine, lidocaine, mexiletine) are effective in controlling positive symptoms (Cianchetti et al., 1999; Sakurai and Kanazawa, 1999) also support a strong role for sodium channels in the generation of ectopic impulses.

A. Triggered Sensations

In some experimentally demyelinated axons it is possible to provoke a "spontaneous" burst of ectopic activity by firing an action potential along the axon; the activity is triggered in an otherwise electrically silent axon as if the burst were waiting to be released (Fig. 11) (Bowe et al., 1987; Huizar et al., 1975; Felts et al., 1995). The underlying mechanism is not certain, but a role for inward potassium currents (Kapoor et al., 1993) is consistent with the observation that the behavior can sometimes be provoked by prior conditioning of the axon with high-frequency stimulation. Such triggered bursts of activity may be related to the observation in patients that light touch may sometimes evoke pain referred to the same receptive field.

B. Impulse Reflection

The duration of the action potential is prolonged as it crosses the demyelinated region; this can sometimes mean that the node preceding the demyelinated region can be reexcited by the action currents generated along the demyelinated axolemma if the node has recovered from its refractory period. In this case a daughter impulse is initiated that conducts in a retrograde fashion back along the same axon, as an apparent "reflection" of the first impulse (Howe et al., 1976). A pair of reflecting sites can set up a reverberating condition in which action potentials shuttle back and forth between the sites, perhaps generating a train of action potentials emerging at each site.

C. Mechanosensitivity

Demyelinated axons may become not only spontaneously active but also mechanosensitive, so that they generate trains of impulses if they are deformed. In this respect, demyelinated axolemma acquires properties similar to those of mechanoreceptors, and the discharge patterns generated resemble the familiar phasic and/or tonic bursts of activity

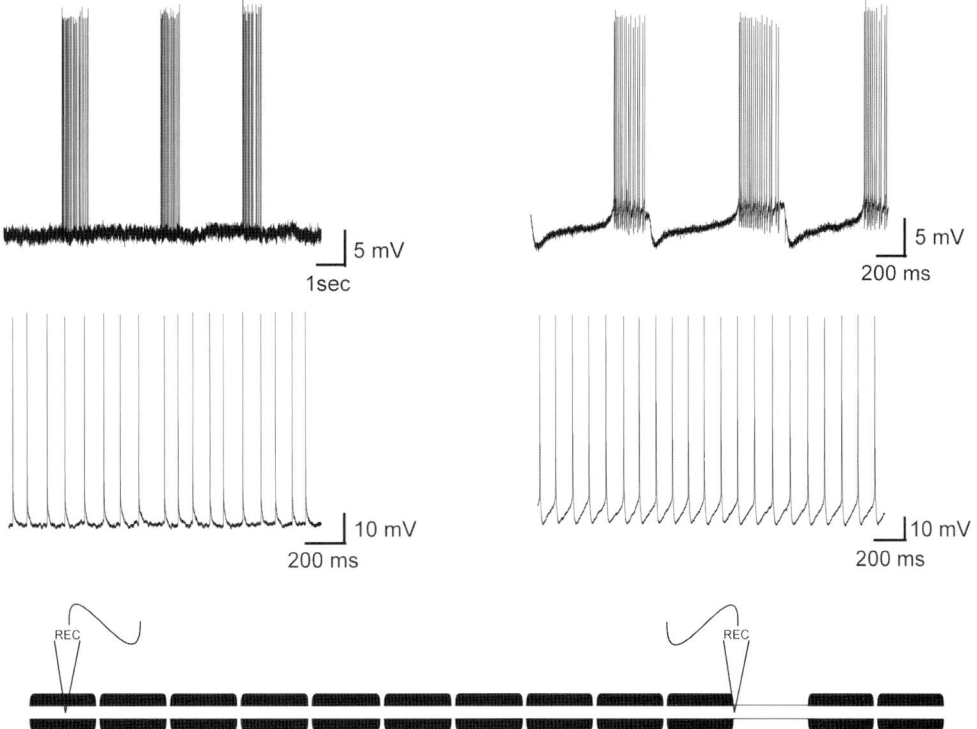

Figure 10 Records obtained using a micropipette positioned in four different central demyelinated axons, showing ongoing activity obtained from sites either remote (*left*) or at (*right*) the location of a demyelinating lesion (indicated). Different axons show either a bursting discharge (*upper records*) or a more even discharge (*lower records*). The changes in membrane potential responsible for generating the impulses can be seen in the records obtained at the lesion. (Redrawn from Felts et al., 1995, and Kapoor et al., 1997.)

recorded from such receptors coincident with the deformation (Smith and McDonald, 1980, 1982). In patients with demyelinating lesions in the optic nerves or the cervical posterior columns of the spinal cord, eye and neck movements, respectively, can deform the demyelinated axons, provoking bursts of activity. This activity is perceived as flashes of light (Davis et al., 1976) or an "electric shock" or tingling sensation that radiates down the limbs and body (i.e., Lhermitte's phenomenon) (Lhermitte et al., 1924; Kanchandani and Howe, 1982). Recordings from cutaneous nerve fascicles have established that the tingling sensations associated with

Lhermitte's sign occur simultaneously with a volley of impulses in sensory axons, presumably representing impulses conducted antidromically following their ectopic generation at a cervical lesion (Fig. 12) (Nordin et al., 1984).

D. Ephaptic Activity

There is evidence that sometimes electrical activity in one axon can excite activity in another axon, which is presumed to lie adjacent to the first. Such cross-excitation at a

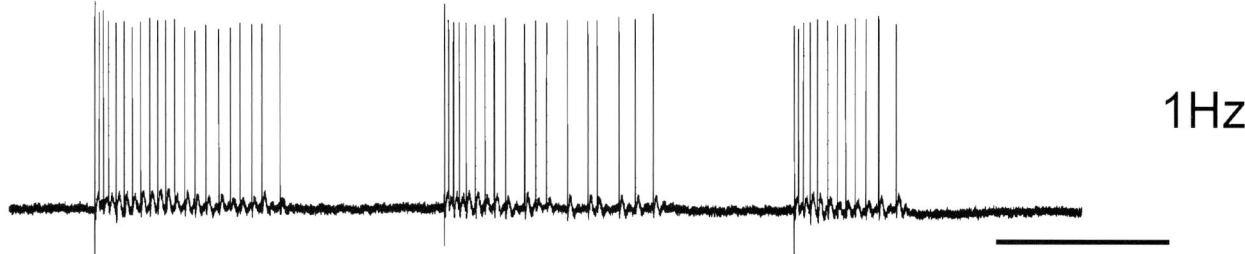

1Hz

Figure 11 Spike triggered bursting record exhibited by the same central demyelinated axon as shown in Fig. 5. After 30 seconds of stimulation at 200 Hz, stimulation at only 1 Hz (indicated by the downward deflections of the stimulus artefacts, which are seemingly superimposed in time with the action potentials they evoked) resulted in the formation of short bursts of impulses triggered by the passage of the first impulse in the train. Calibration bar = 0.5 sec. (Reproduced from Felts et al. 1995.)

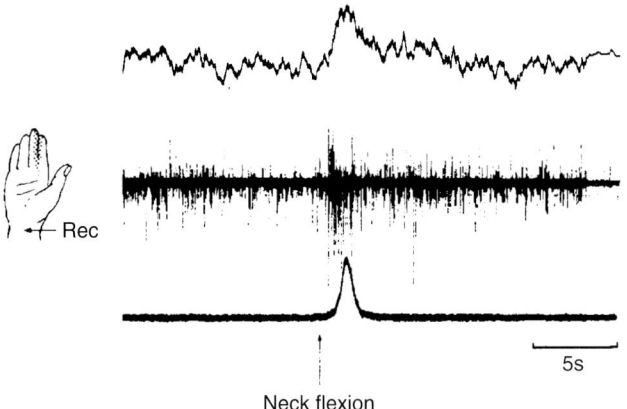

Figure 12 Recording from a cutaneous nerve in the wrist of a patient with MS and Lhermitte's phenomenon. Neck flexion (*vertical arrow*) evoked a nonpainful electric tingling sensation in all the fingers of her hands, indicated by the peak in the lower grip force record. The middle record shows the evoked multiunit burst of activity, which coincides with the paraesthesia, and the upper record shows the integrated neurogram (time constant 0.5 sec). (Reproduced from Nordin et al., 1984.)

site other than a synapse is termed ephaptic transmission, and the phenomenon has been convincingly demonstrated in the "dystrophic" mutant mouse (Rasminsky, 1978, 1980). In this model, impulses traveling in an amyelinated axon ephaptically excited daughter impulses in a normal axon;

the daughter impulses traveled away from the ephapse in both directions (Fig. 13) (Rasminsky, 1980). This demonstration involved peripheral amyelinated axons, but it is reasonable to suppose that a similar phenomenon might occur in central and peripheral demyelinated axons. This view is encouraged by a host of peculiar phenomena in patients (e.g., Kapoor et al., 1992; Hartmann et al., 1999) that have reasonably been attributed to ephaptic transmission occurring by the lateral spread of excitability across different, but anatomically adjacent, spinal or brainstem tracts.

IV. Remyelination

Demyelination can be repaired by remyelination, even in MS (Prineas and Connell, 1979; Prineas et al., 1993), namely by the formation of new internodes of myelin across the demyelinated gap. The new internodes are both thinner and shorter than normal (Gledhill and McDonald, 1977; Harrison et al., 1972), and this latter consideration means that new nodes are formed at sites along the axon that were previously covered by myelin. These sites will, initially at least, lack nodal specializations such as the accumulation of sodium channels, and so it was not inevitable that remyelinated axons would be able to conduct impulses. Indeed, conduction block could theoretically be favored by the thinness of the myelin, especially in the early stages of remyelination,

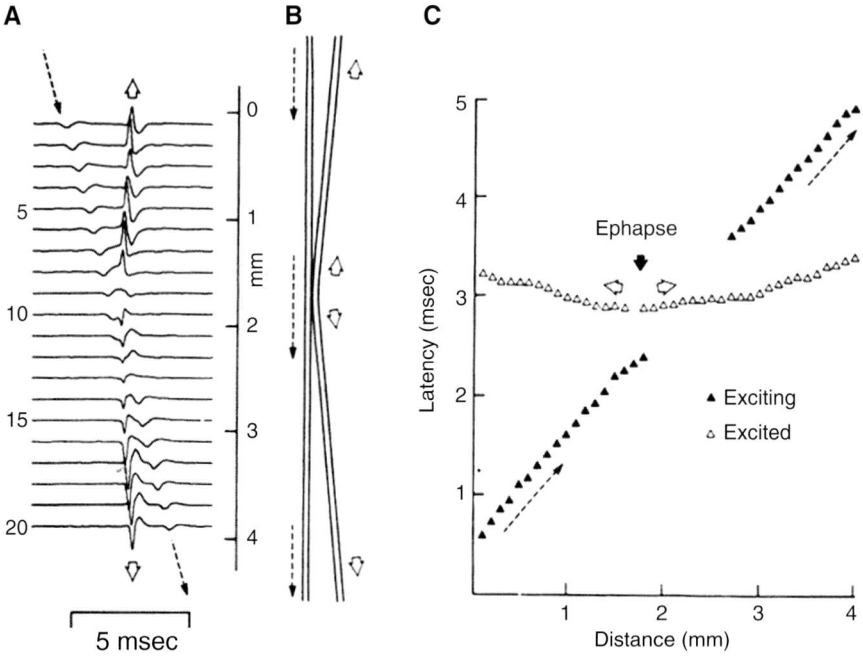

Figure 13 Plots showing ephaptic transmission from a nonmyelinated axon to a myelinated axon in the ventral root of a dystrophic mouse (illustrated in **B**). (**A**) Ladder plot of external longitudinal currents recorded at intervals of 200 μm from proximal (top) to distal. The directions of travel of the exciting and excited action potentials are indicated by the dashed and open arrows, respectively. (**C**) Graph of the latency of the exciting and excited action potentials. The slow conduction velocity of the exciting impulse (*dashed arrows*) indicates the nonmyelinated characteristics of the exciting axon. (Reproduced from Rasminsky, 1980.)

as this will be associated with a raised internodal capacitance and reduced resistance, both of which will impair conduction. However, studies that have serially monitored conduction in central axons as they underwent demyelination and remyelination have established that remyelination is accompanied by the restoration of fast conduction, probably in all remyelinated axons (Fig. 14) (Smith et al., 1979, 1981). The conduction is as secure as in normal axons, as judged by the restoration of the RPT to within normal limits, and the ability of the axons to conduct high frequency trains (Smith et al., 1979, 1981). Studies in peripheral remyelinated axons (Smith et al., 1982) have established that each new node is excited in turn as impulses conduct along remyelinated regions, and it seems safe to assume that a similar pattern will occur in central remyelinated axons. Certainly the new nodes can express high densities of sodium channels (Craner et al., 2003; Dugandzija-Novakovic et al., 1995).

Using different techniques, it has been found that remyelinated axons can conduct when invested with only thin new myelin sheaths, composed of only five lamellae of myelin (Felts et al., 1997). The robustness of conduction in remyelinated axons is in accord with the observation that remyelination is associated with the restoration of function at the behavioral level (Jeffery and Blakemore, 1997), and it is reasonable to assume that remyelination will contribute to remissions in MS.

Given the preceding observations it is not surprising that the promotion of remyelination continues to be a major goal of research in MS (see Chapter 28), and a number of different strategies have been used, including immunological (Warrington et al., 2000; Asakura and Rodriguez, 1998) and, especially, transplantation strategies (Blakemore and Franklin, 2000; Baron-Van et al., 1997). It is encouraging that conduction has now been demonstrated in axons remyelinated primarily by oligodendrocytes (Smith et al., 1979, 1981), Schwann cells (Felts and Smith, 1992), transplanted Schwann cells (Honmou et al., 1996), olfactory ensheathing cells (Imaizumi et al., 1998, 2000; Utzschneider et al., 1994), human neural precursor cells (Akiyama et al., 2001), bone marrow cells (Akiyama et al., 2002), and human frozen Schwann cells (Kohama et al., 2001). Given the wide range of strategies that result in successful conduction, the prospect for achieving meaningful improvements in axonal function in MS is good.

References

Akiyama, Y., Honmou, O., Kato, T., Uede, T., Hashi, K., and Kocsis, J. D. (2001). Transplantation of clonal neural precursor cells derived from adult human brain establishes functional peripheral myelin in the rat spinal cord. *Exp. Neurol.* **167**, 27–39.

Akiyama, Y., Radtke, C., and Kocsis, J. D. (2002). Remyelination of the rat spinal cord by transplantation of identified bone marrow stromal cells. *J. Neurosci.* **22**, 6623–6630.

Andermann, F., Cosgrove, J. B. R., Lloyd-Smith, D. L., Gloor, P., and McNaughton, F. L. (1961). Facial myokymia in multiple sclerosis. *Brain* **84**, 31–44.

Arroyo, E. J. and Scherer, S. S. (2000). On the molecular architecture of myelinated fibers. *Histochemistry* **113**, 1–18.

Asakura, K., and Rodriguez, M. (1998). A unique population of circulating autoantibodies promotes central nervous system remyelination. *Multiple Sclerosis* **4**, 217–221.

Avis, S. P. and Pryse-Phillips, W. E. (1995). Sudden death in multiple sclerosis associated with sun exposure: A report of two cases. *Can. J. Neurol. Sci.* **22**, 305–307.

Baker, M., and Bostock, H. (1992). Ectopic activity in demyelinated spinal root axons of the rat. *J Physiol. (London)* **451**, 539–552.

Baker, M. D. (2000). Axonal flip-flops and oscillators. *Trends Neurosci.* **23**, 514–519.

Barnes, D., Munro, P. M., Youl, B. D., Prineas, J. W., and McDonald, W. I. (1991). The longstanding MS lesion. A quantitative MRI and electron microscopic study. *Brain* **114**, 1271–1280.

Baron-Van, E. A., Avellana-Adalid, V., Lachapelle, F., and Liblau, R. (1997). Schwann cell transplantation and myelin repair of the CNS. *Multiple Sclerosis* **3**, 157–161.

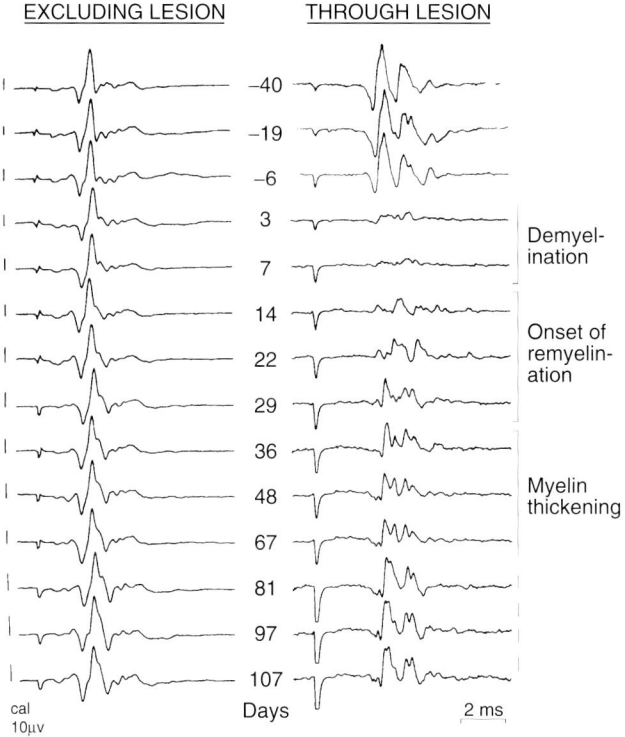

EXCLUDING LESION   THROUGH LESION

−40
−19
−6
3
7   Demyelination
14
22   Onset of remyelination
29
36
48   Myelin thickening
67
81
97
107

cal 10μV   Days   2 ms

Figure 14 Records obtained over 5 months showing the changes in conduction occurring along dorsal columns containing a central demyelinating lesion. On the left are shown records obtained excluding the lesion from the conduction pathway, and these were quite stable throughout. Conduction was also stable (top 3 records on the right) in records obtained including the site of the lesion, but before the lesion was induced. At day 0, the demyelinating lesion was induced by the intraspinal injection of lysolecithin, and this blocked conduction for about 2 weeks in most axons. Conduction was progressively restored during the period of repair by remyelination. Remyelination also restored the security of conduction (not shown). (Reproduced from Smith et al., 1979.)

Berger, J. R. and Sheremata, W. A. (1985). Reply to letter by F. A. Davis. *JAMA* **253**, 203.

Black, J. A., Renganathan, M., and Waxman, S. G. (2002). Sodium channel Na(v)1.6 is expressed along nonmyelinated axons and it contributes to conduction. *Mol. Brain Res.* **105**, 19–28.

Black, J. A., and Waxman, S. G. (1996). Sodium channel expression: A dynamic process in neurons and non-neuronal cells. *Dev. Neurosci.* **18**, 139–152.

Blakemore, W. F., and Franklin, R. J. M. (2000). Transplantation options for therapeutic central nervous system remyelination. *Cell Transplant.* **9**, 289–294.

Blakemore, W. F., and Smith, K. J. (1983). Node-like axonal specializations along demyelinated central nerve fibres: Ultrastructural observations. *Acta Neuropathol.* **60**, 291–296.

Bostock, H. (1984). Internodal conduction along undissected nerve fibers in experimental neuropathy. *In* "Peripheral Neuropathy", P. J. Dyck, P. K. Thomas, E. H. Lambert, and R. Bunge, eds.), pp. 900–910. W.B. Saunders, Philadelphia.

Bostock, H., (1994). The pathophysiology of demyelination. *In* "Multiple Sclerosis: Current Status of Research and Treatment,"(R. M. Herndon, & F. J. Seil, eds.) pp. 89–112, Demos Publications, Inc., New York.

Bostock, H., and Grafe, P. (1985). Activity-dependent excitability changes in normal and demyelinated rat spinal root axons. *J. Physiol.* **365**, 239–257.

Bostock, H., and Sears, T. A. (1978). The internodal axon membrane: electrical excitability and continuous conduction in segmental demyelination. *J. Physiol.* **280**, 273–301.

Bostock, H., Sears, T. A., and Sherratt, R. M. (1981). The effects of 4-aminopyridine and tetraethylammonium ions on normal and demyelinated mammalian nerve fibres. *J. Physiol.* **313**, 301–315.

Bostock, H., Sherratt, R. M., and Sears, T. A. (1978). Overcoming conduction failure in demyelinated nerve fibres by prolonging action potentials. *Nature* **274**, 385–387.

Bowe, C. M., Kocsis, J. D., Targ, E. F., and Waxman, S. G. (1987). Physiological effects of 4-aminopyridine on demyelinated mammalian motor and sensory fibers. *Am. J. Neurol.* **22**, 264–268.

Brinkmeier, H., Aulkemeyer, P., Wollinsky, K. H., and Rudel, R. (2000). An endogenous pentapeptide acting as a sodium channel blocker in inflammatory autoimmune disorders of the central nervous system. *Nature Med.* **6**, 808–811.

Burchiel, K. J. (1981). Ectopic impulse generation in demyelinated axons: Effects of Pa_{CO2}, pH, and disodium edetate. *Am. J. Neurol.* **9**, 378–383.

Caldwell, J. H., Schaller, K. L., Lasher, R. S., Peles, E., and Levinson, S. R. (2000). Sodium channel Na(v)1.6 is localized at nodes of Ranvier, dendrites, and synapses. *Proc. Natl. Acad. Sci.* **97**, 5616–5620.

Cappelen-Smith, C., Kuwabara, S., Lin, C. S. Y., Mogyoros, I., and Burke, D. (2000). Activity-dependent hyperpolarization and conduction block in chronic inflammatory demyelinating polyneuropathy. *Ann. Neurol.* **48**, 826–832.

Chiu, S. Y., and Ritchie, J. M. (1981). Evidence for the presence of potassium channels in the paranodal region of acutely demyelinated mammalian single nerve fibres. *J. Physiol.* **313**, 415–437.

Cianchetti, C., Zuddas, A., Randazzo, A. P., Perra, L., and Marrosu, M. G. (1999). Lamotrigine adjunctive therapy in painful phenomena in MS: Preliminary observations. *Neurology* **53**, 433.

Craner, M. J., Lo, A. C., Black, J. A., and Waxman, S. G. (2003). Abnormal sodium channel distribution in optic nerve axons in a model of inflammatory demyelination. *Brain* **126**, 1552–1561.

Craner, M. J., Newcombe, J., Black, J. A., Hartle, C., Cuzner, M. L., and Waxman, S. G. (2004). Molecular changes in neurons in MS: Altered axonal expression of Nav1.2 and Nav1.6 sodium channels and Na/Ca exchanger, *Proc. Natl. Acad. Sci. U. S. A.* **101**, 8168–8173.

Cummins, T. R., Renganathan, M., Stys, P. K., Herzog, R. I., Scarfo, K., Horn, R., Dib-Hajj, S. D., and Waxman, S. G. (2003). The pentapeptide QYNAD does not block voltage-gated sodium channels. *Neurology* **60**, 224–229.

Davis, F. A., Becker, F. O., Michael, J. A., and Sorensen, E. (1970). Effect of intravenous sodium bicarbonate, disodium edetate (Na2EDTA), and hyperventilation on visual and oculomotor signs in multiple sclerosis. *J. Neurol. Neurosurg. Psychiatry* **33**, 723–732.

Davis, F. A., Bergen, D., Schauf, C., McDonald, I., and Deutsch, W. (1976). Movement phosphenes in optic neuritis: a new clinical sign. *Neurology* **26**, 1100–1104.

Davis, F. A. and Schauf, C. L. (1981). Approaches to the development of pharmacological interventions in multiple sclerosis. *Adv. Neurol.* **31**, 505–510.

Davis, F. A., Schauf, C. L., Reed, B. J., and Kesler, R. L. (1975). Experimental studies of the effects of extrinsic factors on conduction in normal and demyelinated nerve. *J. Neurol. Neurosurg. Psychiatry* **39**, 442–448.

Dugandzija-Novakovic, S., Koszowski, A. G., Levinson, S. R., and Shrager, P. (1995). Clustering of Na⁺ channels and node of Ranvier formation in remyelinating axons. *J. Neurosci.* **15**, 492–503.

Edmund, J., and Fog, T. (1955). Visual and motor instability in multiple sclerosis. *Arch. Neurol. Psychiatry* **73**, 316–323.

England, J. D., Gamboni, F., and Levinson, S. R. (1991). Increased numbers of sodium channels form along demyelinated axons. *Brain Res.* **548**, 334–337.

Felts, P. A., Baker, T. A., and Smith, K. J. (1997). Conduction in segmentally demyelinated mammalian central axons. *J. Neurosci.* **17**, 7267–7277.

Felts, P. A., Kapoor, R., and Smith, K. J. (1995). A mechanism for ectopic firing in central demyelinated axons. *Brain* **118**, 1225–1231.

Felts, P. A., and Smith, K. J. (1992). Conduction properties of central nerve, fibers remyelinated by Schwann cells. *Brain Res.* **574**, 178–192.

Foster, R. E., Whalen, C. C., and Waxman, S. G. (1980). Reorganization of the axon membrane in demyelinated peripheral nerve fibers: morphological evidence. *Science* **210**, 661–663.

Garthwaite, G., Goodwin, D. A., and Garthwaite, J. (1999). Nitric oxide stimulates cGMP formation in rat optic nerve axons, providing a specific marker of axon viability. *Eur. J. Neurosci.* **11**, 4367–4372.

Ghatak, N. R., Hirano, A., Lijtmaer, H., and Zimmerman, H. M. (1974). Asymptomatic demyelinated plaque in the spinal cord. *Arch. Neurol.* **30**, 484–486.

Gilliatt, R. W. (1982). Electrophysiology of peripheral neuropathies: An overview. *Muscle Nerve* **5**, S108–S116.

Gledhill, R. F., and McDonald, W. I. (1977). Morphological characteristics of central demyelination and remyelination: a single-fiber study. *Ann. Neurol.* **1**, 552–560.

Guthrie, T. C. (1951). Visual and motor changes in patients with multiple sclerosis. *Arch. Neurol. Psychiatry* **65**, 437–451.

Halliday, A. M., McDonald, W. I., and Mushin, J. (1973). Visual evoked response in diagnosis of multiple sclerosis. *Br. Med. J.* **4**, 661–664.

Hammarstrom, A. K. M., and Gage, P. W. (1999). Nitric oxide increases persistent sodium current in rat hippocampal neurons. *J. Physiol.* **520**, 451–461.

Harbison, J. W., Calabrese, V. P., and Edlich, R. F. (1989). A fatal case of sun exposure in a multiple sclerosis patient. *J. Emerg. Med.* **7**, 465–467.

Harrison, B. M., McDonald, W. I., and Ochoa, J. (1972). Remyelination in the central diphtheria toxin lesion. *J. Neurol. Sci.* **17**, 293–302.

Hartmann, M., Rottach, K. G., Wohlgemuth, W. A., and Pfadenhauer, K. (1999). Trigeminal neuralgia triggered by auditory stimuli in multiple sclerosis. *Arch. Neurol.* **56**, 731–733.

Hille, B. (1992). *Ionic Channels of Excitable Membranes*, 2nd ed. Sinauer Associates Inc., Sunderland, MA.

Honmou, O., Felts, P. A., Waxman, S. G., and Kocsis, J. D. (1996). Restoration of normal conduction properties in demyelinated spinal cord axons in the adult rat by transplantation of exogenous Schwann cells. *J. Neurosci.* **16**, 3199–3208.

Hopper, C. L., Matthews, C. G., and Cleeland, C. S. (1972). Symptom instability and thermoregulation in multiple sclerosis. *Neurology* **22**, 142–148.

Howe, J. F., Calvin, W. H., and Loeser, J. D. (1976). Impulses reflected from dorsal root ganglia and from focal nerve injuries. *Brain Res.* **116,** 139–144.

Huizar, P., Kuno, M., and Miyata, Y. (1975). Electrophysiological properties of spinal motoneurones of normal and dystrophic mice. *J. Physiol.* **248,** 231–246.

Imaizumi, T., Lankford, K. L., and Kocsis, J. D. (2000). Transplantation of olfactory ensheathing cells or Schwann cells restores rapid and secure conduction across the transected spinal cord. *Brain Res.* **854,** 70–78.

Imaizumi, T., Lankford, K. L., Waxman, S. G., Greer, C. A., and Kocsis, J. D. (1998). Transplanted olfactory ensheathing cells remyelinate and enhance axonal conduction in the demyelinated dorsal columns of the rat spinal cord. *J. Neurosci.* **18,** 6176–6185.

Jeffery, N. D., and Blakemore, W. F. (1997). Locomotor deficits induced by experimental spinal cord demyelination are abolished by spontaneous remyelination. *Brain* **120,** 27–37.

Kaji, R., Happel, L., and Sumner, A. J. (1990). Effect of digitalis on clinical symptoms and conduction variables in patients with multiple sclerosis. *Ann. Neurol.* **28,** 582–584.

Kaji, R., and Sumner, A. J. (1989). Ouabain reverses conduction disturbances in single demyelinated nerve fibers. *Neurology* **39,** 1364–1368.

Kanchandani, R., and Howe, J. G. (1982). Lhermitte's sign in multiple sclerosis: a clinical survey and review of the literature. *J. Neurol. Neurosurg. Psychiatry* **45,** 308–312.

Kapoor, R., Brown, P., Thompson, P. D., and Miller, D. H. (1992). Propriospinal myoclonus in multiple sclerosis. *J. Neurol. Neurosurg. Psychiatry* **55,** 1086–1088.

Kapoor, R., Li, Y. G., and Smith, K. J. (1997). Slow sodium-dependent potential oscillations contribute to ectopic firing in mammalian demyelinated axons. *Brain* **120,** 647–652.

Kapoor, R., Smith, K. J., Felts, P. A., and Davies, M. (1993). Internodal potassium currents can generate ectopic impulses in mammalian myelinated axons. *Brain Res.* **611,** 165–169.

Kazarinova-Noyes, K., and Shrager, P. (2002). Molecular constituents of the node of Ranvier. *Mol. Neurobiol.* **26,** 167–182.

Kiernan, M. C., Guglielmi, J. M., Kaji, R., Murray, N. M., and Bostock, H. (2002). Evidence for axonal membrane hyperpolarization in multifocal motor neuropathy with conduction block. *Brain* **125,** 664–675.

Kohama, I., Lankford, K. L., Preiningerova, J., White, F. A., Vollmer, T. L., and Kocsis, JD. (2001). Transplantation of cryopreserved adult human Schwann cells enhances axonal conduction in demyelinated spinal cord. *J. Neurosci.* **21,** 944–950.

Koles, A. J., and Rasminsky, M. (1972). A computer simulation of conduction in demyelinated nerve fibres. *J. Physiol.* **227,** 351–364.

Lewis, R. A., Sumner, A. J., Brown, M. J., and Asbury, A. K. (1982). Multifocal demyelinating neuropathy with persistent conduction block. *Neurology* **32,** 958–964.

Lhermitte, J., Bollack, J., and Nicholas, M. (1924). Les douleurs à type de décharge électrique consécutives à la flexion céphalique dans la sclérose en plaques. *Revue Neurologique* **2,** 56–62.

Lu, J. L., Sheikh, K. A., Wu, H. S., Zhang, J., Jiang, Z. F., Cornblath, D. R., McKhann, G. M., Asbury, A. K., Griffin, J. W., and Ho, T. W. (2000). Physiologic-pathologic correlation in Guillain-Barré syndrome in children. *Neurology* **54,** 33–39.

Malhotra, A. S., and Goren, H. (1981). The hot bath test in the diagnosis of multiple sclerosis. *JAMA* **246,** 1113–1114.

Matthews, B. (1998). Symptoms and signs of multiple sclerosis. *In* "McAlpine's Multiple Sclerosis" (A. Compston, G. Ebers, H. Lassmann, W. I. McDonald, B. Matthews, and H. Wekerle, eds.) pp. 145–190. Churchill Livingstone, London.

McDonald, I. (1998). Pathophysiology of multiple sclerosis. *In* "McAlpine's Multiple Sclerosis" (A. Compston, G. Ebers, H. Lassmann, I. McDonald, B. Matthews, and H. Wekerle, eds.), pp. 359–378. Churchill Livingstone, London.

McDonald, W. I. (1963). The effects of experimental demyelination on conduction in peripheral nerve: A histological and electrophysiological study. II. Electrophysiological observations. *Brain* **86,** 501–524.

McDonald, W. I. (1975). Mechanisms of functional loss and recovery in spinal cord damage. *In* "Outcome of Severe Damage to the Central Nervous System" pp. 23–33.

McDonald, W. I. (1986). The pathophysiology of multiple sclerosis. *In* "Multiple Sclerosis" (W. I. McDonald and D. H. Silberberg, eds.) pp. 112-133. Butterworth, London.

McDonald, W. I., and Sears, T. A. (1970). The effects of experimental demyelination on conduction in the central nervous system. *Brain* **93,** 583–598.

Meuth, S. G., Budde, T., Duyar, H., Landgraf, P., Broicher, T., Elbs, M., Brock, R., Weller, M., Weissert, R., and Wiendl, H. (2003). Modulation of neuronal activity by the endogenous pentapeptide QYNAD. *Eur. J. Neurosci.* **18,** 2697–2706.

Mogyoros, I., Bostock, H., and Burke, D. (2000). Mechanisms of paresthesias arising from healthy axons. *Muscle Nerve* **23,** 310–320.

Mogyoros, I., Kiernan, M. C., Burke, D., and Bostock, H. (1997). Excitability changes in human sensory and motor axons during hyperventilation and ischaemia. *Brain* **120,** 317–325.

Moreau, T., Coles, A., Wing, M., Isaacs, J., Hale, G., Waldmann, H., and Compston, A. (1996). Transient increase in symptoms associated with cytokine release in patients with multiple sclerosis. *Brain* **119,** 225–237.

Nordin, M., Nystrom, B., Wallin, U., and Hagbarth, K. E. (1984). Ectopic sensory discharges and paresthesiae in patients with disorders of peripheral nerves, dorsal roots and dorsal columns. *Pain* **20,** 231–245.

Paintal, A. S. (1966). The influence of diameter of medullated nerve fibres of cats on the rising and falling phases of the spike and its recovery. *J. Physiol.* **184,** 791–811.

Phadke, J. G., and Best, P. V. (1983). Atypical and clinically silent multiple sclerosis: a report of 12 cases discovered unexpectedly at necropsy. *J. Neurol. Neurosurg. Psychiatry* **46,** 414–420.

Prineas, J. W., Barnard, R. O., Kwon, E. E., Sharer, L. R., and Cho, E. S. (1993). Multiple sclerosis: remyelination of nascent lesions. *Ann. Neurol.* **33,** 137–151.

Prineas, J. W., and Connell, F. (1979). Remyelination in multiple sclerosis. *Ann. Neurol.* **5,** 22–31.

Quasthoff, S., Pojer, C., Mori, A., Hofer, D., Liebmann, P., Kieseier, B. C., and Schreibmayer, W. (2003). No blocking effects of the pentapeptide QYNAD on Na+ channel subtypes expressed in Xenopus oocytes or action potential conduction in isolated rat sural nerve. *Neurosci. Lett.* **352,** 93–96.

Rasminsky, M. (1973). The effects of temperature on conduction in demyelinated single nerve fibers. *Arch. Neurol.* **28,** 287–292.

Rasminsky, M. (1978). Ectopic generation of impulses and cross-talk in spinal nerve roots of "dystrophic" mice. *Ann. Neurol.* **3,** 351–357.

Rasminsky, M. (1980). Ephaptic transmission between single nerve fibres in the spinal nerve roots of dystrophic mice. *J. Physiol.* **305,** 151–169.

Redford, E. J., Kapoor, R., and Smith, K. J. (1997). Nitric oxide donors reversibly block axonal conduction: demyelinated axons are especially susceptible. *Brain* **120,** 2149–2157.

Ritchie, J. M., and Rogart, R. B. (1977). Density of sodium channels in mammalian myelinated nerve fibers and nature of the axonal membrane under the myelin sheath. *Proc. Natl. Acad. Sci.* **74,** 211–215.

Rizzo, M. A., Kocsis, J. D., and Waxman, S. G. (1996). Mechanisms of paresthesiae, dysesthesiae, and hyperesthesiae: Role of Na$^+$ channel heterogeneity. *Eur. Neurol.* **36,** 3–12.

Rosenbluth, J., Tao-Cheng, J.-H., and Blakemore, W. F. (1985). Dependence of axolemmal differentiation on contact with glial cells in chronically demyelinated lesions of cat spinal cord. *Brain Res.* **358,** 287–302.

Rushton, W. A. H. (1937). Initiation of the propagated disturbance. *Proc. R. Soc. Lond. Series B* **124,** 210–243.

Sakurai, M., and Kanazawa, I. (1999). Positive symptoms in multiple sclerosis: Their treatment with sodium channel blockers, lidocaine and mexiletine. *J. Neurol. Sci.* **162,** 162–168.

Scherokman, B. J., Selhorst, J. B., Waybright, E. A., Jabbari, B., Bryan, G. E., and Maitland, C. G. (1985). Improved optic nerve conduction with ingestion of ice water. *Ann. Neurol.* **17,** 418–419.

Sears, T. A., and Bostock, H. (1981). Conduction failure in demyelination: is it inevitable? *Adv. Neurol.* **31,** 357–375.

Sherratt, R. M., Bostock, H., and Sears, T. A. (1980). Effects of 4-aminopyridine on normal and demyelinated mammalian nerve fibres. *Nature* **283,** 570–572.

Shrager, P. (1993). Axonal coding of action potentials in demyelinated nerve fibers. *Brain Res.* **619,** 278–290.

Shrager, P., Custer, A. W., Kazarinova, K., Rasband, M. N., and Mattson, D. (1998). Nerve conduction block by nitric oxide that is mediated by the axonal environment. *J. Neurophysiol.* **79,** 529–536.

Shrager, P., and Rubinstein, C. T. (1990). Optical measurement of conduction in single demyelinated axons. *J. Gen. Physiol.* **95,** 867–890.

Smith, K. J. (1994). Conduction properties of central demyelinated and remyelinated axons, and their relation to symptom production in demyelinating disorders. *Eye* **8,** 224–237.

Smith, K. J., Blakemore, W. F., and McDonald, W. I. (1979). Central remyelination restores secure conduction. *Nature* **280,** 395–396.

Smith, K. J., Blakemore, W. F., and McDonald, W. I. (1981). The restoration of conduction by central remyelination. *Brain* **104,** 383–404.

Smith, K. J., Bostock, H., and Hall, S. M. (1982). Saltatory conduction precedes remyelination in axons demyelinated with lysophosphatidyl choline. *J. Neurol. Sci.* **54,** 13–31.

Smith, K. J., Felts, P. A., and John, G. R. (2000). Effects of 4-aminopyridine on demyelinated axons, synapses and muscle tension. *Brain* **123,** 171–184.

Smith, K. J., Felts, P. A., and Kapoor, R. (1997). Axonal hyperexcitability: mechanisms and role in symptom production in demyelinating diseases. *The Neuroscientist* **3,** 237–246.

Smith, K. J., and Hall, S. M. (1980). Nerve conduction during peripheral demyelination and remyelination. *J. Neurol. Sci.* **48,** 201–219.

Smith, K. J., and McDonald, W. I. (1980). Spontaneous and mechanically evoked activity due to central demyelinating lesion. *Nature* **286,** 154–155.

Smith, K. J., and McDonald, W. I. (1982). Spontaneous and evoked electrical discharges from a central demyelinating lesion. *J. Neurol. Sci.* **55,** 39–47.

Sumner, A. J., Saida, K., Saida, T., Silberberg, D. H., and Asbury, A. K. (1982). Acute conduction block associated with experimental antiserum-mediated demyelination of peripheral nerve. *Ann. Neurol.* **11,** 469–477.

Swadlow, H. A., Waxman, S. G., and Weyand, T. G. (1981). Effects of variations in temperature on impulse conduction along nonmyelinated axons in the mammalian brain. *Exp. Neurol.* **71,** 383–389.

Targ, E. F., and Kocsis, J. D. (1985). 4-Aminopyridine leads to restoration of conduction in demyelinated rat sciatic nerve. *Brain Res.* **328,** 358–361.

Tasaki, I. (1953). "Nervous Transmission." Charles C. Thomas, Springfield, IL.

Titcombe, A. F., and Willison, R. G. (1961). Flicker fusion in multiple sclerosis. *J. Neurol. Neurosurg. Psychiatry* **24,** 260–265.

Utzschneider, D. A., Archer, D. R., Kocsis, J. D., Waxman, S. G., and Duncan, I. D. (1994). Transplantation of glial cells enhances action potential conduction of amyelinated spinal cord axons in the myelin-deficient rat. *Proc. Natl. Acad. Sci.* **91,** 53–57.

Vagg, R., Mogyoros, I., Kiernan, M. C., and Burke, D. (1998). Activity-dependent hyperpolarization of human motor axons produced by natural activity. *J. Physiol.* **507,** 919–925.

van Diemen, H. A., van Dongen, M. M., Dammers, J. W., and Polman, C. H. (1992). Increased visual impairment after exercise (Uhthoff's phenomenon) in multiple sclerosis: therapeutic possibilities. *Eur. Neurol.* **32,** 231–234.

Warrington, A. E., Asakura, K., Bieber, A. J., Ciric, B., Van, K. V., Kaveri, S. V., Kyle, R. A., Pease, L. R., and Rodriguez, M. (2000). Human monoclonal antibodies reactive to oligodendrocytes promote remyelination in a model of multiple sclerosis. *Proc. Natl. Acad. Sci.* **97,** 6820–6825.

Waxman, S. G. (1977). Conduction in myelinated, unmyelinated, and demyelinated fibers. *Arch. Neurol.* **34,** 585–589.

Waxman, S. G. (1981). Clinicopathological correlations in multiple sclerosis and related diseases. *Adv. Neurol.* **31,** 169–182.

Waxman, S. G. (1989). Demyelination in spinal cord injury. *J. Neurol Sci* **91,** 1–14.

Waxman, S. G., Black, J. A., Kocsis, J. D., and Ritchie, J. M. (1989). Low density of sodium channels supports action potential conduction in axons of neonatal rat optic nerve. *Proc. Natl. Acad. Sci.* **86,** 1406–1410.

Waxman, S. G.. and Brill, M. H. (1978). Conduction through demyelinated plaques in multiple sclerosis: computer simulations of facilitation by short internodes. *J. Neurol. Neurosurg. Psychiatry* **41,** 408–416.

Waxman, S. G., and Geschwind, N. (1983). Major morbidity related to hyperthermia in multiple sclerosis. *Ann. Neurol.* **13,** 348.

Weber, F., Rudel, R., Aulkemeyer, P., and Brinkmeier, H. (2002). The endogenous pentapeptide QYNAD induces acute conduction block in the isolated rat sciatic nerve. *Neurosci. Lett.* **317,** 33–36.

Wisniewski, H. M., Oppenheimer, D., and McDonald, W. I. (1976). Relation between myelination and function in MS and EAE. *J. Neuropathol. Exp. Neurol.* **35,** 327.

7

Altered Distributions and Functions of Multiple Sodium Channel Subtypes in Multiple Sclerosis and Its Models

Stephen G. Waxman, M.D., Ph.D.

I. Introduction

Given the essential contribution of voltage-gated sodium (Na) channels to the generation and conduction of action potentials along axons, it is not surprising that these complex molecules play important roles in multiple sclerosis (MS). The contribution of sodium channels to action potential conduction is shaped by their nonuniform spatial distribution within the axon membrane, with a very high density of channels ($\sim 10^3/\mu m^2$) in the axon membrane at the node of Ranvier, and a much lower density ($<25/\mu m^2$) in the paranodal and internodal axon membrane beneath the myelin (see, for example, Waxman 1998; Peles and Salzer, 2000; and elsewhere in this volume). This nonuniform channel distribution focuses the channels where they are needed for normal saltatory conduction, but, after damage to the myelin, current loss through sodium channel-poor (formerly paranodal or internodal) membrane interferes with conduction (Ritchie and Rogart, 1977; Waxman, 1977). After demyelination, the expression of sodium channels in denuded (previously channel-poor) parts of the axon membrane can nonetheless lead to restoration of impulse conduction, which can contribute to clinical remissions (Bostock and Sears, 1978;

Foster et al., 1980). Thus, sodium channels can play an adaptive role in MS.

Emerging evidence also suggests that, under some circumstances, sodium channels can also play maladaptive roles in MS. Axonal degeneration is a major contributor to disability in MS; and recent studies indicate that some sodium channels can support sustained ion fluxes, which can injure axons. Moreover, evidence suggests that switches in sodium channel expression—the deployment of the wrong subtype of sodium channel within a particular class of neurons—can distort firing patterns and thus interfere with neuronal signaling in MS.

Molecular analysis has now shown that at least nine different genes encode distinct voltage-gated sodium channels ($Na_v1.1$–$Na_v1.9$). Molecular identification and characterization of the sodium channel subtypes, or isoforms, that are expressed by neurons in the demyelinating diseases (which channel isoforms are expressed by neurons in MS? Where? What functional roles do the different isoforms play?) is critical to an understanding of the pathophysiology of MS and to the development of therapeutic strategies. Molecular analysis has now begun to identify the channel subtypes that are expressed by neurons in animal models of MS and in human MS, and their functional contributions to molecular pathophysiology are being delineated. This chapter reviews recent progress in this molecular analysis of sodium channels, both in experimental models of MS and in MS.

II. Multiple Sodium Channel Subtypes

The nine isoforms of sodium channels share a common overall structural motif but have different amino acid sequences (Catterall, 1992; Plummer and Meisler, 1999; Goldin et al., 2000). The functional characteristics of many of these channels have now been studied, and these analyses have demonstrated that different sodium channel isoforms can exhibit different voltage-dependences, activation and inactivation kinetics, and recovery properties. Some subtypes of sodium channels open, close, and reprime rapidly; others have slower kinetics; while still others can remain persistently open (see, for example, Dib-Hajj et al., 1997; Cummins et al., 1999, 2001; Herzog et al., 2003). Recent studies have also shown that the selective expression of different ensembles of sodium channels contributes to the different functional properties of different types of neurons. Threshold, refractory period, and the temporal patterning of action potentials are all influenced by the type(s) of sodium channels that are expressed within a given neuron (see, for example, Stuart and Sakmann, 1995; Pennartz et al., 1997; Waxman, 2000; Taddese and Bean, 2002). Thus, it is not unexpected that changes in

sodium channel expression can have significant effects on neuronal function.

III. Sodium Channel Expression: A Dynamic Process

Since this chapter describes changes in sodium channel expression in MS and its models, it is worth pointing out that sodium channel expression is a dynamic process, even within the normal, uninjured nervous system. Levels of transcription for some sodium channels (e.g., $Na_v1.6$) increase during the course of development of some types of neurons, whereas transcription of others (e.g., $Na_v1.3$) falls (Beckh et al., 1989; Brysch et al., 1991; Felts et al., 1997). The mechanisms that control sodium channel transcription, translation, and deployment are not fully understood, although some regulatory influences have been identified. These include neurotrophic factors that exert complex and powerful effects on sodium channel expression. For example, NGF (Black et al., 1997; Dib-Hajj et al., 1998a; Cummins et al., 2000; Fjell et al., 1999a) and GDNF (Cummins et al., 2000; Fjell et al., 1999b; Boucher et al., 2000) upregulate transcription of the $Na_v1.8$ and $Na_v1.9$ sodium channel genes, while downregulating transcription of the $Na_v1.3$ gene in dorsal root ganglion neurons. Electrical activity may also modulate the expression of sodium channels (Offord and Catterall, 1989; Klein et al., 2003; Sashihara et al., 1996, 1997). Regulatory control also occurs at posttranscriptional stages of sodium channel expression. For example, an oligodendrocyte-derived soluble factor contributes to the regulation of clustering of $Na_v1.2$ channels along axons (Kaplan et al., 2001), while myelination is necessary for $Na_v1.6$ clustering (Boiko et al., 2001; Kaplan et al., 2001). The formation of paranodal axoglial junctions (although not of transverse bands) also appears to play a role in the transition from $Na_v1.2$ to $Na_v1.6$ as nodes of Ranvier mature (Rios et al., 2003).

Plasticity in sodium channel expression within the uninjured nervous system is not limited to development. One well-studied example is provided by the magnocellular neurons within the hypothalamic supraoptic nucleus, which are part of an osmoregulatory system that controls water balance. Although relatively quiescent in their basal state where they fire irregularly at low frequencies (<3 impulses per second), these neurons convert to a bursting mode in which they generate high-frequency bursts of action potentials that trigger vasopressin release from their terminals in response to increases in the osmolarity of extracellular milieu (Andrew and Dudek, 1983; Inenaga et al., 1993; Li and Hatton, 1996). Because these neurons exhibit both quiescent and bursting modes of operation, and can be driven from one state to another by noninvasive maneuvers such as oral salt-loading that results in a change in brain osmolarity, they provide a model system in which it is straightforward to ask: When a neuron converts from a quiescent to a bursting state, does it simply use its preexisting sodium channels differently, or is there a change in sodium channel expression? *In situ* hybridization experiments have shown that, in association with the transition to the bursting state, levels of mRNA for the $Na_v1.2$ and $Na_v1.6$ sodium channels (but not for $Na_v1.1$ or $Na_v1.3$) are upregulated in these cells (Tanaka et al., 1999). Immunocytochemical studies showed that the increase in mRNA is accompanied by an increase in channel protein. Patch clamp recordings demonstrated that the newly produced $Na_v1.2$ and $Na_v1.6$ channels are inserted into the neuronal cell membrane and are functional, contributing to the lowering of threshold for action potential generation and to bursting (Tanaka et al., 1999). Thus in association with the transition to the bursting state, these neurons alter their pattern of sodium channel expression so as to increase their electrogenicity. This is an example of *adaptive molecular plasticity within the healthy central nervous system (CNS)*, via the production and deployment of a new repertoire of sodium channels.

IV. Sodium Channel Expression in the Absence of Myelin: Developing and Dysmyelinated Axons

Within the normal adult nervous system, $Na_v1.6$ is the predominant sodium channel that is clustered at mature nodes of Ranvier (Caldwell et al., 2000). The aggregation of sodium channels within the nodal axon membrane, however, is the endpoint of a complex developmental sequence. At early stages before glial ensheathment, premyelinated axons display a low density of sodium channels that are distributed uniformly along the fiber (Black et al., 1982; Waxman et al., 1989). Aggregation of $Na_v1.6$ channels within the nodal axon membrane occurs relatively late within the developmental sequence; $Na_v1.2$ channels are first expressed (initially in a widely distributed, diffuse manner) in the membrane of premyelinated axons and then at immature nodes within CNS white matter, followed by a switch to $Na_v1.6$ at mature nodes of Ranvier with completion of the myelin sheath (Boiko et al., 2001; Kaplan et al., 2001).

As subtype-specific sodium channel antibodies began to be developed, studies on myelin mutants yielded hints of a relationship between myelination and the specification of sodium channel subtype. In an early study on axons lacking myelin within the Shiverer mutant, Westenbroek et al. (1992) observed $Na_v1.2$ along dysmyelinated tracts. In a more recent study on the same mutant model, Boiko et al. (2001) observed a lack of $Na_v1.6$ and retention of $Na_v1.2$ that was distributed along dysmyelinated axons. These studies, however, did not examine the distribution of $Na_v1.2$ and $Na_v1.6$ in *de*myelinated axons.

V. Sodium Channel Expression after Demyelination: Experimental Allergic Encephalomyelitis

What sodium channel subtype(s) is present along demyelinated axons? Early studies using cytochemical (Foster et al., 1980) and immunocytochemical approaches with pan-specific sodium channel antibodies (England et al., 1991; Dugandzija-Novakovic et al., 1995; Novakovic et al., 1998; Vabnick et al., 1997) demonstrated a change in organization of the axon membrane after demyelination, with a loss of nodal sodium channel clustering and appearance of more widely distributed sodium channels that are diffusely deployed along demyelinated axon regions; however, these early studies did not distinguish between the various sodium channel isoforms.

Studies using subtype-specific antibodies have examined sodium channel expression at an isoform-specific level along demyelinated axons within the CNS in experimental allergic encephalomyelitis (EAE) induced with myelin oligodendrocyte glycoprotein, an inflammatory model of demyelination, and have demonstrated altered expression of $Na_v1.6$ and $Na_v1.2$ along demyelinated axons in this model. The first study (Craner et al., 2003a) focused on the optic nerve, a white-matter tract in which virtually all axons are normally myelinated; a subsequent study (Craner et al., 2004a) yielded similar results in the spinal cord. Staining for myelin basic protein demonstrates the presence of demyelination extending throughout the length of the optic nerve and spinal cord from mice with this type of EAE. A significant reduction in the number of nodes flanked by well-defined Caspr staining in EAE is accompanied by an increase in the number of nodes with attenuated Caspr staining, suggesting loss of nodal integrity; a trend toward an increase in the total number of nodes in EAE compared to controls suggests the development of shortened, remyelinated internodes (Craner et al., 2003a).

A. $Na_v1.2$ in Demyelinated Axons in EAE

Figs. 1 and 2 demonstrate an increase in $Na_v1.2$ expression along axons in this animal model of inflammatory demyelination. As shown in Fig. 1, there is a reduction in frequency of $Na_v1.6$-positive nodes (84.5% $Na_v1.6$-immunopositive nodes in controls vs. 32.9% in EAE), and increased frequency of $Na_v1.2$-positive nodes (11.8% $Na_v1.2$ immunopositive nodes in controls vs. 74.9% in EAE). It is not yet clear whether the $Na_v1.2$-expressing nodes are formed by remyelination or by replacement of $Na_v1.6$ with $Na_v1.2$ at preexisting nodes.

There are also a large number of demyelinated axons in EAE, which appear as linear axonal profiles lacking an association with myelin basic protein. Use of the optic nerve as an experimental model permits the unequivocal

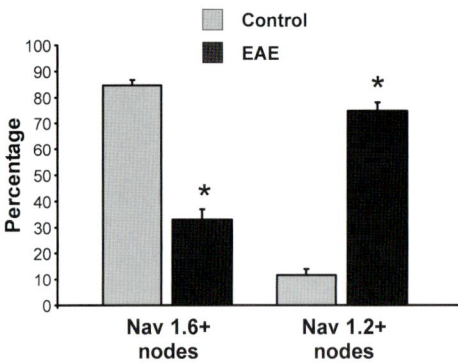

Figure 1 Histogram demonstrating a significant reduction in percentage of Na$_v$1.6-positive nodes with robust Caspr (*left panel*) and increased percentage of Na$_v$1.2-positive nodes with robust Caspr (*right panel*) in EAE. *$P < 0.005$.

identification of demyelinated (as opposed to nonmyelinated) axons, as virtually 100% of the axons in this tract are normally myelinated. Diffuse sodium channel immunostaining for Na$_v$1.2 or Na$_v$1.6 extends for tens of microns along the fiber axis in these demyelinated axons, as illustrated in Fig. 2 (Craner, 2003a). The increase in Na$_v$1.2 immunostaining is accompanied by upregulated levels of Na$_v$1.2 mRNA within

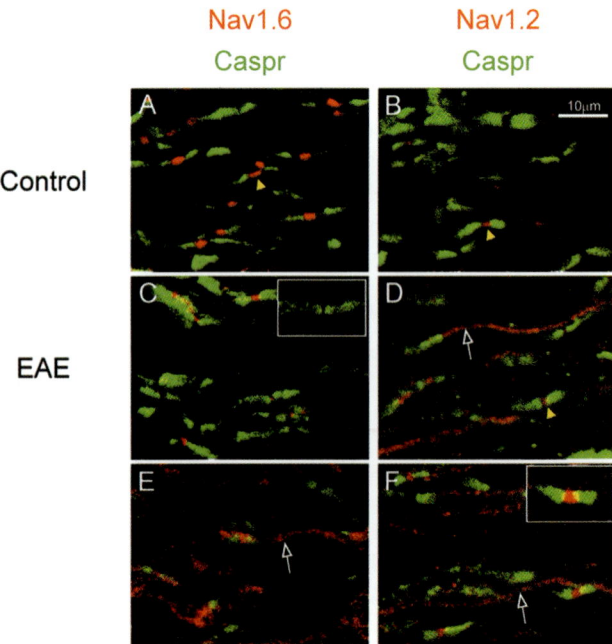

Figure 2 Changes in Na$_v$1.6 and Na$_v$1.2 expression in optic nerve axons in EAE. Representative digital images of sections of optic nerve from control (**A** and **B**) and EAE (**C–F**). **A** and **B** demonstrate nodes with robust Caspr with Na$_v$1.6 (**A**) and, less commonly, (**B**) Na$_v$1.2-positive immunostaining (*yellow arrowhead*) in control optic nerve. **C–E** and **D–F** demonstrate a pattern of progressive nodal disruption. Some nodes show weak and diffuse Caspr immunostaining (*inset*, **C**). There is a loss of Na$_v$1.6 immunostaining (**C** and **E**) and an increase in Na$_v$1.2 immunostaining (**D** and **F**) at nodes. Some demyelinated axonal profiles display diffuse Na$_v$1.6 (**E**) and Na$_v$1.2 (**D**, **F**) immunostaining (*unfilled white arrows*, **D**, **E**, **F**), which can extend for tens of microns along the fiber axis.

the retinal ganglion cells, which give rise to demyelinated optic nerve axons (Fig. 3). Thus the emergence of increased numbers of nodes expressing Na$_v$1.2, and of extensive regions of Na$_v$1.2 along demyelinated axons, appears to reflect upregulated synthesis of Na$_v$1.2 channels.

B. Na$_v$1.6 in Injured Axons in EAE

As documented elsewhere in this volume, there is extensive evidence for axonal degeneration that is a substrate for nonremitting disability in MS. Stys et al. (1992) demonstrated that sodium channels can participate in the production of calcium (Ca)-mediated axonal degeneration of CNS axons by providing a route for sustained sodium influx that drives reverse (calcium-importing) activity of the Na/Ca exchanger. The available evidence indicates that a persistent (noninactivating) sodium conductance carries the sustained sodium influx (Stys et al., 1993). Consistent with this schema, Imaizumi et al. (1997) have provided evidence for involvement of sodium channels and the Na/Ca exchanger in axonal degeneration in the anoxic spinal cord studied in vitro, and sodium channel blockers are protective, preventing axonal degeneration in a number of models of white matter injury *in vivo* (see, for example, Agrawal and Fehlings, 1996; Rosenberg et al., 1999).

There is also more direct evidence that sodium channels contribute to axonal degeneration *in vivo* in neuroinflammatory models of MS (see Waxman, 2003). Lo et al. (2002, 2003) have demonstrated that treatment with the sodium channel blocker phenytoin has a neuroprotective effect, preventing the degeneration of axons within the spinal cord and optic nerve, maintaining axonal conduction, and improving clinical outcome in progressive EAE. Bechtold et al. (2004) have demonstrated a similar protective effect of flecainide in chronic-relapsing EAE.

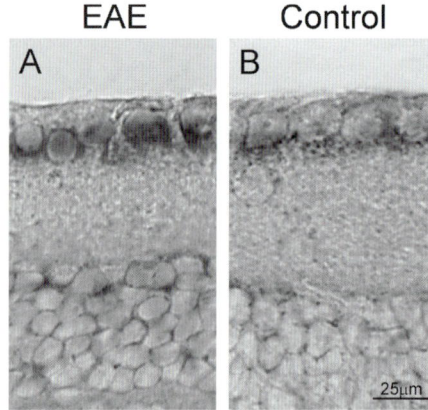

Figure 3 Upregulation of Na$_v$1.2 mRNA within retinal ganglion neurons, which gives rise to demyelinated axons, in EAE. Representative digital images of retinal sections demonstrate upregulation of Na$_v$1.2 mRNA in retinal ganglion neurons in EAE (**A**) compared with control (**B**). From Craner et al. (2003a).

As described previously, Na$_v$1.6 and Na$_v$1.2 sodium channels are both expressed diffusely along demyelinated axon regions that can extend for tens of microns in EAE. This raises the question of whether one, or both, of these sodium channel isoforms might be associated with axonal injury. Interestingly, Na$_v$1.6 channels can produce a persistent current that becomes larger with depolarization (Herzog et al., 2003), which is less prominent in Na$_v$1.1 or Na$_v$1.2 channels (Smith et al., 1998; Raman and Bean, 1997; Tanaka et al., 1999). Reasoning that co-expression of Na$_v$1.6 and the Na/Ca exchanger could predispose these axons to injury, Craner et al. (2004a) studied spinal cord white matter in mice with EAE to determine whether there is a correlation between the expression of Na$_v$1.6 sodium channel immunoreactivity, expression of the Na/Ca exchanger, and immunoreactivity to β-amyloid precursor protein (β-APP), a marker of axonal injury (Cochran et al., 1991; Trapp et al., 1998; Bitsch et al., 2000; Kuhlmann et al., 2002).

β-APP immunostaining demonstrated robust axonal injury in this EAE model. To test the hypothesis that Na$_v$1.6, Na$_v$1.2, or both are associated with axonal injury, Craner et al. (2004a) asked whether β-APP-positive axons tend to express Na$_v$1.6 or Na$_v$1.2. 92% of β-APP-positive axons were observed to be Na$_v$1.6 immunopositive (either expressing Na$_v$1.6 alone, 56.0%; or co-expressing Na$_v$1.6 *and* Na$_v$1.2, 36.2%), compared to only 1.8% of β-APP positive

axons that expressed Na$_v$1.2. Because these findings suggest that Na$_v$1.6 is preferentially associated with axonal injury in EAE, Craner et al. (2004a) next asked whether Na$_v$1.6 and the Na/Ca exchanger are co-localized in β-APP-positive axons, using triple-labeling fluorescence immunohistochemistry. Representative fields are shown in Fig. 4 (right panels), which demonstrates co-localization of Na$_v$1.6 (Fig. 4B) and the Na/Ca exchanger (Fig. 4C) along extensive regions of β-APP positive axons. In all, 73.5% of β-APP-positive axons displayed extensive regions labeled for both Na$_v$1.6 and Na/Ca exchanger, but only 4.4% of β-APP-negative axons displayed immunolabeling for Na$_v$1.6 and the Na/Ca exchanger (Fig. 4, left panel). Thus, Na$_v$1.6 and the Na/Ca exchanger tend to be co-localized within injured axons in this model of MS.

VI. Sodium Channel Expression along Axons in MS

Despite the utility of EAE as an animal model of MS, there is no perfect model that mimics all of the features of the human disorder. Thus the question "what sodium channels are expressed along demyelinated axons in MS?" requires examination of human tissue. Craner et al. (2004b) recently carried out such a study, examining postmortem

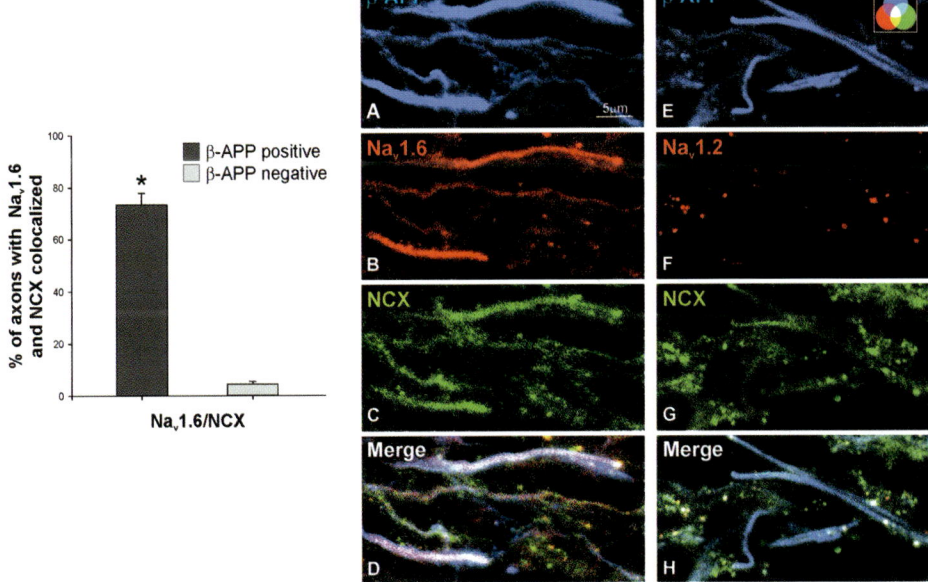

Figure 4 Degenerating spinal cord axons in EAE co-express Na$_v$1.6 and sodium-calcium exchanger over extensive regions. *Left*: Histogram showing co-expression of NCX and Na$_v$1.6 in β-APP-positive axons in EAE. Triple immunolabeling was used to determine the proportion of β-APP-positive axons and β-APP negative axons that co-express NCX and Na$_v$1.6 overextensive regions. The proportion of axons that co-express Na$_v$1.6 and NCX is significantly higher in β-APP positive axons (*filled bar*) compared with β-APP negative axons (light bar). *$^*P < 0.001$. (*Right*): Spinal cord axons in EAE spinal cord immunostained for β-APP (*blue*; **A, E**), sodium channel Na$_v$1.6 (*red*; **B**) and Na$_v$1.2 (*red*; **F**), and sodium-calcium exchanger (NCX) (*green*; **C, G**). Panels **D** and **H** correspond to merged images (*white*). Note the co-expression of Na$_v$1.6, NCX and β-APP, a marker of axonal injury (**A–D**). In contrast, β-APP/NCX-positive profiles do not display Na$_v$1.2 immunoreactivity. (**E–H**). (From Craner et al., 2004a.)

spinal cord and optic nerve tissue from controls without neurological disease and from patients with disabling secondary progressive MS, acquired via a rapid autopsy protocol (Newcombe and Cuzner, 1993). Analysis of acute lesions from this tissue has revealed a pattern of sodium channel expression that is similar to the pattern in EAE. Control white matter, from patients with no neurological disease, displayed abundant myelin basic protein (MBP) and the expected pattern of expression of $Na_v1.6$, which was focally expressed at nodes of Ranvier. $Na_v1.2$ was expressed along unmyelinated axons within control spinal cord tissue (but not within control optic nerves, as there are very few unmyelinated axons within that tract). Within acute MS plaques, which could be identified on the basis of attenuated MPB immunostaining and the presence of substantial numbers of ORO-positive macrophages containing neutral lipids resulting from myelin breakdown, $Na_v1.6$ and $Na_v1.2$ sodium channels were expressed along extensive regions, in many cases extending for tens of microns, along demyelinated axons (Fig. 5C–H). Fig. 5G-J illustrates staining of these profiles for neurofilaments, establishing their identity as axons. In some cases these extensive zones of $Na_v1.6$ or $Na_v1.2$ immunostaining were bounded by Caspr, a protein specifically expressed at the paranodal axoglial junction, further confirming the identity of these profiles as axons, but, as at normal nodes, there was no overlap between $Na_v1.6$ and Caspr immunostaining (Fig. 5E,F).

To examine the relationship of $Na_v1.6$ compared to $Na_v1.2$ expression and axonal injury within MS lesions, Craner et al. (2004b) examined the co-localization of these channel isoforms with β-APP. This analysis demonstrated a large number of β-APP-positive axons within MS plaques, suggesting the presence of approximately 7,500 injured axons per cubic millimeter of tissue within these acute lesions, similar to the value (11,000 per mm³) reported by Trapp et al. (1998). Of importance, β-APP-immunopositive axons within MS lesions tended to express $Na_v1.6$ over extensive regions. A total of 82% of β-APP-immunopositive axons expressed diffuse $Na_v1.6$ sodium channel immunostaining, whereas only 21% of β-APP-immunopositive axons expressed diffuse $Na_v1.2$ sodium channel immunostaining.

This analysis also demonstrated, as shown in Fig. 6, that $Na_v1.6$ and the Na/Ca exchanger tend to be co-localized within β-APP-positive axons within acute MS lesions (Craner et al., 2004b). A total of 60% of β-APP-positive axons (but only 19% of β-APP-negative axons) displayed co-expression of $Na_v1.6$ and the Na/Ca exchanger (Fig. 6, left panel). $Na_v1.2$ and the Na/Ca exchanger tended to be co-expressed within β-APP-negative axons. A total of 56% of β-APP-negative axons co-expressed $Na_v1.2$ and the Na/Ca exchanger, but only 18% of β-APP-positive axons showed this co-expression. Thus, the majority of β-APP-positive axons in these MS lesions display extensive regions where both $Na_v1.6$ and the Na/Ca

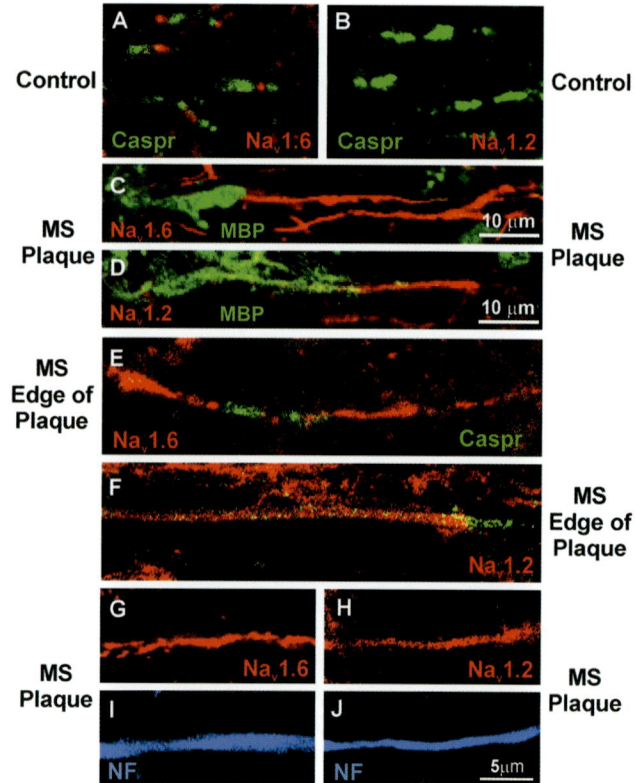

Figure 5 Changes in $Na_v1.6$ and $Na_v1.2$ expression along axons in human spinal cord, from active lesions identified by ORO staining in tissue obtained via a rapid protocol from patients with disabling secondary progressive MS. Note expression of $Na_v1.6$ (panel *A, red*), bounded by Caspr (**A**, *green*), while $Na_v1.2$ (**B**, *red*) is not detectable at nodes from controls without neurological disease. Panels **C** and **D** show the edge of active lesions, where extensive regions of diffuse expression of $Na_v1.6$ (**C**, *red*) and $Na_v1.2$ (**D**, *red*) are present at regions where myelin basic protein (**C**, **D**, *green*) is absent or markedly attenuated. Co-localization of neurofilament immunostaining (**I**, **J**, *blue*) with $Na_v1.6$ (**G**, *red*) and $Na_v1.2$ (**H**, *red*) establishes the identity of these profiles as axons. In some cases extensive regions of $Na_v1.6$ (**E**, *red*) or $Na_v1.2$ (**F**, *red*) are bounded by Caspr (**E**, **F**, *green*), without overlap, consistent with expression of $Na_v1.6$ and $Na_v1.2$ within the axon membrane. (From Craner et al., 2004b.)

exchanger are present, in contrast to β-APP-negative axons, which tend to co-express $Na_v1.2$ and the Na/Ca exchanger. In summary, this recent study of human MS tissue reveals a pattern of sodium channel expression within acute MS lesions that is similar to EAE, with $Na_v1.2$ and $Na_v1.6$ diffusely deployed along extensive regions of axons lacking myelin, and with $Na_v1.6$ (but not $Na_v1.2$) co-expressed together with the Na/Ca exchanger in injured axons.

A. Functional Role of $Na_v1.2$

The widespread expression of $Na_v1.2$, extending for tens of microns along demyelinated axons in EAE and in MS, is similar to the diffuse expression of $Na_v1.2$ immunostaining that has been reported along axons during early development

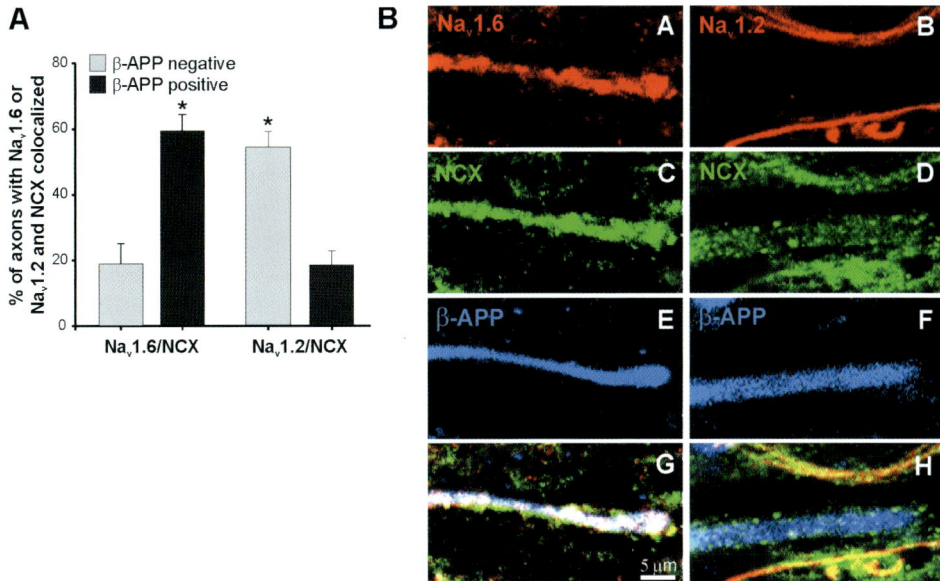

Figure 6 The Na/Ca exchanger and Na$_v$1.6 are co-expressed in β-APP-positive axons in MS. Histogram (*left*) showing the proportions of β-APP-positive axons and β-APP-negative axons that co-express the Na/Ca exchanger and Na$_v$1.6 or the Na/Ca exchanger and Na$_v$1.2, over extensive regions. The proportion of axons that co-express Na$_v$1.6 and the Na/Ca exchanger is significantly higher in β-APP-positive axons than in β-APP-negative axons. *$P < 0.005$. Digital images (*right*) demonstrate representative axons in MS spinal cord white matter immunostained for β-APP (*blue*; **E, F**), Na$_v$1.6 (*red*; **A**) or Na$_v$1.2 (*red*; **B**), and Na/Ca exchanger (*green*; **C, D**). Panels **G** and **H** show merged images (*white*). Panels **A, C, E** and **G** show co-expression of Na$_v$1.6 and Na/Ca exchanger within axons displaying β-APP, a marker of axonal injury. In contrast, panels **B, D, F,** and **H** demonstrate the Na/Ca exchanger but an absence of Na$_v$1.2 within β-APP-positive axons, and co-expression the Na/Ca exchanger and Na$_v$1.2 within β-APP-negative axons. (From Craner at al., 2004b.)

before myelination and in genetic dysmyelination (Boiko et al., 2001). Diffusely distributed Na$_v$1.2 channels are also present along nonmyelinated axons within the CNS (Westenbroek et al., 1989; Gong et al., 1999; Whitaker et al., 2000) where they appear to support action potential conduction.

Na$_v$1.2 and Na$_v$1.6 sodium channels both produce rapidly activating and inactivating currents that can support action potential electrogenesis, but the two channel subtypes exhibit some different functional properties. The rapid repriming kinetics of Na$_v$1.6 channels (Herzog et al., 2003) can support sustained high rates of firing while Na$_v$1.2 channels have slower repriming kinetics, support low-frequency firing, and are more likely to generate activity in response to sustained or slow depolarizations (Zhou and Goldin, 2002; Herzog et al., 2003). As discussed later, Na$_v$1.2 channels produce significantly less persistent current than Na$_v$1.6 channels (Smith et al., 1998; Goldin, 2001), a factor that may permit Na$_v$1.2 to be expressed along premyelinated and demyelinated axons without causing axonal degeneration. The conduction of action potentials, although with slowed conduction velocities, along CNS fibers before maturation of myelin (Foster et al., 1982; Waxman et al., 1989; Rasband et al., 1999) when only Na$_v$1.2 is present, suggests that the expression of Na$_v$1.2 channels may serve to support conduction of action potentials in demyelinated axons. Thus deployment of Na$_v$1.2 channels along demyelinated axons may serve an adaptive function. Nonetheless, the ability of Na$_v$1.2 to sustain high-frequency conduction may be limited, and the sensitivity of Na$_v$1.2 channels to small, slow depolarizations may contribute to ectopic firing or unstable patterns of firing after demyelination.

B. Functional Implications of Na$_v$1.6

These results demonstrate the co-expression of Na$_v$1.6 and the Na/Ca exchanger at regions of axonal injury in EAE and in MS and provide, for the first time, information about the molecular identity of a sodium channel subtype that may drive reverse Na/Ca exchange in neuroinflammatory disorders. Physiological data are consistent with a contribution of Na$_v$1.6 to neuronal injury. Rapidly inactivating sodium current would not be expected to produce the sustained influx of Na that is needed to drive reverse Na/Ca exchange. As described previously, a persistent sodium conductance has been shown to play a prominent role in the triggering of reverse Na/Ca exchange and resultant calcium entry in myelinated axons (Stys et al., 1992, 1993). Baker and Bostock (1997) demonstrated a TTX-sensitive, low-threshold persistent sodium current within large diameter dorsal root ganglion cells that gives rise to myelinated axons.

Na$_v$1.6 is expressed at high levels within these neurons while they express Na$_v$1.2 at only low levels (Black et al., 1996). Na$_v$1.6 is, moreover, known to produce a persistent sodium current that becomes larger with depolarization (see, for example, Smith et al., 1998; Raman and Bean, 1997; Tanaka et al., 1999). Herzog et al. (2003) performed patch clamp analysis on dorsal root ganglion neurons expressing Na$_v$1.6 channels (using tetrodotoxin-resistant recombinant channels, permitting unequivocal identification of Na$_v$1.6 current) and detected persistent Na$_v$1.6 currents in all cells that they studied. Fig. 7 shows a persistent current produced by Na$_v$1.6 when expressed within dorsal root ganglion neurons. Although Na$_v$1.2 may produce a persistent current when co-expressed with G-protein βγ subunits (Ma et al., 1997), Na$_v$1.6 channels produce a much larger persistent current than Na$_v$1.2 (Smith et al., 1998), and in many cells types Na$_v$1.6 is responsible for the majority of persistent current (Maurice et al., 2001).

Collaboration of Na$_v$1.6 and the Na/Ca exchanger in triggering axonal degeneration would suggest that subtype-specific blockade of Na$_v$1.6 (or, preferably, of the persistent component of the current produced by these channels) might have a protective effect, preventing axonal degeneration. The clinical efficacy of such an approach would depend, in part, on the proportion of Na$_v$1.6 channels that would have to be blocked along demyelinated axons and on the safety factor (in terms of the fraction of Na$_v$1.6 channels that are required to remain operable) at normal nodes where Na$_v$1.6 is widely deployed. The development of Na$_v$1.6-specific blockers may make it possible to test this hypothesis. Encouraging results have been provided by the demonstration that the nonspecific sodium channel blockers phenytoin (Lo et al., 2002, 2003) and flecainide (Bechtold et al., 2004) provide neuroprotection in EAE where they prevent axonal degeneration, maintain axonal conduction, and improve clinical outcome without apparent deleterious side effects in animal models.

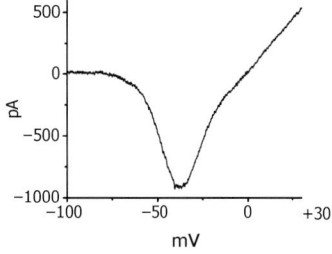

Figure 7 Persistent current produced by Na$_v$1.6. Sodium current elicited in a typical Na$_v$1.8-null DRG neuron expressing Na$_v$1.6r channels by a 500-ms ramp depolarization from −100 to +30 mV. The peak sodium current amplitude elicited in this cell with step depolarizations was 65.1 nA. (From Herzog et al., 2003.)

VII. Dysregulated Sodium Channel Expression and Altered Activity Patterns: Lessons from Nerve Injury

As described later, there is also evidence for dysregulated neuronal sodium channel expression that can result in distorted firing patterns, both in animal models of MS and in MS. Precedent for a role of aberrantly expressed sodium channels in distorting the pattern of neuronal activity is provided by peripheral nerve disorders, another class of disorders involving pathology of axons. A growing body of evidence from animal models and humans indicates that changes in sodium channel transcription occur and contribute to changes in neuronal firing patterns that produce clinically significant phenomena, including paresthesia and neuropathic pain, in peripheral nerve injury and in peripheral neuropathies. The changes triggered by nerve injury within dorsal root ganglion (DRG) neurons include down-regulated expression of some sodium channels (Na$_v$1.8 and Na$_v$1.9) together with upregulated expression of another (Na$_v$1.3) sodium channel (Dib-Hajj et al., 1996; Sleeper et al., 2000; Waxman et al., 1994). Newly formed Na$_v$1.3 mRNA is translated and produces Na$_v$1.3 sodium channel protein that is transported to distal parts of transected axons, which are sites of abnormal impulse generation within neuromas (Black et al., 1999a). The aberrantly expressed Na$_v$1.3 channels produce a rapidly repriming sodium current (i.e., a current with rapid recovery from inactivation) and this, in turn, leads to a decrease in the refractory period that contributes to ectopic activity of DRG neurons that underlies pain and paresthesia after nerve injury (Cummins and Waxman, 1997; Cummins et al., 2001; Dib-Hajj et al., 1999).

The factor(s) that triggers changes in sodium channel expression after nerve injury includes loss of access to peripheral pools of neurotrophic factors such as NGF and GDNF. Experimental delivery of NGF (Dib-Hajj et al., 1998a) and GDNF (Cummins et al., 2000) to peripherally axotomized DRG neurons reestablishes access to these factors and upregulates the levels of Na$_v$1.8 and Na$_v$1.9 mRNA and protein as well as the number of functional channels within the cell membrane (Cummins et al., 2000). These neurotrophic factors also down-regulate Na$_v$1.3 expression in DRG neurons (Black et al., 1997; Boucher et al., 2000; Leffler et al., 2002).

Recent studies have also demonstrated upregulation of Na$_v$1.3 within secondary and tertiary sensory neurons within the spinal cord afternerve injury (Hains et al., 2004). The increase in Na$_v$1.3 occurs with a time course that parallels the onset of a pain syndrome and the development of hyperexcitability in these neurons. Antisense knockdown of Na$_v$1.3 results in attenuation of this hyperexcitability and amelioration of pain-associated behaviors after spinal cord injury (Hains et al., 2004). Thus, axonal injury can trigger changes in the expression of sodium channels and resultant changes in excitability, within central neurons as well as DRG neurons; and these changes in excitability can produce clinical symptoms. In the next section, we describe altered expression of the $Na_V1.8$ sodium channel in MS.

A. Upregulated Expression of $Na_V1.8$ in MS and Its Models

It now appears likely that, in addition to altered expression of $Na_V1.2$ and $Na_V1.6$ along demyelinated axons in MS, there is altered expression of at least one other sodium channel isoform *within neuronal cell bodies* that can give rise to distorted patterns of impulse generation in these cells. This line of research originated with a study by Black et al. (1999b) who examined neuronal sodium channel expression in the *Taiep* rat, a mutant model in which myelin initially ensheaths CNS axons in a normal manner but subsequently degenerates as a result of an abnormality of oligodendrocytes (Duncan et al., 1992). This study focused on expression of the $Na_V1.8$ sodium channel [a slowly-inactivating tetrodotoxin (TTX)-resistant sodium channel which was originally termed SNS, **S**ensory **N**euron **S**pecific, since it is normally detectable only in DRG neurons and trigeminal neurons; (Akopian et al., 1996; Sangameswaren et al., 1996] because the transcription

of $Na_V1.8$ within these neurons changes markedly after axon transection (Dib-Hajj et al., 1996). *In situ* hybridization of the *Taiep* brain showed that, following loss of myelin within the cerebellar white matter, there is markedly enhanced expression of $Na_V1.8$ mRNA within Purkinje cells. Immunocytochemical studies showed that the up-regulation of $Na_V1.8$ mRNA is accompanied by the production of $Na_V1.8$ protein in Purkinje cells (Black et al., 1999b).

A more recent study (Black et al., 2000) used *in situ* hybridization and immunohistochemistry to examine the expression of $Na_V1.8$ in the brains of mice with chronic-relapsing EAE (CR-EAE) and in postmortem brain tissue from humans with MS. As shown in Fig. 8, in situ hybridization and immunocytochemistry demonstrated significantly increased expression of $Na_V1.8$ mRNA and protein within Purkinje cells in CR-EAE (Black et al., 2000). A global up-regulation of all sodium channels could not account for up-regulated expression of $Na_V1.8$ because expression of $Na_V1.9$, another TTX-resistant sodium channel that is normally expressed preferentially, like $Na_V1.8$, in DRG and trigeminal ganglion neurons, was not upregulated.

The increased expression of $Na_V1.8$ within Purkinje cells is not limited to animal models of MS. Study of postmortem human brain tissue (Black et al., 2000) has demonstrated up-regulation of $Na_V1.8$ mRNA and protein within Purkinje cells in patients with disabling progressive MS with cerebellar deficits on neurological examination (Fig. 9).

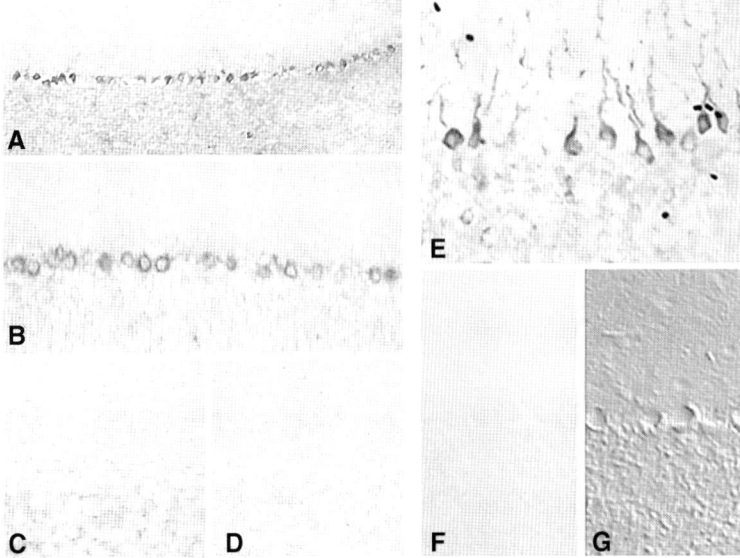

Figure 8 Sodium channel $Na_V1.8$ (originally termed SNS, Sensory Neuron Specific) is abnormally expressed within cerebellar Purkinje neurons in mice with EAE. **A–D**: in situ hybridization showing $Na_V1.8$ mRNA within Purkinje cells in EAE (**A, B**) but not in healthy control mice (**C**) or after hybridization with sense riboprobes (**D**). **E–G**: Immunostaining with $Na_V1.8$-specific antibodies, showing upregulated expression of $Na_V1.8$ protein in EAE (**E**) compared to controls (**F**, bright field; **G**, Nomarski; image). (**A**) 120; (**B–D**)×200; (**E–G**) ×220. (From Black et al., 2000.)

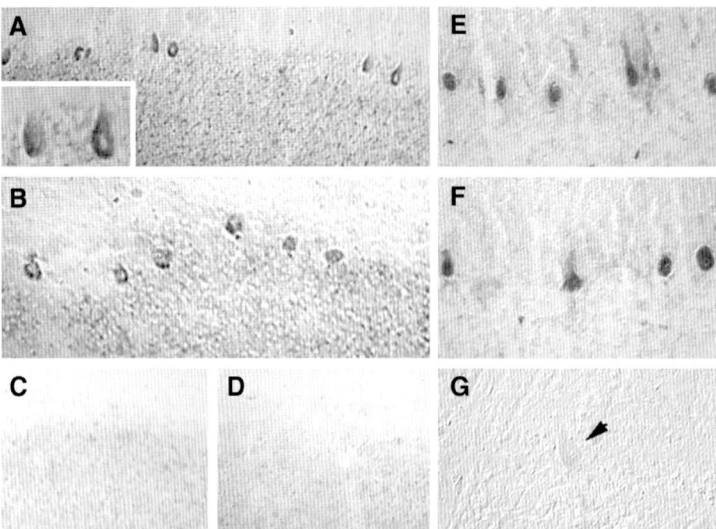

Figure 9 Expression of the Sensory Neuron Specific (SNS) sodium channel Na$_v$1.8 is upregulated in cerebellar Purkinje neurons in patients with MS. *In situ* hybridization demonstrates increased Na$_v$1.8 mRNA in Purkinje cells from two MS patients obtained at postmortem (**A, B**), compared to controls without neurological disease (**C**). No signal is present following hybridization with sense riboprobe (**D**). Immunocytochemistry with Na$_v$1.8-specific antibodies demonstrates upregulation of Na$_v$1.8 channel protein in Purkinje cells from two MS patients (**E, F**) compared to controls (**G**; arrowhead indicates Purkinje cell). (**A**) ×120, inset ×280; (**B, C, D**) ×165; (**E, F, G**) ×175. (From Black et al., 2000.)

These observations in two animal models of MS, and in humans with MS, demonstrate that expression of the Na$_v$1.8 sodium channel is up-regulated at the transcriptional level in Purkinje neurons, producing Na$_v$1.8 sodium channel protein which is not normally present in these cells.

The trigger of up-regulated expression of Na$_v$1.8 is currently under study. The available evidence (Damarjian et al., 2004) demonstrates up-regulated expression of TrkA and p75 receptors for nerve growth factor (NGF, which is known to be present at elevated levels within the CNS in EAE and MS; Laudiero et al., 1991; De Simone et al., 1996), within Na$_v$1.8-immunopositive Purkinje neurons in EAE, and suggests that activation of p75, in particular, may trigger the expression of Na$_v$1.8.

The Na$_v$1.8 sodium channel, like other sodium channels, binds to accessory proteins and at least one of these is up-regulated in a coordinate manner with Na$_v$1.8 in EAE and MS (Craner et al., 2003b). AnnexinII/p11 binds to the N-terminus of Na$_v$1.8 and facilitates the insertion of functional channels into the neuronal cell membrane (Okuse et al., 2002). As shown in Fig. 10 the expression of annexinII/p11 is up-regulated within Purkinje cells, and it is co-localized with Na$_v$1.8, both in EAE and in MS (Craner et al., 2003b).

While a full mapping of the CNS has not yet been completed, other neuronal cell types may show similar abnormalities in MS and its models. Expression of Na$_v$1.8 and annexin11/p11 is also up-regulated in retinal ganglion cells

(which give rise to axons that travel in the optic nerve) in EAE (Craner, Black, and Waxman, unpublished). Na$_v$1.8 protein is not detectable, however, along Purkinje cell axons within the cerebellar white matter (Craner, Black and Waxman, unpublished) or retinal ganglion cell axons within the optic nerve (Craner et al., 2003a).

Although the functional consequences of up-regulated Na$_v$1.8 expression in Purkinje cells have not yet been definitively determined in humans, several studies suggest that it interferes with neuronal signaling. In theory it is possible is that Na$_v$1.8 up-regulation might be an adaptive change, which could support the restoration of action potential conduction along demyelinated Purkinje cell axons. Renganathan et al. (2001) demonstrated that Na$_v$1.8 channels produce a substantial fraction of the inward current that underlies the depolarizing phase of the action potential in the DRG neurons in which these channels are normally present. Thus, if Na$_v$1.8 channels were inserted into the demyelinated axon membrane, they might be expected to contribute to restoration of action potential conduction in demyelinated axons. However, while Na$_v$1.8 is up-regulated in the cell bodies of Purkinje cells and retinal ganglion cells in EAE, Na$_v$1.8 protein has not been detected along demyelinated Purkinje cell or optic nerve axons, in contrast to Na$_v$1.2 and Na$_v$1.6 protein which, as shown in Fig. 2, can be clearly detected (Craner et al., 2003a). An adaptive role of Na$_v$1.8 in restoration of conduction along demyelinated axons thus seems unlikely.

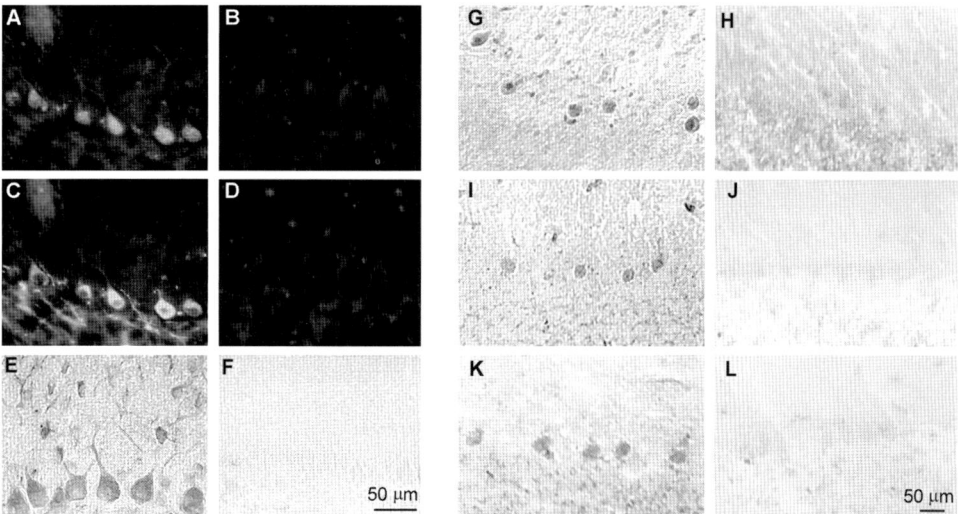

Figure 10 AnnexinII/p11, which facilitates insertion of functional Na$_v$1.8 channels into the cell membrane, is upregulated and co-expressed with Na$_v$1.8 in Purkinje cells in EAE and MS. (**Left panels**) Na$_v$1.8 (**A**) and annexinII/p11 (**C**) are upregulated in Purkinje neurons in EAE as compared to control (**B** and **D**, respectively). Note the co-localization of annexinII/P11 in Na$_v$1.8 in the same neurons (compare panels **A** and **C**). AnnexinII/p11 immunostaining extends along the proximal portion of the dendritic tree in EAE (**E**) but not in control (**F**). (**Right**) Na$_v$1.8 is upregulated in neurons in postmortem MS tissue (**G**) vs. control (**H**). Upregulated expression of annexinII/p11 is shown for two MS cases (**I**, **K**) in comparison to controls (**J**, **L**). (Modified from Craner et al., 2003b.)

A number of observations strongly suggest that upregulated expression of Na$_v$1.8 in EAE and MS is maladaptive. Electrogenesis within Purkinje cells depends, in part, on sodium channel activity (Llinas and Sugimori, 1980; Stuart and Hausser, 1994; Raman and Bean, 1997) and mutations of sodium channels that are expressed in Purkinje cells can produce substantial changes in the patterns of impulse generation in these cells that can result in clinical signs of cerebellar dysfunction such as ataxia (Raman et al., 1997; Kohrman et al., 1996). Na$_v$1.8 displays unique physiological properties including a depolarized voltage-dependence of inactivation, slow development of inactivation (Akopian et al., 1996; Sangameswaren et al., 1996) and rapid recovery from inactivation (Elliott and Elliott, 1993; Dib-Hajj et al., 1997). As a result of these properties Na$_v$1.8 channels are available over a wider range of dynamic activity and membrane potential than other sodium channels (Schild and Kunze, 1997), so that cells expressing Na$_v$1.8 are predicted to be more slowly adapting than cells lacking Na$_v$1.8 (Elliott and Elliott, 1993).

Electrophysiological observations confirm this prediction and demonstrate that Na$_v$1.8 expression can, in fact, substantially alter the temporal pattern of electrical activity. Renganathan et al. (2001) used current-clamp and voltage-clamp recording to examine the pattern of action potential generation in DRG neurons from transgenic Na$_v$1.8 –/– mice in which functional Na$_v$1.8 channels are absent (Akopian et al., 1999) and compared it with electrogenesis in Na$_v$1.8 +/+ neurons. This study showed that the presence

of Na$_v$1.8 channels within DRG neurons markedly influences both the configuration of the action potentials (a change that can effect activation of N-type channels and thus transmitter release [Scroggs and Fox, 1992] if Na$_v$1.8 is deployed to axon terminals) and the temporal pattern of firing in response to depolarizing stimuli. Consistent with the suggestion that cells expressing Na$_v$1.8 should be slowly adapting, Na$_v$1.8 +/+ DRG neurons produce sustained pacemaker-like trains of action potentials in response to depolarizing stimuli, which are not present within Na$_v$1.8 –/– neurons (Renganathan et al., 2001).

In a more recent study, Renganathan et al. (2003) transfected Purkinje cells *in vitro* with Na$_v$1.8. Voltage-clamp recordings demonstrated that functional Na$_v$1.8 channels can be expressed within Purkinje cells where they produce slowly inactivating TTX-resistant Na$_v$1.8 currents at physiological levels (with current amplitudes of approximately 4 to 5 nA, similar to those observed within DRG neurons where Na$_v$1.8 is normally expressed). Current-clamp recordings demonstrated that expression of Na$_v$1.8 produces several physiological changes within Purkinje neurons. First, expression of Na$_v$1.8 increases action potential amplitude and duration (compare Fig. 11B and 11A). Second, Na$_v$1.8 expression decreases the proportion of action potentials that display the conglomerate configuration characteristically observed in Purkinje cells (15% in Na$_v$1.8-transfected neurons compared to 62% in controls) and the number of spikes per conglomerate action potential, which was 2.13 in Na$_v$1.8-transfected neurons compared to 3.38 in controls

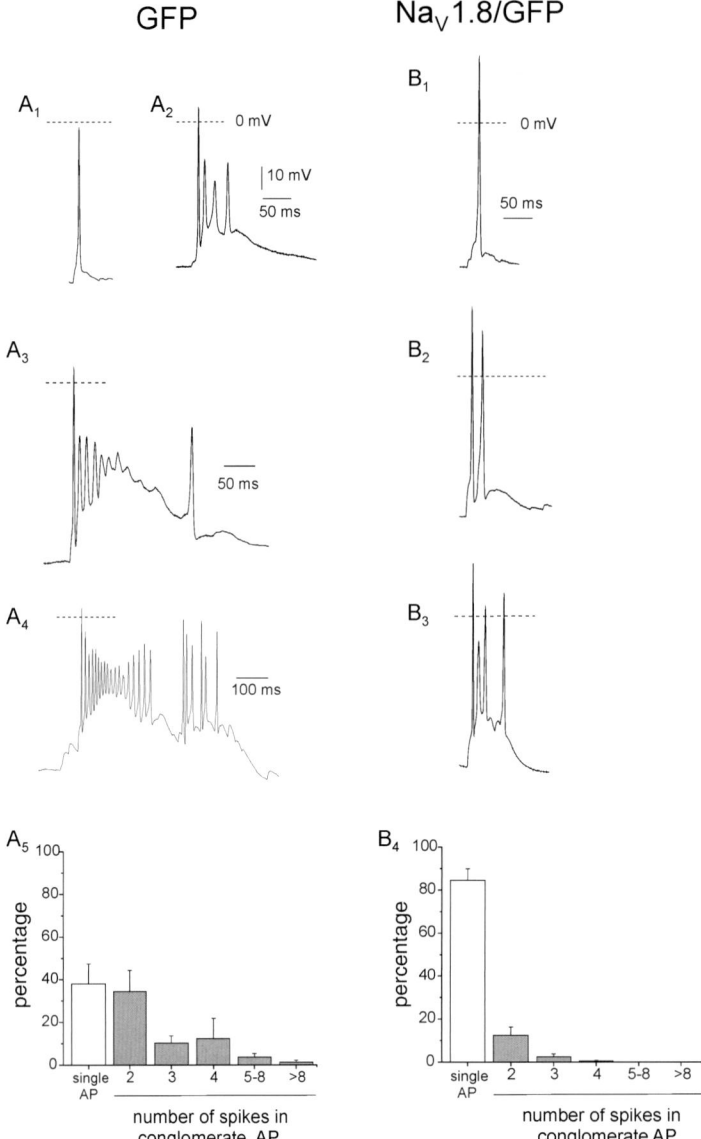

Figure 11 Expression of $Na_V1.8$ alters action potential electrogenesis within Purkinje cells. These current clamp recordings show spontaneous action potentials recorded in Purkinje neurons two days after biolistic expression of GFP that provided a marker of transfection (without $Na_V1.8$) ($A_1 - A_4$) or of $Na_V1.8$/GFP ($B_1 - B_3$). A_1-A_4: Action potentials in control neurons lacking $Na_V1.8$ ($A_1 - A_4$) show little if any overshoot (dotted lines indicate 0 mV) and tend to be conglomerate (62%; $A_2 - A_4$). B_1-B_3: Action potentials in neurons expressing $Na_V1.8$ display larger overshoot. Conglomerate action potentials are less common after expression of $Na_V1.8$ (15%) and, when present, tend to consist of doublets (B_2), only rarely consisting of more than 2 spikes (B_3). Time calibration in A_2 applies to A_1; time calibration in B_1 applies to B_1-B_3. The mV calibration in A_2 applies to all panels. A_5, B_4: Percentage of action potentials that were single, or conglomerate with 2, 3, 4, 5–8 or more spikes, in Purkinje cells lacking $Na_V1.8$ and with $Na_V1.8$, respectively. There is a lower percentage of conglomerate action potentials and a smaller number of spikes per conglomerate action potential in Purkinje neurons expressing $Na_V1.8$. (Modified from Renganathan et al., 2003.)

(compare Fig. 11B and 11A). Third, Na$_v$1.8 expression supports sustained, pacemaker-like impulse trains in response to depolarization, which are not seen in the absence of Na$_v$1.8 (Fig. 12). More recently, Saab et al. (2004) observed similar changes in the firing patterns of Purkinje cells *in vivo* in mice with EAE (Fig. 13). The results of these studies indicate that expression of Na$_v$1.8 within Purkinje neurons *in vitro* distorts the pattern of activity of these cells, a change that could interfere with cerebellar function, and show that similar changes occur *in vivo* in EAE. Whether the upregulated Na$_v$1.8 expression and resultant change in excitability lead to degeneration of Purkinje cells is not known.

Biopsy of the cerebellum is only infrequently performed in MS, and it is therefore difficult to directly establish whether similar physiological changes occur in Purkinje cells in humans with MS. Support for this suggestion nonetheless is provided by the observations on postmortem MS tissue described previously, and by several observations

from the clinic. First, most clinicians have observed occasional patients of MS with cerebellar deficits on clinical examination, but without apparent cerebellar lesions in neuroimaging studies; this observation is consistent with a contribution of molecular changes, too subtle to be detected by currently available imaging techniques, to cerebellar dysfunction. Second, cerebellar signs in MS are often nonremitting even if developing early in the course of the disease (see, for example, Matthews et al., 1991), and this is not readily explained by inflammation or demyelination per se. Craner et al. (2003c) observed that, in relapsing-remitting EAE, the level of Na$_v$1.8 expression within Purkinje cells is correlated with the severity of nonremitting deficits (which include cerebellar dysfunction). Finally, paroxysmal ataxia has been well described in MS and, in many cases, responds to treatment with sodium channel blockers such as carbamazepine (Andermann et al., 1959; Espir et al., 1966). These sudden and brief episodes of ataxia in MS are similar to the paroxysmal attacks that occur in the episodic ataxias (which are known to be inherited channelopathies) and are not easily explained by demyelination or axonal degeneration. The therapeutic response to carbamazepine suggests that sodium channels may participate in their pathogenesis.

The observation of upregulated Na$_v$1.8 expression within retinal ganglion neurons in EAE (Craner, Black, and Waxman, unpublished) may also have implications for MS, as sodium channels contribute significantly to electrogenesis in retinal ganglion cells (Lipton and Tauck, 1986). The electroretinogram provides some evidence for retinal dysfunction in MS, suggestive of an abnormality of retinal neurons even in patients without a history of optic neuritis (Plant et al., 1986; see also Chapter 16). Study of suitably preserved human retinal tissue should make it possible to determine whether Na$_v$1.8 is in fact expressed in retinal ganglion neurons in MS.

The hypothesis that aberrant expression of Na$_v$1.8 channels contributes to symptomatology in MS would be strengthened if it could be shown that Na$_v$1.8 blocking drugs ameliorate ataxia or other clinical abnormalities. Na$_v$1.8-specific channel blocking drugs are not yet available, but the high level of expression of Na$_v$1.8 within nociceptive DRG neurons has made this channel an attractive target for drug screening. When Na$_v$1.8-specific blocking drugs are developed, it will be possible to examine the effect of these drugs on animal models of MS such as EAE and, if indicated, in humans with MS.

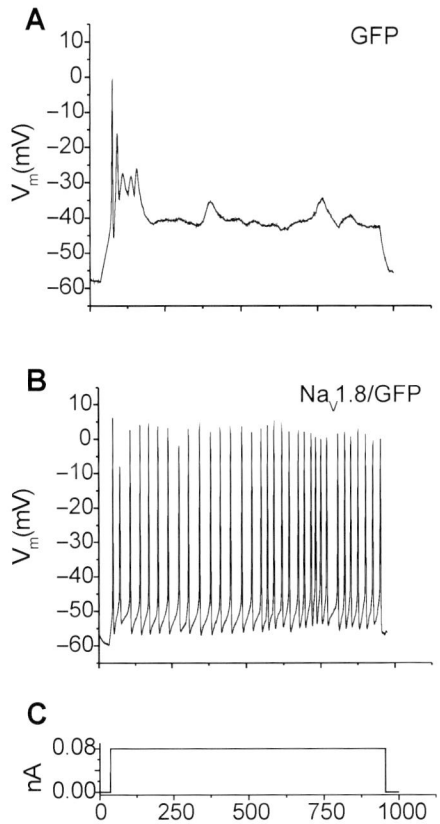

Figure 12 Purkinje neurons transfected with Na$_v$1.8 show sustained repetitive firing, not present in the absence of Na$_v$1.8, on injection of depolarizing current. (**A**) Control Purkinje neuron lacking Na$_v$1.8 produces a conglomerate action potential consisting of five spikes, but no sustained firing, in response to a sustained depolarizing stimulus (80 pA, 1 second). (**B**) Purkinje neuron expressing Na$_v$1.8 produces larger-amplitude action potentials and shows sustained pacemaker-like activity in response to identical stimulus. The current pulse protocol is shown in **C**. (Modified from Renganathan et al., 2003.)

VIII. Is Expression of Other Channels Altered in MS?

Although this chapter has focused on sodium channels, expression of other types of channels may also be altered in MS. Increased expression of K$_v$1.1 and K$_v$1.2 potassium

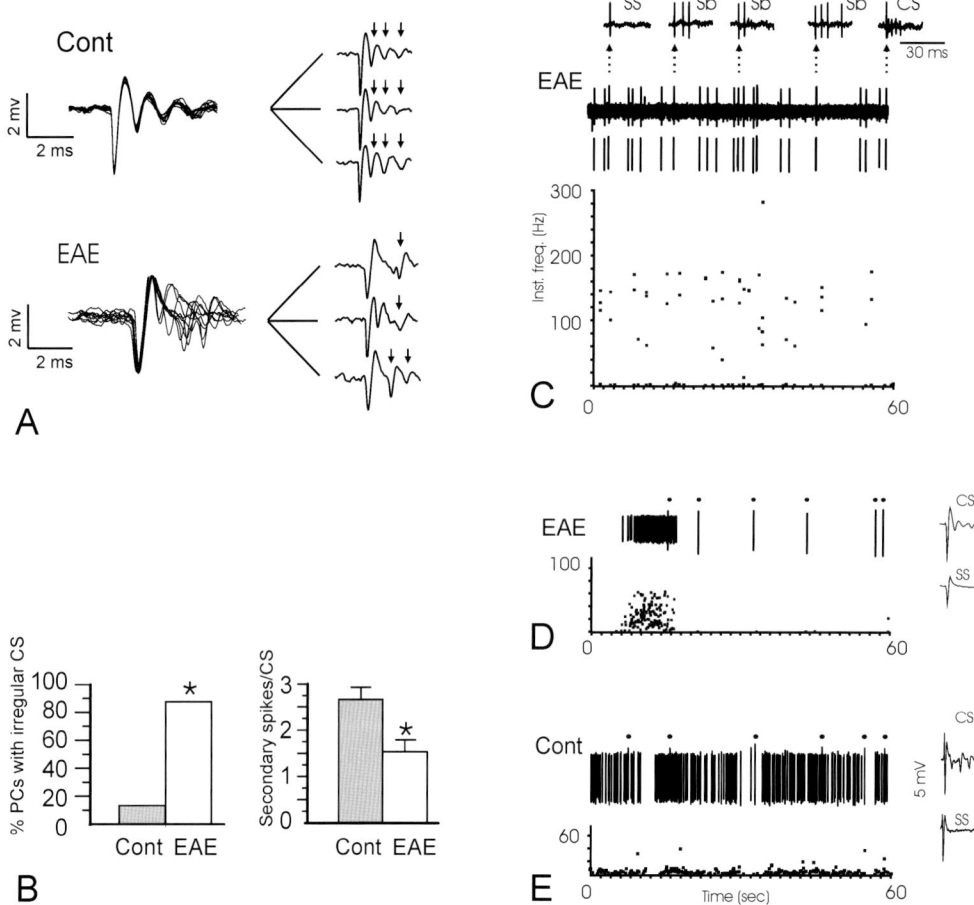

Figure 13 The firing patterns of Purkinje cells within their native cerebellar environment *in vivo* are altered in EAE. (**A**) Conglomerate action potentials in Purkinje cells from control (*upper traces*) and EAE (*lower traces*). Superimposed conglomerate action potentials show regularity of secondary spikes in controls and irregularity in EAE (note the irregularity in latencies of secondary spikes for each cell; *downward arrows on right*). (**B, left panel**) Percentage of Purkinje cells with irregular temporal organization of conglomerate action potentials is higher in EAE ($^*P < 0.001$). (**B, right panel**) Average number of secondary spikes per conglomerate action potential is lower in EAE ($^*P < 0.005$). (**C, D, E**) Abnormal high-frequency bursting in Purkinje cells in EAE. (**C**) Purkinje cells in EAE produced brief bursts (Sb) of repetitive single spikes consisting of doublets, triplets, or quadruplets, not seen in controls, interspersed with isolated single spikes (SS) and conglomerate action potentials. (**C**, *top*). Second and third rows in **C** show a continuous recording; isolated action potentials, plotted using template matching techniques, were used to plot instantaneous frequency (**C–E**, *bottom*). In another Purkinje cell from a mouse with EAE (**D**), sustained high-frequency SS bursts (up to 60 Hz) lasting for >10 seconds are followed by an extended period (more than 3 min) of no recorded SS activity (conglomerate action potentials are indicated by dots; individual conglomerate action potentials and SS are shown to the right). (**E**) These activity patterns were not observed in Purkinje cells recorded in control mice. (Modified from Saab et al., 2004.)

channels (Wang et al., 1999), for example, has been reported along dysmyelinated axons within the brain of the Shiverer mouse. A recent study has suggested the ectopic expression of the α_{1B} pore-forming subunit of N-type calcium channels within dystrophic (presumably degenerating) axons in EAE and MS (Kornek et al., 2001). Another study suggests the presence of mGlu1α-glutamate receptor immunoreactivity along axons in MS (Geurts et al., 2003), although, again, it is not clear whether the receptors are inserted into the axon membrane. If they are, there is the possibility of activation

of signaling cascades that activate injurious intra-axonal processes. Ouardouz et al. (2003) demonstrated, in rat dorsal column axons, that ischemia can trigger a rise in intra-axonal calcium due to ryanodine-sensitive intracellular calcium release that is triggered by L-type calcium channels. This observation raises the possibility that activation of ectopic ion channels may trigger release of calcium from intracellular stores within axons. In summary, there may be changes in expression of multiple channel and receptor mRNAs within neurons whose axons have been demyelinated or subjected to inflammation, and it will be important to determine the full ensemble of channels and receptors that are expressed and their precise pattern of distribution.

IX. Sodium Channels as Therapeutic Targets

The multiplicity of molecularly distinct sodium channel subtypes, and their roles in the pathophysiology in MS and its models, raise the suggestion that it may be possible to therapeutically induce the expression of $Na_v1.2$ channels so as to promote restoration of axonal conduction after demyelination, or to target sodium channels so as to retard axonal degeneration, or reduce symptoms. The ideal sodium channel blocker in this respect would be selective for the offending channel, with no side effects related to channels distributed elsewhere. Block of $Na_v1.6$ sodium channels as a strategy for preventing axonal injury in MS might seem problematical at first sight, as these channels are distributed widely within the CNS. Studies that have already been carried out show that nonspecific sodium channel blockers can provide a degree of protection, preventing axonal degeneration and improving clinical outcome in EAE (Lo et al., 2002, 2003; Bechtold et al., 2004). Therapeutic targeting of $Na_v1.8$ is not yet possible, as selective blockers of this channel subtype are not yet available, but the relatively selective expression of this channel within primary sensory neurons in the normal central nervous system raises the possibility that, when such blockers do become available, they may favorably impact cerebellar symptomatology without significant side effects. Thus the multiplicity of the sodium channel subtypes expressed in MS and its models, while presenting a challenge in the laboratory, may also provide multiple therapeutic opportunities.

Acknowledgments

Research in the author's laboratory has been supported, in part, by grants from the National Multiple Sclerosis Society, the Medical Research Service and Rehabilitation Research Service, Department of Veterans Affairs, and the Nancy Davis Foundation. The Center for Neuroscience and Regeneration Research is a Collaboration of the Paralyzed Veterans of America and the United Spinal Association with Yale University.

References

Agrawal, S. K., and Fehlings, M. G. (1996). Mechanisms of secondary injury to spinal cord axons *in vitro*: role of Na^+, Na^+-K^+-ATPase, the Na^+-H^+ exchanger, and the Na^+-Ca^{2+} exchanger. *J. Neurosci.* **16,** 545–552.

Akopian, A. N., Sivilotti, L., and Wood, J. N. (1996). A tetrodotoxin-resistant voltage-gated sodium channel expressed by sensory neurons. *Nature* **379,** 257–262.

Akopian, A. N., Souslova, V., England, S., Okuse, K., Ogata, N., Ure, J., Smith, A., Kerr, B. J., McMahon, S. B., Boyce, S., Hill, R., Stanfa, L. C.,

Dickenson, A. H., and Wood, J. N. (1999). The tetrodotoxin-resistant sodium channel SNS has a specialized function in pain pathways. *Nat. Neurosci.* **2,** 541–548.

Andermann, F., Cosgrove, J. B. R., Lloyd-Smith, D., and Walters, A. M. (1959). Paroxysmal dysarthria and ataxia in multiple sclerosis. *Neurology* **9,** 21–216.

Andrew, R. D., and Dudek, F. E. (1983). Burst discharge in mammalian neuroendocrine cells involves an intrinsic regenerative mechanism. *Science* **221,** 1050–1052.

Baker, M. D., and Bostock, H. (1997). Low-threshold, persistent sodium current in rat large dorsal root ganglion neurons in culture. *J. Neurophysiol,* **77,** 1503–1513.

Bechtold, D. A., Kapoor, R., and Smith, K. J. (2004). Axonal protection using flecainide in experimental autoimmune encephalomyelitis. *Ann. Neurol.*

Beckh, S., Noda, M., Lubbert, H., and Numa, S. (1989). Differential regulation of three sodium channel messenger RNAs in the rat central nervous system during development, *EMBO J.* **8,** 3611–3616.

Bitsch, A., Schuchardt, J., Bunkowski, S., Kuhlmann, T., and Bruck, W. (2000). Acute axonal injury in multiple sclerosis. Correlation with demyelination and inflammation. *Brain* **123,** 1174–83.

Black, J. A., Foster, R. E., and Waxman, S. G. (1982). Rat optic nerve: freeze-fracture studies during development of myelinated axons. *Brain Research* **258,** 1–10.

Black, J. A., Langworthy, K., Hinson, A. W., Dib-Hajj, S. D., and Waxman, S. G. (1997). NGF has opposing effects on Na^+ channel III and SNS gene expression in spinal sensory neurons. *NeuroReport* **8,** 2331–2335.

Black, J. A., Cummins, T. R., Plumpton, C., Chen, Y. H., Hormuzdiar, W., Clare, J. J., and Waxman, S. G. (1999a). Upregulation of a silent sodium channel after peripheral, but not central, nerve injury in DRG neurons. *J. Neurophysiol.* **82,** 2776–2785.

Black, J. A., Fjell, J., Dib-Hajj, S., Duncan, I. D., O'Connor, L. T., Fried, K., Gladwell, Z., Tate, S., and Waxman, S.G. (1999b). Abnormal expression of SNS/PN3 sodium channel in cerebellar Purkinje cells following loss of myelin in the taiep rat. *NeuroReport* **10,** 913–918.

Black, J. A., Dib-Hajj, S., Baker, D., Newcombe, J., Cuzner, M. L., Waxman, S. G. (2000). Sensory neuron specific sodium channel SNS is abnormally expressed in the brains of mice with experimental allergic encephalomyelitis and humans with multiple sclerosis. *Proc. Natl. Acad. Sci.* **97,** 11598–11602.

Black, J. A., Dib-Hajj, S., McNabola, K., Jeste, S., Rizzo, M. A., Kocsis, J. D., et al. (1996). Spinal sensory neurons express multiple sodium channel alpha-subunit mRNAs. *Mol. Brain Res.* **43,** 117–131.

Boiko, T., Rasband, M. N., Levinson, S. R., Caldwell, J. H., Mandel, G., Trimmer, J. S., and Matthews, G. (2001). Compact myelin dictates the differential targeting of two sodium channel isoforms in the same axon. *Neuron* **30,** 91–104.

Bostock, H., and Sears, T. A. (1978). The internodal axon membrane: electrical excitability and continuous conduction in segmental demyelination. *J. Physiol. (Lond.)* **280,** 273–301.

Boucher, T. J., Okuse, K., Bennett, D. L. H., Munson, J. B., Wood, J. N., and McMahon, S. B. (2000). Potent analgesic effects of GDNF in neuropathic pain states. *Science* **290,** 124–127.

Brysch, W., Creutzfeldt, O. W., Luno, K., Schlingensiepen, R., and Schlingensiepen, K.-H. (1991). Regional and temporal expression of sodium channel messenger RNAs in the rat brain during development. *Exp. Brain Res.* **86,** 562–567.

Caldwell, J. H., Schaller, K. L., Lasher, R. S., Peles, E., and Levinson, S. R. (2000). Sodium channel Na(v)1.6 is localized at nodes of Ranvier, dendrites, and synapses. *Proc. Natl. Acad. Sci. U. S. A.* **97,** 5616–5620.

Catterall, W. A. (1992). Cellular and molecular biology of voltage-gated sodium channels. *Physiol. Rev.* **72,** 515–548.

Cochran, E., Bacci, B., Chen, Y., Patton, A., Gambetti, P., and Autilio-Gambetti, L. (1991). Amyloid precursor protein and ubiquitin immunoreactivity in dystrophic axons is not unique to Alzheimer's disease. *Am. J. Pathol.* **139,** 485–489.

Craner, M. J., Lo, A. C., Black, J. A., and Waxman, S. G. (2003a). Abnormal sodium channel distribution in optic nerve axons in a model of inflammatory demyelination. *Brain* **126**, 1552–1562.

Craner, M. J., Lo, A. C., Black, J. A., Baker, D., Newcombe, J., Cuzner, M. L., and Waxman, S.G. (2003b). Annexin II/p11 is up-regulated in Purkinje cells in EAE and MS. *NeuroReport* **14**, 555–558.

Craner, M. J., Kataoka, Y., Lo, A. C., Black, J. A., Baker, D., and Waxman, S. G. (2003c). Temporal course of upregulation of Nav1.8 in Purkinje neurons parallels the progression of clinical deficit in EAE. *J. Neuropath. Exp. Neurol.* **62**, 968–976.

Craner, M. J., Hains, B. C., Lo, A. C., Black, J. A., and Waxman, S. G. (2004a). Colocalization of sodium channel Nav1.6 and the sodium-calcium exchanger at sites of axonal injury in the spinal cord in EAE. *Brain* **127**, 294–303.

Craner, M. J., Newcombe, J., Black, J. A., Hartle, C., Cuzner, M. L., and Waxman, S. G. (2004b). Molecular changes in neurons in MS: altered axonal expression of $Na_v1.2$ and $Na_v1.6$ sodium channels and Na^+/Ca^{2+} exchanger. *Proc. Natl. Acad. Sci.*

Cummins, T. R., Dib-Hajj, S. D., Black, J. A., Akopian, A. N., Wood, J. N., and Waxman, S. G. (1999). A novel persistent tetrodotoxin-resistant sodium current in SNS-null and wild-type small primary sensory neurons. *J. Neurosci.* **19**, RC 43: 1–16.

Cummins, T. R., Black, J. A., Dib-Hajj, S. D., and Waxman, S. G. (2000). Glial-derived neurotrophic factor upregulates expression of functional SNS and NaN sodium channels and their currents in axotomized dorsal root ganglion neurons. *J. Neurosci.* **20**, 8754–8761.

Cummins, T. R., Aglieco, F., Renganathan, M., Herzog, R. I., Dib-Hajj, S. D., and Waxman, S. G. (2001). Na$_v$1.3 sodium channels: rapid repriming and slow closed-state inactivation display quantitative differences following expression in a mammalian cell line and in spinal sensory neurons. *J. Neurosci.* **21**, 5952–5961.

Cummins, T. R., and Waxman, S. G. (1997). Down-regulation of tetrodotoxin-resistant sodium currents and up-regulation of a rapidly repriming tetrodotoxin-sensitive sodium current in small spinal sensory neurons following nerve injury. *J. Neurosci.* **17**, 3503–3514.

Damarjian, T. A., Craner, M. J., and Waxman, S. G. (2004). Upregulation and colocalization of p75, TrkA and Na$_v$1.8 in Purkinje neurons in EAE.

De Simone, R., Micera, R. A., Terassa, P., and Aloe, L. (1996). mRNA for NGF and p75 in the central nervous system of rats affected by experimental allergic encephalomyelitis. *Neuropathol. Appl. Neurobiol.* **22**, 54–59.

Dib-Hajj, S. D., Black, J. A., Cummins, T. R., Kenney, A. M., Kocsis, J. D., and Waxman, S. G. (1998a). Rescue of alpha-SNS/PN3 sodium channel expression in small dorsal root ganglion neurons after axotomy by nerve growth factor in vivo. *J. Neurophysiol.* **79**, 2668–2676.

Dib-Hajj, S., Black, J. A., Felts, P., and Waxman, S. G. (1996). Down-regulation of transcripts for Na channel α-SNS in spinal sensory neurons following axotomy. *Proc. Natl. Acad. Sci.* **93**, 14950–14954.

Dib-Hajj, S. D., Fjell, J., Cummins, T. R., Zheng, Z., Fried, K., LaMotte, R., Black, J. A., and Waxman, S. G. (1999). Plasticity of sodium channel expression in DRG neurons in the chronic constriction injury model of neuropathic pain. *Pain* **83**, 591–600.

Dib-Hajj, S. D., Ishikawa, I., Cummins, T. R., and Waxman, S. G. (1997). Insertion of an SNS-specific tetrapeptide in the S3-S4 linker of D4 accelerates recovery from inactivation of skeletal muscle voltage-gated Na channel μ1 in HEK293 cells. *FEBS Lett.* **416**, 11–14.

Dugandzija-Novakovic, S., Koszowski, A. G., Levinson, S. R., and Shrager, P. (1995). Clustering of Na$^+$ channels and node of Ranvier formation in remyelinating axons. *J. Neurosci.* **15**, 492–503.

Duncan, I. D., Lunn, K. F., Holmgren, B., Urba-Holmgren, R., and Brignolo-Holmes, L. (1992). The taiep rat: a myelin mutant with an associated oligodendrocyte microtubular defect. *J. Neurocytol.* **21**, 870–884.

Elliott, A. A., and Elliott, J. R. (1993). Characterization of TTX-sensitive and TTX-resistant sodium currents in small cells from adult rat dorsal root ganglia. *J. Physiol. (Lond.)* **463**, 39–56.

England, J. D., Gamboni, F., and Levinson, S. R. (1991). Increased numbers of sodium channels form along demyelinated axons. *Brain Res.* **548**, 334–337.

Espir, M. L. E., Watkins, S. M., and Smith, H. V. (1966). Paroxysmal dysarthria and other transient neurological disturbances in MS. *J. Neurol. Neurosurg. Psychiatry* **29**, 323–330.

Felts, P. A., Yokoyama, S., Dib-Hajj, S., Black, J. A., and Waxman, S. G. (1997). Sodium channel α-subunit mRNAs I, II, III, NaG, Na6 and hNE: Different expression patterns in developing rat nervous system. *Mol. Brain Res.* **45**, 71–83.

Fjell, J., Cummins, T. R., Fried, K., Black, J. A., and Waxman, S. G. (1999a). In vivo NGF deprivation reduces SNS/PN3 expression and TTX-R sodium currents in IB4-negative DRG neurons. *J. Neurophys.* **81**, 803–911.

Fjell, J., Cummins, T. R., Dib-Hajj, S. D., Fried, K., Black, J. A., and Waxman, S. G. (1999b). Differential role of GDNF and NGF in the maintenance of two TTX-resistant sodium channels in adult DRG neurons. *Mol. Brain Res.* **67**, 267–282.

Foster, R. E., Whalen, C. C., and Waxman, S. G. (1980). Reorganization of the axonal membrane of demyelinated nerve fibers: morphological evidence. *Science* **210**, 661–663.

Foster, R. E., Connors, B., and Waxman, S. G. (1982). Rat optic nerve: electrophysiological, pharmacological and anatomical studies during development. *Dev. Brain Res.* **3**, 361–376, 1982.

Geurts, J., Wolswijk G., Bö L., van der Balk, P., Polman, C. H., Troost, D., and Aronica, E. (2003). Altered expression patterns of group I and II metabotropic glutamate receptors in multiple sclerosis. *Brain* **126**, 1755–1766.

Goldin, A. L. (2001) Resurgence of sodium channel research. *Annu. Rev. Physiol.* **63**, 871–894.

Goldin, A. L., Barchi, R. L., Caldwell, J. H., Hofmann, F., Howe, J. R., Hunter, J. C., Kallen, R. G., Mandel, G., Meisler, M. H., Netter, Y. B., Noda, M., Tamkun, M. M., Waxman, S. G., Wood, J. N., and Catterall, W. A. (2000). Nomenclature of voltage-gated sodium channels. *Neuron* **2**, 365–368.

Gong, B., Rhodes, K. J., Bekele-Arcuri, Z., and Trimmer, J. S. (1999). Type I and type II Na$^+$ channel alpha-subunit polypeptides exhibit distinct spatial and temporal patterning, and association with auxiliary subunits in rat brain. *J. Comp. Neurol.* **412**, 342–352.

Hains, B. C., Saab C. Y., Klein, J. P., Craner, M. J., and Waxman, S. G. (2004). Altered sodium channel expression in second-order spinal sensory neurons contributes to pain after peripheral nerve injury. *J. Neurosci.*

Herzog, R. I., Cummins, T. R., Ghassemi, F., Dib-Hajj, S., and Waxman, S. G. (2003). Distinct repriming and closed state inactivation kinetics of Na$_v$1.6 and Na$_v$1.7 sodium channels in spinal sensory neurons. *J. Physiol.* **551**, 741–751.

Imaizumi, T., Kocsis, J. D., and Waxman, S. G. (1997). Anoxic injury in the rat spinal cord: pharmacological evidence for multiple steps in Ca^{2+}-dependent injury of the dorsal columns. *J. Neurotrauma* **14**, 299–311.

Inenaga, K., Nagamoto, T., Kannan, H., and Yamashita, H. (1993). Inward sodium current involvement in regenerative bursting activity of rat magnocellular supraoptic neurons in vitro. *J. Physiol. Lond.* **465**, 289–301.

Kaplan, M. R., Cho, M. H., Ullian, E. M., Isom, L. L., Levinson, S. R., and Barres, B. A. (2001). Differential control of clustering of the sodium channels Na(v)1.2 and Na(v)1.6 at developing CNS nodes of Ranvier. *Neuron* **30**, 105–119.

Klein, J. P., Tendi, E. A., Dib-Hajj, S. D., Fields, R. D., and Waxman, S. G. (2003). Patterned electrical activity modulates sodium channel expression in sensory neurons. *J. Neurosci. Res.* **74**, 192–198.

Kohrman, D. C., Smith, M. R., Goldin, A. L., Harris, J., and Meisler, M. H. (1996). A missense mutation in the sodium channel Scn8a is responsible for cerebellar ataxia in the mouse mutant jolting. *J. Neurosci.* **16**, 5993–5999.

Kornek, B., Storch, M. K., Bauer, J., Djamshidian, A., Weissert, R., Wallstroem, E., Stefferl, A., Zimprich, F., Olsson, T., Linington, C., Schmidbauer, M., and Lassmann, H. (2001). Distribution of a calcium channel subunit in dystrophic axons in multiple sclerosis and experimental autoimmune encephalomyelitis. *Brain* **124**, 1114–1124.

Kuhlmann, T., Lingfeld, G., Bitsch, A., Schuchardt, J., and Bruck, W. (2002). Acute axonal damage in multiple sclerosis is most extensive in early disease stages and decreases over time. *Brain* **125**, 2202–2212.

Laudiero, L. B., Aloe, L., Levi-Montalcini, R., Buttinelli, C., Schilter, D., Gillessen, S., and Otten, U. (1992). Multiple sclerosis patients express increased levels of beta-nerve growth factor in cerebrospinal fluid. *Neurosci. Lett.* **147**, 9–12.

Leffler, A., Cummins, T. R., Dib-Hajj, S. D., Hormuzdiar, W. N., Black, J. A., and Waxman, S. G. (2002). Glial-derived neurotrophic factor and nerve growth factor reverse changes in repriming of TTX-sensitive Na$^+$ currents following axotomy of dorsal root ganglion neurons. *J. Neurophysiol.* **88**, 650–660.

Li, Z., and Hatton, G. I. (1996). Oscillatory bursting of physically firing rat supraoptic neurones in low-Ca^{2+} medium: Na+ influx, cytosolic Ca^{2+} and gap junctions. *J. Physiol. Lond.* **496**, 397–394.

Lipton, S., and Tauck, D. (1986). Voltage-dependent conductances of ganglion cells from rat retina. *J. Physiol.* **385**, 361–391.

Llinas, R., and Sugimori, M. (1980). Electrophysiological properties of in vitro Purkinje cell somata in mammalian cerebellar slices. *J. Physiol.* **305**, 171–195.

Lo, A. C., Black, J. A., and Waxman, S. G. (2002). Neuroprotection of axons with phenytoin in experimental allergic encephalomyelitis. *Neuroreport* **13**, 1909–1912.

Lo, A. C., Saab, C. Y., Black, J. A., and Waxman, S. G. (2003). Phenytoin protects spinal cord axons and preserves axonal conduction and neurological function in a model of neuroinflammation in vivo. *J. Neurophysiol.* **90**, 3566–3572.

Ma, J. Y., Catterall, W. A., and Scheuer, T. (1997). Persistent sodium currents through brain sodium channels induced by G protein betagamma subunits. *Neuron* **19**, 443–52.

Matthews, W. B., Compston, A., Allen, I. V., and Martyn, C. N. (1991). *McAlpine's Multiple Sclerosis*, Churchill Livingstone, New York.

Maurice, N., Tkatch, T., Meisler, M., Sprunger, L. K., and Surmeier, D.J. (2001). D1/D5 dopamine receptor activation differentially modulates rapidly inactivating and persistent sodium currents in prefrontal cortex pyramidal neurons. *J. Neurosci.* **21**, 2268–2277.

Newcombe, J., and Cuzner, M. L. (1993). Organization and research application of the UK Multiple Sclerosis Society tissue bank. *J. Neural Transmission, Suppl.* **39**, 155–163.

Novakovic, S. D., Levinson, S. R., Schachner, M., and Shrager, P. (1998). Disruption and reorganization of sodium channels in experimental allergic neuritis. *Muscle Nerve* **21**, 1019–1032.

Offord, J., and Catterall, W. A. (1989). Electrical activity, cAMP, and cytosolic calcium regulate mRNA encoding sodium channel α? subunits in rat muscle cells. *Neuron* **2**, 1447–1452.

Okuse, K., Malik-Hall, M., Baker, M. D., Poon, W. Y. L., Kong, H., Chao, M. V., and Wood, J. N. (2002). Annexin II light chain regulates sensory neuron-specific sodium channel expression. *Nature* **47**, 653–656.

Ouardouz, M., Nikolaeva, M., Coderre, E., Zamponi, G. W., McRory, J. E., Trapp, B. D., Yin, X., Wang, W., Woulfe, J., and Stys, P. K. (2003). Depolarization-induced Ca^{2+} release in ischemic spinal cord white matter involves L-type Ca^{2+} channel activation of ryanodine receptors. *Neuron* **40**, 53–63.

Peles, E., and Salzer, J. L. (2000). Molecular domains of myelinated axons. *Curr. Opin. Neurobiol.* **10**, 558–565.

Pennartz, C. M. A., Bierlaagh, M. A., and Geurtsen, A. M. S. (1997). Cellular mechanisms underlying spontaneous firing in rat suprachiasmatic nucleus: involvement of a slowly inactivating component of sodium current. *J. Neurophysiol.* **78**, 1811–1825.

Plant, G. T., Hess, R. F., and Thomas, S. J. (1986). The pattern evoked electroretinogram in optic neuritis. A combined psychophysical and electrophysiological study. *Brain* **109**, 469–490.

Plummer, W., and Meisler, M. H. (1999). Evolution and diversity of sodium channel genes. *Genomics* **57**, 323–331.

Raman, I. M., and Bean, B. P. (1997). Resurgent sodium current and action potential formation in dissociated cerebellar Purkinje neurons. *J. Neurosci.* **17**, 4517–4526.

Raman, I. M., Sprunger, L. K., Meisler, M. H., and Bean, B. P. (1997). Altered subthreshold sodium currents and disrupted firing patterns in Purkinje neurons of Scn81 mutant mice. *Neuron* **19**, 881–891.

Rasband, M. N., Peles, E., Trimmer, J. S., Levinson, S. R., Lux, S. E., and Shrager, P. (1999). Dependence of nodal sodium channel clustering on paranodal axo-glial contact in the developing CNS. *J. Neurosci.* **19**, 7516–7528.

Renganathan, M., Cummins, T. R., and Waxman, S. G. (2001). The contribution of Na$_v$1.8 sodium channels to action potential electrogenesis in DRG neurons. *J. Neurophysiol.* **86**, 629–640.

Renganathan, M., Gelderblom, M., Black, J. A., and Waxman, S. G. (2003). Expression of Na$_v$ 1.8 sodium channels perturbs the firing patterns of cerebellar Purkinje cells. *Brain Res.* **959**, 235–243.

Rios, J. C., Rubin, M., St. Martin, M., Downey, R. T., Einheber, S., Rosenbluth, J., Levinson, S. R., Bhat, M., and Salzer, J. L. (2002). Paranodal interactions regulate expression of sodium channel subtypes and provide a diffusion barrier for the node of Ranvier. *J. Neurosci.* **23**, 7001–7011.

Ritchie, J. M., and Rogart, R. B. (1977). The density of sodium channels in mammalian myelinated nerve fibers and the nature of the axonal membrane under the myelin sheath. *Proc. Natl. Acad. Sci. U. S. A.* **74**, 211–215.

Rosenberg, L. J., Teng, Y. D., and Wrathall, J. R. (1999). Effects of the sodium channel blocker tetrodotoxin on acute white matter pathology after experimental contusive spinal cord injury. *J. Neurosci.* **19**, 6122–6133.

Saab, C., Craner, M. J., Kataoka, Y., and Waxman, S. G. (2004). Abnormal Purkinje cell activity *in vivo* in experimental allergic encephalomyelitis. *Exp. Brain Res.*

Sangameswaren, L., Delgado, S. G., Fish, L. M., Koch, B. D., Jakeman, L. B., Stewart, G. R., Sze, P., Hunter, J. C., Eglen, R. M., and Herman, R. C. (1996). Structure and function of a novel voltage-gated tetrodotoxin-resistant sodium channel specific to sensory neurons. *J. Biol. Chem.* **271**, 5953–5956.

Sashihara, S., Greer, C. A., Oh, Y., and Waxman, S. G. (1996). Cell specific differential expression of Na+ channel β1 subunit mRNA in the olfactory system during postnatal development and following denervation. *J. Neurosci.* **16**, 702–714.

Sashihara, S., Waxman, S. G., and Greer, C. A. (1997). Down-regulation of Na+ channel mRNA following sensory deprivation of tufted cells in the neonatal rat olfactory bulb. *NeuroReport* **8**, 1289–1293.

Schild, J. H., and Kunze, D. L. (1997). Experimental and modeling study of Na$^+$ current heterogeneity in rat nodose neurons and its impact on neuronal discharge. *J. Neurophysiol.* **78**, 3198–3209.

Scroggs, R. S., and Fox, A. P. (1992). Multiple Ca^{2+} currents elicited by action potential waveforms in acutely isolated adult rat dorsal ganglion neurons. *J. Neurosci.* **12**, 1789–1801.

Sleeper, A. A., Cummins, T. R., Hormuzdiar, W., Tyrrell, L., Dib-Hajj, S. D., Waxman, S. G, and Black, J. A. (2000). Changes in expression of two tetrodotoxin-resistant sodium channels and their currents in dorsal root ganglion neurons after sciatic nerve injury but not rhizotomy. *J. Neurosci.* **20**, 7279–7289.

Smith, M. R., Smith, R. D., Plummer, N. W., Meisler, M. H., and Goldin, A. L. (1998). Functional analysis of the mouse Scn8a sodium channel. *J. Neurosci.* **18**, 6093–6102.

Stuart, G., and Hausser, M. (1994). Initiation and spread of sodium action potentials in cerebellar Purkinje cells. *Neuron* **13**, 703–712.

Stuart, G., and Sakmann, B. (1995). Amplification of epsps by axosomatic sodium channels in neocortical pyramidal neurons. *Neuron* 1065–1076.

Stys, P. K., Waxman, S. G., and Ransom, B. R. (1992). Ionic mechanisms of anoxic injury in mammalian CNS white matter: role of Na⁺ channels and Na⁺-Ca²⁺ exchanger. *J. Neurosci.* **12,** 430–439.

Stys, P. K., Sontheimer, H., Ransom, B. R., and Waxman, S. G. (1993). Noninactivating, tetrodotoxin-sensitive Na⁺ conductance in rat optic nerve axons. *Proc. Natl. Acad. Sci. U. S. A.* **90,** 6976–6980.

Tanaka, M., Cummins, T. R., Ishikawa, K., Black, J. A., Ibata, I., and Waxman, S. G. (1999). Molecular and functional remodeling of electrogenic membrane of hypothalamic neurons in response to changes in their input. *Proc. Natl. Acad. Sci. U. S. A.* **96,** 1088–1093.

Taddese, A., and Bean, B. P. (2002). Subthreshold sodium current from rapidly inactivating sodium channels drives spontaneous firing of tuberomammillary neurons. *Neuron* **33,** 587–600.

Trapp, B. D., Peterson, J., Ransohoff, R. M., Rudick, R., Mork, S., and Bo, L. (1998). Axonal transection in the lesions of multiple sclerosis. *N. Engl. J. Med.* **338,** 278–285.

Vabnick, I., Messing, A., Chiu, S. Y., Levinson, S. R., Schachner, M., Roder, J., Li, C., Novakovic, S., and Shrager, P. (1997). Sodium channel distribution in axons of hypomyelinated and MAG null mutant mice. *J. Neurosci. Res.* **50,** 321–336.

Wang, H., Allen, M. L., Grigg, J. J., Noebels, J. L., and Tempel, B. L. (1999). Hypomyelination alters K⁺ channel expression in mouse mutants *shiverer* and *Trembler. Neuron* **15,** 1337–1347.

Waxman, S. G. (1977). Conduction in myelinated, unmyelinated, and demyelinated fibers. *Arch. Neurol.* **34,** 585–590.

Waxman, S. G. (1998). Demyelinating diseases: New pathological insights, new therapeutic targets. *N. Engl. J. Med.* **338,** 323–325.

Waxman, S. G. (2000). The neuron as a dynamic electrogenic machine: Modulation of sodium channel expression as a basis for functional plasticity in neurons. *Phil. Trans. Roy. Soc. Lond. B.* **355,** 199–213.

Waxman, S. G. (2001). Transcriptional channelopathies: an emerging class of disorders. *Nature Rev. Neurosci.* **2,** 652–659.

Waxman, S. G. (2003). NO and the axonal death cascade. *Ann. Neurol.* **53,** 150–154.

Waxman, S. G., Black, J. A., Kocsis, J. D., and Ritchie, J. M. (1989). Low density of sodium channels supports action potential conduction in axons of neonatal rat optic nerve. *Proc. Natl. Acad. Sci.* **86,** 1406–1410.

Waxman, S. G., Kocsis, J. D., and Black, J. A. (1994). Type III sodium channel mRNA is expressed in embryonic but not adult spinal sensory neurons, and is re-expressed following axotomy. *J. Neurophysiol.* **72,** 466–471.

Westenbroek, R. E., Merrick, D. K., and Catterall, W. A. (1989). Differential subcellular localization of the RI and RII Na+ channel subtypes in central neurons. *Neuron* **3,** 695–704.

Westenbroek, R. E., Noebels, J. L., and Catterall, W. A. (1992). Elevated expression of type II Na+ channels in hypomyelinated axons of shiverer mouse brain. *J. Neurosci.* **12,** 2259–2257.

Whitaker, W. R., Clare, J. J., Powell, A. J., Chen, Y. H., Faull, R. L., and Emson, P. C. (2000). Distribution of voltage-gated sodium channel alpha-subunit and beta-subunit mRNAs in human hippocampal formation, cortex, and cerebellum. *J. Comp. Neurol.* **422,** 123–139.

Zhou, W., and Goldin, A. L. (2002). Functional differences between the Na$_v$1.6 and Na$_v$1.2 sodium channels. *Soc. Neurosci. Abstr.* **834.4.**

8

Na⁺ Channel Reorganization in Demyelinated Axons

Na$^+$ Channel Reorganization in Demyelinated Axons

Peter Shrager, Ph.D.
William Simon, Ph.D.
Katia Kazarinova-Noyes, Ph.D.

I. Consequences of Demyelination

The concept of saltatory conduction, first defined more than 50 years ago (Tasaki and Takeuchi, 1942; Huxley and Stampfli, 1949), firmly established the fact that in normal myelinated axons, inward current through sodium (Na$^+$) channels occurs uniquely at nodes of Ranvier. Correspondingly, voltage clamp experiments, first on amphibian axons and later on mammalian fibers, demonstrated directly that there is a high density of Na$^+$ channels at these sites (Dodge and Frankenhaeuser, 1959; Chiu et al., 1979). At issue, however, was the possible expression of these channels within internodal regions as well. Na$^+$ channels under myelin are not likely to be activated during action potential propagation, or under voltage clamp, because they would see only a fraction of the resulting depolarization. Thus, other approaches were required to establish with certainty the distribution of these channels. This information is important both to define the steps that neurons must follow during development and because it has functional consequences in demyelinating disease. Some early experiments provided important clues. Nodal regions were found to have biochemically distinct cytoplasmic surfaces, suggesting unique cytoskeletal components (Quick and Waxman, 1977). The more recent demonstration of a specific adapter protein (ankyrin$_G$) and a spectrin isoform (βIV) localized to nodes and initial segments confirms this idea (Kordeli et al., 1995; Berghs et al., 2000; Komada and Soriano, 2002). Freeze-fracture replicas demonstrated high densities of large intramembranous particles in both the node and juxtaparanode, and much lower densities in the axoglial junction region of the paranode and in the remainder of the internode (Rosenbluth, 1976, 1981). The densities of these particles in the nodal gap (~1,300/μm^2) agree with biophysical estimates of Na$^+$ channel density (1,000–1,500/μm^2; reviewed in Hille, (2001). This work suggested a specific clustering of Na$^+$ channels at nodes and initial segments, but left open the possibility of a lower density within internodes.

Direct electrical measurements provide the most sensitive method of detecting voltage-dependent channels. Two groups studied gap-voltage-clamped internodes acutely exposed to lysolecithin to disrupt myelin. Voltage-dependent Na$^+$ and potassium (K$^+$) currents could be recorded concomitant with an increase in membrane capacitance. Grissmer (1986) found the internodal Na$^+$ current density to be only 0.2% of the nodal level. Chiu and Schwarz (1987) measured this ratio to be about 3%, but considered the possibility that the recorded Na$^+$ currents originated from Schwann cell membranes fused to the axolemma by lysolecithin. Schwann cells *in vitro* express voltage-dependent Na$^+$ channels (Chiu et al., 1984; Shrager et al., 1985). However, it was later shown that, *in vivo*, these channels are restricted to nonmyelinating Schwann cells (Wilson and Chiu, 1990; Chiu, 1993).

Studies on axons demyelinated *in vivo* provided more details. Hall and Gregson (1971) introduced a method for focal demyelination that reproduces many aspects of inflammatory demyelinating disease and can be used in amphibian and mammalian species. A small amount of lysolecithin (1 μl, 1% in adult sciatic nerve) is injected surgically directly into a nerve trunk and the animal is allowed to recover. The drug vesiculates the outmost layers of myelin, which initiates an inflammatory response, with macrophages entering the lesion from the blood and removing myelin debris by phagocytosis. Affected internodes are completely stripped of myelin, a process that is completed by 1 week postinjection. At this time, if the nerve is dissected and teased, axons can be found that are devoid of all glial membranes and are surrounded only by a disrupted basal lamina. If the animal is allowed to recover for longer periods, Schwann cells proliferate and begin the process of remyelination (Shrager and Rubinstein, 1990). In the rat sciatic nerve, the earliest signs of repair are seen at about 9 days postinjection, and by 14 days many fibers have thin sheaths of new myelin. In the mouse, all events are speeded by 1 to 2 days. Working with both *Xenopus* and rat sciatic axons, Shrager recorded Na$^+$ currents with the loose patch clamp (Fig. 1) and found an internodal density about 4% of the nodal value (Shrager, 1987, 1988, 1989). Measurements could be made as early as 1 day postinjection, by applying suction to allow the patch pipette to advance through the myelin debris and seal to the axolemma. The internodal density was constant during 2 months postinjection, suggesting that these channels are not introduced as a result of the demyelination.

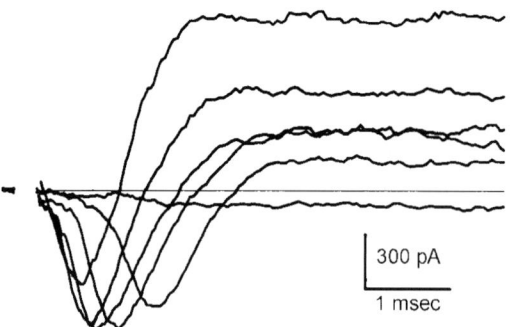

Figure 1 Ionic currents recorded from a rat sciatic demyelinated internode with a loose patch clamp pipette. The membrane potential was held 30 mV negative to the resting value and was depolarized by pulses of 40, 60, 70, 80, 90, and 110 mV. This nerve was 3 days postinjection. (Reprinted from Brain Research [Shrager, 1989], copyright 1989, with permission from Elsevier.)

The measurement also agreed well with that of the acute experiments of Chiu and Schwarz (1987). Since the nodal density of Na$^+$ channels is about 1,000–1,500/μm^2, the internodal density is 40–60/μm^2. This latter figure is significant for two reasons. First, it is close to the value expected for nonmyelinated axons of similar caliber. Thus, in principle, it could support conduction. Second, although it represents only a few percent of the nodal density, since the internodal surface area is about 1,000 times that of nodes, it suggests that more than 95% of the axonal Na$^+$ channels are internodal. Therefore, they constitute a large pool of channels that may be used in repair or replacement. When axons (both peripheral [PNS] and central nervous systems [CNS]) remyelinate they typically form several short internodes within a single previous internodal region. The gaps between these short internodes must function as nodes if saltatory conduction is to be successful through this zone, and they must therefore obtain a high density of Na$^+$ channels from some source. These channels may be synthesized *de novo* in the soma and transported down the fiber, or they may be recruited from the internodal pool.

II. Reorganization of Axonal Na$^+$ Channels after Demyelination

A series of reports from Sears and his colleagues established several important points regarding modes of conduction and localization of functional Na$^+$ channels in demyelinated fibers. Rasminsky and Sears (1972) developed a method in which rat ventral roots were demyelinated by injection of diphtheria toxin and longitudinal currents recorded. By selective stimulation with a microelectrode, it was possible to record propagating signals from single fibers. These authors found axons in which conduction was delayed, but remained saltatory. Bostock and Sears (1978) improved on this technique, increasing spatial resolution, and demonstrated that in addition to saltatory conduction, some fibers exhibited broad stretches of inward current characteristic of continuous conduction through a demyelinated internode. Smith et al. (1982) increased the spatial resolution of this technique even further, and also used lysolecithin to initiate demyelination instead of diphtheria toxin. In contrast with the earlier study, they found that conduction in demyelinated axons proceeded via new foci of inward current at spacings of a few hundred microns. These foci, called φ-nodes, formed before remyelination, and the authors concluded that they were likely to represent aggregates of Na⁺ channels. In the light of later experiments, detailed previously, showing a significant density of Na⁺ channels in the internodal axolemma, one may now conclude that (1) under at least some circumstances the internodal channels can be activated and support conduction and (2) these channels may be reorganized after demyelination.

One disadvantage of the approach used in the previously described work is that the recorded fiber is not seen visually and the extent of demyelination, or association with Schwann cells, is thus not known. Studies on teased sciatic axons circumvent this difficulty and allow a more definitive interpretation. Some early physiological experiments were carried out on *Xenopus* fibers, using the lysolecithin injection system described earlier (Shrager, 1988). At the edges of the injection zone (3 to 5 mm long) one finds heminodes separating normal myelin from the demyelinated region. Applying loose patch clamp pipettes to sites adjacent to these heminodes at about 1 week postinjection resulted in outward currents with a voltage dependence that was very sharp and was in some cases "all-or-none." These currents originated from zones of high Na⁺ channel density just outside the patch (inward through the channels and outward through the patch) and suggested that Na⁺ channels at the original nodes of Ranvier were very stable, remaining clustered even 1 week after myelin disruption. It was also possible to record propagating action potentials with the loose patch clamp because only the external potential is controlled by the pipette. At 2 weeks postinjection, a time when in *Xenopus* new myelin is not yet seen, but Schwann cells have begun to adhere, action potentials invaded the demyelinated zone far more than would have been possible by passive spread alone. This result was confirmed and extended by optical recording utilizing potential-sensitive dyes (Shrager and Rubinstein, 1990). It was possible to record propagating signals from single nodes of Ranvier and from small patches of membrane 10 μm long in demyelinated zones. Before Schwann cell adherence, action potentials were blocked at the heminode border of the demyelinated region (Fig. 2A). However, as soon as Schwann cells associated with the axon, but before remyelination, signals were able to traverse a full demyelinated internode, though with much lower

velocity than in the myelinated regions of the same fiber (Fig 2B). As would be expected, action potentials resumed normal velocity when they emerged from the lesion into the distal myelinated zone. The block at the heminode is due to the high capacitance of the demyelinated zone, which creates an "impedance mismatch" (i.e., the last node cannot supply sufficient current to depolarize the Na⁺ channels at the heminode to the level required for activation) (see Chapter 6). Calculations show that the internodal density of Na⁺ channels is adequate for conduction (but just barely so) if the demyelinated segment can be stimulated. The newly adherent Schwann cells in Fig. 2B improve the passive cable properties, but as will be seen next, this is not the only

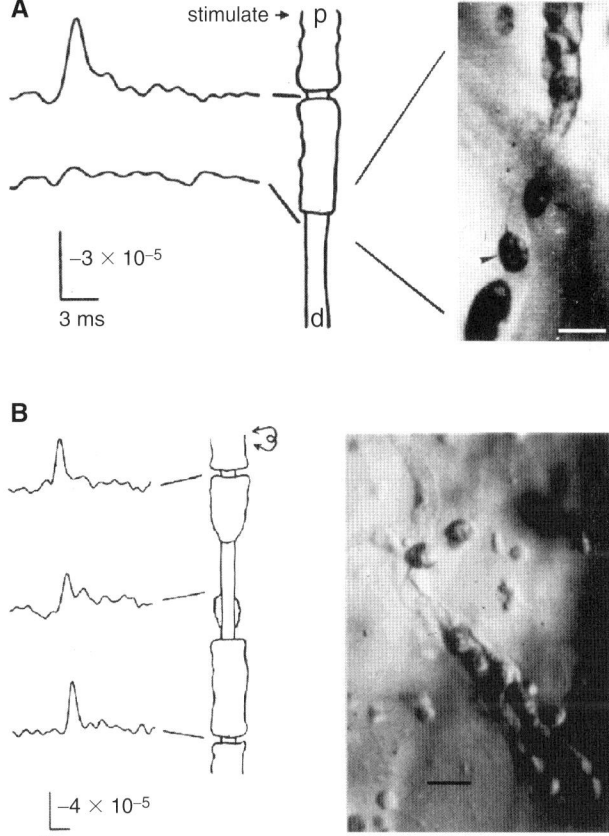

Figure 2 Optical recording of propagating action potentials. *Xenopus* axons were stained with the dye RH155, and changes in the amplitude of transmitted light at 705 ± 25 nm were recorded from a 10 × 10 μm region. (**A**) An action potential reached the last intact node before the demyelinated zone, but was blocked at the proximal heminode. The light micrograph shows the heminode. This nerve was 8 days postinjection (dpi), and macrophages (*arrow*) but no Schwann cells were adherent. (Reproduced from the *Journal of General Physiology* [Shrager and Rubinstein, 1990] by copyright permission of The Rockefeller University Press.) (**B**) At 10 dpi an action potential successfully propagates through a demyelinated internode. Schwann cells are adhering to the demyelinated region, but myelin is not yet seen at the ultrastructural level at this stage. The light micrograph shows the distal heminode. A few macrophages (*dark cells*) are also visible.

consequence of this early stage of repair that is important for restoring function.

III. Clustering of Na⁺ Channels and Formation of New Nodes of Ranvier

The results described thus far suggest that after demyelination conduction may be blocked, but can be restored by just the earliest and most minimal association of Schwann cells with axons (Smith et al., 1982; Shrager, 1988; Shrager and Rubinstein, 1990). The low density of Na⁺ channels in the internode could, in principle, participate in the restoration of conduction, but computational models confirm that without additional restructuring, the high capacitance of the demyelinated axon limits the invading signal to levels insufficient to activate these channels. Immunocytochemical labeling has greatly improved the resolution with which ion channels can be localized, and results shed light on both recovery processes during demyelination and on normal axonal development. An antibody with excellent specificity for vertebrate Na⁺ channels was first made by Levinson (Ellisman and Levinson, 1982; Dugandzija-Novakovic et al., 1995). This antibody was targeted to a region of the intracellular linker between domains III and IV that is conserved in all mammalian voltage-dependent Na⁺ channel subtypes. Normal nodes of Ranvier are brightly labeled with indirect immunofluorescence. After demyelination by lysolecithin injection, Schwann cells proliferate and adhere to axons, and may then begin the process of myelination. At this stage (overlapping ensheathment) their protein expression pattern changes markedly, with NCAM, L1, and the p75 NGF receptor downregulated, and with increased expression of myelin proteins, notably myelin-associated glycoprotein (MAG) (Martini and Schachner, 1986). Initially, MAG appears uniformly over the Schwann cell surface and then becomes increasingly sequestered in cytoplasmic-containing regions, including the paranode, as myelination progresses. The ability to distinguish premyelinating from myelinating Schwann cells was an important step in the development of a general hypothesis regarding the clustering of Na⁺ channels and the formation of nodes of Ranvier. At issue was the question of the controlling influence in determining the ultimate sites of nodes. Were these zones predetermined by the axon at regular intervals, or were they the result of glial influences upon the neuron? The remyelinating axon provided early clues.

At about 1 week postinjection, rat sciatic axons have very few newly adherent Schwann cells, and also very few clusters of Na⁺ channels within the demyelinated zone. The clusters seen are about 1 mm apart and are likely to be at the sites of the original nodes (Fig. 3A). However, just a few days later, Schwann cells appear, and associated with them are new clusters of Na⁺ channels (Fig 3B). In Fig. 3B–E nerves

were labeled with antibodies to MAG (red) to identify Schwann cells committed to myelination and also with antibodies to pan Na⁺ channels (green). The uniform expression of MAG over the glial surface indicates that these cells are just beginning the process of myelination. These Schwann cells are wrapping multiple lamellae and are also growing longitudinally. As they extend processes, they appear to "push" the Na⁺ channel clusters along with them, because these clusters always appear just outside the tips of the MAG-labeled zone, never under it. This was confirmed at the ultrastructural level (Novakovic et al., 1996). In time, clusters associated with neighboring Schwann cells approach each other (Fig. 3C) and, ultimately, appear to fuse (Fig. 3D) to form a new node of Ranvier (Fig. 3E). The sketch in Fig. 3 illustrates the basic hypothesis. A quantitative analysis of the frequency of occurrence of each stage supported the view that this sequence of events is correct (Dugandzija-Novakovic et al., 1995). Further, the distance across remyelinating Schwann cells (between clusters) grows in a roughly exponential fashion over time (Fig. 4). Thus, at least in the lysolecithin model of demyelination, it is the Schwann cells, and not the axon, that determine the location of new nodes of Ranvier. Tzoumaka et al. (1995) demonstrated that at least the early stages of this process could take place even in the absence of communication with the neuronal soma. It is likely, therefore, that the Na⁺ channels that cluster adjacent to the glial processes are derived from the low density internodal pool described earlier. As will be discussed later, in more chronic demyelinating conditions, there is evidence for additional *de novo* synthesis of these channels (see also Chapter 7). Finally, although this chapter is concerned primarily with demyelination, it should be noted that a similar mechanism of node formation has been proposed for development as well (Vabnick et al., 1996).

The initial clustering of Na⁺ channels illustrated in Fig. 3 is likely to represent the basis for the ϕ-nodes seen functionally by Smith et al. (1982). Further, it is also probable that this reorganization is an essential step in the early restoration of conduction seen in Fig. 2B. If the only improvement was in passive cable properties, the intermittent one to two layers of Schwann cell ensheathment would be minimal. By concentrating Na⁺ channels at these sites, conduction is more readily restored. The high level of stability of nodal clusters (seen as late as 9 days after myelin disruption [Custer et al., 2003]) is almost certainly due to the link of Na⁺ channels to the cytoskeleton via ankyrin_G (Kordeli et al., 1995; Bennett and Lambert, 1999). It is not yet clear just what the role of ankyrin_G may be in the initial clustering process. Ankyrin_G appears at new cluster sites virtually simultaneously with Na⁺ channels. On the other hand, in remyelinating axons, the early Na⁺ channel clusters that formed were not as stable as original adult clusters (Custer et al., 2003). It may be that there is an initial sequestration that serves to accumulate a high density of channels at the

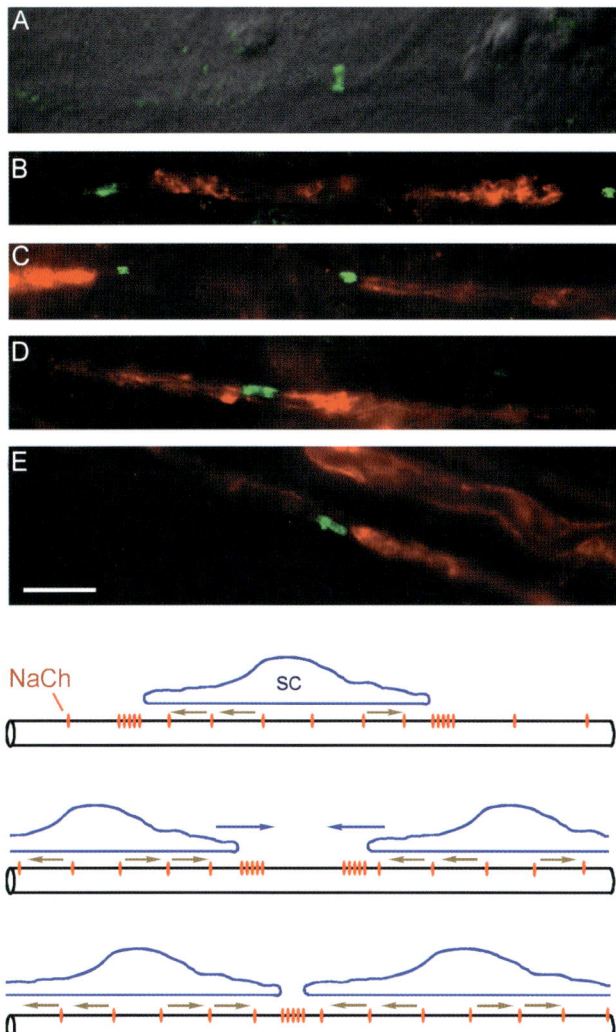

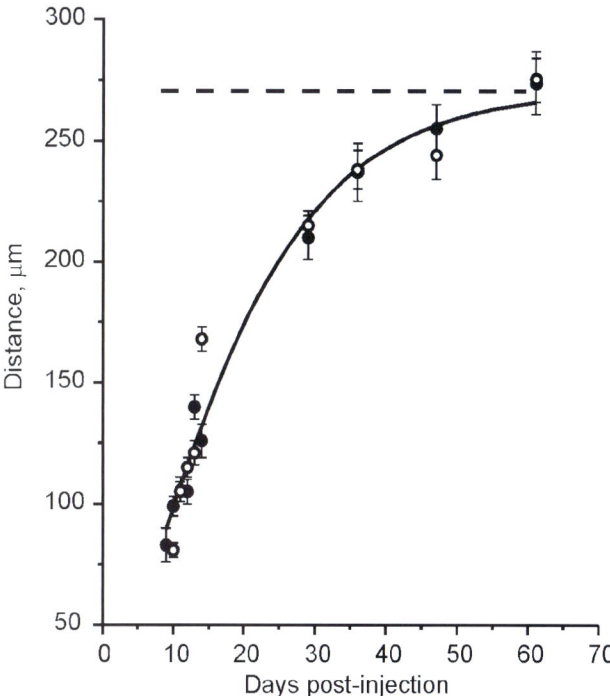

Figure 4 Distance across remyelinating Schwann cells plotted vs. days postinjection. All measurements were made across a MAG-positive Schwann cell. Filled circles show distances between Na+ channel clusters. Open circles show distances between Caspr1-positive sites. The solid curve is drawn to indicate trends. The dashed line is drawn at 270 μm, the distance measured after remyelination is complete. It is thus the prediction if the axon predetermined the location of new nodes of Ranvier, and clearly does not fit the experimental points. That results are virtually the same whether Na⁺ channels or Caspr1 is measured indicates that the loci of the channels are tightly linked to the Schwann cell process edges (if exclusively so the two should agree within a few mm). (Reproduced by permission from the *Journal of Neuroscience* [Custer et al., 2003], copyright 2003 by the Society for Neuroscience.)

Figure 3 Na⁺ channel clustering during demyelination and early remyelination in the PNS. (**A**) An original nodal cluster at 1 week postinjection. (**B–E**) New node formation, 12 to 15 days postinjection. (**B**) New Na⁺ channel clusters forming at the edges of a MAG-positive Schwann cell. (**C**) Na⁺ channel clusters associated with neighboring Schwann cells approaching each other as the Schwann cells lengthen. (**D**) Two clusters appear to fuse. (**E**) A new, broad node of Ranvier. Scale bar, 5 μm. (*Bottom*) Proposed mechanism of node formation.

glial edges, but then further links to ankyrin$_G$ may be forged through multiple binding sites. A hypothesis for cluster formation that incorporates the first step is presented later in this chapter.

Experimental allergic neuritis (EAN) is an autoimmune disease of the PNS that is inducible in rodents and has similarities to human neuropathies, including Guillain-Barré syndrome. When Lewis rats were immunized with purified bovine root myelin, Na⁺ channel immunofluorescence at PNS nodes became more diffuse, and eventually undetectable (Novakovic et al., 1998). The loss of nodal channels corresponded closely with the development of clinical dis-

ease. During recovery, new Na⁺ channel clusters formed at the edges of adherent Schwann cells, and the formation of new nodes paralleled that seen after lysolecithin injection. However, at many sites in EAN, paranodes were retracted but myelin stripping was absent. The nodal Na⁺ channel cluster then split into two parts, each remaining highly focal (Fig. 5) (Novakovic et al., 1998). It thus appeared as though these channels retain their association with an individual Schwann cell even after myelin has formed. This pattern has recently also been seen in lysolecithin-induced demyelination at early stages (Arroyo, 2003). On the other hand, when myelin is retracted by exposure to protease, Na⁺ channels remain as a single cluster at the original nodal site (Dugandzija-Novakovic et al., 1995). Finally, it must be pointed out that all of the discussion thus far has been focused on acute changes in Na⁺ channel organization in peripheral nerves (scale of days or weeks). These events may be responsible for some of the clinical remissions in demyelinating disease that can occur in such a time frame.

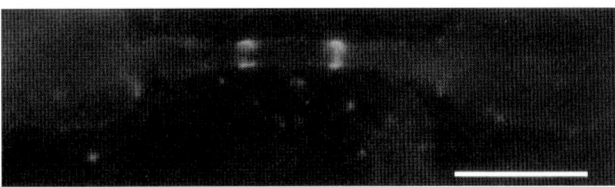

Figure 5 Redistribution of Na⁺ channels in experimental allergic neuritis (EAN). This is a retracted nodal region, 28 days after induction of EAN. Scale bar, 25 mm. (Reproduced by permission from *Muscle and Nerve* [Novakovic et al., 1998], copyright 1998 by Wiley Periodicals Inc.)

Quite different, but equally clinically relevant changes take place in more chronic disease, as discussed later.

IV. Repair Mechanisms in the CNS

Although there is thus extensive evidence for conduction in segmentally demyelinated axons in the PNS, corresponding data in the CNS are much more difficult to obtain. Since experimental and disease-induced lesions typically contain axons with considerable variation in morphologies, ranging from minimal paranodal disruption to frank myelin stripping, it is necessary to make measurements on visually identified fibers. A technologically demanding approach was used successfully by Felts et al. (1997) (see Chapter 6). Dorsal columns were demyelinated by surgical injection of ethidium bromide and examined electrophysiologically at 17 to 37 days (for demyelinated axons) or 300 days (for remyelinated axons). The use of fine micropipettes allowed recording from single axons. By recording signals that propagated either across the lesion or across the uninjected region, it was possible to identify fibers with long refractory periods characteristic of demyelination. These axons were then injected with horseradish peroxidase for later morphological identification. It was found that axons with no cellular contacts for less than 60 μm, or with contact restricted to other demyelinated axons for up to 126 μm, could conduct action potentials, albeit with low velocity and long refractory periods. The remyelinating cells in this lesion are Schwann cells, and it is thus possible that some of the results from peripheral axons are applicable here, namely intermittent ensheathment and Na⁺ channel clustering at the glial process edges. The resulting combination of minimal improvement in passive cable properties and "hot-spots" of regenerative membrane might suffice to maintain conduction. It remains to be determined if conduction along acutely demyelinated CNS axons can occur when only central glia are present. Finally, while the evidence for nodal Na⁺ channel clustering requiring glial contact is strong in the PNS, an alternative view has been presented for CNS axons. When media conditioned by oligodendrocytes is added to retinal ganglion cells in culture, there is an increased incidence of Na⁺ channel-positive sites in axonal processes (Kaplan et al., 1997, 2001). Only $Na_v1.2$ is seen and the progression to $Na_v1.6$ does not take place. These sites could signify an early stage of molecular organization in the axon, but it has been argued that they may not represent axonally determined loci of nodes of Ranvier, and the extent to which node formation in the CNS is governed by soluble factors released by glia remains unresolved (Kazarinova-Noyes and Shrager, 2002; Salzer, 2003).

V. Increased Na⁺ Channel Expression during Persistent Demyelination of the CNS

Beyond the acute reorganization that takes place during remyelination over several days, quite different events are seen if the demyelination persists or is repeated over several weeks to months. It has long been noted that there is a poor correlation between histology and neurological deficits in demyelinating disease, and regions of extensive myelin damage may function, albeit with altered conduction velocities. A possible compensatory mechanism was uncovered in studies of the Shiverer mutation. *Shi/shi* mice are hypomyelinated as a result of a deletion of five exons in the gene for myelin basic protein. Axons are ensheathed by oligodendroglia, and multiple lamellae are present, but are not compacted. Paranodes are highly abnormal, and regions of axoglial junctions have an irregular morphology (Rosenbluth, 1980; Inoue et al., 1981). There are reduced numbers of nodal Na⁺ channel clusters, and many of those that are present are highly irregular (Rasband et al., 1999). Using ³H-saxitoxin (³H-STX) autoradiography, Noebels et al. (1991) found a 2.2- to 4.7-fold increase in Na⁺ channel expression in fiber tracts in *shi/shi* vs. (+/+) controls. In contrast, there was almost no increase in gray matter or in unmyelinated fibers. These authors considered the idea that glial association during myelination decreases expression of Na⁺ channels. During extended periods of demyelination, as can occur in multiple sclerosis, conduction may be restored by a reversion to a high density of Na⁺ channels. This work was later extended, using antibodies to $Na_v1.1$, $Na_v1.2$, and $Na_v1.3$, to probe several regions of the Shiverer CNS (Westenbroek et al., 1992). Of these three isotypes, only $Na_v1.2$ was elevated, and only in myelinated tracts. With the additional resolution, it could be shown definitively that the new channels were neuronal and not glial.

There are 10 known voltage-dependent Na⁺ channel α-subunits expressed in mammals. For a number of years, the identity of the specific isoform(s) present at nodes of Ranvier was unknown. The development of better antibodies for immunofluorescence led to the identification of $Na_v1.6$ at adult nodes in both PNS and CNS axons (Caldwell et al., 2000; Tzoumaka et al., 2000). There is developmental regulation of this channel, and in the optic nerve $Na_v1.2$ is expressed first, but as myelination proceeds, it is replaced by $Na_v1.6$ at nodes, while $Na_v1.2$ remains within the unmyelinated region adjacent to retinal ganglion cell (RGC) bodies (Boiko et al., 2001). In the Shiverer mutant the primary isoform expressed in the region of RGC axons distal to the lamina cribrosa is $Na_v1.2$, and thus the presence of compact myelin seems to determine the axonal switch to $Na_v1.6$ at nodes (Boiko et al., 2001). It is noteworthy that this subtype replacement does occur at the initial segment of Shiverer RGC axons (Boiko et al., 2003), but this is a zone in which the clustering of Na^+ channels is independent of glia. Immunization of Biozzi mice with myelin oligodendrocyte glycoprotein peptide results in relapsing-remitting experimental autoimmune encephalomyelitis (EAE) (Craner et al., 2004). In the dorsal columns of the spinal cord the number of fibers with diffuse labeling of $Na_v1.6$ went up fivefold. There was also a large increase in the number of injured axons, and these were also typically positive for $Na_v1.6$ staining. The Na^+ to Ca^{+2} exchanger (NCX) co-localized with $Na_v1.6$ in most of these injured axons, and the authors suggest that activation of the Na^+ channel could increase $[Na^+]_i$ and this, in turn, might lead to increased $[Ca^{+2}]_i$, leading to cell death (see Chapter 7). Because axonal loss is thought to play a major role in irreversible deficits in multiple sclerosis (Trapp et al., 1998), these ectopic Na^+ channels may be exacerbating the disease. $Na_v1.6$ has unique properties that may contribute to its possible role in disease, and also pose interesting questions concerning its selection as the nodal channel. When a neuron is depolarized, Na^+ channels open rapidly and then inactivate. In most cases, a return of V_m to negative levels does not result in current because the recovery pathway does not pass through open states. $Na_v1.6$, however, produces a resurgent inward current of 100 to 300 pA that decays with a time constant of about 30 msec (Raman and Bean, 1997). This current could produce the increase in $[Na^+]i$ discussed previously, and, in normal axons, could in principle lead to reentry excitation and instability. The latter clearly does not occur, and normal nodes have a complement of ion channels that may ensure smooth propagation. In particular, Shaker-type voltage-dependent K^+ channels are clustered in the juxtaparanode and may participate in damping reentrant depolarizations. Under some limited conditions, it has been possible to demonstrate repetitive firing when these channels are mis-localized, blocked, or genetically deleted (Rasband et al., 1998; Zhou et al., 1998; Vabnick et al., 1999). This is discussed in more detail in Chapter 4.

VI. Molecular Mechanisms Involved in Na⁺ Channel Clustering

The evidence discussed thus far suggests a scheme in which nodes form during remyelination as the low density of axonal internodal Na^+ channels cluster adjacent to the tips of myelinating glia, move laterally as the glial processes elongate, and form nodes of Ranvier by fusing with a neighboring cluster (Dugandzija-Novakovic et al., 1995; Vabnick et al., 1996; Lambert et al., 1997; Ching et al., 1999). We now advance the hypothesis that Na^+ channels are clustered by exclusion from regions of contact with myelinating glial cells (Kazarinova-Noyes and Shrager, 2002) and that this could occur if the rate of lateral diffusion is increased by this association. Evidence suggests a molecular mechanism that might account for such a scheme. Na^+ channels at the node of Ranvier are part of a large complex of transmembrane, extracellular matrix, and intracellular proteins (Kazarinova-Noyes and Shrager, 2002; Poliak and Peles, 2003; Salzer, 2003). Among these are members of the L1-type cell adhesion family, including NrCAM and the 186 kDa form of neurofascin (NF186), whose association with $ankyrin_G$, and hence with the cytoskeleton, is controlled by phosphorylation of a specific intracellular tyrosine in a FIGQY domain (Garver et al., 1997; Jenkins et al., 2001). There is evidence that Na^+ channel β subunits are also linked to $ankyrin_G$ by a phosphorylation-dependent mechanism (Malhotra et al., 2002). Na^+ channels in excitable cell membranes are thought to be normally highly immobile (Stuhmer and Almers, 1982; see also Custer et al., 2003), presumably through the $ankyrin_G$ link to the cytoskeleton. We therefore consider a mechanism of clustering in which glial contact activates an axonal tyrosine kinase that phosphorylates one or more key membrane components, breaking the link to $ankyrin_G$, and thereby increasing the effective coefficient of lateral diffusion. As a Na^+ channel diffuses beyond the axoglial contact zone, it enters a region in which it may be dephosphorylated by the combined absence of the activated kinase and presence of a tyrosine phosphatase. (It should be noted that there is evidence that receptor protein tyrosine phosphatase β associates with Na^+ channels [Ratcliffe et al., 2000]). This sharp change in enzymatic environment may also be mediated by Schwann cell microvilli that are arrayed close to the nodal axolemma. These structures are rich in the ezrin-radixin-moesin (ERM) protein family, appear very early in node formation, and may contain receptors for axonal proteins, including NF186 (Melendez-Vasquez et al., 2001; Scherer et al., 2001). Channels would then cluster at the edge of the myelinating glial cell as their link to $ankyrin_G$ is restored. Although qualitatively plausible, this model requires a quantitative test to judge its applicability. There are several key parameters: the diffusion coefficient of Na^+ channels in axons, rates of tyrosine phosphorylation and dephosphorylation of membrane proteins, the Na^+ channel densities at the node and internode, and the rate of growth of glial processes. Values for all of these have been estimated from published measurements, the last coming from the experiment shown in Fig. 4. Because it is thus possible to construct a quantitative model in which virtually all critical parameters are under tight constraints, we felt that this exercise might serve as a plausibility test to see if the resulting clustering matches can be seen experimentally.

VII. Computational Test of a Model for Na⁺ Channel Clustering

The computational model consists of an axon in contact with an initially nonmyelinating Schwann cell. The idea is to calculate the rate of formation and shape of axonal Na⁺ channel clusters that form at the edges of the Schwann cell after it begins remyelination and compare these with results from immunofluorescence. As discussed earlier, the Na⁺ channel density at adult nodes is about 1,000–1,500/μm^2. The internodal density is much less (40–60/μm^2), but the total number of internodal channels is high (~95% of the axonal population). As mentioned previously, because there is evidence that the nodal channels are derived primarily from an existing axonal pool, we can conclude that the nodal density has a maximum value that cannot be exceeded despite the availability of other channels. From the preceding numbers, we have taken the mean value of 1,250 channels/μm^2 for the normal adult node, and the internodal density is then set at 4% of this value, or 50 channels/μm^2. We set U as the density of unbound channels, B the density of bound or anchored channels, and D the diffusion coefficient. With the chemical reaction (equation 1) approximated by a first order process with rate constants α and β, the system is then described by equation (2) in one dimension (Crank, 1975).

$$(1) \quad U \underset{\beta}{\overset{\alpha}{\rightleftharpoons}} B \qquad (\partial U / \partial t)_{chem} = \beta B - \alpha U$$

$$(2) \quad (\partial U / \partial t)_{total} = D \partial^2 U / \partial x^2 + \beta B - \alpha U$$

Each of the rate constants has two possible values, one in regions covered by a Schwann cell (α_{SC}, β_{SC}) and another in "naked" zones with no Schwann cell (α_N, β_N). Only unbound channels are free to diffuse laterally in the membrane. We took as a starting point for the kinetics of the chemical reaction rate constants derived from data for tyrosine phosphorylation and dephosphorylation of membrane proteins that were available in the literature. The model is illustrated by the sketch in Fig. 6A. Initially, Na⁺ channels are uniformly distributed in the axon at a density of 50/μm^2 and $\alpha = \alpha_N$, $\beta = \beta_N$ everywhere. At t = 0 the Schwann cell commits to myelination, and the rate constants in the region of contact (bounded by the MAG-positive regions shown in red) change abruptly to α_{SC}, β_{SC}. As the Schwann cell grows longitudinally, the rate constants in the newly covered zones also change to α_{SC}, β_{SC}. Just outside the MAG-positive zones (destined to become paranodes) nascent microvilli appear, and in this region and beyond, rate constants remain α_N and β_N.

The axon was 163 μm long, divided initially into a central zone of 83 μm covered by a Schwann cell and two 40-μm uncovered zones on either side of the Schwann cell. The diffusion coefficient of mobile Na⁺ channels in axon membranes has been measured in fluorescence photobleach recovery experiments to be about 10^{-10} cm²/sec (see Custer et al., 2003, for details), and this is assigned to all unbound channels, regardless of location. Because data on Na⁺ channels are not available, we used kinetic data on another membrane protein, the insulin receptor, for plausible starting values of reaction kinetics. The half-time of tyrosine dephosphorylation of the latter protein has been reported in different experiments at 21 sec (Mooney and Anderson, 1989) and 37 sec (Mooney and Bordwell, 1992) at 37°C. Using 30 sec as an intermediate value, we assigned rate constants outside the Schwann cell region of α_N = 1.4 min⁻¹ and β_N = 0.001 min⁻¹. (The half-time gives the sum of the rate constants, and we made the assumption that the reverse reaction rate was much smaller than the forward rate.) Phosphorylation kinetics were similar (Mooney and Anderson, 1989), and we chose for values under the Schwann cell, α_{SC} = 0.001 min⁻¹ and β_{SC} = 1.0 min⁻¹. The longitudinal growth of Schwann cells was approximated by fitting a single exponential function to the data in Fig. 4 (initial length, 83 μm; final length, 274 μm; τ = 17 days). The equations were solved numerically using the method of Euler (Simon, 1986). Accuracy was determined first by varying the distance resolution and the time step. Solutions were stable with x-divisions of 0.2 μm and time steps of 0.15 sec. Final calculations were done with x-divisions of 0.1 μm and time steps of 0.015 sec, but these varied by less than 1% from the former. Further, if the chemical reaction were eliminated, solutions of the diffusion equation alone agreed with the analytical solution (Crank, 1975) within 0.1%.

In Fig. 6B the profile of Na⁺ channel density at the right edge of the Schwann cell is plotted for several times ranging from 1 to 24 hours. An example of typical new clusters of Na⁺ channels forming during remyelination at 13 dpi is shown in panel F. It is not possible to know with certainty the time that has elapsed between the differentiation of a particular Schwann cell to a myelinating phenotype and the appearance of adjacent Na⁺ channel clusters. However, almost all MAG-positive Schwann cells are associated with clusters detected by immunofluorescence during both development and remyelination, and channels must therefore accumulate within hours (Vabnick et al., 1996). Cluster formation is predicted by the model to be correspondingly fast, with significant gradients in density appearing rapidly. However, the shapes of the calculated density profiles do not match the observed immunolabeled sites, especially at shorter times. While some zones of high Na⁺ channel immunofluorescence appear to have a gradient in density, the great majority are more sharply defined, as in Fig. 6F. The model, on the other hand, predicts for short times a

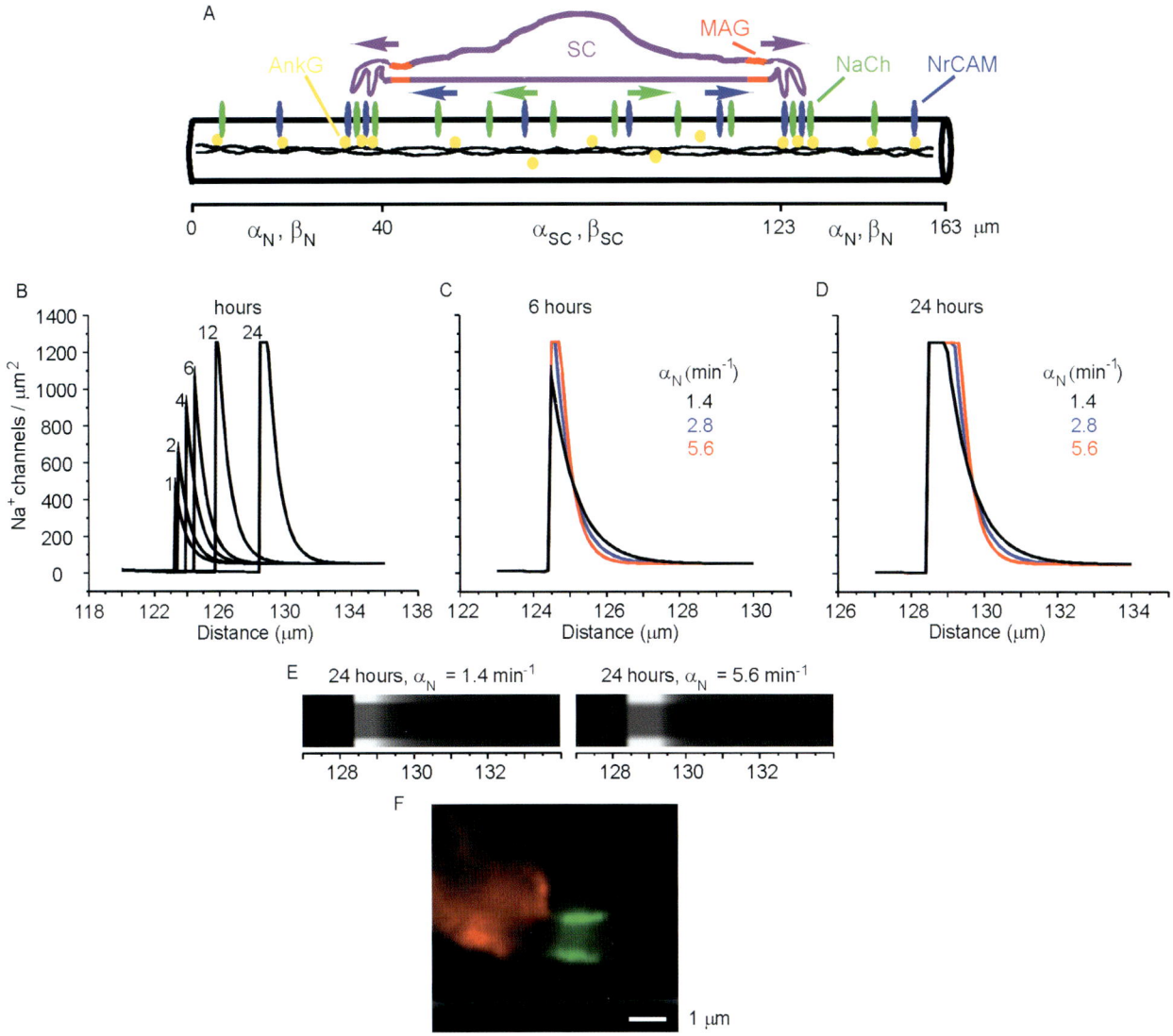

Figure 6 Computational model of Na+ channel clustering. The diagram in (**A**) illustrates the configuration. The x-axis below the sketch gives the distances at time zero. The curves in graph (**B**) plot Na+ channel density vs. distance along the axon at 1, 2, 4, 6, 12, and 24 hours after the Schwann cell reaches a myelinating state. Since the Schwann cell grows longitudinally according to the curve in Fig. 4, the position of the right edge changes with time. (**C** and **D**) Result of varying the rate constant α_N at 6 and 24 hours, respectively. The black curves repeat the calculations in (**B**) on an expanded x-axis. The blue and red curves show results with α_N = 2.8 and 5.6 min^{-1}, respectively. (**E**) Representations of the 24-hour curves with α_N = 1.4 min^{-1} (*left*) and 5.6 min^{-1} (*right*), converted to a gray scale of 15 to 230, which mimics the green immunofluorescence intensity range in the cluster in (**F**). (**F**) A cluster of Na+ channels (green) at the tip of a remyelinating Schwann cell process (MAG, red) 13 days after injection of lysolecithin. (**C, D, E,** and **F**) are all scaled to the same distance calibration.

sharp peak followed by a gradual decrease in density with distance from the glial edge (for example, the 6-hour curve in Fig. 6B), and even at 24 hours the shapes do not match well. This can be seen in Fig. 6E (left) in which the curve at 24 hours in B has been converted to a gray scale plot for comparison with the immunolabeled image (the distance scales in Fig. 6C, D, E, and F are identical).

To judge which property of this system might be responsible for the deficiencies in the fit, we tested the sensitivity of the model to several parameters. NrCAM and NF186 seem to precede Na+ channels at nascent nodes (Lambert

et al., 1997; Custer et al., 2003). At E21 there are relatively few identifiable nodal sites, but at 60% of these, NrCAM was found in the absence of Na+ channels (Custer et al., 2003). Further, in NrCAM null mutant mice, Na+ channel clustering at nodes is delayed by several days, but reaches normal levels by P10. Binding of NrCAM to ankyrin$_G$ would be dependent on similar phosphorylation/dephosphorylation reactions, and clustering mechanisms could thus be similar. Since this protein is smaller than the Na+ channel α-subunit, it might diffuse more rapidly and thus cluster sooner. Could the early presence of these ankyrin$_G$

binding proteins then speed the immobilization reaction of Na⁺ channels either by concentrating an essential phosphatase or by association with $ankyrin_G$, which has multiple membrane-binding domains? In either case, the rate constant for Na⁺ channels to bind at the Schwann cell edge (α_N) would rise. Results of two- and fourfold increases in α_N are shown in the blue and red curves, respectively, in Fig. 6C and D. At 6 hours (Fig. 6C), Na⁺ channel clustering is predicted to be significantly stronger and more focal. At 24 hours (Fig. 6D), the major change is in the cluster shape. Both provide better fits to the immunofluorescence, and the fourfold 24-hour curve is translated to a gray scale plot in Fig. 6E (right). In contrast, results were only minimally sensitive to fivefold changes (up or down) in β_N, and were virtually unaffected by fivefold changes in α_{SC} or β_{SC} because diffusion is much slower than the rate at which channels are released from their cytoskeletal link after conversion of the Schwann cell to a myelinating state. We also modeled the fusion of two clusters to form a node by including two Schwann cells separated by an initial gap of 12 μm. The density profiles matched immunostaining observations quite well (not shown). It should be emphasized that the idea behind development of a computational model is not to prove that a suggested mechanism is correct, but rather the opposite: Should the hypothesis be rejected for lack of consistency with the available data? In this case, the proposed mechanism seems not to be inconsistent with the calculated predictions.

VIII. Summary

In normal myelinated axons, ion channels are localized with a high level of precision in specific regions. Voltage-dependent Na⁺ channels are sequestered at high density at initial segments and within the nodal gap, and their subtype is developmentally regulated. Myelin damage has consequences beyond the resulting deficits in passive cable properties, and reorganization of ion channels takes place in both acute and chronic phases. Na⁺ channel clusters have a high degree of stability, no doubt resulting from their link to the underlying cytoskeleton by $ankyrin_G$, and perhaps the specialized form of spectrin present at these sites. Nonetheless, these channels ultimately disperse or are internalized, and must be restored. The low density internodal pool of Na⁺ channels appears to serve this purpose on short time scales. In more extended periods of demyelination, particularly in the CNS, *de novo* synthesis increases the axonal density. This may partially compensate for the relative paucity of remyelination by oligodendrocytes. In the PNS, remyelination is rapid, and channels are recruited from the existing pool and relocated by Schwann cells as they adhere and grow longitudinally. In both the PNS and CNS, when remyelination takes place, the original structure is not repli-

cated and new nodes of Ranvier are formed in regions that previously were internodal.

Molecular details of the neuron-glial communication that is responsible for ion channel localization are becoming increasingly clear. Much attention is focused on the adapter protein $ankyrin_G$, because it binds several nodal cell adhesion molecules in addition to Na⁺ channels, and thus seems to serve as a coordinating center. $Ankyrin_G$ is not likely, however, to initiate node formation, as it is cytoplasmic, whereas signaling, at least in the PNS, requires contact with glia. L1-family proteins and β subunits are more probable candidates for this role, as all have Ig-type domains, and, perhaps most important, a link to $ankyrin_G$ that can be regulated by phosphorylation. This provides a mechanism for controlling lateral mobility in spatially defined zones, thereby establishing patterns of localization. The reorganization of ion channels that follows demyelination is of prime importance in determining the neurological deficits that result, and perhaps even the survival of the axon itself. Determining the precise mechanism of these events will provide new targets for therapies aimed at restricting and perhaps reversing the functional loss that is a consequence of demyelinating disease.

References

Arroyo, E. J., Chitale, R. and Scherer, S. S. (2003). Paranodal demyelination disrupts the molecular organization of nodes. *Soc. Neurosci. Abs.* **675.5.**

Bennett, V., and Lambert, S. (1999). Physiological roles of axonal ankyrins in survival of premyelinated axons and localization of voltage-gated sodium channels. *J. Neurocytol.* **28**, 303–318.

Berghs, S., Aggujaro, D., Dirkx, R., Jr., Maksimova, E., Stabach, P., Hermel, J. M., Zhang, J. P., Philbrick, W., Slepnev, V., Ort, T., and Solimena, M. (2000). BetaIV spectrin, a new spectrin localized at axon initial segments and nodes of Ranvier in the central and peripheral nervous system. *J Cell Biol.* **151**, 985–1002.

Boiko, T., Rasband, M. N., Levinson, S. R., Caldwell, J. H., Mandel, G., Trimmer, J. S., and Matthews, G. (2001). Compact myelin dictates the differential targeting of two sodium channel isoforms in the same axon. *Neuron* **30**, 91–104.

Boiko, T., Van Wart, A., Caldwell, J. H., Levinson, S. R., Trimmer, J. S., and Matthews, G. (2003). Functional specialization of the axon initial segment by isoform-specific sodium channel targeting. *J. Neurosci.* **23**, 2306–2313.

Bostock, H., and Sears, T. A. (1978). The internodal axon membrane: electrical excitability and continuous conduction in segmental demyelination. *J. Physiol.* **280**, 273–301.

Caldwell, J. H., Schaller, K. L., Lasher, R. S., Peles, E., and Levinson, S. R. (2000). Sodium channel Na(v)1.6 is localized at nodes of Ranvier, dendrites, and synapses. *Proc. Natl. Acad. Sci. U. S. A.* **97**, 5616–5620.

Ching, W., Zanazzi, G., Levinson, S. R., and Salzer, J. L. (1999). Clustering of neuronal sodium channels requires contact with myelinating Schwann cells. *J. Neurocytol.* **28**, 295–301.

Chiu, S. Y. (1993). Differential expression of sodium channels in acutely isolated myelinating and non-myelinating Schwann cells of rabbits. *J. Physiol.* **470**, 485–499.

Chiu, S. Y., Ritchie, J. M., Rogart, R. B., and Stagg, D. (1979). A quantitative description of membrane currents in rabbit myelinated nerve. *J. Physiol.* **292**, 149–166.

Chiu, S. Y., and Schwarz, W. (1987). Sodium and potassium currents in acutely demyelinated internodes of rabbit sciatic nerves. *J. Physiol.* **391**, 631–649.

Chiu, S. Y., Shrager, P., and Ritchie, J. M. (1984). Neuronal-type Na+ and K+ channels in rabbit cultured Schwann cells. *Nature* **311**, 156–157.

Craner, M. J., Hains, B. C., Lo, A. C., Black, J. A., and Waxman, S. G. (2004). Co-localization of sodium channel Nav1.6 and the sodium-calcium exchanger at sites of axonal injury in the spinal cord in EAE. *Brain* **127**, 294–303.

Crank, J. (1975). "The Mathematics of Diffusion." Oxford University Press: London.

Custer, A. W., Kazarinova-Noyes, K., Sakurai, T., Xu, X., Simon, W., Grumet, M., and Shrager, P. (2003). The role of the ankyrin-binding protein NrCAM in node of Ranvier formation. *J. Neurosci.* **23**, 10032–10039.

Dodge, F., and Frankenhaeuser, B. (1959). Sodium currents in the myelinated nerve fibre of Xenopus laevis investigated with the voltage clamp technique. *J. Physiol.* **148**, 188–200.

Dugandzija-Novakovic, S., Koszowski, A. G., Levinson, S. R., and Shrager, P. (1995). Clustering of Na channels and node of Ranvier formation in remyelinating axons. *J. Neurosci.* **15**, 492–502.

Ellisman, M. H., and Levinson, S. R. (1982). Immunocytochemical localization of sodium channel distributions in the excitable membranes of Electrophorus electricus. *Proc. Natl. Acad. Sci. U. S. A.* **79**, 6707–6711.

Felts, P. A., Baker, T. A., and Smith, K. J. (1997). Conduction in segmentally demyelinated mammalian central axons. *J. Neurosci.* **17**, 7267–7277.

Garver, T. D., Ren, Q., Tuvia, S., and Bennett, V. (1997). Tyrosine phosphorylation at a site highly conserved in the L1 family of cell adhesion molecules abolishes ankyrin binding and increases lateral mobility of neurofascin. *J. Cell Biol.* **137**, 703–714.

Grissmer, S. (1986). Properties of potassium and sodium channels in frog internode. *J. Physiol.* **381**, 119–134.

Hall, S. M., and Gregson, N. A. (1971). The *in vivo* and ultrastructural effects of injection of lysophosphatidyl choline into myelinated peripheral nerve fibres of the adult mouse. *J. Cell Sci.* **9**, 769–789.

Hille, B. (2001). "Ionic Channels of Excitable Membranes." Sinauer Associates: Sunderland, MA.

Huxley, A. F., and Stampfli, R. (1949). Evidence for saltatory conduction in peripheral myelinated nerve fibres. *J. Physiol.* **108**, 315–339.

Inoue, Y., Nakamura, R., Mikoshiba, M., and Tsukada, Y. (1981). Fine structure of the central myelin sheath in the myelin deficient mutant Shiverer mouse, with special reference to the pattern of myelin formation by oligodendroglia. *Brain Res.* **219**, 85–94.

Jenkins, S. M., Kizhatil, K., Kramarcy, N. R., Sen, A., Sealock, R., and Bennett, V. (2001). FIGQY phosphorylation defines discrete populations of L1 cell adhesion molecules at sites of cell-cell contact and in migrating neurons. *J. Cell Sci.* **114**, 3823–3835.

Kaplan, M. R., Cho, M. H., Ullian, E. M., Isom, L. L., Levinson, S. R., and Barres, B. A. (2001). Differential control of clustering of the sodium channels Na(v)1.2 and Na(v)1.6 at developing CNS nodes of Ranvier. *Neuron* **30**, 105–119.

Kaplan, M. R., Meyer-Franke, A., Lambert, S., Bennett, V., Duncan, I. D., Levinson, S. R., and Barres, B. A. (1997). Induction of sodium channel clustering by oligodendrocytes. *Nature* **386**, 724–728.

Kazarinova-Noyes, K., and Shrager, P. (2002). Molecular constituents of the node of Ranvier. *Mol. Neurobiol.* **26**, 167–182.

Komada, M., and Soriano, P. (2002). BetaIV-spectrin regulates sodium channel clustering through ankyrin-G at axon initial segments and nodes of Ranvier. *J. Cell Biol.* **156**, 337–348.

Kordeli, E., Lambert, S., and Bennett, V. (1995). AnkyrinG. A new ankyrin gene with neural-specific isoforms localized at the axonal initial segment and node of Ranvier. *J. Biol. Chem.* **270**, 2352–2359.

Lambert, S., Davis, J. Q., and Bennett, V. (1997). Morphogenesis of the node of Ranvier: co-clusters of ankyrin and ankyrin-binding integral proteins define early developmental intermediates. *J. Neurosci.* **17**, 7025–7036.

Malhotra, J. D., Koopmann, M. C., Kazen-Gillespie, K. A., Fettman, N., Hortsch, M., and Isom, L. L. (2002). Structural requirements for interaction of sodium channel beta 1 subunits with ankyrin. *J. Biol. Chem.* **277**, 26681–26688.

Martini, R., and Schachner, M. (1986). Immunoelectron microscopic localization of neural cell adhesion molecules (L1, N-CAM, and MAG) and their shared carbohydrate epitope and myelin basic protein in developing sciatic nerve. *J. Cell Biol.* **103**, 2439–2448.

Melendez-Vasquez, C. V., Rios, J. C., Zanazzi, G., Lambert, S., Bretscher, A., and Salzer, J. L. (2001). Nodes of Ranvier form in association with ezrin-radixin-moesin (ERM)-positive Schwann cell processes. *Proc. Natl. Acad. Sci. U. S. A.* **98**, 1235–1240.

Mooney, R. A., and Anderson, D. L. (1989). Phosphorylation of the insulin receptor in permeabilized adipocytes is coupled to a rapid dephosphorylation reaction. *J. Biol. Chem.* **264**, 6850–6857.

Mooney, R. A., and Bordwell, K. L. (1992). Differential dephosphorylation of the insulin receptor and its 160-kDa substrate (pp160) in rat adipocytes. *J. Biol. Chem.* **267**, 14054–14060.

Noebels, J. L., Marcom, P. K., and Jalilian-Tehrani, M. H. (1991). Sodium channel density in hypomyelinated brain increased by myelin basic protein gene deletion. *Nature* **352**, 431–434.

Novakovic, S. D., Deerinck, T. J., Levinson, S. R., Shrager, P., and Ellisman, M. H. (1996). Clusters of axonal Na+ channels adjacent to remyelinating Schwann cells. *J. Neurocytol.* **25**, 403–412.

Novakovic, S. D., Levinson, S. R., Schachner, M., and Shrager, P. (1998). Disruption and reorganization of sodium channels in experimental allergic neuritis. *Muscle Nerve* **21**, 1019–1032.

Poliak, S., and Peles, E. (2003). The local differentiation of myelinated axons at nodes of Ranvier. *Nat. Rev. Neurosci.* **4**, 968–980.

Quick, D. C., and Waxman, S. G. (1977). Specific staining of the axon membrane at nodes of Ranvier with ferric ion and ferrocyanide. *J. Neurol. Sci.* **31**, 1–11.

Raman, I. M., and Bean, B. P. (1997). Resurgent sodium current and action potential formation in dissociated cerebellar Purkinje neurons. *J. Neurosci.* **17**, 4517–4526.

Rasband, M. N., Peles, E., Trimmer, J. S., Levinson, S. R., Lux, S. E., and Shrager, P. (1999). Dependence of nodal sodium channel clustering on paranodal axoglial contact in the developing CNS. *J. Neurosci.* **19**, 7516–7528.

Rasband, M. N., Trimmer, J. S., Schwarz, T. L., Levinson, S. R., Ellisman, M. H., Schachner, M., and Shrager, P. (1998). Potassium channel distribution, clustering, and function in remyelinating rat axons. *J. Neurosci.* **18**, 36–47.

Rasminsky, M., and Sears, T. A. (1972). Internodal conduction in undissected demyelinated nerve fibres. *J. Physiol.* **227**, 323–350.

Ratcliffe, C. F., Qu, Y., McCormick, K. A., Tibbs, V. C., Dixon, J. E., Scheuer, T., and Catterall, W. A. (2000). A sodium channel signaling complex: modulation by associated receptor protein tyrosine phosphatase beta. *Nature Neurosci.* **3**, 437–444.

Rosenbluth, J. (1976). Intramembranous particle distribution at the node of Ranvier and adjacent axolemma in myelinated axons of the frog brain. *J. Neurocytol.* **5**, 731–745.

Rosenbluth, J. (1980). Central myelin in the mouse mutant Shiverer. *J. Comp. Neurol.* **194**, 639–648.

Rosenbluth, J. (1981). Freeze-fracture approaches to ionophore localization in normal and myelin-deficient nerves. *Adv. Neurol.* **31**, 391–418.

Salzer, J. L. (2003). Polarized domains of myelinated axons. *Neuron* **40**, 297–318.

Scherer, S. S., Xu, T., Crino, P., Arroyo, E. J., and Gutmann, D. H. (2001). Ezrin, radixin, and moesin are components of Schwann cell microvilli. *J. Neurosci. Res.* **65**, 150–164.

Shrager, P. (1987). The distribution of sodium and potassium channels in single demyelinated axons of the frog. *J. Physiol.* **392,** 587–602.

Shrager, P. (1988). Ionic channels and signal conduction in single remyelinating frog nerve fibres. *J. Physiol.* **404,** 695–712.

Shrager, P. (1989). Sodium channels in single demyelinated mammalian axons. *Brain Res.* **483,** 149–154.

Shrager, P., Chiu, S. Y., and Ritchie, J. M. (1985). Voltage-dependent sodium and potassium channels in mammalian cultured Schwann cells. *Proc. Natl. Acad. Sci. U. S. A.* **82,** 948–952.

Shrager, P., and Rubinstein, C. T. (1990). Optical measurement of conduction in single demyelinated axons. *J. Gen. Physiol.* **95,** 867–889.

Simon, W. (1986) "Mathematical Techniques for Biology and Medicine." Dover Publications, Inc.: New York

Smith, K. J., Bostock, H., and Hall, S. M. (1982). Saltatory conduction precedes remyelination in axons demyelinated with lysophosphatidyl choline. *J. Neurol. Sci.* **54,** 13–31.

St:uhmer, W., and Almers, W. (1982). Photobleaching through glass micropipettes: sodium channels without lateral mobility in the sarcolemma of frog skeletal muscle. *Proc. Natl. Acad. Sci. U. S. A.* **79,** 946–950.

Tasaki, I., and Takeuchi, T. (1942). Weitere Studien uber den Aktionsstrom der markhaltigen Nervensfasern und uber die elektrosaltatorische Ubertragung des Nervenimpulses. *Pflugers Arch.* **245,** 764–782.

Trapp, B. D., Peterson, J., Ransohoff, R. M., Rudick, R., Mork, S., and Bo, L. (1998). Axonal transection in the lesions of multiple sclerosis. *N. Engl. J. Med.* **338,** 278–285.

Tzoumaka, E., Novakovic, S. D., Levinson, S. R., and Shrager, P. (1995). Na+ channel aggregation in remyelinating mouse sciatic axons following transection. *Glia* **15,** 188–194.

Tzoumaka, E., Tischler, A. C., Sangameswaran, L., Eglen, R. M., Hunter, J. C., and Novakovic, S. D. (2000). Differential distribution of the tetrodotoxin-sensitive rPN4/NaCh6/Scn8a sodium channel in the nervous system. *J. Neurosci. Res.* **60,** 37–44.

Vabnick, I., Novakovic, S. D., Levinson, S. R., Schachner, M., and Shrager, P. (1996). The clustering of axonal sodium channels during development of the peripheral nervous system. *J. Neurosci.* **16,** 4914–4922.

Vabnick, I., Trimmer, J. S., Schwarz, T. L., Levinson, S. R., Risal, D., and Shrager, P. (1999). Dynamic potassium channel distributions during axonal development prevent aberrant firing patterns. *J. Neurosci.* **19,** 747–758.

Westenbroek, R. E., Noebels, J. L., and Catterall, W. A. (1992). Elevated expression of type II Na+ channels in hypomyelinated axons of shiverer mouse brain. *J. Neurosci.* **12,** 2259–2267.

Wilson, G. F., and Chiu, S. Y. (1990). Ion channels in axon and Schwann cell membranes at paranodes of mammalian myelinated fibers studied with patch clamp. *J. Neurosci.* **10,** 3263–3274.

Zhou, L., Zhang, C. L., Messing, A., and Chiu, S. Y. (1998). Temperature-sensitive neuromuscular transmission in Kv1.1 null mice: role of potassium channels under the myelin sheath in young nerves. *J. Neurosci.* **18,** 7200–7215.

9

Ion Currents and Axonal Oscillators: A Possible Biophysical Basis for Positive Signs and Symptoms in Multiple Sclerosis

Mark D. Baker, B.Sc., Ph.D.

I. Introduction

This chapter draws on the documented changes in axonal properties occurring in experimental demyelination in both peripheral and central axons, and assumes that the biophys-ical changes in axonal function in models of demyelination provide an insight into the symptomatology of multiple sclerosis (MS).

MS is an inflammatory disease of the central nervous system (CNS) usually associated with negative symptoms, including loss of motor function and sensation. The negative symptoms result from damage to white-matter tracts, including loss of axons, and loss of myelin leading to nerve impulse conduction failure. Normal action potential conduction in myelinated axons is saltatory, where only the nodes of Ranvier generate sodium (Na^+) currents (Huxley and Stämpfli, 1949). The myelin sheaths provide a low capacitance conduit for action current between adjacent nodes (Barrett and Barrett, 1982). Damage or removal of the myelin greatly increases the effective electrical capacity of the non-excitable internodes and exposes internodal voltage-gated potassium (K^+) channels, stabilizing the axonal membrane potential. The increased capacitative load and the depolarization activated outward current generated by K^+ channels are understood to prevent action potential propagation through a demyelinated region. Axonal conduction failure caused by myelin loss is potentially reversible. Formerly myelinated axons respond to loss of the sheath by exhibiting a changed distribution of Na^+ channels, where the normally inexcitable internodal membrane gains Na^+ channels and continuous conduction can become possible (Bostock and Sears, 1978). The slowly propagating action potentials exhibited by demyelinated axons are generated by long-action currents, leading to another pathological property of functional diseased axons, namely their inability to conduct trains of nerve impulses. This inability to conduct trains is caused, in part, by a substantial fall in excitability during impulse activity, leading to use-dependent conduction failure, and may contribute to the clinically important phenomenon of fatigue. The fall in excitability is due to an Na^+/K^+ adenosine triphosphatase (ATPase)-induced electrogenic hyperpolarization, triggered by Na^+ influx, that can be counteracted by the application of an external depolarizing current in experimental demyelination (Bostock and Grafe, 1985).

Positive symptoms, including chronic paresthesia and pain, are also apparent in MS and they can be both unpleasant and debilitating. Given the fact that conduction failure is associated with demyelination, how axons could become a source of pathological impulse generation was for many years a mystery, although this mystery has now been at least partially solved by sophisticated electrophysiological techniques. Experimental demyelination has shown that aberrant sensations in demyelinating disease are probably associated with ectopic impulse generation in axons (Rasminsky, 1981). Normal impulses arise at the initial segments of central axons. In contrast, ectopic impulses arise at sites normally involved only in impulse transmission. Somehow damage to myelin and its sequelae allow some injured axons to become ectopically active, and this presents a serious clinical problem. Although some pain in MS may be generated as a secondary consequence of muscular spasm, recent hypotheses concerning the mechanism by which neuropathic pain states are initiated include the involvement of ectopic activity in non-nociceptive axons (Boucher et al., 2000), followed by changes in central nociceptive processing. Similarities between the underlying mechanisms of neuropathic pain states and the positive symptoms of MS are further suggested by the drugs used to treat both conditions. The anticonvulsants carbamazepine and gabapentin, the former a known Na^+ channel blocker (Willow et al., 1985), are commonly used to treat the positive symptoms of MS, as well as pain states that occur after other forms of nerve injury.

It has yet to be determined how the aberrant activity underlying spasticity and tremor in MS is generated, although demyelination might damage central circuitry involved in generating motor programs, and loss of connectivity (resulting in disinhibition, for example) or ectopic activity could be involved. MS sufferers who experience pain and spasticity are pursuing the use of delta9-tetrahydrocannabinol (delta9-THC) to ameliorate painful symptoms, an effect apparently mediated by CB1 receptors (reviewed by Smith, 2002), activation of which may, remark-

ably, more generally antagonize the progression of inflammatory degenerative disease in the CNS (Pryce et al., 2003).

II. Distribution of Ion Channels in Myelinated Axons

Experiments involving isolated nodal voltage-clamping, isolated internodal voltage-clamping (following the acute removal of myelin by detergents such as lysolethicin), patch-clamping demyelinated axons, recordings of electrotonus from normal axons and immunocytochemistry of peripheral and central axons have elucidated and confirmed the normal distribution of ion channel types in myelinated nerve (Chiu et al., 1979; Baker et al., 1987; Röper and Schwarz, 1989; Reid et al., 1999; Rasband and Shrager, 2000). The patterns in the peripheral nervous system (PNS) and CNS appear similar. Normally, transiently opening Na^+ channels are confined to the nodes of Ranvier, and are present at densities of around 2,000 per μm^2 (estimated from nonstationary noise analysis, gating current measurements, and by counting freeze-fracture particles, reviewed by Ritchie, 1995). A far lower density of several tens of channels per μm^2 is thought to be present in the internode (Chiu and Schwarz, 1987), insufficient to confer excitability on the internodal membrane (although in absolute terms the node and internode may have similar numbers of channels, as the internodal membrane area is three orders of magnitude larger than that of a node). The normal peripheral axon also has kinetically fast and slow delayed rectifier K^+ channels (GK_f and GK_s, respectively), corresponding well with the fast and slow K^+ current kinetics originally described in frog axons by J.-M. Dubois (Dubois, 1981). The fast and slow K^+ channels in the mammal exhibit a complementary distribution. The fast channels are present at the juxtaparanodal regions under the myelin (Ritchie and Chiu, 1981; Röper and Schwarz, 1989; Rasband and Shrager, 2000), whereas the slow K^+ channels contribute to nodal conductance (Baker et al., 1987; Röper and Schwarz, 1989) activating during a train of action potentials, and providing a major component of axonal accommodation. In normal adult mammalian axons, the contribution of fast K^+ channels to nodal repolarization after an action potential is minimal (Chiu et al., 1979). Repolarization after an action potential takes place by way of a circuit incorporating the relatively vast internodal capacity (Barrett and Barrett, 1982, and Baker et al., 1987; reviewed by Baker, 2000a). Any loosening or retraction of myelin thus exposes kinetically fast K^+ channels, which will stabilize the nodal membrane potential, potentially compromising conduction. The normal distribution of conductances with Na^+ channels at the nodes and fast K^+ channels under the myelin is summarized in Fig. 1.

During the few days after diphtheritic demyelination (e.g., 5 to 7 days), the electrophysiological properties of

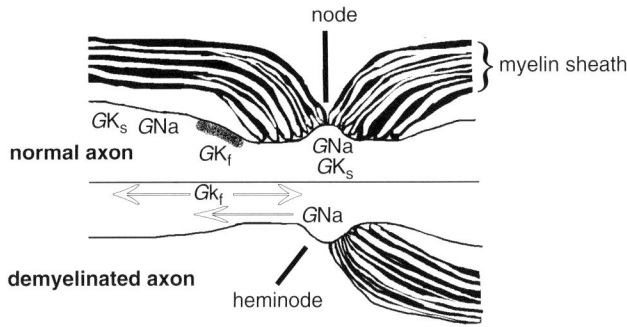

Figure 1 Simplified distribution of Na⁺ and K⁺ conductances in a myelinated axon. In the normal axon (*upper distribution*), the node possesses a Na⁺ conductance (GNa) and kinetically slow K⁺ channels (GK_s). The highest density of both these channel types is found at the node of Ranvier. Kinetically fast K⁺ channels (GK_f) have their highest density under the myelin in a band at the juxtaparanodal region (*shading*). There is a much lower density of Na⁺ channels and slow K⁺ channels in the internodal membrane (GNa, GK_s). After segmental demyelination, the original node becomes a heminode and a Na⁺ channel distribution is established with a higher than normal density of channels in the exposed internodal membrane. This is indicated by a movement of Na⁺ channels away from the node. In addition, the punctate distribution of fast K⁺ channels breaks down, and they are distributed away from the juxtaparanode, indicated by a movement into the node and internode.

axons can be substantially altered by a redistribution of Na⁺ and K⁺ channels. Impulse conduction can be restored by an increase in the number of Na⁺ channels expressed in the normally electrically unexcitable internode (Bostock and Sears, 1978), allowing continuous conduction and thus the restoration of function (Fig. 1), albeit with prolonged conduction times. The same authors (Sherratt et al., 1980; Bostock et al., 1981) also showed that blockade of axonal fast K⁺ channels exposed by myelin withdrawal, using the channel blocker 4-aminopyridine, could help overcome conduction failure after demyelination. This provided a clinical strategy for the symptomatic treatment of MS that has met with some success (e.g., Schwid et al., 1997, and Sheean et al., 1998), although it is limited by the nonspecific effects of K⁺ channel blockers on nervous system function. Craner et al. (2003) reported that in allergic encephalomyelitis, apparently demyelinated optic nerve axons express $Na_V1.6$ and $Na_V1.2$, the channels being present diffusely and continuously over many tens of microns. These Na⁺ channel subtypes are therefore likely to contribute to the conferment of excitability on internodal membrane. In demyelinated lesions of rat sciatic nerve, Rasband et al. (1998) described a redistribution of kinetically fast K⁺ channels ($K_V1.1$ and $K_V1.2$) away from the normal juxtaparanodal sites to a more diffuse distribution, including nodes. Moreover, some damaged axons were devoid of immunostaining for fast K⁺ channels, a situation that could potentially encourage ectopic activity. These authors also reported that with remyelination, the K⁺ channel distribution was only partially restored. After

spinal cord injury that included demyelination, the punctuate distribution of $K_V1.1$ in central axons was lost, and a more diffuse distribution of channels became evident (Nashmi et al., 2000). Thus, although conduction may be restored by the remodeling of axonal membrane properties after demyelination, axons can become ectopic impulse generators, and the clinical use of K⁺ channel blocking agents would be expected to make this more likely.

III. What Forms of Activity Arise in Axons?

When mammalian axons are injured, they can generate spontaneous activity. The characteristics of such ectopic activity in isolated nerve were studied by Adrian (1930). He described both high frequency (>150 Hz) regular and low frequency irregular activity, and a third type consisting of bursts of impulses repeating at a lower frequency (<10 Hz). However, these forms of injury-induced discharge differ from the low frequency, regular discharge seen in experimental demyelination.

Adrian's third type of activity is similar to that known to arise in human nerve fibers *in situ* after a period of ischemia (Culp et al., 1983). Kapoor et al. (1993) reported very similar burst discharges induced by loading myelin with a solution containing a high concentration of K⁺ ions., This finding provides a clue as to how postischemic activity is generated. It seems that to generate these burst discharges, the axonal membrane potential must be able to acquire two stable values (i.e.. it must become *bistable*) and an internode loaded with K⁺ is necessary to allow a bistable membrane potential to exist. David et al. (1992) recorded membrane bistability in lizard axons with K⁺-loaded internodes and demonstrated that regenerative K⁺ currents were responsible for producing long-lasting depolarizing events. Before these findings were published, Bostock deduced that the explanation for muscle fasciculation after peripheral nerve ischemia depends on the membrane potential of myelinated motor axons becoming bistable in the postischemic state. A depolarized value of membrane potential is associated with raised external K⁺ (expected to result from ischemia) and a hyperpolarized value independent of the K⁺ equilibrium potential (E_K) where the K⁺ channels are closed and a high Na⁺/K⁺ ATPase current operates (Bostock et al., 1991). Any movement between the two values from the hyperpolarized to depolarized state would be relatively rapid (i.e., a *flip*) and associated with ectopic impulse generation. Such a *flip* could be triggered by changes in Na⁺/K⁺ ATPase current, or by the arrival of an independently generated propagated action potential. Journeying back to the hyperpolarized state (i.e., a *flop*) silences activity and potentially reprimes the axon to generate more impulses.

With transection of peripheral nerve, regenerative sprouting occurs that fails to achieve reconnection with the peripheral target and may result in neuroma formation. The afferent endings trapped within the nerve end are a source of spontaneous activity (e.g., Lisney and Devor, 1987) and are pathologically mechanosensitive (e.g., Welk et al., 1990). The latter is also a characteristic of demyelinating lesions (Smith and McDonald, 1980; Calvin et al., 1982). Neuromas in humans can be a source of chronic pain, and surgical excision runs the risk of further neuroma formation. The hyperexcitability and ectopic impulse generation at diseased terminals are plausibly related to the accumulation of Na$^+$ channels, which has been demonstrated by using specific Na$^+$ channel antibodies in peripheral nerve of fish, *Apteronotus* (Devor et al., 1989) and in rat (Devor et al., 1993). Consistent with Na$^+$-channel involvement, ectopic activity can be attenuated and inhibited by agents that block Na$^+$ channels, such as the marine toxin tetrodotoxin (TTX) (Matzner and Devor, 1994). It is also silenced by low concentrations of local anesthetic (Devor et al., 1992), insufficient to prevent normal impulse transmission but consistent with the block of low-threshold Na$^+$ channels that do not undergo fast inactivation (Baker, 2000b). (Low concentrations of local anesthetic also increase the fraction of inactivated transient Na$^+$ channels at the resting potential [for example, Hille, 1977], and will tend to quench high frequency burst discharges, by promoting transient channel inactivation.) The underlying mechanisms of such spontaneous activity in neuromas may be related to those involved in promoting ectopic activity in demyelinated or partially demyelinated axons, because abnormal Na$^+$ currents are probably responsible for initiating and maintaining the activity in both cases.

IV. The Importance of Persistent Na$^+$ Current

Although ectopic discharges after experimental demyelination had been recorded previously (Smith and McDonald, 1980; Burchiel, 1980, 1981; Calvin et al., 1982), I assisted Hugh Bostock to make the first and only membrane potential and membrane current recordings from the site of impulse initiation in ectopically active demyelinated axons (Baker and Bostock, 1992). The active fibers were spinal root axons that had undergone diphtheritic demyelination. The importance of these recordings were twofold. First, they showed that ectopic impulses were generated at heminodes, where the myelin was missing or loosened on one side of a node of Ranvier (Fig. 2), although the node maintained a more focused population of Na$^+$ channels and was the site at which regenerative inward current was initiated. Second, our records clearly indicated that a pacemaker potential was responsible for initiating and maintaining highly rhythmic discharge, where the pacemaker was generated by a sustained inward current operating within the subthreshold potential range. At the time, we did not know what channel

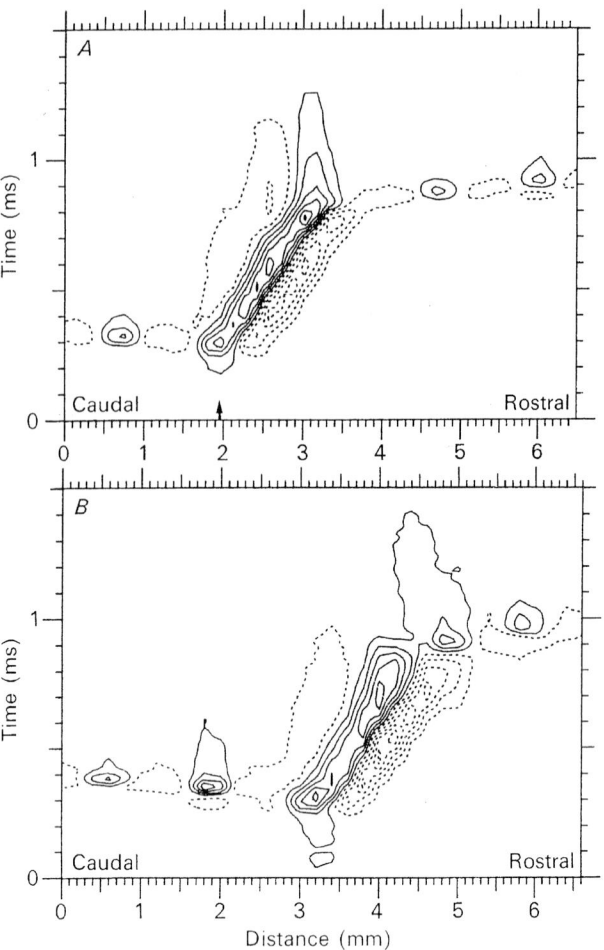

Figure 2 Membrane current contour maps recorded for two spontaneously active rat spinal root axons, previously demyelinated after exposure to diphtheria toxin. Regular discharges were induced by 4-aminopyridine (1 mM). Continuous lines represent inward current, and broken lines outward current. The outward currents are largely capacitive, the magnitude of late active outward current in the demyelinated internode reduced by the presence of the K$^+$ channel blocker. (**A**) Sensory fiber 6 days after exposure to the toxin. (**B**) Motor fiber 7 days after exposure. Arrow in (**A**) indicates the point along the axon at which inward current is first recorded, and represents the ectopic site. Inward current in (**B**) can be seen to precede the initiation of the action potential. In both recordings, action potentials propagate away from the ectopic site, in a saltatory fashion caudally, but much more slowly and continuously in the rostral direction over a whole demyelinated internode. The ectopic sites are heminodes, where the myelin is functional on only one side. (Figure reproduced, with permission, from Baker and Bostock, 1992.)

type provided the sustained inward current, although more recent experiments are consistent with a persistent Na$^+$ current (Baker and Bostock, 1997, 1998; Bostock and Rothwell, 1997). Action-potential firing frequency was low, on the order of 10 to 20 Hz, and the firing frequency was increased by exposure to tetraethyl-ammonium ions, indicating that axonal slow K$^+$ channels control the discharge frequency (Baker and Bostock, 1992) by modifying the slope of the pacemaker potential. Subsequently, subthreshold and barely suprathreshold membrane potential oscillations at a similar frequency were recorded by Kapoor et al. (1997), using intra-axonal electrodes in dorsal column axons, focally demyelinated by exposure to ethidium bromide. These oscillations could occur without action potential generation and could thus be studied alone. The oscillations were eliminated by exposure to TTX, providing strong evidence that a TTX-sensitive (TTX-s) form of persistent Na^+ current was responsible for the depolarizing phase of the cycle, and that, in at least some diseased axons, the current is large enough to drive a membrane potential oscillation (reviewed by Baker, 2000a).

Usually, when activated by a suprathreshold depolarization, Na^+ channels generate a brief inward current that underlies the upswing of an action potential. The channels that contribute to membrane excitability in this way are referred to as *transient* Na^+ channels. Eight of the nine functionally described mammalian Na^+ channel subtypes generate a transient current, although the current kinetics are variable. Of these, the TTX-resistant (TTX-r) sensory neuron-specific channel ($Na_V1.8$) has activation and inactivation kinetics four to five times slower than those of TTX-s channels, and this may be related to its function in small diameter and unmyelinated afferents. The transient nature of a Na^+ current is brought about by an inactivation mechanism that plugs the channel and prevents persistent opening (reviewed by Catterall, 2000). The inactivation mechanism appears voltage-dependent and becomes more complete with increasing depolarization. A highly conserved motif of three amino acids (IFM; isoleucine-phenylalanine-methionine), located on the intracellular loop between the third and fourth membrane-spanning domains of the protein, is associated with the inactivation gate; these residues are known to be involved in blocking the channel pore from the inside.

We now know, however, that Na^+ channel gating is more complicated than this, and that individual Na^+ channels can exhibit a range of gating behaviors. Thus Na^+ channel gating, even of a supposedly uniform population of channels, can be nonhomogeneous. Unitary-current studies of muscle Na^+ channels by Patlak and Ortiz (1985, 1986) indicated that apparently normal cardiac and frog skeletal muscle Na^+ channels could sporadically lose their ability to inactivate and thus produce sustained Na^+ currents. Some of the most convincing recordings of apparently normal cardiac Na^+ channels undergoing a series of sporadic behavioral changes or "modal-gating switches" were provided by the studies of Böhle and Bendorff (1995). A range of Na^+ channel behaviors were recorded by Baker and Bostock (1998) in primary sensory neurons, including brief, sporadic, openings that were increased in number (but unaffected in duration) by depolarization (Fig. 3). (One possibility is that these openings correspond with a

second Na^+ channel open-state; see for example, Keynes and Elinder, 1998.) Such openings (present even at −80 mV) and other types of openings appearing throughout long duration voltage-clamp protocols might be expected to contribute to persistent Na^+ current in sensory neurons over a wide range of membrane potentials.

Nonhomogeneous Na^+ channel gating behavior in squid axons was reported by Chandler and Meves (1970), who observed persistent Na^+ currents when F^- ions were introduced to the inside of the axon. The persistent Na^+ current activated with a more negative voltage-dependence than the transient current and had the same voltage dependence as steady-state inactivation, leading the authors to suggest that a second open state could be reached once the channel had undergone fast inactivation. The channel openings attained either with loss of fast inactivation or the attainment of a second open channel state are limited in duration by other, slower inactivation processes (Patlak and Ortiz, 1986). The second open state is incorporated in the model of the squid axon Na^+ channel subsequently developed by Keynes and Elinder (1998). One important characteristic predicted by a second open state exhibiting the same voltage dependence as fast inactivation is that persistent openings will occur at more negative membrane potentials than transient openings, and this is the case for persistent Na^+ currents in large-diameter dorsal root ganglion (DRG) neurons, recorded without F^- (Baker and Bostock, 1997, 1998). This is also a necessary characteristic of the currents driving spontaneous activity in demyelinated nerve. Thus, the ability of a single subtype of Na^+ channel to generate a variety of Na^+ currents has been considered to be caused by the loss of fast inactivation or the attainment of a second open state, through the fast-inactivated state. While the molecular mechanisms underlying these behaviors or gating modes are not fully understood, the reduction/oxidation state of axonal Na^+ channels (Mitrović et al., 1993) modifiable by glutathione, and whether or not neuronal Na^+ channels are co-associated with βγ G-protein subunits (for $Na_V1.2$, Ma et al., 1997) are two possible contributing factors. Normally, Na^+ channel α-subunits are complexed with accessory β-subunits and heterologous expression studies have shown that the co-expression of β-subunits can substantially speed inactivation (i.e., reduce channel open-times) (for example, for $Na_V1.6$ [Smith et al., 1998]). Channel gating behavior may thus also be affected by the gain (and perhaps loss) of β-subunits.

Persistent Na^+ current almost certainly operates in normal human peripheral nerves. Data obtained on sensory nerves in normal subjects using the technique of threshold-tracking have shown that current threshold responds to the application of a brief hyperpolarizing current as though a persistent inward membrane current is switched off by the resulting change in membrane potential (Bostock and

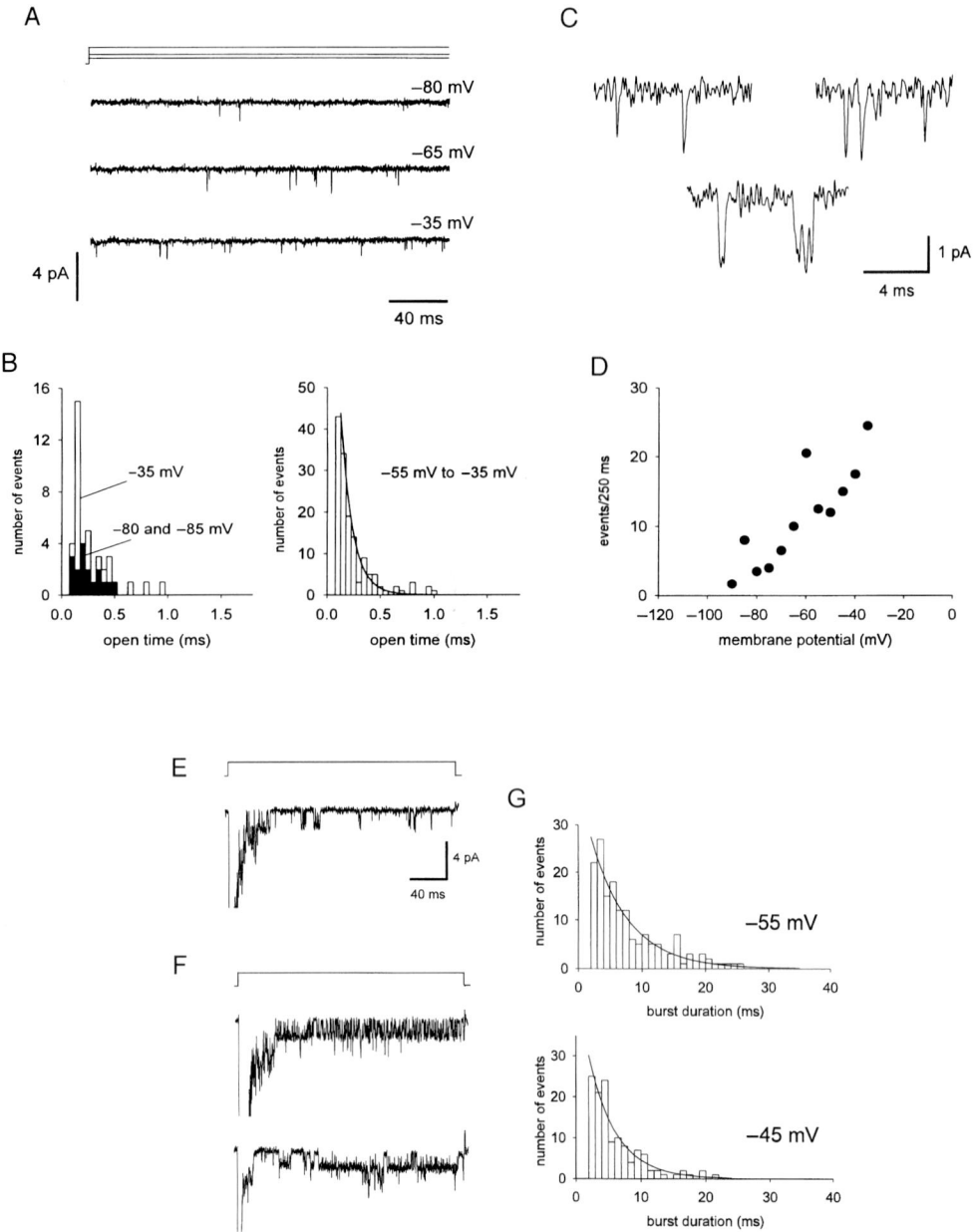

Figure 3 **TTX-s Na⁺ channels in primary sensory neurons exhibit a variety of gating behaviors.** (**A**) Brief sporadic channel openings recorded from an outside-out patch, pulled from a large diameter DRG neuron. (**B**) In this patch, channel open-time does not depend on membrane potential (open-time distribution at −80 and −85 mV shown as solid bars, distribution at −35 mV shown as open bars). Right hand panel, frequency histogram of pooled measurements made between −55 and −35 mV is well described by a single exponential, indicating a mean open-time of 100 μs. (**C**) Example openings recorded at −60 mV. (**D**) The number of channel openings increases with depolarization, revealing that channel activation is voltage-dependent. (**E**) Recordings from outside-out patches also exhibit burst-opening Na⁺ channels. Example bursts lasting up to a few 10s of milliseconds. (**F**) In the same patch as shown in (**E**), much longer burst openings were recorded, at −55 (*upper trace*) and −35 mV (*lower trace*). At −35 mV, the intraburst flicker is less apparent. (**G**) Estimates of burst duration from single best-fit exponentials to burst duration histograms are 5.8 ms at −55 mV and 4.2 ms at −45 mV. None of these behaviors can be explained by transient channel activation-inactivation gating overlap. (Figure reproduced, with permission, from Baker and Bostock, 1998.)

Rothwell, 1997). Consistent with this interpretation, Tokuno et al. (2003) have presented direct evidence for a steady-state depolarization of rat axons *in vitro* in both sensory and motor nerve, near rest, by a TTX-s Na⁺ current. In addition, optic nerve axons are known to have a steady-state TTX-s Na⁺ conductance that must contribute to the pathological influx of Na⁺ that precipitates white matter damage during ischemia (Stys et al., 1993).

V. Na⁺ Channel Subtypes Involved in Generating Persistent Na⁺ Current in Myelinated Nerve

Which Na^+ channel subtypes generating persistent Na^+ current are present in myelinated axons? The evidence already discussed suggests that TTX-s currents play a leading role. The explanation as to how TTX-s persistent currents are generated is probably that at least some Na^+ channels can lose their ability to undergo fast inactivation and/or exhibit a second open state.

While all transient Na^+ channels are expected to generate a small, steady-state activation-inactivation gating (*mh*) overlap current, some subtypes seem particularly adept at generating a persistent current at negative membrane potentials. The persistent currents found in primary afferents have been attributed to $Na_V1.9$ (NaN) (Cummins et al., 1999; Dib-Hajj et al., 2002) and surmised to be generated by $Na_V1.6$ (Baker and Bostock, 1998). Whereas $Na_V1.9$ is a Na^+ channel found in small diameter axons, $Na_V1.6$ is probably the major Na^+ channel isoform in both normal peripheral and central myelinated axons (Caldwell et al., 2000). $Na_V1.6$ is a TTX-s channel, known to generate persistent and "resurgent" currents in central neurons during relatively brief voltage-clamp protocols (Raman et al., 1997). Resurgence is a kinetic property seen in voltage-clamp, characteristic of $Na_V1.6$, in which channels apparently open from the inactivated state (into which they have previously entered during a positive prepulse) within a narrow range of membrane potentials close to the activation threshold for the current, rather than remaining nonconducting.

These properties of $Na_V1.6$ contribute to the spontaneous and burst-firing of cerebellar Purkinje neurons (Kahliq et al., 2003). $Na_V1.6$, when transfected and expressed in $Na_V1.8$ null neurons, may well generate a persistent current over a wider potential range than $Na_V1.7$ (data presented by Herzog et al. 2003a). Baker and Bostock (1997, 1998) found a low-threshold, persistent TTX-s Na^+ current in large diameter DRG neurons in the rat, and Kiernan et al. (2003) found a similar current in about one third of small (<25 μm, apparent diameter) neurons. This current also exhibited "resurgence" in large neurons (unpublished observation). $Na_V1.6$ appears to be the predominant Na^+ channel at peripheral nodes of Ranvier and in optic nerve (Caldwell et al., 2000). It is also found in unmyelinated axons in the retina and the parallel fibers of the cerebellum (Caldwell et al., 2000; Schaller and Caldwell, 2003). Black et al. (2002) have provided evidence that $Na_V1.6$ is present in unmyelinated corneal afferents and probably contributes to conduction in unmyelinated sciatic nerve axons. The distribution of $Na_V1.6$ mRNA expression in primary sensory neurons indicates that it is widely expressed in both myelinated and unmyelinated axon cell bodies (Black et al., 1996). The channel gene includes the *med* locus, where *med*

(motor end-plate disease) is associated with loss of action potential invasion of the mouse motor nerve terminal (Duchen and Stefani, 1971). In *med* mutants, immunostaining for $Na_V1.6$ is lost at nodes of Ranvier (Caldwell et al., 2000). The failure of action potential propagation into motor nerve terminals may simply reflect a reduced safety factor for action potential invasion after a general fall in Na^+ channel density. Alternatively, where there is compensation for the functional loss of $Na_V1.6$ in axons, allowing axonal conduction to continue, it is conceivable that a low-threshold, persistent current may be important in initiating an action potential within this unmyelinated, high-capacitance structure at the end of a motor nerve, and that such a current is lost in the mutant. Herzog et al. (2003b) reported that the expression of mutant $Na_V1.6$ in peripheral neurons (from an $Na_V1.8$ null) is dependent on calmodulin binding to the channel C-terminus, and that raised internal $[Ca^{2+}]$ can slow the macroscopic inactivation kinetics, indicating that channel open-time is probably increased by Ca^{2+} binding with the channel-calmodlin complex. Thus Ca^{2+} influx might increase the amount of persistent current by modifying channel gating.

Recently, Craner et al. (2003) have reported that in allergic encephalomyelitis, optic nerve axons not only express $Na_V1.6$, but also $Na_V1.2$ along apparently demeylinated internodes. These findings suggest that in central axons, $Na_V1.6$ and $Na_V1.2$ could contribute to the conferment of excitability in denuded internodes, although the authors believe that $Na_V1.2$ becomes the most commonly expressed channel in demyelinated axons.

VI. Selective Blockers of Persistent Na⁺ Current

Low concentrations of local anesthetics block persistent current selectively and thus are far more effective against ectopic activity than in blocking normal action potential transmission (e.g., Devor et al., 1992). This selectivity arises because of channel-state-dependent drug binding. Block by charged local anesthetics and other anticonvulsants, such as carbamazepine, have an open-channel requirement, and hence show "use-dependence." Individual channels that are predisposed to open, and subsequently reopen, near the resting potential are affected by local anesthetic at concentrations an order of magnitude less than that effective against the much larger transient current present in the same neuron (Baker, 2000b). The uncharged local anesthetic, benzocaine, appeared to be able to block closed persistent channels in large diameter DRG neurons, whereas the transient channels, even in the continuous presence of drug, had to be activated before block became evident (Baker, 2000b). Block of persistent Na^+ current, as predicted from its negative voltage dependence, has a major effect on neuronal excitability (Fig. 4).

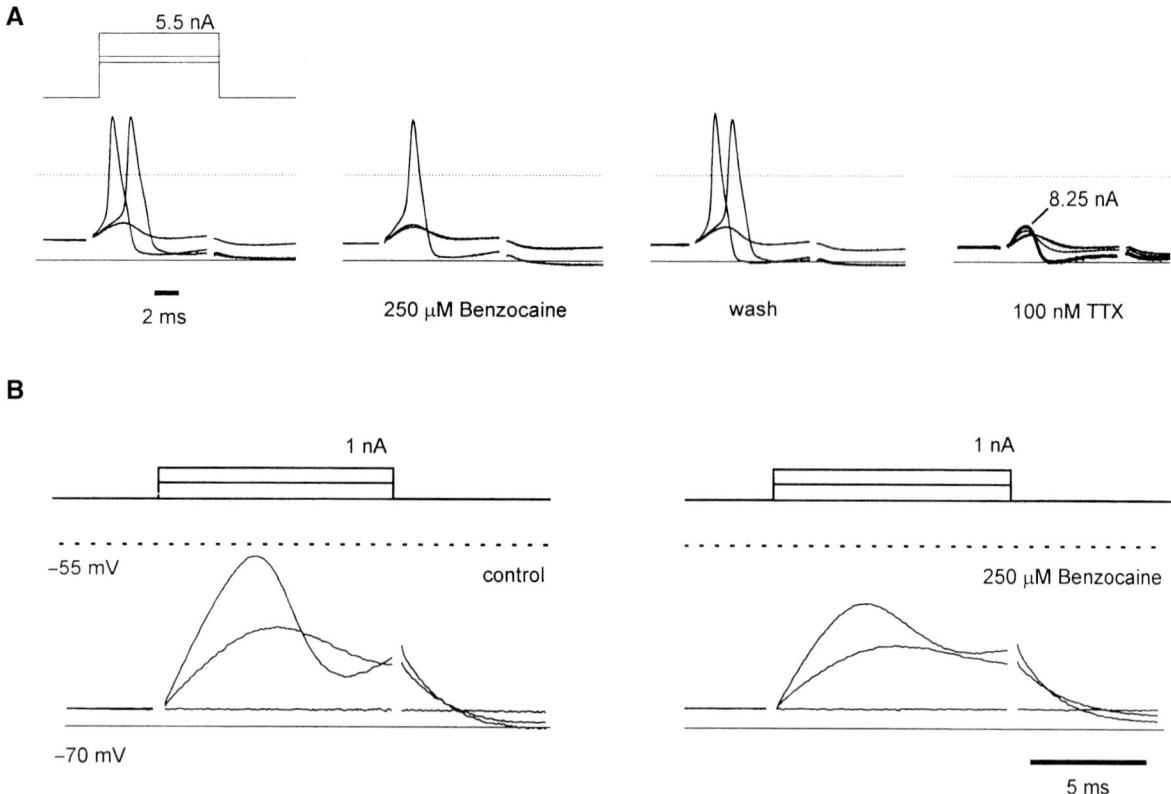

Figure 4 Low-threshold persistent Na+ current in a large DRG neuron contributes to excitability and is selectively blocked by the local anesthetic benzocaine. (**A**) large diameter neuron exhibits subthreshold and suprathreshold responses to incrementing applied currents (*left hand panel*). Superfusion of 250 µM benzocaine (that blocks persistent Na+ current by more than 90%) reversibly increases the current threshold, but fails to prevent action potential generation (*center two panels*). A matched concentration of TTX, expected to block persistent Na+ current to a closely similar degree, does not select between transient and persistent Na+ current and anesthetizes the neuron (*right hand panel*). The neuron is inexcitable even when the stimulus current is increased to 8.25 nA. (**B**) In another large-diameter neuron 250 µM benzocaine eliminates the contribution of persistent Na+ current to the subthreshold electrotonic responses to applied currents, thus reducing them in amplitude. Left hand panel control recordings, right hand panel in the presence of benzocaine. (Reproduced, with permission, from Baker, 2000b.)

In small-diameter DRG neurons, µ-conotoxin PIIIA selectively blocks TTX-s currents and can be used to discriminate different subtypes of Na+ channel (Safo et al., 2000). The toxin also blocks transient Na+ current in isolated hippocampal neurons (Nielsen et al., 2002). In experiments in which hippocampal neurons were exposed to a truncated analog of PIIA (PIIIA-(2-22)), the persistent Na+ current found in these neurons was preferentially blocked by modified toxin (by 70 % with 1 µM), implying a submicromolar IC50 for the persistent current (Nielsen et al., 2002). When activated from a negative holding potential of −80 mV, the transient current amplitude in the same neurons was unaffected at 1 µM, but reduced close to 80% by 10 µM. This selectivity for persistent current is intriguing because it shows that the truncated toxin is able to discriminate between persistent and transient Na+ channels. For this reason conotoxins or their derivatives may represent a novel pharmacological approach to the control of ectopic activity that is dependent on TTX-s persistent Na+ current.

VII. Modifiers of Persistent Na+ Current in Neurons in Primary Culture

A. Extracellular pH

The persistent Na+ current found in large DRG neurons has an apparent pKa close to 7. Extracellular alkalinization increases the current, acidification reduces it (Baker and Bostock, 1999). This effect was found to be caused by a combination of the pH dependence of single-channel conductance and channel gating. The pH-dependent activity in single A-fibers on shifting external pH from 7.2 to 7.3 to 7.9 to 8.0 is slow (6.5 to 7 Hz) and highly rhythmic, consistent with an underlying just suprathreshold membrane potential oscillation (Baker, 2002) of a type similar to that found for ectopically active demyelinated units. Thus, ectopic activity in demyelinated axons that is driven by persistent Na+ current would be expected to be sensitive to plasma pH over the physiological range. The obvious prediction is that lowering extracellular pH should reduce ectopic activity. Rebreathing expired air might therefore be expected to suppress ectopic activity by raising end-tidal CO_2 and lowering plasma pH, but this technique is not generally used for the control of organic disease.

B. Hypoxia

Conditions within MS plaques could actually promote ectopic activity. In some lesions, a dying-back oligodendropathy has been described that is consistent with ischemic injury and similar to white matter damage in stroke (reviewed by Lassmann, 2003). In active plaques, inducible nitric oxide synthase is found in macrophages and microglia (DeGroot et al., 1997; Liu et al 2001), along with reactive oxygen species (likely to cause mitochondrial damage) and nitric oxide intermediates. In hippocampal neurons, hypoxia or exposure to metabolic inhibitors or to nitric oxide (NO) donors increase persistent Na^+ current, whereas the reducing agent dithiothreitol has the opposite effect (Hammarström and Gage, 1998, 1999). Conversely, exposure of small dorsal root ganglion neurons to NO donors has been reported to reversibly inhibit all forms of Na^+ current, including persistent current (Renganathan et al., 2002), and this is hypothesized to be due to S-nitrosylation of the channel resulting in block. However, in peripheral nerve, unitary Na^+ channel openings in patch-clamp recordings from axonal patches are sensitive to changes in their reduction-oxidation state by glutathione. Reduced channels (i.e., where cystine-cystine disulphide bridges are broken) give rise to shorter openings that contribute less to persistent current than do oxidized channels (Mitrović et al., 1993), and this is similar to the findings in the hippocampus. Compromised metabolism and anoxia might upregulate persistent Na^+ current, and thus could potentially encourage the generation of ectopic activity. Hammarström and Gage (2002) have concluded that anoxia acts on persistent Na^+ current in a way similar to oxidizing agents. Provided that the hypoxia within a lesion was not severe enough to produce a depolarizing block, axonal excitability might be increased by a lowered membrane potential and a predisposition of Na^+ channels to gate in a persistent manner, both of which might contribute to ectopic discharge.

VIII. Numerical Model of Ectopically Active Axon

Although it seems almost intuitive that a rapidly activating, persistent Na^+ current and kinetically slow K^+ channels may conspire together to generate a slow rhythmic discharge, a numerical simulation can help to more objectively rule-in persistent Na^+ current as a candidate for the bio-

physical basis of ectopic activity. A numerical model of a space-clamped, lumped node and demyelinated internode from a large axon, was written in Visual Basic (Microsoft). The simulations contained the same channel types as those included in the axon model of Bostock et al. (1991), with voltage-dependent gating parameters taken from Schwarz et al. (1995), but omitted inward rectification. They also included a persistent Na^+ current that activated 20 mV more negative than transient Na^+ current (c.f., Bostock and Rothwell, 1997), where the value of persistent Na^+ conductance was 1.5% that of the transient Na^+ conductance. The model output could be made to mimic the low-frequency, regular discharge recorded in demyelinated axons (although the balance of Na^+ and slow K^+ channels was critical).

Although real discharge cannot be generated by a depolarization elicited by raised external K^+ alone, the discharge frequency in the model was increased by raising external K^+, because GK_s becomes a less efficient check on the excitatory influence of persistent Na^+ current. This effect is similar to the effect of blocking GK_s (Baker and Bostock, 1992). Using the kinetic gating parameters published by Schwarz et al. (1995) for 20°C and running the model at a higher temperature, it did not seem possible to get 10 Hz activity at 37°C, whereas at 20 or 30°C, it was possible (at the higher temperature, a higher frequency discharge occurred with sufficient Na^+ current). Increasing the temperature tends to stabilize the membrane potential, preventing the lowest frequency ectopic activity through an action on the kinetics of GK_s. Thus, while this model clearly demonstrates the probable role of persistent Na^+ current in generating ectopic activity, it is too simple. Two shortcomings were a poor reproduction of ectopic activity at 37°C (probably related to the kinetics of GK_s), and the lack of a Na^+/K^+ ATPase, that would normally tend to reduce the frequency of discharge and contribute to burst discharges interspersed with quiet periods.

Typical output of the model can be seen in Fig. 5A and B, along with the effects of very slightly raising external $[K^+]$. Action potentials were generated at 10.5 Hz, a slow and similar frequency to that of real ectopic activity. As in real activity, this was close to the lowest frequency attainable. The pacemaker potential was caused by the low-threshold persistent Na^+ current, whose presence meant that the membrane current was inward (and never zero) after the repolarization phase of an action potential (Fig. 5D).

A. Parameters of the Model

Capacity = 350 pF (Bostock et al., 1991)
Input resistance = 450 MΩ
GNa (transient) = 10.4 μS (a node of 30 μm², with 2,000 Na channels per μm² would be expected to have a conductance around 0.9 μS [c.f., McIntyre et al., 2002])
GN$_a$ (persistent) = 0.15 μS

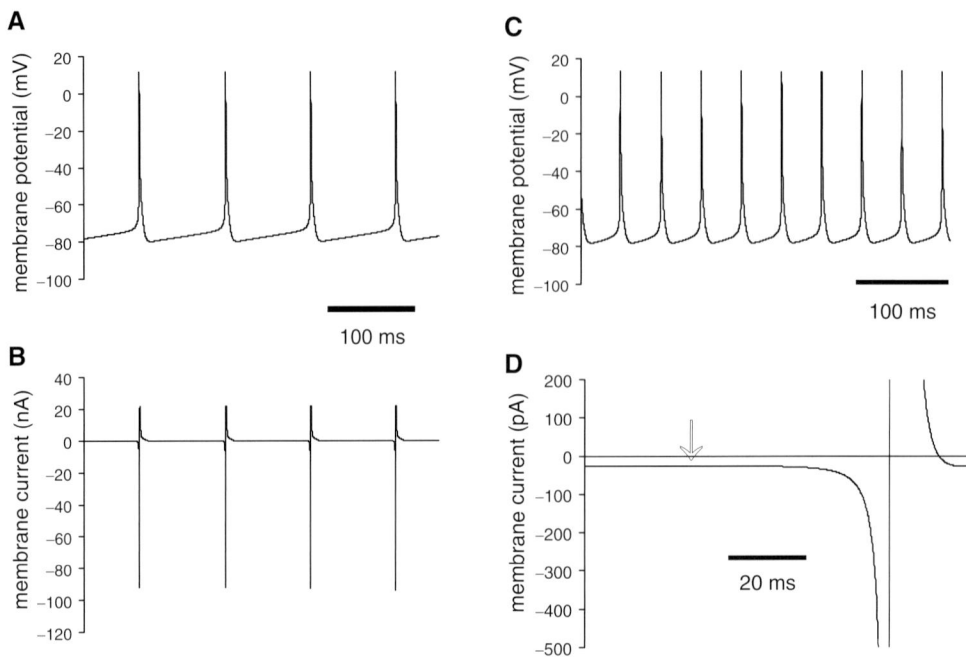

Figure 5 **Numerical simulation of an ectopically active site.** (**A**) Membrane potential and (**B**) simultaneous membrane current records from a space-clamped heminode/internode. A dynamic equilibrium was reached with ectopic action potentials generated at a steady 10.5 Hz. The simulation was sufficiently long to be independent of initial conditions. (**A**) A pacemaker potential can be clearly seen preceding each action potential. Time calibration same in (**A**) and (**B**). (**C**) Changing the value of E_K from −83 to −82 mV (e.g., equivalent to an increase in external [K⁺] by 0.2 mM if internal [K⁺] is taken as 120 mM) causes an increase in the discharge frequency to 22.5 Hz. (**D**) A more detailed plot of the pacemaker current (*arrow*) that precedes the large regenerative inward current seen in (**B**) (that is truncated in the panel). The pacemaker current is small (upwards of a few 10s of pA) and provided by a low-threshold, persistent Na⁺ current.

$GK_f = 0.4\ \mu S$
$GK_s = 0.9\ \mu S$
$ENa = +69\ \text{mV}$
$EK = -83\ \text{mV}$
$E\text{leak} = 0\ \text{mV}$

Integration was by the Euler method, and the integration time step was 1 µs. Calculation of rate constants at 30°C assumed a Q_{10} of 2 for α_m and β_m (for both transient and persistent Na⁺ current), α_h and β_h, α_n and β_n, and a Q_{10} of 1.5 for α_s and β_s. Voltage-dependent rate constants were the same as those published in Schwarz et al. (1995), except that the persistent Na⁺ current activation parameters α_m and β_m were half the value of the same parameters for the transient current (Bostock and Rothwell, 1997), and they incorporated a 20 mV voltage offset. Persistent Na⁺ current also did not inactivate (c.f., Bostock and Rothwell, 1997), whereas real persistent Na⁺ currents are subject to voltage-dependent slow inactivation (e.g., Patlak and Oritiz, 1986; Baker and Bostock, 1998).

IX. Summary

MS is characterized by negative symptoms, including loss of sensation and muscular weakness, caused by loss of central axons and loss of axonal function through demyelination. Positive symptoms are also generated, almost certainly related to the adaptive changes that follow demyelination, and are probably caused by the generation of ectopic activity in demyelinated axons. The remarkable adaptive changes involving the production of new ion channel distributions along axons and the conferment of excitability on the normally inexcitable internodal membrane are thought to be involved in functional recovery from demyelination, but unfortunately must also be involved in the generation of positive symptoms.

This chapter has presented the argument that persistent Na⁺ current is a good candidate for the biophysical cause of membrane potential oscillations and ectopic activity in diseased axons. Na⁺ channel subtypes that normally gate in a transient fashion can apparently enter gating modes in which fast inactivation is lost, and thus generate a persistent current, most crucially at potentials more negative than the threshold for transient Na⁺ current activation. Na$_V$1.6 is the Na⁺ channel subtype believed to be most important for conduction in peripheral and central myelinated fibers, and it is likely to play a role in generating persistent Na⁺ current in axons. The characteristics of Na⁺ channel gating that give rise to persistent Na⁺ current, namely reopening, may offer at least a part of the explanation as to why activation (or use)-

dependent Na$^+$ channel blockers are useful in treating positive symptoms. Persistent Na$^+$ current can be targeted pharmacologically in both PNS and CNS *in vitro* systems, and these studies may provide a rationale for the development of selective blockers or modulators of such currents, which could potentially be useful in treating both the symptoms of demyelinating disease and neuropathic pain.

Acknowledgments

Matthew Kiernan, Hugh Bostock, and Liam Drew have contributed valuable comments in the preparation of this manuscript.
Supported by the Medical Research Council U.K.

References

Adrian, E. D. (1930). The effects of injury on mammalian nerve fibres. *Proc. Roy. Soc.* **B, 106,** 596–618.

Baker, M. D. (2000a). Axonal flip-flops and oscillators. *Trends. Neurosci.* **23,** 514–519.

Baker, M. D. (2000b). Selective block of late Na$^+$ current by local anaesthetics in rat large sensory neurones. *Br. J. Pharmacol.* **129,** 1617–1626.

Baker, M. D. (2002). Function and local anaesthetic block of late Na$^+$ current in sensory neurones. *In* "Molecular and Basic Mechanisms of Anesthesia" (B. W. Urban and M. Barann, eds.), pp. 214–218. Pabst Science Publishers: Lengerich.

Baker, M., and Bostock, H. (1992). Ectopic activity in demyelinated spinal root axons of the rat. *J. Physiol.* **451,** 539–552.

Baker, M. D., and Bostock, H. (1997). Low-threshold, persistent sodium current in rat large dorsal root ganglion neurons in culture. *J. Neurophysiol.* **77,** 1503–1513.

Baker, M. D., and Bostock, H. (1998). Inactivation of macroscopic late Na$^+$ current and characteristics of unitary late Na$^+$ currents in sensory neurons. *J. Neurophysiol.* **80,** 2538–2549.

Baker, M. D., and Bostock, H. (1999). The pH dependence of late sodium current in large sensory neurons. *Neuroscience* **92,** 1119–1130.

Baker, M., Bostock, H., Grafe, P., and Martius, P. (1987). Function and distribution of three types of rectifying channel in rat spinal root myelinated axons. *J. Physiol.* **383,** 45–67.

Barrett, E. F., and Barrett, J. N. (1982). Intracellular recording from vertebrate myelinated axons: Mechanism of the depolarizing afterpotential. *J. Physiol.* **323,** 117–144.

Black, J. A., Dib-Hajj, S., McNabola, K., Jeste, S., Rizzo, M. A., Kocsis, J. D., and Waxman, S. G. (1996). Spinal sensory neurons express multiple sodium channel α-subunit mRNAs. *Brain Res. Mol. Brain Res.* **43,** 117–131.

Black, J. A., Renganathan, M., and Waxman, S. G. (2002). Sodium channel Na$_V$1.6 is expressed along nonmyelinated axons and it contributes to conduction. *Brain Res. Mol. Brain Res.* **105,** 19–28.

Böhle, T., and Benndorf, K. (1995). Multimodal action of single Na$^+$ channels in myocardial mouse cells. *Biophys. J.* **68,** 121–130.

Bostock, H., Baker, M. D., and Reid, G. (1991). Changes in excitability of human motor axons underlying post-ischaemic fasciculations. Evidence for two stable states. *J. Physiol.* **441,** 537–557.

Bostock, H., and Grafe, P. (1985). Activity-dependent excitability changes in normal and demyelinated rat spinal root axons. *J. Physiol.* **365,** 239–257.

Bostock, H., and Rothwell, J. C. (1997). Latent addition in motor and sensory fibres of human peripheral nerve. *J. Physiol.* **498,** 277–294.

Bostock, H., and Sears, T. A. (1978). The internodal axon membrane: Electrical excitability and continuous conduction in segmental demyelination. *J. Physiol.* **280,** 273–301.

Bostock, H., Sears, T. A., and Sherratt, R. M. (1981). The effects of 4-aminopyridine and tetraethylammonium ions on normal and demyelinated mammalian nerve fibres. *J. Physiol.* **313,** 301–315.

Boucher, T. J., Okuse, K., Bennett, D. L., Munson, J. B., Wood, J. N., and McMahon, S. B. (2000). Potent analgesic effects of GDNF in neuropathic pain states. *Science* **290,** 124–127.

Burchiel, K. J. (1980). Abnormal impulse generation in focally demyelinated trigeminal roots. *J. Neurosurg.* **53,** 674–683.

Burchiel, K. J. (1981). Ectopic impulse generation in demyelinated axons: Effects of PaCO$_2$, pH, and disodium edetate. *Ann. Neurol.* **9,** 378–383.

Caldwell, J. H., Schaller, K. L., Lasher, R. S., Peles, E., and Levinson, S. R. (2000). Sodium channel Na$_V$1.6 is localized at nodes of Ranvier, dendrites, and synapses. *Proc. Natl. Acad. Sci. U. S. A.* **97,** 5616–5620.

Calvin, W. H., Devor, M., and Howe, J. F. (1982). Can neuralgias arise from minor demyelination? Spontaneous firing, mechanosensitivity, and afterdischarge from conducting axons. *Exp. Neurol.* **75,** 755–763.

Catterall, W. A. (2000). From ionic currents to molecular mechanisms: The structure and function of voltage-gated sodium channels. *Neuron* **26,** 13–25.

Chandler, W. K., and Meves, H. (1970). Evidence for two types of sodium conductance in axons perfused with sodium fluoride solution. *J. Physiol.* **211,** 653–678.

Chiu, S. Y., Ritchie, J. M., Rogart, R. B., and Stagg, D. (1979). A quantitative description of membrane currents in rabbit myelinated nerve. *J. Physiol.* **292,**149–166.

Chiu, S. Y., and Schwarz, W. (1987). Sodium and potassium currents in acutely demyelinated internodes of rabbit sciatic nerves. *J. Physiol.* **391,** 631–649.

Craner, M. J., Lo, A. C., Black, J. A., and Waxman, S. G. (2003). Abnormal sodium channel distribution in optic nerve axons in a model of inflammatory demyelination. *Brain* **126,** 1552–1561.

Culp, W. J., Ochoa, J., and Torebjörk, E. (1983). Ectopic impulse generation in myelinated sensory nerve fibres in man. *In* "Abnormal Nerves and Muscles as Impulse Generators" (W. J. Culp et al., eds.), pp. 490–512, OUP: New York.

Cummins, T. R., Dib-Hajj, S. D., Black, J. A., Akopian, A. N., Wood, J. N., and Waxman, S. G. (1999). A novel persistent tetrodotoxin-resistant sodium current in SNS-null and wild-type small primary sensory neurons. *J. Neurosci.* **19,** RC43.

David, G., Barrett, J. N., and Barrett, E. F. (1992). Evidence that action potentials activate an internodal potassium conductance in lizard myelinated axons. *J. Physiol.* **445,** 277–301.

De Groot, C. J., Ruuls, S. R., Theeuwes, J. W., Dijkstra, C. D., and Van der Valk, P. (1997). Immunocytochemical characterization of the expression of inducible and constitutive isoforms of nitric oxide synthase in demyelinating multiple sclerosis lesions. *J. Neuropathol. Exp. Neurol.* **56,** 10–20.

Devor, M., Keller, C. H., Deerinck, T. J., Levinson, S. R., and Ellisman, M. H. (1989). Na$^+$ channel accumulation on axolemma of afferent endings in nerve end neuromas in Apteronotus. *Neurosci. Lett.* **102,** 149–154.

Devor, M., Wall, P. D., and Catalan, N. (1992). Systemic lidocaine silences ectopic neuroma and DRG discharge without blocking nerve conduction. *Pain* **48,** 261–268.

Devor, M., Govrin-Lippmann, R., and Angelides, K. (1993). Na$^+$ channel immunolocalization in peripheral mammalian axons and changes following nerve injury and neuroma formation. *J. Neurosci.* **13,** 1976–1992.

Dib-Hajj, S., Black, J. A., Cummins, T. R., and Waxman, S. G. (2002). NaN/Na$_V$1.9: A sodium channel with unique properties. *Trends Neurosci.* **25,** 253–259.

Dubois, J. M. (1981). Evidence for the existence of three types of potassium channels in the frog Ranvier node membrane. *J. Physiol.* **318,** 297–316.

Duchen, L. W., and Stefani, E. (1971). Electrophysiological studies of neuromuscular transmission in hereditary "motor end-plate disease" of the mouse. *J. Physiol.* **212,** 535–548.

Hammarström, A. K., and Gage, P. W. (1998). Inhibition of oxidative metabolism increases persistent sodium current in rat CA1 hippocampal neurons. *J. Physiol.* **510,** 735–741.

Hammarström, A. K., and Gage, P. W. (1999). Nitric oxide increases persistent sodium current in rat hippocampal neurons. *J. Physiol.* **520,** 451–461.

Hammarström, A. K., and Gage, P. W. (2002). Hypoxia and persistent sodium current. *Eur. Biophys. J.* **31,** 323–330.

Herzog, R. I., Cummins, T. R., Ghassemi, F., Dib-Hajj, S. D., and Waxman, S. G. (2003a). Distinct repriming and closed-state inactivation kinetics of $Na_V1.6$ and $Na_V1.7$ sodium channels in mouse spinal sensory neurons. *J. Physiol.* **551,** 741–750.

Herzog, R. I., Liu, C., Waxman, S. G., and Cummins, T. R. (2003b). Calmodulin binds to the C terminus of sodium channels $Na_V1.4$ and $Na_V1.6$ and differentially modulates their functional properties. *J. Neurosci.* **23,** 8261–8270.

Hille, B. (1977). Local anesthetics: hydrophilic and hydrophobic pathways for the drug-receptor reaction. *J. Gen. Physiol.* **69,** 497–515.

Huxley, A. F., and Stämpfli, R. (1949). Evidence for saltatory conduction in peripheral myelinated nerve fibres. *J. Physiol.* **108,** 315–339.

Khaliq, Z. M., Gouwens, N. W., and Raman, I. M. (2003). The contribution of resurgent sodium current to high-frequency firing in Purkinje neurons: an experimental and modeling study. *J. Neurosci.* **23,** 4899–4912.

Kapoor, R., Smith, K. J., Felts, P. A., and Davies, M. (1993). Internodal potassium currents can generate ectopic impulses in mammalian myelinated axons. *Brain. Res.* **611,** 165–169.

Kapoor, R, Li, Y. G., and Smith, K. J. (1997). Slow sodium-dependent potential oscillations contribute to ectopic firing in mammalian demyelinated axons. *Brain* **120,** 647–652.

Keynes, R. D., and Elinder, F. (1998). Modelling the activation, opening, inactivation and reopening of the voltage-gated sodium channel. *Proc. R. Soc. Lond. B Biol. Sci.* **265,** 263–270.

Kiernan, M. C., Baker, M. D., and Bostock, H. (2003). Characteristics of late Na^+ current in adult rat small sensory neurons. *Neuroscience* **119,** 653–660.

Lassmann, H. (2003). Hypoxia-like tissue injury as a component of multiple sclerosis lesions. *J. Neurol. Sci.* **206,** 187–191.

Lisney, S. J., and Devor, M. (1987). Afterdischarge and interactions among fibers in damaged peripheral nerve in the rat. *Brain Res.* **415,** 122–136.

Liu, J. S., Zhao, M. L., Brosnan, C. F., and Lee, S. C. (2001). Expression of inducible nitric oxide synthase and nitrotyrosine in multiple sclerosis lesions. *Am. J. Pathol.* **158,** 2057–2066.

Ma, J. Y., Catterall, W. A., and Scheuer, T. (1997). Persistent sodium currents through brain sodium channels induced by G protein βγ subunits. *Neuron* **19,** 443–452.

Matzner, O., and Devor, M. (1994). Hyperexcitability at sites of nerve injury depends on voltage-sensitive Na^+ channels. *J. Neurophysiol.* **72,** 349–359.

McIntyre, C. C., Richardson, A. G., and Grill, W. M. (2002). Modelling the excitability of mammalian nerve fibers: Influence of afterpotentials on the recovery cycle. *J. Neurophysiol.* **87,** 995–1006.

Mitrović, N., Quasthoff, S., and Grafe, P. (1993). Sodium channel inactivation kinetics of rat sensory and motor nerve fibres and their modulation by glutathione. *Pflugers Arch.* **425,** 453–461.

Nashmi, R., Jones, O. T., and Fehling, M. G. (2000). Abnormal axonal physiology associated with altered expression and distribution of $K_V1.1$ and $K_V1.2$ K^+ channels after chronic spinal cord injury. *Eur. J. Neurosci.* **12,** 491–506.

Nielsen, K. J., Watson, M., Adams, D. J., Hammarstrom, A. K., Gage, P. W., Hill, J. M., Craik, D. J., Thomas, L., Adams, D., Alewood, P. F., and Lewis, R. J. (2002). Solution structure of μ-Conotoxin PIIIA, a preferential inhibitor of persistent tetrodotoxin-sensitive sodium channels. *J. Biol. Chem.* **30,** 27247–27255.

Patlak, J. B., and Ortiz, M. (1985). Slow currents through single sodium channels of the adult rat heart. *J. Gen. Physiol.* **86,** 89–104.

Patlak, J. B., and Oritiz, M. (1986). Two modes of gating during late Na^+ channel currents in frog sartorius muscle. *J. Gen. Physiol.* **87,** 305–326.

Pryce, G., Ahmed, Z., Hankey, D. J., Jackson, S. J., Croxford, J. L., Pocock, J. M., Ledent, C., Petzold, A., Thompson, A. J., Giovannoni, G., Cuzner, M. L., and Baker, D. (2003). Cannabinoids inhibit neurodegeneration in models of multiple sclerosis. *Brain* **126,** 2191–202.

Raman, I. M., Sprunger, L. K., Meisler, M. H., and Bean, B. P. (1997). Altered subthreshold sodium currents and disrupted firing patterns in Purkinje neurons of *Scn8a* mutant mice. *Neuron* **19,** 881–891.

Rasband, M. N., Trimmer, J. S., Schwarz, T. L., Levinson, S. R., Ellisman, M. H., Schachner, M., and Shrager, P. (1998). Potassium channel distribution, clustering and function in remyelinating rat axons. *J. Neurosi.* **18,** 36–47.

Rasband, M. N., and Shrager, P. (2000). Ion channel sequestration in central nervous system axons. *J. Physiol.* **525,** 63–73.

Rasminsky, M. (1981). Hyperexcitability of pathologically myelinated axons and positive symptoms in multiple sclerosis. *Adv. Neurol.* **31,** 289–297.

Reid, G., Scholz, A., Bostock, H., and Vogel, W. (1999). Human axons contain at least five types of voltage-dependent potassium channel. *J. Physiol.* **518,** 681–696.

Renganathan, M., Cummins, T. R., and Waxman, S. G. (2002). Nitric oxide blocks fast, slow, and persistent Na^+ channels in C-type DRG neurons by S-nitrosylation. *J. Neurophysiol.* **87,** 761–775.

Ritchie, J. M. (1995). Physiology of axons. *In* "The Axon, Structure, Function and Pathophysiology" (S. G. Waxman et al., eds.) pp. 68–96. OUP: New York.

Ritchie, J. M., and Chiu, S. Y. (1981). Distribution of sodium and potassium channels in mammalian myelinated nerve. *In* "Demyelinating Diseases, Basic and Clinical Electrophysiology" (S. G. Waxman and J. M. Ritchie, eds.), *Advances in Neurology* Vol. 31, pp. 324–329. Raven Press: New York.

Röper, J., and Schwarz, J. R. (1989). Heterogeneous distribution of fast and slow potassium channels in myelinated rat nerve fibres. *J. Physiol.* **416,** 93–110.

Safo, P., Rosenbaum, T., Shcherbatko, A., Choi, D. Y., Han, E., Toledo-Aral, J. J., Olivera, B. M., Brehm, P., and Mandel, G. (2000). Distinction among neuronal subtypes of voltage-activated sodium channels by μ-conotoxin PIIIA. *J. Neurosci.* **20,** 76–80.

Schaller, K. L., and Caldwell, J. H. (2003). Expression and distribution of voltage-gated sodium channels in the cerebellum. *Cerebellum* **2,** 2–9.

Schwarz, J. R., Reid, G., and Bostock, H. (1995). Action potentials and membrane currents in the human node of Ranvier. *Pflugers Arch.* **430,** 283–292.

Schwid, S. R., Petrie, M. D., McDermott, M. P., Tierney, D. S., Mason, D. H., and Goodman, A. D. (1997). Quantitative assessment of sustained-release 4-aminopyridine for symptomatic treatment of multiple sclerosis. *Neurology* **48,** 817–821.

Sheean, G. L., Murray, N. M., Rothwell, J. C., Miller, D. H., and Thompson, A. J. (1998). An open-labeled clinical and electrophysiological study of 3,4 diaminopyridine in the treatment of fatigue in multiple sclerosis. *Brain* **121,** 967–975.

Sherratt, R. M., Bostock, H., and Sears, T. A. (1980). Effects of 4-aminopyridine on normal and demyelinated mammalian nerve fibres. *Nature* **283,** 570–572.

Smith, M. R., Smith, R. D., Plummer, N. W., Meisler, M. H., and Goldin, A. L. (1998). Functional analysis of the mouse *Scn8a* sodium channel. *J. Neurosci.* **18,** 6093–6102.

Smith, P. F. (2002). Cannabinoids in the treatment of pain and spasticity in multiple sclerosis. *Curr. Opin. Investig. Drugs* **3,** 859–864.

Smith, K. J., and McDonald, W. I. (1980). Spontaneous and mechanically evoked activity due to a central demyelinating lesion. *Nature* **286,** 154–156.

Stys, P. K., Sontheimer, H., Ransom, B. R., and Waxman, S. G. (1993). Noninactivating, tetrodotoxin-sensitive Na⁺ conductance in rat optic nerve axons. *Proc. Natl. Acad. Sci. U. S. A.* **90,** 6976–6980.

Tokuno, H. A., Kocsis, J. D., and Waxman, S. G. (2003). Noninactivating, tetrodotoxin-sensitive Na⁺ conductance in peripheral axons. *Muscle Nerve* **28,** 212–217.

Welk, E., Leah, J. D., and Zimmermann, M. (1990). Characteristics of A- and C-fibers ending in a sensory nerve neuroma in the rat. *J. Neurophysiol.* **63,** 759–766.

Willow, M., Gonoi, T., and Catterall, W. A. (1985). Voltage clamp analysis of the inhibitory actions of diphenylhydantoin and carbamazepine on voltage-sensitive sodium channels in neuroblastoma cells. *Mol. Pharmacol.* **27,** 549–558.

10

Clinical Pharmacology of Abnormal Potassium Channel Organization in Demyelinated Axons

Christopher T. Bever, Jr., M.D.

I. Introduction

Clinical observations suggested that some deficits in patients with multiple sclerosis (MS) were due to physiological abnormalities rather than structural loss and were potentially reversible. A series of authors reported changes in symptoms and signs in patients with MS who had temperature elevation and depression (Simons, 1937; Guthrie, 1951; Nelson and McDowell, 1959; Watson, 1959). Also supportive of this idea were changes in symptoms induced by procedures that lowered serum ionized calcium (Davis et al., 1970). Together, these observations supported the idea that some neurological deficits in MS patients were physiologically reversible.

Studies examining action potential propagation in normal and demyelinated nerves demonstrated a reorganization of axolemmal ion channels, which results in conduction disturbances and provides a likely basis for physiologically reversible neurological deficits (reviewed in Waxman, 1982). In 1979 Chiu and co-workers showed that action potential propagation in normal myelinated nerve fibers involves currents generated by the opening of voltage-sensitive sodium channels at nodes of Ranvier (see Chapters 4 and 5). Sherratt and co-workers (1980) then showed that in areas of demyelination, sodium channel densities are decreased and voltage-sensitive potassium channels, which are not active on normal myelinated nerve fibers, become detectable. This reorganization leads to a reduction in axon-potential amplitude and duration, resulting in abnormal conduction including conduction block. Bostock and co-workers (1981) showed that the potassium channel blockers dendrotoxin and 4-aminopyridine improved conduction abnormalities in experimentally demyelinated nerves and provided the rationale for studies of potassium channel blockers in patients with MS.

II. Early Clinical Trials

A. Demonstration of Concept Studies

A series of early clinical trials sought to provide evidence that potassium channel blockers could improve neurological deficits in MS patients. The first report of the use of a potassium channel blocker in multiple sclerosis patients was from Jones and co-workers (1983). They conducted a placebo-controlled, open-label study of the potassium channel blocker, 4-aminopyridine (AP). They enrolled ten MS patients, five with visual impairment caused by MS and five with chronic stable MS. The five patients with visual deficits were treated with intravenous and oral doses of AP. Visual acuity, formal visual field, and visual-evoked response (VER) testing were carried out before and during treatment. Improvements in visual acuity and visual fields were seen in all five patients. No changes were seen in VER P-100 latencies or amplitudes. Side effects included only paresthesias. The five patients with chronic spastic paraparesis were treated with oral AP in divided doses up to 60 mg per day. Patients were examined neurologically. The investigators reported improved ambulation in one and improved sensation in a second patient. Side effects included paresthesias and confusion. This study suggested that AP treatment might improve symptoms in some patients with MS.

A second "demonstration of concept" study was published in 1987 by Stefoski and co-workers who reported a dose titration study of intravenous AP in 12 men with MS. Patients were selected for study based on a history of functionally significant neurological deficits made worse by temperature elevation and were enrolled in a placebo-controlled, crossover design trial. Patients were given either increasing doses of AP or saline by intravenous injection by a treating neurologist. Evaluations focused on the temperature-sensitive study deficit and included visual acuity, flicker-fusion frequency, quantitative perimetry, and videotaped neurological evaluations scored by a blinded rater. Reversible improvements related to treatment with active drug were seen in selected deficits in 10 of 12 patients including improvements in vision (7 of 9), eye movements (5 of 6), and motor function (5 of 9) including improved ambulation. The only reported side effect was paresthesia. This study confirmed the results of the earlier study on visual impairment and extended them by using blinded outcome measures in other areas.

A second chemically related potassium channel blocker, 3,4 diaminopyridine (DAP), attracted interest because it was a more potent potassium channel blocker but had less convulsant activity (Molgo et al., 1980). In 1990, Bever and co-workers reported a preliminary trial of DAP in 10 male patients with MS. Patients were treated with increasing single doses of DAP up to 100 mg and then with DAP in divided dosage for up to 21 days. Evaluations included patient-subjective responses, neurological examination findings, and P-100 latencies and amplitudes on VER testing. Five patients reported reversible subjective improvement (primarily in leg strength) and all patients had reversible improvements on neurological examination (primarily leg strength and spasticity). Reversible improvements in VER P-100 latencies were seen in two of six patients with baseline abnormalities. Dose-related abdominal pain was reported by all patients and was dose limiting in six. All patients reported dose-related paresthesias. Electroencephalograms were monitored in all patients and although increases in baseline slowing were seen in three patients, no epileptiform activity was reported. This study suggested that DAP might also be useful as a symptomatic treatment for MS deficits but that toxicity might be limiting. It further supported the clinical utility of potassium channel blockers in patients with MS.

B. Exploratory Studies

Several studies were conducted to explore issues of dosing, toxicity, patient selection criteria, drug selection, and outcome measurement. Although intravenous administration of AP was adequate for a demonstration of concept study, it was recognized that the drug would have to be orally active to be clinically useful. In 1990, Davis and co-workers reported a placebo-controlled trial of short-term, orally administered AP. A total of 20 men with MS who had temperature-sensitive neurological deficits were assigned to single oral doses of up to 25 mg of AP (15 patients) or placebo (5 patients). Outcome measures again focused on the patient's predefined study deficit and included visual acuity, flicker-fusion frequency, quantitative perimetry, VER testing, and videotaped neurological examinations scored by a blinded rater. Improvements were seen in all of 15 patients who received active drug and in none of those who received placebo. Vision improved in 11 of 13, oculomotor function in 1 of 2, and motor function in 9 of 13. Improvements in VER P-100 latencies were seen in 4 of 11 patients with baseline abnormalities. Side effects of treatment included light-headedness or dizziness in 10 and paresthesias in 5. This study demonstrated short-term benefit of orally administered AP.

In 1991, Stefoski and co-workers published a study designed to address several of the shortcomings of earlier studies. Initial trials of AP and DAP were limited to men because of U.S. Food and Drug Administration concerns about teratogenicity. Nine women were included in this study. Previous studies had been unblinded or single-blind; in this study there was an attempt to blind the patients as to treatment. Seventeen temperature-sensitive MS patients (9 women and 8 men) received from 2 to 5 days of treatment with AP or placebo three times a day. Eight patients received AP only; nine patients received both AP and placebo at different times. AP doses were as high as 52.5 mg/day. The responses of predefined temperature-sensitive study deficits were monitored using flicker-fusion frequency testing, VER testing, and videotaped neurological examinations scored by a blinded rater. A total of 13 of 17 patients had what the investigators considered clinically significant improvements while on AP treatment, but only 3 of 9 patients on placebo had comparable improvements. Improvements were seen in motor function (13), vision (11), and oculomotor function (3). VER improved in four of five patients with baseline abnormalities. Side effects included dizziness (13), paresthesias (5), nausea (5), and anxiety (4). This study demonstrated a beneficial effect in men and women with an improved study design.

C. Proof of Concept Studies

Two single-center randomized, double-blind, placebo-controlled crossover design studies sought to establish "proof of concept" using well-accepted clinical trial designs and widely accepted outcome measures. Van Diemen and co-workers reported the first such study in 1992. In all, 70 patients with clinically definite MS were randomly assigned to two 12-week treatment periods of AP and placebo. Side-effect evaluations were carried out on all patients who received any drug treatment (69 patients), and efficacy evaluations were carried out on all patients who received at least 2 weeks of drug treatment (67 patients). A total of 57 patients completed the treatment protocol. Disability as measured by the Expanded Disability Status Scale (EDSS) (Kurtzke, 1983) was evaluated at baseline and at weeks 2, 6, and 12 of each treatment period. The mean EDSS improved during the AP treatment period and worsened during the placebo treatment period in each group, and overall the mean EDSS of patients on AP on week 12 improved by 0.28 compared to the mean at the end of the placebo period (P = 0.001). Ten patients improved by 1 or more points on AP; none had comparable improvement on placebo ($P < 0.05$). Significant improvements were seen in the pyramidal system functions of the EDSS ($P < 0.01$) and not in other areas. Quantitative testing of visual and oculomotor function showed improvements in VER P-100 latency, smooth pursuit eye movement gain, and saccadic eye movement V_{max}. Subjective improvement was reported by 18 patients on AP; only 1 patient reported improvement on placebo ($P < 0.05$). An analysis of responders showed that patients with longer disease durations, progressive disease, and more pyramidal impairment were more likely to respond. Side effects were reported by 48 patients during AP treatment. Most were mild but in 14 cases dose reductions were required, and in 5 cases the patients withdrew because of side effects. A total of 16 patients had side effects on placebo, and one patient withdrew because of placebo-related side effects. Side effects included paresthesias (15 on AP and 10 on placebo), dizziness (36 on AP and 4 on placebo), gait instability (11

on AP and 1 on placebo), nausea (9 on AP), anxiety (4 on AP), abdominal pain (5 on AP), obstipation (1 on AP), and headache (1 on placebo). Blinding was not maintained, with 41 patients able to identify their treatment. No seizures occurred, but in one patient epileptiform activity was seen on EEG during AP treatment. Although conclusions were limited by the unblinding of patients, this study suggested that AP treatment could improve function in patients with MS with acceptable toxicity.

In 1996, Bever et al. reported a single-center, randomized, placebo-controlled, double-blind crossover design trial of orally administered DAP. A total of 36 patients with MS who had a prospectively defined study deficit were randomized to two 30-day treatment periods separated by a 30-day washout period. Patients were treated during one treatment period with escalating doses of DAP, and during the other, with escalating doses of nicotinic acid, which was chosen as a placebo to reduce unblinding. Outcome measures included evaluation of the prospectively defined study deficit (primary), patient subjective response, manual motor testing of leg strength, videotaped neurological examination scored by a blinded rater, quantitative quadriceps and hamstrings strength measured by isometric dynamometry, ambulation index, expanded disability status scale score, and neuropsychological testing using the Brief Repeatable Battery of Neuropsychological Tests (BRBN) (Rao et al., 1990). The study deficit (leg weakness and spasticity) improved in 24 patients, 22 on DAP and 2 on placebo (P = 0.0005). In all, 17 patients reported subjective improvement, 14 on DAP, 2 on placebo, and 1 on both (P = 0.009). Manual motor testing of leg strength and quantitative testing of quadriceps and hamstrings strength by isometric dynamometry improved on DAP compared to placebo. Videotaped ratings of leg strength and ambulation index improved. No significant changes were seen in global rating of the videotaped neurological examination, the EDSS, or in cognitive functioning on neuropsychological testing. A total of 31 of 36 patients reported adverse events that included paresthesias (25 on DAP and 5 on placebo), abdominal pain (19 on DAP and 2 on placebo), and confusion (3 on DAP). One patient had a grand mal seizure while on DAP. Dose reductions were required in five patients as a result of abdominal pain and treatment was discontinued in three (2 for abdominal pain and 1 because of seizure). This study suggested that DAP might lead to symptomatic improvements in patients with MS, but that toxicity was limiting in many patients.

III. Later Clinical Trials

A. Trials Addressing Formulation Issues

In the trial described previously, Van Diemen and co-workers (1933) examined the relationship between serum levels, efficacy, and toxicity. Their data suggested that efficacy was related to total exposure to AP while toxicity was related to peak serum levels. To further explore this issue, Bever and co-workers (1994) conducted a serum concentration-controlled trial of AP in eight temperature-sensitive MS patients. Two target serum concentration ranges, low (30–59 ng/ml) and high (60–100 ng/ml), were compared to placebo in a randomized, double-blind crossover trial. Treatment periods lasted 36 hours and were separated by a washout period of at least 5 days. Serum AP levels were measured every 4 to 6 hours during the treatment period, and Bayesian estimation was used to construct serum concentration curves for each patient. Outcome measures included measurement of visual contrast sensitivity, flicker fusion frequency, VER P-100 latencies, leg strength by manual motor testing, quadriceps and hamstrings strength by isometric dynamometry, EDSS, Ambulation Index, and neurological impairment by scoring of videotaped neurological examinations by blinded raters. Visual contrast sensitivity, leg strength by manual motor testing, quadriceps and hamstrings strength measured by isometric dynamometry, and scores on videotaped examinations all improved with treatment; and improvements were related to the area under the serum AP level curve (total AP exposure) rather than peak levels achieved. Patients were observed during treatment and the timing of adverse events was recorded. All patients experienced side effects during the high serum concentration arm, which correlated with peak serum levels. One patient had a grand mal seizure, with a peak serum level of 104 ng/ml, and one patient had an episode of confusion at 114 ng/ml. This study supported the idea that peak levels contributed to toxicity without enhancing efficacy and suggested that a controlled release formulation of AP might be better tolerated than the immediate release formulation in use at the time.

The pharmaceutical company, Elan Pharmaceutical Research Corporation, developed a controlled release formulation of AP and in 1994 organized a 10-center randomized, double-blind, placebo-controlled parallel design trial. Only a brief summary of the results has been published (Schwid et al., 1997). A total of 161 patients with stable deficits were randomized to AP or placebo. The primary outcome measure was overall disability as measured by EDSS. No significant treatment effect was seen because of a larger-than-expected placebo response. Because of concern that the change in formulation might have reduced the efficacy of the drug, a small crossover study was conducted by Schwid and co-workers (1997) with the new controlled release formulation. A total of 10 MS patients were randomized to AP, 17.5 mg two times a week, or placebo for 1 week. Outcome measures included timed ambulation, timed stair climbing, quantitative isometric motor power, manual motor testing, grip strength, EDSS, and patient subjective response. Timed 8-meter ambulation improved on AP com-

pared to placebo in 9 of 10 patients ($P = 0.02$). The other outcome measures had less than significant improvements with AP compared to placebo. Seven patients preferred AP and only one patient preferred placebo. No serious adverse events occurred, but minor side effects, including nausea, dizziness, paresthesias, and insomnia, occurred in some patients. This study showed that the controlled release formulation could improve neurological deficits in patients with MS who have minimal side effects and no significant toxicity.

B. Comparison of AP and DAP

One study directly compared the efficacy and tolerability of AP and DAP in patients with MS (Polman et al., 1994b). A total of 24 patients with MS, who had completed an earlier trial of AP, were enrolled in a head-to-head comparison trial. In all, 14 patients who had not responded to AP were treated with DAP for 4 weeks in an open-label study with doses up to 1 mg/kg. Ten patients who had responded to AP were enrolled in a 6-week, double-blind, randomized, crossover comparative study of AP and DAP. Outcome measures included measurement of contrast sensitivity, VER P-100 amplitudes and latencies, saccadic and pursuit eye movements, and EDSS. In the nonresponder group, there were no significant changes in contrast sensitivity, VER measures, eye movement measures, or EDSS. The side effect profile for DAP was different from AP, with paresthesias, nausea, and abdominal pain being more common and dizziness and gait instability less common. Two patients withdrew from the study because of abdominal pain. In the responder group, improvements were seen in contrast sensitivity, VEP measurements, and eye movement measurements that were not significantly different from the improvements seen on AP. Six of seven patients in this group who completed the study reported clinically meaningful improvements on AP, but only two reported comparable changes on DAP. Three patients in the responder group withdrew from the study because of lack of efficacy. All withdrew during DAP treatment. Side effects were less common than in the responder group, but again abdominal pain was seen during DAP treatment but not during AP treatment. The authors concluded that AP produced more clinically meaningful improvements in patients who will respond to treatment. In general, AP was better tolerated than DAP, with abdominal pain being the limiting side effect with DAP. There was no evidence that a subpopulation of patients who did not respond to AP would respond to treatment wDAP.

C. Safety and Efficacy of Long-Term Treatment

Experience with receptor blockers raised the possibility that prolonged drug exposure might lead to loss of efficacy as a result of the upregulation of potassium channel synthesis. Two studies have addressed the long-term effects of AP in patients with MS. Polman and co-workers (1994a) enrolled 23 patients with MS who had treatment-related improvement during a double-blind, placebo-controlled, crossover trial of AP in an open-label study. Patients were treated for 6 to 32 months, with 20 of the 23 patients reporting sustained benefit. In general, side effects were mild, but two patients had grand mal seizures. One patient developed elevated liver function tests that improved when treatment was stopped. Bever and co-workers (1997) enrolled 22 patients with MS who had participated in studies of the pharmacokinetics of AP in an open-label safety study of the controlled release formulation of AP described previously (see Trials Addressing Formulation Issues). Patients were treated for 6 to 42 months with a total of 52 patient-years of exposure. Sixteen patients reported sustained benefit. One grand mal seizure occurred after 24 months of treatment. These studies provide no support for the idea that upregulation of potassium channel synthesis is occurring. They do show that the risk of seizures persists even after many months of treatment without side effects and that AP may have rare hepatotoxicity. The subjective benefits of AP persist in many patients with long-term treatment.

D. The Effects of Potassium Channel Blockers on Cognitive Impairment

Rao and co-workers (1991) demonstrated that mild cognitive impairment can appear early in MS and that it does not correlate with overall neurological impairment. They identified a series of tests that were sensitive to the cognitive changes typically seen early in MS patients and published them as the BRBN (Rao et al., 1990). The BRBN consisted of the five standard tests of memory and attention, the Selective Reminding, 10/36 Spatial Recall, Symbol Digits Modalities, Paced Auditory Serial Addition, and Word List Generation tests.

Because of anecdotal reports of improved memory and concentration while on potassium channel blockers, two studies examined the effects of potassium channel blockers on cognitive dysfunction in patients with MS using the BRBN. Smits and co-workers (1994) reported a randomized, double blind, placebo-controlled, crossover design trial examining the effects of oral AP given over a 14-day period. They found trends toward improvement in some measures but no statistically significant changes. Bever and co-workers (1997) included the BRBN in their evaluation of 36 patients treated with DAP in a randomized, placebo-controlled, double-blind, crossover design trial. No significant differences were found. Despite anecdotal reports of improved cognition in patients receiving AP and DAP, these well-designed trials using a neuropsychological testing battery designed to be sensitive to the deficits typically seen in early MS patients found no improvement.

Rossini and co-workers (2001) reported a study of the effects of AP on neurocognitive dysfunction using a larger, more generalized battery of tests. A total of 60 primary and secondary progressive patients with MS were randomized in a double-blind, placebo-controlled, crossover trial of oral AP using 6-month treatment periods. A total of 49 patients completed the study. The testing battery included tests for sustained attention (the Auditory Attention test), short-term memory (the Forward Digit and Corsi's Block Span tests), long-term memory (the 15' Delayed Recall of Rey's 15-Words List and the 15' Delayed Recall of Rey's Figure A tests), visual perception (Benton's Line Orientation test), language (Token test), executive function (Wisconsin Card Sorting test), general intelligence (Raven's Progressive Maticies test), and depression (Hamilton's scale). Neither the study group as a whole nor a subgroup analysis based on serum AP levels showed any treatment-related changes. Studies to date fail to demonstrate any effect of AP or DAP on cognition.

E. The Effects of Potassium Channel Blockers on Fatigue

Fatigue is one of the most common and disabling symptoms in patients with MS (Murray, 1985; Krupp et al., 1988). It has little relationship to neurological impairment and has been one of the most difficult MS symptoms to document objectively. A number of scoring methodologies have been developed for quantifying subjective fatigue for pharmaceutical trials (Murray, 1985; Canadian Multiple Sclerosis Research Group, 1987; Cohen and Fisher, 1989). Krupp and co-workers (1989) introduced the Fatigue Severity Scale (FSS), which was designed to measure MS fatigue in patients with MS and has been validated in a number of clinical trials. Motor fatigue has been quantitated in patients with MS by monitoring motor power output using prolonged or repetitive isometric contractions (Schwid et al., 1999). Mental fatigue has been quantitated by measuring neuropsychological performance before and after mentally taxing activities (Schwid et al., 2002). One study of central motor conduction suggested that some MS-related fatigue may be central in origin (Sheean et al., 1997). That objective measures of fatigue have not correlated strongly with subjective fatigue suggests that the causes of subjective fatigue may vary from patient to patient and that multiple causes may contribute in a single patient.

Anecdotal reports of improved fatigue in patients with MS receiving potassium channel blockers led to two studies designed to examine the effect of DAP and AP on fatigue. Sheean and co-workers (1998) conducted an open-label study of DAP in eight MS patients who complained of fatigue. Patients were treated with 20 to 60 mg of oral DAP in divided dosage for 3 weeks. Outcome measures included the FSS, as well as electrophysiological measures of fatigue. FSS scores improved in seven patients and statistically significant improvements were seen in physiological measures of maximum voluntary contraction (central activation, physiological fatigue index, and twitch force). Rossini and co-workers (2001) reported the results of a randomized, double-blind, placebo-controlled, crossover design trial of 6 months of treatment with oral AP. In all, 49 of 60 patients with primary and secondary progressive MS who were enrolled completed the study. Fatigue, quantitated with the FSS, improved during both treatment periods, with no difference between AP and placebo. A subgroup analysis based on serum AP levels showed a slight statistically significant improvement in fatigue in the patients with serum levels above 30 ng/ml ($P = 0.05$). A separate analysis of the correlation of motor-evoked potential morphology (see next section), and fatigue scores showed a significant correlation ($P = 0.01$). Although these studies did not provide very compelling support for an effect of DAP and AP on MS fatigue, they leave open this possibility, which would have to be addressed in larger trials. It is unlikely that the development of DAP or AP will be pursued for the indication of fatigue in view of the potential side effects and the alternative therapies already available.

F. The Effects of Potassium Channel Blockers on Motor-Evoked Potentials and Central Conduction

Transcranial magnetic stimulation has been suggested as a methodology that could be used to objectively document the effect of potassium-channel blockers in patients with MS. The methodology is based on the finding that a strong, focused magnetic field applied to the scalp over the motor cortex can depolarize pyramidal motor neurons, resulting in a motor response in specific muscles in the arms and legs. The motor response can be detected electrophysiologically and is called a motor-evoked potential (MEP). The latency and amplitude of the resulting muscle depolarization can be characterized and central motor conduction times (CMCTs) calculated. CMCTs are frequently slowed in patients with MS (Britton, 1991; Jones et al., 1991), and CMCTs improve in parallel with clinical improvement when patients with MS are treated with corticosteroids (Kandler et al., 1991). If potassium channel blockers improve conduction in demyelinated motor pathways, it could lead to changes in MEP latencies, amplitudes, or morphologies.

In the first study that examined MEPs in patients with MS who were treated with potassium channel blockers, already reviewed in the preceding section, Sheean and co-workers (1998) studied eight patients with MS enrolled in an open-label study of the effect of DAP treatment on fatigue.

A statistically significant ($P < 0.05$) treatment-related reduction in MEP amplitude was found, but there was no change in MEP area or in CMCT. There was no correlation between MEP changes and changes in reported fatigue, so the investigators concluded that the improvements in subjective fatigue did not involve improved conduction in the pathways tested.

A second study reported by Fujihara and Miyoshi (1998) examined the effect of AP on central motor conduction in six patients with MS. Transcranial magnetic stimulation was used to study MEP in the upper and lower extremities before and after treatment with intravenous AP. Mean amplitudes of MEPs increased significantly after treatment ($P = 0.008$), with a reduction in onset latency variability without any change in mean or shortest onset latencies. In four limbs of three patients in whom there were no detectable baseline MEP responses, MEPs were detectable after treatment. The authors concluded that the increase in MEP amplitude and reduction in onset latency variability were consistent with restored conduction and/or increased conduction velocities in a subset of demyelinated nerve fibers.

In the most recent study reported by Rossini and co-workers (2001), 62 patients with primary or secondary progressive MS were enrolled in a randomized, double-blind, placebo-controlled, crossover trial of AP administered orally for 6 months. At baseline 90% of MEPs studied were markedly abnormal. No significant treatment-related changes in amplitude or latencies were found. Examination of waveform morphology showed that more normal, less complex morphologies were found during AP treatment, which reversed after treatment was discontinued. Together these studies provide some objective confirmation of the effects of potassium channel blockers on the motor conduction pathways in patients with MS.

IV. A Recent Multicenter Parallel Design Trial of AP

Goodman and co-workers (2002) reported the results of a four-center randomized, double-blind, placebo-controlled parallel group study of controlled release AP in 31 patients with MS. Patients were treated with escalating doses of 20 to 80 mg of AP per day in divided doses. A total of 25 patients received active drug and 11 patients received placebo. Outcome measures included timed ambulation, manual testing of leg strength, paced auditory serial addition task, 9-hole peg test, and a fatigue diary. There was a statistically significant and dose-related improvement in timed ambulation (approximately 18% improvement in the AP-treated patients vs. 2% in the placebo-treated patients, $P = 0.04$). A significant improvement in leg strength was also seen (approximately 11% improvement in the AP-treated group compared with a 4% worsening in the placebo treated group, $P = 0.01$).

Side effects were similar to those in earlier studies, with dizziness, insomnia, paresthesias, nausea, asthenia, headache, tremor, pain, and anxiety being reported by more than 10% of patients on AP. Two patients had seizures on daily doses of 60 and 70 mg. This trial is the first multicenter, randomized, placebo-controlled, parallel design trial to demonstrate statistically significant benefits of AP treatment in patients with MS.

V. The Mechanisms of Potassium Channel Blockers in MS

Felts and Smith (1994) suggested that some of the beneficial effects of potassium channel blockers in patients with MS might be due to synaptic rather than axonal effects. They first noted the failure of some direct attempts to demonstrate improved nerve conduction in patients. They then pointed out that drug levels attainable in patients were lower than the levels needed to produce changes in several of the experimental models used. They noted that the one model in which improvements were seen at attainable levels of AP was probably not a good model of the changes that occur in MS. A subsequent study (Smith et al., 2000) described a series of experimental studies that demonstrating that, at the serum AP levels seen in patients with MS, some of the effects of AP could be explained by presynaptic effects leading to enhanced neurotransmitter release and direct effects on muscle. They argued that these effects might be responsible for some of the neurological improvements reported in patients with MS.

VI. Conclusion

Treatment with the potassium channel blocking drugs, 4-aminopyridine and 3,4 diaminopyridine, can improve some symptoms in some patients with MS. Minor side effects include paresthesias, dizziness, anxiety, abdominal pain, nausea, and insomnia, with abdominal pain being more common with DAP and confusion with AP. Major side effects, which occur rarely, include encephalopathy and seizures. Several crossover design trials have demonstrated improvements in motor function in the legs and in ambulation ability. Conclusions from these trials are limited by the fact that side effects may disclose treatment assignment to patients. Two parallel design trials have been completed but have not yet been published in full.

References

Bever, C. T., Katz, E., Tierney, D., Johnson, K. P. (1995). Experience with slow release 4-aminopyridine in multiple sclerosis patients: Long term tolerability and safety. *J. Neuroimmuno.* 56–63 (Supplement 1), 58 (Abstract 192).

Bever, C. T., Leslie, J., and Camenga, D., et al. (1990). Preliminary trial of 3,4 diaminopyridine in patients with multiple sclerosis. *Ann. Neurol.* **27**, 421–427.

Bever, C. T. Jr., Anderson, P. A., Leslie, J., et al. (1996). Treatment with oral 3,4 diaminopyridine improves leg strength in multiple sclerosis patients: results of a randomized double-blind, placebo-controlled, crossover trial. Neurology **47**, 1457–1462.

Bever, C. T., Young, D., Anderson, P. M., et al. (1994). The effects of 4-aminopyridine in multiple sclerosis patients: Results of a randomized, placebo-controlled, double-blind, concentration-controlled, crossover trial. *Neurology* **44**, 1054–1059.

Bostock, H., Sears, T. A., and Sherratt, R. M. (1981). The effects of 4-aminopyridine and tetraethylammonium ions on normal and demyelinated mammalian nerve fibers. *J. Physiol. (London)* **313**, 301–315.

Britton, T. C., Meyer, B. U., and Benecke, R. (1991). Variability of cortically evoked motor responses in multiple sclerosis. *Electroencephalogr. Clin. Neurophysiol.* **81**, 186–194.

Canadian MS Research Group. (1987). A randomized controlled trial of amantadine in fatigue associated with multiple sclerosis. *Can. J. Neurol. Sci.* **14**, 273–278.

Chiu, S. Y., Ritchie, J. M., Rogart, R. B., and Staff, D. (1979). A quantitative description of membrane currents in rabbit myelinated nerve. *J. Physiol. (London)* **292**, 149–166.

Cohen, R. A., and Fisher, M. (1989). Amantadine treatment of fatigue associated with multiple sclerosis. *Arch. Neurol.* **46**, 676–680.

Davis, F. A., Becker, F. O., Michael, J. A., and Sorensen, E. (1970). Effect of intravenous sodium bicarbonate edetate (Na2EDTA), and hyperventilation on visual and oculomotor signs in multiple sclerosis. *J. Neurol. Neurosurg. Psychiatry* **33**, 723–732.

Davis, F. A., Stefoski, D., and Schauf, C. L. (1990). Orally administered 4-aminopyridine improves clinical signs in multiple sclerosis. *Ann. Neurol* **27**, 186–192.

Felts, P. A., and Smith. K. J. (1994). The use of potassium channel blocking agents in the therapy of demyelinating diseases. *Ann. Neurol.* **36**, 454.

Fujihara, K, and Miyoshi, T. (1998). The effects of 4-aminopyridine on motor evoked potentials in multiple sclerosis. *J. Neurol. Sci.* **159**, 102–106.

Goodman, A. D., Blight, A., Cohen, J. A., Cross, A. H., Katz, M., Rizzo, M. A., and Vollmer, T. (2002). Placebo-controlled double-blinded dose ranging study of Fampridine-SR in multiple sclerosis. *Multiple Sclerosis* **8**(Supplement 1), S116 (P308).

Guthrie, T. C. (1951). Visual and motor changes in patients with multiple sclerosis. A result of induced changes in environmental temperature. *Arch. Neurol. Psychiatry,* **65**, 437–451.

Jones, R. E., Heron, J. R., Foster, D. H., Snelgar, R. S., and Mason, R. J. (1983). Effects of 4-aminopyridine in patients with multiple sclerosis. *J. Neurol. Sci.* **60**, 353–362.

Jones, S. M., Streletz, L. J., Raab, V. E., et al. (1991). Lower extremity motor evoked potentials in multiple sclerosis. *Arch. Neurol.* **48**, 944–948.

Kandler, R. H., Jarrett, J. A., Davies-Jones, G. A., et al. (1991). The role of magnetic stimulation as a quantifier of motor disability in patients with multiple sclerosis. *J. Neurol. Sci.* **106**, 25–34.

Krupp, L. B., Alvarez, L. A., LaRocca, N. G., and Scheinberg, L. C. (1988). Fatigue in multiple sclerosis. *Arch. Neurol.* **45**, 435–437.

Krupp, L. B., LaRocca, N. G., Muir-Nash, J., and Steinberg, A. D. (1989). The fatigue severity scale: Application to patients with multiple sclerosis and systemic lupus erythematosus. *Arch. Neurol.* **46**, 1121–1123.

Kurtzke, J. F. (1983). Rating neurologic impairment in multiple sclerosis: An expanded disability status scale (EDSS). *Neurology* **33**, 1444–1452.

Molgo, J., Lundh, H., and Thesleff, S. (1980). Potency of 3,4 diaminopyridine and 4-aminopyridine on mammalian neuromuscular transmission and the effect of pH changes. *Eur. J. Pharmacol.* **61**, 25–34.

Murray, N. M., and Newsom-Davis, J. (1981). Treatment with oral 4-aminopyridine in disorders of neuromuscular transmission. *Neurology* **31**, 265–271.

Murray, T. J. (1985). Amantadine therapy for fatigue in multiple sclerosis. *Can. J. Neurol. Sci.* **12**, 251–254.

Nelson, D. A., and McDowell, F. (1959). The effects of induced hyperthermia on patients with multiple sclerosis. *J. Neurol. Neurosurg. Psychiatry* **22**, 113–116.

Polman, C. H., Bertelsmann, F. W., vanLoenen, A. C., and Koetsier, J. C. (1994a). 4-aminopyridine in the treatment of patients with multiple sclerosis: long term efficacy and safety. *Arch. Neurol.* **51**, 292–296.

Polman, C. H., Bertelsmann, F. W., de Waal, R., et al. (1994b). 4-aminopyridine is superior to 3,4 diaminopyridine in the treatment of multiple sclerosis. *Arch. Neurol.* **51**, 1136–1139.

Rao, S. M., and Cognitive Function Study Group, NMSS. (1990). "A Manual for the Brief Repeatable Battery of Neuropsychological Tests in Multiple Sclerosis." National Multiple Sclerosis Society, New York.

Rao, S. M., Leo, G. J., Ellington, L., et al. (1991). Cognitive dysfunction in multiple sclerosis. I. Frequency, patterns and prediction. *Neurology* **41**, 685–691.

Rossini, P. M., Pasqualetti, P., Pozzilli, C., et al. (2001). Fatigue in progressive multiple sclerosis: results of a randomized, double-blind, placebo-controlled, crossover trial of oral 4-aminopyridine. *Multiple Sclerosis* **7**, 354–358.

Schwid, S. R., Petrie, M. D., McDermott, M. P., et al. (1997). Quantitative assessment of sustained-release 4-aminopyridine for symptomatic treatment of multiple sclerosis. *Neurology* **48**, 817–821.

Schwid, S. R., Thornton, C. A., Pandya, S., et al. (1999). Quantitative assessment of motor fatigue and strength in MS. *Neurology* **53**, 743–750.

Schwid, S. R., Weinstein, A., Goodman, A. E., et al. (2002). Cognitive fatigue during a test requiring sustained attention. *Multiple Sclerosis* **8** (Suppl 1), S26 (P14).

Sheean, G. L., Murray, N. M., Rothwell, J. C., et al. (1997). An electrophysiological study of the mechanism of fatigue in multiple sclerosis. *Brain* **120**, 299–315.

Sheean, G. L., Murray, N. M. F., Rothwell, J. C., et al. (1998). An open labeled clinical and electrophysiological study of 3,4 diaminopyridine in the treatment of fatigue in multiple sclerosis. *Brain* **121**, 967–975.

Sherrat, R. M., Bostock, H., and Sears, T. A. (1980). Effects of 4-aminopyridine on normal and demyelinated mammalian nerve fibers. *Nature* **283**, 570–572.

Simons, D. J. (1937). A note on the effect of heat and cold upon certain symptoms of multiple sclerosis. *Bull. Neurol. Inst. NY* **6**, 385–386.

Smith, K. J., Felts, P. A., and John., G. R. (2000). Effects of 4-aminopyridine on demyelinated axons, synapses and muscle tension. *Brain* **123**, 171–184.

Smits, R. C. F., Emmen, H. H., Bertelsmann, F. W., et al. (1994). The effects of 4-aminopyridine on cognitive function in patients with multiple sclerosis: A pilot study. *Neurology* **44**, 1701–1705.

Stefoski, D., Davis, F. A., Faut, M., and Schauf, C. L. (1987). 4-aminopyridine in patients with multiple sclerosis. *Ann. Neurol.* **27**, 71–75.

Stefoski, D,, Davis, F. A., Fitzsimmons, W. E., et al. (1991). 4-aminopyridine in multiple sclerosis: Prolonged administration. *Neurology* **41**, 1344–1348.

Van Diemen, H. A. M., Polman, C. H., Koetsier, J. C., et al. (1993). 4-aminopyridine in patients with multiple sclerosis: dosage and serum level related to efficacy and safety. *Clin. Neuropharmacol.* **16**, 195–204.

Van Diemen, H. A. M., Polman, C. H., van Dongen, M. M. M., et al. (1993). 4-aminopyridine induces functional improvement in multiple sclerosis patients: A neurophysiological study. *J. Neurol. Sci.* **116**, 220–226.

Van Diemen, H. A. M., Polman, C. H., van Dongen, M. M. M., et al. (1992). The effect of 4-aminopyridine on clinical signs in multiple sclerosis: a randomized placebo-controlled, double-blind, crossover study. *Ann. Neurol.* **32**, 123–130.

Watson, C. (1959). Effect of lowering body temperature on the symptoms and signs of multiple sclerosis. *N. Engl. J. Med.* **261**, 1253–1259.

Waxman, S. G. (1982). Membranes, myelin and the pathophysiology of multiple sclerosis. *N. Engl. J. Med.* **306**, 1529–1533.

11

Pathology of Neurons in Multiple Sclerosis

Hans Lassmann, M.D.

I. Introduction

Multiple sclerosis (MS) is the most common neurological disease of young adults in Western countries. It is a chronic inflammatory disease of the central nervous system, in which myelin sheaths are the main target of tissue injury (Charcot, 1968). This leads to the formation of focal demyelinated plaques, which are randomly distributed throughout the white matter of the brain and spinal cord (Babinski, 1885; Marburg, 1906). Demyelination, although less obvious on gross inspection of the brain, is also present in the gray matter, in particular in the cerebral and cerebellar cortex but also in the brainstem and the spinal cord (Brownell and Hughes, 1962; Lumsden, 1970). Although the disease primarily affects myelin, axons too are injured in and lost from the lesions. While the functional consequences of inflammation and demyelination are at least in part reversible, the deficit due to axonal loss is irreversible (Kornek and Lassmann, 1999; Bjartmar et al., 2000, 2003). Thus axonal destruction in MS is a major correlate of permanent neurological deficit in the patients. MS lesions can also in part be repaired spontaneously by remyelination. This can be quite extensive at early stages of the disease, where large plaques become completely remyelinated and remain in the CNS as so-called shadow plaques (Lassmann, 1983; Prineas, 1985). At late stages of the disease and in particular in patients with progressive disease, the remyelinating capacity is low and remyelination is mostly restricted to small rims at the lesion edges.

Multiple sclerosis is a disease with heterogeneous clinical course and pathology (Noseworthy et al., 2000; Lucchinetti et al., 2000). In most patients the disease starts with relapses and remissions but converts after several years of duration into a state of slow uninterrupted progression (the secondary progressive stage of MS). About 20% of the patients miss the relapsing-remitting stage of the disease but

153

start with continuous disease progression from the onset. This type of disease is called primary progressive MS. More rare variants of multiple sclerosis are acute MS (Marburg's type; Marburg, 1906) or benign MS. In addition, special disease variants exist. Devic's type of neuromyelitis optica in most instances takes an acute and rapidly progressive course and is characterized by the selective or dominant involvement of the spinal cord and the optic nerves (Devic, 1894). Balo's concentric sclerosis, too, is an acute variant of MS, which is defined by the appearance of large demyelinated plaques with concentric layering of myelinated and demyelinated areas (Baló, 1928).

When actively demyelinating lesions are analyzed in a large sample of patients with MS, distinctly heterogeneous patterns of demyelination can be identified (Lucchinetti et al., 2000). These patterns suggest that in different patients different immunological mechanisms are involved in demyelination and tissue destruction. Although in some patients demyelination seems to be mainly mediated by T-lymphocytes and activated macrophages or microglia, in others a prominent involvement of antibodies and complement is apparent. In another subgroup active lesions display features of a hypoxia-like tissue injury (Aboul-Enein et al., 2003). Finally in a small number of patients, an unusually severe involvement of oligodendrocytes is present, suggesting an increased susceptibility of these cells for immune-mediated injury. This pathological heterogeneity may in part reflect differences in the stage of the disease or the severity of the lesions and clearly segregates in the extreme variants of the disease, such as Devic's (Lucchinetti et al., 2002) and Balo's disease. More importantly, however, it may reflect the highly polygenic nature of the disease.

For many years research in MS focused on mechanisms of inflammation and demyelination. Only recently has the importance of axonal involvement in the disease been recognized (Ferguson et al., 1997; Trapp et al., 1998). Since axonal loss is associated with permanent functional deficit, neuroprotective and axonoprotective therapeutic strategies may become increasingly important. A prerequisite for their design, however, is to understand where and when axons are destroyed in MS and the mechanisms of axonal destruction.

II. Pathology of Axonal Injury in Multiple Sclerosis

A. History

When MS pathology was defined at the end of the nineteenth century, whether the primary lesion in the central nervous system (CNS) affects myelin or axons was controversial. Fromann (1878), mainly concentrating on spinal cord lesions, emphasized axonal transection and loss within lesions and tract degeneration. In contrast, Charcot

(1880), focusing more on brain lesions, defined MS as a demyelinating disease, although he, too, acknowledged the presence of axonal injury and loss. In detailed morphological studies performed at the turn of the nineteenth century, it became clear that primary demyelination is the key and most characteristic pattern of tissue damage in MS lesions (Babinski, 1885; Charcot, 1880); however, this did not imply that axons are unaffected in this disease. As clearly pointed out by Marburg (1906), the hallmark of the MS lesions is primary demyelination with *relative* sparing of axons. Remarkable progress in the understanding of the fate of axons in MS was achieved during the next three decades. It became clear that axonal injury is most pronounced during the phase of active demyelination, occurring already during the earliest bouts of the disease (Doinikov, 1915) and that a close association of macrophages to degenerating axons suggests the active role of these cells in the destructive process (Fraenkel and Jakob, 1913). The detection of axonal end bulbs with sproutlike processes suggested attempts of regeneration (Doinikov, 1915; Jakob, 1915). Finally, even in these early studies, it was proposed that axonal injury may be an important substrate for permanent functional deficit in patients with MS (Charcot, 1880). Thus, most of the aspects of axonal injury in MS lesions, which are the main focus of research at present, were described and discussed in detail about 100 years ago (for details on historical aspects, see Kornek and Lassmann, 1999). Why has this knowledge been forgotten or even suppressed for so many years?

In the neuropathology community, this knowledge was alive, but not regarded as terribly important. It was clear also from other diseases that primary demyelination invariably is associated with axonal injury, but the clinical importance of this association was ignored. For researchers outside the neuropathology community, axonal pathology just did not fit the concept of MS being an autoimmune disease against myelin. Only detailed clinical studies with magnetic resonance imaging (MRI) and spectroscopy followed by detailed quantitative morphological investigations (Ferguson et al., 1997; Trapp et al., 1998) shed light on the clinical importance of axonal injury in patients with MS and stimulated major research efforts to understand the underlying mechanisms and to find therapeutic clues to prevent permanent axonal damage in this disease.

B. Extent and Timing of Axonal Injury in MS Lesions

The extent of axonal loss in established MS lesions is highly variable between different plaques within a single brain and even more variable between MS plaques from different patients (Fig.1). Some axonal loss is present in all MS lesions; the extent of axonal density reduction in plaques, however, may range from 20% to nearly 100%. Analysis of axonal density in relation to lesion development shows in

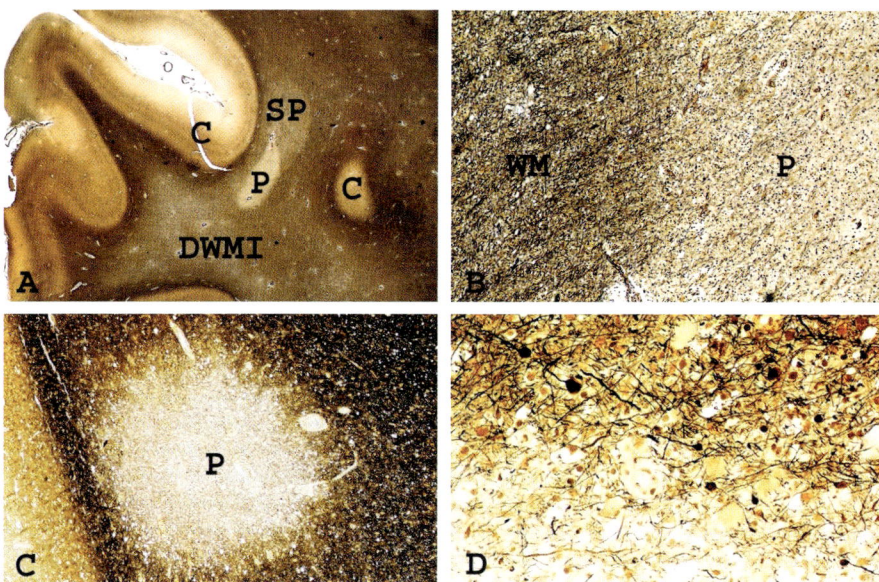

Figure 1 **Axonal loss in multiple sclerosis lesions.** (**A**) Subcortical white matter in a patient with primary progressive multiple sclerosis, stained for axons with Bieschowsky's silver impregnation. A small subcortical plaque (P) shows marked reduction in axonal staining, while an adjacent remyelinated shadow plaque (SP) reveals much higher axonal density; in addition there is diffuse axonal loss within the whole white matter (DWMI = diffuse white matter injury; C = cortex) (× 2). (**B**) Edge of the plaque shown in (**A**); note the profound reduction in axonal profiles in the plaque (P) compared to the adjacent white matter (WM) (× 100). (**C**) Small subcortical plaque in a patient with acute multiple sclerosis; extensive reduction in axonal density within the plaque (P). Bielschowsky's silver impregnation (× 5). (**D**) Edge of the plaque shown in (**C**); massive reduction of axonal profiles in the plaque and numerous axonal spheroids (acute axonal injury) at the plaque edge (× 300).

initial actively demyelinating lesions an average reduction of 30% to 40%. This reduction is only due in part to axonal loss, but also mediated by local edema and inflammatory infiltration of the tissue. Thus, in later stages of active lesions, as well as in remyelinated shadow plaques, axonal density in general is higher compared to that in acute lesions. In contrast, in permanently demyelinated lesions the reduction of axonal density is on average much more pronounced compared to fresh lesions, reaching average levels of 50% to 70% (Mews et al., 1998). The reason for this further reduction of axonal density in old demyelinated plaques may be twofold. First, the same areas in the CNS may become the target for repeated demyelinating attacks (Prineas et al., 1993), each bout leading not only to new demyelination, but also to further axonal injury and loss. In addition there is a slow burning axonal injury within old inactive demyelinated lesions, which in the long term may contribute to a major extent to the final axonal loss in established plaques (Kornek et al., 2000).

All these studies are based on simple determination of axonal density within a given tissue area; however, this only partially reflects true axonal loss and may lead to false estimates of axonal loss in acute lesions due to tissue edema or in old established plaques due to tissue atrophy. This problem was recently overcome by counting axons within defined tract systems (Bjartmar et al., 2000; Evangelou et al., 2000a). This method allows the determination of true axonal loss, independent from changes due to edema or atrophy. Overall, the values for axonal loss determined by this method were similar to those established by simple determination of axonal density, also showing an average axonal loss in established lesions in the range of 50% to 70%. This indicates that the variation in the extent of axonal loss between plaques of different stages or from different patients is larger than the effect of tissue edema or atrophy.

Another way to determine the extent of axonal damage in MS lesions is to study acute axonal injury at different stages of plaque formation (Ferguson et al., 1997). Earliest signs of axonal injury are reflected by a disturbance of fast axonal transport. Thus proteins or other molecules trafficking along the axons by fast axonal transport accumulate at the sites of axonal injury. A very reliable marker for the disturbance of axonal transport is the focal accumulation of amyloid precursor protein (β-APP). Disturbed axonal transport also leads to the formation of focal axonal swelling, which may occur either at sites of axonal transsection or uninterrupted axons (Fig. 2).

Using these tools to study acute axonal injury in MS plaques, it was found that massive axonal damage occurs during the phase of active demyelination in fresh lesions (Ferguson et al., 1997; Trapp et al., 1998; Kornek et al,. 2000; Bitsch et al., 2000). Thus, axonal loss and damage take place in every newly formed lesion, regardless of whether it develops during the earliest or at late stages of the disease. Analysis of brain biopsies taken in patients at the first bout of the disease even suggested that axonal injury at this stage may be more severe compared to that in lesions formed in the chronic stage (Kuhlmann et al., 2002). This, however, seems to be due to a sampling bias, as biopsies in patients with MS are rare and generally restricted to patients with very severe and atypical disease.

Besides the profound axonal injury, which occurs in actively demyelinating lesions, there is an additional slow burning axonal injury and loss, which is present in inactive demyelinated plaques (Kornek et al., 2000). Although the extent of axonal injury at a given time in these chronic lesions is more than hundred times lower compared to that in active plaques, it may be of major significance. Acute lesions develop within a few days to weeks, whereas chronic demyelinated plaques may persist in the CNS for many years. Thus even a smoldering ongoing axonal injury within chronic lesions may contribute a large share to the total axonal loss in the MS brain. This slow burning chronic axonal injury is absent when plaques are remyelinated.

Axonal injury and loss in MS brains are not restricted to demyelinated plaques (Evangelou et al., 2000b; Bjartmar et al., 2001). In particular in patients with primary or secondary progressive MS, a diffuse inflammatory process is found throughout the whole brain and spinal cord, thus also affecting the so-called normal white matter. This diffuse inflammatory process is associated with diffuse axonal injury and loss, which leads to fiber degeneration and secondary myelin destruction. This process is reflected by diffuse myelin pallor throughout the whole white matter. The extensive activation of local microglia and their expression of inducible nitric oxide synthase suggests that the diffuse white matter damage in chronic MS is mainly mediated through reactive oxygen and nitrogen intermediates.

Within the plaques not all axons are destroyed to the same extent. Thick axons are much better preserved than thin fibers (Evangelou et al., 2001). This could in part be explained by changes in axonal caliber in the course of demyelination. Indeed, it has been shown by light microscopy more than 100 years ago (Marburg, 1906), and later been confirmed by electron microscopy (Shintaku et al., 1988), that demyelinated internodes in MS lesions have thicker calibers than their respective myelinated axonal portions. In addition to a dominant reduction of thin fibers that has been found within the plaques, however, there is also a preferential loss of small neurons at the sites of axonal origin (Evangelou et al., 2001). This can most clearly be seen in the retina in patients with demyelinated plaques in the optic nerve. It thus seems that overall thin axons, originating from small neurons, are more vulnerable in MS lesions compared to thick axons. As discussed later, one major factor responsible for axonal disintegration within plaques seems to be mitochondrial dysfunction and energy failure (Smith and Lassmann, 2002). In such a situation, it is likely that small axons, which contain fewer mitochondria compared to thick ones, are affected more severely.

III. Consequences of Axonal Injury Within Demyelinated Plaques

Disruption of the axonal continuity within a demyelinated plaque has necessarily to result in degenerations of the distal portion of the nerve fiber. In addition, axon disruption may also lead to retrograde degeneration, affecting the proximal axon and the neuron of origin. It has thus to be expected that degenerative alterations occur in MS brain outside the classical plaques.

Many studies have shown the presence of secondary (Wallerian) tract degeneration in MS brains (see Kornek and Lassmann, 1999). As an example, the extent of fiber degeneration and atrophy in the corpus callosum correlated well with the size and destructiveness of demyelinated plaques in the adjacent cerebral hemispheres (Evangelou et al., 2000a). The situation is even more impressive in the spinal cord. In this area of the CNS, loss of axons in defined tract systems is similar within demyelinated plaques compared to that in spinal cord areas not affected by focal demyelinated lesions (Lovas et al., 2000; Ganter et al., 1999). This is at first glance a paradox, which resolves when it is considered that axonal degeneration in a single plaque in a defined tract sys-

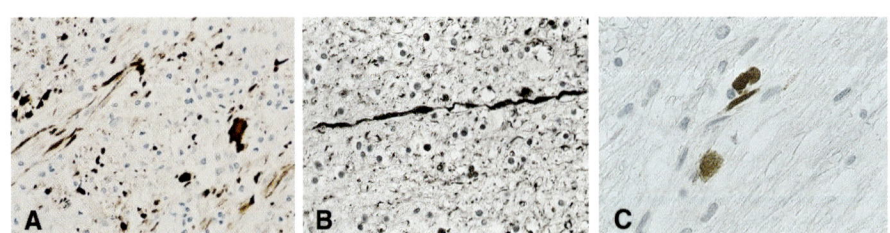

Figure 2 Acute axonal injury in active multiple sclerosis plaques. (**A**) Multiple large axonal swellings (spheroids) reactive for nonphosphorylated neurofilament (× 600). (**B**) Longitudinal section of an axon within an active demyelinating plaque; multiple small beadlike swellings within the course of the axon, suggesting disturbance of axonal transport; immunocytochemistry for nonphosphorylated neurofilament (× 600). (**C**) Small axonal spheroids, reactive for Alzheimer amyloid precursor protein, as a sign of disturbed axonal transport (× 600).

tem has inevitably to result in secondary Wallerian degeneration of the whole distal portion.

Much less evidence is available for retrograde degeneration of axons and neurons in MS. Only a few studies described swollen "chromatolytic" neurons suggestive of a retrograde reaction due to axonal injury (Lumsden, 1970). In our experience this may occur sometimes in the cortex of patients with very destructive lesions, located in the subcortical white matter (Fig. 3). Whether the recently described signs of neuronal apoptosis in the cerebral cortex (Peterson et al., 2001) are related to retrograde degeneration or to active demyelinating lesions in the cerebral cortex is unresolved. In addition, in a single case neuronophagia by microglia cells was described and regarded as evidence for profound neuronal damage (Fraenkel and Jakob, 1913). In this particular case, however, it remained open whether the pronounced neuronal degeneration in the cortex was due to a superimposed meningoencephalitis. Whether the cortical atrophy, seen in quantitative MRI studies at later stages of the disease (Bozzali et al., 2002), is mainly due to cortical demyelination or to secondary retrograde degeneration, is currently unresolved.

These alterations, secondary to axonal degeneration in the plaques, which affect the brain as a whole, have been summarized under the term *multiple sclerosis encephalopathy* (Jellinger, 1969). This condition is characterized by tissue atrophy, which is more pronounced in the white than in the gray matter, and reflected by the progressive dilation of the lateral cerebral ventricles with increasing disease duration. On a fine structural basis, this diffuse brain damage is associated with chronic activation of microglia and a diffuse astrocytic scarring in the "normal" white matter.

For a long time, it has been believed that all diffuse abnormalities in the "normal" white matter of patients with

MS are secondary to axonal degeneration within the plaques; however, this seems not to be the case. In particular, in patients with primary progressive MS, a massive diffuse damage of the whole "normal" white matter is seen, which frequently occurs in spite of only very few local plaques. Such diffuse changes cannot be explained by secondary alterations occurring as a consequence of axonal degeneration in the plaques (Pelletier et al., 2003).

A. Changes in Axons in the Course of and After Demyelination

When axons lose their myelin sheaths, sodium channels primarily remain located at the former nodes of Ranvier. After some days, sodium channels redistribute along the whole internode. Thus conduction is temporarily blocked in acutely demyelinated axons, but is restored later. This has also been directly shown to happen in MS plaques, where sodium channels have been found throughout the whole internode in established demyelinated lesions (Moll et al., 1991). In addition, changes in the expression patterns of sodium channel subtypes may occur, which may disturb the functional properties of demyelinated axons (Waxman, 2001; Craner et al., 2003, 2004; see Chapter 7).

Besides sodium channels, other molecules located at the myelin/axon interface, too, show abnormalities in their expression in demyelinated MS plaques. The axonal glycoprotein contactin-associated protein (Caspr), which is normally expressed in paranodal regions of myelinated fibers, is lost from demyelinated axons in the plaques, but reappears when remyelination is initiated. In addition, however, more subtle alterations in Caspr expression occur in the periplaque white matter, suggesting myelin abnormalities that extend beyond the borders of demyelinated plaques (Wolswijk and Balesar, 2003).

In addition, axonal transport is disturbed in acutely injured axons. Thus, ion channels, which are transported within the axons to reach the synaptic terminals, may accumulate at the sites of acute damage. In MS lesions, for instance, the accumulation of N-type voltage-gated calcium channels at sites of acute axonal injury has been shown, and ultrastructural studies in demyelinating lesions of autoimmune encephalitis have found that these channels are even inserted in the axonal membrane (Kornek et al., 2001). Although it has not been shown that these channels are functionally active, aberrantly expressed calcium channels in the axolemma could further increase influx of calcium in sublethally injured axons within the plaques and may further augment the damage.

Axons that survive the acute injury during the active phase of demyelination are profoundly abnormal. At least in early and active lesions, the axonal caliber changes at the site of the first demyelinated internode (Marburg, 1906). The axons in the demyelinated portions are generally thicker compared to their myelinated segments and cytoskeletal

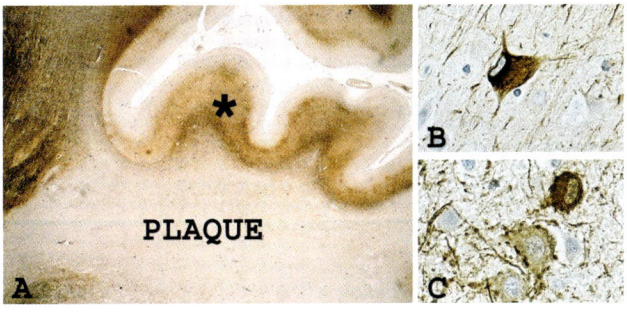

Figure 3 Retrograde neuronal reaction in the cerebral cortex in multiple sclerosis. (**A**) Large demyelinated subcortical plaque in a patient with acute multiple sclerosis. The staining by Bielschowsky's silver impregnation shows massive reduction of axonal density in the subcortical plaque. The alterations in the superimposed cortex (*arrow*) are shown in **B** and **C** (× 2). (**B, C**) Neuronal reaction in the cortex, superimposed over a plaque with massive axonal injury; the neurons show an enlarged pericaryon, eccentric positioning of the nucleus and massive expression of phosphorylated neurofilament epitopes, features which are typical for a retrograde reaction following axotomy (× 500).

proteins appear deranged (Shintaku et al., 1988). This difference is also associated with profound changes in the composition and functional state of cytoskeletal proteins. The degree of phosphorylation of neurofilament subunits decreases (Trapp et al., 1998). Finally, the expression of ubiquitin within the demyelinated axons in MS plaques has been reported (Giordana et al., 2003), indicating proteolytic cleavage of intra-axonal proteins.

Some demyelinated plaques are rapidly remyelinated, whereas remyelination is sparse or absent in others, in spite of the presence of large numbers of oligodendrocyte progenitor cells (Chang et al., 2002). Thus, in some patients, axons within the demyelinated plaques seem to be nonpermissive for remyelination. PSA-NCAM, a molecule that is present on the axonal surface during development before myelination and that may inhibit the axon-oligodendrocyte interaction in the myelinating process, is reexpressed on demyelinated axons in such lesions (Charles et al., 2002).

IV. Mechanisms of Axonal Damage in MS

When discussing the mechanisms of axonal damage in MS lesions, two different phases of axonal destruction have to be distinguished. The trigger of axonal injury most likely depends on cells or mediators of the activated immune system and may be heterogeneous, depending on the genetic background of the patients. This immune response triggers downstream events, which finally lead to the complete dissolution of the axon. As it appears now, the downstream events in axonal degeneration seem to be conserved between different patients and may even be similar in different diseases, such as MS, stroke, or brain trauma.

A. Triggers of Axonal Injury in Patients with MS

In principle, axons can be attacked through antigen-specific interactions with T-lymphocytes or antibodies, as well as through antigen-independent events, mediated by toxic products of macrophages or microglia cells. *In vitro* studies show that not only the nerve cell bodies, but also the axons can be selectively attacked by cytotoxic T-lymphocytes, in a reaction that depends on the recognition of specific antigen in the context of class I MHC molecules (Medana et al., 2001). In MS lesions, there is a weak, but significant correlation between the number of Class I MHC restricted CD8[+] T-lymphocytes and the extent of acute axonal injury (Bitsch et al., 2000). This correlation was not found for total T-cells or CD4[+] T-cells. Neurons and axons may express Class I MHC molecules in MS lesions (Höftberger et al., 2004). These structures are, thus, potential targets for a direct T-cell-mediated attack. By studying lesions of Marburg's type of acute MS, a direct interaction between

cytotoxic T-cells and axons can sometimes be observed. In this situation T-lymphocytes, which express granzyme B as a marker for their cytotoxic potential, are found in close contact with acutely demyelinated axons (Neumann et al., 2002). In addition, these lymphocytes form zones of contact with the axon, which are characterized by a polar orientation of cytotoxic granules toward the contact zone. Such structural features of T-cell contact with axons closely resemble the formation of immunological synapses, which can be seen *in vitro*, when cytotoxic T-cells interact with their target cells. Thus, direct T-cell-mediated injury of axons seems to play a role at least in some MS lesions (Neumann et al., 2002).

Axons could also possibly be damaged by specific antibodies through the activation of complement or the interaction with activated macrophages. Although deposition of activated complement at sites of active demyelination is a specific feature of a subtype of MS lesions (Lucchninetti et al., 2000), clear-cut evidence of a dressing of axonal surfaces with antibodies and activated complement has up to now not been provided. Furthermore, antibodies against axonal components, detected in serum or cerebrospinal fluid (CSF) of patients with MS, are mainly directed against intracytoplasmic determinants, which are not accessible on the intact axonal surface.

Although, as described previously, there is some correlation between the numbers of CD8[+] T-cells and acute axonal injury in MS lesions, this correlation is very weak in comparison to that with activated macrophages and microglia cells. The close association between degenerating axons and macrophages was noted nearly 100 years ago in a study by Fraenkel and Jakob (1913) and has recently been confirmed in more detailed quantitative studies (Ferguson et al., 1997; Trapp et al., 1998; Kornek et al., 2000). Several different toxic products of macrophages have been identified, which may mediate axonal injury *in vitro* or *in vivo* in experimental models. Proteases, directly applied into the CNS parenchyma, may not only trigger demyelination, but also axonal injury (Anthony et al., 1998). Other molecules that are likely to be involved in axonal injury are reactive oxygen or nitrogen species (see Chapter 18). Nitric oxide, applied on demyelinated nerve fibers *in vitro*, can induce acute conduction block, thus being responsible for temporary and reversible functional deficit (Redford et al., 1997). Furthermore, nitric oxide may induce irreversible axonal destruction when acting on electrically active nerve fibers (Smith et al., 2001). Since nitric oxide impairs mitochondrial function (Bolanos et al., 1997), the degeneration of electrically active axons may at least in part be due to a disturbance in their energy metabolism (Kalman and Leist, 2003). Such a disturbance may impair clearance of intra-axonally accumulated calcium ions.

Other possible candidates for initiation of axonal damage in MS lesions are excitotoxins (Pitt et al., 2000; Smith et al., 2000). Experimental data have shown that axonal and neuronal destruction can be ameliorated *in vivo* through the blockade of AMPA-type glutamate receptors. Pathological studies in MS lesions indicate that there may be a disturbance of glutamate homeostasis within actively demyelinating plaques. These data suggest an increased synthesis of glutamate within the lesions, which may occur in parallel with a decreased detoxification of glutamate by astrocytes (Werner et al., 2001). Although in experimental studies an axonoprotective effect of AMPA receptor blockers has been described (Pitt et al., 2000), direct evidence for the expression of the respective glutamate receptors on demyelinated axons is lacking. It is not clear, therefore, whether axonal damage is mediated through a glutamate effect on the axon itself or through damage of neuronal cell bodies leading to secondary axonal degeneration.

All these data suggest that various different immunological mechanisms may trigger axonal injury in inflammatory demyelinating lesions and that these triggers may be heterogeneous between patients, depending on the dominant immunological mechanism responsible for tissue damage. It thus seems unlikely that interference with a single one of these mechanisms will be of major therapeutic value in all patients.

B. Execution Pathways of Axonal Destruction

Although the initial triggers of axonal damage may be heterogenous between different MS patients, the consecutive steps leading to axonal dissolution appear to be more uniform. A key event occurring at the earliest stages of axonal degeneration appears to be the uncontrolled influx of sodium ions into the axoplasm. For instance, this may be responsible for axonal depolarization and conduction block, induced by nitric oxide toxicity (Redford et al., 1997). In a consecutive step axoplasmic sodium ions appear to be replaced by Ca^{2+} through a reverse operation of the Na^+/Ca^{2+} exchanger (Waxman, 2002; see Chapter 19). Intra-axonal accumulation of Ca^{2+} may then activate proteases, which will initiate the degradation of cytoskeletal proteins. The result of this process is an acute disturbance of fast axonal transport, which is reflected by the focal accumulation of proteins such as, for instance, amyloid precursor protein or N-type voltage-gated calcium channels (Kornek et al., 2001). The latter can aberrantly be incorporated into the axonal membrane at the site of axonal injury, which may further increase influx of Ca^{2+} into the axolemma. The final result of the Ca^{2+} overload will then be the complete dissolution of intra-axonal proteins and axonal disruption. Blockade of Na^+/Ca^{2+} exchanger and of N-type voltage-gated calcium channels has been shown to inhibit axonal degeneration (Stys et al., 1992; Kapoor et al., 2003).

As discussed previously, these mechanisms have so far been identified and defined in experimental models *in vitro* and *in vivo*. Direct evidence for their involvement in axonal

destruction in MS lesions is lacking. Future studies are needed to show whether axonal degeneration can be inhibited in patients with MS through therapeutic interference with these mechanisms.

V. Gray Matter Involvement in Patients with Multiple Sclerosis

Multiple sclerosis is generally perceived as a disease that affects the white matter of the CNS. Indeed on gross inspection of the brain, demyelinated plaques can easily be identified in the white matter and are hardly seen in the cortex or the gray matter of deep cerebral nuclei. However, early microscopic studies of MS brains clearly documented that demyelination may also affect the cerebral cortex or the brainstem nuclei (Brownell and Hughes, 1962; Lumsden, 1970). In addition, MRI of the brain of patients with MS shows profound atrophy of the gray matter, in particular of the cerebral cortex, which is mainly present in patients with long-standing progressive disease (Bozzali et al., 2002). Gray matter atrophy also appears to be a better correlate of cognitive dysfunction in patients with MS, compared with lesion load in the white matter (Rovaris et al., 2000; Charil et al., 2003). Thus, the cerebral cortex in patients with MS can be affected in two distinctly different ways, by general cortical atrophy and by focal demyelinated plaques.

A. Cortical Atrophy

Cortical atrophy in MS has not been systematically addressed in neuropathological studies. A global reduction of cortical thickness, associated with decreased volumes of cortical gyri and widening of sulci, can be seen in patients with long-standing disease. For two reasons, however, neuropathological data on cortical atrophy are so far inconclusive. First, they are based only on subjective observations derived from single patients and have not been substantiated by exact, quantitative morphometric investigations. Second, most patients in whom such cortical changes have been observed were in an advanced age group, where age-related neuropathological changes are also present.

Diffuse cortical atrophy appears at least in part to be a consequence of axonal destruction in the white matter, which occurs either within demyelinated plaques or diffusely in the so-called "normal" white matter. This view is supported by the occasional presence of chromatolytic cortical neurons, which is a characteristic alteration of retrograde reaction or degeneration (Fig. 3). This is particularly the case in patients with destructive subcortical plaques. Thus, neuronal degeneration in the cortex of MS patients may occur as a reaction to axonal injury within the white matter. How extensive it is, and to what extent it is the pathological substrate of cortical atrophy seen in quantitative MRI studies, remains to be determined.

B. Cortical Plaques

The subcortical white matter has been identified as one of the predilection sites for MS lesions (Lumsden, 1970). Many of them are leukocortical lesions; thus they affect both the cortex and the white matter. In addition, pure intracortical lesions have been described. Detailed studies on cortical plaques, performed during the last years, have identified three different types of lesions, which are distinct in several important aspects (Kidd et al., 1999; Peterson et al., 2001; Bo et al., 2003).

Leuko-cortical plaques (compound plaques): These lesions are located at the cortico-subcortical junction and thus affect both the gray and white matter.

Focal intracortical plaques: These are small demyelinated lesions located entirely within the cortex and generally centered by a small vein or venule.

Bandlike (CSF-oriented) demyelination of the outer cortical layers: These lesions are characterized by a bandlike demyelination, which affects the outer three to five layers of the cortex. They may extend over large distances of the cortical surface, even involving more than one gyrus (Fig. 4).

Whereas leukocortical and focal intracortical lesions, like their counterparts in the white matter, are centered by small veins or venules, the bandlike lesions show a topographical orientation, which is clearly related to inflammation in the meninges. Furthermore, the fine structural changes within these bandlike cortical lesions strongly suggest that they are induced by mediators that are produced within meningeal inflammatory cells and diffuse into the cortex from the meningeal surface.

C. Structural Features of Cortical Lesions in MS

The structural features of cortical lesions differ in several aspects from those of white matter plaques. Although, as in white matter plaques (Trebst et al., 2001), microglia activation is always associated with active demyelination in the cortex, the density of perivascular and diffuse inflammation by T-lymphocytes and B-cells is very low (Bo et al., 2003). Thus classical perivascular inflammatory infiltrates are rare, and the diffuse infiltration of T- and B-cells is sparse and not significantly different from that in the adjacent normal cortex. This difference in the degree of inflammation between gray and white matter lesions can be directly seen in active leukocortical plaques, where the cortico-subcortical border sharply demarcates the profound inflammation in the white matter compared to the minimal inflammation in the gray matter (Fig. 5). This is also reflected in the sparse or absent blood-brain barrier leakage in cortical plaques (Fig. 5). Furthermore, microglia cells in the cortex generally main-

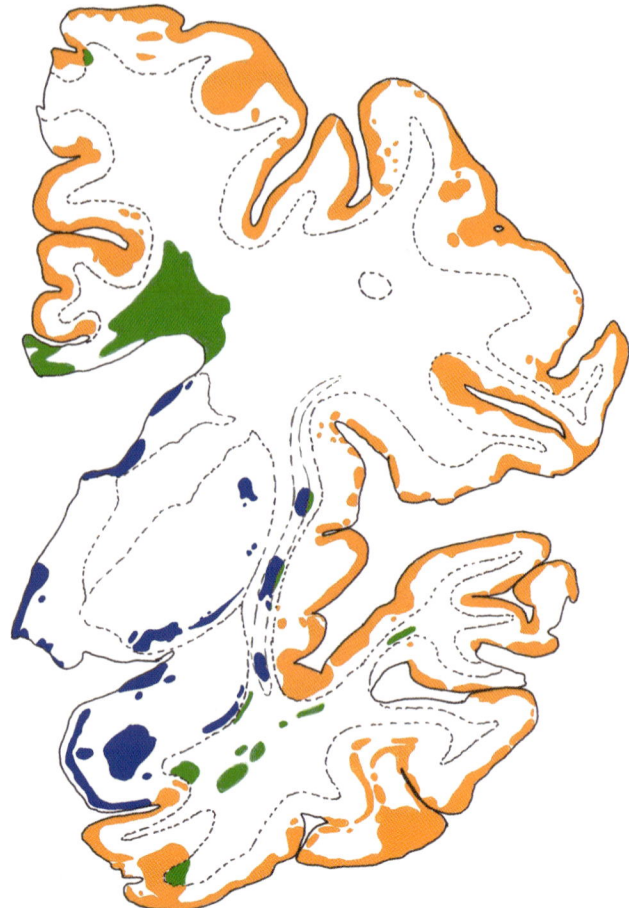

Figure 4 Distribution of demyelinating lesions in the brain of a patient with secondary progressive multiple sclerosis. Large lesions are present in the white matter, in particular in periventricular location (*green lesions*); in addition there is massive demyelination in the cerebral cortex (*orange lesions*); most of the cortical lesions are bandlike areas of demyelination, which affect the outermost layers of the cortex; furthermore, lesions can also be found in the deep gray matter, such as for instance the basal ganglia (*blue lesions*).

tain the ramified phenotype (Bo et al., 2003), while in white matter plaques, they are rapidly transformed into a macrophage phenotype (Trebst et al., 2001). The low intensity of the inflammatory reaction within active cortical plaques may explain why they are not detected as enhancing lesions in MRI.

A second feature that distinguishes cortical plaques from those in the white matter is the degree of selectivity of the pathological process. As mentioned previously, demyelination in the white matter is associated with quite extensive axonal loss. This results in a massive increase in the volume of the extracellular space, which renders the plaques easily detectable in conventional MRI sequences. Demyelination in the cortex is also associated with some acute axonal injury and some neuronal degeneration or alterations of dendrites (Peterson et al., 2001). Overall, however, this neuronal and axonal degeneration is minor compared to that occurring in the white matter, and the loss of cells does not lead to a major expansion of the cortical extracellular space (Fig. 5). Considering further the

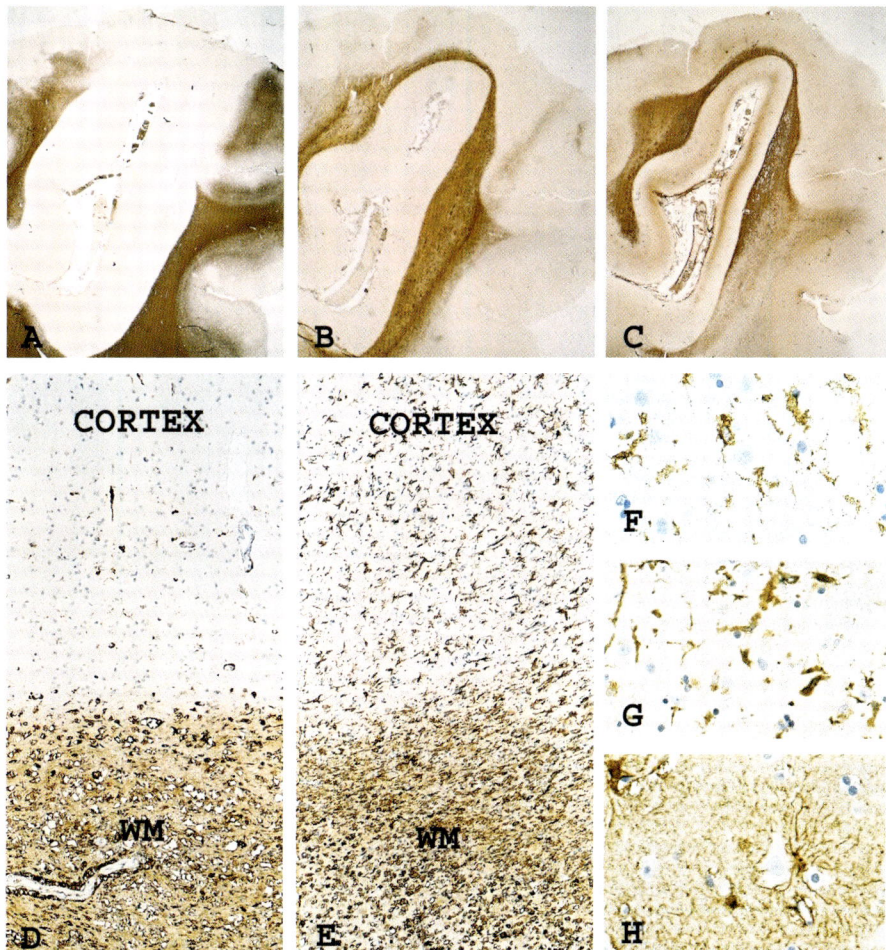

Figure 5 **Demyelinated plaques in the cerebral cortex in a patient with secondary progressive multiple sclerosis.** (A) Staining for myelin shows widespread demyelination, affecting all cortical areas and extending into the subcortical white matter; the meninges in the center of the lesion show massive inflammation (×2) (B) Immunocytochemistry for HLA-D (activated microglia and macrophages) shows massive expression in the white matter areas of the plaques, but very little in the gray matter areas (× 2). (C) A similar distribution is also found by immunocytochemistry for immunoglobulins, which shows massive blood-brain barrier leakage in the white matter areas, but very little in the cortical areas (× 2). (D) Inactive demyelinated plaque affecting the white as well as the gray matter (cortex); immunocytochemistry for HLA-D shows profound residual macrophage infiltration in the white matter areas (WM), but very little in the gray matter (CORTEX) (× 80). (E) Actively demyelinating lesion in the cortex and subcortical white matter; in the white matter most HLA-D-positive cells show a macrophage phenotype, while in the cortex, most HLA-D-positive cells are activated microglia cells (× 80). (F, G) Actively demyelinating lesions in the cortex express inducible nitric oxide synthase (i-NOS) in activated microglia cells (× 300). (H) Demyelinated cortical lesions show profound expression of glia fibrillary acidic protein (GFAP) in reactive astrocytes (× 300).

fact that myelin sheaths occupy only a small fraction of the total cortical volume, it is not surprising that most cortical plaques escape detection by conventional MRI.

D. Cortical Lesions are a Discriminative Variable between Acute/Relapsing MS and Progressive MS

One of the most characteristic differences between acute or relapsing MS and secondary or primary progressive MS is the affection of the cerebral and cerebellar cortex. Cortical

plaques are very rare in patients with acute or early relapsing-remitting MS, and when present their size is very small. This is fundamentally different in patients with secondary or primary progressive MS, where demyelination on average affects 20% to 30% of the total cortical area. Most of the cortical plaques in progressive MS are bandlike lesions, oriented toward the outer surface of the brain. Furthermore, in patients with progressive MS, there is no relation between the lesion load in the white matter and the presence of cortical plaques. This is most dramatically seen in patients with primary progressive MS, where the incidence and size of white matter plaques may be very low, while demyelination may affect up to 50% of the cerebral and cerebellar cortical area.

It is not clear to what extent demyelination in the cortex contributes to clinical disability in the patients. Because of the relatively minor destruction and loss of cortical neurons and axons, it is unlikely that there is a major contribution to focal deficits. The diffuse nature of the demyelinated lesions in the cerebral and cerebellar cortex, however, may contribute to the development of cognitive deficits and cerebellar disturbances, which are generally prominent in patients with primary and secondary progressive MS. Furthermore, cortical lesions may be involved in the generation of epileptic seizures which are present in patients with MS patients in higher frequency than in the normal population (Spatt et al., 2001; Poser and Brinar, 2003).

E. Mechanisms of Demyelination and Tissue Injury in Cortical Plaques

Most cortical lesions are based on the outer surface of the brain and extend in variable depth into the cortical ribbon (Peterson et al., 2001; Bo et al., 2003). Active cortical lesions are always associated with the presence of meningeal inflammatory infiltrates in the respective regions (Fig. 5). Furthermore, their topography suggests that they may arise in areas where the CSF flow is impaired. This is reflected by their location in the cerebral sulci and the deep invaginations of the brain surface, such as the insular region, the cingulate gyrus, and the indentation in the temporal lobe (Fig. 4). On a structural basis, cortical lesions are characterized by demyelination, which is associated with microglia activation, but by very sparse or absent T- and B-cell infiltrates around cortical vessels or within the parenchyma of the lesion itself (Bo et al., 2003). The only way to explain the topography, shape, and structure of such a lesion is to postulate that inflammatory cells within the meninges—possibly T-cells or B-cells—produce factors that diffuse into the cortex and mediate tissue damage, either directly or indirectly through the activation of microglia cells. What could these factors be?

One factor could be the production of autoreactive antibodies within the meningeal compartment. Such antibodies could then mediate demyelination and/or tissue damage either through complement activation or through the interaction with activated microglia. Indeed, intrathecal production of antibodies is a typical feature of MS and is particularly prominent in patients with progressive MS. Furthermore, high numbers of B-cells in the CSF of MS patients appears to be associated with a severe disease course and pronounced disease progression (Cepok et al., 2001). With a single exception, our own immunopathological studies did not provide evidence for a local precipitation of immunoglobulins or activated complement on degenerating cortical myelin. It may, however, be that current methods are not sensitive enough to detect antibody-mediated

demyelination in a slowly burning demyelinating process, as it is characteristic for cortical lesions.

Another way to explain the formation of such lesions is that meningeal inflammatory cells produce inflammatory mediators that are either directly toxic for myelin or that activate cortical microglia to produce myelinotoxic molecules. As discussed before regarding mechanisms of axonal injury, nitric oxide may play a major role in the induction of cortical tissue injury (Smith and Lassmann, 2002). In actively demyelinating cortical lesions all microglia cells express inducible nitric oxide synthase (Fig. 5). Nitric oxide together with oxygen radicals may exert a direct toxic effect by the formation of peroxynitrite, and oligodendrocytes seem to be particularly vulnerable. In addition, it may also affect mitochondrial function and may thus potentiate the toxic effect in cells or cell processes that have either low numbers of mitochondria or are exposed to energy-demanding stress situations. The latter mechanisms may be particularly important in the induction of axonal and neuronal damage. However, if microglia cells are the prime source of toxic mediators, such as for instance nitric oxide, the question as to what T- or B-cell-derived factors are responsible for microglia activation in cortical plaques remains open.

VI. Conclusion

Although MS is generally considered to be a demyelinating disease, the importance of axonal and neuronal pathology cannot be overestimated. Although inflammation and demyelination lead to clinical deficit, which is at least in principle reversible, the consequences of axonal and neuronal loss can be compensated only by reorganization of CNS function, but not by repair. Axonal and neuronal pathology is undoubtedly an important feature of MS pathology and may already occur at early stages of the disease. Therapeutic strategies to prevent axonal and neuronal degeneration are thus urgently warranted.

The extent and importance of axonal and neuronal destruction and loss in patients with MS have only recently been acknowledged. Since current immunological therapies of MS have little effect on disease progression and the development of axonal loss and atrophy in patients' brains, it has been suggested that the basic problem in MS may even be a neurodegenerative process, which may be superimposed and aggravated in its consequences by the inflammatory reaction (Bjartmar et al., 2003; Owens, 2003; Kalman and Leist, 2003; Zamvil and Steinman, 2003). Although such a scenario cannot be ruled out at the present time, the data discussed in this chapter are more consistent with the notion that all aspects of MS pathology, including axonal and neuronal injury, are driven by an immune-mediated inflammatory response.

References

Aboul-Enein, F., Rauschka, H., Kornel, B., Stadelmann, C., Stefferl, A., Brück, W., Lucchinetti, C. F., Schmidbauer, M., Jellinger, K., and Lassmann, H. (2003). Preferential loss of myelin associated glycoprotein reflects hypoxia-like white matter damage in stroke and inflammatory brain diseases. *J. Neuropathol. Exp. Neurol.* **62**, 25–33.

Anthony, D. C., Miller, K. M., Fearn, S., Townsend, M. J., Opdenakker, G., Wells, G. M., Clements, J. M., Chandler, S., Gearing, A. J., and Perry, V. H. (1998). Matrix metalloproteinase expression in an experimentally-induced DTH model of multiple sclerosis in the rat CNS. *J. Neuroimmunol.* **87**, 62–72.

Babinski, J. (1885). Recherches sur l'anatomie pathologique de la sclerose en plaque et etude comparative des diverses varietes de la scleroses de la moelle. *Arch. Physiol. (Paris)* **5-6**, 186–207.

Baló, J. (1928). Encephalitis periaxialis concentrica. *Arch. Neurol. Psychiatry* **19**, 242–264.

Bitsch, A., Schuchardt, J., Bunkowski, S., Kuhlmann, T., and Bruck, W. (2000). Acute axonal injury in multiple sclerosis. Correlation with demyelination and inflammation. *Brain* **123**, 1174–1183.

Bitsch, A., Kuhlmann, T., Stadelmann, C., Lassmann, H., Lucchinetti, C., and Brück, W. (2001). A longitudinal MRI study of histopathologically defined hypointense multiple sclerosis lesions. *Ann. Neurol.* **49**, 793–796.

Bjartmar, C., Kidd, G., Mork, S., Rudick, R., and Trapp, B. D. (2000). Neurological disability correlates with spinal cord axonal loss and reduced N-acetyl aspartate in chronic multiple sclerosis patients. *Ann. Neurol.* **48**, 893–901.

Bjartmar, C., Kinkel, R. P., Kidd, G., Rudick, R. A., and Trapp, B. D. (2001). Axonal loss in normal-appearing white matter in a patient with acute MS. *Neurology* **57**, 1248–1252.

Bjartmar, C., Wujek, J. R., Trapp, B. D. (2003). Axonal loss in the pathology of MS: consequences for understanding the progressive phase of the disease. *J. Neurol. Sci.* **206**, 165–171.

Bo, L., Vedeler, C. A., Nyland, H. I., Trapp, B. D., and Mork, S. J. (2003). Subpial demyelination in the cerebral cortex of multiple sclerosis patients. *J. Neuropathol. Exp. Neurol.* **62**, 723–732.

Bolanos, J. P., Almeida, A., Stewart, V., Peuchen, S., Land, J. M., Clark, J. B., and Heales, S. J. (1997). Nitric oxide-mediated mitochondrial damage in the brain: Mechanisms and implications for neurodegenerative diseases. *J. Neurochem.* **68**, 2227–2240.

Bozzali, M., Cercignani, M., Sormani, M. P., Comi, G., and Filippi, M. (2002). Quantification of brain grey matter damage in different MS phenotypes by use of diffusion tensor MR imaging. *Am. J. Neuroradiol.* **23**, 985–988.

Brownell, B., and Hughes, J. T. (1962). The distribution of plaques in the cerebrum in multiple sclerosis. *J. Neurol. Neurosurg. Psychiatry* **25**, 315–320.

Cepok, S., Jacobsen, M., Schock, S., Omer, B., Jaekel, S., Böddeker, I., Oertel, W. H., Sommer, N., and Hemmer, B. (2001). Patterns of cerebrospinal fluid pathology correlate with disease progression in multiple sclerosis. *Brain* **124**, 2169–2176.

Charcot, J. M. (1868). Histologie de la sclerose en plaque. *Gaz Hopital (Paris)* **41**, 554–566.

Charcot, J. M. (1880). Lecons sur les maladies du systeme nerveux faites a la Salpetriere. Tome 1, 4e ed. Paris, 1880.

Charil, A., Zijdenbos, A. P., Taylor, J., Boelman, C., Worsley, K. J., Evans, A. C., and Dagher, A. (2003). Statistical mapping analysis of lesion location and neurological disability in multiple sclerosis: Application to 452 patient data sets. *Neuroimage* **19**, 532–544.

Charles, P., Reynolds, R., Seilhean, D., Rougon, G., Aigrot, M. S., Niezgoda, A., Zalc, B., and Lubetzki, C. (2002). Re-expression of PSA-NCAM by demyelinated axons: An inhibitor or remyelination in multiple sclerosis? *Brain* **125**, 1972–1979.

Chang, A., Tourtellotte, W. W., Rudick, R., and Trapp, B. D. (2002). Premyelinating oligodendrocytes in chronic lesions of multiple sclerosis. *N. Engl. J. Med.* **346**, 165–173.

Craner, M. J., Haines, B. C., Lo, A. C., Black, J. A., and Waxman, S. G. (2004). Co-localization of sodium channel $Na_v1.6$ and the sodium-calcium exchanger at sites of axonal injury in the spinal cord in EAE. *Brain* **127**, 294–303.

Craner, M. J., Lo, A. C., Black, J. A., and Waxman, S. G. (2003). Abnormal sodium channel distribution in optic nerve axons in a model of inflammatory demyelination. *Brain* **126**, 1552–1562.

Devic, E. (1894). Myelite subaigua compliquee de nevrite optique. *Bulletin Medical (Paris)* **8**, 1033.

Doinikow, B. (1915). Über De-und Regenerationserscheinungen an Achsenzylindern bei der multiplen Sklerose. *Z ges Neurol. Psychiat.* **27**, 151–178.

Evangelou, N., Esiri, M. M., Smith, S., Palace, J., and Matthews, P. M. (2000b). Quantitative pathological evidence for axonal loss in normal appearing white matter in multiple sclerosis. *Ann. Neurol.* **47**, 391–395.

Evangelou, N., Konz, D., Esiri, M. M., Smith, S., Palace, J., and Matthews, P. M. (2000a). Regional axonal loss in the corpus callosum correlates with cerebral white matter lesion volume and distribution in multiple sclerosis. *Brain* **123**, 1845–1849.

Evangelou, N., Konz, D., Esiri, M. M., Smith, S., Palace, J., Matthews, P. M. (2001). Size-selective neuronal changes in the anterior optic pathways suggest a differential susceptibility to injury in multiple sclerosis. *Brain* **124**, 1813–1820.

Ferguson, B., Matyszak, M. K., Esiri, M. M., and Perry, V. H. (1997). Axonal damage in acute multiple sclerosis lesions. *Brain* **120**, 393–399.

Filippi, M., Bozzali, M, Rovaris, M., Gonen, O., Kesavadas, C., Ghezzi, A., Martinelli, V., Grossman, R., Scotti, G., Comi, G., and Falini, A. (2003). Evidence for widespread axonal damage at the earliest clinical stage of multiple sclerosis. *Brain* **126**, 433–437.

Fisher, E., Rudick, R. A., Cutter, G., Baier, M., Miller, D., Weinstock-Guttman, B., Mass, M. K., Dougherty, D. S., and Simonian, N. A. (2000). Relationship between brain atrophy and disability: an 8-year follow-up study of multiple sclerosis patients. *Multiple Sclerosis* **6**, 373–377.

Fraenkel, M., and Jakob, A. (1913). Zur Pathologie der multiplen Sklerose mit besonderer Berücksichtigung der akuten Formen. *Z. Neurol.* **14**, 565–603.

Fromann, C. (1878). Untersuchungen über die Gewebsveränderungen bei der multiplen Sklerose des Gehirns und Rückenmarks. Jena.

Ganter, P., Prince, C., and Esiri, M. M. (1999). Spinal cord axonal loss in multiple sclerosis: A post-mortem study. *Neuropathol. Appl. Neurobiol.* **25**, 459–467.

Girodana, M. T., Richiardi, P., Trevisan, E., Boghi, A., and Palmucci, L. (2003). Abnormal ubiquitination of axons in normally myelinated white matter in multiple sclerosis brain. *Neuropathol. Appl. Neurobiol.* **28**, 35–41.

Höftberger, R., Aboul-Enein, F., Brück, W., Lucchinetti, C., Rodriguez, M., Schmidbauer, M., Jellinger, K., and Lassmann, H. (2004). Expression of major histocompatibility complex class I molecules on the different cell types in multiple sclerosis lesions. *Brain Pathol.* **14**, 43–50.

Jakob, A. (1915). Zur Pathologie der diffusen infiltrativen Enzephalomyelitis in ihren Beziehungen zur diffusen und multiplen Sklerose. *Z. ges Neurol. Psychiat.* **27**, 290–320.

Jellinger, K. (1969). Einige morphologische Aspekte der Multiplen Sklerose. *Wien Z. Nervenheilk (Suppl) II*, 12–37.

Kalman, B., and Leist, T. P. (2003). A mitochondrial component of neurodegeneration in multiple sclerosis. *Neuromolecular Med.* **3**, 147–158.

Kapoor, R., Davies, M., Blaker, P. A., Hall, S. M., and Smith, K. J. (2003). Blockers of sodium and calcium entry protect axons from nitric oxide-mediated degeneration. *Ann. Neurol.* **53**, 174–180.

Kidd, T., Barkhof, F., McConnell, R., Algra, P. R., Allen, I. V., and Revesz, T. (1999). Cortical lesions in multiple sclerosis. *Brain* **122**, 17–26.

Kornek, B., Storch, M., Weissert, R., Wallstroem, E., Stefferl, A., Olsson, T., Linington C., Schmidbauer, M., and Lassmann, H. (2000). Multiple sclerosis and chronic autoimmune encephalomyelitis: A comparative quantitative study of axonal injury in active, inactive and remyelinated lesions. *Am. J. Pathol.* **157**, 267–276.

Kornek, B., Storch, M. K., Bauer, J., Djamshidian, A., Weissert, R., Wallstrom, E., Stefferl, A., Zimprich F., Olsson, T., Linington, C., Schmidbauer, M., and Lassmann, H. (2001). Distribution of calcium channel subunit in dystrophic axons in multiple sclerosis and experimental autoimmune encephalomyelitis. *Brain* **124**, 1114–1124.

Kornek, B., and Lassmann, H. (1999). Axonal pathology in multiple sclerosis: a historical note. *Brain Pathol.* **9**, 651–656.

Kuhlmann, T., Lingfeld, G., Bitsch, A., Schuchardt, J., and Brück, W. (2002). Acute axonal damage in multiple sclerosis is most extensive in early disease stages and decreases over time. *Brain* **125**, 2202–2212.

Lassmann, H. (1983). Comparative neuropathology of chronic experimental allergic encephalomyelitis and multiple sclerosis. *Springer Schriftenr. Neurol.* **25**, 1–135.

Lovas, G., Szilagyi, N., Majtenyi, K., Palkovits, M., and Komoly, S. (2000). Axonal changes in chronic demyelinated cervical spinal cord plaques. *Brain* **123**, 308–317.

Lucchinetti, C., Brück, W., Parisi, J., Scheithauer, B., Rodriguez, M., and Lassmann, H. (2000). Heterogeneity of multiple sclerosis lesions: Implications for the pathogenesis of demyelination. *Ann. Neurol.* **47**, 707–717.

Lucchinetti, C. F., Mandler, R., McGavern, D., Brück, W., Gleich, G., Ransohoff, R. M., Trebst, C., Weinshenker, B., Wingerchuck, D., Parisi, J., and Lassmann, H. (2002). A role for humoral mechanisms in the pathogenesis of Devic's neuromyelitis optica. *Brain* **125**, 1450–1461.

Lumsden, C. E. (1970). The neuropathology of multiple sclerosis. *In:* "Handbook of Clinical Neurology" (P. I. Vinken, and G. W. Eds.) Vol . 9, pp. 217–309, Elsevier, New York.

Marburg, O. (1906). Die sogenannte "akute Multiple Sklerose" *Jahrb Psychiatrie* **27**, 211–312.

Medana, I., Martinic, M. A., Wekerle, H., and Neumann, H. (2001). Transection of major histocompatibility complex class I-induced neurites by cytotoxic T lymphocytes. *Am. J. Pathol.* **159**, 809–815.

Mews, I., Bergmann, M., Bunkowski, S., Gullotta, F., and Brück, W. (1998). Oligodendrocyte and axon pathology in clinically silent multiple sclerosis lesions. *Multiple Sclerosis* **4**, 55–62.

Moll, C., Mourre, C., Lazdunski, M., and Ulrich, J. (1991). Increase of sodium channels in demyelinated lesions of multiple sclerosis. *Brain Res.* **556**, 311–316.

Neumann, H., Medana, I., Bauer, J., and Lassmann, H. (2002). Cytotoxic T lymphocytes in autoimmune and degenerative CNS diseases. *Trend Neurosci.* **25**, 313–319.

Noseworthy, J. H., Lucchinetti, C., Rodriguez, M., and Weinshenker, B. G. (2000). Multiple sclerosis. *N. Engl. J. Med.* **343**, 938–952.

Owens, T. (2003). The enigma of multiple sclerosis: inflammation and neurodegeneration causes heterogenous dysfunction and damage. *Curr. Opin. Neurol.* **16**, 259–265.

Pelletier, D., Nelson, S. J., Oh, J., Antel, J. P., Kita, M., Zamvill, S. S., and Goodkin, D. E. (2003). MRI lesion volume heterogeneity in primary progressive MS in relation with axonal damage and brain atrophy. *J. Neurol. Neurosurg. Psychiatry* **74**, 950–952.

Peterson, J. W., Bo, L., Mork, S., Chang, A., and Trapp, B. D. (2001). Transsected neurites, apoptotic neurons and reduced inflammation in cortical multiple sclerosis lesions. *Ann. Neurol.* **50**, 389–400.

Pitt, D., Werner, P., and Raine, C. S. (2000). Glutamate excitotoxicity in a model of multiple sclerosis. *Nature Med.* **6**, 67–70.

Poser, C. M., and Brinar, V. V. (2003). Epilepsy and multiple sclerosis. *Epilepsy Behav.* 4, 6–12.

Prineas, J. W. (1985). The neuropathology of multiple sclerosis. *In:* "Handbook of Clinical Neurology" (J.C. Koetsier, Ed.). Vol. 47, pp. 337–395, Elsevier, New York.

Prineas, J. W., Barnard, R. O., Revesz, T., Kwon, E. E., Sharer, L., and Cho, E. S.(1993a). Multiple sclerosis. Pathology of recurrent lesions. *Brain* **116**, 681–693.

Redford, E. J., Kapoor, R., and Smith, K. J. (1997). Nitric oxide donors reversibly block axonal conduction: demyelinated axons are especially susceptible. *Brain* **120**, 2149–2157.

Rovaris, M., Filippi, M., Minicucci, L, Ianucci, G, Santuccio, G., Possa, F., and Comi, G. (2000). Cortical/subcortical disease burden and cognitive impairment in patients with multiple sclerosis. *Am. J. Neuroradiol.* **21**, 402–408.

Shintaku, M., Hirano, A., and Llena, J. F. (1988). Increased diameter of demyelinated axons in chronic multiple sclerosis of the spinal cord. *Neuropathol. Appl. Neurobiol.* **14**, 505–510.

Smith, K. J., and Lassmann, H. (2002). The role of nitric oxide in multiple sclerosis. *Lancet Neurol.* **1**, 232–241.

Smith, K. J., Kapoor, R., Hall, S. M., and Davies, M. (2001). Electrically active axons degenerate when exposed to nitric oxide. *Ann. Neurol.* **49**, 470–476.

Smith, T., Groom, A., Zhu, B., and Turski, L. (2000). Autoimmune encephalomyelitis ameliorated by AMPA antagonists. *Nature Med.* **6**, 62–66.

Spatt, J., Chaix, R., and Mamoli, B. (2001). Epileptic and non-epileptic seizures in multiple sclerosis. *J. Neurol.* **248**, 2–9.

Stys, P. K., Waxman, S. G., and Ransom, B. R. (1992). Ionic mechanisms of anoxic injury in mammalian CNS white matter: Role of Na+ channels and Na+-Ca2+ exchanger. *J. Neurosci.* **12**, 430–439.

Trapp, B. D., Peterson, J., Ransohoff, R. M., Rudick, R., Mork, S., and Bo, L. (1998). Axonal transection in the lesions of multiple sclerosis. *N. Engl. J. Med.* **338**, 278–285.

Trebst, C., Sorensen, T. L., Kivisakk, P., Cathcart, M. K., Hesselgesser, J., Horuk, R., Sellebjerg, F., Lassmann, H., and Ransohoff, R. M. (2001). CCR1+/CCR5+ mononuclear phagocytes accumulate in the central nervous system of patients with multiple sclerosis. *Am. J. Pathol.* **159**, 1701–1710.

Waxman, S. G. (2002). Sodium channels as molecular targets in multiple sclerosis. *J. Rehabil. Res. Dev.* **39**, 233–242.

Waxman, S. G. (2001). Acquired channelopathies in nerve injury and MS. *Neurology* **56**, 1621–1627.

Werner, P., Pitt, P., and Raine, C. S. (2001). Multiple sclerosis: altered glutamate homeostasis in lesions correlates with oligodendrocyte and axonal damage. *Ann. Neurol.* **50**, 169–180.

Wolswijk, G., and Balesar, R. (2003). Changes in the expression and localization of the paranodal protein Caspr on axons in chronic multiple sclerosis. *Brain* **126**, 1638–1649.

Zamvil, S. S., and Steinman, L. (2003). Diverse targets for intervention during inflammatory and neurodegenerative phases of multiple sclerosis. *Neuron* **38**, 685–688.

12

Axonal Degeneration in Multiple Sclerosis: The Histopathological Evidence

John W. Peterson, Ph.D.
Grahame J. Kidd, Ph.D.
Bruce D. Trapp, Ph.D.

I. Introduction

Multiple sclerosis (MS) is an inflammatory neurodegenerative disease of the central nervous system (CNS). Approximately 1 million people worldwide have MS, with females outnumbering males 2:1 (Weinshenker, 1996; Noseworthy et al., 2000). As a result of its high prevalence, MS is the leading cause of nontraumatic neurological disability in young adults in the United States and Europe. Although MS is most widely considered an autoimmune disease triggered in susceptible individuals by an environmental agent, the cause of MS remains unknown. The majority of MS patients exhibit a relapsing-remitting disease course (RR-MS) (Fig. 1) (Weinshenker, 1996; Noseworthy et al., 2000). After 8 to 15 years, most patients with RR-MS convert to a secondary-progressive disease course (SP-MS) characterized by persistent increasing neurological disability (Fig. 1) (Weinshenker et al., 1989; Noseworthy et al., 2000).

Currently available drugs for the treatment of patients with MS are predominantly anti-inflammatory or immunomodulatory in nature. During the RR phase of the disease, patients often benefit clinically from anti-inflammatory therapeutics. However, during the SP phase of the disease, the efficacy of anti-inflammatory therapeutics is of little clinical benefit. Unfortunately, few clinically beneficial therapies are available for SP-MS patients. The biphasic nature and refractory response to therapeutics raises questions regarding the mechanisms responsible for progression of neurological disability in MS. Therefore, of keen interest is the elucidation of the pathophysiological mechanisms responsible for conversion of RR-MS to SP-MS.

Although the cause of MS remains unknown, recent work has provided insight into the pathological basis of permanent disability in patients with MS. The identification of axonal loss as the biological substrate underlying permanent disability in MS has proved challenging. The stochastic distribution

165

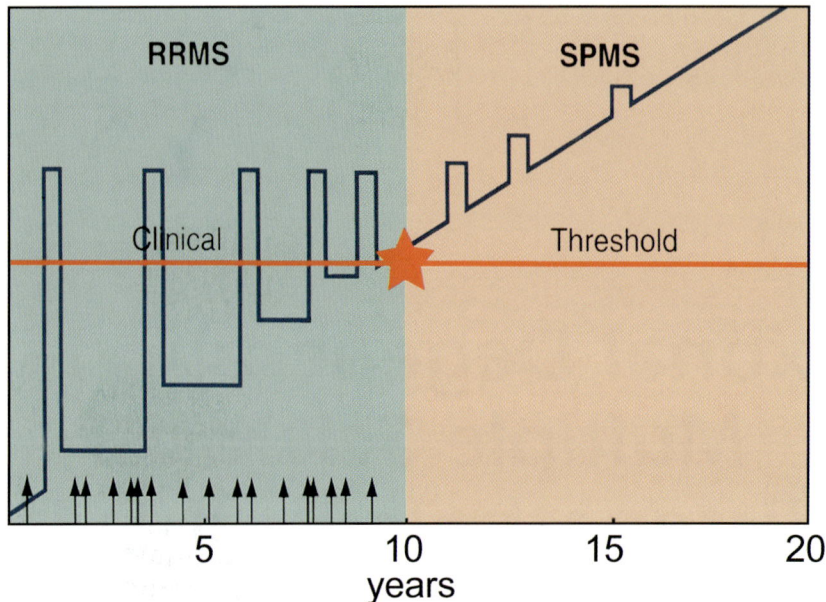

Figure 1 The etiology of the most common form of MS is biphasic. Initially MS patients exhibit relapsing-remitting disease (RR-MS) (*blue background*) characterized by alternating periods of clinical disability punctuated by periods of recovery (*blue line*). Neurological disability is detected clinically when severity of disability exceeds clinical threshold (*red line*). After about a decade, conversion of RR-MS to secondary progressive MS (SP-MS) (*pink background*) occurs when clinical disability becomes progressive without remission. During RR-MS (*blue background*) inflammatory activity (*arrows*) is prominent while during SP-MS (*pink background*) inflammatory activity is negligible. Inflammatory activity refers to the presence of gadolinium-enhancing lesions or the appearance of new lesions on T_2-weighted MRI scans. Once axonal loss surpasses the compensatory capacity of the CNS, RR-MS converts to SP-MS (*star*). (Reproduced from Trapp et al., 1999b, with permission.)

of lesions within the CNS, variability of lesion pathology, and our inability to identify and monitor all lesions often make it impossible to assign specific neurological disabilities to specific lesions. In addition, the chronic nature of MS amplifies the difficulty of retrospectively matching neuropathological changes with specific neurological symptoms by increasing the time between symptom onset and the identification of the potential pathological changes responsible. Thus, clarification of the relationship between MS pathology and neurological disability is extremely complex.

The histopathological hallmarks of MS lesions include multifocal inflammation, breakdown of the blood-brain barrier, demyelination, oligodendrocyte loss, reactive astrogliosis, and axonal pathology (Prineas, 2001). Historically the most salient pathological features of MS lesions were inflammation and demyelination, which, to date, have been the major focus of MS research. Although MS is considered primarily an immune-mediated disease of CNS myelin, axonal loss is now widely accepted as the major cause of persistent neurological disability (Trapp et al., 1999b; Bjartmar et al., 2003; Bruck and Stadelmann, 2003). Clear evidence of axonal loss as the cause of irreversible neurological disability in MS was provided by new insights into

the timing and functional consequences of axonal loss identified using various approaches including magnetic resonance imaging (MRI) (van Waesberghe et al., 1999; Stevenson and Miller, 1999; De Stefano et al., 2003), magnetic resonance spectroscopy (MRS) (Narayana et al., 1998; Matthews et al., 1998; Arnold, 1999), functional MRI (Reddy et al., 2000; Pantano et al., 2002; Parry et al., 2003; Rocca et al., 2003), and morphological analysis of MS tissue (Ferguson et al., 1997; Trapp et al., 1998).

This chapter focuses on the histopathological evidence for axonal pathology based on morphological analyses of CNS tissue from patients with MS and studies of animal models for MS pertinent to progression of neurological disability in patients with MS. Collectively, the studies identify cumulative axonal loss as the pathobiological substrate responsible for progressive irreversible neurological disability in patients with MS.

A. Neurological Disability in MS

The onset of neurological symptoms in MS is rapid while demyelination is a relatively slow process. Neurological symptoms therefore are hypothesized to initially result from impairment of normal neuronal function by inflammation and edema. Increases in the numbers of immune cells and levels of specific cytokines in cerebral spinal fluid (CSF) often precede the occurrence of relapses. More recently, gadolinium-enhanced MRI has been correlated with active inflammation and has been associated with the onset of relapses in patients with MS of short duration (Fig. 1) (Harris et al., 1991; McFarland et al., 1992; Miller et al., 1993; Koudriavtseva et al., 1997; Khoury et al., 2000; Weiner et al., 2000; Wang et al., 2002). Possible mechanisms for the onset or renewal of impaired axonal conduction include the production of inflammatory substances (Hohlfeld, 1997), putative conduction blocking factors (Brinkmeier et al., 2000; but see Chapter 22), and disruption of the normal ionic milieu induced by breakdown of the blood-brain barrier and resulting edema.

Demyelination is thought to contribute to extended periods of disability. Although remyelination certainly occurs early in the disease, it is a slow process and often incomplete. Demyelinated plaques in patients often occur in multiple areas disrupting the function of many systems and may also occur at multiple levels within the same functional system. In addition, demyelination of several separate segments along axons can occur, especially in the long tracts of the ascending sensory and descending motor systems, such as the dorsal column-medial lemniscal and the lateral-corticospinal systems, respectively. This may cause conduction block at multiple points within a functional system and even along single axons. As the disease progresses, repeated episodes of inflammatory demyelination result in the accumulation of lesions, which increasingly fail to remyelinate. In addition, progression of disability in SP-MS may result from the continued expansion of chronic active lesions (Prineas et al., 2001). Historically, permanent neurological disability in MS had been attributed to decreased axonal conduction and conduction block secondary to the failure of the CNS to remyelinate and the resulting state of chronic demyelination (Fig. 2).

This concept of MS was sufficient for explaining reversible neurological disability during RR-MS, but it failed to adequately explain the progressive persistent neurological disability seen in SP-MS patients (Waxman, 1998; Trapp et al., 1999a). Chronically demyelinated axons can compensate for conduction block by an altered distribution of axolemmal ion channels, which allow them to conduct impulses relatively well, albeit at reduced velocities (Fig. 2) (Bostock and Sears, 1978; Foster et al., 1980; Felts et al., 1997; see also Chapter 7). In addition, in many SP-MS patients, inflammatory activity is no longer prominent and lesion load is relatively stable (Fig. 1). Inflammation, edema, and ongoing demyelination would not be expected to be major contributors to increasing neurological disability. Therefore, progression of neurological disability must occur by other mechanisms. A number of early, as well as more recent, reports describe substantial axonal loss in MS lesions.

Destruction of axons provides a biological mechanism sufficient for explaining irreversible disability in SP-MS patients.

B. Historical Observations of Axonal Pathology

Some reports of axonal degeneration in MS date back over a century (for review see Kornek and Lassmann, 1999). Despite some early descriptions of axonal loss, inflammation, demyelination, and gliosis attracted most research efforts. Several early studies clearly identified axonal pathology by the presence of axonal swellings, axonal transection, and Wallerian degeneration in MS lesions (Kornek and Lassmann, 1999). Controversy existed, however, over the extent and timing of axonal loss. For example, two histological studies published in 1936 analyzed the extent of axonal loss in the spinal cords of patients with MS and reported opposite findings. The first study reported a 50% loss of axons in MS lesions from 11 patients (Putnam, 1936). In contrast, the other study reported normal axon densities in more than 90% of the MS lesions from 13 patients (Greenfield and King, 1936). The discrepancies in axonal loss between these studies were suggested to result from more sensitive axonal staining in the latter study. Although several studies in the MS literature described axonal pathology, it was not widely accepted as a significant pathological feature. Emphasis continued to be placed on the preservation of axon cylinders in MS lesions, and axonal preservation continued as a defining pathological feature of MS. With the exception of chronic stage highly sclerotic lesions (Barnes et al., 1991) or lesions from fulminant cases of MS, the presence of axon damage in MS was considered unusual. Concurrently, evidence for MS being an inflammatory demyelinating disease against myelin proteins was demonstrated by accident when individuals given a vaccine containing whole-brain homogenate developed a disease similar to MS (Peters, 1968) and the subsequent demonstration of immune recognition of specific myelin antigens in patients with MS (Sobel et al., 1994). The focus of MS research shifted to mechanisms of inflammatory demyelination. Consequently, the axonal component of MS pathogenesis received less attention, and the questions regarding the extent and timing of axonal damage in MS remained unresolved.

II. Axonal Transection Occurs during Inflammatory Demyelination

A. Axonal Injury Disrupts Axonal Transport

Disruption of axonal transport is a common response to axonal injury. Thus, the abnormal accumulation of axonally transported proteins along axons can be used to identify axonal damage. Axonal injury in MS has been identified by

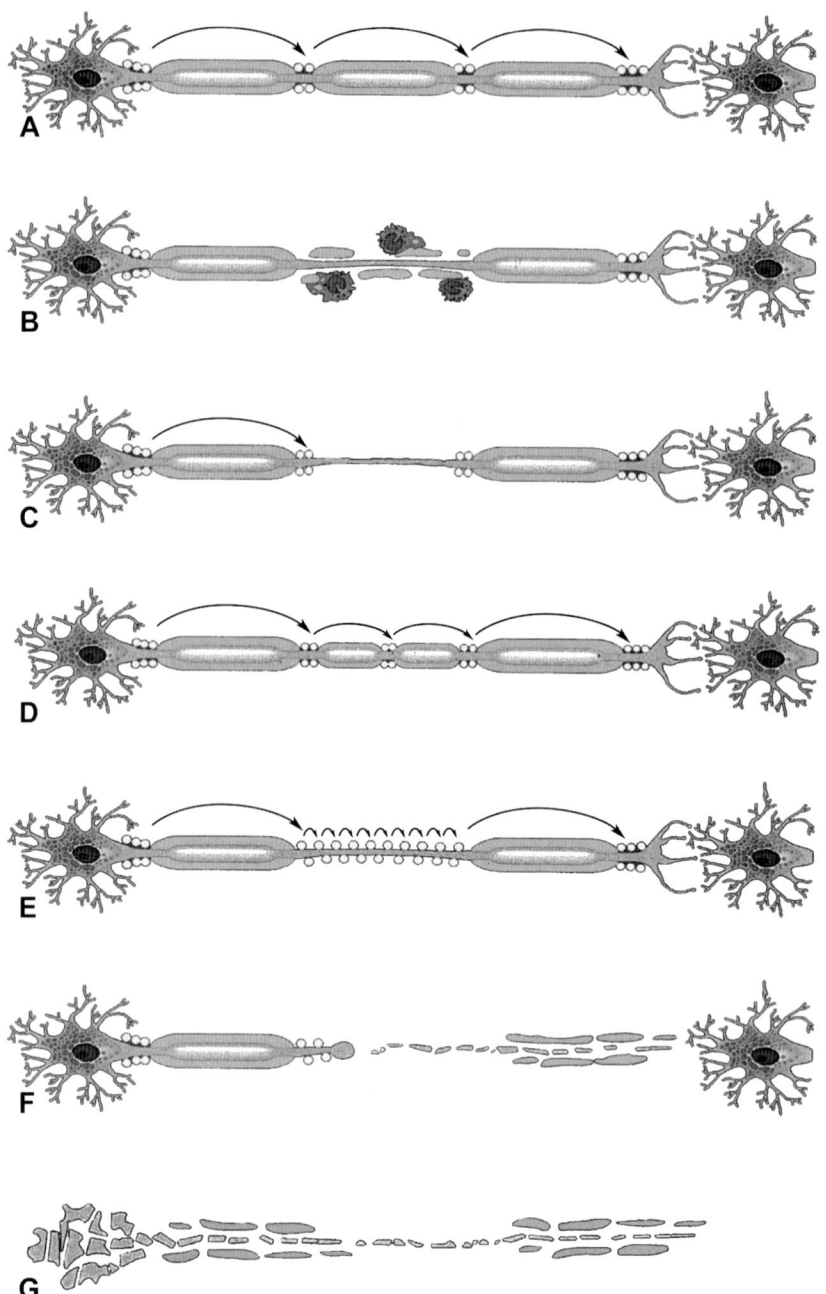

Figure 2 Concepts on pathogenesis of neurological disability in patients with multiple sclerosis (MS). Historically, permanent disability occurred when normal myelinated axons (**A**) underwent immune-mediated demyelination (**B**) resulting in chronic demyelination and persistent conduction block (**C**). Restoration of impulse conduction and neurological function may occur as a result of remyelination (**D**) or redistribution of Na+ channels along chronically demyelinated axonal segments (**E**). Conceptually, permanent disability is now associated with axonal transection (**F**) that occurs during inflammatory demyelination (**B**) and is clinically silent during relapsing-remitting MS because of CNS compensation for axonal loss. Recent evidence suggests that chronic demyelination (**C, E**) leads to axonal degeneration (**G**). (Adapted from Trapp et al., 1999a, with permission.)

the abnormal accumulation of amyloid precursor proteins (APP) (Gehrmann et al., 1995; Ferguson et al., 1997), non-phosphorylated neurofilament proteins (Trapp et al., 1998), the pore-forming subunit of N-type calcium channels (Kornek et al., 2001), and metabotropic glutamate receptors (Geurts et al., 2003) along axons in active lesions and at the borders of chronic active lesions. Additional studies have confirmed correlations between inflammatory activity of lesions and APP-positive axons in MS and experimental autoimmune encephalomyelitis (EAE) (Kornek et al., 2000, 2001; Bitsch et al., 2000). The aforementioned studies establish that axonal damage occurs during inflammatory demyelination and correlates with the degree of inflammation in cerebral MS lesions.

While accumulation of axonally transported proteins is a reliable indicator of disrupted axonal transport and therefore axonal injury, the extent and timing to which injured axons either degenerate or functionally recover is unknown. For example, *N*-acetyl aspartate (NAA) is used as an *in vivo* marker of axonal function with decreased levels indicating axonal injury and loss in MS (Bjartmar and Trapp, 2001). However, increased levels of NAA in regions previously identified with reduced NAA indicate that injured axons can survive and axonal injury is reversible (De Stefano et al., 1995). The observations of axonal injury in MS lesions were extended, and the occurrence of permanent axonal damage in the form of transected axons were substantiated for the first time in acute MS lesions by an

immunocytochemical study using confocal microscopy (Trapp et al., 1998). Using nonphosphorylated neurofilaments, axonal dilations and axonal ovoids indicative of axonal injury were identified in active and chronic active cerebral MS lesions from patients with disease durations ranging from 2 weeks to 27 years (Fig. 3A, B). Accumulation of axonal proteins and formation of axonal ovoids are highly suggestive of transected axons, as terminal ovoids are formed by the accumulation of proteins by anterograde transport at the proximal ends of transected axons (Fig. 2). However, not all axonal ovoids occur at the terminal ends of transected axons. The formation of *en passant* axonal ovoids also occurs along damaged axons that remain intact. Whether axons with *en passant* axonal ovoids degenerate or axonal transport is restored, allowing resumption of normal axonal function, is unknown. Therefore, to accurately determine the extent of axonal transection, quantification of terminal ovoids is required. Further analyses of the nonphosphorylated neurofilament-positive axonal ovoids in MS lesions using three-dimensional reconstruction of

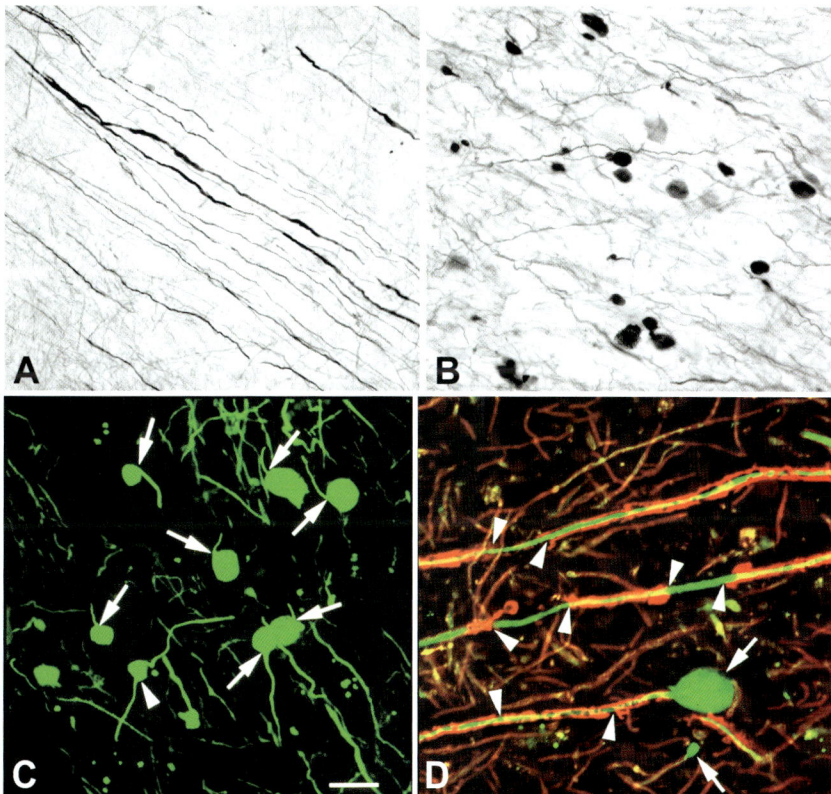

Figure 3 Axonal damage identified in multiple sclerosis lesions by immunostaining for nonphosphorylated neurofilaments (**A–D**) and visualized by DAB immunohistochemistry (**A, B**) or immunofluorescence (**C, D**, *green*). Demyelinated axons and axonal ovoids suggestive of axonal transection were detected in chronic active (**A**) and active MS lesions (**B**). While most axonal ovoids had single axonal connections indicative of axonal transection (**C**, *arrows*), some had dual axonal connections (**C**, *arrowhead*). Nonphosphorylated-neurofilament-positive axons (**D**, *green*) are undergoing active demyelination (*arrowheads, red is myelin basic protein*). Two axons end in terminal ovoids (*arrows*). (Panels C and D reproduced from Trapp et al., 1998, with permission.)

confocal microscopy images provided conclusive evidence that many of the axonal ovoids contained a single axonal connection and therefore were the proximal ends of transected axons (Fig. 3C). Quantification of terminal ovoids identified a strong correlation between axonal transection and the inflammatory activity of lesions. On average, more than 11,000 terminal ovoids/mm^3 were detected in active lesions, more than 3,000/mm^3 were identified at the edge of chronic active lesions, and approximately 900/mm^3 were detected within the core of chronic active lesions. In contrast, control white matter contained less than 1 transected axon/mm^3. The correlation of significant amounts of axonal transection with inflammation in patients with short disease duration when inflammatory demyelination is predominant helped establish the occurrence of axonal loss at disease onset in MS (Fig. 3D).

B. Immune-Mediated Mechanisms of Axonal Loss

The exact molecular mechanisms of axonal loss in MS are unknown. The development of future neuroprotective therapies is not only critically dependent on our elucidating the cellular and molecular mechanisms of axonal loss in MS, but also on comprehending the interplay of these mechanisms with disease progression. Complicating our ability to interpret the pathophysiology of axonal injury is the probability that there are multiple mechanisms of axonal degeneration, which are dependent on the stage of the disease (Kornek and Lassmann, 1999; Bjartmar and Trapp, 2003). The link between disease activity and CNS inflammation is highly correlated, even when the disease is subclinical (Rudick et al., 1999b). Further, evidence supporting a link between inflammation and axonal pathology in MS patients was indicated by the positive correlation between inflammatory activity of cerebral MS lesions and axonal damage (Ferguson et al., 1997; Trapp et al., 1998; Kornek et al., 2000, 2001; Bitsch et al., 2000; Geurts et al., 2003). Additionally, axonal damage identified by increased levels of the light subunit of neurofilament proteins was detected in 78% of the CSF samples from RR-MS patients and demonstrated to correlate with clinical disability (Lycke et al., 1998). MRI studies provide further support for the dependence of axonal pathology on inflammation. For example, gadolinium-enhancing lesions on MRI scans have linked progressive brain atrophy with inflammation in RR-MS patients (Zivadinov and Zorzon, 2002). Previous reports have correlated CNS atrophy, as measured by MRI, with clinical disability suggesting that atrophy may represent axonal loss (Losseff and Miller, 1998). Of interest are the findings of progressive atrophy and persistent inflammation identified as gadolinium-enhancing lesions on MRI scans, which can be documented on subsequent MRI examinations, occurring even in the absence of clinical symptoms in patients

with RR-MS (Simon et al., 1998, 1999; Rudick et al., 1997). These observations indicate that even during so-called stages of clinical remission, MS is progressing silently.

The strong correlation between inflammation and axonal transection suggests that axonal transection is immune-mediated. Specific immunological attack on the axon has been considered as a possible mechanism of axonal degeneration in MS. Macrophages and activated microglia have been detected in close association with the end bulbs of transected axons in MS lesions using confocal microscopy (Fig. 4A, B) (Trapp et al., 1998). In addition, these cells sometimes contain neurofilament-positive inclusions (Fig. 4A). These observations suggest that macrophages and activated microglia may be targeting axons. Whether these cells are directly attacking axons or only removing axonal debris remains to be determined. Direct immunological targeting of axons is not without precedence. In acute motor axonal neuropathy (AMAN), a variant of Guillain-Barré syndrome (GBS), which is an autoimmune disease of the peripheral nervous system, primary immune-mediated attack on axons has been identified as the mechanism responsible for axonal degeneration (Ho et al., 1998). Antibody binding to an axolemmal protein has been demonstrated by the identification of immunoglobulins and the complement activation marker C3d at the nodes of Ranvier (Hafer-Macko et al., 1996). Macrophages then target the nodes of Ranvier, possibly in response to complement-derived chemoattractant signals such as C5a, and invade the periaxonal space, displacing myelin internodes and promoting axonal degeneration. Unlike AMAN, localization of antibodies specific to axonal components in the CNS has not been identified in MS lesions (Hafer-Macko et al., 1996; Ho et al., 1998).

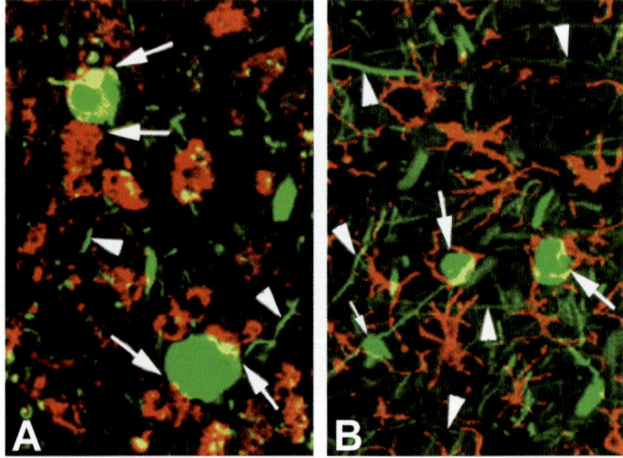

Figure 4 Macrophages and microglia associate with transected axons (*green*) in active MS lesions. Macrophages (*red*, **A**) and microglia (*red*, **B**) surround and engulf terminal axonal swellings (*large arrows*), but have no consistent association with normal-appearing axons (*arrowheads*) or swellings in nontransected axons (*small arrow*). (Confocal micrographs reproduced from Trapp et al., 1998, with permission.)

In addition, an immunological attack directed at axons seems unlikely since most axons survive the acute demyelinating process. However, recent observations implicating cytotoxic CD8+ T-cells as mediators of axonal transection in inflammatory lesions were made in MS tissue (Babbe et al., 2000; Skulina et al., 2004), in EAE mice (Huseby et al., 2001), and in vitro (Medana et al., 2001; Giuliani et al., 2003). Other recent studies have reported that immune-mediated mechanisms might target axonal subpopulations (Ganter et al., 1999; Lovas et al., 2000; Evangelou et al., 2001). In addition, antibodies to enriched fractions of axolemma have been detected in the CSF and serum of MS patients (Rawes et al., 1997). While evidence supporting direct immunological attack of axons in MS is scant, we should not overlook the possibility that it contributes to axon loss in MS.

Although evidence for cell-mediated mechanisms of axonal transection is inconclusive, loss of axons may be caused by nonspecific damage resulting from the inflammatory process. The inflammatory microenvironment contains a multitude of substances produced by activated immune and glial cells that potentially injure axons, including proteolytic enzymes such as matrix metalloproteases, cytokines, oxidative products, and free radicals (Hohlfeld, 1997). In addition to the direct effects of inflammatory mediators, recent studies have indicated that inflammation induces aberrant glutamate homeostasis (Piani et al., 1991; Werner et al., 2001) and production of nitric oxide (NO) (Bö et al., 1994; Smith and Lassmann, 2002) in MS. Damage to mitochondrial DNA and impaired activity of mitochondrial enzyme complexes of the electron transport chain mediated by oxidative radicals in MS lesions indicate that inflammation can affect energy metabolism, adenosine triphosphate (ATP) synthesis, and the viability of affected cells (Lu et al., 2000). Treatment with NBQX, an AMPA/kinate glutamate receptor antagonist, resulted in increased oligodendrocyte survival and reduced axonal damage in EAE, an animal model of MS (Pitt et al., 2000). The reduced axonal damage and increased oligodendrocyte survival were not due to reductions in inflammatory activity because NBQX has no anti-inflammatory effects; therefore NBQX's beneficial effects suggest that glutamate may also be involved in tissue damage in acute lesions.

Acute axonal damage may also occur via mechanical compression caused by increased extracellular pressure from inflammation-induced edema. Severe swelling in the CNS can lead to herniation or compression damage. Spinal cord axons may be more susceptible to compression damage, because they are anatomically located on the outside of the cord and have less space in the vertebrae to expand compared to the brain in the skull. In relapsing-remitting EAE mice, there was a 9% increase in spinal cord cross-sectional area during the first attack, which returned to normal at end-stage disease (Wujek et al., 2002). Inflammation would also result in the disruption of normal vascular function, which could lead to ischemic-mediated axonal damage. An analogous mechanism for ischemic-induced axonal damage is proposed in GBS. Edema in GBS is thought to cause increased endoneurial fluid pressure and disruption of the nerve's vascular supply, resulting in ischemia-mediated axonal degeneration (Powell and Myers, 1996). Intriguing evidence for the activation of molecules involved in protecting against hypoxia/ischemia in MS brains has been reported (Graumann et al., 2003; Lassmann, 2003). The exact mechanism of inflammatory-mediated axonal loss is unknown; however, inflammation strongly correlates with axonal transection and is likely a major contributor responsible for accumulating axonal pathology during early stages of MS. Therefore, in addition to reducing inflammation and demyelination, aggressive anti-inflammatory treatment during RR-MS should also prevent axonal transection.

C. Axonal Loss in EAE Correlates with Inflammation and Disability

The use of animal models has provided valuable insights regarding the pathophysiological mechanisms and functional consequences of axonal injury during immune-mediated demyelination. Axonal transection has been described in mouse (Brown et al., 1982; Craner et al., 2004), guinea pig (Raine and Cross, 1989), and primate (Raine et al., 1999; Mancardi et al., 2001) models of EAE as indicated by the presence of both axonal dystrophy and swellings.

Induction of EAE in SWXJ mice by immunization with the 139-151 peptide of PLP produces consistent progression from relapsing disease to chronic disability (Yu et al., 1996). The neurological disability or clinical score for each animal was correlated with inflammation and axonal loss at first attack and at end-stage disease (Wujek et al., 2002). Initiation of axonal pathology and progressive axonal loss in spinal cord white matter occurred early in the disease course and was detected on immunohistochemical examination (Wujek et al., 2002). Clinical scores correlated with spinal cord inflammation, but not axon loss, which is low after initial attack. In contrast, during the chronic end-stage of relapsing EAE, clinical scores correlated highly with axon loss in both cervical ($P < 0.0001$) and lumbar spinal cords ($P < 0.004$) (Fig. 5), but not inflammation. The end-stage mice with permanent limb paralysis had average spinal cord axonal losses of 59% at cervical and 43% at lumbar levels. The number of symptomatic relapses varied between one and five. Regression analysis verified a significant correlation between number of relapses and axonal loss, which was stronger for the cervical cord ($\rho = 0.75$) than for the lumbar cord ($\rho = 0.63$). The number of relapses for each mouse was significantly related to clinical score, as predicted from the relationship between episode number and axonal loss (Wujek et al., 2002).

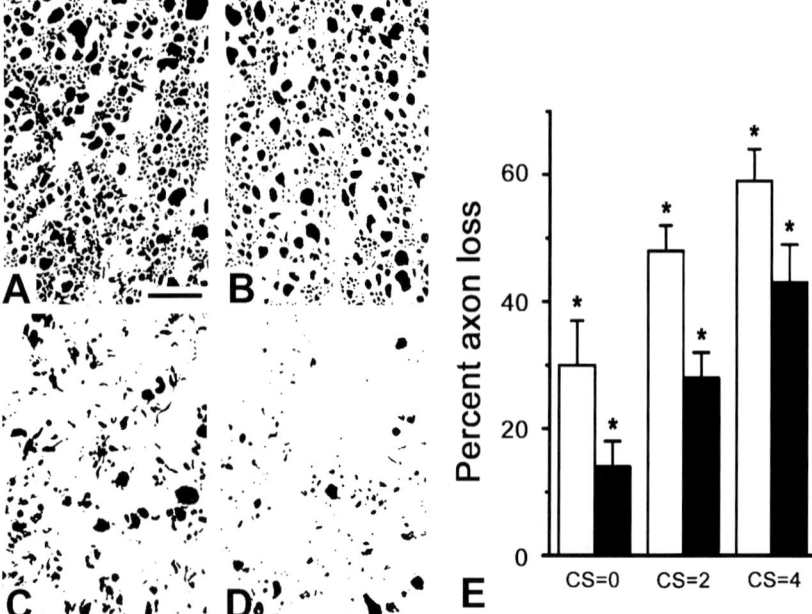

Figure 5 Spinal cord axonal loss correlates with permanent neurological disability in mice with chronic EAE. Neurofilament-positive axons in dorsolateral region of spinal cord from control (**A**) and EAE mice with clinical scores of 0 (**B**), 2 (**C**), and 4 (**D**). Increasing axonal loss in cervical (*white bars*) and lumbar (*black bars*) spinal cord correlated with increasing clinical score (**E**). Asterisks indicate significant correlation between axon loss and clinical score. Spearman's rank correlation test was used to test for significance (cervical cord: $\rho = 0.75$; $P = 0.0001$; lumbar cord: $\rho = 0.63$; $P = 0.004$). (Reproduced from Wujek et al., 2002, with permission.)

A causal relationship between number of inflammatory attacks, axonal loss, and permanent neurological disability in mice with relapsing EAE is indicated and related to the stage of EAE by these data (Wujek et al., 2002). The correlation between clinical disability and the extent of axonal loss was poor after the initial exacerbation. During the stable chronic end-stage of the disease, however, mice showed signs of irreversible functional impairment of varying severity, which had a strong correlation with spinal cord axonal loss. For example, during the chronic EAE stage, relatively modest white-matter axon loss was detected in mice with minimal or no clinical signs, whereas extensive axonal loss was detected in the severely disabled animals. Specifically, in end-stage mice with no observable symptoms (clinical score 0), axonal loss was 30% in the cervical and 15% in the lumbar spinal cord compared to controls. Curiously, the amount of axonal loss was substantially higher than in first attack mice with a reversible clinical score of 4 (limb paralysis). The 43% to 59% axonal loss measured in irreversibly paralyzed chronic end-stage EAE mice is of similar extent to the 68% reduction in axons detected in paralyzed MS patient spinal cord lesions (Bjartmar et al., 2000). Mice with a clinical score of 2 exhibited poor righting reflex with the extent of axonal loss midway between the amounts of axonal loss detected in mice

with scores of 0 and 4 (Fig. 5). Analysis of spinal cords collected from the most disabled end-stage mice identified some lesions consisting predominantly of damaged axons with extremely few normal axons (Wujek et al., 2002).

These data have two important ramifications for our understanding of neurological disability. First, these data indicate that acute reversible disability in relapsing EAE results from inflammation and edema not axonal transection, as functional disability did not strongly correlate with early axonal loss. Second, these data indicate that at chronic stages, when axonal degeneration highly correlates with disability, axonal loss is the cause of neurological disability in these EAE mice. Data from this animal model support the hypothesis that irreversible neurological disability occurs in MS once axonal loss surpasses a certain threshold. Suitable animal models will be required for the development of new neuroprotective drugs for MS. This relapsing EAE model recapitulates many pathological and functional aspects of MS. These mice also benefit from interferon-β treatment, exhibiting milder symptoms and fewer relapses (Yu et al., 1996). Finally, the spinal cord axonal loss measured in the chronic paralyzed mice is of similar magnitude as the axonal loss observed in spinal cord lesions of severely disabled patients with chronic MS (Ganter et al., 1999; Lovas et al.,

2000; Bjartmar et al., 2000). Thus, this particular EAE model may be useful for testing the efficacy of novel neuroprotective therapeutics being developed for patients with MS.

III. Degeneration of Chronically Demyelinated Axons

Recent studies indicate that although significant axonal loss often occurs early during RR-MS in association with inflammation, permanent disability is not clinically evident because of the compensatory capacity of the CNS. In addition most symptoms are transitory because they are caused predominantly by inflammation, edema, and demyelination. Once axonal loss surpasses the reserve compensatory capacity of the CNS, however, irreversible neurological disability becomes clinically evident and the disease transitions to the SP-MS phase (Fig. 1). During the SP-MS stage of the disease, active inflammation is no longer prominent, as indicated by MRI and suggested by the lost efficacy of anti-inflammatory therapeutics. Although inflammation is no longer prominent during SP-MS, there is a steady progression of irreversible neurological disability. Also, CNS atrophy and axonal loss continue as indicated by MRI measurements (Rudick et al., 1999a; Miller et al., 2002) and MRS measurements (De Stefano et al., 1998; Matthews et al., 1998; Gonen et al., 2000). Therefore, progression of irreversible neurological disability during SP-MS is caused by continued axonal loss, which occurs by mechanisms independent of active inflammation.

A. Loss of Normal Oligodendrocyte/Myelin-Axon Interactions Cause Axonal Degeneration

The accumulation of axonal loss in chronic MS likely occurs by several mechanisms. In the later stages of MS, lesions often remain chronically demyelinated. Axonal degeneration in SP-MS may be caused by mechanisms triggered by chronic demyelination (Scherer, 1999; Bjartmar et al., 1999). Although proof that chronic demyelination causes axonal degeneration in MS patients is difficult to demonstrate, the concept is supported by animal models with abnormal axon-myelin interactions (Bjartmar et al., 1999), estimates of total axonal loss (De Stefano et al., 1998; Matthews et al., 1998; Gonen et al., 2000), and measures of CNS atrophy (Rudick et al., 1999a; Miller et al., 2002) in patients with long-term MS. Studies on axonal degeneration secondary to disruption of normal axon-myelin interactions suggest that myelin-forming cells influence axonal morphology and long-term viability. Chronic demyelination of axons results in alterations in neurofilament spacing as a result of changes in phosphorylation status and axolemmal redistribution of ion channels.

In MAG-deficient mice, myelination progresses normally and formation of compact myelin appears normal (Li et al., 1994; Yin et al., 1998). However, at 35 days, changes in axonal caliber are detected and by 3 months, progressive axonal atrophy characterized by reduced neurofilament phosphorylation, reduced neurofilament spacing, and reduced axonal caliber was detected and preceded axonal degeneration (Fig. 6) (Li et al., 1994; Yin et al., 1998). Similar changes in neurofilament phosphorylation status and axonal transection were detected in chronically demyelinated lesions from patients with SP-MS (Trapp et al., 1998). The development of late-onset axonal degeneration, which preferentially affects the long tracts and results in the development of neurological disability, occurs in PLP-null mice that have a dysmyelinating phenotype (Griffiths et al., 1998; Klugmann et al., 1997). Similar length-dependent axonal losses were identified in patients deficient for PLP1 histologically and *in vivo* by MRS measurements of NAA in (Garbern et al., 2002). CNP-null mice exhibit a similar, but even more severe axonal phenotype than the PLP-null mice (Lappe-Siefke et al., 2003). Compact myelin formation appeared normal in both the MAG- and CNP-null mice, indicating that axonal degeneration was not secondary to dysmyelination as may be the case in the PLP-null mice. The MAG- and CNP-null mice data imply that myelin-forming cells provide trophic support necessary for axonal survival independent of the formation of compact myelin. MAG may exert direct or indirect long-term modulating effects on the cytoskeleton via axonal kinases or phosphatases (Yin et al., 1998).

B. Axonal Degeneration in Chronically Demyelinated MS Lesions

Ten chronically demyelinated inactive spinal cord lesions, from five paralyzed patients with MS (EDSS $\geq$7.5) with disease duration ranging from 12 to 39 years, were analyzed to quantify total axon numbers and axonal density (Bjartmar et al., 2000). Substantial axonal loss was identified in these lesions (Fig. 7A, B). In one lesion, axonal loss was as great as 84%, with a mean axonal loss of 68% (range 45–84%) for all the lesions analyzed (Fig. 7C). Measures of the average axonal density for these lesions identified decreases in axon densities by 58%, corroborating the substantial axonal loss determined by quantification of axons. In another study, similar reductions in average axonal density of 61% were found in spinal cord lesions from patients with SP-MS (Lovas et al., 2000). These studies analyzed patients with considerable disability; therefore, these results support axonal degeneration as the main cause of irreversible neurological impairment during chronic progressive stages of MS. The observations on these lesions suggest that axonal loss in SP-MS may result from chronic demyelination (Bjartmar et al., 1999; Trapp et al., 1999a). Thus, loss of axon-myelin and axon-oligoden-

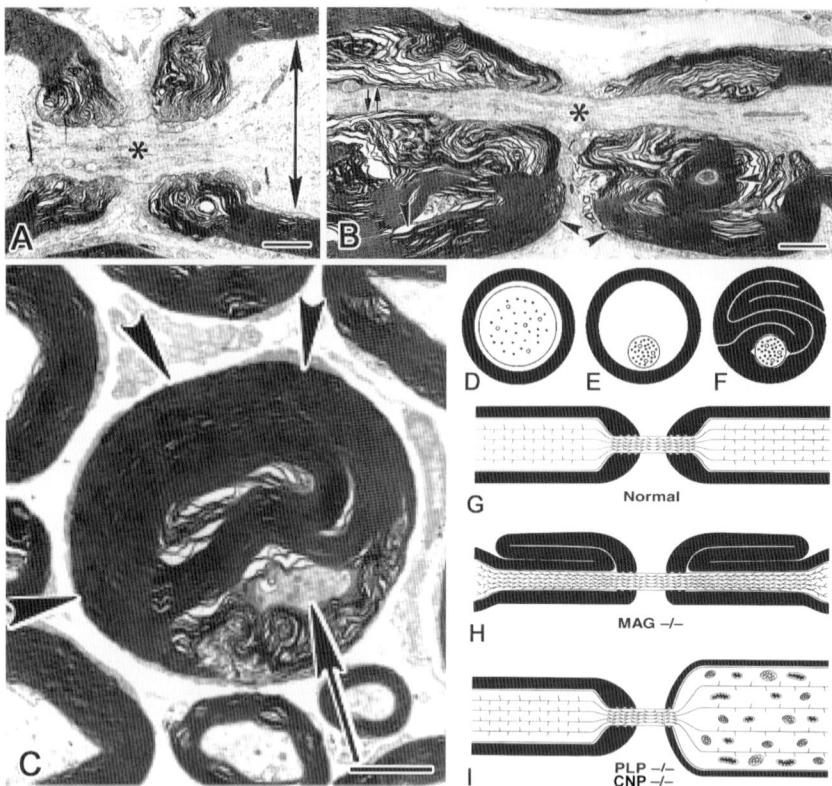

Figure 6 Pathology precedes axonal degeneration in myelinated nerve fibers from mice expressing myelin protein gene defects. By electron microscopy, paranodal axonal caliber is much greater in control (**A**) than in MAG-deficient (**B**) fibers. In transverse orientation, thick redundant myelin (**C**, *arrowheads*) partially surrounds an axon (**C**, *arrow*) with remarkably small caliber. Schematic representation of myelin and axonal pathology in MAG-, PLP-, and CNP-deficient fibers (**D–I**). In MAG-deficient mice, paranodes develop normally (**D, G**), but with time, they develop late-onset axonal degeneration preceded by paranodal axon atrophy with reduced neurofilament spacing (**E, H**), resulting in myelin sheath collapse and tomacula formation (**F, H**). PLP-, and CNP-deficient mice develop late-onset paranodal axonal swellings caused by apparent defects in axonal transport (**I**). (Reproduced from Yin et al., 1998 (**A-F**) and Trapp et al., 1999a (G-I), with permission.)

drocyte interactions is another pathological aspect responsible for inducing changes that may cause axonal degeneration.

C. Axonal Degeneration Induced by Altered Redistribution of Ion Channels

Another mechanism of chronic demyelination-induced axonal degeneration may be triggered by the compensatory changes axons undergo to restore impulse conduction. Demyelination results in conduction block. An altered distribution of sodium channels along demyelinated axonal segments compensates for loss of myelin internodes permitting the resumption of action potential conduction and neurological function (Bostock and Sears, 1978; Foster et al., 1980; Felts et al., 1997). Change in channel distribution, however, can also make these axons more susceptible to degeneration by increasing energy demand when energy production may be compromised (see Chapter 7). The greatest consumption of ATP in the CNS is by Na/K ATPases for the maintenance

of ionic gradients necessary for neurotransmission (Ames, III, 2000). When axons are demyelinated, energy consumption is greatly increased as a result of the redistribution of Na channels and the resulting increased influx of sodium. As mentioned earlier, ATP production may be compromised by oxidative damage to the mitochondrial enzyme complexes. In addition, slowing of axonal transport resulting from demyelination and decreased ATP availability may decrease rates of mitochondrial renewal. Collectively, all these factors will eventually result in the axon operating with an energy deficit leading to ionic imbalances (Stys et al., 1992; Leppanen and Stys, 1997). Several recent reports in EAE indicate axonal degeneration is Ca-mediated (Craner et al., 2003, 2004). Excess axonal Ca may result from reversal of Na/Ca exchangers caused by increased axonal Na levels as a result of insufficient ATP to run the Na/K ATPases (Stys et al., 1992; Agrawal and Fehlings, 1996; Li et al., 2000).

Collectively, the aforementioned studies indicate that myelin-forming glia exert trophic effects on axons at a local

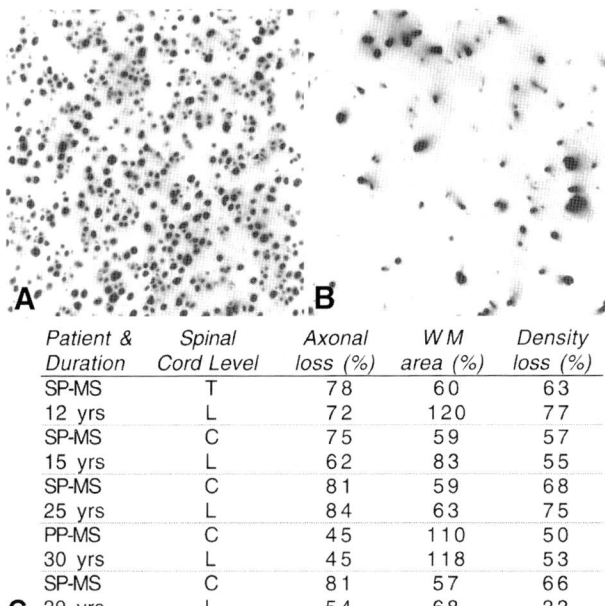

Patient & Duration	Spinal Cord Level	Axonal loss (%)	WM area (%)	Density loss (%)
SP-MS	T	78	60	63
12 yrs	L	72	120	77
SP-MS	C	75	59	57
15 yrs	L	62	83	55
SP-MS	C	81	59	68
25 yrs	L	84	63	75
PP-MS	C	45	110	50
30 yrs	L	45	118	53
SP-MS	C	81	57	66
39 yrs	L	54	68	33

Figure 7 Axonal loss and spinal cord atrophy in paralyzed MS patients. Reduced neurofilament staining indicates significantly decreased axonal density in a demyelinated area of the gracile fascicle from MS cervical spinal cord (**B**) compared to matching control sample (**A**). Measures of axonal loss in spinal cords from 5 chronic MS patients at cervical (C5), thoracic (T5), and lumbar (L5) levels averaged 68% (**C**). Whole spinal cord cross sections (mm²) from controls and chronic MS patients with severe neurological impairment were measured at cervical (C5–C7) and lumbar (L1–L3) levels to determine the percent change in area between MS and control (**C**). Average MS spinal cord area was reduced, significantly at the cervical level ($P = 0.02$). (Reproduced from Bjartmar et al., 1999 (**A, B**) and Bjartmar et al., 2001 (**C**) with permission.)

level, and that disruption of the axonal cytoskeleton plays a critical role in mediating the pathogenesis of axonal degeneration secondary to demyelination. Consequently, the effects of chronic demyelination may drive late axonal degeneration in SP-MS by inducing deleterious compensatory changes by the axolemma and altering axonal transport. Further, chronic demyelination results in unresolved loss of trophic support from myelin-forming cells. Therefore, remyelination is important not just for restoring normal impulse conduction, but as a neuroprotective event for ameliorating mechanisms of late axonal degeneration.

IV. Cortical Lesions in Multiple Sclerosis

Do mechanisms other than loss of white matter axons contribute to neurodegeneration in MS? The cerebral cortex contains myelin, as many axons originating from and terminating on cortical neurons are myelinated. Although MS has traditionally been regarded as a white matter disease, demyelinated lesions also occur in the gray matter (Brownell and Hughes, 1962; Lumsden, 1970; Kidd et al., 1999; Peterson et al., 2001; Bo et al., 2003b). A recent pathological

study identified axonal transection, dendritic transection, and neuronal apoptosis in cortical lesions (Peterson et al., 2001). In addition, Peterson et al., (2001) observed striking differences in the inflammatory cell character and density between white matter lesions and cortical lesions. These findings establish the occurrence of significant irreversible neuronal damage in cortical MS lesions and raise questions regarding the etiology of neurological disability in MS patients, the regulation of inflammation in MS, and the potential treatment of MS. Compared to white matter lesions, however, cerebral cortical lesions are less obvious macroscopically, histologically, and on conventional T_2-weighted MRI scans.

A. Incidence and Types of Cortical Lesions

Several studies have described the incidence of cerebral cortical lesions in MS. A histological study by Brownell and Hughes (1962) reported that 26% of the brain lesions in MS involved the gray matter. The majority of gray matter lesions (~65%) was located at the leukocortical junction and affected both the cortex and white matter. The remaining 35% of the lesions were located either in the central gray matter (15%) or completely within in the cortex (~19%). Another histological study of 60 MS brains reported cortical lesions in 93% of cases, with 59% of the cerebral lesions affecting the cortex (Lumsden, 1970). In one brain there was extensive involvement of the cerebral cortex, which contained an incredible 465 gyral plaques.

Despite the identification of cortical involvement, which can be quite extensive in some patients with MS, this aspect of the disease has been overlooked for the last 30 years. Recently, there has been renewed interest in the involvement of cerebral cortex in MS (Filippi, 2001). MRI allows the *in vivo* detection of white matter lesions, which sometimes correlate with neurological symptoms; however, MS patients often display neurological symptoms that cannot be explained by the identified white matter pathology. A recent immunocytochemical study identified and characterized 112 cortical lesions in 110 tissue blocks from 50 MS brains (Peterson et al., 2001). Based on the distribution of the demyelinated areas, three general types of cortical lesions were described (Fig. 8). Type I lesions, which demyelinated both white matter and cortex, made up 34% of the cortical lesions. Demyelinating lesions that were intracortical were called Type II lesions and consisted of 16% of the cortical lesions. The remaining 50% of the cortical lesions extended into the cortex from the pial surface and were defined as Type III lesions. All three lesion types were often identified in tissue from the same MS brains. Although no single pattern of cortical demyelination appears to predominate in individual patients, it remains to be determined whether subgrouping patients with variable pathogenesis (Lucchinetti et al., 2000) can identify a prevalence of subtypes. Each subtype may be informative regarding mechanisms of demyelination and characteristics of the immune response or demyelinating inflammatory environment. Cortical lesions were identified in

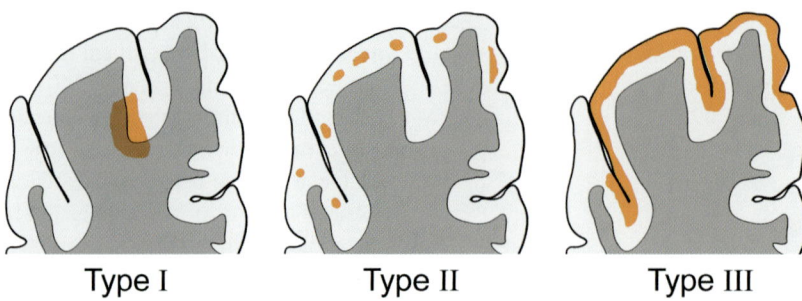

Type I   Type II   Type III

Figure 8 **Three types of cortical demyelination are prominent in MS.** Type I lesions occur at the leukocortical junction affecting both white and gray matter. Type II lesions are small, circular intracortical lesions most often centered around vessels. Type III lesions extend from the pial surface midway into the cortex and often involve multiple gyri. Cortex is white, white matter is gray, and orange represents demyelination.

tissue samples from all 50 of the MS brains, suggesting that cortical involvement in MS is common. The extent of cortical demyelination was more carefully analyzed in another recent immunocytochemical study that prospectively selected the frontal, parietal, and temporal cortices along with cingulate gyrus for analysis from postmortem MS brains. The study determined that on average approximately 27% of the sampled cortices was demyelinated, indicating significant involvement of the cortices in MS (Bo et al., 2003b).

Although these studies suggest that cortical demyelination is significant in MS brains, the precise incidence and dynamics of cortical demyelination remain to be elucidated. Cortical lesions are often missed in sections stained histologically for myelin with luxol fast blue (LFB) because the protocol recommends destaining LFB sections until the cerebral cortex is no longer blue. This may explain why the earlier histological studies (Brownell and Hughes, 1962; Lumsden, 1970) identified fewer cortical only lesions, which would be harder to detect than lesions that also affected the white matter. However, myelin protein immunocytochemistry has proven to be highly sensitive and reliable for identifying cortical lesions in paraffin, free floating, and frozen tissue sections (Peterson et al., 2001; Bo et al., 2003b). A more practical approach to determine the cortical lesion load is the possibility of using MRI scans. In a combined MRI/histology study the use of gadolinium-enhancement increased the detection of cortical lesions on MRI scans by 140% (Kidd et al., 1999). In addition, 26% of all active brain lesions identified in this study were within or adjacent to the cerebral cortex. Although the use of gadolinium with T_2-weighted MRI scans improved detection of cortical lesions, histological examination of the same brains revealed that MRI analysis still underestimated the presence of cortical lesions. Although standard MRI and MRS protocols are relatively insensitive for detection of cortical lesions (Kidd et al., 1999; Sharma et al., 2001), specialized pulse sequences or spec-

troscopy with 3 Tesla scanners may provide the higher resolution necessary for detection of cortical lesions.

B. Reduced Inflammation of Cortical Lesions

Fewer inflammatory cells are present in Type I cortical lesions compared to white matter lesions (Peterson et al., 2001). The cortical portion of Type I lesions contained 6 times less CD68-positive microglia/macrophages and 13 times less CD3-positive lymphocytes than the white matter portion of the lesions. Another recent immunocytochemical study of Type I and Type II lesions also identified reduced inflammation in the cortex compared to the white matter (Bo et al., 2003a). In addition, perivascular cuffs were rare in cortical lesions and when present contained few cells (Peterson et al., 2001; Bo et al., 2003a). Cortical lesions appear normal in routine histological analyses (e.g., hematoxylin and eosin) that rely on nuclear stains as a result of the paucity of inflammatory cells. The lack of inflammatory cells and perivascular cuffs in cortical lesions suggest that trafficking of leukocytes may be differentially regulated in the cortices than in the white matter. It is possible that cortical endothelial cells express decreased or increased levels of molecules that either promote or inhibit leukocyte-endothelial adhesion, respectively. The molecular regulation of leukocyte entry into inflammatory brain lesions has been partially characterized (Hickey, 1991; Lassmann et al., 1991; Perry et al., 1993; von Andrian and Mackay, 2000). Antigen-specific lymphocytes produce pro-inflammatory cytokines inducing a cascade of cytokine and chemokine expression by resident astrocytes and microglia (Lo et al., 1999). The recruitment of lymphocytes and monocytes is promoted by the activation and increased expression of adhesion molecules on the luminal surface of endothelial cells (Springer, 1994; von Andrian and Mackay, 2000). Therefore, endothelial cells, astrocytes, and microglia modulate the inflammatory signals in cortex and white matter lesions determining the inflammatory cell character of the immune response. Because Type I lesions affect both the cortex and white matter simultaneously, they eliminate the confounding variable of matching lesion stages between samples. The identification, quantification, and characterization of chemokines, pro-inflammatory cytokines, and cell adhesion molecules on endothelial cells expressed in cortical and white matter portions of Type I lesions may provide a molecular explanation for the reduced inflammation of cortical MS lesions.

The paucity of leukocytic infiltration in the cortical lesions of MS brains establishes that demyelination can occur in the absence of extensive inflammatory cell infiltration. This suggests that induction of demyelination may not require a large influx of leukocytes and that the large influx of leukocytes in white matter lesions may be related to phagocytosis of myelin debris rather than primary destruction of myelin. Type III lesions, which represented approximately 50% of the total cortical lesions identified, are the most interesting pattern of demyelination (Peterson et al., 2001). Many Type III lesions extended from the pial surface to cortical layers three or four, often extending over multiple gyri with the depth of the demyelinated area remarkably constant. This pattern of demyelination indicates that demyelination or loss of oligodendrocytes in Type III lesions may be linked with a factor or factors that diffused from the brain surface. There are reports of demyelinating factors in the CSF of patients with MS (Alcazar et al., 2000) or serum from rodents with EAE (Bornstein and Appel, 1965), although such observations have been rare. Of interest is that the progression of demyelination was stopped at cortical layer 5 in many Type III lesions. This suggests that the mechanisms of demyelination may differ in Type III cortical lesions from those in Types I and II cortical lesions.

C. Neuronal Pathology in Cortical Lesions

Transected axons, transected dendrites, and neuronal apoptosis were identified in cortical MS lesions obtained from patients with clinical disease ranging from 2 weeks to 27 years (Peterson et al., 2001). Despite reduced cortical inflammation, significant amounts of neuronal injury occur in cortical lesions. Similar to axons in the white matter, neurofilament-positive swellings were detected along dendrites and axons suggesting disruption of normal cellular transport. Many of these swellings were identified by confocal analysis as the terminal ends of axons and dendrites (Fig. 9A, B). The density of transected neurites (axons and dendrites) in cortical lesions correlated with the degree of microglial activation, numbering $4,119/mm^3$ in active, $1,107/mm^3$ in chronic active, and $25/mm^3$ in chronic inactive lesions. In contrast, myelinated cortex from MS and control brains contained an average of 8 and 1 transected neurite/ mm^3, respectively. The correlation between neuritic transection and microglial activation of the lesion suggests that

dendrites and demyelinated axons are vulnerable to microglial activation associated with cortical demyelination.

Decreased synaptic input into the cortex caused by loss of dendritic arborization is a previously unidentified pathological change in MS that can contribute to neurological disability. Depending on which axons are transected, the functional deficit induced by axonal transection will vary. Efferent axonal inputs transected close to their targets may have the ability to sprout and reinnervate postsynaptic densities. Proximal transection of afferent axonal outputs of cortical neurons (Fig. 9B), however, will result in the irreversible functional loss of the neuron. Axonal transection often results in apoptosis or atrophy of the affected neuron depending on the extent of remaining target-derived support (Meyer et al., 2001; Ginsberg and Martin, 2002; al Abdulla and Martin, 2002; Hains et al., 2003). Thus it was not surprising when apoptotic neurons were significantly increased in cortical lesions compared to myelinated cortex in MS brains (Peterson et al., 2001). In addition, as cortical neurons are lost this will reduce the trophic support for the afferent neurons projecting to them and eventually these target-deprived neurons may die (al Abdulla and Martin, 2002). Neuronal or axonal assaults unrelated to axonal transection may also cause apoptotic neuronal death. CSF collected from a primary progressive MS patient during ongoing inflammatory activity induced apoptosis of neurons in vitro (Alcazar et al., 2000). This study suggests the existence of a diffusible factor in the CSF, which can mediate neuronal damage and death.

If demyelination, deafferentation, or inflammatory mediators secreted by activated microglia cause neuronal apoptosis, then therapeutic intervention may help preserve the neuron and maintain the neuronal circuitry. Significant neuronal apoptosis was identified in chronic active and chronic inactive lesions indicating that neuronal loss may result from chronic insults to neurons, dendrites, or axons in addition to direct immune attack during the demyelinating process (Peterson et al., 2001). While the number of apoptotic neurons appears small, clearance of apoptotic cells is known to occur within 24 hours (al Abdulla et al., 1998; Olanow and Tatton, 1999) and the apoptotic neurons were prevalent in chronic lesions that existed for years. Therefore over time, neuronal loss by apoptosis could be significant. In some cases considerable areas of cortex were partially remyelinated, suggesting that additional neuritic and neuronal loss may have occurred in areas not analyzed.

D. Microglial Response in Cortical MS Lesions

The resident immune cells of the CNS are the microglia, which monitor pathological changes locally and also at sites distant to their location (Gonzalez-Scarano and Baltuch, 1999; Streit et al., 1999). In cortical MS lesions a striking association between microglia and neurons was identified (Peterson et al., 2001). Double-labeling confocal microscopy

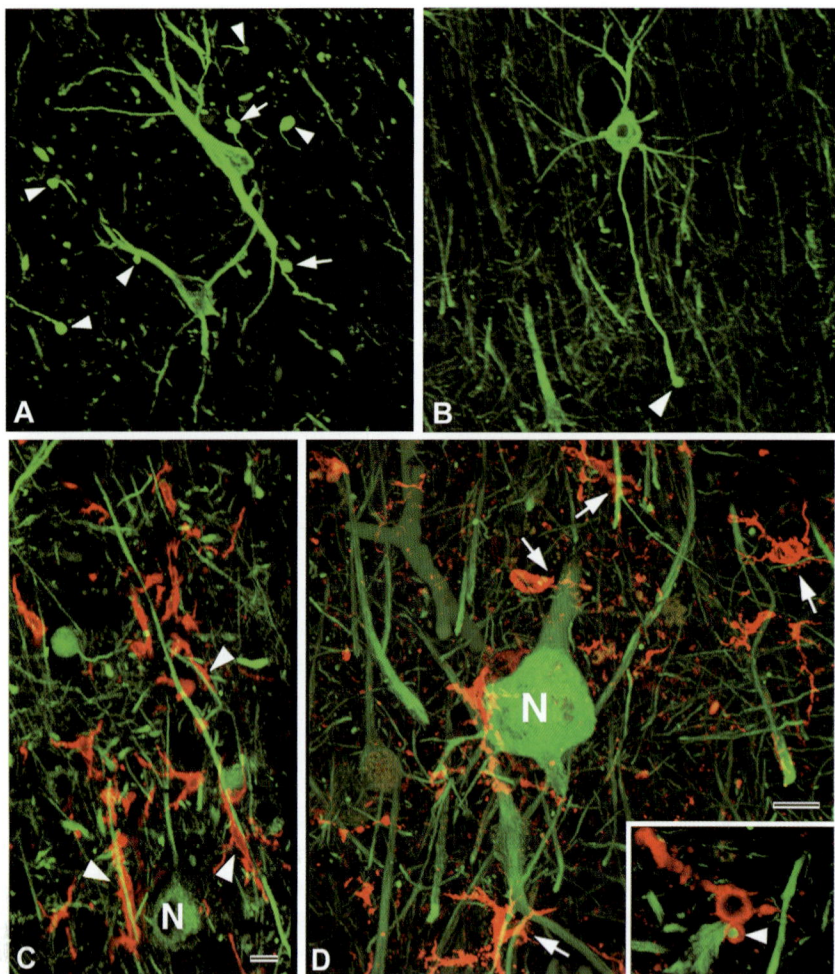

Figure 9 Neuronal pathology in cortical lesions. Nonphosphorylated neurofilament-positive ovoids are abundant in cortical lesions (**A, B,** *green*). Confocal microscopy confirmed most of these ovoids as terminal ends of neurites (**A,** *arrowheads*) and some as *en passant* swellings (**A,** *arrows*). Some ovoids close to neuronal perikarya could be identified as axonal (**B,** *arrowhead*) or dendritic (not shown). Microglial (*red*) targeting of neuronal perikarya and processes (*green*) (**C, D**). Confocal microscopy detected ferritin-positive microglia with elongated shapes ensheathing neurites (**C,** *arrowheads*). More stellate-shaped microglia were detected in close apposition to neuronal perikarya and extending processes to and around neurofilament-positive neurites (**D,** *arrows*). High magnification image of microglial process (*red, arrowhead*) ensheathing a branch of an apical dendrite (*green*) (*inset*). N = neuron. (Reproduced from Peterson et al., 2001, with permission.)

detected elongated microglia oriented perpendicular to the pial surface, closely apposed, and ensheathing apical dendrites and axons in active and chronic active cortical lesions (Fig. 9C, D). In addition, other more ramified stellate-shaped microglia often extended processes to neuronal perikarya and ensheathed dendrites or axons (Fig. 9D). Unlike microglia/macrophages in white matter lesions which often apposed the terminal ends of transected axons (Trapp et al., 1998) microglia in cortical lesions did not consistently associate with the terminal ends of transected neurites in the cortical lesions (Fig. 9C).

The targeting of neurons and neuronal processes by microglia is suggestive of the process of synaptic stripping.

Microglia in cortical lesions morphologically resemble microglia in an animal model of synaptic stripping (Blinzinger and Kreutzberg, 1968; Graeber et al., 1988). After distal regions of the facial nerve are transected, microglia become activated and target neurons of the affected VII cranial nerve nucleus within a day. By electron microscopy, the microglial processes were detected separating presynaptic and postsynaptic terminals (Blinzinger and Kreutzberg, 1968). Whether microglia in cortical lesions actively target synaptic terminals remains to be determined. It is unknown whether this association between microglia and neurons is destructive or protective. It is likely that the microglia are targeting neurons already functionally impaired. For example, in

Alzheimer's disease (AD), activated microglia are associated with damaged neurites and neuronal loss (Haga et al., 1989; McGeer et al., 1992; Mochizuki et al., 1996). Some of the most promising AD therapeutics are anti-inflammatory therapies targeting activated microglia (Breitner, 1996; Combs et al., 2000). Thus, similar anti-inflammatory therapies, which reduce microglial activation in the cerebral cortex, may benefit patients with MS.

E. Cortical Lesions Contribute to Disease Burden in MS

These studies indicate that cortical lesions should be considered major contributors to disease burden in patients with MS, considering the substantial amount of neuronal pathology that occurs in cortical lesions. It is possible that ambulatory decline is modulated significantly by neuronal damage in motor and sensory cortex. Further, 40% to 70% of all individuals diagnosed with MS exhibit various aspects of cognitive deficits (Rao et al., 1991; Beatty et al., 1995). Functions most commonly affected involve learning, memory, and information processing (Rao et al., 1991). Correlation between decreased cerebral metabolism and increased MRI lesion load with cognitive dysfunction in MS was demonstrated by positron emission tomography studies (Blinkenberg et al., 2000). Although cognitive impairment in MS patients has been attributed to subcortical white matter lesions, reconciliation between the anatomical location of the subcortical lesions and the identified cognitive deficits is often problematic because they do not match. It is probable given the extent and nature of damage to cortical neurons in many MS brains, however, cortical lesions provide an additional biological substrate for functional impairment.

V. Functional Consequences

What are the short- and long-term functional consequences of cumulative axonal degeneration during the course of MS? The evolving concept of MS having an inflammatory-mediated neurodegenerative component provides a conceptual framework explaining disease progression and development of permanent neurological disability in MS patients. Acute inflammatory activity and demyelination cause reversible disability during RR-MS. However, it is well documented that axolemmal remodeling of denuded axons allows them to regain the ability to conduct impulses (Bostock and Sears, 1978; Foster et al., 1980; Felts et al., 1997); therefore it is unlikely that demyelination alone causes chronic disability in MS (Matthews et al., 1998; Bjartmar et al., 1999; Trapp et al., 1999b). Even in the absence of overt inflammatory disease activity, most MS patients display continuous functional deterioration from moderate to severe disability (Bjartmar et al., 1999). This observation indicates that different mechanisms of neurological disability occur during different stages of the disease. Early in MS when neurological disability is minimal to moderate, symptoms in most MS patients are caused predominantly by conduction block mediated by inflammation, edema, and demyelination (Fig. 2). Neurological function not recovered during remission in the initial stages of MS are likely caused by early axonal transection in pathways with poor compensatory reserve such as the long tracks that make up the corticospinal motor system. In addition, loss of myelin-derived trophic support and induction of axolemmal compensatory mechanisms may initiate a deleterious cascade causing chronically demyelinated axons to degenerate contributing to disability (Fig. 2) (Scherer, 1999; Bjartmar et al., 1999; Waxman, 2001). Axonal and neuronal degeneration, which occur by the previously described mechanisms, will have cumulative effects on remaining neurons.

An epidemiological study reported the time from onset of MS to EDSS 4 varied between 1 and 33 years, in contrast to the time from EDSS 4 to EDSS 7, which was strikingly similar among the patients (Confavreux et al., 2000). These observations indicate that once a pathological threshold is surpassed, most patients with MS progress along a final common pathway of preprogrammed neuronal degeneration. The progression of neurological disability from EDSS 4 to EDSS 7 occurs by neurodegenerative mechanisms other than inflammatory-mediated axonal transection, which most likely contributes to severe neurological decline during later stages of the disease (Trapp et al., 1999b; Confavreux et al., 2000; Noseworthy et al., 2000; Bjartmar and Trapp, 2001). Neuronal pathology results in the loss of both pre-synaptic and/or post-synaptic trophic support. It is possible the lack of trans-synaptic trophic support will further induce anterograde and retrograde propagation of trans-synaptic neurodegenerative changes in the remaining neurons. In addition, mechanisms of neuronal loss similar to those in post-polio syndrome (PPS) may be involved. In PPS, motor neurons that survive the polio infection compensate for the lost motor neurons. The motor neurons undergo axonal sprouting and innervate muscles denervated by the dying α motor neurons, enabling patients with polio to recover functionally. It is hypothesized that after several decades, these motor neurons begin to die prematurely from the years of increased workload. These preprogrammed, neurodegenerative changes dissociate acute inflammatory damage observed early in the disease from progressive tissue degeneration during chronic stages of MS. The histopathological identification of neuronal pathology in MS, specifically the destruction of axons and dendrites along with neuronal cell death, provides a pathological substrate for the progressive disability many patients with chronic MS experience and suggests a mechanism by which early inflammatory activity may initiate a state of preprogrammed neuronal degeneration.

Why is neuronal pathology subclinical during RR-MS if it begins at disease onset? All neurodegenerative diseases have an initial silent stage of neuronal cell loss. The CNS has a remarkable capacity to compensate for neuronal damage. For example, it has been estimated that 50% to 80% of target neurons in amyotrophic lateral sclerosis and Parkinson's disease, respectively, are lost before presentation of neurological symptoms (Lloyd, 1977; Bradley, 1987). In RR-MS, lesions outnumber clinical relapses by as many as 10:1 (McFarland et al., 1992). Indeed, correlations are usually weak between clinical status and T2 lesion load on MRI scans (Simon et al., 1998; Filippi et al., 1995). Additionally, clinical features during RR-MS are poor predictors of subsequent disability progression (Rudick et al., 1999b). However, there is positive correlation between progressive disability and increasing brain atrophy in individual patients that likely parallels accumulating axonal loss (Losseff et al., 1996). Clinical symptoms are reversible during RR-MS because they are primarily associated with acute inflammatory lesions in articulate parts of the CNS. Once resolution of inflammation and edema, redistribution of axolemmal sodium channels, remyelination, and/or compensatory cortical adaptation occurs, there is clinical remission (Waxman, 1998; Bjartmar and Trapp, 2001). A recent report identified patients with MS who had undiagnosed neurological symptoms; they had an astounding average axonal loss of 64% within sampled lesions (Mews et al., 1998). The lack of clinical signs was attributed to lesion site, neuronal redundancy, low levels of total axon loss, and remyelination. In a study using both functional MRI and MRS, RR-MS patients, without overt permanent functional disability, demonstrated a fivefold increase in sensorimotor cortex activation with simple hand movements compared to individuals who did not have MS (Reddy et al., 2000). These data indicate that maintained motor function during early stages of MS may result from adaptive cortical changes, such as the reorganization of functional pathways, which could compensate for axonal damage.

The data presented collectively suggest that axonal injury begins at disease onset, and cumulative neuronal pathology most adequately accounts for permanent disability in patients with MS. Based on the identification of neuronal pathology as a major feature, MS can be considered an inflammatory neurodegenerative disease, which has several important implications. It is probable that different mechanisms contribute to neuronal damage during different stages of disease; therefore it is crucial to clarify the pathophysiology of neurodegeneration in MS. In contrast to most neurodegenerative diseases, MS patients are more likely to be identified at initial stages of the disease by the presentation of symptoms caused by inflammatory demyelination. Therefore MS may provide a tractable disease for testing neuroprotective therapies, as patients can be treated early before substantial neurodegeneration has occurred.

The prevention of persistent neurological disability is the main goal when treating neurological diseases. Because tissue destruction begins at disease onset and inflammatory-mediated tissue damage may occur in the absence of clinical symptoms during RR-MS, early aggressive proactive application of disease-modifying therapeutics is warranted to prevent and delay accumulating neuronal damage. Accumulation of demyelination and neuronal damage during RR-MS triggers the subsequent unrelenting progression of neurological disability during SP-MS (Rudick et al., 1999b). During RR-MS, response is reasonable to current anti-inflammatory and immunomodulatory drugs. In contrast, SP-MS is characterized by negligible response to anti-inflammatory therapeutics with few satisfactory therapies available. Therefore, inflammation remains a major therapeutic target and use of anti-inflammatory drugs is most prudent during early MS, where early aggressive anti-inflammatory treatment may have indirect neuroprotective effects. In addition, patients with MS may benefit from the use of neuroprotective therapies along with current anti-inflammatory and immunomodulatory treatments. The development of neuroprotective drugs applicable to MS is an urgent goal for MS researchers. Remyelination would also be considered neuroprotective. Promotion of remyelination restores conduction and oligodendrocyte-derived trophic support, and may prevent axonal degeneration.

VI. Conclusion

This chapter summarizes data indicating that neuronal injury is an integral part of MS, and that loss of axons, dendrites, and neurons contributes to the irreversible functional impairment observed in affected individuals. Recent reports describe various aspects and potential mechanisms of neuronal injury in MS. Through different methods and use of various animal models, our understanding of neuropathological mechanisms involved in the development of permanent symptoms during the disease course has increased. Several lines of evidence indicate that primary inflammatory demyelination underlies early axonal loss during RR-MS; however, this axonal loss is clinically silent. The transition from RR-MS to SP-MS has been suggested to occur when a threshold of axonal loss is reached, and the compensatory capacity of the CNS is surpassed, resulting in the subsequent development of permanent neurological symptoms. The level of inflammatory activity during RR-MS determines the rate of neurodegeneration and the point at which a patient is said to have SP-MS.

The inflammatory neurodegenerative disease concept of MS has several clinical implications. Surrogate markers of axonal loss are needed to monitor neurodegeneration. Early aggressive anti-inflammatory and immunomodulatory treatment should be provided to prevent and delay disability. Neuroprotective therapeutics should be developed for MS.

Finally, further elucidation of the molecular mechanisms behind axonal injury and their relation to disease stage in MS is essential for the development of novel therapeutic strategies.

Acknowledgments

Supported by NIH grant NS35058.

The authors thank Dr. Xinghua Yin for helpful discussions, Susan De Stefano for assistance with preparation of the manuscript, and Rosalia Yacubova for assistance with the illustrations and figures.

References

Agrawal, S. K., and Fehlings, M. G. (1996). Mechanisms of secondary injury to spinal cord axons in vitro: Role of Na+, Na(+)-K(+)-ATPase, the Na(+)-H+ exchanger, and the Na(+)-Ca2+ exchanger. *J. Neurosci.* **16**, 545–552.

al Abdulla, N. A., and Martin, L. J. (2002). Projection neurons and interneurons in the lateral geniculate nucleus undergo distinct forms of degeneration ranging from retrograde and transsynaptic apoptosis to transient atrophy after cortical ablation in rat. *Neuroscience* **115**, 7–14.

al Abdulla, N. A., Portera-Cailliau, C., and Martin, L. J. (1998). Occipital cortex ablation in adult rat causes retrograde neuronal death in the lateral geniculate nucleus that resembles apoptosis. *Neuroscience* **86**, 191–209.

Alcazar, A., Regidor, I., Masjuan, J., Salinas, M., and Alvarez-Cermeno, J. C. (2000). Axonal damage induced by cerebrospinal fluid from patients with relapsing-remitting multiple sclerosis. *J. Neuroimmunol.* **104**, 58–67.

Ames, A., III. (2000). CNS energy metabolism as related to function. *Brain Res. Brain Res. Rev.* **34**, 42–68.

Arnold, D. L. (1999). Magnetic resonance spectroscopy: imaging axonal damage in MS. *J. Neuroimmunol.* **98**, 2–6.

Babbe, H., Roers, A., Waisman, A., Lassmann, H., Goebels, N., Hohlfeld, R., Friese, M., Schroder, R., Deckert, M., Schmidt, S., Ravid, R., and Rajewsky, K. (2000). Clonal expansions of CD8(+) T cells dominate the T cell infiltrate in active multiple sclerosis lesions as shown by micromanipulation and single cell polymerase chain reaction. *J. Exp. Med.* **192**, 393–404.

Barnes, D., Munro, P. M., Youl, B. D., Prineas, J. W., and McDonald, W. I. (1991). The longstanding MS lesion. A quantitative MRI and electron microscopic study. *Brain* **114**, 1271–1280.

Beatty, W. W., Paul, R. H., Wilbanks, S. L., Hames, K. A., Blanco, C. R., Goodkin, D. E. (1995). Identifying multiple sclerosis patients with mild or global cognitive impairment using the Screening Examination for Cognitive Impairment (SEFCI). *Neurology* **45**, 718–723.

Bitsch, A., Schuchardt, J., Bunkowski, S., Kuhlmann, T., and Bruck, W. (2000). Acute axonal injury in multiple sclerosis. Correlation with demyelination and inflammation. *Brain* **123**, 1174–1183.

Bjartmar, C., Kidd, G., Mork, S., Rudick, R., and Trapp, B. D. (2000). Neurological disability correlates with spinal cord axonal loss and reduced *N*-acetyl aspartate in chronic multiple sclerosis patients. *Ann. Neurol.* **48**, 893–901.

Bjartmar, C., and Trapp, B. D. (2001). Axonal and neuronal degeneration in multiple sclerosis: mechanisms and functional consequences. *Curr. Opin. Neurol.* **14**, 271–278.

Bjartmar, C., and Trapp, B. D. (2003). Axonal degeneration and progressive neurologic disability in multiple sclerosis. *Neurotox. Res.* **5**, 157–164.

Bjartmar, C., Wujek, J.R., and Trapp, B. D. (2003). Axonal loss in the pathology of MS: Consequences for understanding the progressive phase of the disease. *J. Neurol. Sci.* **206**, 165–171.

Bjartmar, C., Yin, X., and Trapp, B. D. (1999). Axonal pathology in myelin disorders. *J. Neurocytol.* **28**, 383–395.

Blinkenberg, M., Rune, K., Jensen, C. V., Ravnborg, M., Kyllingsbaek, S., Holm, S., Paulson, O. B., and Sorensen, P. S. (2000). Cortical cerebral metabolism correlates with MRI lesion load and cognitive dysfunction in MS. *Neurology* **54**, 558–564.

Blinzinger, K., and Kreutzberg, G. (1968). Displacement of synaptic terminals from regenerating motor neurons by microglial cells. *Z. Zellforsch. Mikrosk. Anat.* **85**, 145–157.

Bö, L., Dawson, T. M., Wesselingh, S., Mörk, S., Choi, S., Kong, P. A., Hanley, D., and Trapp, B. D. (1994). Induction of nitric oxide synthase in demyelinating regions of multiple sclerosis brains. *Ann. Neurol.* **36**, 778–786.

Bo, L., Vedeler, C. A., Nyland, H., Trapp, B. D., and Mork, S. J. (2003a). Intracortical multiple sclerosis lesions are not associated with increased lymphocyte infiltration. *Multiple Sclerosis* **9**, 323–331.

Bo, L., Vedeler, C. A., Nyland, H. I., Trapp, B. D., and Mork, S. J. (2003b). Subpial demyelination in the cerebral cortex of multiple sclerosis patients. *J. Neuropathol. Exp. Neurol.* **62**, 723–732.

Bornstein, M. B., and Appel, S. H. (1965) Tissue culture studies of demyelination. *Ann. N. Y. Acad. Sci.* **122**, 280–286.

Bostock, H., and Sears, T. A. (1978). The internodal axon membrane: Electrical excitability and continuous conduction in segmental demyelination. *J. Physiol.* **280**, 273–301.

Bradley, W. G. (1987). Recent views on amyotrophic lateral sclerosis with emphasis on electrophysiological studies. *Muscle Nerve* **10**, 490–502.

Breitner, J. C. (1996). The role of anti-inflammatory drugs in the prevention and treatment of Alzheimer's disease. *Annu. Rev. Med.* **47**, 401–411.

Brinkmeier, H., Aulkemeyer, P., Wollinsky, K. H., and Rudel, R. (2000). An endogenous pentapeptide acting as a sodium channel blocker in inflammatory autoimmune disorders of the central nervous system. *Nat. Med.* **6**, 808–811.

Brown, A., McFarlin, D. E., and Raine, C. S. (1982). The chronologic neuropathology of relapsing experimental allergic encephalomyelitis in the mouse. *Lab. Invest.* **46**, 171–185.

Brownell, B., and Hughes, J. T. (1962). Distribution of plaques in the cerebrum in multiple sclerosis. *J. Neurol. Neurosurg. Psychiatry* **25**, 315–320.

Bruck, W., and Stadelmann, C. (2003). Inflammation and degeneration in multiple sclerosis. *Neurol. Sci.* **24 Suppl. 5**, S265–S267.

Combs, C. K., Johnson, D. E., Karlo, J. C., Cannady, S. B., and Landreth, G. E. (2000). Inflammatory mechanisms in Alzheimer's disease: Inhibition of beta-amyloid-stimulated proinflammatory responses and neurotoxicity by PPARgamma agonists. *J. Neurosci.* **20**, 558–567.

Confavreux, C., Vukusic, S., Moreau, T., and Adeleine, P. (2000). Relapses and progression of disability in multiple sclerosis. *N. Engl. J. Med.* **343**, 1430–1438.

Craner, M. J., Hains, B. C., Lo, A. C., Black, J. A., and Waxman, S. G. (2004). Co-localization of sodium channel Nav1.6 and the sodium-calcium exchanger at sites of axonal injury in the spinal cord in EAE. *Brain* **127**, 294–303.

Craner, M. J., Lo, A. C., Black, J. A., and Waxman, S. G. (2003) Abnormal sodium channel distribution in optic nerve axons in a model of inflammatory demyelination. *Brain* **126**, 1552–1561.

De Stefano, N., Guidi, L., Stromillo, M. L., Bartolozzi, M. L., and Federico, A. (2003). Imaging neuronal and axonal degeneration in multiple sclerosis. *Neurol. Sci.* **24 Suppl. 5**, S283–S286.

De Stefano, N., Matthews, P. M., and Arnold, D. L. (1995). Reversible decreases in *N*-acetylaspartate after acute brain injury. *Magn. Reson. Med.* **34**, 721–727.

De Stefano, N., Matthews, P. M., Fu, L., Narayanan, S., Stanley, J., Francis, G. S., Antel, J. P., and Arnold, D. L. (1998). Axonal damage correlates with disability in patients with relapsing-remitting multiple sclerosis. Results of a longitudinal magnetic resonance spectroscopy study. *Brain* **121**, 1469–1477.

Evangelou, N., Konz, D., Esiri, M. M., Smith, S., Palace, J., and Matthews, P. M. (2001). Size-selective neuronal changes in the anterior optic pathways suggest a differential susceptibility to injury in multiple sclerosis. *Brain* **124**, 1813–1820.

Felts, P. A., Baker, T. A., and Smith, K. J. (1997). Conduction in segmentally demyelinated mammalian central axons. *J. Neurosci.* **17**, 7267–7277.

Ferguson, B., Matyszak, M. K., Esiri, M. M., and Perry, V. H. (1997). Axonal damage in acute multiple sclerosis lesions. *Brain* **120**, 393–399.

Filippi, M. (2001). Multiple sclerosis: a white matter disease with associated gray matter damage. *J. Neurol. Sci.* **185**, 3–4.

Filippi, M., Paty, D. W., Kappos, L., Barkhof, F., Compston, D. A., Thompson, A. J., Zhao, G. J., Wiles, C. M., McDonald, W. I., and Miller, D. H. (1995). Correlations between changes in disability and T2-weighted brain MRI activity in multiple sclerosis: a follow-up study. *Neurology* **45**, 255–260.

Foster, R. E., Whalen, C. C., and Waxman, S. G. (1980). Reorganization of the axon membrane in demyelinated peripheral nerve fibers: morphological evidence. *Science* **210**, 661–663.

Ganter, P., Prince, C., and Esiri, M. M. (1999). Spinal cord axonal loss in multiple sclerosis: A post-mortem study. *Neuropathol. Appl. Neurobiol.* **25**, 459–467.

Garbern, J. Y., Yool, D. A., Moore, G. J., Wilds, I. B., Faulk, M. W., Klugmann, M., Nave, K. A., Sistermans, E. A., van der Knaap, M. S., Bird, T. D., Shy, M. E., Kamholz, J. A., Griffiths, I.R. (2002). Patients lacking the major CNS myelin protein, proteolipid protein 1, develop length-dependent axonal degeneration in the absence of demyelination and inflammation. *Brain* **125**, 551–561.

Gehrmann, J., Banati, R. B., Cuzner, M. L., Kreutzberg, G. W., and Newcombe, J. (1995). Amyloid precursor protein (APP) expression in multiple sclerosis lesions. *Glia* **15**, 141–151.

Geurts, J. J., Wolswijk, G., Bo, L., van der Valk, P., Polman, C. H., Troost, D., and Aronica, E. (2003). Altered expression patterns of group I and II metabotropic glutamate receptors in multiple sclerosis. *Brain* **126**, 1755–1766.

Ginsberg, S. D., and Martin, L. J. (2002). Axonal transection in adult rat brain induces transsynaptic apoptosis and persistent atrophy of target neurons. *J. Neurotrauma* **19**, 99–109.

Giuliani, F., Goodyer, C. G., Antel, J. P., and Yong, V. W. (2003). Vulnerability of human neurons to T cell-mediated cytotoxicity. *J. Immunol.* **171**, 368–379.

Gonen, O., Catalaa, I., Babb, J. S., Ge, Y., Mannon, L. J., Kolson, D. L., and Grossman, R. I. (2000). Total brain N-acetylaspartate: a new measure of disease load in MS. *Neurology* **54**, 15–19.

Gonzalez-Scarano, F., and Baltuch, G. (1999). Microglia as mediators of inflammatory and degenerative diseases. *Annu. Rev. Neurosci.* **22**, 219–240.

Graeber, M. B., Streit, W. J., and Kreutzberg, G. W. (1988) Axotomy of the rat facial nerve leads to increased CR3 complement receptor expression by activated microglial cells. *J. Neurosci. Res.* **21**, 18–24.

Graumann, U., Reynolds, R., Steck, A. J., and Schaeren-Wiemers, N. (2003). Molecular changes in normal appearing white matter in multiple sclerosis are characteristic of neuroprotective mechanisms against hypoxic insult. *Brain Pathol.* **13**, 554–573.

Greenfield, J. G., and King, L. S. (1936). Observations on the histopathology of the cerebral lesions in disseminated sclerosis. *Brain* **59**, 445–458.

Griffiths, I., Klugmann, M., Anderson, T., Yool, D., Thomson, C., Schwab, M. H., Schneider, A., Zimmermann, F., McCulloch, M., Nadon, N., and Nave, K.-A. (1998). Axonal swellings and degeneration in mice lacking the major proteolipid of myelin. *Science* **280**, 1610–1613.

Hafer-Macko, C., Hsieh, S.-T., Li, C. Y., Ho, T. W., and Sheikh, K. A. (1996). Acute motor axonal neuropathy: an antibody-mediated attack on axolemma. *Ann. Neurol.* **40**, 635–644.

Haga, S., Akai, K., and Ishii, T. (1989). Demonstration of microglial cells in and around senile (neuritic) plaques in the Alzheimer brain. An immunohistochemical study using a novel monoclonal antibody. *Acta Neuropathol.* **77**, 569–575.

Hains, B. C., Black, J. A., and Waxman, S. G. (2003). Primary cortical motor neurons undergo apoptosis after axotomizing spinal cord injury. *J. Comp. Neurol.* **462**, 328–341.

Harris, J. O., Frank, J. A., Patronas, N., McFarlin, D. E., and McFarland, H. F. (1991). Serial gadolinium-enhanced magnetic resonance imaging scans in patients with early, relapsing-remitting multiple sclerosis: implications for clinical trials and natural history. *Ann. Neurol.* **29**, 548–555.

Hickey, W. F. (1991). Migration of hematogenous cells through the blood-brain barrier and the initiation of CNS inflammation. *Brain Pathol.* **1**, 97–105.

Ho, T. W., McKhann, G. M., and Griffin, J. W. (1998). Human autoimmune neuropathies. *Annu. Rev. Neurosci.* **21**, 187–226.

Hohlfeld, R. (1997). Biotechnological agents for the immunotherapy of multiple sclerosis. Principles, problems and perspectives (invited review). *Brain* **120**, 865–916.

Huseby, E. S., Liggitt, D., Brabb, T., Schnabel, B., Ohlen, C., and Goverman, J. (2001). A pathogenic role for myelin-specific CD8(+) T cells in a model for multiple sclerosis. *J. Exp. Med.* **194**, 669–676.

Khoury, S. J., Guttmann, C. R., Orav, E. J., Kikinis, R., Jolesz, F. A., and Weiner, H. L. (2000). Changes in activated T cells in the blood correlate with disease activity in multiple sclerosis. *Arch. Neurol.* **57**, 1183–1189.

Kidd, D., Barkhof, F., McConnell, R., Algra, P. R., Allen, I. V., and Revesz, T. (1999). Cortical lesions in multiple sclerosis. *Brain* **122**, 17–26.

Klugmann, M., Schwab, M. H., Puhlhofer, A, Schneider, A., Zimmermann, F., Griffiths, I. R., and Nave, K. A. (1997). Assembly of CNS myelin in the absence of proteolipid protein. *Neuron* **18**, 59–70.

Kornek, B., and Lassmann, H. (1999). Axonal pathology in multiple sclerosis. A historical note. *Brain Pathol.* **9**, 651–656.

Kornek, B., Storch, M. K., Bauer, J., Djamshidian, A., Weissert, R., Wallstroem, E., Stefferl, A., Zimprich, F., Olsson, T., Linington, C., Schmidbauer, M., and Lassmann, H. (2001). Distribution of a calcium channel subunit in dystrophic axons in multiple sclerosis and experimental autoimmune encephalomyelitis. *Brain* **124**, 1114–1124.

Kornek, B., Storch, M. K., Weissert, R., Wallstroem, E., Stefferl, A., Olsson, T., Linington, C., Schmidbauer, M., and Lassmann, H. (2000). Multiple sclerosis and chronic autoimmune encephalomyelitis: a comparative quantitative study of axonal injury in active, inactive, and remyelinated lesions. *Am. J. Pathol.* **157**, 267–276.

Koudriavtseva, T., Thompson, A. J., Fiorelli, M., Gasperini, C., Bastianello, S., Bozzao, A., Paolillo, A., Pisani, A., Galgani, S., and Pozzilli, C. (1997). Gadolinium enhanced MRI predicts clinical and MRI disease activity in relapsing-remitting multiple sclerosis. *J. Neurol. Neurosurg. Psychiatry* **62**, 285–287.

Lappe-Siefke, C., Goebbels, S., Gravel, M., Nicksch, E., Lee, J., Braun, P. E., Griffiths, I. R., and Nave, K. A. (2003). Disruption of Cnp1 uncouples oligodendroglial functions in axonal support and myelination. *Nat. Genet.* **33**, 366–374.

Lassmann, H. (2003). Hypoxia-like tissue injury as a component of multiple sclerosis lesions. *J. Neurol. Sci.* **206**, 187–191.

Lassmann, H., Zimprich, F., Rossler, K., and Vass, K. (1991). Inflammation in the nervous system. Basic mechanisms and immunological concepts. *Rev. Neurol.* **147**, 763–781.

Leppanen, L. L., and Stys, P. K. (1997). Ion transport and membrane potential in CNS myelinated axons. II: Effects of metabolic inhibition. *J. Neurophysiol.* **78**, 2095–2107.

Li, C., Tropak, M. B., Gerial, R., Clapoff, S., Abramow-Newerly, W., Trapp, B., Peterson, A., and Roder, J. (1994). Myelination in the absence of myelin-associated glycoprotein. *Nature* **369**, 747–750.

Li, S., Jiang, Q., and Stys, P. K. (2000). Important role of reverse Na(+)-Ca(2+) exchange in spinal cord white matter injury at physiological temperature. *J. Neurophysiol.* **84**, 1116–1119.

Lloyd, K. G. (1977). CNS compensation to dopamine neuron loss in Parkinson's disease. *Adv. Exp. Med. Biol.* **90**, 255–266.

Lo, D., Feng, L., Li, L., Carson, M. J., Crowley, M., Pauza, M., Nguyen, A., and Reilly, C. R. (1999). Integrating innate and adaptive immunity in the whole animal. *Immunol. Rev.* **169**, 225–239.

Losseff, N. A., Wang, L., Lai, H. M., Yoo, D. S., Gawne-Cain, M. L., McDonald, W. I., Miller, D. H., and Thompson, A. J. (1996). Progressive cerebral atrophy in multiple sclerosis. A serial MRI study. *Brain* **119**, 2009–2019.

Losseff, N. A., and Miller, D. H. (1998). Measures of brain and spinal cord atrophy in multiple sclerosis. *J. Neurol. Neurosurg. Psychiatry.* May; 64 Suppl: S102–105.

Lovas, G., Szilagyi, N., Majtenyi, K., Palkovits, M., and Komoly, S. (2000). Axonal changes in chronic demyelinated cervical spinal cord plaques. *Brain* **123**, 308–317.

Lu, F., Selak, M., O'Connor, J., Croul, S., Lorenzana, C., Butunoi, C., and Kalman, B. (2000). Oxidative damage to mitochondrial DNA and activity of mitochondrial enzymes in chronic active lesions of multiple sclerosis. *J. Neurol. Sci.* **177**, 95–103.

Lucchinetti, C., Bruck, W., Parisi, J., Scheithauer, B., Rodriguez, M., and Lassmann, H. (2000). Heterogeneity of multiple sclerosis lesions: Implications for the pathogenesis of demyelination. *Ann. Neurol.* **47**, 707–717.

Lumsden, C. E. (1970). The neuropathology of multiple sclerosis. *In:* "Handbook of Clinical Neurology" (Vinken PJ, and Bruyn GW, Eds.), pp. 217–309. Amsterdam: Elsevier Science.

Lycke, J. N., Karlsson, J. E., Andersen, O., and Rosengren, L. E. (1998). Neurofilament protein in cerebrospinal fluid: a potential marker of activity in multiple sclerosis. *J. Neurol. Neurosurg. Psychiatry* **64**, 402–404.

Mancardi, G., Hart, B., Roccatagliata, L., Brok, H., Giunti, D., Bontrop, R., Massacesi, L., Capello, E., and Uccelli, A. (2001). Demyelination and axonal damage in a non-human primate model of multiple sclerosis. *J. Neurol. Sci.* **184**, 41–49.

Matthews, P. M., De Stefano, N., Narayanan, S., Francis, G. S., Wolinsky, J. S., Antel, J. P., and Arnold, D. L. (1998). Putting magnetic resonance spectroscopy studies in context: axonal damage and disability in multiple sclerosis. *Semin. Neurol.* **18**, 327–336.

McFarland, H. F., Frank, J. A., Albert, P. S., Smith, M. E., Martin, R., Harris, J. O., Patronas, N., Maloni, H., and McFarlin, D. E. (1992). Using gadolinium-enhanced magnetic resonance imaging lesions to monitor disease activity in multiple sclerosis. *Ann. Neurol.* **32**, 758–766.

McGeer, P. L., Kawamata, T., Walker, D. G., Akiyama, H., Tooyama, I., and McGeer, E. G. (1992). Microglia in degenerative neurological disease. *Glia* **7**, 84–92.

Medana, I., Martinic, M. A., Wekerle, H., and Neumann, H. (2001). Transection of major histocompatibility complex class I-induced neurites by cytotoxic T lymphocytes. *Am. J. Pathol.* **159**, 809–815.

Mews, I., Bergmann, M., Bunkowski, S., Gullotta, F., and Bruck, W. (1998). Oligodendrocyte and axon pathology in clinically silent multiple sclerosis lesions. *Multiple Sclerosis* **4**, 55–62.

Meyer, R., Weissert, R., Diem, R., Storch, M. K., de Graaf, K. L., Kramer, B., and Bahr, M. (2001). Acute neuronal apoptosis in a rat model of multiple sclerosis. *J. Neurosci.* **21**, 6214–6220.

Miller, D. H., Barkhof, F., Frank, J. A., Parker, G J., and Thompson, A. J. (2002). Measurement of atrophy in multiple sclerosis: Pathological basis, methodological aspects and clinical relevance. *Brain* **125**, 1676–1695.

Miller, D. H., Barkhof, F., and Nauta, J. J. (1993). Gadolinium enhancement increases the sensitivity of MRI in detecting disease activity in multiple sclerosis. *Brain* **116 (Pt 5)**, 1077–1094.

Mochizuki, A., Peterson, J. W., Mufson, E. J., and Trapp, B. D. (1996). Amyloid load and neural elements in Alzheimer's disease and nondemented individuals with high amyloid plaque density. *Exp. Neurol.* **142**, 89–102.

Narayana, P. A., Doyle, T. J., Lai, D., and Wolinsky, J. S. (1998) Serial proton magnetic resonance spectroscopic imaging, contrast-enhanced magnetic resonance imaging, and quantitative lesion volumetry in multiple sclerosis. *Ann. Neurol.* **43**, 56–71.

Noseworthy, J. H., Lucchinetti, C., Rodriguez, M., and Weinshenker, B. G. (2000) Multiple sclerosis. *N. Engl. J. Med.* **343**, 938–952.

Olanow, C. W., and Tatton, W. G. (1999). Etiology and pathogenesis of Parkinson's disease. *Annu. Rev. Neurosci.* **22**, 123–144.

Pantano, P., Iannetti, G. D., Caramia, F., Mainero, C., Di Legge, S., Bozzao, L., Pozzilli, C., and Lenzi ,G. L. (2002). Cortical motor reorganization after a single clinical attack of multiple sclerosis. *Brain* **125**, 1607–1615.

Parry, A. M., Scott, R. B., Palace, J., Smith, S., and Matthews, P. M. (2003). Potentially adaptive functional changes in cognitive processing for patients with multiple sclerosis and their acute modulation by rivastigmine. *Brain* **126**, 2750–2760.

Perry, V. H., Andersson, P. B., and Gordon, S. (1993). Macrophages and inflammation in the central nervous system [Review]. *TINS* **16**, 268–273.

Peters, G. (1968). Multiple sclerosis. *In:* "Pathology of the Nervous System." McGraw-Hill, New York.

Peterson, J. W., Bo, L., Mork, S., Chang, A., and Trapp, B. D. (2001). Transected neurites, apoptotic neurons and reduced inflammation in cortical MS lesions. *Ann. Neurol.* **50**, 389–400.

Piani, D., Frei, K., Do, K. Q., Cuenod, M., and Fontana, A. (1991). Murine brain macrophages induced NMDA receptor mediated neurotoxicity in vitro by secreting glutamate. *Neurosci. Lett.* **133**, 159–162.

Pitt, D., Werner, P., and Raine, C. S. (2000). Glutamate excitotoxicity in a model of multiple sclerosis. *Nat. Med.* **6**, 67–70.

Powell, H. C., and Myers, R. R. (1996). The axon in Guillain-Barre syndrome: Immune target or innocent bystander? Editorial. *Ann. Neurol.* **39(1)**, 4–5.

Prineas, J. (2001). Pathology of multiple sclerosis. *In:* "Handbook of Multiple Sclerosis" (S. Cook, Ed), pp. 289–324. Basel, NY: Marcel Dekker.

Prineas, J. W., Kwon, E. E., Cho, E. S., Sharer, L. R., Barnett, M. H., Oleszak, E. L., Hoffman, B., and Morgan, B. P. (2001). Immunopathology of secondary-progressive multiple sclerosis. *Ann. Neurol.* **50**, 646–657.

Putnam, T. J. (1936). Studies in multiple sclerosis. *Arch. Neurol. Psychiatry* **35**, 1289–1308.

Raine, C. S., Cannella, B., Hauser, S. L., and Genain, C. P. (1999). Demyelination in primate autoimmune encephalomyelitis and acute multiple sclerosis lesions: A case for antigen-specific antibody mediation. *Ann. Neurol.* **46**, 144–160.

Raine, C. S., and Cross, A. H. (1989). Axonal dystrophy as a consequence of long-term demyelination. *Lab. Invest.* **60**: 714–725.

Rao, S. M., Leo, G. J., Bernardin, L., and Unverzagt, F. (1991). Cognitive dysfunction in multiple sclerosis. I. Frequency, patterns, and prediction. *Neurology* **41**, 685–691.

Rawes, J. A., Calabrese, V. P., Khan, O. A., and DeVries, G. H. (1997). Antibodies to the axolemma-enriched fraction in the cerebrospinal fluid and serum of patients with multiple sclerosis and other neurological diseases. *Multiple Sclerosis* **3**, 363–369.

Reddy, H., Narayanan, S., Arnoutelis, R., Jenkinson, M., Antel, J., Matthews, P. M., and Arnold, D. L. (2000). Evidence for adaptive functional changes in the cerebral cortex with axonal injury from multiple sclerosis. *Brain* **123 (Pt 11)**, 2314–2320.

Rocca, M. A., Mezzapesa, D. M., Falini, A., Ghezzi, A., Martinelli, V., Scotti, G., Comi, G., and Filippi, M. (2003). Evidence for axonal pathology and adaptive cortical reorganization in patients at presentation with clinically isolated syndromes suggestive of multiple sclerosis. *Neuroimage* **18**, 847–855.

Rudick, R. A., Cohen, J. A., Weinstock-Guttman, B., Kinkel, R. P., and Ransohoff, R. M. (1997). Management of multiple sclerosis. *N. Engl. J. Med.* **337**, 1604–1611.

Rudick, R. A., Fisher, E., Lee, J. C., Simon, J.,and Jacobs, L. (1999a). Use of the brain parenchymal fraction to measure whole brain atrophy in relapsing-remitting MS. Multiple Sclerosis Collaborative Research Group. *Neurology* **53**, 1698–1704.

Rudick, R. A., Goodman, A., Herndon, R. M., and Panitch, H. S. (1999b). Selecting relapsing remitting multiple sclerosis patients for treatment: The case for early treatment. *J. Neuroimmunol.* **98,** 22–28.

Scherer, S. (1999). Axonal pathology in demyelinating diseases. *Ann. Neurol.* **45,** 6–7.

Sharma, R., Narayana, P. A., and Wolinsky, J. S. (2001). Grey matter abnormalities in multiple sclerosis: Proton magnetic resonance spectroscopic imaging. *Multiple Sclerosis* **7,** 221–226.

Simon, J. H., Jacobs, L. D., Campion, M., Wende, K., Simonian, N., Cookfair, D. L., Rudick, R. A., Herndon, R. M., Richert, J. R., Salazar, A. M., Alam, J. J., Fischer, J. S., Goodkin, D. E., Granger, C. V., Lajaunie, M., Martens-Davidson, A. L., Meyer, M., Sheeder, J., Choi, K., Scherzinger, A. L., Bartoszak, D. M., Bourdette, D. N., Braiman, J., Brownscheidle, C. M., and Whitham, R. H. (1998). Magnetic resonance studies of intramuscular interferon beta-1a for relapsing multiple sclerosis. The Multiple Sclerosis Collaborative Research Group. *Ann. Neurol.* **43,** 79–87.

Simon, J. H., Jacobs, L. D., Campion, M. K., Rudick, R. A., Cookfair, D. L., Herndon, R. M., Richert, J. R., Salazar, A. M., Fischer, J. S., Goodkin, D. E., Simonian, N., Lajaunie, M., Miller, D. E., Wende, K., Martens-Davidson, A., Kinkel, R. P., Munschauer, F. E., III, and Brownscheidle, C. M. (1999). A longitudinal study of brain atrophy in relapsing multiple sclerosis. The Multiple Sclerosis Collaborative Research Group (MSCRG). *Neurology* **53,** 139–148.

Skulina, C., Schmidt, S., Dornmair, K., Babbe, H., Roers, A., Rajewsky, K., Wekerle, H., Hohlfeld, R., and Goebels, N. (2004). Multiple sclerosis: brain-infiltrating CD8+ T cells persist as clonal expansions in the cerebrospinal fluid and blood. *Proc. Natl. Acad. Sci. U. S. A.* **101,** 2428–2433.

Smith, K. J., and Lassmann, H. (2002). The role of nitric oxide in multiple sclerosis. *Lancet Neurology* **1,** 232–241.

Sobel, R. A., Greer, J. M., and Kuchroo, V. K. (1994). Minireview: Autoimmune responses to myelin proteolipid protein. *Neurochem. Res.* **19,** 915–921.

Springer, T. A. (1994). Traffic signals for lymphocyte recirculation and leukocyte emigration: The multistep paradigm. *Cell* **76,** 301–314.

Stevenson, V. L., and Miller, D. H. (1999). Magnetic resonance imaging in the monitoring of disease progression in multiple sclerosis. *Multiple Sclerosis* **5,** 268–272.

Streit, W. J., Walter, S. A., and Pennell, N. A. (1999). Reactive microgliosis. *Prog. Neurobiol.* **57,** 563–581.

Stys, P. K., Waxman, S. G., and Ransom, B. R. (1992). Ionic mechanisms of anoxic injury in mammalian CNS white matter: role of Na+ channels and Na(+)– Ca2+ exchanger. *J. Neurosci.* **12,** 430–439.

Trapp, B. D., Peterson, J., Ransohoff, R. M., Rudick, R., Mork, S., and Bo, L. (1998). Axonal transection in the lesions of multiple sclerosis. *N. Engl. J. Med.* **338,** 278–285.

Trapp, B. D., Ransohoff, R. M., Fisher, E., and Rudick, R. A. (1999a). Neurodegeneration in multiple sclerosis: Relationship to neurological disability. *The Neuroscientist* **5,** 48–57.

Trapp, B. D., Ransohoff, R., and Rudick, R. (1999b). Axonal pathology in multiple sclerosis: relationship to neurological disability. *Current Opinion Neurology* **12:**295–302.

van Waesberghe, J. H., Kamphorst, W., De Groot, C. J., van Walderveen, M. A., Castelijns, J. A., Ravid, R., Nijeholt, G. J., van der Valk, P., C. H., Thompson, A. J., and Barkhof, F. (1999). Axonal loss in multiple sclerosis lesions: magnetic resonance imaging insights into substrates of disability. *Ann. Neurol.* **46,** 747–754.

von Andrian, U. H., and Mackay, C. R. (2000). T-cell function and migration. Two sides of the same coin. *N. Engl. J. Med.* **343,** 1020–1034.

Wang, H. Y., Matsui, M., and Saida, T. (2002). Immunological disturbances in the central nervous system linked to MRI findings in multiple sclerosis. *J. Neuroimmunol.* **125,** 149–154.

Waxman, S. G. (1998). Demyelinating diseases—new pathological insights, new therapeutic targets. *N. Engl. J. Med.* **338,** 323–325.

Waxman, S. G. (2001). Acquired channelopathies in nerve injury and MS. *Neurology* **56,** 1621–1627.

Weiner, H. L., Guttmann, C. R., Khoury, S. J., Orav, E. J., Hohol, M. J., Kikinis, R., and Jolesz, F. A. (2000). Serial magnetic resonance imaging in multiple sclerosis: correlation with attacks, disability, and disease stage. *J. Neuroimmunol.* **104,** 164–173.

Weinshenker, B. G. (1996). Epidemiology of multiple sclerosis. *Neurol. Clin.* **14,** 291–308.

Weinshenker, B. G., Bass, B., Rice, G. P., Noseworthy, J., Carriere, W., Baskerville, J., and Ebers, G. C. (1989). The natural history of multiple sclerosis: a geographically based study. I. Clinical course and disability. *Brain* **112,** 133–146.

Werner, P., Pitt, D., and Raine, C. S. (2001). Multiple sclerosis: Altered glutamate homeostasis in lesions correlates with oligodendrocyte and axonal damage. *Ann. Neurol.* **50,** 169–180.

Wujek, J. R., Bjartmar, C., Richer, E., Ransohoff, R. M., Yu, M., Tuohy, V. K., and Trapp, B. D. (2002). Axon loss in the spinal cord determines permanent neurological disability in an animal model of multiple sclerosis. *J. Neuropathol. Exp. Neurol.* **61,** 23–32.

Yin, X., Crawford, T O., Griffin, J W., Tu, P.-H., Lee, V. M. Y., Li, C., Roder, J., and Trapp, B. D. (1998). Myelin-associated glycoprotein is a myelin signal that modulates the caliber of myelinated axons. *J. Neurosci.* **18,** 1953–1962.

Yu, M., Nishiyama, A., Trapp, B. D., and Tuohy, V. K. (1996). Interferon-beta inhibits progression of relapsing-remitting experimental autoimmune encephalomyelitis. *J. Neuroimmunol.* **64,** 91–100.

Zivadinov, R., and Zorzon, M. (2002). Is gadolinium enhancement predictive of the development of brain atrophy in multiple sclerosis? A review of the literature. *J. Neuroimag.* **12,** 302–309.

13

Natural History of Multiple Sclerosis: When Do Axons Degenerate?

David Miller, M.B., Ch.B., M.D.

I. Introduction

In trying to learn about the natural history of axonal loss in multiple sclerosis (MS), it is appropriate to consider what can be gleaned from both direct studies of tissue pathology and from indirect observations that use surrogate markers of axonal loss in vivo. The former serves as the gold standard but access to pathological tissue in the earlier stages of disease is limited and potentially biased. Few patients die within the first 5 years of onset of MS—thus post mortem studies of early MS are quite limited. Those who undergo brain biopsy in early disease usually have large and/or atypical lesions that raise concern that there is some other (non-demyelinating) pathology, especially cerebral tumor; only a small minority of MS patients is investigated in this manner.

Much more is of course known about axonal loss in patients with longstanding and progressive MS and there has been more opportunity to investigate the findings in lesions with acute inflammatory features as these may be found even in longer duration disease. Since there is limited information in early disease, and because the neuropathological findings of axonal loss are comprehensively reviewed elsewhere in this volume, this chapter will mainly concentrate on the insights provided using in vivo surrogate markers. Specifically, there will be a detailed account of the findings obtained using putative magnetic resonance (MR) markers of axonal loss, since this modality has become the most sensitive way of monitoring MS pathology noninvasively and in vivo.

The chapter begins with a consideration of the importance of timing of axonal loss followed by a short account of pathological findings. It then discusses putative MR methods for measuring axonal loss. Technical aspects of the various methods are reviewed along with a consideration of their robustness as measures of axonal loss. There is a discussion of the findings when such techniques—most particularly atrophy—have been applied at different stages of disease from onset with a first clinical attack (clinically isolated syndrome) through to advanced progressive forms of disease. In addition to axonal loss, which is predominantly (though not exclusively) located in white matter, there is a consideration of neuronal loss, as inferred from application of MR neuroaxonal surrogates to gray matter structures. There is a review of the evidence for neuroaxonal loss in white matter lesions, normal appearing white matter (NAWM) and gray matter (where lesions are common but almost never detected on conventional MRI), along with an evaluation of the relationship between MR surrogate markers of inflammation (gadolinium enhancing and T_2-weighted lesions) and axonal loss. The results of treatment trials using MR surrogate markers of neuroaxonal loss are summarized. Concluding remarks include a consideration of how surrogate measures of neuroaxonal loss might be applied in the future in order to better characterize its natural history and mechanisms, as well as to monitor and detect effective neuroprotective treatments.

II. Importance of Timing of Axonal Loss

Given the evident potential for demyelinated axons to restore nerve conduction, it seems probable that axonal loss rather than demyelination per se is the single most important pathological substrate of irreversible disability in MS. In human adult CNS, axonal loss is in essence an irreversible process. Once there is a sufficient extent of axonal loss within a clinically eloquent pathway, it is likely that irreversible disability will ensue. Although the threshold of axonal loss that results in permanent disability may take many years to develop (as is typically the case in MS), it may be accumulating steadily or in a stepwise fashion over a long period before irreversible clinical dysfunction is manifest. It is therefore important to know when it starts, the rate at which it develops, and the mechanisms that underlie it. Such insights will be fundamental in developing rational and timely therapeutic interventions aimed at its prevention. Since direct study of pathology is not possible in early disease, the introduction of validated surrogate measures of axonal loss will not only help to elucidate its natural history but will also provide a measure of the efficacy of neuroprotective therapies at a time when axonal loss is minor and has not yet reached the extent of being clinically apparent.

III. Neuropathology Findings

Although the classical neuropathological descriptions of multiple sclerosis has been of a disease in which complete loss of myelin is accompanied by relative sparing of axons, it was clear even from early reports that considerable axonal loss had occurred by the time patients had died from the disease (Charcot, 1868). The early observations have been amply confirmed and extended during the last 10 years, a period during which interest in axonal damage in MS has abounded. The renewed attention to axonal pathology has come about in part because neurophysiological research had shown that demyeli-

nation per se might not be an adequate explanation of irreversible disability and partly because of the evidence from studies using putative MR markers that axonal loss was extensive. In patients coming to postmortem (usually with longstanding secondary progressive disease), marked axonal loss has been reported in lesions in the cerebral white matter (Lassmann et al., 1994) and spinal cord (Lovas et al., 2000); furthermore, extensive loss if axons also is seen in the NAWM in both regions (Evangelou et al., 2000; Lovas et al., 2000). It has also been shown that marked neuronal loss occurs in the thalamus in secondary progressive MS (Cifelli et al., 2002) and that cortical gray matter lesions are abundant in MS (Kidd et al., 1999) and are associated with evidence of axonal transection (Petersen et al., 2001) . Naturally, observations at the early stages of MS are relatively scarce, although it is clear that signs of axonal damage and death can be marked in acute inflammatory lesions (Trapp et al., 1998), and one study reported that inflammation-related axonal loss occurs more often in patients with a disease duration of less than one year (Kuhlmann et al., 2002).

IV. MR Markers of Neuroaxonal Loss

It has been possible to begin to compose a picture of the natural history of axonal loss in MS by the application of putative MR neuroaxonal markers in vivo at all stages of the disease. The insights obtained will be summarized but first it should be emphasized that there are three general limitations that should be recognized when interpreting the existing data. First, none of the putative imaging surrogates provides a precise and direct measure of axonal loss—the potential limitations will be considered for each method, and inherent in the discussion are certain assumptions between the imaging measure and axonal loss that may not always prove to be reliable. Secondly, in order to obtain a complete picture of natural history, very long-term follow-up studies are needed in individual subjects, ideally followed from onset of disease—so far, almost all serial studies have been limited to at most only a few years. Thirdly, many different methodologies have been employed to evaluate the surrogate markers, and comparison between studies is therefore often difficult. It follows that the present understanding of the natural history of neuroaxonal loss is incomplete. Although it is based in part on consistently observed data, it also involves assumptions and extrapolations some of which may not be verified when more definitive data is available. Nevertheless, the considerable information already generated provides a useful basis for describing the natural history of neuroaxonal damage and loss in MS.

Atrophy

Of all the proposed MR measures of the neurodegenerative component of MS, measurement of tissue loss (atrophy) is the most attractive and robust and to date is the most widely used in studies of MS natural history and treatment trials (Table 1). Axons make the largest bulk contribution to white matter volume (45%), followed by myelin (25%) and other tissue elements—glial and vascular tissues and water (Miller et al., 2002). Neuronal cell bodies and axons contribute the bulk of gray matter volume although there is also myelin in gray matter, albeit to a lesser extent than white matter. It follows that atrophy of white or gray matter in MS is likely to predominantly reflect axonal and neuronal loss. In a study of the spinal cord of five MS cases, in which atrophy and axonal loss were studied (Bjartmar et al., 2000), there was axonal loss within spinal cord lesions of between 45% to

85% and atrophy was more marked in the cervical than the lumbar area and affected gray and white matter equally.

Axonal loss is not the sole cause of atrophy and loss of myelin *per se* will contribute. Variation in glial bulk, inflammation, and tissue water content will also affect global or regional volume measures in MS: acute inflammation will increase volume, whereas a decrease in tissue water and inflammation due to treatment, dehydration, or other factors will decrease volume. Gliosis might increase volume by adding tissue bulk or decrease volume through retraction. It is likely that the use of atrophy to measure progressive neurodegeneration in MS will be made less sensitive because of the volumetric fluctuations due to inflammation. It should

Table 1　Clinical Studies of Atrophy in MS

Atrophy detected			Method	Comments
Clinically isolated syndromes				
Dalton 2002	(55)	+	Ventricular volume	Significant increase in those developing MS or with T2 lesions
Brex 2001	(43)	+	C2 area	Atrophy at presentation in those with brain lesions but no change over 1 year
Hickman 2002	(17)	+	Optic nerve area	Atrophy increases over months to years after an attack of optic neuritis
Dalton 2004	(58)	+	GMF and WMF	Progressive gray matter atrophy over 3 years in those developing MS
Filippi 2004	(263)	+	PBVC	30% reduction in atrophy over two years in BIFN versus placebo-treated patients
Relapsing-remitting MS				
Losseff 1996b	(29)	+	Central cerebral volume	Strong correlation with disability but not with lesions over 18 months
Rudick 1999	(85)	+	BPF	Slowing of atrophy during year 2 of BIFN therapy
Rovaris 2001	(239)	+	Central cerebral volume	No effect of glatiramer acetate over 9 months
Jones 2001	(519)	+	WBR	No effect of BIFN on atrophy
Zidavinov 2001	(88)	−	Brain volume	Absence of atrophy over 5 years in patients treated with regular IV steroids
Chard 2002a	(26)	+	GMF and WMF	Gray and white matter atrophy in early RR MS
Fisher 2002	(138)	+	BPF	Atrophy over two years relates to disability 8 years later
Gasperini 2002	(52)	+	Regional brain volumes	Enhancing lesions over 6 months corrrelated with atrophy in next 2 yrs
de Stefano 2003	(90[+])	+	Cortex volume	Cortical atrophy in RRMS and PPMS of short disease duration
Chard 2004	(13)	+	GMF and WMF	Progressive gray matter atrophy over 18 months in early RRMS
Frank 2004	(30)	+	Brain volume	Decreased rate of atrophy in second and third year after starting beta interferon
Secondary progressive MS				
Losseff 1996a	(60[γ])	+	C2 area	Atrophy correlated with disability
Coles 1999	(27)	+	Central cerebral volume	Progressive atrophy associated with increasing disability
Molyneux 2000	(95)	+	Central cerebral volume	No effect of BIFN on atrophy
Ge 2000	(36*)	+	Parenchymal brain volume	Correlated with disability in SP but not RRMS
Filippi 2000	(159[@])	+	Whole brain volume	No effect of cladribine on atrophy
Wolinsky 2000	(718*)	+	Normalized CSF volume	Higher CSF volume in more disabled patients
Kalkers 2001	(137[γ])	+	BVF	Atrophy correlates better with disability than lesion load
Lin 2003	(38*)	+	Upper cervical cord area	Progressive cord atrophy over 4 years
Primary progressive MS				
Stevenson 2000	(167)	+	Central cerebral slices	Progressive atrophy over 1 year
Kalkers 2002	(16)	+	C2 area	Riluzole may slow cord atrophy
Ingle 2003	(41)	+	Brain andcord measures	Progressive cerebral and cord atrophy over 5 years

Glossary of terms for Table 1

+: atrophy detected　　　　　BPF: brain parenchymal fraction　　　　BIFN: beta interferon
(): number of patients studied　BVF: brain volume fraction　　　　　　GMF: gray matter fraction
WBR: whole brain ratio　　　　CSF: cerebrospinal fluid volume　　　　WMF: white matter fraction
RR: relapsing-remitting　　　　SP: secondary progressive　　　　　　PP: primary progressive
C2 area: cross-sectional area of cervical cord at C2 level　　　　　　　IV: intravenous
PBVC: percentage brain volume change

*includes RR & SPMS; [+]Includes RR & PPMS; [γ]includes RR, SP, & PPMS; [@]includes SP & PPMS.

also be borne in mind that anti-inflammatory therapies (e.g., high-dose corticosteroids or beta interferon) may reduce brain volume without there having been axonal loss. If such an effect is anticipated, it would seem wise to wait for a period of time after receiving such therapy—for the anti-inflammatory volume reduction effect to occur—before using ongoing atrophy as a presumed measure of axonal loss. Three months is a sufficient interval after a course of intravenous steroids, as this therapy has only a short-term effect on brain volume (Rao et al., 2002).

The optimal technique for detecting atrophy should be reproducible, sensitive to change, accurate, and practical to implement, although small errors of accuracy are probably insignificant, as long as they are constant between subjects and over time. The two distinct methodological aspects involved in measuring tissue volumes are data acquisition and data analysis.

Data Acquisition

The ability to reduce partial volume errors with high resolution scans means that 3-D acquisitions are attractive, although 2-D sequences have also been used successfully to derive volume measures in the CNS. For whole-brain atrophy measurements segmentation of the brain is necessary, and suppression of CSF helps to generate a sharp distinction in signal between cerebral and extra-cerebral matter. The most widely used 3-D sequence is a T1-weighted gradient echo, with or without added CSF suppression, the latter provided by an inversion recovery pre-pulse, allowing $1 \times 1 \times 1$mm resolution. Specific study of white or gray matter requires good contrast between white matter, gray matter, CSF, and lesions and may be aided by multiple-contrast acquisitions e.g. T_1, T_2 and proton-density.

Data Analysis Methods

Manual outlining or linear measurements provide the simplest approach to measuring changes in volume. An experienced observer is required, who is familiar with normal neuroanatomy and pathology. Manual segmentation is useful in small structures or regions, e.g., third ventricle, where significant atrophy is reported in MS (Simon et al., 1999). Disadvantages of manual segmentation include operator bias, long analysis time and poor reproducibility when compared with automated techniques.

Semiautomated methods improve speed and reproducibility. Regional segmentation algorithms—e.g., seed growing, contouring—outline lesions, spinal cord, optic nerves and ventricles. Measurement reproducibility improves from ~3–5% for manual outlining to ~1–3% for semi-automated approaches for measuring spinal cord and ventricles.

A considerable number of automated methods exist for segmentation (and thus volume measurement) of the whole brain. Both single contrast and multi-spectral data have been utilized for whole-brain segmentation. Usually the difference in signal intensity between brain parenchyma and CSF on a single contrast acquisition is enough to drive the segmentation process. Segmentation of gray and white matter may also be accomplished with either single-contrast or multi-spectral data, although additional sophistication is required to separate the two tissue types. Methods include Statistical Parametric Mapping-based segmentation and the fuzzy C-means algorithm. Masking of MS lesions is necessary to avoid their misclassification.

As atrophy is the measurement of change in volume, measurements of absolute volumes at separate time points are not necessarily needed; information may be obtained by looking for differences between serial scans (Smith et al., 2001). Non-linear registration of such scans produces deformation fields that yield information concerning regional and global atrophy. Rigid body registration can be used to track the displacement of the surface of the brain during atrophy. Using the inner table of the skull as a standard of reference, Freeborough and Fox (1997) have developed a method to quantify atrophy with high sensitivity in many neurological diseases. Changes in the whole brain or in the ventricles can be investigated.

Comparisons between groups of patients are confounded by the presence of substantial inter-subject variations in head size that can mask differences attributable to atrophy. Normalizing the brain volume to head size reduces these variations. Relative volumes also remove variability in volume data due to scanner instability. A number of normalization methods have emerged: the scalp, total intracranial capacity determined by the sum of the volumes of gray matter, white matter, and CSF, or the sum of the brain and ventricular and sulcal CSF, have all been used to create volumes for normalization.

Tissue Volume Changes Produced by Individual Inflammatory/Demyelinating Lesions

The amount of atrophy that is produced by *individual* inflammatory/demyelinating lesions can best be investigated by studying the optic nerve of patients who have an attack of optic neuritis. Quantitation of optic nerve size is made difficult by its small size, liability to motion during imaging, and close proximity to CSF in the optic nerve sheath and also to orbital fat. Suppression of signal from orbital fat is required in order to avoid a chemical shift artifact at the interface between nerve and fat. This is achieved either by using a short tau inversion recovery sequence (STIR) or a fat suppressed sequence. Additional water suppression can be added to the latter by using a fluid attenuated inversion recovery sequence (FLAIR). The latter provides the most reliable assessment of the cross-sectional area of the nerve itself, being unhindered by signal from CSF in the sheath. A short TE fat suppressed fast FLAIR sequence (sTEfFLAIR) combined with semiautomated contouring on coronal images has proved sufficiently reproducible to detect and quantify the extent of optic nerve atrophy following a single episode of optic neuritis (Hickman et al., 2001a). Atrophy of about 10% to 15% has also been observed in the optic nerve following such an attack, and evidence has emerged to suggest that atrophy may continue to develop for several months or even years after the episode (Hickman et al., 2002).

A systematic investigation of the effect of unilateral optic neuritis lesions on the size of the nerve from the acute to the chronic stage has been undertaken with up to 7 MRI scans obtained using the sTEfFLAIR sequence over one year (Hickman et al., 2004). The first study was obtained within 4 weeks of onset of visual symptoms, at which time 27 of 28 acutely symptomatic lesions displayed gadolinium enhancement, indicating the presence of acute inflammation. At this stage, compared with the clinically unaffected companion optic nerve and with nerves of healthy control subjects, the cross-sectional area of the symptomatic nerve was increased by a mean of 20%. Subsequent studies showed a gradual resolution of swelling over several months and by one year there was a mean decrease in optic nerve area of 12% compared to healthy nerves. Almost all cases had a good recovery to normal or near normal visual acuity.

These observations of individual lesions have implications for interpretation of studies of atrophy in the brain, which reflect the global effects of the disease including both old and new lesions (as well as normal-appearing tissues). The observation of swelling in the acute inflammatory lesion and atrophy in the more chronic postinflammatory lesion suggest that the concurrent presence of lesions of differing ages—as is often seen in the brain of patients with relapsing forms of MS—may introduce noise when using the measure of progressive brain atrophy as a surrogate marker of axonal loss.

There is probably considerable potential to use optic neuritis as a model for the mechanisms of development of atrophy following single inflammatory demyelinating lesions. By obtaining, in parallel, visual evoked potentials (to monitor nerve conduction), detailed clinical measures of function and other MR techniques that investigate intrinsic aspects of the pathology (e.g., gadolinium enhancement to study inflammation; magnetization transfer imaging to study myelination), it should be possible to develop a picture of pathophysiological events as atrophy develops. It is also now possible to obtain a more direct assessment of axonal damage following optic neuritis by investigating the retinal nerve fiber layer thickness using noninvasive measures such as ocular coherence tomography (Parisi et al., 1999); combining this technique with MR imaging of the optic nerve should help to understand the relationship between the MR measures and axonal damage.

A further implication of the demonstration of atrophy from single inflammatory/demyelinating lesions is that disease modifying therapies for preventing acute inflammation have the potential to decrease the extent of tissue damage and axonal loss in MS and that optic neuritis is a good model for evaluating new treatments which are given during the acute inflammatory episode with the aim of preventing or reducing subsequent tissue loss. Using STIR imaging, it has

been reported that high dose intravenous methylprednisolone failed to prevent optic nerve atrophy 6 months after an attack of optic neuritis (Hickman et al., 2003), a finding consistent with the evidence that long-term clinical outcome for vision is not affected (Beck and Cleary, 1993). Novel therapies for preventing axonal loss and permanent disability associated with acute MS inflammatory lesions and relapses are therefore required. In future trials of such agents, inclusion of patients with optic neuritis and the use of combined clinical, electrophysiological, and quantitative MRI measures including optic nerve size would be useful in assessing the response to treatment.

Clinically Isolated Syndromes (CIS)

Fifty to 70% of patients presenting with a CIS (i.e., a single relapse of the sort seen in MS) affecting the optic nerve, brain stem, or spinal cord already have disseminated cerebral white matter lesions typical of MS and most such individuals will develop clinically definite MS with follow-up (Brex et al., 2002, Beck et al., 2003). A cohort of 55 CIS patients has been followed over a one year period to investigate ventricular enlargement (Dalton et al., 2002). Significant enlargement was seen in the 18 patients who developed clinical MS (i.e., experienced a second clinical relapse) and in the 40 patients with abnormal brain MRI at presentation (Fig. 1). There was no change in ventricular volume in the 15 patients with normal imaging. Significant but generally modest correlations were observed between ventricular enlargement and lesion load measures. Thus, brain atrophy occurs at the earliest clinical stage of MS and appears to be partly independent of lesions.

More recently, Dalton et al. (2004a) have investigated the location of progressive atrophy in the first 3 years following presentation with a CIS. Of 58 patients who were studied, 31 had developed multiple sclerosis according to the new McDonald criteria (McDonald et al., 2001). Statistical Parametric Mapping was used to segment gray matter from white matter on the baseline and 3-year follow-up scans after the lesions had been segmented and masked using a semi-automated local contour method. The subjects who developed MS displayed significant progressive gray matter atrophy (mean decrease in the gray matter fraction [normalized to intracranial volume] was $-.3.3\%$, $p = 0.001$). In contrast the white matter fraction did not decrease and actually showed a marginal increase ($+1.1\%$, $p = 0.023$). There was also a smaller decrease in the gray matter fraction in those subjects who did not develop MS during the 3 years (Fig. 2).

While the study by Dalton (2004a) suggests that neuro-axonal loss is occurring in gray matter in the earliest clinical stages of MS, the lack of atrophy in white matter does not exclude the possibility that there is also axonal loss occurring in this tissue. It is possible that other bulk tissue changes compensate for axonal loss, e.g., gliosis and inflammation. Inflammatory white matter lesions are often observed in early relapsing MS and may temporarily increase tissue bulk. The NAWM may also be affected by such processes. A recent

Baseline ventricular volume = 5.6cm³   One year ventricular volume = 12.8cm³

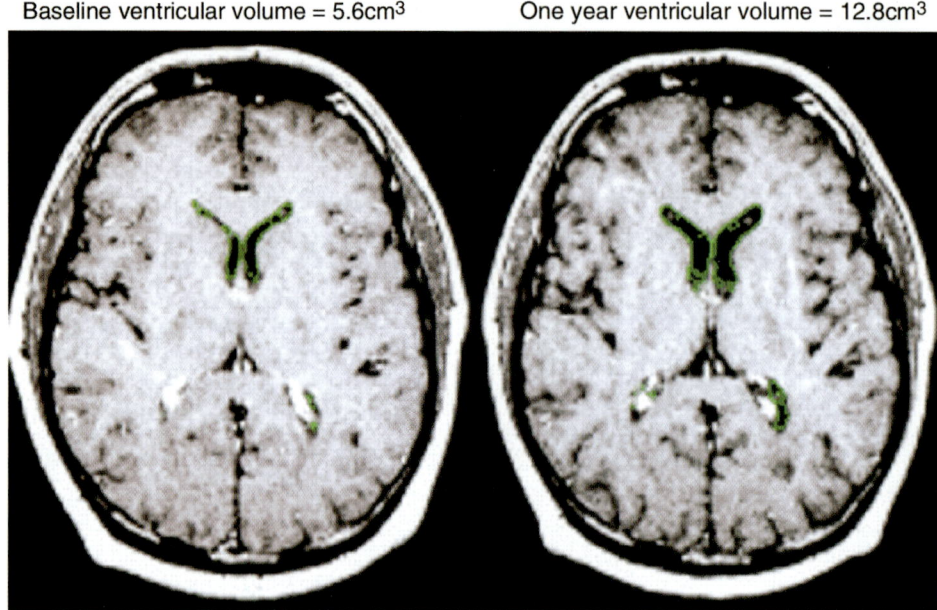

Figure 1 Ventricular enlargement over 1 year in a patient who presented with isolated optic neuritis and who had three further relapses during the 1-year follow-up period, leading to a diagnosis of clinically definite MS. (From Dalton et al. (2002), *J. Neurol. Neurosurg. Psychiatry* **73**, 141–147.)

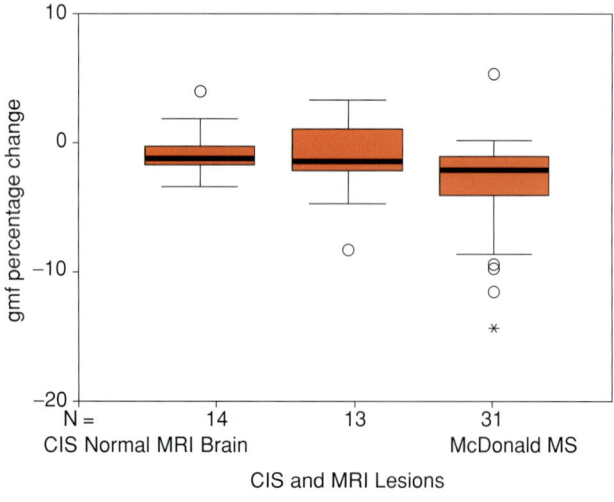

Figure 2 Changes in gray matter fraction seen at 3-year follow-up evaluation in patients with a clinically isolated syndrome. Box plot showing the medians, interquartile ranges (*box*), highest and lowest values, excluding outliers (*whiskers*), outliers (*circles*), and extreme value (*asterisk*) for gray matter fraction percentage change in patients with CIS, with and without MRI lesions, and patients with MS. (From Dalton et al. (2004), *Brain* **117**, 49–58.)

study using proton MR spectroscopy has observed an increase in myoinositol in the NAWM of patients within 6 months of presenting with a CIS (Fernando et al., 2004). This metabolite is produced by astroglia and potentially by other cell types involved in inflammation, e.g., microglia, and

the increase was most evident in those subjects who already had MS according to the McDonald criteria at the time spectroscopy was performed. In comparison to white matter lesions, gray matter lesions in MS show less inflammation (Peterson et al., 2001; Bo et al., 2003). Gray matter atrophy may therefore be a more sensitive measure of neuroaxonal loss in early relapse onset MS where the effect of inflammation on white matter volume may be more prominent.

One of the recurring limitations of studies that explore the relationship between inflammatory lesions and axonal loss is that they have a relatively short duration of follow-up. This shortcoming has been partly addressed in a recent study that investigated the extent of brain atrophy in 28 subjects who had developed MS 14 years after presenting with a CIS (Chard et al., 2003). Because the patients had undergone T2-weighted brain imaging at presentation and subsequently every 5 years, it was possible to investigate—over the 14 years—the extent to which T2-lesion load changes were related to subsequent atrophy. In this context, T2-lesion load was considered as an approximate surrogate marker for prior inflammation since almost all T2 lesions undergo an initial phase of gadolinium enhancement in relapse-onset MS. The main finding was a moderate correlation between T2-lesion load increase during the first 5 years and atrophy at year 14 (Spearman correlation = −0.53). This suggests that early inflammation has a modest link with much later neurodegeneration, although the mechanism for such a link is uncertain. The relatively low magnitude of the correlation emphasizes that factors unrelated to visible MRI lesions probably play an even larger role on the development of atrophy.

Relapsing Remitting MS

Recent studies have shown that both white matter and gray matter brain atrophy are evident in established relapsing remitting MS even within 3 to 5 years of symptom onset (Chard et al., 2002a; de Stefano et al., 2003). A serial study over 18 months of 13 patients compared with 9 healthy controls showed that at baseline there was significant white matter but not gray matter atrophy, but over the follow-up period, there was a significant loss of tissue in the gray matter but not white matter (Chard et al., 2004). This suggests that the temporal dynamics of atrophy in the two tissue types are different, possibly that white matter atrophy is present earlier but increases more slowly than gray matter atrophy.

Whereas brain atrophy is clearly present and increasing from clinical onset, the situation is less clear in the spinal cord. Using a 3-dimensional T1-weighted sequence to measure cross-sectional area of the upper cervical cord, Losseff and colleagues (1996a) found no evidence for atrophy in 15 patients with relapsing remitting MS compared with healthy controls (Fig. 3). On the other hand, Brex et al. (2001a) observed a small but significant degree of atrophy in CIS patients who also had T2 lesions on brain MRI. However, there was no change in cord size over one year of follow-up. In this study, there was a slightly higher proportion of females in the patients versus controls and the scans in patients (but not controls) were obtained after administration of contrast; whether these factors have influenced the result is uncertain.

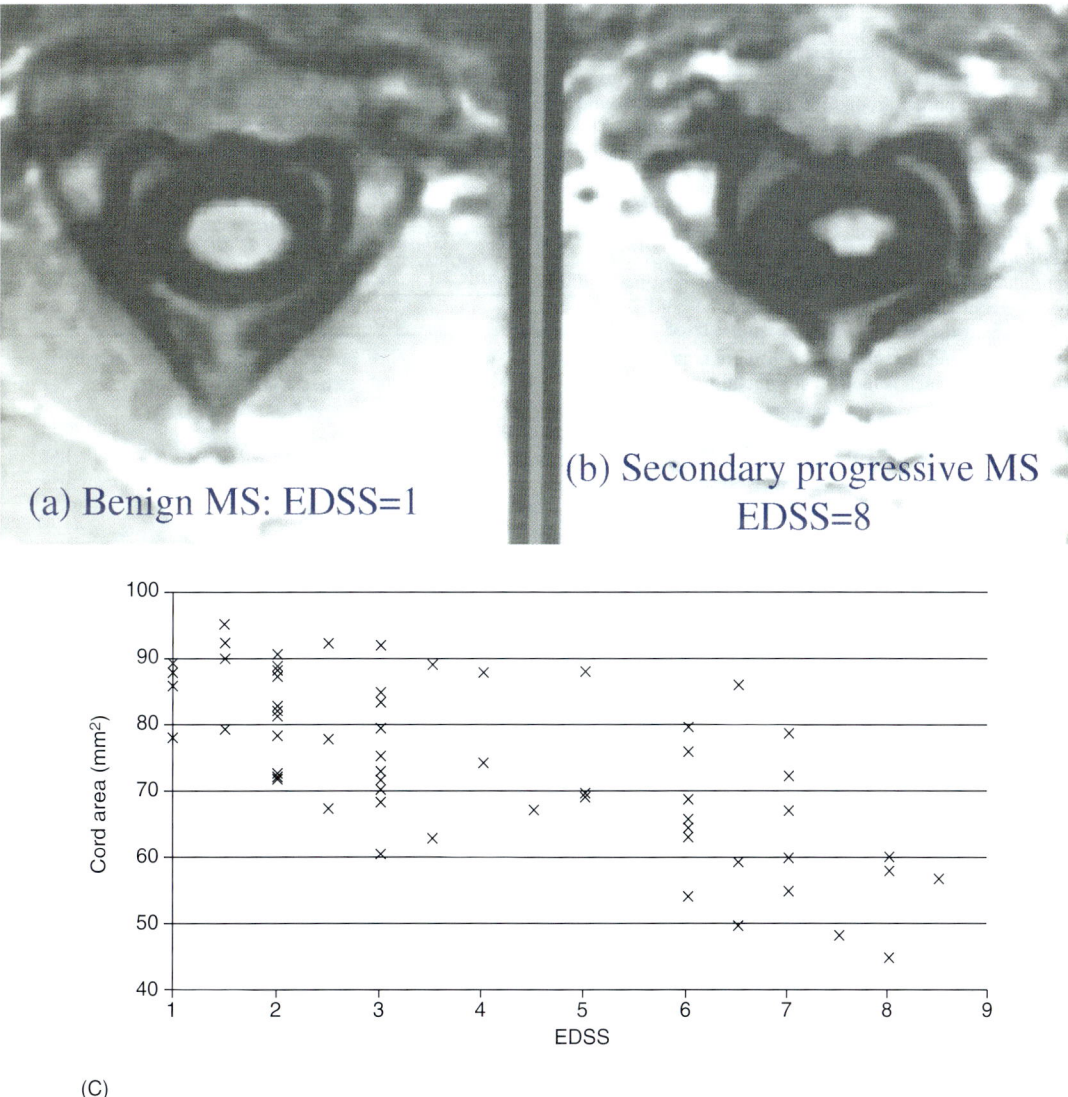

Figure 3 Upper cervical spinal cord atrophy and its relationship to disability in multiple sclerosis: (a) Normal cord size in a patient without disability; (b) Marked cord atrophy in a patient with severe disability; (c) Correlation between cord area and EDSS (r = 0.7). (From Losseff et al. (1996a), *Brain* **199,** 701–708.)

With the evidence for brain atrophy in relapsing remitting disease, measures of brain volume have not surprisingly been applied in several clinical trials at this stage of disease. Using a whole brain ratio (WBR) method, brain atrophy was assessed over two years in a placebo-controlled trial of beta interferon in relapsing remitting MS (Jones et al., 2001). Atrophy measures were available in 519 patients, 172 of whom were on placebo. Significant brain atrophy was seen in the total cohort over two years: the mean WBR decreased by 1.4%. The baseline WBR was weakly correlated with T2-lesion load. No difference in the rate of atrophy was seen between treatment arms.

Cerebral atrophy has been evaluated from 52 relapsing remitting patients for 6 months prior to and 24 months following beta interferon treatment and correlated with other MRI lesion and clinical parameters (Gasperini et al., 2002). During the two years of treatment there was a significant reduction of brain volume (mean −2.2%) that was correlated weakly with the mean number of enhancing lesions on monthly scans during the 6 months pre-treatment. During the two years of treatment, 26 patients exhibited significant atrophy and 26 did not; in the former group, 13 experienced an increase in disability whereas in the latter group only 3 became more disabled. This confirms other studies in showing a link between increasing atrophy and disability (Losseff et al., 1996b; Coles et al., 1999).

In a 2-year placebo controlled trial of beta interferon in relapsing remitting MS, atrophy was measured from yearly scans using the brain parenchymal fraction (BPF). The mean BPF decrease was similar in both arms in year 1, but was smaller in the beta interferon arm in year 2 (Rudick et al., 1999). The changes in BPF during this 2-year period showed little or no correlation with lesion measures. Prolonged 8-year follow-up of some of the placebo cohorts from this trial assessed the longer term relationship between earlier BPF change and later disability (Fisher et al., 2002). Comparison of patient quartiles based on change in BPF over the first two years revealed a greater likelihood of developing severe disability (EDSS of 6 or more at follow-up) in those with the most atrophy during the initial two years.

A recent uncontrolled study of 30 patients with relapsing remitting MS treated with beta interferon reported a −1.35% decrease in brain volume during the first year, but a much smaller reduction of −0.165%/year for the next two years (Frank et al., 2004). The authors proposed that the year one decrease in brain volume was accentuated by a treatment associated decrease in inflammation, and that the much lower rate of atrophy subsequently indicated a positive therapeutic effect.

A 5-year follow-up study has reported comparisons of outcome for patients treated with regular 3 monthly high dose methylprednisolone compared with a group who received steroids only as required for relapses (Zidavinov et al., 2001). The group on regular steroid treatment had a slowing in the rate of cerebral atrophy, in spite of an increase in T2 lesion volume. This surprising result has not been replicated, and is not sufficient to endorse such a treatment

approach, especially bearing in mind the morbidity that could be anticipated from it.

A 9-month, placebo-controlled trial of glatiramer acetate in 239 relapsing remitting MS revealed a mean 0.7%–0.8% reduction in central cerebral volume with no significant differences between the patient groups (Rovaris et al., 2001). The study showed a weak association between enhancing lesion numbers and atrophy. Bearing in mind the evidence suggesting that an effect of beta interferon on atrophy in relapsing remitting MS might be delayed for up to a year (Rudick et al., 1999; Frank et al., 2004), the study may have been too short to definitively evaluate the treatment effect on this outcome.

Progressive Forms of MS

Atrophy is seen in both the brain and spinal cord in secondary and primary progressive MS. The most marked atrophy occurs in secondary progressive disease and correlates with disability (Losseff et al., 1996a, 1996b; Lycklana et al., 1998; Wolinsky et al., 2000; Kalkers et al., 2001; Ge et al., 2000; Lin et al., 2003) but weakly if at all with lesion load and activity (Figs. 3 and 4). In primary progressive MS, significant atrophy of brain and cord over one year was evident in a large cohort of primary progressive patients drawn from six European centers (Stevenson et al., 2000). Change in cerebral volume over one year correlated only weakly with change in T1 and T2 brain load. More recently, progressive cerebral and cervical cord atrophy have been observed over 5 years of follow-up in a cohort of 41 primary progressive MS patients (Ingle et al., 2003). The rates of atrophy appeared to be relatively constant within individual patients but varied between subjects.

A study of 16 patients with primary progressive MS evaluated riluzole, a neuroprotective glutamate antagonist, using change in cervical cord area as a putative measure of progressive axonal loss (Kalkers et al., 2002). During one year pre-treatment, there was a 2% reduction in mean cord area whereas during one year on treatment the cord area was stable (mean decrease of 0.2% only), but the difference was not significant. This preliminary study indicates the potential of using tissue volume measures in larger cohorts to study the efficacy of neuroprotective agents.

Therapeutic trials have evaluated the effect of three immunomodulatory agents in secondary progressive MS— beta interferon (Molyneux et al., 2000), Campath-1H (Coles et al., 1999), and cladribine (Filippi et al., 2000). In spite of all three therapies suppressing inflammatory MRI lesions, there was no evidence for a significant slowing in the rate of ongoing cerebral atrophy. In the beta interferon trial there was ~1% loss of central cerebral volume per year in the treated and placebo arms (Molyneux et al., 2000).

Time Course Issues for Measuring Atrophy

While it is clear that significant tissue loss can be detected in MS within as little as 12 months, little work has been done to determine the optimal sample sizes and length of study required to demonstrate significant slowing of

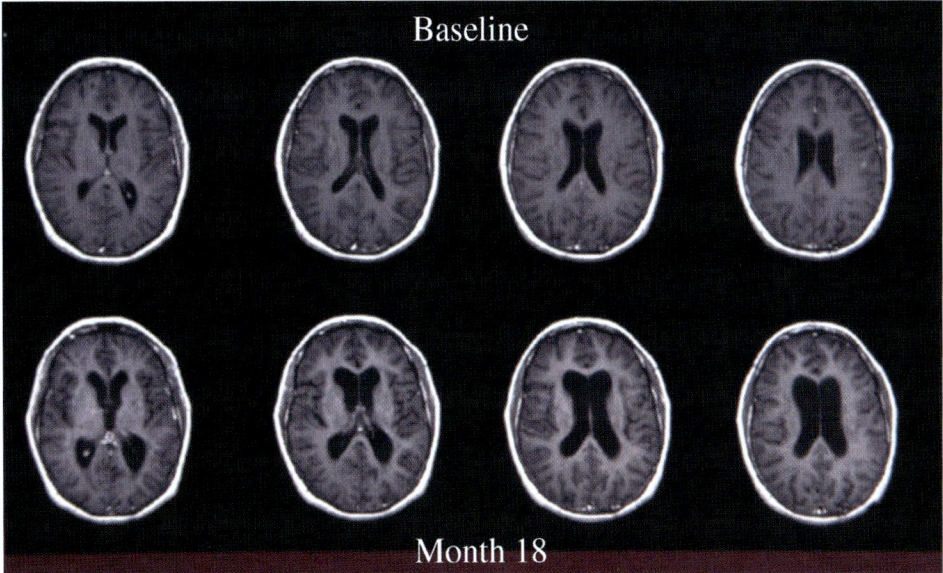

Figure 4 Patient with secondary progressive MS and increasing disability and cerebral atrophy over 18 months in spite of a paucity of inflammation (the volume of gadolinium-enhancing lesions was only 0.4 ml). (From Losseff et al. (1996b), *Brain* **199**, 2009–2019.)

progressive atrophy as a result of therapeutic intervention. This is a priority area for further research, which should include a consideration of the stage of disease (e.g. relapsing remitting, secondary progressive), the type of acquisition and image analysis method, the region of CNS being studied (e.g. whole brain, regional brain, spinal cord etc), the frequency of scanning, and other potential confounding factors (e.g. atrophy due to anti-inflammatory therapy).

Summary of Atrophy as a Surrogate Marker in MS

For several reasons, atrophy has emerged as a preferred method for monitoring the neurodegenerative process in MS: (i) robust methods for detecting tissue loss are available; (ii) it is progressive from onset and increases with increasing disability; (iii) it correlates only modestly with inflammatory lesions, thus providing additional information in therapeutic monitoring and natural history studies; (iv) whereas a number of existing therapies have shown good suppression of inflammatory lesions, an effect on progressive atrophy has been less evident. A recent review discusses in-depth methodological and clinical aspects of atrophy in MS (Miller et al., 2002).

MR Spectroscopy: N-Acetyl Aspartate (NAA)

The main peak in the proton MR spectrum from human adult CNS is *N*-acetyl aspartate (NAA), an amino acid contained almost exclusively in neurones and axons. A reduction in NAA provides evidence of axonal dysfunction or loss and has been consistently reported in MS lesions and NAWM (Fu et al., 1998). Neuroaxonal loss *per se* is not a sufficient explanation for all instances where a decrease in NAA is observed. In acute gadolinium enhancing lesions, decreased NAA is consistently present during the acute phase but frequently increases with follow-up in subsequent months (Davie et al., 1994). This suggests that there is a partly reversible element to the decrease indicating dysfunction but not death of neurones and axons. A possible mechanism is mitochondrial dysfunction during acute inflammation, which reduces the normal production and metabolism of NAA (that is closely linked to mitochondrial function). There is evidence from a study of acute experimental allergic encephalomyelitis that decreased NAA and ultrastructural mitochondrial abnormalities occur in the absence of axonal loss (Brenner et al., 1993). Follow-up of acute MS lesions has nevertheless revealed that the recovery of NAA is incomplete; persistent decrease in postinflammatory lesions would be consistent with axonal loss, although a persistent disturbance of mitochondrial function in the presence of demyelination may also be a possible explanation.

Two approaches have been used to measure NAA: (i) an absolute measure of concentration and using an external standard reference of known concentration and (ii) a ratio of NAA/Cr which assumes that Cr (creatine/phosphocreatine) remains stable in pathological situations. Although both approaches have produced robust evidence that NAA is reduced in MS lesions and normal appearing tissues, abnormalities of Cr may also occur (Fernando et al., 2004). Therefore absolute measures are preferable. A methodological approach of recent interest is the quantitation of whole brain NAA (Gonen et al., 2000). As a global marker of the progressive neurodegenerative process in MS it appears promising, although any changes observed are not anatomically localized and could represent abnormality in lesions,

NAWM, or gray matter. The resonance for whole brain NAA is broad and requires manual delineation for quantification—its analysis is potentially subject to bias and poor reproducibility. The narrow NAA resonances from small voxels—obtained as a single region or as part of a spectroscopic imaging slice—can be automatically identified and quantified with a model that uses as reference a solution with a known concentration of NAA (Provencher, 1993).

There have been several studies of NAA in cohorts with CIS or early relapsing remitting MS, which are of interest in understanding when neuroaxonal dysfunction or loss begins. Tourbah and colleagues (1999) reported a normal NAA/Cr ratio from the NAWM in a group of patients with isolated optic neuritis compared with controls. Recently, Fernando et al. (2004) have investigated NAWM NAA in 96 patients within 6 months of a CIS; compared to 44 healthy controls they reported a mean −2.2% decrease in NAA but this difference was not significant. Another recent study—in patients with clinically definite relapsing-remitting MS and a disease duration less than 3 years—reported that compared to controls, there was a significant reduction in MS NAWM NAA (mean −5%; Chard et al., 2002b). Taking these findings together suggests that axonal loss or dysfunction in NAWM is minimal at MS onset with a CIS but becomes apparent within a few years.

These findings of limited or no abnormality of NAWM NAA contrasts with another recent study of CIS patients, which reported a −22.3% decrease in whole brain NAA of patients versus controls (Filippi et al., 2003). The difference in findings may have several explanations: (i) the whole brain study included lesions and gray matter as well as white matter; (ii) the cohort studied was smaller and restricted to those with evidence fulfilling the McDonald criteria of dissemination in space; (iii) there are fundamental differences in the methodologies used. Based on evidence from a cross-sectional study of patients with relapsing-remitting MS compared with controls that the extent of decrease in whole brain NAA is greater than that of brain atrophy, it has been suggested that neuronal/axonal dysfunction (decrease in NAA) precedes parenchymal tissue loss (atrophy) (Ge et al., 2004). Further studies are needed that specifically explore disease effects upon gray matter and white matter metabolite profiles in patients with CIS.

A greater reduction of NAWM NAA is observed in secondary progressive than in relapsing-remitting MS (Fu et al., 1998), and disability has been correlated with reduced NAA in both cerebral (Sarchielli et al., 1999) and cerebellar white matter (Davie et al., 1995) NAWM (Fig. 5). The observation that there is a significant correlation between increasing atrophy and decreasing NAA in both cerebral hemispheres (Coles

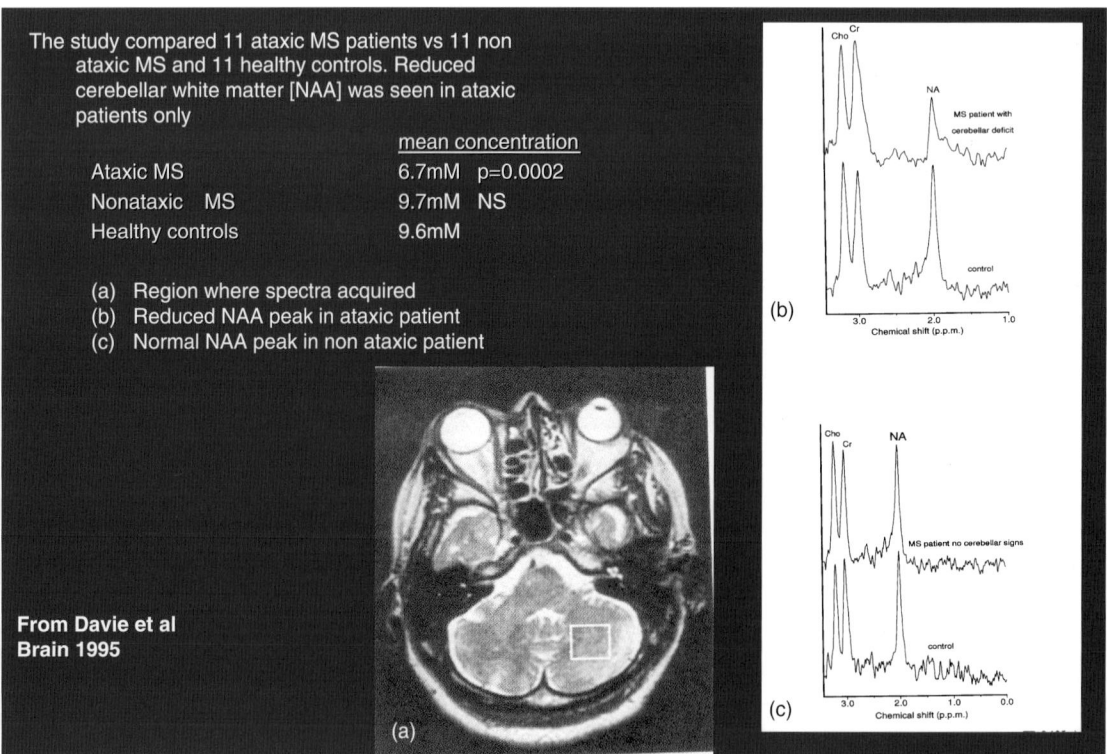

Figure 5 MR spectroscopy evidence of cerebellar white matter axonal loss and disability in MS. (From Davie et al. (1995), *Brain* **118,** 1583–1592.)

et al., 1999) and cerebellum (Davie et al., 1995) supports their role as measures of axonal loss. Decreased NAA has also been observed in cortical gray matter in early relapsing-remitting MS (−7%) suggesting that early neuronal cell body damage is occurring (Chard et al., 2002b). It is reduced by ~20% in thalamic gray matter in secondary progressive MS and in a postmortem study, the decrease in NAA (accompanied by atrophy) was associated with decreased numbers of neurones (Cifelli et al., 2002). In primary progressive MS, NAWM NAA is decreased (Leary et al., 1999) and reduction of NAA and atrophy appear to be relatively independent of T2-lesion load (Pelletier et al., 2003).

Additional studies comparing relapsing-remitting versus secondary progressive MS have yielded valuable information. A cross-sectional analysis using a large single slab of tissue acquired through the cerebral hemispheres above the level of the lateral ventricles reported a similar reduction in the NAA/Cr ratio in both subgroups although a larger proportion of the region of interest was occupied by lesions in the relapsing-remitting group (Matthews et al., 1996). Subsequent investigation using single-slice spectroscopic imaging revealed that NAWM NAA was reduced in both groups but more so in those with secondary progressive MS (Fu et al., 1998). The reduction in NAWM NAA was not as great as that seen in lesions (Fu et al., 1998), but is potentially of more functional importance since the NAWM constitutes a much larger proportion of the CNS. A follow-up study after an interval of two years reported a further reduction of NAWN NAA/Cr in the relapsing remitting but not secondary progressive cohort (Fu et al., 1998). Taken together, these studies point to a dynamic process of progressive axonal dysfunction or loss in cerebral NAWM that contributes to disease progression, although its contribution may diminish with increasing disease duration.

A lower level of cerebral hemisphere NAA was recently reported in a subgroup of 19/72 MS patients who had the epsilon4 allele of apolipoprotein E (Enzinger et al., 2003). Among 44 patients followed up for an average of 34 months, there was a greater ongoing decline in NAA in epsilon4 carriers. This study points to the potential for genetic factors to influence the susceptibility to axonal loss and, by implication, the clinical prognosis.

A limitation of spectroscopy is the low signal-to-noise ratio and modest reproducibility of the measured metabolite concentrations. For this reason, it has been little used in multi-center therapeutic trials. Two small single-center studies of patients treated with beta interferon have produced conflicting results. One study showed an increase in NAA suggesting a therapy-induced reversal of axonal dysfunction (Narayanan et al., 2001). The other showed a decrease in NAA suggesting that progressive axonal loss continues in spite of treatment (Parry et al., 2003). In spite of methodological difficulties, more vigorous efforts to investigate NAA as a surrogate outcome in trials of neuro-

protection in MS would seem warranted, given that this metabolite provides specific information on axonal survival and function.

Diffusion Tensor Imaging

Diffusion tensor imaging offers a potentially specific investigation of the integrity of white matter tracts. Fractional anisotropy (FA) indicates the orientation of diffusion and is high along well-defined pathways such as the corpus callosum, pyramidal tracts, and optic radiations. A reduction in FA in such pathways is therefore a potential marker of axonal structural integrity. Most recently, algorithms have been developed for identifying individual white matter tracts. Diffusion tractography can be performed using several approaches (Parker et al., 2002). Problems arise in areas of crossing tracts or where there are sharp bends in a tract. However, using tractography algorithms it is now possible to quantify—with moderate reproducibility— the size and FA of major pathways in the brain such as optic radiation and pyramidal tract (Ciccarelli et al., 2003).

AU: ok?

In a study of 7 patients with isolated optic neuritis, A. Toosy et al. (unpublished observations) have found a significant reduction in the volume and FA of the optic radiations when compared with the findings in healthy controls. These abnormalities may reflect a more disseminated pathological process that includes the optic radiations; an alternative mechanism is trans-synaptic degeneration secondary to the primary optic nerve lesion. Decreased FA in the NAWM in MS has been observed most notably in patients with progressive forms of MS (Ciccarelli et al., 2001; Rovaris et al., 2002), but not in early relapsing remitting disease (Griffin et al., 2001). Sequences have been developed that allow measurement of FA in the spinal cord (Wheeler-Kingshott et al., 2002) and optic nerve (Wheeler-Kingshott et al., 2004). With the increasing availability of higher field scanners (3 Tesla and above), the resolution of diffusion tensor imaging and tractography will improve and this in turn should allow more detailed investigation of structural abnormalities in white matter tracts.

T_1 Hypointense Lesions

About 20%–30% of T2 lesions appear hypointense on T1-weighted MRI. In serial studies, some of these so-called "black holes" are reversible, first appearing during the phase of acute inflammation associated with gadolinium enhancement and resolving over subsequent months. Such a course reflects initial edema and demyelination with subsequent resolution of edema and remyelination (Barkhof et al., 2003). Other lesions persist as chronic stable "black holes" and these have been shown to have greater axonal loss than those T2 lesions which are T1 isointense (van Walderveen et al., 1998; van Waesberghe et al., 1999). A recent study investigated the relationship of prior radiological features and persistence of T1-hypointensity in lesions, and concluded that the longer the duration of gadolinium enhancement, the greater the duration of subsequent persistence of T1-hypointensity (Bagnato et al., 2003).

Correlations have been found between T1-hypointense lesion load in the brain and the development of cerebral atrophy (Sailer et al., 2001). This has been noted even in the first years after presentation with a CIS (Dalton et al., 2002). Compared to T1-isointense lesions, T1-hypointense lesions exhibit a lower NAA (van Walderveen et al., 1999; Brex et al., 2000) indicating more severe axonal damage or loss. They have also been shown to have more prolonged T1 relaxation time and a higher concentration of myoinositol (Brex et al., 2000)—as already discussed, the latter may indicate increased glial cellularity either as a response or a contributory mechanism to tissue damage.

There is evidence that the ratio of T1-hypointense to T2 lesions increases with increasing disease duration and disability (van Walderveen et al., 2001). T1-hypointense lesion load is typically very small in patients with CIS and is most marked in secondary progressive MS. These observations suggest that there is a propensity for greater axonal loss to develop within focal white matter lesions in secondary progressive that relapsing remitting MS.

As for T2 lesion load, the T1-hypointense lesion load has in general only a modest correlation with disability in cross-sectional studies of MS cohorts. There are paradoxically fewer T1-hypointense lesions in regions of the CNS where pathology often leads to the major locomotor disabilities. Thus, there are very few markedly T1-hypointense lesions seen in the posterior fossa (Gass et al., 1998; although the load of such lesions has been correlated with disability [Hickman et al., 2001b]), and almost no such lesions are seen in the spinal cord; it appears that increasing atrophy rather than T1 hypointensity is the predominant effect of axonal loss in lesions within the cord.

Because there is a strong correlation between T2- and T1-hypointense lesion loads (O'Riordan et al., 1998), the latter probably adds only modestly to the former when monitoring treatment effect on total lesion load. For example, beta interferon has been shown to substantially diminish the increase in both T2- and T1-lesion load compared to placebo-treated patients with secondary progressive MS (Miller et al., 1999; Barkhof et al., 2001). It is potentially more useful to monitor the evolution of individual gadolinium enhancing lesions into persistent black holes. A reduction in such evolution could perhaps be considered as the surrogate marker for improved recovery from acute relapses (i.e., there is less residual axonal loss due to acute inflammation). Such a treatment effect has been demonstrated for glatiramer acetate (Filippi et al., 2001) and natalizumab (Dalton et al., 2004b) but not beta interferon (Brex et al., 2001).

Given the abundant evidence for neuroaxonal loss in the white matter and gray matter beyond MR visible lesions, *global* MR measures such as atrophy are more plausible than T1-hypointense lesions as a surrogate marker for irreversible and progressive disability.

Other Measures

Many other quantitative MR measures have been applied to study MS, e.g., magnetization transfer ratio (MTR), T1 relaxation time, and the apparent diffusion coefficient. Such measures are sensitive in depicting subtle abnormalities in NAWM and gray matter and convincing evidence has emerged that increasing abnormality in these tissues is associated with clinical progression (Filippi et al., 1999; Traboulsee et al., 2003). However, these subtle MR changes are pathologically nonspecific and could potentially represent the effects of inflammation, gliosis, or axonal loss, all of which occur in NAWM. Although they may be valuable for monitoring clinically relevant disease progression they should not be considered as specific markers of neurodegeneration.

Serial measurements of MTR and diffusion indicate that changes in NAWM may precede and perhaps even trigger focal white matter lesion formation (Filippi et al., 1998; Werring et al., 2000), or subsequently appear as a consequence of such lesions (Werring et al., 2000). Another abnormality reported in MS is a decrease in signal on T2-weighted images of deep gray matter structures (Grimaud et al., 1995; Bakshi et al., 2002), which probably reflects increased iron deposition; whether this correlates with neuronal loss is unclear.

MTR has shown initial promise for monitoring clinically relevant disease progression in clinical trials. In a recent placebo-controlled trial of beta interferon in secondary progressive disease, there was a significant increase in whole brain MTR abnormality in both the treated and placebo arms but no beneficial effect of treatment (Inglese et al., 2003); this finding is concordant with the lack of effect of this therapy on progressive disability. A caveat to remember is that progressive MTR abnormality may not be specific for neurodegeneration, although a recent postmortem study indicates that it may reflect the extent of tissue myelination (Schmierer et al., 2004).

V. Conclusion and Implications for Therapy

When the extensive MR imaging and spectroscopy literature is considered as a whole, it can be concluded that neuroaxonal damage and loss is present from the earliest clinical stages of MS, although frank axonal loss and atrophy is probably mild or minimal in patients with a first clinical episode (CIS). The process of neuroaxonal degeneration involves white matter lesions, NAWM, and gray matter and becomes increasingly prominent with increasing disability and the progressive phase of MS. The two most specific MR methods for detecting neuroaxonal loss are atrophy and decreased NAA. The former has been preferred in clinical trials because more reproducible and sensitive methods are available to detect it. To date, no therapy has been shown to have a robust and consistent effect in slowing the rate of tissue atrophy, although some studies have suggested that there may be a partial delayed effect of beta interferon in relapsing-remitting MS.

Fractional anisotropy measured from diffusion tensor images has potential to provide distinctive information on the structural integrity of white matter pathways. Although other MR markers of diffuse disease are not specific for axonal loss (e.g., MTR, T1, diffusion coefficient), they do provide—along with atrophy—a sensitive measure of a diffuse, progressive underlying process that appears relevant to clinical progression and MTR may reflect myelination.

The generally modest correlation of atrophy and intrinsic NAWM and gray matter abnormalities with lesion load, even in the earliest clinical stages of disease, suggests that these diffuse processes are at least partly independent of focal lesions. They may nevertheless also be partly related in providing a trigger for (Werring et al., 2000) or being a consequence of focal inflammation (the latter, by causing axonal transection [Trapp et al., 1998], will lead to secondary Wallerian degeneration in the NAWM). The potential importance of atrophy, NAWM, and gray matter measures for predicting future disability—although not yet confirmed—is readily apparent. It is therefore recommended that atrophy should be measured in trials aiming to prevent disability at all stages of disease (CIS, relapsing-remitting, primary, and secondary progressive) and where feasible, NAA should also be measured along with other techniques to monitor progressive NAWM and gray matter abnormality (e.g. MTR).

It is nevertheless important to remember that the MR surrogates for neuroaxonal loss and diffuse disease are not yet proven beyond doubt as predicting future disability and its prevention by treatment. Long-term follow-up studies of well characterized cohorts, including those participating in controlled clinical trials, will be needed to clarify the relationship. Meanwhile, definitive trials should continue to measure an appropriate clinical endpoint.

Acknowledgment

The author would like to thank all of his colleagues in the MS NMR Research Unit for their excellent work and collaboration, and the MS Society of Great Britain and Northern Ireland for their continued support of the Unit.

References

Bagnato, F., Jeffries, N, Richert, N. D., et al. (2003). Evolution of T1 black holes in patients with multiple sclerosis imaged monthly for four years. *Brain* **126**, 1782–1789.

Bakshi, R., Benedict, R. H. B., Bermel, R. A. , et al. (2002). T2 hypointensity in the deep gray matter of patients with multiple sclerosis. *Arch. Neurol.* **59**, 62–68.

Barkhof, F., van Waesberghe, J. H. T. M., Filippi, M., et al. (2001). T1 hypointense lesions in secondary progressive MS: Effect of interferon beta-1b. *Brain* **124**, 1396–1402.

Barkhof, F., Bruck, W., de Groot, J. C., et al. (2003). Remyelinated lesions in multiple sclerosis: Magnetic resonance image appearance. *Arch. Neurol.* **60**, 1073–1081.

Beck, R. W., and Cleary, PA. (1993). Optic neuritis treatment trial. One-year follow-up results. *Arch. Ophthalmol.* **111**, 773–775.

Beck, R. W., Trobe, J. D., Moke, P. S., et al. (2003). High and low risk profiles for the development of multiple sclerosis within 10 years after optic neuritis: experience of the optic neuritis treatment trial. *Arch. Ophthalmol.* **121**, 944–949.

Bjartmar, C., Kidd, G., Mork, S., et al. (2000). Neurological disability correlates with spinal cord axonal loss and reduced *N*-acetyl aspartate in chronic multiple sclerosis patients. *Ann. Neurol.* **48**, 893–901.

Bo, L., Vedeler, C. A., Nyland, H., et al. (2003). Intracortical multiple sclerosis lesions are not associated with increased lymphocyte infiltration. *Multiple Sclerosis* **9**, 323–331.

Brenner, R. E., Munro, P. M., Williams, S. C., et al. (1993). The proton NMR spectrum in acute EAE: The significance of the change in the Cho:Cr ratio. *Magn. Reson. Med.* **29**, 737–745.

Brex, P. A., Parker, G. J M., Leary, S. M., et al. (2000). Lesion heterogeneity in MS: A study of the relations between appearances on T1 weighted images, T1 relaxation times and metabolite concentrations. *J. Neurol. Neurosurg. Psychiatry* **68**, 627–632.

Brex, P. A., Leary, S. M., O'Riordan, J. I., et al. (2001). Measurement of spinal cord area in clinically isolated syndromes suggestive of multiple sclerosis. *J. Neurol. Neurosurg. Psychiatry* **70**, 544–547.

Brex, P. A., Molyneux, P. D., Smiddy, P., et al. (2001). The effect of interferon beta-1b on the size and evolution of enhancing lesions in secondary progressive MS. *Neurology* **57**, 2185–2190.

Brex, P. A., Ciccarelli, O., O'Riordan, J. I., et al. (2002). A longitudinal study of abnormalities on MRI and disability from multiple sclerosis. *N. Engl. J. Med.* **346**, 158–164.

Charcot, M. (1868). Histologie de la sclerose en plaques. *Gaz. Hosp.* 141:554–555, 557–558.

Chard, D. T., Griffin, C M., Parker, G J. M., et al. (2002a). Brain atrophy in clinically early relapsing-remitting multiple sclerosis. *Brain* **125**, 327–337.

Chard, D., Griffin, C. M., McLean, M. A., et al. (2002b). Brain metabolite changes in cortical grey matter and normal appearing white matter in clinically early relapsing remitting multiple sclerosis. *Brain* **125**, 2342–2352.

Chard, D. T., Brex, P. A., Ciccarelli, O., et al. (2003). The longitudinal relation between brain lesion load and atrophy in multiple sclerosis: a 14-year follow-up study. *J. Neurol. Neurosurg. Psychiatry* **74**, 1551–1554.

Chard, D. T., Griffin, C. M., Rashid, W., Davies, G. R., Altmann, D. R., Kappor, R., Barker, G. J., Thompson, A. J., and Miller, D. H. (2004). Progressive grey matter atrophy in clinically early relapsing-remitting multiple sclerosis. *Multiple Sclerosis* **10**, 387–391.

Ciccarelli, O., Werring, D. J., Wheeler-Kingshott, C. A., et al. (2001). Investigation of MS normal-appearing brain using diffusion tensor MRI with clinical correlations. *Neurology* **56**, 926–933.

Ciccarelli, O., Toosy, A. T., Parker, G. J. M., et al. (2003). Diffusion tractography based group mapping of major white-matter pathways in the human brain. *NeuroImage* **19**, 1545–1555.

Cifelli, A., Arridge, M., Jezzard, P., et al. (2002). Thalamic neurodegeneration in multiple sclerosis. *Ann. Neurol.* **52**, 650–653.

Coles, A J., Wing, M. G., Molyneux, P., et al. (1999). Monoclonal antibody treatment exposes three mechanisms underlying the clinical course of multiple sclerosis. *Ann. Neurol.* **46**, 296–304.

Dalton, C. M., Brex, P A., Jenkins, R., et al. (2002). Progressive ventricular enlargement in patients with clinically isolated syndromes is associated with the early development of multiple sclerosis. *J. Neurol. Neurosurg. Psychiatry* **73**, 141–147.

Dalton, C. M., Chard, D. T., Davies, G. R., et al. (2004a). Early development of multiple sclerosis is associated with progressive grey matter atrophy in patients presenting with clinically isolated syndromes. *Brain* **127**, 1101–1107.

Dalton, C. M., Miszkiel, K. A., Barker, G J., et al. (2004b). Effect of natalizumab on conversion of gadolinium enhancing lesions to T1 hypointense lesions in relapsing multiple sclerosis. *J. Neurol.* **251**, 407–413.

Davie, C., Hawkins, C. P., Barker, G. J., et al. (1994). Serial proton magnetic resonance spectroscopy of multiple sclerosis lesions. *Brain* 117, 49–58.

Davie, C., Barker, G. J., Webb, S., et al. (1995). Persistent functional deficit in multiple sclerosis and autosomal dominant cerebellar ataxia is associated with axon loss. *Brain* **118**, 1583–1592.

de Stefano, N., Matthews, P. M., Filippi, M., et al. (2003). Evidence of early cortical atrophy in MS: relevance to white matter changes and disability. *Neurology* **60**, 1157–1162.

Enzinger, C., Ropele, S., Strasser-Fuchs, S., et al. (2003). Lower levels of *N*-acetyl aspartate in multiple sclerosis patients with the apolipoprotein E epsilon4 allele. *Arch. Neurol.* **60**, 65–70.

Evangelou, N., Esiri, M. M., Smith, S., Palace, J., Mathews, P. M. (2000). Quantitative pathological evidence for axonal loss in normal appearing white matter in multiple sclerosis. *Ann. Neurol.* **47**, 391–395.

Fernando, K. T. M., McLean, M. A., Chard, D. T., MacManus, D. G., Dalton, C. M., Miszkiel, K. A., Gordon, R. M., Plant, G. T., Thompson, A. J., and Miller, D. H. (2004). Elevated white matter *myo*-inositol in clinically isolated syndromes suggestive of multiple sclerosis. *Brain* **127**, 1361–1369.

Filippi, M., Rocca, M. A., Martino, G., et al. (1998). Magnetization transfer changes in the normal appearing white matter precede the appearance of enhancing lesions in patients with multiple sclerosis. *Ann. Neurol.* **43**, 809–814.

Filippi, M., Iannucci, G., Tortorella, C., Minicucci, L., Horsfield, M. A., Colombo, B., Sormani, M. P., and Comi, G. (1999). Comparison of MS clinical phenotypes using conventional and magnetization transfer MRI. *Neurology* **52**, 588–594.

Filippi, M., Rovaris, M., Iannucci, G., Mennea, S., Sormani, M. P., and Comi, G. (2000). Whole brain volume changes in progressive MS patients treated with cladribine. *Neurology* **55**, 1714–1718.

Filippi, M., Rovaris, M., Rocca, M. A., Sormani, M. P., Wolinsky, J. S., Comi, G., et al. (2001). Glatiramer acetate reduces the proportion of new MS lesions evolving in to "black holes". *Neurology* **57**, 731–733.

Filippi, M., Bozzali, M., Rovaris, M., Gonen, O., Kesavadas, C., Ghezzi, A., et al. (2003). Evidence for widespread axonal damage at the earliest clinical stage of multiple sclerosis. *Brain* **126**, 433–437.

Filippi, M., Rovaris, M., Barkhof, F., de Stefano, N., Smith, S., and Comi, G., for the ETOMS Study Group (Interferon beta-1a for brain tissue loss in patients at presentation with syndromes suggestive of multiple sclerosis: a randomised, double-blind, placebocontrolled trial. *Lancet* **364**, 1489–1496.

Fisher, E., Rudick, R. A., Simon J. H., Cutter, G., Baier, M., Lee, J.C., et al. (2002). Eight year follow up study of brain atrophy in patients with MS. *Neurology* **59**, 1412–1420.

Frank, J. A., Richert, N., Bash, C., et al. (2004). Interferon β-1b slows progression of atrophy in RRMS. *Neurology* **62**, 719–725.

Freeborough, P. A., and Fox, N. C. (1997). The boundary shift integral: An accurate and robust measure of cerebral volume changes from registered repeat MRI. *IEEE Trans Med Imag* **16**, 623–629.

Fu, L., Matthews, P. M., De Stefano, N., Worsley, K. J., Narayanan, S., Francis, G. S., et al. (1998). Imaging axonal damage of normal-appearing white matter in multiple sclerosis. *Brain* **121**, 103–113.

Gasperini, C., Paolillo, A., Giugni E, Galgani, S., Bagnato, F., Mainero, C., et al. (2002). MRI brain volume changes in relapsing remitting multiple sclerosis patients treated with interferon beta-1a. *Multiple Sclerosis* **8**, 119–123.

Gass, A., Filippi, M., Rodegher, M. E., et al. (1998). Characteristics of chronic MS lesions in the cerebrum, brainstem, spinal cord and optic nerve on T1-weighted MRI. *Neurology* **50**, 548–550.

Ge, Y., Grossman, R. I., Udupa, J. K., Wei, L., Mannon, L. J., Polansky, M., and Kolson, D. L. (2000). Brain atrophy in relapsing-remitting multiple sclerosis and secondary progressive multiple sclerosis: Longitudinal data analysis. *Radiology* **214**, 665–670.

Ge, Y., Gone,n O., Inglese, M., et al. (2004). Neuronal cell injury precedes brain atrophy in multiple sclerosis. *Neurology* **62**, 624–627.

Gonen, O., Catalaa, I., Babb, J. S., Ge, Y., Mannon, L. J., Kolson, D. L., and Grossman, R. I. (2000). Total brain N-acetylaspartate: a new measure of disease load in MS. *Neurology* **54**, 15–19.

Griffin, C., Chard, D. T., Ciccarelli O, Kapoor R, Barker GJ, Thompson AJ, Miller DH. Diffusion tensor imaging in early relapsing remitting multiple sclerosis. *Multiple Sclerosis.* 2001; 7:290–297.

Grimaud J, Millar J, Thorpe, J. W., Moseley, I. F., McDonald, W. I., and Miller, D. H. (1995). Signal intensity on MRI of basal ganglia in multiple sclerosis. *J. Neurol. Neurosurg. Psychiatry* **59**, 306–308.

Hickman, S. J., Brex, P. A., Brierley, C. M. H., Silver, N. C., Barker, G. J., Scolding, N. J., et al. (2001a). Detection of optic nerve atrophy following a single episode of unilateral optic neuritis by MRI using a fat-saturated short-echo fast FLAIR sequence. *Neuroradiology* **43**, 123–128.

Hickman, S. J., Brierley, C. M. H., Silver, N. C., Moseley, I. F., Scolding, N. J., Compston, D. A. S., and Miller, D. H. (2001b). Infratentorial hypointense lesion volume on T1-weighted magnetic resonance imaging correlates with disability in patients with chronic cerebellar ataxia due to multiple sclerosis. *J. Neurol. Sci.* **187**, 35–39.

Hickman, S. J., Brierley, C. M. H., Brex, P. A., MacManus, D. G., Scolding, N. J., Compston, D. A. S., and Miller, D. H. (2002). Continuing optic nerve atrophy following optic neuritis: A serial MRI study. *Multiple Sclerosis* **8**, 339–342.

Hickman, S. J., Kapoor, R., Jones, S. J., Altmann, D. R., Plant, G. T., and Miller, D. H. (2003). Corticosteroids do not prevent optic nerve atrophy following optic neuritis. *J. Neurol. Neurosurg. Psychiatry* 74, 1139–1141.

Hickman, S. J., Tousy, A. T., Jones, S. J., Altmann, D. R., Miszkiel, K. A., MacManus, D. G., Barker, G. J., Plant, G. T., Thompson, A. J., and Miller, D. H. (2004). A serial MRI study following optic nerve mean area in acute optic neuritis. *Brain* **127**, 2498–2505.

Ingle, G. T., Stevenson, V. L., Miller, D. H., and Thompson, A. J. (2003). Primary progressive multiple sclerosis: A 5-year clinical and MR study. *Brain* **126**, 2528–2536.

Inglese, M., van Waesberghe, J. H. T. M., Rovaris, M., Beckmann, K., Barkhof, F., Hahn, D., Kappos, L., Miller, D. H., Polman, C., Pozzilli, C., Thompson, A. J., Yousry, T. A., Wagner, K., Comi, G., and Filippi, M. (2003). The effect of interferon B-1b on quantities derived from MT MRI in secondary progressive MS. *Neurology* **60**, 853–860.

Jones, C. K., Riddehough, A., Li, D. K. B., Zhao, G. J., and Paty, D. W. (2001). MRI cerebral atrophy in relapsing remitting MS: Results of the PRISMS trial. *Neurology* **56 (suppl 3)**, A379.

Kalkers, N. F., Bergers, L., Castelijns, J. A., van Walderveen, M. A. A., Bot, J. C. J., Ader, H. J., Polman, C. H., and Barkhof, F. (2001). Optimizing the association between disability and biological markers in MS. *Neurology* **57**, 1253–1257.

Kalkers, N. F., Barkhof, F., Bergers, E., van Schijndel, R., and Polman, C. H. (2002). The effect of the neuroprotective agent riluzole on MRI parameters in primary progressive multiple sclerosis. *Multiple Sclerosis* 8, 532–533.

Kidd, D., Barkhof, F., McConnell, R., et al. (1999). Cortical lesions in multiple sclerosis. *Brain* **122**, 17–26.

Kuhlmann, T., Lingfield, G., Bitsch, A., et al. (2002). Acute axonal damage in multiple sclerosis is most extensive in early disease stages and decreases over time. *Brain* **125**, 2202–2212.

Lassmann, H., Suchanek, G., and Ozawa, K. (1994). Histopathology and the blood-cerebrospinal fluid barrier in multiple sclerosis. *Ann. Neurol.* **36 (suppl)**, S42–46.

Leary, S., Davie, C., Parker, G., Stevenson, V. L., Wang, L. Q., Barker, G. J., et al. (1999). H magnetic resonance spectroscopy of normal appearing white matter in primary progressive multiple sclerosis. *J. Neurol.* **246**, 1023–1026.

Lin, X., Tench, C. R., Turner, B., Blumhardt, L. D., and Constantinescu, C. S. (2003). Spinal cord atrophy and disability in multiple sclerosis over four years: Application of a reproducible automated technique in monitoring disease progression in a cohort of the interferon β-1a (Rebif) treatment trial. *J. Neurol. Neurosurg. Psychiatry* **74**, 1090–1094.

Losseff, N. A., Webb, S. L., O'Riordan, J. I., Page, R., Wang, L., Barker, G. J., et al. (1996a). Spinal cord atrophy and disability in multiple sclerosis. A new reproducible and sensitive MRI method with potential to monitor disease progression. *Brain* **119**, 701–708.

Losseff, N. A., Wang, L., Lai, H. M., Yoo, D. S., Gawne-Cain, M. L., McDonald, W. I., et al. (1996b). Progressive cerebral atrophy in multiple sclerosis. A serial study. *Brain* **119**, 2009–2019.

Lovas, G., Szilagyi, N., Majtenyi, K., et al. (2000). Axonal changes in chronic demyelinated cervical spinal cord plaques. *Brain* **123**, 308–317.

Lycklamaà Nijeholt, G. J., van Walderveen, M. A., Castelijns, J. A., van Waesberghe, J. H. T. M., Polman, C., Scheltens, P., et al. (1998). Brain and spinal cord abnormalities in multiple sclerosis. Correlation between MRI parameters, clinical subtypes and symptoms. *Brain* **121**, 687–697.

Matthews, P. M., Pioro, E., Narayanan, S., et al. (1996). Assessment of lesion pathology in multiple sclerosis using quantitative MRI morphometry and magnetic resonance spectroscopy. *Brain* **119**, 715–722.

McDonald, W. I., Compston, A., Edan, G., Goodkin, D., Hartung, H.-P., Lublin, F. D., et al. (2001). Recommended diagnostic criteria for multiple sclerosis: guidelines from the international panel on the diagnosis of multiple sclerosis. *Ann. Neurol.* **50**, 121–127.

Miller, D. H., Molyneux, P. D., Barker, G. J., MacManus, D. G., Moseley, I. F., Wagner, K., and European study group. (1999). Effect of Interferon Beta1b on magnetic resonance imaging outcomes in secondary progressive multiple sclerosis: Results of a European multicenter, randomized, double-blind, placebo-controlled trial. *Ann. Neurol.* **46**, 850–859.

Miller, D. H., Barkhof, F., Frank, J. A., Parker, G. J. M., and Thompson, A. J. (2002). Measurement of atrophy in multiple sclerosis: Pathological basis, methodological aspects and clinical relevance. *Brain* **125**, 1676–1695.

Molyneux, P. D., Kappos, L., Polman, C., Pozzilli, C., Barkhof, F., Filippi, M., et al. (2000). The effect of interferon beta-1b treatment on MRI measures of cerebral atrophy in secondary progressive multiple sclerosis. *Brain* **123**, 2256–2263.

Narayanan, S., De Stefano, N., Francis, G. S., Arnouetelis, R., Caramanous, Z., Collins, L. D., et al. (2001). Axonal metabolic recovery in multiple sclerosis patients treated with interferon beta-1b. *J. Neurol.* **249**, 979–986.

O'Riordan, J. I., Gawne-Cain, M., Coles, A., Wang, L., Compston, D. A. S., and Miller, D. H. (1998). T1 hypointense lesion load in secondary progressive multiple sclerosis: a comparison of pre versus post contrast loads and of manual versus semi automated threshold techniques for lesion segmentation. *Multiple Sclerosis* **4**, 408–412.

Parisi, V., Manni, G., Spadaro, M., et al. (1999). Correlation between morphological and functional retinal impairment in multiple sclerosis patients. *Invest. Ophthalmol.Vis. Sci.* **40**, 2520–2527.

Parker, G. J., Wheeler-Kingshott, C. A., and Barker, G. J. (2002). Estimating distributed anatomical brain connectivity using fast marching methods and diffusion tensor imaging. IEEE *Trans. Med. Imaging* **21**, 505–512.

Parry, A., Corkill, R., Blamire, A. M., Palace, J., Narayanan, S., Arnold, D., et al. (2003). Beta-interferon does not always slow the progression of axonal injury in multiple sclerosis. *J. Neurol.* **250**, 171–178

Pelletier, D., Nelson, S. J., Oh, .J, Antel, J. P., Kita, M., Zamvil, S. S., and Goodkin, D. E. (2003). MRI lesion volume heterogeneity in primary progressive MS in relation with axonal damage and brain atrophy. *J. Neurol. Neurosurg. Psychiatry* **74**, 950–952.

Peterson, J. W., Bo, L., Mork, S., Chang, A., and Trapp, B. D. (2001). Transected neuritis, apoptotic neurons, and reduced inflammation in cortical multiple sclerosis lesions. *Ann. Neurol.* **50**, 389–400.

Provencher, S. W. (1993). Estimation of metabolite concentrations from localized in vivo proton NMR spectra. *Magn. Reson. Med.* **30**, 672–679.

Rao, S., Richert, N., Howard, T., et al. (2002). Methylprednisolone effect on brain volume and enhancing lesions in MS before and during IFN beta-1b. *Neurology* **59**, 688–694.

Rovaris, M., Comi, G., Rocca, M., Wolinsky, J., Filippi, M., and the European/Canadian Glatiramer Acetate Study Group. (2001). Short term brain volume change in relapsing-remitting multiple sclerosis: effect of glatiramer acetate and implications. *Brain* **124**, 1803–1812.

Rovaris, M., Bozzali, M., Iannucci, G., et al. (2002). Assessment of normal appearing white and gray matter in patients with primary progressive multiple sclerosis: a diffusion tensor magnetic resonance imaging study. *Arch. Neurol.* **59**, 1406–1412.

Rudick, R. A., Fischer, E., Lee, J.-C., Simon, J., and Jacobs, L. (1999). Use of brain parenchymal fraction to measure whole brain atrophy in relapsing-remitting MS. *Neurology* **53**, 1698–1704.

Sailer, M., Losseff, N. A., Wang, L., Gawne-Cain, M. L., Thompson, A. J., and Miller, D. H. (2001). T1 lesion load and cerebral atrophy as a marker for clinical progression in patients with multiple sclerosis. A prospective 18 months follow-up study. *Eur. J. Neurol.* **8**, 37–42.

Sarchielli, P., Presciutti, O., Pelliciolli, G. P., Tarducci, R., Gobbi, G., Chiarini, P., et al. (1999). Absolute quantification of brain metabolites by proton magnetic spectroscopy of normal appearing white matter of patients with multiple sclerosis. *Brain* **122**, 513–522.

Schmierer, K., Scaravilli, F., Altmann, D. R., Barker, G. J., and Miller, D. H. (2004). Magnetization transfer ratio and myelin in post mortem multiple sclerosis brain. *Ann. Neurol.* **56**, 407–415.

Simon, J. H., Jacobs, L. D., Campion, M. K., Rudick, R. A., Cookfair, D. L., Herndon, R. M., et al. (1999). A longitudinal study of brain atrophy in relapsing multiple sclerosis. *Neurology* **53**, 139–148.

Smith, S., de Stefano, N., Jenkinson, M., and Matthews, P. (2001). Normalised accurate measurement of longitudinal brain change. *J. Comput. Assist. Tomogr.* **25**, 466–475.

Stevenson, V. L., Miller, D. H., Leary, S. M., Rovaris, M., Barkhof, F., Brochet, B., et al. (2000). One year follow up study of primary and transitional progressive multiple sclerosis. *J. Neurol. Neurosurg. Psychiatry* **68**, 713–718.

Tourbah, A., Stievenart, J. L., Gout, O., Fontaine, B., Liblau, R., Lubetzki, C. et al. (1999). Localized proton magnetic resonance spectroscopy in relapsing remitting versus secondary progressive multiple sclerosis. *Neurology* **53**, 1091–1097.

Traboulsee, A., Dehmeshki, J., Peters, K. R., Griffin, C. M., Brex, P. A., Silver, N., et al. (2003). Disability in multiple sclerosis is related to normal appearing brain tissue MTR histogram abnormalities. *Multiple Sclerosis* **9**, 566–573.

Trapp, B. D., Peterson, J., Ransohoff, R. M., Rudick, R., Mork, S., and Bo, L. (1998). Axonal transection in the lesions of multiple sclerosis. *N. Engl. J. Med.* **338**, 278–285.

van Waesberghe, J. H., Kamphorst, W., De Groot, C. J., et al. (1999). Axonal loss in multiple sclerosis lesions: magnetic resonance imaging insights into substrates of disability. *Ann. Neurol.* **46**, 747–754.

van Walderveen, M. A., Kamphorst, W., Scheltens, P., van Waesberghe, J. H., Ravid, R., Valk, J., et al. (1998). Histopathological correlate of hypointense lesions on T1-weighted spin echo MRI in multiple sclerosis. *Neurology* **50**, 1282–1288.

van Walderveen, M. A., Barkhof, F., Pouwels, P. J., et al. (1999). Neuronal damage in T1 hypointense multiple sclerosis lesions demonstrated in vivo using proton magnetic resonance spectroscopy. *Ann. Neurol.* **46**, 79–87.

van Walderveen, M. A.A., Lycklama, A., Nijeholt, G. J., Ader, H. J., et al. (2001). Hypointense lesions on T1-weighted spin echo magnetic resonance imaging: relation to clinical characteristics in subgroups of patients with multiple sclerosis. *Arch. Neurol.* **58,** 76–81.

Werring, D. J., Brassat, D., Droogan, A. G., Clark, C. A., Symms, M. R., Barker, G. J., MacManus, D. G., Thompson, A. J., and Miller, D. H. (2000). The pathogenesis of lesions and normal-appearing white matter changes in multiple sclerosis. A serial diffusion MRI study. *Brain* **123,** 1667–1676.

Wheeler-Kingshott, C. W., Hickman, S. J., Parker, G. J. M., Ciccarelli, O., Symms, M. R., Miller, D. H., and Barker, G. J. (2002). Investigating cervical spinal cord structure using axial diffusion tensor imaging. *NeuroImage* **16,** 93–102.

Wheeler-Kingshott, C. A., Trip, S. A., Symms, M. R., et al. (2004). In vivo anisotropy and diffusivity of the optic nerve: pilot study. *Proc. Int. Soc Magn. Reson. Med.*, e-poster.

Wolinsky, J. S., Narayana, P. A., Noseworthy, J. H., et al. (2000). Linomide in relapsing remitting and secondary progressive multiple sclerosis: MRI results. *Neurology* **54,** 1734–1741.

Zidavinov, R., Rudick, R. A., De Masi, R., et al. (2001). Effects of IV methylprednisolone on brain atrophy in relapsing remitting MS. *Neurology* **57,** 1239–1247.

14

Brain Atrophy as a Measure of Neurodegeneration and Neuroprotection

Richard A. Rudick, M.D.
Elizabeth Fisher, Ph.D.

I. Introduction

A. Multiple Sclerosis as a Neuronal Disease

The view that multiple sclerosis (MS) may be predominantly a neuronal disease is controversial, even though the pathological process has long been known to affect neurons and axons. Recent emphasis on axons and neurons as central to the neuropathology is supported by incontrovertible evidence for axonal transaction and axonal degeneration in the central nervous system (CNS) of patients with the disease. Moreover, consensus has developed that progressive axonal pathology best explains the progressive neurological disability experienced by large numbers of MS patients. Accompanying the view that MS is a "neurodegenerative disease" are the clinical implications. How should the process of neurodegeneration be monitored for clinical care and clinical trials? This chapter is one of several in this book addressing imaging modalities that may provide such a tool.

B. Outcome Measures Used to Measure MS Disease Severity

Magnetic resonance imaging (MRI) is a sensitive tool for measuring MS pathology *in vivo*. Lesions on T_2-weighted and contrast-enhanced T_1-weighted MRIs are used routinely as indicators of disease activity for diagnosis and to measure the effects of therapeutic intervention. However, gadolinium-enhanced lesions and T_2 lesions reflect pathological processes that are potentially reversible and reflect variable amounts of tissue injury. Furthermore, lesion measurements fluctuate over time and do not account for diffuse pathology

201

in the normal-appearing white matter. These factors limit the usefulness of conventional lesion measurements. MRI measures are needed that more reliably reflect progression of MS. One straightforward approach is the estimation of atrophy of CNS structures. In contrast to lesions, atrophy reflects the end result of destructive, irreversible pathological processes operant in MS patients. Axonal loss, demyelination, and gliosis may result in reduced volume of CNS parenchymal tissue and a corresponding increase in the volume of cerebrospinal fluid (CSF) spaces. Although loss of CNS tissue is not specific to the underlying pathology in MS patients, it is likely to reflect axonal pathology, simply because axons contribute a large proportion of normal parenchymal volume (Fig. 1).

Brain atrophy was generally mentioned but not emphasized in early descriptions of MS pathology. Historically, it was associated with late stages of MS, but this may be an artifact of the nature of cases coming to autopsy. In a chapter on the pathological features of MS, John Prineas (1990) commented, "Inspection of coronal slices of the fixed brain in patients with severe long-standing disease will usually show some ventricular enlargement, which may be marked." There is no discussion of the pathological evolution of this change.

Computed tomography (CT) scanning was the first informative *in vivo* imaging modality used for MS. In the first reported series of MS cases using CT scanning, brain atrophy was noted in 4 of 19 patients with MS (Cala and Mastaglia, 1976). The application of MRI to patients with MS was first reported 5 years later (Young et al., 1981). MRI detected many more brain lesions than did CT scanning, and it was immediately apparent that MRI would supersede CT scanning for this disease because of its sensitivity in detecting brain lesions.

Nearly all of the early MRI literature on MS focused on the highly conspicuous T_2 bright parenchymal lesions. In 1987, however, Simon and colleagues published an impor-

tant early MRI study of CNS atrophy in patients with MS (Simon et al., 1987). Atrophy affecting the corpus callosum was quantified by measuring the callosal area in the midsagittal plane in 41 patients with definite MS and 48 controls with normal MR scans. Mean midsagittal callosal area was significantly higher in the brains of the control patients compared with the patients with MS. The degree of corpus callosum atrophy paralleled estimated volumes of periventricular and corpus callosum T_2-hyperintense lesions, suggesting a possible cause-effect relationship. This study suggested that atrophy was much more prevalent than previously thought, and led to a prospectively defined study, which was incorporated into a clinical trial of interferon β-1a (IFNβ-1a, Avonex) initiated in 1989 (Jacobs et al., 1996). Patients in that study were relatively early in the course of MS, with average age of 36 years, average disease duration of 6 years, and mild to moderate disability. Significant increases were detected in third ventricle width at year 2 and lateral ventricle width at years 1 and 2; significant decreases were observed in corpus callosum area and brain width at 1 and 2 years (Simon et al., 1999). Regression analyses showed that the number of gadolinium-enhancing lesions at baseline correlated significantly with change in third ventricle width. Greater disability increments over 1 and 2 years were associated with more severe third ventricle enlargement. This study generated considerable interest when it was presented at the American Academy of Neurology in 1996, because it clearly documented that progressive brain atrophy occurred much earlier in the course of MS than generally appreciated. The study focused attention on brain atrophy as an important measure of the disease process.

By the end of the 1990s, groups from around the world were working on methods to quantify CNS atrophy in MS, and reports were appearing at an increasing rate in the literature. As a result, an international workshop was convened in London, England, in November 2001. At that workshop, it was noted that atrophy was an attractive disease measure because it reflected a global marker of the adverse outcome of MS pathology. The workshop attendees reached the consensus that atrophy in MS probably reflects both inflammation-induced axonal loss followed by wallerian degeneration and postinflammatory neurodegeneration that may be partly due to failure of remyelination. It was concluded that "atrophy provides a sensitive measure of the neurodegenerative component of multiple sclerosis and should be measured in trials evaluating potential anti-inflammatory, remyelinating or neuroprotective therapies" (Miller et al., 2002).

II. Atrophy Measures in MS

Loss of parenchymal volume can be estimated using standard MRIs and a wide range of approaches to image analysis. Different groups have proposed various methods

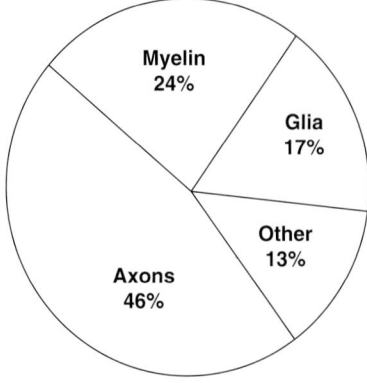

Figure 1 Proportion of normal adult CNS contributed by CNS components. Axons constitute about 46% of brain volume; myelin 24%. (Modified from Esiri (in Miller et al. 2002.))

for atrophy assessment, and results from cross-sectional and longitudinal studies have accumulated. Techniques vary according to the extent of automation or user interactivity, and by the structures measured. For example, the degree of operator interaction that is required ranges from completely subjective rating scales to fully automated volumetric calculations. The structures measured range from highly localized measurements of third ventricular width (on the order of 3 mm) to global measurements of whole brain volume (on the order of 1,000 cm^3). The conceptual approach to measurement also varies widely, from estimating total atrophy since disease onset from a single image, to determining the shift in the edges of a structure between serially acquired images.

One of the most important aspects of CNS atrophy measurements is reliability, because the rate of atrophy in MS patients is relatively slow. Measurement errors can exceed biological change in longitudinal studies, even with follow-up durations of several years. Measurement reliability is usually expressed as reproducibility or inter-rater agreement. This is commonly expressed as a coefficient of variation (CV), defined as the standard deviation of the mean, divided by the mean. Repeated measurements performed on scan-rescan data simulate conditions in serial studies and therefore provide a better estimate of measurement variability than repeated measurements on the same image data.

A. Manual Methods

Several different studies have reported on atrophy in MS patients using manual estimates (Simon et al., 1999; Rao et al., 1985; Janardhan and Bakshi 2000; Leist et al., 2001; Turner et al., 2001; Liu et al., 1999; Edwards et al., 2001; Kidd et al., 1993; Filippi et al., 1998). An advantage of manual methods is that there is no need for specialized software. Subjective rating of atrophy on an ordinal scale (Rao et al., 1985; Janardhan and Bakshi, 2000) has been used and demonstrated very good intraobserver agreement ($\kappa = 0.9$) and interobserver agreement ($\kappa = 0.8$). However, the ordinal rating scale approach is not very useful in detecting changes over time, because it is relatively insensitive. Another technique that does not require specialized software is measurement of the distance between anatomical landmarks on films using graded calipers. This approach was applied to estimate ventricular enlargement and demonstrated good agreement with volumetric digital image analysis ($r^2 = 0.84$, $P = 0.009$); a significant shortcoming is the need for precise and consistent patient positioning in the MRI scanner (Leist et al., 2001).

Use of image analysis software allows for quantitative estimation of widths, areas, and/or volumes of CNS structures directly from digital images. The calculation of distances between manually selected anatomical landmarks has been used to estimate the sizes of particular structures, such as the third ventricle width, lateral ventricle width, and brain width (Simon et al., 1999; Turner et al., 2001). Intrarater variability ranged from 1% (CV for brain width) to 7% (CV for third ventricle width). Stereology, an approach used to calculate volumes by randomly overlaying a grid on an image and counting the number of grid intersection points, has been applied to measure various CNS structures (Liu et al., 1999; Edwards et al., 2001). Intraoperator variability of this method has been reported to be 2.8% for cerebral volume and 6.9% for ventricular volume (Filippi et al., 1998). Another manual approach is to use tracing tools included in image analysis packages to delineate structures of interest (Kidd et al., 1993; Filippi et al., 1998). Manual tracing by an expert observer yields accurate segmentation, but it is also the most time-consuming approach and measurement variability is relatively high.

B. Semiautomated and Automated Methods

Semiautomated and automated segmentation programs offer more rapid assessment of areas and volumes. Such programs have been used to calculate spinal cord cross-sectional area (Losseff et al., 1996b), lateral ventricle volume (Matthews et al., 1996; Lycklama et al., 1998; Brex et al., 2000; Kalkers et al., 2001), CSF volume (Wolinsky et al., 2000; Dastidar et al. 1999), and whole or partial brain volumes (DeCarli et al., 1992; Losseff et al., 1996a; Bedell and Narayana, 1996; Hohol et al., 1997; Fisher et al., 1997; Goldszal et al., 1998; Alfano et al., 1998; Phillips et al., 1998; Rovaris et al., 2000; Collins et al., 2001). There are many different site-specific segmentation algorithms and programs currently in use for MS applications.

One example of a semiautomated technique is a threshold-based algorithm that was developed to measure spinal cord cross-sectional area (Losseff et al., 1996b). An operator selects regions of interest to determine an intensity threshold midway between CSF and spinal cord tissue. To minimize axial repositioning errors, the cord is segmented in five adjacent image slices, and the area is determined as the mean cross-sectional area. Scan-rescan tests resulted in mean CVs ranging from 0.79% to 1.6%. A similar threshold-based approach has been applied for semi-automated segmentation of the lateral ventricles in T_1-weighted images (Brex et al., 2000; Luks et al., 2000). First, the mean intensity of brain parenchyma is determined from automated segmentation or operator-selected regions of interest, and then the threshold is determined as 60% of the brain intensity. The intrarater CV for this technique is 0.13% (Brex et al., 2000) and the intraclass correlation coefficient is 0.99 (Luks et al., 2000).

Various methods have also been applied to measure brain parenchymal volume. Brain segmentation typically consists of two steps: (1) separation of tissue from CSF and background, usually by intensity thresholding; and (2) separation of the brain tissue from other cranial structures, usually by connectivity and morphological operations, manual interaction, and/or knowledge-based anatomical operations. An example of a semiautomated algorithm allows the user to interactively choose low and high thresholds that cover the intensity range of brain parenchyma, and then select a seed point within the parenchyma on a slice-by-slice basis (Rovaris et al., 2000). A region is automatically grown around the seed point that includes all connected pixels within the given range of intensities. Boundaries are drawn manually when necessary to prevent the region from growing outside the brain and into other structures. The intraobserver CV for this technique calculated from resegmentation of 10 images is 1.9% for whole brain volume.

Another approach is to perform the same steps automatically (Fig. 2): (1) Automatically determine the optimal threshold for separation of parenchyma and CSF based on histogram analysis or multispectral classification; (2) apply morphological operations to erode small connections between the brain and other cranial structures; and (3) use connectivity principles to identify the largest connected component within the image. Variations on these steps have been implemented by several groups to generate an initial segmentation of the brain (Losseff et al., 1996a; Bedell et al., 1996; Hohol et al., 1997; Fisher et al., 1997; Goldszal et al., 1998; Collins et al., 2001). In general, however, after the third step there are still some nonbrain structures included in the segmentation, and additional processing is required. In one variation on this approach, the segmentation is restricted to a central 20-mm thick slab of tissue selected by the radiologist (Losseff et al., 1996a). Manual editing is performed after automated segmentation, if necessary. The CV is 0.56%, as determined by a scan-rescan test. The same basic approach has also been applied to whole brain segmentation (Bedell and Narayana, 1996; Fisher et al., 1997; Goldszal et al., 1998; Collins et al., 2001; Udupa et al., 1997; Kikinis

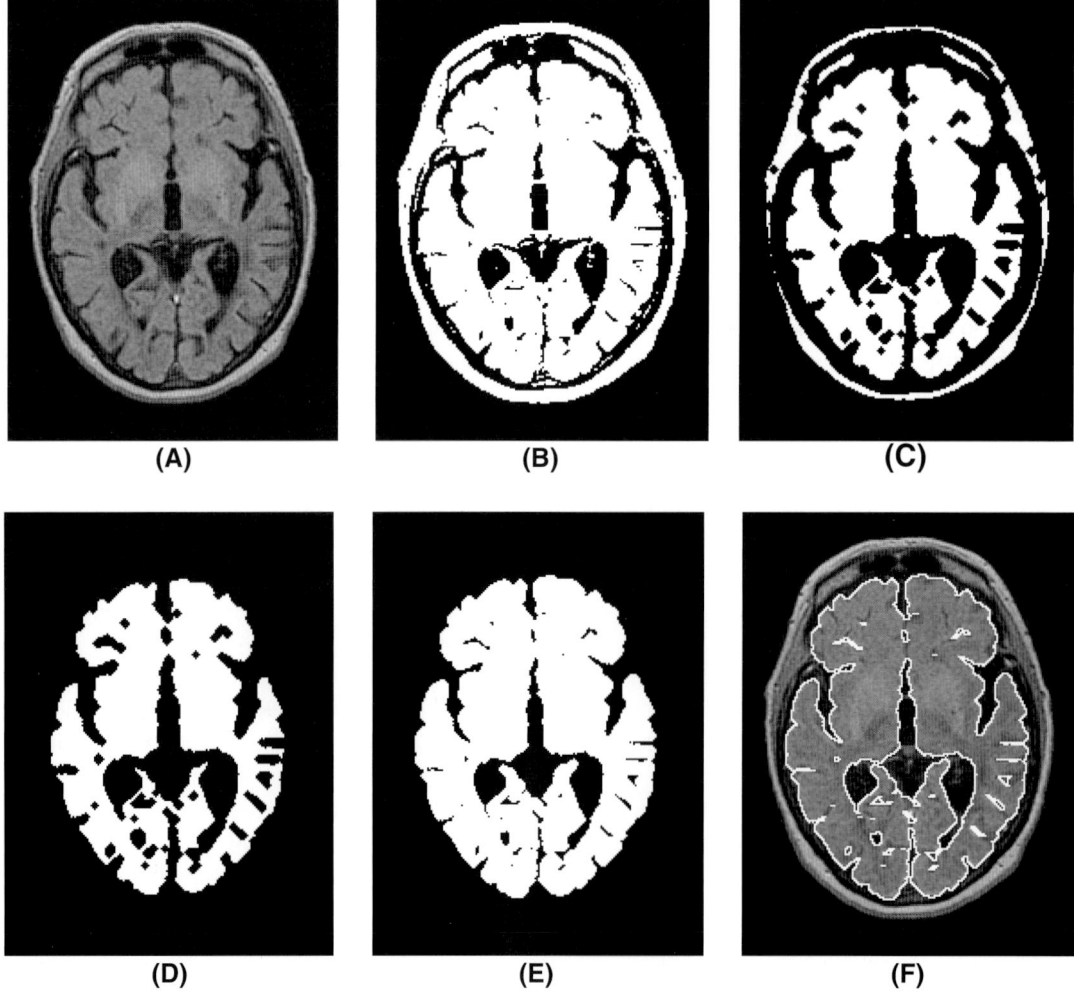

(A)   (B)   (C)

(D)   (E)   (F)

Figure 2 Generic automated brain segmentation algorithm: (**A**) slice from the original PD/T2 dual echo image (early echo minus late echo); (**B**) optimal thresholding to separate tissue from background and CSF; (**C**) morphological erosion with a 5 × 5 × 5 diamond-shaped kernel to disconnect connected structures; (**D**) identification of the largest connected component, the brain parenchyma; (**E**) morphological dilation with a 5 × 5 × 5 diamond-shaped kernel to recover the original shape; (**F**) boundaries of final segmentation superimposed on the original image.

et al., 1999) and implemented as semiautomated programs (with only minor editing requirements) or fully automated programs. Measurement variability with these techniques is consistently below 1%.

An important distinction between volumetric methods of atrophy measurements is whether the structure size is reported as the actual volume (e.g., in milliliters) or as a normalized volume. Normalized measures of whole brain atrophy are calculated as the brain parenchymal volume divided by an estimate of the intracranial volume to correct for head size. Normalized brain volume calculated in this way is referred to as the brain-to-intracranial-cavity volume ratio (Hohol et al., 1997), percent brain parenchyma volume (PBV) (Phillips et al., 1998), brain parenchymal fraction (BPF) (Rudick et al., 1999), brain-to-intracranial-cavity ratio (Collins et. al. 2001), or parenchymal fraction (Kalkers et al., 2001). CVs for normalized brain volume range from 0.2% to 2%, depending on the level of automation in the segmentation (Kalkers et al., 2001; Rudick et al., 1999). Head-size normalization is particularly important in cross-sectional studies in which normal biological variation in head size can easily obscure subtle disease-related volume differences. In normal healthy controls, normalized brain volume is fairly consistent between the ages of 20 and 55 years (Pfefferbaum et al., 1994). Therefore, normalized brain volumes also provide a means to estimate the total amount of atrophy that has occurred up to the time of the scan compared to an age-matched healthy control group. Normalization is also important in placebo-controlled longitudinal trials, where it is necessary to establish that two groups of patients are comparable at baseline. Using absolute brain volumes, it is not possible to ensure that the placebo group and the treated groups do not have different amounts of atrophy at the start of a trial.

Another type of whole brain atrophy estimation calculates brain atrophy directly from images acquired serially over time (Fox et al., 2000; Smith et al., 2001). These techniques require accurate co-registration of the images to determine changes in the brain-CSF boundaries over time. The mean error in atrophy measurement using this technique is approximately 0.2% (Fox et al., 2000).

It is important to note that atrophy measurements based on MRIs may be affected by factors unrelated to MS disease processes. Technical factors include patient positioning, scanner hardware and software upgrades, partial volume effects, motion artifacts, dental artifacts, voxel size calibration, intensity inhomogeneities, protocol or sequence variations, and the like. The measurement strategy may circumvent some of these problems. For example, one- and two-dimensional measures require precise patient repositioning. Volumetric, or three-dimensional techniques that use image registration to the baseline scan, on the other hand, reduce the effects of patient repositioning on atrophy measurements. Scanner upgrades and voxel size drift can be

partially corrected using phantoms and consistent calibration procedures during longitudinal studies, or by using normalized measures of atrophy. Decreasing slice thickness or accounting for partial volume effects in volume calculations may minimize partial volume effects. Atrophy measures are affected by aging, with decreasing brain volumes observed in populations of healthy individuals over age 50. Atrophy measures may also be affected by alcohol ingestion, dehydration, concurrent CNS disease (e.g., cerebral vascular disease), and medications (e.g., steroids, diuretics). It is important that groups be age-matched, and that exclusion criteria include confounding medication and coexisting brain disease.

III. Atrophy During the Course of MS

Recent studies have shown that atrophy begins early in MS and progresses throughout the course of the disease. Axonal transection and severe damage occur in early inflammatory lesions (Trapp et al., 1998). MR spectroscopy of patients whose disease duration is less than 5 years demonstrates reduced N-acetyl aspartate (NAA) indicative of axonal damage or loss (DeStefano et al., 2001). In a longitudinal study of patients with clinically isolated syndromes suggestive of MS (Brex et al., 2000), ventricular enlargement was significantly higher in the patients who progressed to clinically definite MS after 1 year compared with patients who did not develop MS. Similarly, brain atrophy was also detected in 6 of 15 patients with early relapsing-remitting (RR) MS within 18 months of diagnosis (Luks et al., 2000).

In patients with RR-MS with longer disease duration, normalized volumes and, in some studies, absolute volumes of CNS structures have been shown to be significantly lower than in age-matched healthy controls (Liu et al., 1999; Filippi et al., 1998; Kalkers et al., 2001; Phillips et al., 1998; Rudick et al., 1999; Paolillo et al., 2000; Ge et al., 2000b, 2001). Atrophy is not confined to particular CNS structures, even at this stage of disease. Significant differences between RR-MS and controls have been found in whole brain (Kalkers et al., 2001; Phillips et al., 1998; Rudick et al., 1999; Ge et al., 2000b), central slab volume (Paolillo et al., 2000), ventricular volume (Kalkers et al., 2001), corpus callosum (Paolillo et al., 2000), brainstem (Liu et al., 1999; Filippi et al., 1998), cerebellum (Liu et al., 1999), and upper cervical cord (Liu et al., 1999). The differences are due primarily to a decrease in white matter volume in RR-MS (Liu et al., 1999; Ge et al., 2000b).

There has been significant interest in measuring cortical pathology in MS. Atrophy of the cerebral cortex is difficult to measure because of its complex structure. A novel method has been developed to estimate cortical thickness from high-resolution MRIs (Sailer et al., 2003). This method was applied to brain scans obtained from 20 patients with clinically definite MS and 15 age-matched normal subjects. The thickness of the cortical ribbon was reduced in patients with MS compared to controls (2.30 mm vs. 2.48 mm). Disability, disease duration, and T_2 and T_1 lesion volumes were correlated with the differences between patients and controls. This study also showed that there was a characteristic distribution of focal thinning of the cerebral cortex in addition to diffuse cortical atrophy.

Longitudinally, the rate of atrophy in RR-MS patients has been compared to that in age-matched, normal healthy controls (Rovaris et al., 2000; Fox et al., 2000; Stevenson et al., 1998). The rate of decrease in cord cross-sectional area (Stevenson et al., 1998) and whole brain net volume loss (Rovaris et al., 2000; Fox et al., 2000) over 1 year is significantly higher in RR-MS than in controls. For whole brain atrophy measurements, the mean rate of atrophy in RR-MS is approximately 0.6% to 1.5% per year (Rovaris et al., 2000; Rudick et al., 1999; Fox et al., 2000; Ge et al., 2000b), but is highly variable between patients (Table 1).

Most longitudinal studies of patients with secondary progressive MS indicate that brain atrophy continues to progress in secondary progressive multiple sclerosis (SP-MS) at about the same rate as in RR-MS, when subgroups of patients are compared directly (Fox et al., 2000; Ge et al., 2000b; Filippi et al., 2000; Molyneux et al., 2000). However, some have found significantly lower rates of atrophy in SP-MS (Redmond et al., 2000). The rate of spinal cord atrophy may also be less in SP-MS than in RR-MS (Sailer et al., 2003). Comparative reports have included small numbers of patients; rates of atrophy in RR-MS patients have been compared with rates in separate patient groups with SP-MS in

these studies. Further investigation is needed to determine the kinetics of atrophy over the life span of MS.

Brain and spinal cord atrophy is also evident in patients with PP-MS (Losseff et al., 1996b; Kalkers et al., 2001; Fox et al., 2000; Sailer et al., 2003; Filippi et al., 2000; Redmond et al., 2000; Rovaris et al., 2001a; Stevenson et al., 1999; Pelletier et al., 2003). In cross-sectional studies that compare atrophy across MS subtypes, patients with PP-MS appear to have approximately the same amount of brain atrophy as patients with SP-MS of the same disease duration (Kalkers et al., 2001) or similar disability levels (Rovaris et al., 2001a), despite the significantly lower lesion load in patients with PP-MS. So far, only a limited amount of information is available on the rate of atrophy in patients with PP-MS measured longitudinally (Fox et al., 2000; Sailer et al., 2003; Redmond et al., 2000). It appears, however, that spinal cord atrophy may progress at a faster rate in PP-MS than in other MS subgroups (Sailer et al., 2003), whereas brain atrophy may progress at a rate similar to SP-MS and RR-MS (Fox et al., 2000).

IV. Relationship between MRI Parameters and Atrophy

A. Lesions

The major pathologic substrates of atrophy in MS are believed to be demyelination and axonal loss; therefore, it is reasonable to hypothesize that the amount of tissue loss is related to MRI markers of focal pathology, such as lesions

Table 1 Annualized Percent Decrease in Brain Volume Measurements

Study	Atrophy Measure	RR-MS	SP-MS
Losseff (1996a)	4-slice volume	1.12 (n = 13 RRMS, 16 SPMS)	
Rudick (1999)	BPF	0.61 (n = 72)	–
Ge (2000b)	Whole brain volume	1.5 (n = 27)	2.0 (n = 9)
Fox (2000)	Net brain volume loss	0.8 (n = 6)	0.6 (n = 6)
Rovaris (2000)	Whole brain volume	1.3 (n = 50)	–
Molyneaux (2000)	4-slice volume	–	1.3 (n = 46)
Saindane (2000)	PBV	0.92 (n = 24)	
Zivadinov (2001)	Whole brain volume	1.2 (n = 42)	–
Rovaris (2001b)	7-slice volume	0.9 (n = 114)	–

RR-MS, relapsing-remitting multiple sclerosis; SP-MS, secondary progressive multiple sclerosis.

visible on T_2-weighted, T_1-weighted, or contrast-enhanced MRIs. Results from correlational analyses, however, have been inconsistent across studies, particularly in regard to the relationship between enhancing lesions and atrophy. Gadolinium-enhancing lesions on T_1-weighted MRIs indicate acute inflammatory activity accompanied by a breakdown in the blood-brain barrier. Enhancing lesions have been implicated as the initiating events that lead to severe tissue damage and atrophy in MS (Simon, 1999a). This hypothesis is supported by evidence that the presence, number, or volume of enhancing lesions at baseline is predictive of subsequent atrophy (Simon, 1999; Simon et al. 1999; Leist et al., 2001; Luks et al., 2000; Molyneux et al., 2000; Rovaris et al., 2001a; Lin and Blumhardt, 2001; Paolillo et al., 1999; Fisher et al., 2001). In a Phase III clinical trial of IFNβ-1a in RR-MS (Simon et al. 1999), the number of enhancing lesions at baseline was the only significant predictor of change in third ventricle width over 2 years ($r^2 = 0.19$). Similarly, in a trial of glatiramer acetate (Copaxone) in RR-MS (Rovaris et al., 2001b), there was a modest correlation between number of enhancing lesions at baseline and brain volume change over 9 months in the placebo group ($r = -0.34$, $P = 0.0002$). A long-term, follow-up study demonstrated that the number of enhancing lesions at baseline was a significant predictor of brain atrophy over the subsequent 6 years (Fisher et al., 2001).

Other studies, however, have failed to find a relationship between enhancing lesions and atrophy (Losseff et al., 1996a; Filippi et al., 2000; Saindane et al., 2000). The discrepancies in findings may be due to several factors. One explanation is that a reduction in brain volume or an enlargement of ventricles after active inflammation may be due, in part, to the resolution of inflammation and reduction in edema (Molyneux et al., 2000). This may lead to a variable effect on atrophy measurements depending on the degree of associated edema. Another possibility is that enhancing lesions represent a range of underlying lesion types, and different studies may have a different mix of destructive vs. nondestructive lesions included in the enhancing lesion counts. Patients with more enhancing lesions typically have a higher relapse rate and, therefore, a greater number of steroid treatments, which may have an effect on atrophy measurements. It has also been hypothesized that atrophy may stem from disease processes not linked to inflammation such as diffuse, primary axonal damage (Saindane et al., 2000). On the other hand, it could be that inflammation truly is a precursor of the tissue damage that causes atrophy, but that a single snapshot is an insufficient measure of disease activity as changes in blood-brain barrier permeability are relatively rapid. Furthermore, if atrophy is the final step in a pathological cascade initiated by inflammation, then the optimal time to compare inflammation and atrophy would be dependent on the time course of these processes, which is not yet known and may be highly variable. The relationship between inflammation and atrophy may also vary over the course of disease. These issues are important questions for ongoing research.

Lesions on T_2-weighted scans are nonspecific markers of MS pathology and may be due to edema, inflammation, demyelination, axonal loss, and/or gliosis. Correlations between T_2 lesions and atrophy have been demonstrated (Liu et al., 1999; Kalkers et al., 2001; Phillips et al., 1998; Paolillo et al., 2000; Ge et al., 2000b; Rudick et al., 2000; Zivadinov et al., 2001) despite the lack of pathological specificity. An explanation for these findings may be that, to some extent, T_2-lesion volume represents the sum of current and previous focal tissue damage, whereas atrophy is the sum of all previous damage. Significant correlations with concurrent atrophy measures range from −0.24 (between central slab volume and T_2-lesion volume) (Rovaris et al., 2001a) to −0.75 (between PBV and T_2-lesion volume) (Phillips et al., 1998). In several longitudinal studies of patients with RR-MS, T_2 lesions and changes in T_2 lesions were correlated to subsequent atrophy (Simon et al., 1999; Rudick et al., 1999; Rovaris et al., 2001a; Fisher et al., 2001), possibly reflecting the evolution from focal tissue damage to atrophy.

It would be expected that T_1-hypointense lesions ("black holes"), which represent regions of severe tissue damage and axonal loss (van Walderveen et al., 1998), would correlate more strongly with atrophy than nonspecific T_2 lesions. The relationship between T_1 lesions and atrophy, however, appears to be very similar to that between T_2 lesions and atrophy in most studies (Kalkers et al., 2001; Paolillo et al., 2000; Rovaris et al., 2001a; Saindane et al., 2000; Zivadinov et al., 2001). In the Campath 1H study (Paolillo et al., 1999; Sailer et al., 2001), change in T_1-lesion volume was significantly correlated to change in brain volume ($r = 0.49$, $P = 0.006$), but change in T_2-lesion volume was not.

B. Measures of Whole Brain Integrity

Magnetization transfer ratio (MTR), diffusion tensor imaging (DTI), and whole brain NAA measurements provide information on the integrity of normal-appearing brain tissue. The relationships between atrophy and whole brain measures of tissue integrity have not been as extensively studied as the relationship between atrophy and lesions. Decreased MTR is mainly due to demyelination, axonal loss, and diffuse abnormalities in the normal-appearing white matter (Brochet and Dousset, 1999), which are the same factors believed to be responsible for atrophy. Various MTR parameters, including mean MTR; histogram peak height; and first, second, and third MTR histogram quartiles, have been shown to be significantly correlated to central slab volume ($r = 0.4$ to 0.5) (Rovaris et al., 1999). Mean MTR in normal-appearing brain tissue is correlated in cross-section with whole brain atrophy (Richert et al., 2001; Traboulsee et al., 2001; Kalkers et al., 2002). These correlations with atrophy are relatively strong (r = 0.6 to 0.7) compared to correlations with lesions, which is consistent with the hypothesis that both MTR and atrophy are sensitive to diffuse damage in normal-appearing tissue and possibly have common pathological substrates.

DTI and whole brain NAA are other MR methods for measurement of damage in normal-appearing brain tissue. Demyelination and damage to axons lead to alterations in the properties of random water diffusion in brain tissue that can be detected with DTI (Werring et al., 1999). Whole brain NAA is a relatively new MR proton spectroscopy technique that provides an estimate of the total amount of the neuronal injury in the brain (Gonen et al., 2002). A few studies have shown that measures of diffuse tissue damage are correlated with atrophy in cross-section (Phillips et al., 1998; Kalkers, 2002), but their predictive value for subsequent tissue loss has not been studied extensively. Lesions only account for a relatively small amount of variance in subsequent atrophy (Fisher et al., 2002; therefore, diffuse tissue damage in the normal-appearing brain tissue measurable with MTR, DTI, and/or whole brain NAA may account for a substantial portion of brain atrophy. Additional longitudinal studies are needed to clarify the relationship between diffuse tissue damage and atrophy in MS patients.

V. Relationship Between Disease Severity and Brain Atrophy

A. Correlations Between Atrophy and Disability

Measures of atrophy are more closely related to neurological disability in patients with MS than conventional lesion measurements (Table 2). The strength of the correlations depends on the type of atrophy measure, type of disability measure, and possibly, type of MS. In cross-section, correlations between Expanded Disability Status Scale (EDSS) and brain atrophy are typically modest (r = 0.2 to 0.5) (Liu et al., 1999; Kalkers et al., 2001; Rudick et al., 1999; Paolillo et al., 2000; Ge et al., 2000b; Molyneux et al., 2000; Stevenson et al., 1999), while correlations between EDSS and spinal cord atrophy are stronger (r = 0.5 to 0.7) (Losseff et al., 1996b; Lycklama et al., 1998; Stevenson et al., 1999). This may be related to characteristics of the EDSS, which is primarily a measure of ambulation. Correlations between brain atrophy and the MS Functional Composite (MSFC) (Rudick et al., 1997; 2001) are stronger than the atrophy/EDSS correlations (Kalkers et al., 2001; Fisher et al., 2001). The MSFC consists of a walking score (timed 25-meter walk), an arm function score (9-hole peg test), and a cognitive score (paced serial addition test).

By comparison of results across studies, normalized atrophy measures, which correct for head size, appear to be more strongly correlated to disability than absolute volume measurements. Several longitudinal studies indicate that patients with greater rates of atrophy are more likely to worsen clinically (Losseff et al., 1996a; Molyneux et al., 2000; Fisher et al., 2002) and vice versa (Fisher et al., 2000). In an 8-year follow-up study of 172 patients originally enrolled in the Phase III trial of IFNβ-1a in RR-MS, 52% of patients in the quartile with the highest rate of atrophy in the first 2 years had reached an EDSS score of 6 or greater at the 8-year follow-up. In contrast, only 12% of patients in the quartile with the lowest rate of atrophy in the first 2 years had reached an EDSS score of 6 or greater at the time of follow-up visit (Fisher et al., 2002). As with the relationships between atrophy and lesions, the relationship between atrophy and disability may be complicated by a possible time lag between when tissue injury occurs and when this injury is detectable as atrophy on MRI. Furthermore, the brain may be able to compensate for tissue injury early in the disease when there is still sufficient functional reserve and capacity for tissue repair, leading to a dissociation between atrophy and disability. Data demonstrating higher atrophy-disability correlations later on in the disease or in SP-MS as compared to RR-MS support this hypothesis (Ge et al., 2000b; Fisher et al., 2000).

Brain atrophy has also been shown to be related to cognitive impairment (Rao et al., 1985; Edwards et al., 2001; Hohol et al., 1997) in MS patients. An early study of patients with chronic progressive MS (Rao et al., 1985) demonstrated that performance on memory and intelligence tests was correlated to degree of ventricle enlargement. In patients monitored for more than 1 year, cognitive change was related to baseline normalized brain atrophy measures (Hohol et al., 1997).

B. Correlations Between Atrophy and Quality of Life

Health-related quality of life (HRQOL) declines as a consequence of MS; thus significant correlations between brain disease defined by MRI and HRQOL would be expected. This correlation was evaluated in 60 consecutive patients with MS treated in an MS specialty clinic. The Multiple Sclerosis Quality of Life-54 Instrument was used to measure HRQOL, and results were compared with EDSS, clinical course, and MRI findings. Atrophy was rated visually in comparison to healthy control MRI scans, and categorized as normal, mild, moderate, or severe atrophy evident to the examiner. In this study, the severity of brain atrophy correlated significantly with reduced HRQOL scores (Janardhan and Bakshi, 2000).

The relationship between MRI parameters and depression was assessed in 48 MS patients. Patients included in the analysis had an average disease duration of 8.9 years, and were 41 years of age on average. In all, 19 (40%) of these patients were found to be depressed. Compared with patients with MS who were not depressed, the depressed patients had

Table 2 Correlations between Atrophy and Disability

Study	Atrophy Measure	n MS type[*]	Disability Measure	r	P
Losseff (1996b)	Cord area	30 RR 15 SP 15 PP	EDSS	−0.7	< 0.001
Stevenson (1998)	Cord area	10 RR 6 SP 12 PP	EDSS	−0.52	0.005
Lycklama à Nijeholt (1998)	Cord area	28 RR 32 SP 31 PP	EDSS	−0.34	0.001
Stevenson (1999)	Cord area	158 PP 33 TP	EDSS	−0.30	< 0.001
Liu (1999)	Cord area	20 RR 20 SP	EDSS	−0.37	0.023
Lycklama à Nijeholt (1998)	Vetricle volume	28 RR 32 SP 31 PP	EDSS	No correlation	
Losseff (1996a)	4-slice volume	13 RR 16 SP	EDSS	No correlation	
Stevenson (1999)	4-slice volume	158 PP 33 TP	EDSS	−0.20	0.006
			Timed walk	−0.39	< 0.001
Molyneaux (2000)	4-slice volume	95 SP	EDSS	0.18	0.018
Liu (1999)	Cerebral WM	20 RR 20 SP	EDSS	−0.37	0.018
Filippi (2000)	Whole brain volume	11 RR 4 SP	EDSS	No correlation	
Fox (2000a)	Net brain volume loss	6 RR 6 SP 9 PP	EDSS	No correlation	
Ge (2000b)	PBV	27 RR	EDSS	No correlation	
Ge (2000b)	PBV	9 SP	EDSS	−0.69	0.004
Fisher (2000b)	BPF	134 RR	EDSS	−0.29 to −0.42	< 0.001
			MSFC	0.42 to 0.50	< 0.0001
Paolillo (2000)	Infratentorial/supratentorial ratio	52 RR	EDSS	−0.49	0.004
Kalkers (2001)	PF and VF	80 RR 36 SP 21 PP	EDSS	0.24 to −0.25	< 0.01
			MSFC	0.36 to −0.40	< 0.01

EDSS, Expanded Disability Status Scale; MSFC, MS Functional Composite; PBV, brain parenchymal fraction; PF, VF.
[*]RR = relapsing-remitting MS, SP = secondary progressive MS, TP = transitional progressive MS, PP = primary progressive MS.

higher EDSS scores (4.2 vs. 2.9) and had significantly greater ventricular enlargement (Jones et al., 2001).

Health-Related Quality of Life was evaluated in patients who participated in a randomized, double-blind, placebo-controlled trial of IFNβ-1a (Avonex) for RR-MS. The patients who were in the trial for at least 2 years were reexamined an average of 8 years after randomization to the trial. The relationship between Sickness Impact Profile (SIP) scores and the MSFC, EDSS, and BPF were evaluated. SIP Physical and SIP Total scores significantly worsened from baseline to follow-up evaluation. Brain atrophy progression between baseline and year 2, and atrophy progression between year 2 and year 8, were both significantly correlated to SIP Physical scores and SIP Total scores at the 8 year follow-up evaluation (Miller et al., 2003). In an extension of this study, Marrie and colleagues (2004) analyzed the relationship between self-report measures of fatigue and brain atrophy. Fatigue was measured using the SIP Sleep and Rest Scale (SIPSR) and the Fatigue Severity Scale at baseline and year 2. Correlation, linear regression, and logistic regression analyses were used to assess the relationship between changes in fatigue and subsequent atrophy progression. An increase in fatigue on the SIPSR during the initial 2 years was significantly associated with progressive brain atrophy during the subsequent 6 years, and with increased risk of having the greatest amount of atrophy progression during the length of the study. The relationship between increasing fatigue and progressive brain atrophy was independent of changes in disability or baseline MRI characteristics. These results suggest that the subjective complaint of fatigue is linked to atrophy progression in patients with RR-MS.

VI. What Does Atrophy Teach Us about the Pathogenesis of MS?

Studies on brain atrophy that have emerged during the last 5 years showed that the rate of brain atrophy in patients with MS is more than fivefold higher than in age- and gender-matched controls. While the rate of atrophy varies between individual patients with MS, atrophy appears to progress at about the same rate in groups of RR-MS and SP-MS patients. This indicates that the destructive pathological process progresses inexorably over many years during the course of MS.

In most patients with RR-MS, brain atrophy progresses without obvious clinical manifestations; however, the rate of brain atrophy progression predicts long-term disability status. This suggests that progressive brain tissue destruction is clinically silent in patients with MS until a threshold is surpassed, beyond which compensatory mechanisms are exhausted and disability progression ensues. This strongly supports the "threshold" hypothesis of disability progression in MS.

Brain atrophy progression predicts future disability progression better than MRI-defined MS lesions predict disability progression. At the present time, brain atrophy is the best currently validated imaging "biomarker" of MS-related destructive brain pathology; however, measurable factors associated with brain atrophy progression are largely undefined. Typical MRI-defined MS lesions correlate with future brain atrophy progression only weakly, accounting for less than 25% of the variance in future brain atrophy. Therefore, there is an urgent need to identify measurable factors more closely linked to brain atrophy progression in MS.

Finally, preliminary studies reviewed in the next section suggest that anti-inflammatory therapy may slow the rate of brain atrophy progression during RR-MS, but thus far no study has demonstrated a beneficial effect of anti-inflammatory therapy on atrophy progression in SP-MS. These findings are consistent with the view that atrophy progression is driven to some degree by the inflammatory process in early stages of MS.

VII. Atrophy as an Outcome Measure in Clinical Trials

A. Relapsing-Remitting MS

The effects of MS treatments on atrophy have been investigated in several clinical trials, including those for IFNβ-1a (Avonex) (Rudick et al., 1999), Campath 1H (Paolillo et al., 1999), cladribine (Filippi et al., 2000), linomide (Wolinsky et al., 2000), glatiramer acetate (Copaxone) (Rovaris et al.,

2001a; Ge et al., 2000a), IFNβ-1b (Betaseron) (Molyneux et al., 2000), pulsed intravenous methylprednisolone (IVMP) (Zivadinov et al., 2001), and IFNβ-1a (Rebif) (Wolinsky et al., 2001) (Table 3). Many of these drugs have been shown to be effective in reducing the number of gadolinium-enhancing lesions, but their effects on atrophy are not well understood. A 2-year Phase III trial of IFNβ-1a in RR-MS (Rudick et al., 1999) demonstrated a significant treatment effect on atrophy in the second year of the trial. Similar rates of atrophy were observed in the European dose comparison study of IFNβ-1a in RR-MS (Freitag et al., 2001), where the brain atrophy rate in the second and third years was about half of that of the first year. The delay in effectiveness may be due to a continuation of destructive processes initiated by pretrial inflammatory activity. A treatment effect on brain volume change was also observed in a subset of 27 patients from the 2-year Phase III trial of glatiramer acetate in RR-MS (Ge et al., 2000a), but not in the larger, but shorter term European trial of glatiramer acetate (Rovaris et al., 2001b). A 5-year study of pulse IVMP in RR-MS (Zivadinov et al., 2001) resulted in a significantly reduced rate of atrophy in the treated group compared to a group who received steroids only for relapses. In a 3-year European trial of IFNβ-1b in SP-MS (Molyneux et al., 2000), there was no treatment effect for the group overall, but stratification by the presence of gadolinium-enhancing lesions at baseline revealed that in the subgroup without enhancing lesions, the treated group had significantly less atrophy than the placebo group. Other trials (Filippi et al,. 2000; Wolinsky et al., 2001; Jones et al., 2001) have found no treatment effects on atrophy. Results are not easy to compare across trials because each used a different type of atrophy measure and studied patients with different baseline characteristics. The durations of the controlled trials also varied considerably from 9 months to 5 years, and time may be an important factor to consider in studies of brain tissue loss resulting from MS. Atrophy measurement is attractive as an outcome measure for MS treatment trials because it may provide a means to test the ability of a particular therapy to halt tissue destruction.

Results have been more encouraging with RR-MS trials, where some but not all trials show therapeutic benefits on the rate of atrophy progression. To date, no studies in progressive MS have shown a therapeutic effect of anti-inflammatory therapy on atrophy progression. These results are consistent with the view that inflammation drives atrophy during early stages of MS to a greater degree than later in the disease (Fig. 3).

VIII. Future Directions

A. Factors Driving Atrophy

The factors that drive destructive brain pathology, manifest as atrophy, are largely undefined. It has been assumed

Table 3 Atrophy Outcomes in Clinical Trials

Study	Atrophy Measure	Subjects	Duration	Study Design	Atrophy Results
Rudick 1999 IFNβ-1a	BPF	140 RR-MS	24 months	Double-blind, placebo-controlled	Treatment effect on atrophy in second year (P = 0.03)
Ge 2000a GA	Whole brain volume	27 RR-MS	24 months	Double-blind, placebo-controlled	Treatment effect on atrophy
Rovaris 2001b GA	7-slice volume	227 RR-MS	18 months	9m blind, placebo-controlled, + 9 m open label	No treatment effect on atrophy
Zivadinov 2001 IVMP	Whole brain volume	88 RR-MS	60 months	Single-blind controlled	Treatment effect on atrophy (P = 0.003)
Wolinsky 2000 Linomide	CSF volume	718 RRMS SP-MS	<12 months	Double-blind, placebo-controlled	Study stopped because of toxicity
Molyneux 2000 IFNβ-1b	4-slice volume	95 SP-MS	36 months	Double-blind, placebo-controlled	No treatment effect on atrophy overall. In subgroup without gad lesions at baseline, there was significantly more atrophy in placebo (P = 0.003)
Paolillo 1999	4-slice volume	29 SP-MS	18 months	Crossover	No treatment effect on atrophy
Campath 1H					Atrophy strongly correlated to gad lesions pretreatment
Filippi 2000	Whole brain volume	159 SP PP	12 months	Double-blind, placebo-controlled	No treatment effect on atrophy
Cladribine					

IFNβ-1a, interferon β-1a; BPF, brain parenchymal fraction; RR-MS, relapsing-remitting multiple sclerosis; SP-MS, secondary progressive multiple sclerosis.

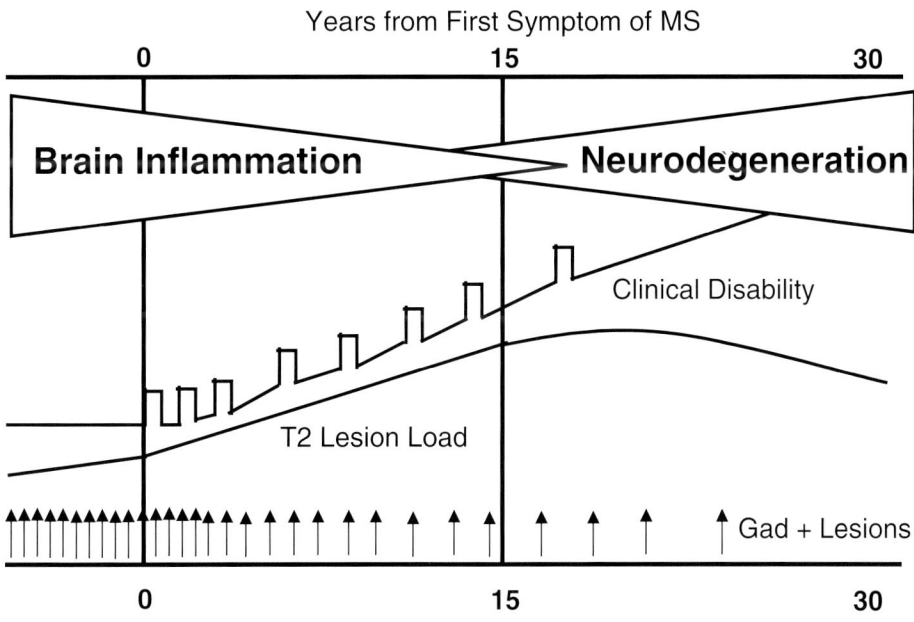

Figure 3 Course of MS over 30 years. The diagram shows new MRI lesions (Gad+ lesions) occur frequently during the preclinical and early clinical phase of MS, declining in frequency as the disease progresses. T2 lesion burden gradually increases as a consequence of the occurrence of new lesions. Clinical symptoms consist primarily of relapses followed by remissions in the early disease phase, followed by gradually worsening disability in the later stages. The diagram shows the current view of MS pathogenesis: Inflammation dominates early in the disease, while neurodegeneration ensues and progressively dominates the pathogenesis during later stages. Neurodegeneration may become disconnected from the inflammatory process as the disease progresses. This could explain why anti-inflammatory therapy is more effective in RR-MS than SP-MS.

211

that inflammation initiates the pathological process that plays out as tissue loss. This is a logical interpretation from studies documenting irreversible axonal injury localized to sites of inflammation in MS brain, even in young patients with very short disease durations. However, correlational studies have shown only weak correlations between MRI markers of inflammation (e.g., new T_2 lesions or gadolinium-enhancing lesions) and brain atrophy. There are two interpretations of this: (1) our measures of brain inflammation are very insensitive; if we had more sensitive markers of brain inflammation, perhaps the correlation between MRI-defined inflammation and subsequent atrophy would be stronger; and (2) atrophy is driven to a limited degree by inflammation, but there are factors, currently not defined, that are not inflammation-dependent. It also remains possible that inflammation drives atrophy predominantly at the earlier stages of the disease. Clinical trial data are consistent with this possibility.

B. Novel Uses of Atrophy for Clinical Trials

Is it possible to monitor atrophy progression in relatively short trials, in a manner similar to Phase II trials targeted at gadolinium-enhancing lesions? This possibility was suggested by Hardmeier and colleagues (2003). In their study, 138 untreated patients with RR-MS had three MRI studies within a 3-month period before randomization into a controlled clinical trial. BPF was determined at all time points. An annualized atrophy rate was estimated by calculating a regression slope. The BPF decreased significantly by −0.22% from scan 1 to scan 3. The estimated annualized atrophy rate was −1.06% (95% confidence interval, −1.50% to −0.62%). The BPF change was only weakly correlated to the volume of gadolinium-enhancing lesions on the baseline MRI (r = −0.185). The authors concluded that measurements of BPF allow detection of atrophy over short time intervals, and that this might form the basis for future Phase II studies with an expected effect on tissue-destructive pathological mechanisms of MS.

References

Alfano, B., Quarantelli, M., Brunetti, A., et al. (1998). Reproducibility of intracranial volume measurement by unsupervised multispectral brain segmentation. *Magn Reson Med* **39**, 497–99.

Bakshi, R., Carnecki, D., Shaikh, Z. A., Priore, R. L., Janardhan, V., Kaliszky, Z., and Kinkel, P. R. (2000). Brain MRI lesions and atrophy are related to depression in multiple sclerosis. *Neuroreport* **11**, 1153–1158.

Bedell, B. J., and Narayana, P. A. (1996). Automatic removal of extrameningeal tissues from MR images of human brain. *J. Magn. Reson. Imaging* **6**, 939–943.

Brex, P. A., Jenkins, R., Fox, N. C., et al. (2000). Detection of ventricular enlargement in patients at the earliest clinical stage of MS. *Neurology* **54**, 1689–1691.

Brochet, B., and Dousset, V. (1999) Pathological correlates of magnetization transfer imaging abnormalities in animal models and humans with multiple sclerosis. *Neurology* **53**, S12–17.

Cala, L. A., and Mastaglia. E. L. (1976). Computerized axial tomography in multiple sclerosis. *Lancet* **1**, 689.

Collins, D. L., Montagnat, J., Zijdenbos, A. P., Evans, A. C., and Arnold, D. L. (2001). Automated estimation of brain volume in multiple sclerosis with BICCR. *In: "Proc of the Annual Symposium on Information Processing in Medical Imaging"* (M. F. Insana and R. M. Leahy, eds.) pp. 1411–1447, Springer, Berlin.

Dastidar, P., Heinonen, T., Lehtimäki, T., et al. (1999). Volumes of brain atrophy and plaques correlated with neurological disability in secondary progressive multiple sclerosis. *J. Neurol. Sci.* **165**, 36–42.

De Stefano, N., Narayanan, S., Francis, G. S., et al. (2001). Evidence of axonal damage in the early stages of multiple sclerosis and its relevance to disability. *Arch. Neurol.* **58**, 65–70.

DeCarli, C., Maisog, J., Murphy, D. G. M., et al. (1992). Method for quantification of brain, ventricular, and subarachnoid CSF volumes from MR images. *J. Comput. Assist. Tomogr.* **16**, 274–284.

Edwards, S. G. M., Liu, C., and Blumhardt, L. D. (2001). Cognitive correlates of supratentorial atrophy on MRI in multiple sclerosis. *Acta Neurol. Scand.* **104**, 214–223.

Filippi, M., Mastronardo, G., Rocca, M. A., Pereira, C., and Comi, G. (1998). Quantitative volumetric analysis of brain magnetic resonance imaging from patients with multiple sclerosis. *J. Neurol. Sci.* **158**, 148–153.

Filippi, M., Rovaris, M., Iannucci, G., Mennea, S., Sormani, M. P., and Comi, G. (2000). Whole brain volume changes in patients with progressive MS treated with cladribine. *Neurology* **55**, 1714–1718.

Fisher, E., Cothren, R. M., Tkach, J. A., Masaryk, T. J., and Cornhill, J. F. (1997). Knowledge-based 3D segmentation of MR images for quantitative MS lesion tracking. *Proc. SPIE (Medical Imaging: Image Processing)* **3034**, 19–25.

Fisher, E., Rudick, R. A., Cutter, G., et al. (2000). Relationship between brain atrophy and disability: An 8-year follow-up study of multiple sclerosis patients. *Multiple Sclerosis* **6**, 373–377.

Fisher, E., Rudick, R. A., Simon, J. H., Cutter, G., Baier, M., Lee, J.-C., Miller, D., Weinstock-Guttman, B., Mass, M. K., Dougherty, D., and Simonian, N. A. (2002). An 8-year follow-up study of brain atrophy in multiple sclerosis patients. *Neurology* **59**, 1412–1420.

Fox, N. C., Jenkins, R., Leary, S. M., et al. (2000). Progressive cerebral atrophy in MS: A serial study using registered, volumetric MRI., *Neurology* **54**, 807–812.

Freitag, P., Hardmeier, M., Fisher, E., et al. (2001). Time course of annual brain atrophy rates in the dose comparison-study of rIFN beta-1a (Avonex) in relapsing multiple sclerosis. *Multiple Sclerosis* **7(Suppl 1)**, S42.

Ge, Y., Grossman, R. I., Udupa, J. K., et al. (2000a). Glatiramer acetate (Copaxone) treatment in relapsing-remitting MS. Quantitative MR assessment. *Neurology* **54**, 813–817.

Ge, Y., Grossman, R. I., Udupa, J. K., et al. (2000b). Brain atrophy in relapsing-remitting multiple sclerosis and secondary progressive multiple sclerosis. Longitudinal quantitative analysis. *Radiology* **214**, 665–670.

Ge, Y., Grossman, R. I., Udupa, J. K., et al. (2001). Brain atrophy in relapsing-remitting multiple sclerosis: Fractional volumetric analysis of gray matter and white matter. *Radiology* **220**, 606–610.

Goldszal, A. F., Davatzikos, C., and Pham, D. L. (1998). An image-processing system for qualitative and quantitative volumetric analysis of brain images. *J. Comp. Assist. Tomogr.* **22**, 827–837.

Gonen, O., Moriarty, D. M., Li, B. S., Babb, J. S., He, J., Listerud, J., Jacobs, D., Markowitz, C. E., and Grossman, R. I. (2002). Relapsing-remitting multiple sclerosis and whole-brain *N*-acetylaspartate measurement: Evidence for different clinical cohorts initial observations. *Radiology* **225**, 261–268.

Hardmeier, M., Wagenpfeil, S., Freitag, P., Fisher, E., Rudick, R. A., Kooijmans-Coutinho, M., et al. (2003). European rIFN beta-1a in Relapsing MS Dose Comparison Trial Study Group. Atrophy is detectable within a 3-month period in untreated patients with active relapsing remitting multiple sclerosis. *Arch. Neurol.* **60,** 17361739.

Hohol, M. J., Guttmann, C. R. G., Orav, J., et al. (1997). Serial neuropsychological assessment and magnetic resonance imaging analysis in multiple sclerosis. *Arch. Neurol.* **54,** 1018–1025.

Jacobs, L. D., Cookfair, D. L., Rudick, R. A., Herndon, R. M., Richert, J. R., Salazar, A. M., et al. (1996). Intramuscular interferon beta-1a for disease progression in relapsing multiple sclerosis. *Ann. Neurol.* **39,** 285–294.

Janardhan, V., and Bakshi, R. (2000). Quality of life and its relationship to brain lesions and atrophy on magnetic resonance images in 60 patients with multiple sclerosis. *Arch. Neurol.* **57,** 1485–1491.

Jones, C. K., Riddehough, A., Li, D. K. B., et al. (2001). MRI cerebral atrophy in relapsing-remitting MS: Results from the PRISMS trial. *Neurology* **56 (Suppl 3),** A379.

Kalkers, N. F., Bergers, E., Castelijns, J. A., et al. (2001). Optimizing the association between disability and biological markers in MS. *Neurology* **57,** 1253–1258.

Kalkers, N. F., Vrenken, H., Uitdehaag, B. M., Polman, C. H., and Barkhof, F. (2002). Brain atrophy in multiple sclerosis: Impact of lesions and of damage of whole brain tissue. *Multiple Sclerosis* **8,** 410–414.

Kidd, D., Thorpe, J. W., Thompson, A. J., et al. (1993). Spinal cord MRI using multi-array coils and fast spin echo II. Findings in multiple sclerosis, *Neurology* **43,** 2632–2637.

Kikinis, R., Guttmann, C. R. G., Metcalf, D., et al. (1999). Quantitative follow-up of patients with multiple sclerosis using MRI: Technical aspects, *J. Magn. Reson. Imaging* **9,** 519–530.

Leist, T. P., Gobbini, M. I., Frank, J. A., and McFarland, H. F. (2001). Enhancing magnetic resonance lesions and cerebral atrophy in patients with relapsing multiple sclerosis. *Arch. Neurol.* **58,** 57–60.

Lin, X., and Blumhardt, L. D. (2001) Inflammation and atrophy in multiple sclerosis: MRI associations with disease course, *J. Neurol. Sci.* **189,** 99–104.

Liu, C., Edwards, S., Gong, Q., Roberts, N., and Blumhardt, L. D. (1999). Three dimensional MRI estimates of brain and spinal cord atrophy in multiple sclerosis. *J. Neurol. Neurosurg. Psychiatry* **66,** 323–330.

Losseff, N. A., Wang, L., Lai, H. M., et al. (1996a). Progressive cerebral atrophy in multiple sclerosis—A serial MRI study. *Brain* **119,** 2009–2019.

Losseff, N. A., Webb, S. L., O'Riordan, J. I., et al. (1996b). Spinal cord atrophy and disability in multiple sclerosis. A new reproducible and sensitive MRI method with potential to monitor disease progression. *Brain* **119,** 701–708.

Luks, T. L., Goodkin, D. E., Nelson, S. J., Majumdar, S., Bacchetti, P., Protnoy, D., and Sloan, R. (2000). A longitudinal study of ventricular volume in early relapsing-remitting multiple sclerosis. *Multiple Sclerosis* **6,** 332–337.

Lycklama à Nijeholt, G. J., van Walderveen, M. A. A., Castelijns, J. A., et al. (1998). Brain and spinal cord abnormalites in multiple sclerosis: Correlation between MRI parameters, clinical subtypes and symptoms. *Brain* **121,** 687–697.

Marrie, R. A., Fisher, E., Miller, D. M., Lee, J.-C., and Rudick, R. A. (2003). Association of Fatigue and Brain Atrophy in Multiple Sclerosis Patients. *Arch. Neurol.* submitted 2004 *J. Neurol. Sci.,* In press.

Matthews, P. M., Pioro, E., Narayanan, S., et al. (1996). Assessment of lesion pathology in multiple sclerosis using quantitative MRI morphometry and magnetic resonance spectroscopy, *Brain* **119,** 715–722.

Miller, D. H., Barkhof, F., Frank, J. A., Parker, G. J., and Thompson, A. J. (2002). Measurement of atrophy in multiple sclerosis: Pathological basis, methodological aspects and clinical relevance. *Brain* **125,** 1676–1695.

Miller, D. M., Rudick, R A., Baier, M., Cutter, G., Doughtery, D. S., Weinstock-Guttman, B., Mass, M. K., Fisher, E., and Simonian, N. (2003). Factors that predict health-related quality of life in patients with relapsing-remitting multiple sclerosis *Multiple Sclerosis* **9,** 1–5.

Molyneux, P. D., Kappos, L., Polman, C., et al. (2000). The effect of interferon beta-1b treatment on MRI measures of cerebral atrophy in secondary progressive multiple sclerosis. *Brain* **123,** 2256–2263.

Paolillo, A., Coles, A. J., and Molyneux, P. D. (1999). Quantitative MRI in patients with secondary progressive MS treated with monoclonal antibody Campath 1H. *Neurology* **53,** 751–757.

Paolillo, A., Pozzilli, C., Gasperini, C., et al. (2000). Brain atrophy in relapsing-remitting multiple sclerosis: Relationship with "black holes," disease duration and clinical disability. *J. Neurol. Sci.* **174,** 85–91.

Pelletier, D., Nelson, S. J., Oh, J., Antel, J. P., Kita, M., Zamvil, S. S., and Goodkin, D. E. (2003). MRI lesion volume heterogeneity in primary progressive MS in relation with axonal damage and brain atrophy. *J. Neurol. Neurosurg. Psychiatry* **74,** 950–952.

Pfefferbaum, A., Mathalon, D. H., Sullivan, E. V., et al. (1994). A quantitative magnetic resonance imaging study of changes in brain morphology from infancy to late adulthood. *Arch. Neurol.* **51,** 874–887.

Phillips, M. D., Grossman, R. I., Miki, Y., et al. (1998). Comparison of T2 lesion volume and magnetization transfer ratio histogram analysis and of atrophy and measures of lesion burden in patients with multiple sclerosis. *Am J Nuclear Reson* **19,** 1055–1060.

Prineas, J. (1990). Pathology of multiple sclerosis. In "Handbook of Multiple Sclerosis." (S.D. Cook, Ed.). pp.187–219, Marcel Dekker, Inc, New York.

Rao, S M., Glatt, S., Hammeke, T. A., et al. (1985). Chronic progressive multiple sclerosis. Relationship between cerebral ventricular size and neuropsychological impairment. *Arch. Neurol.* **42,** 678–82.

Redmond, I. T., Barbosa, S., Blumhardt, L. D., and Roberts, N. (2000). Short-term ventricular volume changes on serial MRI in multiple sclerosis. *Acta Neurol. Scand.* **102,** 99–105.

Richert, N., Fisher, E., Frank, J., McFarland, H., and Stone, L. (2001). Contrast enhancing lesions predict magnetization transfer ratios (MTR) and cerebral atrophy in relapsing-remitting MS patients: Preliminary results of an 8-year follow-up study. Presented at the *Annual Meeting of the American Neurological Association.*

Rovaris, M., Bozzali, M., Rodegher, M., Tortorella, C., Comi, G., and Filippi, M. (1999). Brain MRI correlates of magnetization transfer imaging metrics in patients with multiple sclerosis. *J. Neurol. Sci.* **166,** 58–63.

Rovaris, M., Inglese, M., van Schijndel, R. A., et al. (2000). Sensitivity and reproducibility of volume change measurements of different brain portions on magnetic resonance imaging in patients with multiple sclerosis. *J. Neurol.* **247,** 960–965.

Rovaris, M., Bozzali, M., Santuccio, G., et al. (2001a). In vivo assessment of the brain and cervical cord pathology of patients with primary progressive multiple sclerosis. *Brain* **124,** 2540–2549.

Rovaris, M., Comi, G., Rocca, M. A., Wolinsky, J. S., Filippi, M., and the European/Canadian Glatiramer Acetate Study Group. (2001b). Short-term brain volume change in relapsing-remitting multiple sclerosis: Effect of glatiramer acetate and implications. *Brain* **124,** 1803–1812.

Rudick, R., Antel, J., Confavreux, C., et al. (1997). Recommendations from the National Multiple Sclerosis Society Clinical Outcomes Assessment Task Force. *Ann. Neurol.* **42,** 379–382.

Rudick, R. A., Fisher, E., Lee, J. C., et al. (1999). Use of the brain parenchymal fraction to measure whole brain atrophy in relapsing-remitting MS. *Neurology* **53,** 1698–1704.

Rudick, R. A., Fisher, E., Lee, J.-C., Duda, J. T., and Simon, J. (2000). Brain atrophy in relapsing multiple sclerosis: relationship to relapses, EDSS and treatment with interferon beta-1a. *Multiple Sclerosis* **6,** 365–372.

Rudick, R. A., Cutter, G., Baier, M., et al. (2001). Use of the Multiple Sclerosis Functional Composite to predict disability in relapsing MS. *Neurology* **56,** 1324-1330.

Sailer, M., Losseff, N. A., Wang, L., Gawne-Cain, M. L., Thompson, A. J., and Miller, D. H. (2001). T1 lesion load and cerebral atrophy as a marker for clinical progression in patients with multiple sclerosis. A prospective 18 months follow-up study, *Eur. J. Neurol.* **8,** 37–42.

Sailer, M., Fischl, B., Salat, D., Tempelmann, C., Schonfeld, M. A., Busa, E., et al. (2003). Focal thinning of the cerebral cortex in multiple sclerosis. *Brain* **126,** 1734–1744.

Saindane, A. M., Ge, Y., Udupa, J. K., Babb, J. S., Mannon, L. J., Grossman, R. I. (2000). The effect of gadolinium-enhancing lesions on whole brain atrophy in relapsing-remitting MS. *Neurology* **55,** 61–65.

Simon, J. H., Schiffer, R. B., Rudick, R. A., and Herndon, R. M. (1987). Quantitative determination of MS-induced corpus callosum atrophy in vivo using MR imaging. *Am. J. Neuroradiol.* **8,** 599–604

Simon, J. H. (199a). From enhancing lesions to brain atrophy in relapsing MS. *J. Neuroimmunol.* **98,** 7–15.

Simon, J. H., Jacobs, L. D., Campion, M. K., et al. (1999). A longitudinal study of brain atrophy in relapsing multiple sclerosis. *Neurology* **53,** 39–48.

Smith, S. S., De Stefano, N., Jenkinson, M., and Matthew, P. M. (2001). Normalized accurate measurement of longitudinal brain change. *J. Comp. Assist. Tomogr.* **25,** 466–75.

Stevenson, V. L., Leary, S. M., Losseff, N. A., et al. (1998). Spinal cord atrophy and disability in MS: a longitudinal study. *Neurology* **51,** 234–238.

Stevenson, V. L., Miller, D. H., Rovaris, M., et al. (1999). Primary and transitional progressive MS: A clinical and MRI cross-sectional study. *Neurology* **52,** 839–845.

Traboulsee, A., Demeshki, J., Griffin, C. M. B., et al. (2001). Normal appearing brain MTR and atrophy in multiple sclerosis. *Multiple Sclerosis* **7 (Suppl 1),** S12.

Trapp, B., Peterson, J., Ransohoff, R. M., et al. (1998). Axonal transection in the lesions of multiple sclerosis. *N. Engl. J. Med.* **338,** 278–285.

Turner, B., Ramli, N., Blumhardt, L. D., Jaspan, T. (2001). Ventricular enlargement in multiple sclerosis: A comparison of three-dimensional and linear MRI estimates. *Neuroradiology* **43,** 608–614.

Udupa, J., Wei, L., Samarasekera, S., Miki, Y., van Buchem, M., and Grossman, R. (1997). Multiple sclerosis lesion quantification using fuzzy connectedness principles. *IEEE Trans. Med. Imaging* **16,** 598–609.

van Walderveen, M. A. A., Kamphorst, W., Scheltens, P., et al. (1998). Histopathologic correlates of hypointense lesions on T1-weighted spin-echo MRI in multiple sclerosis. *Neurology* **50,** 1282–1288.

Werring, D. J., Clark, C. A., Barker, G. J., Thompson, A. J., and Miller, D. H. (1999). Diffusion tensor imaging of lesions and normal-appearing white matter in multiple sclerosis. *Neurology* **52,** 1626–1632.

Wolinsky, J. S., Narayana, P. A., Johnson, K. P., and the Copolymer 1 Multiple Sclerosis Study Group, and the MRI Analysis Center. (2001). United States open-label glatiramer acetate extension trial for relapsing multiple sclerosis. MRI and clinical correlates. *Multiple Sclerosis* **7,** 33–41.

Wolinsky, J. S., Narayana, P. A., Noseworthy, J. H., et al. (2000). Linomide in relapsing and secondary progressive MS, Part II: MRI results. *Neurology* **54,** 1734–1741.

Young, I. R., Hall, A. S., Pallis, C. A., et al. (1981). Nuclear magnetic resonance imaging of the brain in multiple sclerosis. *Lancet* **318,** 1063–1066.

Zivadinov, R., Rudick, R. A., De Masi, R., et al. (2001). Effects of IV methylprednisolone on brain atrophy in relapsing-remitting MS. *Neurology* **57,** 1239–1247.

15

MRI-Clinical Correlations in Multiple Sclerosis: Implications for Our Understanding of Neuronal Changes

Massimo Filippi, M.D.
Maria A. Rocca, M.D.

I. Introduction

Although conventional magnetic resonance imaging (cMRI) is widely used for diagnosing multiple sclerosis (MS) and for monitoring its activity and evolution (Rovaris and Filippi, 1999), the correlation between cMRI and clinical findings of MS is limited (Rovaris and Filippi, 1999; Molyneux et al., 2001). This clinical/MRI discrepancy is likely to be the result of the inability of cMRI to quantify the extent of the irreversible tissue damage and loss which is associated to MS.

Pathological (Lumdsen, 1970; Kidd et al., 1999; Peterson et al., 2001) and neurophysiological (McDonald, 1994) studies have indeed shown that MS is not exclusively a demyelinating disease and that demyelination alone is not sufficient to explain the neurological deficits of MS. There are compelling pieces of evidence that axonal damage, which may be represented either by axonal loss or dysfunction, is one of the main contributors to the clinical manifestations of the disease and to its clinical worsening over time. Pathologically, marked axonal transection in inflamed MS lesions has been demonstrated by several authors (Ferguson et al., 1997; Trapp et al., 1998). Focal damage to an axon may lead to wallerian degeneration of the distal segment separated from the cell body, whereas the proximal axon segment may die because of the lack of connections to other neurons (Coleman and Perry, 2002). Loss of neurons may induce further loss of neurons that have lost their connections by retrograde or anterograde transneuronal degeneration and, as a consequence, may lead to degeneration of axons and neurons in areas distant from the primary site of inflammatory lesions (Evangelou et al., 2000a). In addition, lesions located in the gray matter, which may cause a direct damage to neurons and their processes, have also been described in MS (Lumdsen, 1970; Kidd et al., 1999; Peterson et al., 2001). Although MS cortical lesions are characterized by the paucity of inflammatory changes, they are associated with neuronal injury, including neuritic swelling and dendritic and axonal transections (Peterson et al., 2001).

Several structural and metabolic MR-based techniques with increased specificity to the heterogeneous pathological substrates of MS have the potential to detect such abnormalities or, at least, their gross consequences, and thus to improve our understanding of how MS evolves. Quantification of brain atrophy provides a rather coarse but objective measure of overall tissue loss in MS (Miller et al., 2002). Magnetization transfer (Filippi et al., 1999) and diffusion-weighted (Filippi and Inglese, 2001) MRI can quantify the extent and pathological severity of structural changes occurring within and outside cMRI-visible lesions of MS. Proton MR spectroscopy (Filippi et al., 2001) can add information on the biochemical nature of such changes. Functional MRI (fMRI) (Filippi and Rocca, 2003) can provide new insights into the role of cortical adaptive changes in limiting the clinical consequences of irreversible structural damage resulting from MS.

This chapter summarizes the main results obtained by the application of modern MR technology to the study of MS, with the ultimate goal of highlighting how they are changing our understanding of MS, which is now viewed as a diffuse condition affecting both white and gray matter of the central nervous system (CNS) and which causes irreversible clinical disability mainly through axonal/neuronal damage.

II. Brain Atrophy

The progressive development of brain atrophy is a well-known feature of patients with MS (Miller et al., 2002) (Fig. 1). As a consequence, measurement of brain atrophy is viewed as a potentially useful marker of destructive and irreversible MS tissue damage.

Considering that axons represent a large proportion of white matter, axonal loss is likely to be an important contributor to atrophy in MS. Plaques in MS are not limited to the white matter, but they are also located, diffusely, in the cortical (Lumdsen, 1970; Kidd et al., 1999; Peterson et al., 2001) and deep (Cifelli et al., 2002) gray matter, whose neurons might also be affected by retrograde and trans-synaptic degeneration secondary to white matter damage. Therefore, loss of myelin and axons in these lesions might also contribute to brain atrophy in MS. An additional and compelling *in vivo* evidence that brain atrophy might reflect irreversible axonal loss derives from multiparametric MRI studies (Coles et al., 1999; Sailer et al., 2001) that have demonstrated a strong correlation between measures of brain atrophy and (1) the reduction of the level of N-acetylaspartate (NAA) (Coles et al., 1999), a metabolite that is considered a marker of axonal/neuronal loss/dysfunction (Simmons et al., 1991); and (2) the amount of T_1-hypointense lesions (Sailer et al., 2001), which are characterized pathologically by marked axonal loss (van Walderveen et al., 1998). Nevertheless, it is likely that other pathological substrates, such as myelin loss, astrocytosis and inflammation can influence brain volume measures. Therefore, caution should be taken when considering this metric as a measure of axonal/neuronal damage in MS.

Several cross-sectional and longitudinal MRI studies have investigated the magnitude of the correlation between brain volume decrease and clinical findings in MS. The main results of these studies can be summarized as follows:

1. Brain atrophy can develop in the early, relapsing-remitting (RR) phase of MS (Simon et al., 1999; Ge et al., 2000; Chard et al., 2002a), as well as in patients with

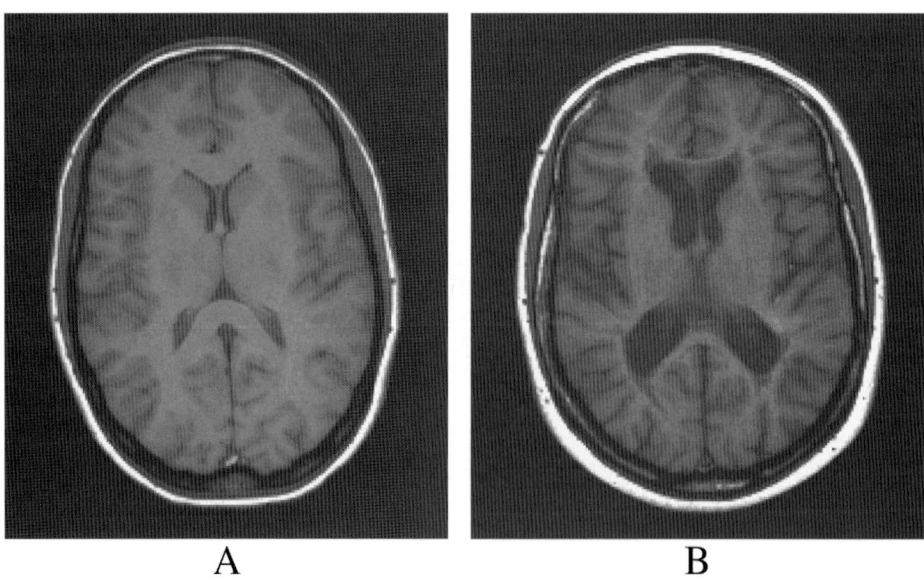

A   B

Figure 1 Axial T_1-weighted magnetic resonance (MR) images of the brain from a normal control (**A**) and from a patient with secondary progressive multiple sclerosis (MS) (**B**). In the patient with MS, an enlargement of the lateral ventricles and of the brain sulci is evident.

clinically isolated syndromes (CIS) suggestive of MS (Dalton et al., 2002; Filippi et al., 2003b)

2. The amount of tissue loss increases with increasing disability and disease duration (Losseff et al., 1996; Stevenson et al., 1999; Kalkers et al., 2001)

3. Brain volume measurements correlate better with clinical disability than other cMRI metrics, particularly in patients with the progressive phenotypes of the disease (Kalkers et al., 2002; Miller et al., 2002)

III. Magnetization Transfer and Diffusion-Weighted MRI

Magnetization transfer (MT) MRI is based on the interactions between protons in a relatively free environment and those where motion is restricted. Off-resonance irradiation is applied, which saturates the magnetization of the less mobile protons, but this is transferred to the mobile protons, thus reducing the signal intensity from the observable magnetization. Thus, a low MT ratio (MTR) indicates a reduced capacity of the macromolecules in the CNS to exchange magnetization with the surrounding water molecules, reflecting damage to myelin or to the axonal membrane (Fig. 2). The most compelling evidence indicating that markedly decreased MTR values correspond to areas where severe and irreversible tissue loss has occurred comes from a postmortem study showing a strong correlation of MTR values from MS lesions and normal-appearing white matter (NAWM) with the percentage of residual axons and the degree of demyelination (van Waesberghe et al., 1999).

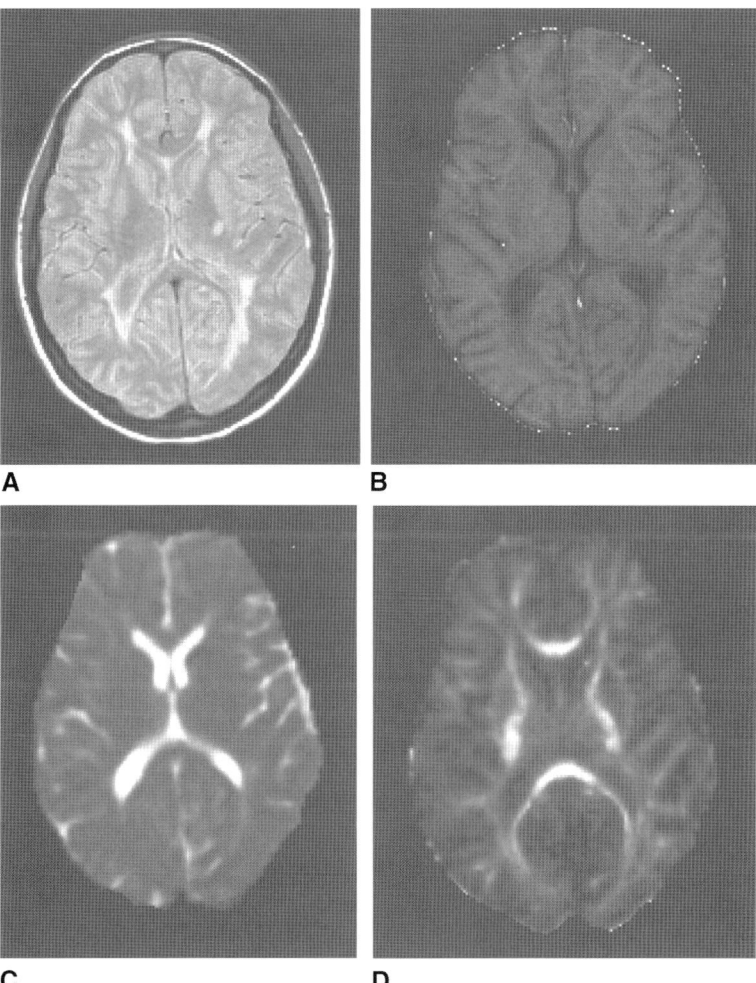

Figure 2 Axial magnetic resonance (MR) images from a patient with multiple sclerosis (MS). The proton–density-weighted scan (**A**) shows multiple lesions. On the magnetization transfer (MT) map (**B**), lesions appear as hypointense areas. The degree of hypointensity is related to decrease in MT ratio and indicates damage to the myelin or to the axonal membranes. On the mean diffusivity (MD) map (**C**), lesions appear as hyperintense areas. The degree of hyperintensity is related to increase in MD and indicates a loss of structural barriers to water molecular motion. On the fractional anisotropy (FA) map (**D**), white matter pixels are bright because of the directionality of the white matter fiber tracts. Dark areas corresponding to macroscopic lesions indicate a loss of FA and suggest the presence of structural disorganization.

Diffusion is the microscopic random translational motion of molecules in a fluid system. Water molecular diffusion can be measured *in vivo* using DW MRI in terms of an apparent diffusion coefficient (Filippi and Inglese, 2001). Although diffusion is inherently a three-dimensional process, in some tissues with an oriented microstructure such as brain white matter (WM), the molecular mobility is not the same in all directions. This property is called anisotropy and results in a variation of the measured diffusivity with tissue measurement direction. White matter fiber tracts consist of aligned myelinated axons; therefore, hindrance of water diffusion is much greater across rather than along the major axis of axonal fibers. Under these conditions, a full characterization of diffusion can be found only in terms of a tensor, a 3×3 matrix, where the on-diagonal elements represent the diffusion coefficients along the axes of the reference frame, and the off-diagonal elements account for the correlations between molecular displacement along orthogonal directions (Basser et al., 1994). From the tensor, it is possible to derive some scalar indices (Filippi and Inglese, 2001). These include the mean diffusivity (MD) (equal to one third of the trace of the diffusion tensor), which is affected by cellular size and integrity, and the fractional anisotropy (FA), which reflects the degree of alignment of cellular structures within fiber tracts, as well as their structural integrity (Fig. 2). Studies on neurodegenerative conditions, such as Alzheimer's disease (Bozzali et al., 2001, 2002b; van der Flier et al., 2002, 2003), have shown increased MD and decreased FA both in the gray matter (as a possible direct consequence of neuronal loss) and in the white matter (as a possible consequence of secondary fiber degeneration) of these patients.

Both MT and DW MRI have substantial advantages over cMRI in the study of MS (Filippi et al., 1999; Filippi and Inglese, 2001). First, they provide quantitative information with increased specificity to the heterogeneous substrates of MS pathology. Second, they enable us to quantify the diffuse damage occurring in brain tissues that appear normal on cMRI. Third, with the application of histogram analysis, they can provide multiple parameters influenced by both the cMRI-visible and cMRI-"occult" lesion burdens.

On average, in new enhancing MS lesions (Filippi et al., 1999; Filippi and Inglese, 2001), the MTR drops and the MD increases dramatically when the lesions start to enhance and can show a complete or partial recovery in the subsequent 1 to 6 months (van Waesberghe et al., 1998). These relatively rapid modifications of MTR and MD suggest demyelination and remyelination as the most likely pathological substrate of such short-term changes. In chronic lesions, MT and DW MRI studies have shown variable degrees of MTR and FA reduction and MD increase in T_2-visible lesions (Filippi et al., 1999; Filippi and Inglese, 2001). These abnormalities are more pronounced in lesions that appear hypointense on T_1-weighted images and in

patients with the most disabling courses of the disease (Filippi et al., 1999; Filippi and Inglese, 2001), thus suggesting axonal loss as one of the main possible pathological substrates of intrinsic lesion changes measured using MT and DW MRI. The variability of MTR, MD, and FA values seen in MS lesions also suggests that different proportions of lesions with different degrees of structural changes might contribute to the evolution of the disease. This concept is supported by a 3-year follow-up study (Rocca et al., 1999) showing that newly formed lesions from secondary progressive (SP)-MS patients have more severe MTR deterioration than those from patients with mildly-disabling RR-MS.

Postmortem studies have shown subtle changes in the NAWM from patients with MS, which include diffuse astrocytic hyperplasia, patchy edema, and perivascular cellular infiltration, as well as axonal damage (Allen and McKeown, 1979; Evangelou et al., 2000b; Bjartmar et al., 2001). Consistent with this finding, reduced MTR and FA values and increased MD values have been found in the NAWM of patients with MS independent of their disease phenotypes (Filippi et al., 1999, 2003a; Filippi and Inglese, 2001). Although all these processes might reduce FA and MTR, myelin and axonal loss should be responsible for the increased MD. Permanent and marked MTR reductions might also correspond to axonal loss as shown by a recent study of the optic nerves of MS patients (Inglese et al., 2002). In this study, very low MTR values were seen in patients with a previous episode of acute optic neuritis (ON) followed by poor clinical recovery. Similar MTR values were also measured from the optic nerve of patients with Leber's hereditary optic neuropathy (Inglese et al., 2002).

The severity of MR-measured NAWM damage has been shown to be associated with increased levels of physical disability and cognitive impairment and to evolve at different rates in the different patient groups, being more pronounced in patients with the progressive forms of the disease (Filippi and Inglese, 2001; Filippi et al., 1999, 2000, 2003a). In patients at presentation with CIS, the extent of normal-appearing brain tissue changes has been found to be an independent predictor of subsequent evolution to clinically definite MS (Iannucci et al., 2000). NAWM-MTR reduction has also been shown to predict the accumulation of clinical disability over the subsequent 5 years in patients with definite MS (Rovaris et al., 2003).

Consistent with postmortem studies (Lumdsen, 1970; Kidd et al., 1999; Peterson et al., 2001; Cifelli et al., 2002), recent studies have shown reduced MTR and increased MD values of the gray matter from patients with MS (Cercignani et al., 2001; Ge et al., 2001; Bozzali et al., 2002a). In patients with RR-MS, these changes worsen over time (Oreja-Guevara et al., 2003) and, as a consequence, they have been found to be more pronounced in patients with the most disabling and progressive disease phenotypes (Bozzali et al., 2002; Ge et al., 2002a). This suggests a progressive accumulation of gray matter damage already in the RR phase of the disease, which was previously unrecognized and which might be one of the factors responsible for the development of brain atrophy (Miller et al., 2002) and for some of the clinical manifestations of the disease, such as neuropsychological impairment (Rao et al., 1989). Recent studies have indeed found a correlation between the severity of cognitive impairment and the degree of MTR (Rovaris et al., 2000) and MD (Rovaris et al., 2002) changes in the gray matter of patients with MS. All of this fits with the notion that gray matter pathology might be an additional factor contributing to the worsening of clinical disability in patients with progressive MS, as a possible consequence of neuronal/axonal damage.

IV. Proton Magnetic Resonance Spectroscopy

Water-suppressed, proton MR spectra of normal human brain at long echo times reveal four major resonances: one at 3.2 ppm from tetramethylamines (mainly from choline-containing phospholipids [Cho]), one at 3.0 ppm from creatine and phosphocreatine (Cr), one at 2.0 ppm from *N*-acetyl groups (mainly NAA), and one at 1.3 ppm from the methyl resonance of lactate (Lac). NAA is a marker of axonal integrity; Cho and Lac are considered as chemical correlates of acute inflammatory/demyelinating changes (Filippi et al., 2001). ^{1}H-MRS studies with shorter echo times can detect additional metabolites, such as lipids and myoinositol (mI), which are also regarded as markers of ongoing myelin damage.

^{1}H-MRS of acute MS lesions reveals increases of metabolites such as Cho and Lac (De Stefano et al., 1995a; Filippi et al., 2001), which reflect the releasing of membrane phospholipids and the metabolism of inflammatory cells, respectively. Short echo time spectra can detect transient increases in visible lipids released during myelin breakdown and mI (Narayana et al., 1998). All these changes are usually followed by a decrease in NAA. Since, NAA is a metabolite detected almost exclusively in neurons and their processes in the normal adult brain, a decrease in NAA is considered to be secondary to neuronal/axonal dysfunction. After the acute phase and over a period of days to weeks, there is a progressive reduction of raised Lac resonance intensities to normal levels. Resonance intensities of Cr also return to normal within a few days. Cho, lipid, and mI resonance intensities return to normal over months. The signal intensity of NAA may remain decreased or show partial recovery, starting soon after the acute phase and lasting for several months (Arnold et al., 1992; De Stefano et al., 1995a). These reversible decreases in NAA are strongly correlated with reversal of functional impairment (De Stefano et al., 1995a). Recovery of NAA may be related to resolution of edema,

increases in the diameter of previously shrunken axons secondary to remyelination and clearance of inflammatory factors, and reversible metabolic changes in neurons. In line with the notion that NAA reduction reflects irreversible axonal loss, NAA concentration has been found to be lower in severely T_1-hypointense MS lesions than in T_1-isointense or hypointense lesions (van Walderveen et al., 1999) and in chronic lesions from patients with SP-MS than in those from patients with benign MS (Falini et al., 1998).

The application of ^{1}H-MRS imaging (MRSI) (De Stefano et al., 1998; Narayana et al., 1998) has enabled spectra from large volumes of interest to be obtained and has improved our ability to interrogate brain NAWM pathology separately. This has led to the demonstration that decreases in NAA are not restricted to MS lesions, but also occur in the NAWM adjacent to or distant from them (Sarchielli et al., 1999; De Stefano et al., 1999, 2002). Although NAA reduction might also reflect transient sublethal axonal injury (Davie et al., 1994; De Stefano et al., 1999), NAA levels of the NAWM tend to decline over time (Fu et al., 1998). Consistent with this finding is the demonstration that NAA reduction is more pronounced in the NAWM of patients with SP-MS and primary progressive (PP)-MS than in those with a RR course (Fu et al., 1998, Suhy et al., 2000). Nevertheless, reduced NAWM-NAA can also be detected in patients with MS in the early phase of the disease (De Stefano et al., 2001; Filippi et al., 2003b) and in patients with very short disease durations and low T_2-visible disease burdens (De Stefano et al., 2002).

Metabolite changes, including decrease of NAA and increase of Cho and mI, have also been shown in the cortical gray matter of patients with MS (Kapeller et al., 2001; Sharma et al., 2001; Chard et al., 2002b; Sarchielli et al., 2002). These abnormalities are more pronounced in patients with SP-MS than in those with RR-MS (Adalsteinsson et al., 2003). More recently, NAA reductions associated with a considerable amount of tissue loss have also been demonstrated in the thalamus of SP-MS (Cifelli et al., 2002) and RR-MS patients (Wylezinska et al., 2003).

De Stefano and co-workers (1998) found a decrease of NAA/Cr ratio with increasing disability, whereas such a correlation was not found with the amount of T_2-visible lesions. Of interest, the relationship between disability and changes of NAA levels has been found to be stronger in patients with RR-MS than in those with SP-MS (Fu et al., 1998), where brain atrophy development progresses at a more rapid pace (De Stefano et al., 2001). These observations have been confirmed by a postmortem study (Bjartmar et al., 2000) where a strong correlation between neurological impairment and both axonal density and NAA reduction in the spinal cord of patients with MS has been found.

NAA levels have also been quantified in specific brain regions, whose damage has been related to the impairment of the corresponding functional systems. Davie et al. (1995)

showed a significant reduction of NAA concentration in the cerebellar white matter of patients with MS and severe ataxia compared with those having little or no cerebellar deficits. Lee et al. (2000a) demonstrated an association between reduction of NAA in the internal capsule and selective motor impairment. Pan et al. (2001) found a relation between cognitive function and NAA levels in the periventricular white matter. More recently, Gadea et al. (2003) found a relationship between attentional dysfunction in early RR-MS patients and NAA/Cr values in the locus coeruleus nuclei of the pontine ascending reticular activation system.

V. Functional MRI

Although the resolution of acute inflammation, remyelination, redistribution of voltage-gated sodium-channels in persistently demyelinated axons, and recovery from sublethal axonal injury are all factors likely to limit the clinical impact of damaging MS pathology (Waxman and Ritchie, 1993; De Stefano et al., 1995b), other mechanisms have been recently recognized as potential contributors to the recovery or to the maintenance of function in the presence of irreversible MS-related axonal damage. Brain plasticity is a well-known feature of the human brain that is likely to have several pathological substrates, including an increased axonal expression of sodium channels (Waxman, 1998), synaptic changes, increased recruitment of parallel existing pathways or "latent" connections, and reorganization of distant sites. All these changes might have a major adaptive role in limiting the functional consequences of axonal loss. The signal changes seen during fMRI studies depend on the blood oxygenation level-dependent mechanism, which in turn involves changes of the transverse magnetization relaxation time—either T_2^* in a gradient echo sequence, or T_2 in spin echo sequence. These changes are attributable to differences in deoxyhemoglobin subsequent to variations of neuronal activity (Ogawa et al., 1993). The application of fMRI to the study of the motor, visual, and cognitive systems in patients with MS has provided new insights into the mechanisms contributing to the progressive clinical worsening of these patients.

Functional cortical changes have been demonstrated in all MS phenotypes, using different fMRI paradigms. A study of the visual system (Werring et al., 2000) in patients who had recovered from a single episode of acute optic neuritis demonstrated that such patients had an extensive activation of the visual network (including the claustrum, lateral temporal, and posterior parietal cortices and thalamus in addition to the primary visual cortex) compared to healthy volunteers. An altered brain pattern of movement-associated cortical activations, characterized by an increased recruitment of the contralateral primary sensorimotor cortex during the performance of simple tasks (Rocca et al., 2003a;

Filippi et al. , 2004a) (Fig. 3) and by the recruitment of additional "classical" and "higher-order" sensorimotor areas during the performance of more complex tasks (Filippi et al., 2004a), has been demonstrated in patients with CIS. An increased recruitment of several sensorimotor areas, mainly located in the cerebral hemisphere ipsilateral to the limb which performed the task has also been demonstrated in patients with early MS and a previous episode of hemiparesis (Pantano et al., 2002a). Interestingly, in patients with similar characteristics, but who presented with an optic neuritis, this increased recruitment involved sensorimotor areas which were mainly located in the contralateral cerebral hemisphere (Pantano et al., 2002b). In patients with established MS and an RR course, functional cortical changes have been shown during the performance of visual (Rombouts et al., 1998), motor (Lee et al., 2000b; Reddy et al., 2000a, 2000b; Filippi et al., 2002a; Rocca et al., 2002a), and cognitive (Staffen et al., 2002; Hillary et al., 2003; Parry et al., 2003) tasks. Movement-associated cortical changes, characterized by the activation of highly specialized cortical areas, have also been described in patients with SP-MS (Rocca et al., 2003b) during the performance of a simple motor task (Fig. 4). Two fMRI studies of the motor system (Filippi et al., 2002b; Rocca et al., 2002b) of patients with PP-MS suggested a lack of "classical" adaptive mechanisms as a potential additional factor contributing to the accumulation of disability in this unusual phenotype of the disease.

The results of all these studies suggest that there might be a "natural history" of the functional reorganization of the cerebral cortex in MS patients, which might be characterized, at the beginning of the disease, by an increased recruitment of those areas "normally" devoted to the performance of a given task, such as the primary sensorimotor cortex and the supplementary motor area in case of a motor task. At a later stage, bilateral activation of these regions is first seen, followed by a widespread recruitment of additional areas, which are usually recruited in normal people to perform novel/complex tasks. This notion has been supported by the results of a study (Filippi et al., 2004b) that has provided a direct demonstration that, during the performance of a simple motor task, patients with MS activate some regions that are part of a frontoparietal circuit, whose activation occurs typically in healthy subjects during object manipulation (Filippi et al., 2004b).

Such functional cortical changes are likely to be adaptive (or maladaptive) phenomena more than to be a mere reflection of a different task performance between patients and controls. If performance factor was, in fact, not controlled in preliminary fMRI studies (Lee et al., 2000b; Reddy et al., 2000a, 2000b), more recent studies have taken into account this confounder either by studying patients with no overt clinical involvement of the investigated system (Filippi et al., 2002a, 2002b; Rocca et al., 2002a, 2003a, 2003b, 2003c) or by assessing the performance of passive tasks

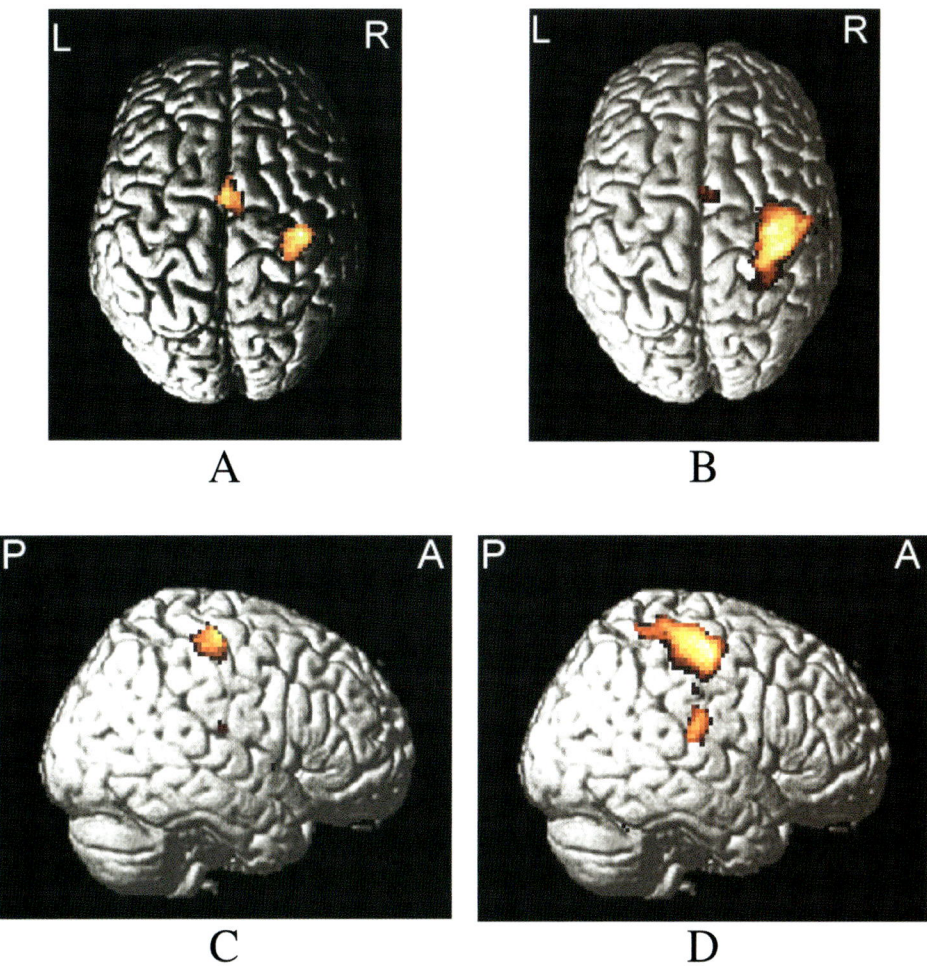

Figure 3 Brain patterns of cortical activations on a rendered brain in right-handed healthy subjects (**A** and **C**) and patients at presentation with clinically isolated syndromes suggestive (CIS) of multiple sclerosis (**B** and **D**) during the performance of a simple motor task with their clinically-unimpaired and fully normal functioning upper left hands. In patients with CIS, an increased activation of the right primary sensorimotor cortex is visible (**B** and **D**).

(Reddy et al., 2002). The following are the main findings supporting the adaptive role of functional cortical changes in MS:

1. The activity of some cortical areas may be influenced by the extent and the severity of T_2-visible lesion damage. Several studies have found a strong correlation between the increased cortical activation of several areas with increasing T_2-lesion load in patients with relapsing MS (Lee et al. , 2000b; Pantano et al., 2002b; Rocca et al., 2002a, 2002b), as well as in those with SP-MS (Rocca et al., 2003b) (Fig. 4) and PP-MS (Rocca et al., 2002b). Some studies also found increased sensorimotor cortex recruitment with increasing lesion damage of the corticospinal tracts, measured on T_1-weighted images (Pantano et al., 2002b), or with whole brain intrinsic lesion damage, measured on MTR and MD maps (Rocca et al., 2002a).

2. The severity of normal-appearing brain tissue damage, measured using MRS (Reddy et al., 2000a; Rocca et al., 2003a), MT MRI, or DW MRI (Filippi et al., 2002b; Rocca et al. , 2002a, 2003b), is another important factor that modulates movement-associated cortical reorganization, as shown by studies of patients with various disease phenotypes and different levels of disability (Reddy et al., 2000a), patients at presentation with CIS suggestive of MS (Rocca et al., 2003a), patients with RR-MS and no clinical disability (Rocca et al., 2002a), and patients with PP-MS and SP-MS with different degrees of clinical involvement (Filippi et al., 2002b; Rocca et al., 2003b).

3. Subtle gray matter damage, not detected when using cMRI, may play a role in modulating cortical excitability, as demonstrated in patients with SP-MS (Rocca et al., 2003b) and in patients with clinically definite MS and

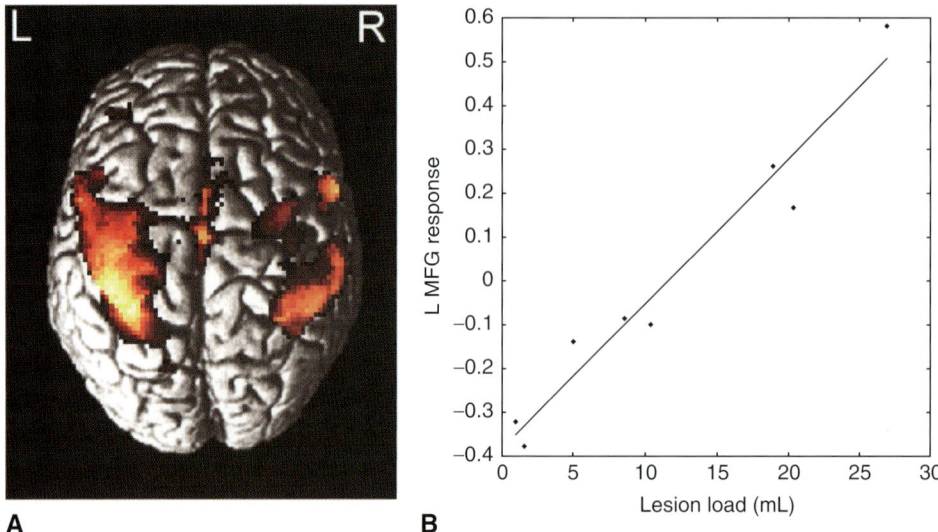

Figure 4 Brain patterns of cortical activations on an axial rendered brain (**A**) from right-handed patients with secondary progressive multiple sclerosis (MS) during the performance of a simple motor task with their clinically unimpaired and fully normal functioning upper right hands. The activity of the contralateral middle frontal gyrus (MFG) was significantly correlated (r = 0.87, *P* < 0.001) with brain dual-echo lesion load (**B**).

nonspecific (less than three lesions) cMRI findings (Rocca et al., 2003c).

4. The demonstration of strong correlations between cortical activations and cervical cord damage, quantified using MT MRI, in patients with PP-MS (Rocca et al., 2002b), patients with a previous episode of acute myelitis of probable demyelinating origin (Rocca et al., 2003d) (Fig. 5), and patients with Devic's neuromyelitis optica (Rocca et al. , 2004) suggests that not only brain, but also spinal cord pathology can induce cortical changes with the potential to limit the functional impact of the disease.

Although the actual role of cortical reorganization on the clinical manifestations of MS remains unclear, the demonstration that patients with MS may have a normal level of performance despite the presence of diffuse tissue damage suggests that cortical adaptive changes are likely to contribute in limiting the clinical consequences of MS-related structural damage (Filippi and Rocca, 2003). The most compelling evidence that cortical reorganization may have a role in recovery from axonal damage derives from the study by Reddy et al. (2000b), who, with serial MRS and fMRI examinations, evaluated a patient after the onset of an acute

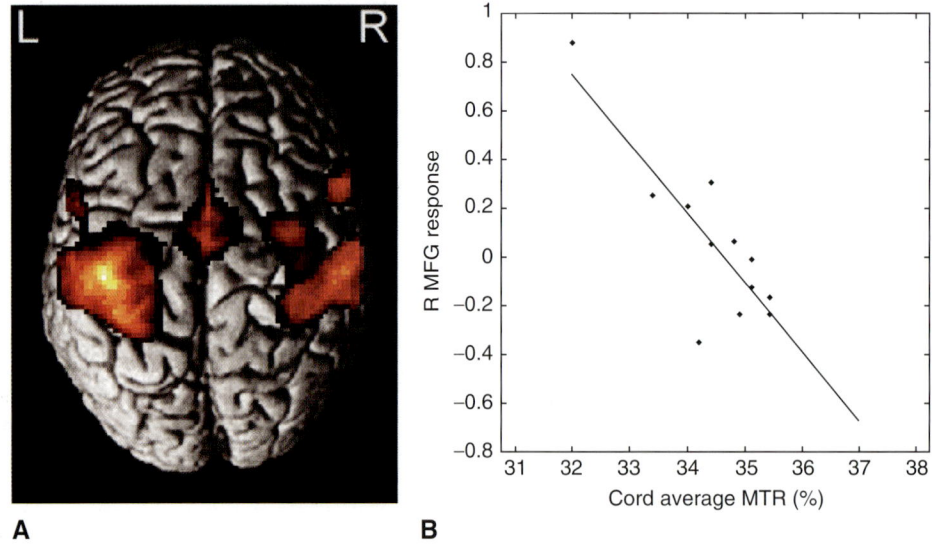

Figure 5 Brain patterns of cortical activations on an axial rendered brain (**A**) from right-handed patients with a previous isolated acute myelitis during the performance of a simple motor task with their clinically unimpaired and fully normal functioning upper right hands. The activity of the ipsilateral middle frontal gyrus (MFG) was significantly correlated (r = –0.80, *P* < 0.001) with average cervical cord magnetization transfer ratio (MTR) (**B**).

hemiparesis and a new, large demyelinating lesion located in the corticospinal tract. In this patient, clinical recovery preceded complete normalization of NAA and was accompanied by increased recruitment of ipsilateral primary sensorimotor cortex and supplementary motor area. In line with these findings, in a group of patients who complained of fatigue when compared to matched nonfatigued patients with MS, there was a reduced activation of a complex movement-associated cortical/subcortical network, including the cerebellum, the rolandic operculum, the thalamus, and the middle frontal gyrus (Filippi et al., 2002a). In these patients, a strong correlation between the reduction of thalamic activity and the clinical severity of fatigue was found, indicating that a less marked cortical recruitment might be associated with the appearance of clinical symptomatology in MS.

VI. Conclusion

Axonal/neuronal loss is an important feature of MS pathology, and it is likely to represent one of the main factors responsible for the accumulation of irreversible disability. The application of modern MR techniques to the *in vivo* study of MS is providing important insights into the pathophysiology of the disease, and it is establishing new markers to understand and monitor MS evolution. None of the quantitative MR-based techniques taken in isolation is likely to be able to provide a complete picture of the complexity of the MS process, and this should call for the definition of aggregates of MR measurements thought to reflect different aspects of MS pathology. This approach is likely to enhance our ability to monitor the disease and to improve the correlation between MRI metrics and disability.

References

Adalsteinsson, E., Langer-Gould, A., Homer, R. J., et al. (2003). Gray matter *N*-Acetyl aspartate deficits in secondary progressive but not relapsing-remitting multiple sclerosis. *AJNR Am J Neuroradiol* **24**, 1941–1945.

Allen, I. V., and McKeown, S. R. (1979). A histological, histochemical and biochemical study of the macroscopically normal white matter in multiple sclerosis. *J. Neurol. Sci.* **41**, 81–91.

Arnold, D. L., Matthews, P. M., Francis, G. S., O'Connor, J., and Antel, J. P. (1992). Proton magnetic resonance spectroscopic imaging for metabolic characterization of demyelinating plaques. *Ann. Neurol.* **31**, 235–241.

Basser, P. J., Mattiello, J., and Le Bihan, D. (1994). Estimation of the effective self-diffusion tensor from the NMR spin-echo. *J. Magn. Reson. B* **103**, 247–254.

Bjartmar, C., Kidd, G., Mork, S., Rudick, R., and Trapp, B. D. (2000). Neurological disability correlates with spinal cord axonal loss and reduced N-acetyl aspartate in chronic multiple sclerosis patients. *Ann. Neurol.* **48**, 893–901.

Bjartmar, C., Kinkel, R. P., Kidd, G., Rudick, R. A., and Trapp, B. D. (2001). Axonal loss in normal-appearing white matter in a patient with acute MS. *Neurology* **57**, 1248–1252.

Bozzali, M., Franceschi, M., Falini, A., et al. (2001). Quantification of tissue damage in AD using diffusion tensor and magnetization transfer MRI. *Neurology* **57**, 1135–1137.

Bozzali, M., Cercignani, M., Sormani, M. P., Comi, G., Filippi, M. (2002a). Quantification of brain gray matter damage in different MS phenotypes by use of diffusion tensor MR imaging. *AJNR Am. J. Neuroradiol.* **23**, 985–988.

Bozzali, M., Falini, A., Franceschi, M., et al. (2002b). White matter damage in Alzheimer's disease assessed in vivo using diffusion tensor magnetic resonance imaging. *J. Neurol. Neurosurg. Psychiatry* **72**, 742–746.

Cercignani, M., Bozzali, M., Iannucci, G., Comi, G., and Filippi, M. (2001). Magnetisation transfer ratio and mean diffusivity of normal-appearing white and gray matter from patients with multiple sclerosis. *J. Neurol. Neurosurg. Psychiatry* **70**, 311–317.

Chard, D. T., Griffin, C. M., Parker, G. J., et al. (2002a). Brain atrophy in clinically early relapsing-remitting multiple sclerosis. *Brain* **125**, 327–337.

Chard, D. T., Griffin, C. M., McLean, M. A., et al. (2002b). Brain metabolite changes in cortical grey and normal-appearing white matter in clinically early relapsing-remitting multiple sclerosis. *Brain* **125**, 2342–2352.

Cifelli, A., Arridge, M., Jezzard, P., Esiri, M. M., Palace, J., and Matthews, P. M. (2002). Thalamic neurodegeneration in multiple sclerosis. *Ann. Neurol.* **52**, 650–653.

Coleman, M. P., and Perry, V. H. (2002). Axon pathology in neurological disease: A neglected therapeutic target. Review. *Trends Neurosci.* **25**, 532–537.

Coles, A. J., Wing, M. G., Molyneux, P., et al. (1999). Monoclonal antibody treatment exposes three mechanisms underlying the clinical course of multiple sclerosis. *Ann. Neurol.* **46**, 296–304.

Dalton, C. M., Brex, P. A., Jenkins, R., et al. (2002). Progressive ventricular enlargement in patients with clinically isolated syndromes is associated with the early development of multiple sclerosis. *J. Neurol. Neurosurg. Psychiatry* **73**, 141–147.

Davie, C. A., Hawkins, C. P., Barker, G. J., et al. (1994). Serial proton magnetic resonance spectroscopy in acute multiple sclerosis lesions. *Brain* **117**, 49–58.

Davie, C. A., Barker, G. J., Webb, S., et al. (1995). Persistent functional deficit in multiple sclerosis and autosomal dominant cerebellar ataxia is associated with axon loss. *Brain* **118**, 1583–1592.

De Stefano, N., Matthews, P. M., Antel, J. P., Preul, M., Francis, G., and Arnold, D. L. (1995a). Chemical pathology of acute demyelinating lesions and its correlation with disability. *Ann. Neurol.* **38**, 901–909.

De Stefano, N., Matthews, P. M., and Arnold, D. L. (1995b). Reversible decreases in *N*-acetylaspartate after acute brain injury. *Magn. Reson. Med.* **34**, 721–727.

De Stefano, N., Matthews, P. M., Fu, L., et al. (1998). Axonal damage correlates with disability in patients with relapsing-remitting multiple sclerosis. Results of a longitudinal magnetic resonance spectroscopy study. *Brain* **121**, 1469–1477.

De Stefano, N., Narayanan, S., Matthews, P. M., Francis, G. S., Antel, J. P., and Arnold, D. L. (1999). In vivo evidence for axonal dysfunction remote from focal cerebral demyelination of the type seen in multiple sclerosis. *Brain* **122**, 1933–1939.

De Stefano, N., Narayanan, S., Francis, G. S., et al. (2001). Evidence of axonal damage in the early stages of multiple sclerosis and its relevance to disability. *Arch. Neurol.* **58**, 65–70.

De Stefano, N., Narayanan, S., Francis, S. J., et al. (2002). Diffuse axonal and tissue injury in patients with multiple sclerosis with low cerebral lesion load and no disability. *Arch. Neurol.* **59**, 1565–1571.

Evangelou, N., Konz, D., Esiri, M. M., Smith, S., Palace, J., and Matthews, P. M. (2000a). Regional axonal loss in the corpus callosum correlates with cerebral white matter lesion volume and distribution in multiple sclerosis. *Brain* **123**, 1845–1849.

Evangelou, N., Esiri, M. M., Smith, S., Palace, J., and Matthews, P. M. (2000b). Quantitative pathological evidence for axonal loss in normal appearing white matter in multiple sclerosis. *Ann. Neurol.* **47**, 391–395.

Falini, A., Calabrese, G., Filippi, M., et al. (1998). Benign versus secondary progressive multiple sclerosis: The potential role of ¹H MR spectroscopy in defining the nature of disability. *AJNR Am. J. Neuroradiol.* **19**, 223–229.

Ferguson, B., Matyszak, M. K., Esiri, M. M., and Perry, V. H. (1997). Axonal damage in acute multiple sclerosis lesions. *Brain* **120**, 393–399.

Filippi, M., and Inglese, M. (2001). Overview of diffusion-weighted magnetic resonance studies in multiple sclerosis. *J. Neurol. Sci.* **186 (Suppl. 1),** S37–S43.

Filippi, M., and Rocca, M. A. (2003). Disturbed function and plasticity in multiple sclerosis as gleaned from functional magnetic resonance imaging. Review. *Curr. Opin. Neurol.* **16**, 275–282.

Filippi, M., Grossman, R. I., and Comi, G. (Eds). (1999). Magnetization transfer in multiple sclerosis. *Neurology* **53 ([Suppl 3])**.

Filippi, M., Arnold, D. L., Comi, G. (Eds.). (2001). Magnetic Resonance Spectroscopy in Multiple Sclerosis. Springer-Verlag, Milan.

Filippi, M., Tortorella, C., Rovaris, M., et al. (2000). Changes in the normal appearing brain tissue and cognitive impairment in multiple sclerosis. *J. Neurol. Neurosurg. Psychiatry* **68**, 157–161.

Filippi, M., Rocca, M. A., Colombo, B., et al. (2002a). Functional magnetic resonance imaging correlates of fatigue in multiple sclerosis. *NeuroImage* **15**, 559–567.

Filippi, M., Rocca, M. A., Falini, A., et al. (2002b). Correlations between structural CNS damage and functional MRI changes in primary progressive MS. *NeuroImage* **15**, 537–546.

Filippi, M., Rocca, M. A., and Comi, G. (2003a). The use of quantitative magnetic-resonance-based techniques to monitor the evolution of multiple sclerosis. *Lancet Neurol* **2**, 337–346.

Filippi, M., Bozzali, M., Rovaris, M., et al. (2003b). Evidence for widespread axonal damage at the earliest clinical stage of multiple sclerosis. *Brain* **126**, 433–437.

Filippi, M., Rocca, M. A., Mezzapesa, D. M., et al. (2004a). Simple and complex movement-associated functional MRI changes in patients at presentation with clinically isolated syndromes suggestive of MS. *Human Brain Mapping* **21**, 108–117.

Filippi, M., Rocca, M. A., Mezzapesa, D. M., et al. (2004b). A functional MRI study of cortical activations associated with object manipulation in patients with MS. *NeuroImage* **21**, 1147–1154.

Fu, L., Matthews, P. M., De Stefano, N., et al. (1998). Imaging axonal damage of normal-appearing white matter in multiple sclerosis. *Brain* **121**, 103–113.

Gadea, M., Martinez-Bisbal, M. C., Marti-Bonmati, L., et al. (2003). Spectroscopic axonal damage of the right locus coeruleus relates to selective attention impairment in early stage relapsing-remitting multiple sclerosis. *Brain* [published online 2003 Sep 23].

Ge, Y., Grossman, R. I., Udupa, J. K., et al. (2000). Brain atrophy in relapsing-remitting multiple sclerosis and secondary progressive multiple sclerosis: Longitudinal quantitative analysis. *Radiology* **214**, 665–670.

Ge, Y., Grossman, R. I., Udupa, J. K., Babb, J. S., Kolson, D. L., and McGowan, J. C. (2001). Magnetization transfer ratio histogram analysis of gray matter in relapsing-remitting multiple sclerosis. *AJNR Am. J. Neuroradiol.* **22**, 470–475.

Ge, Y., Grossman, R. I., Udupa, J. K., Babb, J. S., Mannon, L. J., and McGowan, J. C. (2002). Magnetization transfer ratio histogram analysis of normal-appearing gray matter and normal-appearing white matter in multiple sclerosis. *J. Comput. Assist. Tomogr.* **26**, 62–68.

Hillary, F. G., Chiaravalloti, N. D., Ricker, J. H., et al. (2003). An investigation of working memory rehearsal in multiple sclerosis using fMRI. *J. Clin. Exp. Neuropsychol.* **25**, 965–978.

Iannucci, G., Tortorella, C., Rovaris, M., Sormani, M. P., Comi, G., and Filippi, M. (2000). Prognostic value of MR and magnetization transfer imaging findings in patients with clinically isolated syndromes suggestive of multiple sclerosis at presentation. *AJNR Am. J. Neuroradiol.* **21**, 1034–1038.

Inglese, M., Ghezzi, A., Bianchi, S., et al. (2002). Irreversible disability and tissue loss in multiple sclerosis: A conventional and magnetization transfer magnetic resonance imaging study of the optic nerves. *Arch. Neurol.* **59**, 250–255.

Kalkers, N. F., Bergers, E., Casteljins, J. A., et al. (2001). Optimizing the association between disability and biological markers in MS. *Neurology* **57**, 1253–1258.

Kapeller, P., McLean, M. A., Griffin, C. M., et al. (2001). Preliminary evidence for neuronal damage in cortical grey matter and normal appearing white matter in short duration relapsing-remitting multiple sclerosis: a quantitative MR spectroscopic imaging study. *J. Neurol.* **248**, 131–138.

Kidd, D., Barkhof, F., McConnell, R., Algra, P. R., Allen, I. V., and Revesz, T. (1999). Cortical lesions in multiple sclerosis. *Brain* **122**, 17–26.

Lee, M. A., Blamire, A. M., Pendlebury, S., et al. (2000a). Axonal injury or loss in the internal capsule and motor impairment in multiple sclerosis. *Arch. Neurol.* **57**, 65–70.

Lee, M., Reddy, H., Johansen-Berg, H., et al. (2000b). The motor cortex shows adaptive functional changes to brain injury from multiple sclerosis. *Ann. Neurol.* **47**, 606–613.

Losseff, N. A., Wang, L., Lai, H. M., et al. (1996). Progressive cerebral atrophy in multiple sclerosis: A serial MRI study. *Brain* **119**, 2009–2019.

Lumdsen, C. E. (1970). The neuropathology of multiple sclerosis. *In*: "Handbook of Clinical Neurology" (P J. Vinken and G W. Bruyn, Eds), Vol. 9, pp. 217–309. North-Holland, Amsterdam.

McDonald, W. I. (1994). Rachelle Fishman-Matthew Moore Lecture. The pathological and clinical dynamics of multiple sclerosis. Review. *J. Neuropathol. Exp. Neurol.* **53**, 338–343.

Miller, D. H., Barkhof, F., Frank, J. A., Parker, G. J., and Thompson, A. J. (2002). Measurement of atrophy in multiple sclerosis: pathological basis, methodological aspects and clinical relevance. Review. *Brain* **125**, 1676–1695.

Molyneux, P. D., Barker, G. J., Barkhof, F., et al. (2001). Clinical-MRI correlations in a European trial of interferon beta-1b in secondary progressive MS. *Neurology* **57**, 2191–2197.

Narayana, P. A., Doyle, T. J., Lai, D., and Wolinsky, J. S. (1998). Serial proton magnetic resonance spectroscopic imaging, contrast-enhanced magnetic resonance imaging, and quantitative lesion volumetry in multiple sclerosis. *Ann. Neurol.* **43**, 56–71.

Ogawa, S., Menon, R. S., Tank, D. W., et al. (1993). Functional brain mapping by blood oxygenation level-dependent contrast magnetic resonance imaging. A comparison of signal characteristics with a biophysical model. *Biophys. J.* **64**, 803–812.

Oreja-Guevara, C., Rovaris, M., Caputo, D., et al. (2003). Changes in cortical gray matter in untreated relapsing-remitting MS patients: A follow up study. *Neurology* **60 (Suppl 1)**, A297

Pan, J. W., Krupp, L. B., Elkins, L. E., and Coyle, P. K. (2001). Cognitive dysfunction lateralizes with NAA in multiple sclerosis. *Appl. Neuropsychol.* **8**, 155–160.

Pantano, P., Iannetti, G. D., Caramia, F., et al. (2002a). Cortical motor reorganization after a single clinical attack of multiple sclerosis *Brain* **125**, 1607–1615.

Pantano, P., Mainero, C., Iannetti, G. D., et al. (2002b). Contribution of corticospinal tract damage to cortical motor reorganization after a single clinical attack of multiple sclerosis. *NeuroImage* **17**, 1837–1843.

Parry, A. M., Scott, R. B., Palace, J., Smith, S., and Matthews, P. M. (2003). Potentially adaptive functional changes in cognitive processing for patients with multiple sclerosis and their acute modulation by rivastigmine. *Brain* **126**, 2750–2760.

Peterson, J. W., Bo, L., Mork, S., Chang, A., and Trapp, B. D. (2001). Transected neurites, apoptotic neurons, and reduced inflammation in cortical multiple sclerosis lesions. *Ann. Neurol.* **50**, 389–400.

Rao, S. M., Leo, G. J., Haughton, V. M., St. Aubin-Faubert, P., and Bernardin, L. (1989). Correlation of magnetic resonance imaging with neuropsychological testing in multiple sclerosis. *Neurology* **39**, 161–166.

Reddy, H., Narayanan, S., Arnoutelis, R., et al. (2000a). Evidence for adaptive functional changes in the cerebral cortex with axonal injury from multiple sclerosis. *Brain* **123**, 2314–2320.

Reddy, H., Narayanan, S., Matthews, P. M., et al. (2000b). Relating axonal injury to functional recovery in MS. *Neurology* **54**, 236–239.

Reddy, H., Narayanan, S., Woolrich, M., et al. (2002). Functional brain reorganization for hand movement in patients with multiple sclerosis: defining distinct effects of injury and disability. *Brain* **125**, 2646–2657.

Rocca, M. A., Mastronardo, G., Rodegher, M., Comi, G., and Filippi, M. (1999). Long-term changes of magnetization transfer-derived measures from patients with relapsing-remitting and secondary progressive multiple sclerosis. *AJNR Am. J. Neuroradiol.* **20**, 821–827.

Rocca, M. A., Falini, A., Colombo, B., Scotti, G., Comi, G., and Filippi, M. (2002a). Adaptive functional changes in the cerebral cortex of patients with non-disabling MS correlate with the extent of brain structural damage. *Ann. Neurol.* **51**, 330–339.

Rocca, M. A., Matthews, P. M., Caputo, D., et al. (2002b). Evidence for widespread movement-associated functional MRI changes in patients with PPMS. *Neurology* **58**, 866–872.

Rocca, M. A., Mezzapesa, D. M., Falini, A., et al. (2003a). Evidence for axonal pathology and adaptive cortical reorganisation in patients at presentation with clinically isolated syndromes suggestive of MS. *NeuroImage* **18**, 847–855.

Rocca, M. A., Gavazzi, C., Mezzapesa, D. M., et al. (2003b). A functional magnetic resonance imaging study of patients with secondary progressive multiple sclerosis. *NeuroImage* **19**, 1770–1777.

Rocca, M. A., Pagani, E., Ghezzi, A., et al. (2003c). Functional cortical changes in patients with MS and non-specific conventional MRI scans of the brain *NeuroImage* **19**, 826–836.

Rocca, M. A., Mezzapesa, D. M., Ghezzi, A., et al. (2003d). Cord damage elicits brain functional reorganization after a single episode of myelitis. *Neurology* **61**, 1078–1085.

Rocca, M. A., Agosta, F., Mezzapesa, D. M., et al. (2004). A functional MRI study of movement-associated cortical changes in patients with Devic's neuromyelitis optica. *NeuroImage.* **21**, 1061–1068.

Rombouts, S. A., Lazeron, R. H., Scheltens, P., et al. (1998). Visual activation patterns in patients with optic neuritis: an fMRI pilot study. *Neurology* **50**, 1896–1899.

Rovaris, M., and Filippi, M. (1999). Magnetic resonance techniques to monitor disease evolution and treatment trial outcomes in multiple sclerosis. *Curr. Opin. Neurol.* **12**, 337–344.

Rovaris, M., Filippi, M., Minicucci, L., et al. (2000). Cortical/subcortical disease burden and cognitive impairment in multiple sclerosis. *AJNR Am. J. Neuroradiol.* **21**, 402–408.

Rovaris, M., Iannucci, G., Falautano, M., et al. (2002). Cognitive dysfunction in patients with mildly disabling relapsing-remitting multiple sclerosis: An exploratory study with diffusion tensor MR imaging. *J. Neurol. Sci.* **195**, 103–109.

Rovaris, M., Agosta, F., Sormani, M. P., et al. (2003). Conventional and magnetization transfer MRI predictors of clinical multiple sclerosis evolution: A medium-term follow-up study. *Brain* **126**, 2323–2332.

Sailer, M., Losseff, N. A., Wang, L., Gawne-Cain, M. L., Thompson, A. J., and Miller, D. H. (2001). T1 lesion load and cerebral atrophy as a marker for clinical progression in patients with multiple sclerosis. A prospective 18 months follow-up study. *Eur. J. Neurol.* **8**, 37–42.

Sarchielli, P., Presciutti, O., Pelliccioli, G. P., et al. (1999). Absolute quantification of brain metabolites by proton magnetic resonance spectroscopy in normal-appearing white matter of multiple sclerosis patients. *Brain* **122**, 513–521.

Sarchielli, P., Presciutti, O., Tarducci, R., et al. (2002). Localized (1) H magnetic resonance spectroscopy in mainly cortical gray matter of patients with multiple sclerosis. *J. Neurol.* **249**, 902–910.

Sharma, R., Narayana, P. A., and Wolinsky, J. S. (2001). Grey matter abnormalities in multiple sclerosis: Proton magnetic resonance spectroscopic imaging. *Multiple Sclerosis* **7**, 221–226.

Simmons, M. L., Frondoza, C. G., and Coyle, J. T. (1991). Immunocytochemical localization of *N*-acetyl-aspartate with monoclonal antibodies. *Neuroscience* **45**, 37–45.

Simon, H. J., Jacobs, L. D., Campion, M. K., et al. (1999). A longitudinal study of brain atrophy in relapsing multiple sclerosis. *Neurology* **53**, 139–148.

Staffen, W., Mair, A., Zauner, H., et al. (2002). Cognitive function and fMRI in patients with multiple sclerosis: Evidence for compensatory cortical activation during an attention task. *Brain* **156**, 1275–1282.

Stevenson, V. L., Miller, D. H., Rovaris, M., et al. (1999). Primary and transitional progressive MS. A clinical and MRI cross-sectional study. *Neurology* **52**, 839–845.

Suhy, J., Rooney, W. D., Goodkin, D. E., et al. (2000). 1H MRSI comparison of white matter and lesions in primary progressive and relapsing-remitting MS. *Multiple Sclerosis* **6**, 148–155.

Trapp, B. D., Peterson, J., Ransohoff, R. M., Rudick, R., Mork, S., and Bo, L. (1998). Axonal transection in the lesions of multiple sclerosis. *N. Engl. J. Med.* **338**, 278–285.

van der Flier, W. M., van den Heuvel, D. M., Weverling-Rijnsburger, A. W., et al. (2002). Magnetization transfer imaging in normal aging, mild cognitive impairment, and Alzheimer's disease. *Ann. Neurol.* **52**, 62–67.

van der Flier, W. M., van Buchem, M. A., and van Buchem, H. A. M. (2003). Volumetric MRI predicts rate of cognitive decline related to AD and cerebrovascular disease. *Neurology* **60**, 1558–1559.

van Waesberghe, J. H. T. M., van Walderveen, M. A., Castelijns, J. A., et al. (1998). Patterns of lesion development in multiple sclerosis: longitudinal observations with T1-weighted spin-echo and magnetization MR. *AJNR Am. J. Neuroradiol.* **19**, 675–683.

van Waesberghe, J. H., Kamphorst, W., De Groot, C. J., et al. (1999). Axonal loss in multiple sclerosis lesions: Magnetic resonance imaging insights into substrates of disability. *Ann. Neurol.* **46**, 747–754.

van Walderveen, M. A., Kamphorst, W., Scheltens, P., et al. (1998). Histopathologic correlate of hypointense lesions on T1-weighted spin-echo MRI in multiple sclerosis. *Neurology* **50**, 1282–1288.

van Walderveen, M. A., Barkhof, F., Pouwels, P. J., van Schijndel, R. A., Polman, C. H., and Castelijns, J. A. (1999). Neuronal damage in T1-hypointense multiple sclerosis lesions demonstrated in vivo using proton magnetic resonance spectroscopy. *Ann. Neurol.* **46**, 79–87.

Waxman, S. G. (1998). Demyelinating diseases: New pathological insights, new therapeutic targets. *N. Engl. J. Med.* **338**, 323–326

Waxman, S. G., and Ritchie, J. M. (1993). Molecular dissection of the myelinated axon. *Ann. Neurol.* **33**, 121–136.

Werring, D. J., Bullmore, E. T., Toosy, A. T., et al. (2000). Recovery from optic neuritis is associated with a change in the distribution of cerebral response to visual stimulation: A functional magnetic resonance imaging study. *J. Neurol. Neurosurg. Psychiatry* **68**, 441–449.

Wylezinska, M., Cifelli, A., Jezzard, P., Palace, J., Alecci, M., and Matthews, P. M. (2003). Thalamic neurodegeneration in relapsing-remitting multiple sclerosis. *Neurology* **60**, 1949–1954.

16

Electrophysiological Correlates of Relapse, Remission, Persistent Sensorimotor Deficit, and Long-Term Recovery Processes in Multiple Sclerosis

Steve Jones, Ph.D.

I. Introduction

Many of the pathophysiological consequences of multiple sclerosis (MS) are manifested in abnormal evoked potentials (EPs), rapid changes of electrical potential, recorded from the scalp or the body surface after the application of a sensory stimulus. EPs are conventionally labeled according to their polarity (positive or negative) and the approximate time in milliseconds that normally elapses before a peak is reached (e.g., N20, P100). For clinical purposes, the most useful sensory EPs are those generated in central afferent pathways, subcortical nuclei, and the primary sensory cortex. Motor EPs, on the other hand, are the responses of efferent axons and skeletal muscles to electrical or magnetic stimulation of the motor cortex or the corticospinal tracts.

In patients with MS, cortically generated EPs are characteristically delayed and frequently also attenuated. This accords with the established view that during periods of relapse, factors associated with blood-brain barrier leakage and inflammation cause destruction of the myelin sheath, leaving the axonal membrane intact but vulnerable to further insult. During remission it is possible for partially demyelinated fibers to conduct action potentials, albeit at reduced velocity. During the progressive stage of the disease, degeneration of demyelinated axons is probably the main factor responsible for long-term disability. However, pathological evidence increasingly suggests that axonal damage may be extensive, even in the early stages of a relapse (Ferguson et al., 1997). There is a clear case to be argued that MS is a neuronal disease in the sense that neurons suffer direct injury from outside the cell membrane. A more radical hypothesis is that intraneuronal degenerative processes may play a role, with shedding of the myelin sheath as a secondary consequence.

The aim of this chapter is to review the phenomenology of EP abnormalities in MS, to consider to what extent the electrophysiological data reflect the pattern of neurological impairment and are explicable in terms of temporary conduction block due to inflammation, persistent conduction delay due to demyelination, and subsequent axonal and neuronal degeneration. It may be that by drawing attention to the anomalies, other significant extraneuronal and intraneuronal processes may be uncovered.

II. Visual and Retinal Potentials in Optic Neuritis and Multiple Sclerosis

A. Evolution of Cortical Visual-Evoked Potential Abnormalities after Optic Neuritis

A typical episode of optic neuritis entails acute monocular visual impairment, ranging in severity from mild cloudiness to complete blindness. This is usually associated with the appearance of a local region of high T_2 signal in magnetic resonance imaging (MRI) of the optic nerve that shows enhancement with gadolinium (Youl et al., 1991) and is believed to reflect blood-brain barrier leakage and inflammation. If cortical visual-evoked potentials (VEPs) are recorded at this time, in response to the sudden reversal of a high-contrast grating or checkerboard pattern, they are usually found to be attenuated, roughly in proportion to the visual acuity deficit (reviewed by Halliday, 1993). That the period of VEP attenuation coincides approximately with that during which gadolinium enhancement occurs (Youl et al., 1991), and that VEPs recorded immediately after that period are typically delayed, suggest a likely mechanism of temporary axonal conduction block resulting from factors associated with inflammation and/or demyelination. Furthermore, the observation that both visual acuity and VEP amplitude usually recover to near-normal values within a period of a few weeks indicates that neither axonal transection nor primary neurodegeneration is the prime cause of acute visual failure in optic neuritis.

In a minority of cases, visual function remains persistently impaired and VEPs remain attenuated, even after the resolution of inflammation. This can probably be ascribed to axonal damage, although whether it occurs as an intraneuronal process or as a consequence of demyelination and inflammation is unclear. Attempts have been made to discover electrophysiological or anatomical (MRI) factors that may predict a good or poor recovery (Kapoor et al., 1998), so that patients with a poor prognosis might be targeted for treatment, but so far no such indices have been found. In any case, the bulk of evidence suggests that the benefits of anti-inflammatory treatment are transitory, causing an acceler-

ated recovery but with few if any positive consequences in the longer term (Beck and Cleary, 1993; Kapoor et al., 1998).

Once the visual acuity has improved to some degree and the VEP amplitude has recovered sufficiently for a response to be measured, the latency of the major positive peak (P100) is usually found to be prolonged, typically by between 10 and 40 ms (10% to 40%; Halliday et al., 1972). It seems reasonable to assume that the magnitude of the delay should reflect the longitudinal extent of demyelination, although to date no significant correlation has been demonstrated between VEP latency and the length of the lesion seen on MRI. For a typical lesion length on the order of 30 mm, and assuming that the extent of increased T_2 signal reflects the length of the demyelinated axons, a VEP delay of 30 ms would imply a conduction velocity through the lesion of approximately 1 m/sec. This velocity is comparable to the conduction velocity of normally unmyelinated fibers, although their mechanism of action potential propagation may not be entirely the same. It also seems reasonable to assume that the velocity of conduction through the lesion should be related to the thickness of the individual myelin sheaths. The conduction velocity of normal nerve fibers is roughly proportional to both axonal diameter and myelin thickness, but these two parameters are closely associated and there is no directly relevant evidence as to how conduction velocity may be affected when they become dissociated by disease.

Both acutely and in the longer term, the degree of VEP amplitude reduction is loosely related to the severity of visual acuity impairment (e.g., Jones, 1993a); however, no such correlation has been shown between the severity of the visual deficit and the magnitude of the VEP latency delay (e.g., Sanders et al., 1987; Jones, 1993a). The latency may remain prolonged for months or years, even after the visual acuity has recovered virtually to normal. It appears that, as long as axons of the optic nerve remain in functional continuity, the time required to conduct impulses from the retina to the brain is virtually irrelevant as far as the spatial resolving power of vision (at least for static objects) is concerned. The tendency for VEP delay to persist after the partial or complete recovery of visual acuity is one important reason why VEPs remain a useful diagnostic test for a past episode of optic neuritis. It is also a clear sign that the myelin sheath may be affected independently of the optic nerve axon.

Despite the fact that the VEP usually remains delayed long after the visual acuity has recovered, however, there is a tendency for its latency to decrease over the ensuing months and years (Fig. 1). In a minority of the MS cases studied serially by Matthews and Small (1979, 1983), initially prolonged VEP latencies returned to normal, sometimes after several years. Normalization has since been shown to be the prevalent tendency, although it is not seen in every individual (Hely et al., 1986).

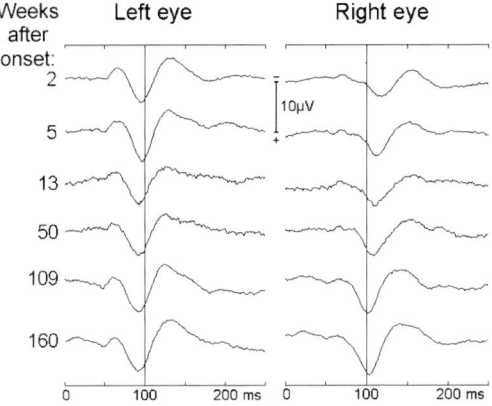

Figure 1 Serial VEPs to central field (4-degree radius) stimulation after an episode of right optic neuritis showing progressive shortening of the P100 latency, particularly between 50 and 109 weeks after onset. The right eye responses obtained after 109 and 160 weeks were within normal latency limits in absolute terms, although the interocular latency difference was still abnormal. For guidance the vertical bar is placed at 100 ms; the upper limit of "normal" for this system is approximately 108 ms.

In the cross-sectional data of Jones (1993a), more than 70% of patients had delayed VEPs when tested more than 2 years after the onset of symptoms, compared with more than 90% whose responses were delayed during the first 6 months. Latency reduction is not usually apparent during the first 3 months after the onset of symptoms (during which time any such effect may be masked by changes resulting

from the resolution of inflammation), but is most clearly manifested between 3 and 12 months (Jones, 1993a) (Fig. 2). Latency shortening has also been found to be significant during the second year (Brusa et al., 2001), associated with only a mild improvement in visual acuity. In a small patient group monitored for 3 years, latencies were on average still shorter in the final examination (Brusa et al., 1999).

Although other possible mechanisms need to be considered, it seems reasonable to suppose that, if the VEP latency delay reflects the degree of demyelination, a gradual reduction of that delay may reflect a long-term process of remyelination. There seems to be no way in which such a change can be ascribed to axonal regeneration. Alteration in the distribution of sodium channels may be an important adaptive process enabling conduction to be restored in demyelinated axons (Craner et al., 2003) (see Chapter 7), but would not be expected to result in a complete normalization of conduction velocity. Latency normalization is also extremely difficult to explain in terms of other adaptive mechanisms such as cortical reorganization (Werring et al., 2000).

B. Retinotopic Variation of VEP Abnormalities

The use of a high-contrast stimulus (checkerboard or grating) is essential to demonstrate dependably a VEP delay in patients with a past history of optic neuritis. The cortical responses to diffuse flash are, on the one hand, more

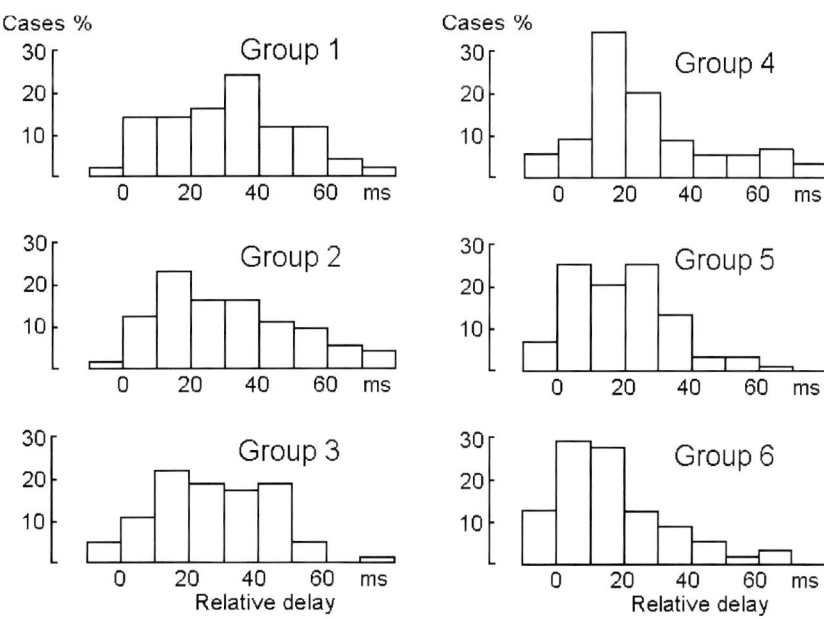

Figure 2 Distribution of VEP delays (affected minus unaffected eye latencies) in six groups of patients divided according to the time elapsed between the onset of symptoms and the VEP recording. Group 1: 1–4 weeks; Group 2: 5–8 weeks; Group 3: 9–13 weeks; Group 4: 14–26 weeks; Group 5: 27–104 weeks; Group 6: >104 weeks. There were at least 55 patients in each group. (Adapted from Jones, 1993a.)

difficult to characterize in terms of their wave structure and, on the other hand, usually delayed to a lesser degree than the pattern-evoked responses when recorded in the same patients (Halliday et al., 1972). The reasons for this remain a matter for debate, one possibility being the apparently greater susceptibility of axons projecting to the "parvocellular" layer of the lateral geniculate nucleus (Evangelou et al., 2001) and thus presumably concerned with the perception of spatial contrast.

However, in patients recently recovered from the acute stage of optic neuritis, the P100 to a reversing checkerboard pattern was found to be significantly (by almost 100%) more delayed when recorded to stimulation of the central portion of the visual field, subtending 8 degrees at the eye, than to stimulation of the surrounding regions out to 13 degrees eccentricity (Rinalduzzi et al., 2001). Virtually no pattern VEP can be recorded to stimuli of greater eccentricity than about 15 degrees, so it appears that even within the visual field area associated with the macula, there is a tendency for the degree of VEP delay to decrease as the degree of retinal eccentricity increases. In a control group there was little or no latency difference between the VEPs from the same macular regions, so it does not seem likely that optic nerve axons deriving from the central area are of markedly smaller diameter. Consequently, the identification of the latter with the "parvocellular" and the more peripheral macular fibers with the "magnocellular" system does not seem to be a valid or relevant distinction.

The most plausible explanation for the greater delay of VEPs to stimulation of the central 8 degrees of the visual field may be that the most affected fibers run centrally in the optic nerve. Elsewhere in the central nervous system, it is known that vigorous remyelination occurs during the first few weeks after the acute episode, most extensively around the edge of the plaques (Prineas et al., 1993). It is plausible, therefore, that initially all optic nerve fibers may be affected to a similar degree (as suggested by the ophthalmological findings of Fang et al., 1999), but that those deriving from more peripheral retinal regions (including those that contribute proportionately more to the VEP when a diffuse flash is used) are rapidly remyelinated and may soon be restored to a condition close, if not identical, to their prepathological state.

In a minority of optic neuritis cases, VEPs are not measurably delayed but show changes suggestive of a central scotoma (Halliday, 1993). This pattern, where the P100 from the central visual field area is selectively attenuated, seems to suggest a preferential loss of axons deriving from retinal ganglion cells located in the center of the macula. As argued previously, these also appear to be the axons that are most prone to persistent demyelination, and it is plausible that this may leave them more vulnerable to spontaneous or inflammation-induced degeneration. On the electrophysiological evidence there is no way of distinguishing between a neurodegenerative pathology causing some demyelinated axons to fail, and one in which transection and/or degeneration occurs as a consequence of further inflammation.

In addition to their latency prolongation, VEPs frequently (although not always) fail to recover to fully normal amplitude after the acute stage of optic neuritis, even in patients whose visual acuity recovers to normal. It has been suggested (Diem et al., 2003) that this amplitude reduction might constitute evidence of axonal degeneration. However, VEP amplitudes cannot be considered a reliable measure of the number of optic nerve axons in functional continuity, as in addition to axonal degeneration and conduction block there are at least two further mechanisms by which amplitudes may be reduced. The VEP consists of a sequence of negative and positive peaks, and the tendency for that portion of the response deriving from the central area of the visual field to be delayed to a greater degree would cause a substantial degree of phase cancellation and a consequent reduction in the recorded amplitude. Sometimes there may be more diffuse temporal dispersion of the response as a result of patchy optic nerve demyelination, such that the volley arrives incoherently at the lateral geniculate nucleus and subsequently the visual cortex. A further possibility may be that demyelination causes an increase in the degree of temporal "jitter" between successive volleys. This would result in a reduction of the recorded amplitude when the responses to a number of stimuli are averaged together. Therefore, there are a number of reasons why the VEP amplitude cannot be considered an accurate reflection of the number of optic nerve axons in functional continuity.

C. VEP Abnormalities in the Absence of Visual Symptoms

One of the most striking early observations in patients with clinically definite MS was that the incidence of VEP abnormalities was scarcely lower among those who exhibited no current signs or past history of visual impairment, as compared with those whose clinical history included one or more episodes of optic neuritis (Halliday et al., 1973). Although subsequent studies tended to report somewhat lower incidences in visually asymptomatic cases (reviewed by Halliday, 1993), it is clear that electrophysiological defects may occur "subclinically." That clinically eloquent and subclinical VEP abnormalities are of a similar nature, the most characteristic feature being latency prolongation, suggests that in both circumstances the pathological processes involve demyelination.

In a follow-up study of 12 patients with monocular optic neuritis, we (Brusa et al., 1999) found that the latencies of "whole field" VEPs to stimulation of the acutely unaffected fellow eyes were significantly increased when recorded 3 years, as compared with 6 months, after the onset of symptoms in the affected eye. The mean latency increase of 3 ms (of which less than 1 ms could plausibly be ascribed to aging) was in marked contrast to the mean decrease of 8 ms in the affected eyes over the same period. In the initial recordings, four of the fellow eye responses were outside normal latency limits. At follow-up evaluation only one further case was certifiably "abnormal," but all 12 showed a latency increase of between 1 and 12 ms. That VEP amplitudes were not significantly altered might suggest a process of demyelination unaccompanied by axonal degeneration. In the same study, however, a significant deterioration was detected in the contrast sensitivity of the fellow eyes, which would not be expected if all axons remained in functional continuity. VEP amplitudes are more variable than latencies, both within and between individuals, so a minor degree of axonal degeneration would be more difficult to detect on electrophysiological study. Further studies are clearly needed to substantiate this finding. It must be noted that we ourselves failed to reproduce the effect in a 2-year follow-up evaluation of 31 cases (Brusa et al., 2001).

D. Postchiasmal Inflammatory Lesions

"In contrast to the high incidence of VEP delays that are recorded after optic neuritis, in a group of 13 patients presenting with partial or complete homonymous hemianopia resulting from a postchiasmal inflammatory lesion, only 5 were found to have relatively delayed or attenuated VEPs to stimulation of the affected hemifields (Plant et al., 1992). At follow-up, persistent hemifield VEP abnormalities were seen in only 3 patients. The frequent absence of latency prolongation might suggest a different pathological process in postchiasmal as compared with prechiasmal lesions. An alternative possibility may be that, since optic nerve fibers are concentrated in a smaller volume than the fibers of the optic radiation, demyelinating lesions of similar size may affect a greater proportion of fibers in the optic nerve. Also, the circumstances of optic nerve inflammation (particularly when this occurs within the optic canal) may entail an additional element of compression, leading to more severe demyelination."

E. Effects of Repetitive Stimulation

Apart from conduction delay, another possible neurophysiological consequence of demyelination is impairment in the ability of the affected axons to transmit rapid trains of impulses. It was reported by Cohen et al. (1980) that the fastest rate of flash stimulation capable of evoking distinct VEP deflections (the "critical frequency of photic driving") was reduced in a high proportion of patients with MS, but that these were not necessarily the same patients as those showing delayed responses to single patterned stimuli. The reliability of this test has been called in question (Ramani et al., 1984), but Mitchell et al. (1983) reported that the second of two responses to patterned stimuli separated by between 10 and

100 ms was abnormally delayed in about 20% of eyes, irrespective of whether or not the response to a single stimulus was delayed. These authors speculated that involvement of more posterior segments of the visual pathway might specifically delay the responses to rapidly repeated stimuli, although why this should be the case is unclear. Alternatively, it may be appropriate to consider the possible effects of pathological changes occurring within the retina.

F. Retinal Involvement in Optic Neuritis and Multiple Sclerosis

A large proportion of the pattern electroretinogram (PERG), which is recorded from the surface of the cornea or the infraorbital skin in response to a similar grating or checkerboard stimulus as is used to evoke the cortical VEP, is believed to be due to the activity of retinal ganglion cells. When recorded at a fast rate, the PERG is usually found to be attenuated in patients with a past history of optic neuritis (e.g., Plant et al., 1986; Bradshaw, 1992), although not significantly in every individual. When recorded to "transient" stimuli presented at a relatively low rate, it is found to be the final negative component (N95), rather than the preceding positivity (P50), which is most affected (Holder, 1991) (Fig. 3). In the acute phase of optic neuritis the P50 may also be temporarily attenuated, recovering in parallel with the recovery in visual acuity (Berninger and Heider, 1990). The P50 component can also be chronically attenuated in patients with long-standing optic nerve lesions or after optic nerve section, presumably as a result of retrograde degeneration of the ganglion cell layer, but the mechanism of its brief attenuation during acute optic neuritis is unclear. A 28% incidence of retinal vascular abnormalities (retinal venous sheathing and/or evidence of inflammation) was noted in a group of patients in the early stages of optic neuritis (Lightman et al., 1987), but it was not determined whether this was associated with PERG changes. Among patients with clinically definite MS, similar ocular inflammatory changes were seen in 18% (Graham et al., 1989), suggesting that vascular lesions in the retina may occur independently of optic neuritis. These usually appear to be asymptomatic, but it is possible they may contribute to electrophysiological abnormalities such as delayed VEPs to repetitive stimulation (Mitchell et al., 1983).

In patients who had made a good functional recovery from optic neuritis a relationship was found between the PERG and the thickness of the nerve fiber layer (NFL), seen in optical coherence tomography of the retina (Parisi et al., 1999). Remarkably, the NFL was on average almost 50% thinner in the patients as compared with the controls, suggesting that it may be possible to retain a near-normal visual acuity even when there has been a marked degree of axonal degeneration. The N95 amplitude was directly correlated with the NFL thickness and the P50 latency inversely so,

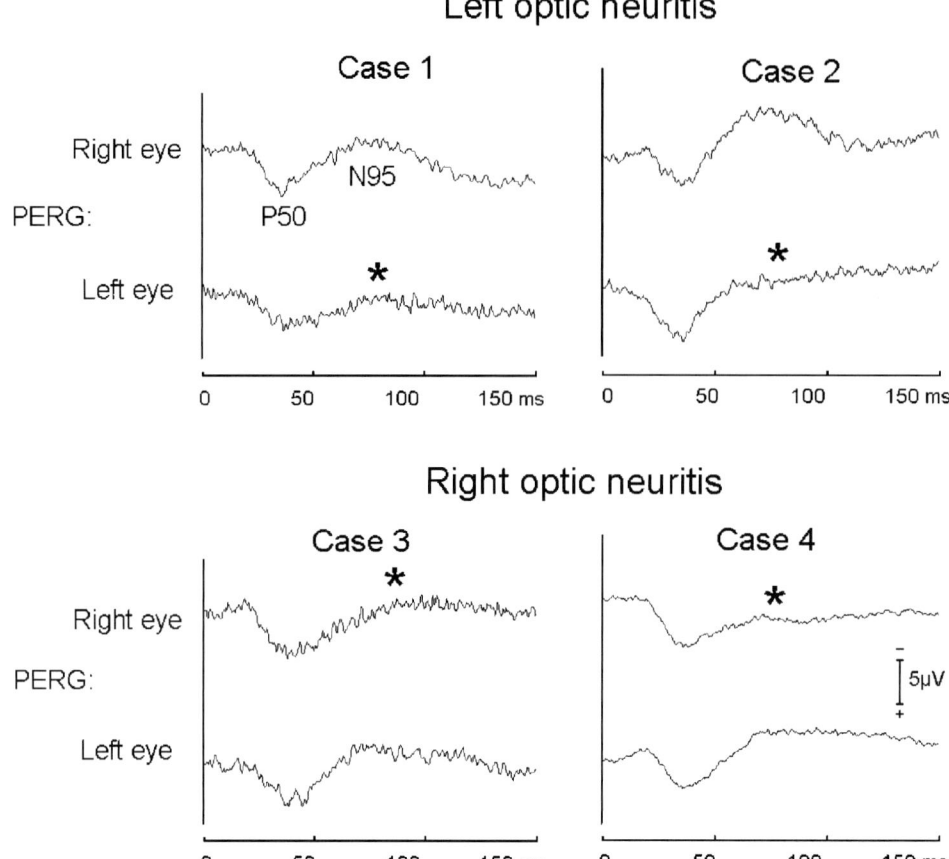

Figure 3 Abnormal pattern ERGs in four patients with a past history of optic neuritis. In every case the N95 peak recorded from the cornea of the affected eye is relatively attenuated (*asterisks*). In Case 1 the P50 also appears relatively attenuated and broadened.

suggesting that the degree of retinal ganglion cell degeneration was related to the extent of axonal loss. This group of patients was tested at least 12 months after the optic neuritis episode, so there had been ample time for retrograde degeneration to occur subsequent to demyelination and (presumably) axonal transection.

It was reported by Falsini et al. (1992) that the PERGs were also significantly affected in the eyes of patients with MS but no history of optic neuritis, this time in terms of phase (latency) but not of amplitude. However, they did not report how many of these patients also had delayed cortical VEPs, which might indicate that the PERG changes were due to subclinical optic nerve demyelination rather than a primary retinal lesion. Among a group of patients with MS who did have a past history of optic neuritis, Porciatti and Sartucci (1996) found that PERGs to color-contrast gratings reversed at a fast rate were significantly attenuated in the affected, but not the fellow, eyes. When presented at a slower rate, the responses of the fellow eyes were also smaller on average than those of normal controls,

although it was not stated whether the difference was statistically significant. The cortical VEPs were also apparently abnormal to stimulation of the fellow eyes, so the PERG changes might represent a similar process of retrograde ganglion cell degeneration, secondary to subclinical, insidious demyelination.

In a later study (Falsini et al., 1999), significant PERG amplitude attenuation was noted in response to sinusoidally modulated, monochromatic gratings reversing at a fast rate in the eyes of patients with MS but without any history of optic neuritis. Although the most marked effects tended to be associated with delayed cortical potentials and measurable psychophysical defects, suggesting subclinical demyelination and axonal loss, the PERGs were also significantly attenuated (albeit only at relatively high spatial frequencies) in eyes for which all other investigations, including VEPs, were normal. This appears to be the most suggestive electrophysiological evidence for changes in the properties of retinal ganglion cells that apparently cannot be explained as a secondary consequence of optic nerve demyelination. Also consistent with a change in the firing properties of retinal ganglion cells, there is evidence for expression of an abnormal ensemble of sodium channels within these retinal neurons in experimental autoimmune encephalomyelitis, a model of MS, and this would be expected to alter the firing pattern of these cells (see Chapter 7).

From the 1960s to the 1980s, there was a small but not inconsiderable literature (reviewed by Halliday, 1993) suggesting that the flash electroretinogram, generated in more peripheral retinal layers as compared with the PERG, may also be affected in some patients with MS. Papakostopoulos et al. (1989) reported a significant amplitude reduction of the b wave recorded under photopic conditions in two groups of patients, one with clinically isolated optic neuritis of recent onset and the other with a past history of optic neuritis in the context of MS. Since it is generally agreed that the b wave has a preganglionic origin, this might suggest a process of retrograde, trans-synaptic degeneration occurring relatively early during the episode of optic neuritis. No evidence was found for involvement of the asymptomatic fellow eyes; hence there was no suggestion of a primary retinal defect occurring independently of optic neuritis.

III. Somatosensory-Evoked Potentials

Cortical somatosensory evoked potentials (SEPs) to stimulation of major nerve trunks in the arm or the leg are abnormal in a large proportion of patients with established MS (reviewed by Jones, 1993b). During periods of acute sensory relapse, the distribution of SEP abnormalities tends to coincide quite closely with that of the clinical sensory deficit. Most SEP abnormalities are therefore presumed to be due to discrete lesions of sensory pathways of the spinal cord and the brain, although there has been only one pub-

lished case study demonstrating an apparent relationship between abnormal SEPs and a cervical cord lesion seen at autopsy (Matthews and Esiri, 1979). Lower limb SEPs tend to be more often affected than upper, which may be a simple consequence of the greater length of the pathway and the consequently greater likelihood that a plaque will be situated in an appropriate location.

The first cortically generated potentials, N20 to median nerve stimulation and P40 to stimulation of the posterior tibial nerve, may sometimes be delayed by 10 ms or more. This suggests a similar slow conduction velocity through the plaque as was suggested for the optic nerve lesions causing VEP delays. An earlier subcortical component of the median nerve SEP (N13), recorded from the dorsum of the neck with reference to an electrode on the scalp, is not usually straightforwardly delayed but may be attenuated, fragmented, or even apparently absent (Fig. 4). This occurs mainly because more than one structure between the dorsal root entry zone and the cuneate nucleus contributes to the N13, partially through far-field activity picked up at the reference site. Also, the absence of any recordable activity is probably attributable to temporal dispersion and phase cancellation. With the reference electrode at an electrically indifferent site away from the head, it is sometimes possible to recognize a response pattern in which that part of the N13 generated more rostrally, at or above the foramen magnum (sometimes termed N14), is delayed, whereas the "true" N13, which arises in the dorsal horns at low cervical level, is apparently unaffected. Such a pattern would seem to be entirely consistent with conduction delay caused by a demyelinating lesion affecting the cuneate tract of the spinal cord at cervical level.

Occasionally, the cervical N13 to median nerve stimulation may be abnormally attenuated while the cortical N20 is apparently unaffected (e.g., Fig. 4, Case 3) (Jones, 1982). By

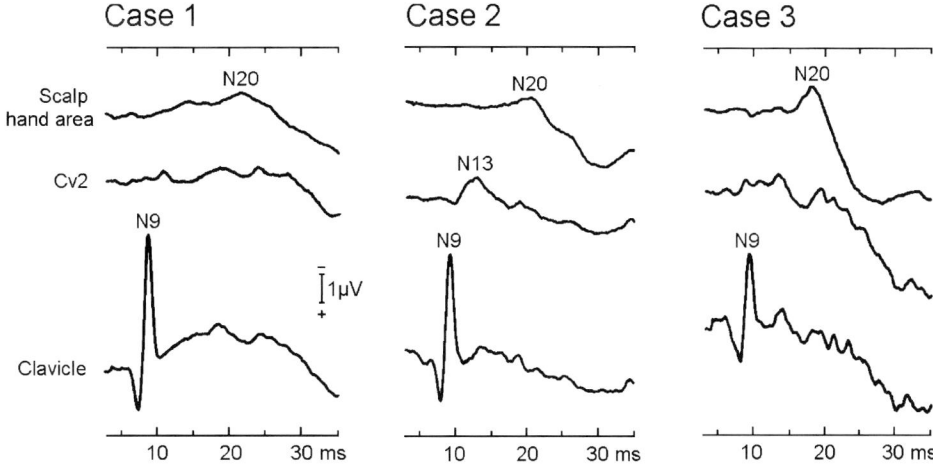

Figure 4 SEPs to median nerve stimulation showing three response patterns occurring in MS. Case 1: delayed N20, absent N13, normal N9. Case 2: delayed N20 (prolonged N9-N20 interpeak latency), normal N13, normal N9. Case 3: normal N20, attenuated N13, normal N9. (Adapted from Jones, 1982.)

use of a local reference electrode on the anterior side of the neck, this can sometimes be shown to be due to selective involvement of the "true" N13, generated in internuncial neurons of the dorsal horn close to the root entry zone at low cervical level. This pattern is more frequently seen in association with herniation of the cord resulting from syringomyelia (Restuccia and Mauguière, 1991). That the cervical potential is attenuated rather than delayed suggests damage to neurons within the dorsal horn rather than demyelination of presynaptic axons, although more likely as a result of extraneuronal inflammation than intrinsic neurodegeneration.

The peripheral N9 potential recorded from the region of the clavicle or Erb's point to stimulation of the median nerve is generally, perhaps even universally, found to be normal in patients with MS, with or without sensory impairment in the appropriate limb. In a group comparison of 75 patients with MS and normal controls, we discovered no significant delay or attenuation of the N9 (Jones, unpublished). The greater part of the N9, probably at least 90%, is due to stimulation of peripheral sensory fibers whose cell bodies reside in the dorsal root ganglia. A much smaller proportion of the N9 is likely to be due to antidromic activation of motor fibers, with their cell bodies in the ventral horns. Although it is conceivable that plaques involving the ventral horns might lead to degeneration of some peripheral motor axons contributing to the N9, given the wide normal variability of its amplitude and the preponderance of sensory fascicles in the median nerve, it is not surprising that no such effect has been detected. When lesions in the cervical region cause delay of the cortical N20, it is presumably the central axons of the primary sensory neurons that are demyelinated. The absence of any evidence for electrophysiological changes in the N9, generated in the peripheral branch of the same neurons, implies no primary degenerative process involving the sensory neuron itself. There must also be little or no retrograde degeneration of the dorsal root ganglia resulting from demyelination and/or transection of the central axons in the dorsal columns.

In a study where SEPs were recorded in conjunction with MRI of the cervical cord in MS patients with sensorimotor symptoms in the upper limbs (Turano et al., 1991), an association was noted between SEP abnormalities and MRI defects in the dorsal rather than the ventral, and the ipsilateral rather than the contralateral quadrants of the cord. This confirms that SEPs depend on the dorsal sensory tracts of the cord that project ipsilaterally as far as the dorsal column nuclei of the brainstem. In accordance with this model, when MS patients exhibit a dissociated sensory deficit, abnormal SEPs tend to be recorded from limbs with sensory impairment of the "dorsal column" type (joint-position and/or vibration sense) rather than the "spinothalamic" modalities of temperature and pain (as first described by Halliday and Wakefield, 1963).

In our own experience, most patients with abnormal SEPs complain of some degree of numbness in the affected limb(s), which is probably a reflection of diminished light touch sensitivity rather than insensitivity to pain. Positive sensory symptoms such as paresthesias and Lhermitte's phenomenon tend not to be associated with abnormal SEPs. As in the visual system, one would not expect to find overt sensory deficits resulting from lesions that cause only delayed conduction without interruption of axonal continuity. It is probably the case, therefore, that the sensory impairment usually associated with abnormal SEPs ("clinically silent" SEP abnormalities being relatively rare) reflects a degree of conduction block, axonal transection, or neuronal degeneration. Regarding the electrophysiological evidence, there would seem to be no way of deciding between a primary degenerative process and a secondary effect of inflammation and demyelination, but the tendency of cord lesions not to respect the anatomical boundaries between fiber tracts and white vs. gray matter argues in favor of the latter.

IV. Motor-Evoked Potentials

Motor-evoked potentials (MEPs)—compound muscle action potentials to transcranial magnetic or electrical stimulation of motor areas of the brain—are frequently found to be abnormal in patients with MS, resulting either from attenuation of amplitude or prolongation of the central motor conduction time (CMCT) (reviewed by Mills, 1999). A strong association exists between MEP abnormalities and clinical signs of damage to the corticospinal tracts, in accordance with the general understanding that transcranial electrical brain stimulation directly activates the pyramidal cells of the motor cortex, whereas magnetic stimulation achieves the same end indirectly through prior activation of cortical interneurons.

There is some evidence that the axons of the corticospinal tracts may be unable to sustain the same high rate of firing in patients with MS as in normal individuals. In the latter, it appears that a single transcranial stimulus of sufficient intensity will evoke a brief train of corticospinal volleys with a separation of 1.5 to 2 ms. In patients with MS, Boniface et al. (1991) found evidence for a doubling of that interval, as if alternate volleys were missing. Sheean et al. (1997) attempted to discover whether the symptoms of muscular fatigue often experienced by patients with MS might be due to frequency-dependent conduction block of corticospinal tract axons. They found that MS patients were indeed unable to sustain maximal voluntary contraction of their hand muscles for as long as healthy individuals, starting from a similar baseline force, and that the CMCT was significantly prolonged to single transcranial stimuli. However, they did not find any greater MEP amplitude decrement in the second of two responses to paired transcranial stimuli. Their preferred explanation was that the fatiguing effect originates in the brain "upstream" of the pyramidal neurons. Alternatively, it might be suggested that frequency-dependent conduction block may become more marked under natural circumstances, when the fibers are required to conduct long trains of impulses rather than double volleys. A third possibility might be that the ability to sustain maximal contraction for long periods depends on the redundancy of corticospinal axons, some of which were transected or had degenerated in the patient group.

V. Auditory-Evoked Potentials

Brainstem auditory-evoked potentials (BAEPs) are frequently abnormal in patients with clinically definite MS, although in a somewhat lower percentage as compared with visual and somatosensory EPs (reviewed by Chiappa, 1997). When present, BAEP abnormalities range from a delay or absence of wave V only (this peak being generated at mid-upper pontine level, probably in the tracts of the lateral lemnisci connecting the nuclei of the superior olivary complex with the inferior colliculus) to absence of all waves after wave I, which originates in distal segments of the eighth nerve (Fig. 5). It may be possible to define the level of a brainstem lesion more specifically, according to whether or not wave III is affected in addition to wave V. An abnormality including wave III is most likely to be due to a lesion at

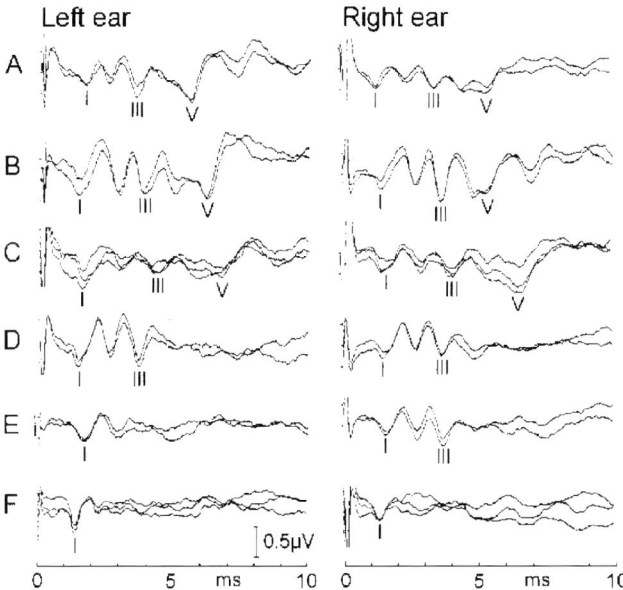

Figure 5 **Examples of BAEP waveforms in MS patients.** (**A**) Normal. (**B**) Delayed wave V with increased I–V and III–V interpeak latencies on the left. (**C**) Delayed wave V on the right; delayed waves III and V on the left with all interpeak latencies increased. (**D**) Bilateral absence of wave V; wave IV also absent on the left. (**E**) Bilateral absence of waves IV and V; wave III also absent on the left. (**F**) Bilateral absence of all waves except wave I. None of these patients complained of auditory symptoms.

lower pontine level, adjacent to the cochlear nucleus on the side of stimulation or within the decussating tracts of the trapezoid body that project to the contralateral superior olivary complex. When latencies are prolonged, with concomitant increase in the I-III, III-V, or I-V interpeak latencies, the conclusion of a demyelinating process would seem to be justified, although there are many other conditions causing minor latency delays of this sort.

In contrast to the somatosensory modality where SEP abnormalities are frequently associated with sensory deficits, a remarkable discrepancy exists between the high incidence of abnormal BAEPs and the low incidence of reported auditory symptoms in MS. Although subtle deficits may be demonstrated by sophisticated hearing tests, even patients with gross BAEP abnormalities tend not to report hearing difficulties and usually have normal or near-normal audiograms. How it is possible for hearing to remain virtually unimpaired, sometimes in the complete absence of recordable potentials supposedly reflecting the integrity of brainstem auditory pathways, remains a matter of conjecture. One partial explanation may be that the absence of particular peaks is usually not due to conduction block, axonal transection, or neuronal degeneration but rather to demyelination-related temporal dispersion. Impulses that are normally temporally coherent and give rise to strong electrical fields on the scalp may become spread out and overlap in time with activity at other levels of the pathway. As long as the acoustic spectral information carried in the affected fibers is securely place-encoded, disruption of their timing patterns may result in a relatively minor degree of perceptual degradation.

It would surely be expected, however, that temporally based auditory processes that depend on the precise timing of neuronal impulses in the brainstem should be impaired by lesions causing BAEP abnormalities. One such process is that by which interaural time differences (ITD) are used to localize sound sources in the horizontal plane. In animals, and presumably also humans, the first binaurally responsive neurons are in the superior olivary complex, and many of these are found to be sensitive to ITD. In a group of 28 patients with MS selected for clinical brainstem involvement (van der Poel et al., 1988), 23 were found to have a defect of sound lateralization by ITD discrimination. In a forced-choice design, clicks were played through headphones, either simultaneously to both ears or within a certain range of ITD; the patients were required to say only whether the sound appeared to come from the left or right of the midline. Some patients would consistently mislateralize the sounds, and might require ITD well outside the normally occurring range to produce a midline sensation; others appeared to have a general blurring of the sound image. BAEPs were abnormal in 21 patients, and all of those whose abnormalities involved wave III as well as wave V had impaired ITD discrimination. Because wave III is probably generated mostly by the decussating axons of the trapezoid body, projecting from the cochlear nucleus to the contralateral superior olivary complex, it seems understandable that the patients with ITD defects should be those in whom the timing of input to the first center for binaural processing was disrupted by demyelination. That patients with brainstem lesions affecting only wave V sometimes had preserved ITD perception suggests that ITD may be securely place-encoded by the activity of specific superior olivary complex neurons, with the effect that temporal disruption resulting from demyelination at higher levels of the pathway may be of lesser functional consequence.

The potentials immediately after wave V and presumed to be generated between the inferior colliculus and the thalamus are generally too inconsistent to determine their patterns of involvement in MS. The so-called middle-latency auditory-evoked potentials (MLAEP), generated between the midbrain and the auditory cortex, are reportedly abnormal in a fairly high proportion of cases (e.g., Versino et al., 1992), not necessarily those exhibiting abnormal brainstem components. As with the BAEPs, abnormality might be defined by latency prolongation or absence of individual waves. MLAEP latencies were found to be significantly prolonged when the patients with MS were considered as a group, so demyelination would seem to be the most parsimonious explanation. Later auditory cortical potentials, on the other hand, have frequently been reported not to be significantly delayed in MS patients. This apparent anomaly is considered in the context of long-latency event-related potentials next.

VI. Long Latency Event-Related Potentials

In contrast to the high incidence of brainstem and MLAEP abnormalities, the cortical N100 potential (or N1) evoked by the onset of sounds is seldom found to be abnormal, either in individual patients with MS or in intergroup comparison with normal controls (e.g., Newton et al., 1989; Honig et al., 1992; Sailer et al., 2001). This might possibly be accounted for by the multiplicity of pathways by which auditory input may arrive at the cortex, such that sufficient fibers to produce a normal-appearing response are practically always spared. With the additional assumption that many functions are likely to be duplicated in the auditory cortices of the two hemispheres, this may also explain why auditory sensation is considerably more robust than the other sensory modalities to the kind of lesions that occur in MS.

In our own study (Jones et al., 2002), we distinguished two different forms of the N1 resulting from modulation of a continuous complex tone, one due to infrequent step-changes in the spectral composition and the other reflecting a different type of change, when a period of rapid, regularly occurring frequency modulations suddenly came to an end. In a group of patients with definite MS, the N1 to infrequent frequency changes (as well as the conventional response to the onset of the tone) was not delayed, although the following P2 was apparently (nonsignificantly) attenuated. At the end of a period of rapid frequency modulation, however, the N1 appeared marginally delayed and the following P2 significantly so (Fig. 6). This seems inexplicable by damage to the afferent auditory pathways, but suggests involvement of corticocortical connections or corticothalamic circuits responsible for analyzing the temporal sound pattern and generating a response when the expected frequency modulation, predicted on the basis of extrapolating the preceding few seconds, suddenly fails to occur. The prolonged latencies would suggest diffuse demyelination of these circuits, rather than axonal transection or neurodegeneration.

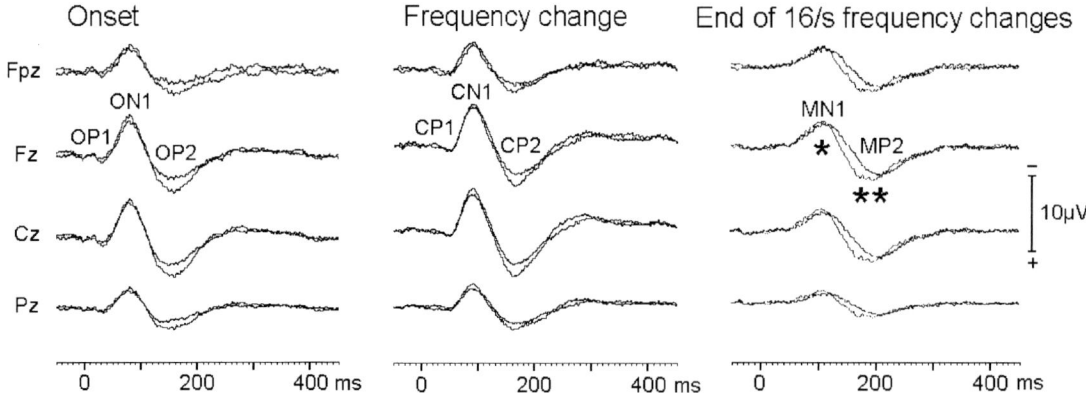

Figure 6 Group mean waveforms of long-latency AEPs to the onset of a complex harmonic tone, to frequency change of the same continuous tone by 12.3% every 2 seconds, and on resumption of steady frequencies after 2 seconds of 16-second frequency changes, left ear stimulation. The responses of the patients with MS (*darker lines*) are superimposed on those of normal controls. In the responses to onset and frequency change only the P2 amplitude is relatively (nonsignificantly) attenuated in the patients. At the end of the 16-second frequency changes the responses of the patient group are relatively delayed, significantly so for the MN1 ($^*P < 0.05$) and MP2 ($^{**}P < 0.001$). (Adapted from Jones et al., 2002.)

Still later peaks in the AEP waveform, termed event-related potentials (ERPs), reflect brain processes that are less "sensory" in nature but more concerned with conscious perception and cognition. In common with many other conditions causing mild or severe dementia, patients with MS may have delayed and/or attenuated ERPs, particularly the P300, when infrequent stimuli requiring an active response are interspersed with more frequent stimuli that are to be ignored. On average, the P300 tends to be delayed by 20 to 40 ms as compared with age-matched controls. The incidence or degree of P300 abnormality has been shown to be correlated with the MRI lesion load (Newton et al., 1989; Sailer et al., 2001), the degree of cognitive impairment (Giesser et al., 1992; Honig et al., 1992), and the duration of illness (Gil et al., 1993).

In one group of patients with MS of relatively recent onset (Sailer et al., 2001), the ERPs to auditory stimulation were apparently normal. However, Barrett et al. (1999) reported a 57% incidence of ERP abnormalities to auditory stimulation (similar to that found in other ERP studies of MS patients) among 21 patients who presented with clinically isolated optic neuritis. The P300 amplitude was shown to be lower in patients with a higher MRI lesion load (Fig. 7), but 4 of 7 patients with apparently normal MRI scans of the brain had abnormal ERPs. It was noted that in these patients, optic neuritis had occurred less than 1 month before the ERP test. It may be speculated, therefore, that factors associated with an active demyelinating lesion could have influenced the distributed brain processes responsible for the P300, in some cases exacerbated by preexisting, subclinical lesions.

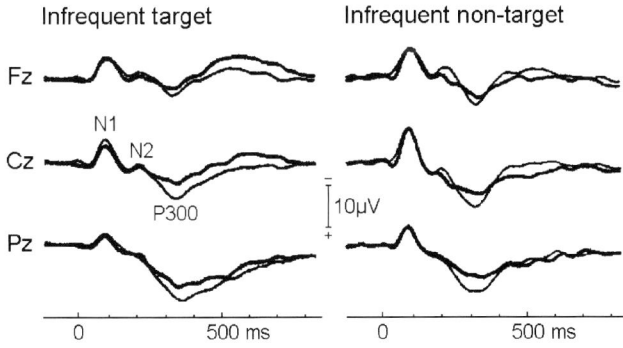

Figure 7 Group mean ERP waveforms to infrequent "target" and "nontarget" stimuli of 21 patients with clinically isolated optic neuritis, divided according to a high (*thicker lines*, 9 patients) or low (*thinner lines*, 12 patients) lesion load on T_2-weighted MRI of the brain. The difference in P300 amplitude was statistically significant at Pz, the patients with the higher lesion load having the lower amplitudes. Additionally, four of the patients with entirely normal MRI had ERPs that were outside normal limits. (Adapted from Barrett et al., 1999.)

VII. Disease Prognosis and Progression

The prognostic value of "clinically silent" VEP, SEP, and BAEP abnormalities in patients with suspected MS was assessed by Deltenre et al. (1984). The risk of progression to clinically definite MS after 5 or more years was 76% for patients with clinically silent VEP and SEP abnormalities, and as high as 86% for BAEP abnormalities, although VEPs were by far the most likely to demonstrate a clinically silent defect. In the study of Hume and Waxman (1988), 71% of patients suspected of having MS and who had clinically silent EP abnormalities had deteriorated clinically after a mean of 2.5 years; 48% had progressed to clinically definite MS. Of those without clinically silent EP abnormalities, only 16% deteriorated and 4% developed MS.

Mention has already been made of serial studies of patients with optic neuritis in which, over a follow-up period of 2 to 4 years, the prevalent tendency was for the VEPs of the acutely affected eye to recover. One of our own studies (Brusa et al., 1999) found a significant tendency for the responses of the fellow eye to deteriorate. In the longer term, there would seem to be little doubt that the overall tendency would be of deterioration. It would be interesting to discover whether specific lesions that are first detected while in a "subclinical" state eventually become symptomatic, and if so whether this occurs suddenly as a result of further inflammation or insidiously.

VIII. Conclusion

Much of the electrophysiological literature on the pathophysiology of MS has used optic neuritis as a model. The evidence generally supports the conventional view of MS as a disease in which episodes of acute, usually temporary conduction block are associated with local regions of inflammation. These are followed by longer periods of remission during which continuity of conduction is restored, although at reduced velocity, consistent with demyelination. There is also considerable evidence for long-term recovery of conduction delay in optic nerve axons, which can best be accounted for by remyelination.

A somewhat different pathophysiological process is perhaps suggested by the frequent finding of delayed conduction in optic nerves (or other pathways) for which there seems to be no evidence of an acute inflammatory attack. Evidence is limited as to whether such delays are due to macroscopic, circumscribed lesions, similar to those causing clinically eloquent effects but in which the phase of acute conduction block has somehow been bypassed, or to diffusely distributed lesions of much smaller scale whose acute effects were minimal and whose chronic manifestations happen, in sum, to mimic those of macroscopic plaques. The possibility cannot be excluded that such "clinically silent" lesions may involve entirely different pathological processes, perhaps originating within the affected neurons themselves.

In various regions of the nervous system, clinical and electrophysiological phenomena have been described that are difficult to account for in conventional terms of temporary conduction block as a result of inflammation, plaques of demyelination, and secondary axonal degeneration. These include the evidence for retinal ganglion cell dysfunction in the acute stage of optic neuritis and involvement of middle retinal layers in the longer term. The prevalence of fatigue as a symptom of MS lacks a convincing explanation in electrophysiological terms, and it remains a mystery why functional auditory impairment tends to be mild and infrequent, even in patients who have clear electrophysiological evidence for lesions in the auditory pathways of the brainstem. Finally, long-latency event-related potentials support the increasing evidence for diffuse cognitive impairment, even in the early stages of MS when MRI evidence for disseminated brain lesions is minimal. Although the macroscopic lesions seen in MRI are the most visible signs of disease in the early stages, and the most clinically and electrophysiologically eloquent when situated in sensorimotor structures, they should not cause us to neglect the subtle evidence for more diffuse changes of the normal-appearing white matter. At present, EPs are still the most effective way of demonstrating and investigating the neurophysiological defects responsible for neurological impairment; however, we have probably come close to the limit of their capabilities. In the future, we should be looking to refined functional imaging methods to better understand the neurophysiological correlates of MS symptomatology.

References

Barrett, G., Feinstein, A., Jones, S., Turano, G., and Youl, B. (1999). Event-related potentials in the assessment of cognitive function in multiple sclerosis. *In:* "Clinical Neurophysiology: From Receptors to Perception" (G. Comi, C. H. Lucking, J. Kimura, and P. M. Rossini, Eds.). *Electroenceph. Clin. Neurophysiol.*, Suppl. 50 , pp. 469–479. Elsevier, Amsterdam.

Beck, R. W., and Cleary, P. A. (1993). Optic Neuritis Treatment Trial. One year follow-up results. *Arch. Ophthalmol.* **111**, 773–775.

Berninger, T. A., and Heider, W. (1990). Pattern electroretinograms in optic neuritis during the acute stage and after remission. *Graefe's Arch. Clin. Exp. Ophthalmol.* **228**, 410–414.

Boniface, S. J., Mills, K. R., and Schubert, M. (1991). Responses of single spinal motoneurones to magnetic brain stimulation in healthy subjects and patients with multiple sclerosis. *Brain,* **114**, 643–662.

Bradshaw, K. (1992). Early onset of abnormality of the pattern-evoked ERG in patients with optic neuritis. *Clin. Vis. Sci.* **7**, 313–-325.

Brusa, A., Jones, S. J., and Plant, G. (2001). Long-term remyelination after optic neuritis: A 2-year visual evoked potential and psychophysical serial study. *Brain* **124**, 468–479.

Brusa, A., Jones, S. J., Kapoor, R., Miller, D. H., and Plant, G. T. (1999). Long term recovery and fellow eye deterioration after optic neuritis, determined by serial visual evoked potentials. *J. Neurol.* **246**, 776–782.

Chiappa, K. H. (Ed.). (1997). "Evoked Potentials in Clinical Medicine," 3rd edition, Lippincott-Raven, Philadelphia.

Cohen, S. N., Syndulko, K., Tourtelotte, W. W., and Potvin, A. R. (1980). Critical frequency of photic driving in the diagnosis of multiple sclerosis. *Arch. Neurol.* **37**, 80–83.

Craner, M. J., Lo, A. C., Black, J. A., and Waxman, S. G. (2003). Abnormal sodium channel distribution in a model of inflammatory demyelination. *Brain* **126**, 1552–1561.

Deltenre, P., van Nechel, C., Strul, S., and Ketelaer, P. (1984). A five-year prospective study on the value of multimodal evoked potentials and blink reflex, as an aid to the diagnosis of multiple sclerosis. *In:* "Evoked Potentials II" (R.H. Nodar and C. Barber, Eds), pp. 603–608. Butterworth, Boston.

Diem, R., Tschirne, A., and Bärn, M. (2003). Decreased amplitudes in multiple sclerosis patients with normal visual acuity: a VEP study. *J. Clin. Neurosci.* **10**, 67–70.

Evangelou, N., Konz, D., Esiri, M. M., Smith, S., Palace, J., and Matthews, P. M. (2001). Size-selective neuronal changes in the anterior optic pathways suggest a differential susceptibility to injury in multiple sclerosis. *Brain* **124**, 1813–1820.

Falsini, B., Bardocci, A., Porciatti, V., Bolzani, R., and Piccardi, M. (1992). Macular dysfunction in multiple sclerosis revealed by steady-state flicker and pattern ERGs. *Electroenceph. Clin. Neurophysiol.* **82**, 53–59.

Falsini, B., Porrello, G., Porciatti, V., Fadda, A., Salgarello, T., and Piccardi, M. (1999). The spatial tuning of steady state pattern electroretinogram in multiple sclerosis. *Eur. J. Neurol.* **6**, 151–162.

Fang, J. P., Donahue, S. P., and Lin, R. H. (1999). Global visual field involvement in optic neuritis. *Am. J. Ophthalmol.* **128**, 554–565.

Ferguson, B., Matyszak, M. K., Esiri, M. M., and Perry, V. H. (1997). Axonal damage in acute multiple sclerosis lesions. *Brain* **120**, 393–399.

Giesser, B. S., Schroeder, M. M., LaRocca, N. G., Kurtzberg, D., Ritter, W., Vaughan, H. G., and Scheinberg, L. C. (1992). Endogenous event-related potentials as indices of dementia in multiple sclerosis. *Electroenceph. Clin. Neurophysiol.* **82**, 820–329.

Gil, R., Zai, L., Neau, J. P., Jonveaux, T., Agbo, C., Rosolacci, T., Burbaud, P., and Ingrand, P. (1993). Event-related auditory evoked potentials and multiple sclerosis. *Electroenceph. Clin. Neurophysiol.* **88**, 182–187.

Graham, E. M., Francis, D. A., Sanders, M. D., and Rudge, P. (1989). Ocular inflammatory changes in established multiple sclerosis. *J. Neurol. Neurosurg. Psychiatry* **52**, 1360–1363.

Halliday, A. M. (1993). The visual evoked potential in the investigation of diseases of the optic nerve. *In:* "Evoked Potentials in Clinical Testing" (A. M. Halliday, Ed.), 2nd edition, pp.195–278. Churchill-Livingstone, Edinburgh.

Halliday, A. M., and Wakefield, G. S. (1963). Cerebral evoked potentials in patients with dissociated sensory loss. *J. Neurol. Neurosurg. Psychiatry* **26**, 211–219.

Halliday, A. M., McDonald, W. I., and Mushin, J. (1972). Delayed visual evoked response in optic neuritis. *Lancet* **I**, 982–985.

Halliday, A. M., McDonald, W. I., and Mushin, J. (1973). Visual evoked responses in diagnosis of multiple sclerosis. *Br. Med. J.* **4**, 661–664.

Hely, M. A., McManis, P. G., Walsh, J. C., and McLeod, J. G. (1986). Visual evoked responses and ophthalmological examination in optic neuritis. A follow-up study. *J. Neurol. Sci.* **75**, 275–283.

Holder, G. E. (1991). The incidence of abnormal pattern electroretinography in optic nerve demyelination. *Electroenceph. Clin. Neurophysiol.* **78**, 18–26.

Honig, L. S., Ramsay, R. E., and Sheremata, W. A. (1992). Event-related P300 in multiple sclerosis. Relation to magnetic resonance imaging and cognitive impairment. *Arch Neurol.* **49**, 44–50.

Hume, A. L., and Waxman, S. (1988). Evoked potentials in suspected multiple sclerosis: Diagnostic value and prediction of clinical course. *J. Neurol. Sci.* **83**, 191–210.

Jones, S. J. (1982). Clinical applications of short-latency somatosensory evoked potentials. *Ann. N. Y. Acad. Sci.* **388**, 369–386.

Jones, S. J. (1993a). Visual evoked potentials after optic neuritis. Effect of time interval, age and disease dissemination. *J. Neurol.* **240**, 489–494.

Jones, S. J. (1993b). Somatosensory evoked potentials II: Clinical observations and applications. *In:* "Evoked Potentials in Clinical Testing" (A. M. Halliday, Ed.), 2nd edition, pp. 421–466. Churchill-Livingstone, Edinburgh.

Jones, S. J., Sprague, L., and Vaz Pato, M. (2002). Electrophysiological evidence for a defect in the processing of temporal sound patterns in multiple sclerosis. *J. Neurol. Neurosurg. Psychiatry* **73**, 561–567.

Kapoor, R., Miller, D. H., Jones, S. J., Plant, G. T., Brusa, A., Gass, A., Hawkins, C. P., Page, R., Wood, N. W., Compston, D. A. S., Moseley, I. F., and McDonald, W. I. (1998). Effects of intravenous methylprednisolone on outcome in MRI-based prognostic subgroups in acute optic neuritis. *Neurology* **50**, 230–237.

Lightman, S., McDonald, W. I., Bird, A. C., Francis, D. A., Hoskins, A., Batchelor, J. R., and Halliday, A. M. (1987). Retinal venous sheathing in multiple sclerosis. *Brain* **110**, 405–414.

Matthews, W. B., and Esiri, M. (1979). Multiple sclerosis plaque related to abnormal somatosensory evoked potentials. *J. Neurol. Neurosurg. Psychiatry* **42**, 940–942.

Matthews, W. B., and Small, D. G. (1979). Serial recording of visual and somatosensory evoked potentials in multiple sclerosis. *J. Neurol. Sci.* **40**, 11–21.

Matthews, W. B., and Small, M. (1983). Prolonged follow-up of abnormal visual evoked potentials in multiple sclerosis: evidence for delayed recovery. *J. Neurol. Neurosurg. Psychiatry* **46**, 639–643.

Mills, K. R. (1999). "Magnetic Stimulation of the Human Nervous System." Oxford University Press, Oxford.

Mitchell, J. D., Hansen, S., McInnes, A., and Campbell, F. W. (1983). The recovery cycle of the pattern visual evoked potential in normal subjects and patients with multiple sclerosis. *Electroenceph. Clin. Neurophysiol.* **56**, 309–315.

Newton, M. R., Barrett, G., Callanan, M. M., and Towell, A. D. (1989). Cognitive event-related potentials in multiple sclerosis. *Brain* **112**, 1637–1660.

Papakostopoulos, D., Fotiou, F., Dean Hart, J. C., and Banerji, N. K. (1989). The electroretinogram in multiple sclerosis and demyelinating optic neuritis. *Electroenceph. Clin. Neurophysiol.* **74**, 1–10.

Parisi, V., Manni, G., Spadaro, M., Colacino, G., Restuccia, R., March, S., Bucci, M. G., and Pierelli, F. (1999). Correlation between morphological and functional retinal impairment in multiple sclerosis patients. *Invest. Ophthalmol. Vis. Sci.* **40**, 2520–2527.

Plant, G. T., Hess, R. F., and Thomas, S. J. (1986). The pattern evoked electroretinogram in optic neuritis: A combined psychophysical and electrophysiological study. *Brain* **109**, 469–490.

Plant, G. T., Kermode, A. G., Turano, G., Moseley, I. F., Miller, D. H., MacManus, D. G., Halliday, A. M., and McDonald, W. I. (1992). Symptomatic retrochiasmal lesions in multiple sclerosis: Clinical features, visual evoked potentials, and magnetic resonance imaging. *Neurology* **42**, 68–76.

Porciatti, V., and Sartucci, F. (1996). Retinal and cortical evoked responses to chromatic contrast stimuli. Specific losses in both eyes of patients with multiple sclerosis and unilateral optic neuritis. *Brain* **119**, 723–740.

Prineas, J. W., Barnard, R. O., Kwon, E. E., Sharer, L. R., and Cho, E.-S. (1993). Multiple sclerosis: remyelination of nascent lesions. *Ann. Neurol.* **33**, 137–155.

Ramani, V., Torres, F., and Lowenson, R. (1984). Critical frequency of photic driving in the diagnosis of multiple sclerosis. *Arch. Neurol.* **41**, 752–755.

Restuccia, D., and Mauguière, F. (1991). The contribution of median nerve SEPs in the functional assessment of the cervical spinal cord in syringomyelia. A study of 24 patients. *Brain* **114**, 361–380.

Rinalduzzi, S., Brusa, A., and Jones, S. J. (2001). Variation of visual evoked potential delay to stimulation of central, nasal and temporal regions of the macula in optic neuritis. *J. Neurol. Neurosurg. Psychiatry* **70**, 28–35.

Sailer, M., Heinze, H. J., Tendolkar, I., Decker, U., Kreye, O., von Rolbicki, U., and Munte, T. F. (2001). Influence of cerebral lesion volume and lesion distribution on event-related potentials in multiple sclerosis. *J. Neurol.* **248**, 1049–1055.

Sanders, E. A., Volkers, A. C., van der Poel, J. C., and van Lith, G. H. (1987). Visual function and pattern visual evoked response in optic neuritis. *Br. J. Ophthalmol.* **71**, 602–608.

Sheean, G. L., Murray, N. M. F., Rothwell, J. C., Miller, D. H., and Thompson, A. J. (1997). An electrophysiological study of the mechanism of fatigue in multiple sclerosis. *Brain* **120**, 299–315.

Turano, G., Jones, S. J., Miller, D. H., Kakigi, R., du Boulay, G. H., and McDonald, W. I. (1991). Correlation of SEP abnormalities with brain and cervical cord MRI in multiple sclerosis. *Brain* **114**, 663–681.

Van der Poel, J. C., Jones, S. J., and Miller, D. H. (1988). Sound lateralization, brainstem auditory evoked potentials and magnetic resonance imaging in multiple sclerosis. *Brain* **111**, 1453–1474.

Versino, M., Bergamaschi, R., Romani, A., Banfi, P., Callieco, R., Citterio, A., Gerosa, E., and Cosi, V. (1992). Middle latency auditory evoked potentials improve the detection of abnormalities along auditory pathways in multiple sclerosis patients. *Electroenceph. Clin. Neurophysiol.* **84**, 296–299.

Werring, D. J., Bullmore, E. T., Toosy, A. T., Miller, D. H., Barker, G. J., MacManus, D. G., Brammer, M. J., Giampietro, V. P., Brusa, A., Brex, P. A., Mosely, I. F., Plant, G. T., McDonald, W. I., and Thompson, A. J. (2000). Recovery from optic neuritis is associated with a change in the distribution of cerebral response to visual stimulation: a functional magnetic resonance imaging study. *J. Neurol. Neurosurg. Psychiatry* **68**, 441–449.

Youl, B. D., Turano, G., Miller, D. H., Towell, A. D., MacManus, D. G., Moore, S. G., Jones, S. J., Barrett, G., Kendall, B. E., Moseley, I. F., Tofts, P. S., Halliday, A. M., and McDonald, W. I. (1991). The pathophysiology of acute optic neuritis. *Brain* **114**, 2437–2450.

17

Inflammation and Axon Degeneration

V. Hugh Perry, M.A., D.Phil.

I. Introduction

Multiple sclerosis (MS) is the archetypal inflammatory demyelinating disease of the central nervous system (CNS). It is widely believed to be an autoimmune disease in which the immune system attacks specific elements of the CNS after breakdown of immune tolerance. The major targets for this immune system assault are thought to be components of the myelin sheath, or the oligodendrocytes themselves. A complex interaction of genetic and environmental factors leads to disease onset in affected individuals, but the etiology of the disease remains unknown (Compston and Coles, 2002).

For several decades before the 1990s, pathological investigations into CNS tissue damage in MS focused on the mech-

anisms of damage to the oligodendrocyte and myelin sheath by cells of the immune system. Relatively little attention was paid to axon damage despite the fact that axon injury had been described as early as the 1880s (Korneck and Lassmann, 1999). Whatever the influences that resulted in the relative neglect of axon pathology in MS, it is now abundantly clear that axon injury occurs early in the disease process and that it is a significant part of the pathology. It seems possible, as suggested by Kornek and Lassmann (1999), that the recent studies added a new dimension to the understanding of this problem by providing accurate quantitative data of the timing and extent of axon injury. Critical data that have triggered this renascence of interest in axon injury have come from a number of different lines of investigation.

Tissue loss and white matter damage can be detected *in vivo* in patients with MS by imaging modalities including magnetic resonance imaging (MRI) (Loseff et al., 1996), magnetic resonance spectroscopy (Davie et al., 1994), and magnetization transfer imaging (Filippi, 2003). The early studies applying these techniques provided a clear impetus for the application of modern histopathological techniques to reinvestigate axon injury in MS. Evidence of ongoing axon injury can be detected in MS postmortem tissue samples using sensitive immunocytochemical detection of axon end-bulbs (Fig. 1), a hallmark of axon injury.

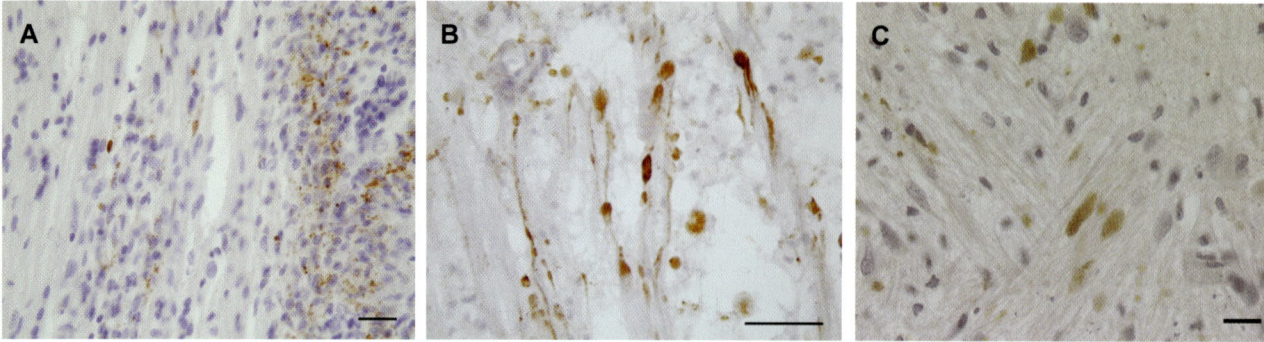

Figure 1 Axon end-bulbs as revealed by immunocytochemistry for amyloid precursor protein present in (**A**) a rat EAE lesion 30 days after the initiation of disease, (**C**) in fiber tracts of brain tissue from an MS patient. (**B**) End-bulbs after a traumatic transection injury to rat spinal cord. Scale bar = 50 μm.

The number of injured axons, many presumed to be actual transections, was correlated with the intensity of the inflammatory response (Ferguson et al., 1997; Trapp et al., 1998). There were large numbers of injured axons in acute and chronic acute lesions, although few in chronic lesions.

The degree of axon injury has now been quantified in several major fiber tracts and is extensive in the corpus callosum (Evangelou et al., 2000) and spinal cord (Bjartmar et al., 2003). Axon injury is also present in animal models of MS (Korneck et al., 2000; Bjartmar et al., 2003). Furthermore, imaging studies have shown that there is significant loss of tissue and/or axons from the brains of person with MS and the loss of tissue correlates with clinical disability (Brex et al., 2002).

In short, it is now apparent that axon injury occurs early in the evolution of MS pathology, continues throughout the evolution of the disease, is a significant part of the pathology, and likely contributes to the irreversible accumulation of neurological deficits. These observations raise many important new questions in MS research, and indeed the outcomes of this research will likely impact on other neurological diseases. We need to understand the cellular and molecular events by which inflammation in the CNS leads to axon injury. We need to identify the secondary consequences of axon injury distal to the site of injury. Our understanding of the events of axon injury in MS are rudimentary and indeed axon injury has been somewhat neglected in many neurological diseases (Coleman and Perry, 2002; Medana and Esiri, 2003). In stroke, for example, after many years of research focused on protection of the neuronal cell soma, there is now recognition that preservation of axons injured by the ischemic insult is one of the major challenges (Dewar et al., 1999).

II. Mechanisms of Axon Injury

The cellular components in MS pathology that result in axon injury include not only the contribution of the various

inflammatory cells, and the inflammatory mediators that they secrete, but also different cellular and molecular components of the target itself. We consider first each of the inflammatory cells that may be involved in axon injury.

A. Cellular Immune Components

1. T-Cells

It is widely held that MS is an autoimmune disease in which immunological tolerance to one or more CNS antigens is broken down, or dysregulated (Wekerle et al., 1994). Thus, T-cells play a central role in the targeting of the immune system to the CNS, and it is thought that the immune assault is directed at myelin antigens. It is not known whether during the evolution of MS, or in experimental models of MS, the axons eventually become a specific immunological target. As tissue, including axons, degenerates, there may be epitope spreading (Tuohy et al., 1998) leading to the generation of axon antigen-specific T-cell populations. In this regard, the role of both Th1 and Th2 cells needs to be considered. Although the Th1 component of the inflammatory response is usually believed to lead to tissue damage and the Th2 component to a protective response, it is clear that Th2 cytokines have a profound influence on the macrophage phenotype (Gordon, 2003). Macrophages activated by Th1 cytokines, such as interferon-γ, secrete molecules known to cause tissue damage (see later), whereas macrophages activated by Th2 cytokines have an enhanced capacity for antigen presentation and promoting humoral immunity (Gordon, 2003). Enhanced antigen presentation and humoral immunity may both contribute to axon injury.

Previous studies have demonstrated that the degree of axon injury within the plaque is related to the intensity of the inflammatory response (Ferguson et al., 1997; Trapp et al., 1998). It is known that as MS plaques mature, the proportions of T-cells and macrophages change, but it is not known how this impacts on axon injury. In a Th1 delayed-type-hypersensitivity (DTH) lesion in the CNS directed against the mycobacterium bacillus Calmette-Guérin, and thus in the absence of an immunologically specific attack on axons *per se*, the axons are injured in a bystander fashion (Matyszak and Perry 1995; Matyszak et al., 1997) possibly releasing novel axon antigens.

There is some evidence to suggest that CD8 T-cells may have a particular capacity to damage axons (Bitsch et al., 2000). Direct evidence implicating populations of CD8 T-cells specific for axon antigens have not been described.

2. B-lymphocytes

The potential role of the B-lymphocyte in axon injury in the CNS has received little attention. Identification of myelin oligodendrocyte glycoprotein (MOG) as a target for antibody-mediated demyelination in rodent and primate models of experimental autoimmune encephalomyelitis (EAE) (Genain et al., 1995; Linington et al., 1988) has provided a clear example of the role of B-cells in immune-mediated pathologies in the CNS. Although antibodies are not directed against the axon in MOG-induced EAE, there is evidence to suggest that these antibodies can exacerbate the axon injury by activating the complement cascade (Mead et al., 2002, 2004).

Antibodies directed against components of axons have been detected in the cerebrospinal fluid and serum of individuals with MS (Eikelenboom et al., 2003), but it is wholly unclear whether these antibodies are pathogenic or simply a secondary consequence of the tissue damage. There is a now well-described precedent for antibody-mediated axon injury in the peripheral nervous system disease acute motor axon neuropathy (Hafer-Macko et al., 1996) (see Chapter 25). The mechanisms by which these antibodies cause injury are discussed next.

3. Macrophages

Macrophages attack and kill cells through both contact-dependent and contact-independent mechanisms (Kreutz et al., 2002) and are thus likely key players in axon injury. It should be recognized, however, that the development of cytotoxic macrophages is a multistep process requiring several steps, possibly sequential steps, in their activation. Monocytes entering the CNS microenvironment under the influence of the relevant chemokines (Trebst et al., 2001) differentiate to macrophages and may then be activated by T-cell-derived cytokines (e.g., interferon-γ), by the phagocytosis of myelin debris through the Fc receptor, and also by complement products. The evidence that macrophages are significant players in axon injury comes from studies showing that the number of injured axons in MS lesions correlates with the number of macrophages present within acute, acute chronic, and chronic lesions (Ferguson et al., 1997; Trapp et al., 1998). In these studies, no attempt was made to distinguish between the contribution of macrophages derived from the resident microglia or the recently recruited monocytes. In a model of EAE, it has been suggested that lesions infiltrated by monocyte-derived macrophages have a greater degree of axon damage than lesions dominated by microglia (Storch et al., 2002). There is also considerable heterogeneity in the morphology and phenotype of mononuclear phagocytes within demyelinating lesions, and it has been suggested that CD8+ macrophages and microglia play a specific role in myelin and axon damage (Schroeter et al., 2003).

Although axon injury has been detected in both acute and chronic acute lesions and associated with large numbers of inflammatory cells, it is not known how ongoing axon injury in a patient with MS relates to disease activity as detected by MRI gadolinium-enhancing lesions, or other imaging techniques. There is evidence from an experimental focal DTH lesion within the brain (Matyszak and Perry, 1995) that these Th1 T-cell and macrophage-dominated lesions continue to grow in size and to generate axon injury in the absence of detectable gadolinium enhancement (Newman et al., 2001). Thus, lesion activity including axon injury may persist behind the intact blood-brain barrier. The poor correlation between the load of enhancing lesions and the clinical score, or progression, is consistent with these observations (Giovannoni et al., 2000).

Molecules that have been shown to cause axon injury include secretory products of macrophages (see later), but it is unlikely that the full spectrum has been identified, or their relative importance established. It is not known whether macrophages make, or need to make, direct contact with axons to cause injury to them. The possible role of activated macrophages in white matter injury in the brain has recently been reviewed with regard to diseases as diverse as HIV-dementia, HTLV-1-associated myelopathy, cerebral malaria, and other white matter diseases (Medana and Esiri, 2003).

4. Dendritic Cells

In the normal CNS parenchyma there are no dendritic cells (Matyszak and Perry, 1996), but they are recruited in small numbers to inflammatory lesions in the CNS in both experimental models and MS (Matyszak and Perry, 1996; Plumb et al., 2003). As has been discussed elsewhere (Perry, 1998), if these cells have the capacity to migrate out of the CNS carrying neoantigens released from ongoing axon damage, then they may contribute to epitope spreading and an immune assault on axons. At the present time, however, there is no direct evidence that dendritic cells migrate from parenchymal lesions to peripheral tissues.

B. Cellular Axon Components

1. Axon Heterogeneity

The majority of axons in the human CNS are myelinated and the thickness of the myelin sheath is proportional to the diameter of the axon (Hirano and Llena, 1995). Intuitively one might expect that the myelin sheath would act to "protect" the axon from the potentially damaging effects of inflammatory cells and their secretory products. Axons are not uniform along their length, however, and different axon populations may differ in their susceptibility to injury. All myelinated axons of the CNS have nodes of Ranvier where the myelin sheath is absent. The node of Ranvier could be a susceptible site for injury (Fig. 2) in an inflammatory milieu; it appears to be particularly susceptible to injury after axon stretch (Maxwell and Graham, 1997) and also in the peripheral nervous system (PNS) to antibody-mediated injury (Griffin et al., 1996). The thinning of the axon, the lack of the myelin sheath, and the accumulation of mitochondria may all predispose the nodal region to injury. Another region of the axon that might also be important in this regard is the axon terminal region where the axon loses its myelin sheath as it branches to form the profuse ending typical of many axons (Fig. 2). Whether the terminals or their branch points are susceptible regions is not known. The axon hillock is also exposed and may be susceptible to injury in lesions that border or lie within the gray matter. There is evidence that small-caliber axons are more susceptible to injury than large-caliber axons (Medana and Esiri, 2003).

In addition to heterogeneity of axon size and possible focal points of susceptibility, axons have intrinsic differences in that they arise from different neuron populations, each of which has its own molecular phenotype. An example of this heterogeneity is to be found in the different neu-

rotransmitters that axons transport to their terminals. The potential significance of this variable is raised by recent studies investigating the impact of inflammation on neurons of the substantia nigra. A focal innate inflammatory response, induced by the local injection of endotoxin into the normal brain, does not lead to significant neuronal degeneration except when the endotoxin is injected into the substantia nigra (Herrera et al., 2000) when large numbers of the tyrosine hydroxylase containing neurons die. Whether the susceptibility of the dopaminergic cell bodies is reflected in their axonal response to an inflammatory challenge is not known, and whether this susceptibility is to be found in other populations during different forms of inflammation is also unknown.

2. Demyelinated Axons

It is a *sine qua non* of MS pathology that there are regions of CNS fiber tracts that are demyelinated. It is a matter of considerable importance to discover whether the loss of the myelin sheath makes axons more susceptible to injury, and how large this effect may be since strategies to promote remyelination may turn out to be also axon protective (Franklin, 2002). There have been a number of suggestions that the severity of demyelination and axon degeneration are related. However, it has not yet been demonstrated with any degree of confidence that for a given degree of inflammation, the axon degeneration is more likely in a demyelinated region than in a myelinated region. Whether populations of unmyelinated fibers are more or less susceptible to inflam-

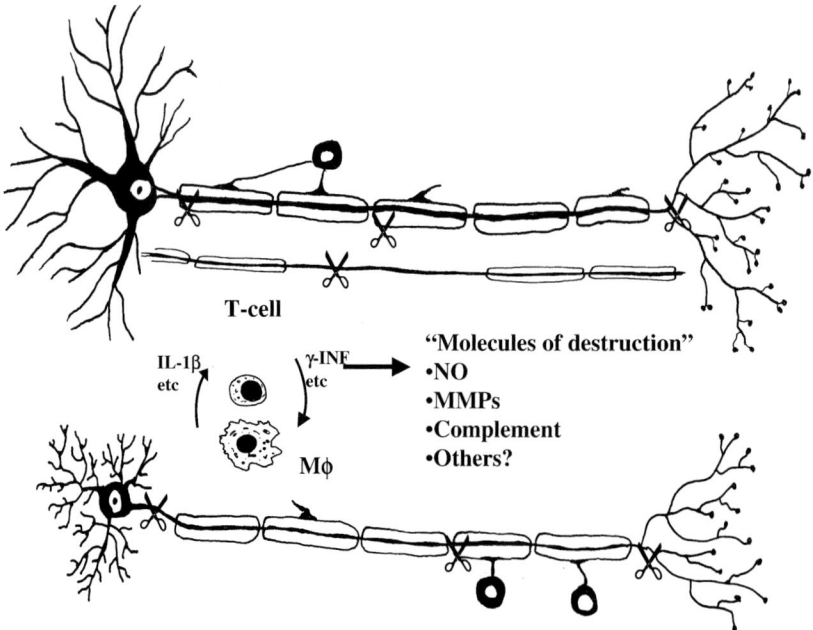

Figure 2 Possible sites of axon injury sensors during an immune mediated assault on the CNS by T-cells and macrophages. Axon injury may occur at the nodes of Ranvier, the axon terminal, or the axon hillock. Fine-caliber axons appear to be more susceptible than large-caliber axons to injury. It has been suggested that demyelinated axons may be more susceptible to injury by inflammatory cells.

mation-mediated injury has also not been investigated. This is of some importance given that unmyelinated fibers are to be found throughout the CNS including superficial cortical layers where large lesions may occur in MS (Peterson et al., 2001).

Axon injury and degeneration are a consequence of the inflammatory response around the axons, but an alternative view has also prevailed for many years. This view suggests that it is the consequences of demyelination *per se* that leads to axon degeneration. It is well established that the myelin-forming cells have a profound effect upon the axon, influencing the axon cytoskeleton and distribution of ion channels (Salzer, 1995) (see Chapter 8), and genetic abnormalities of the myelin sheath may lead to axon degeneration. Although it is not immediately clear how loss of myelin from only a relatively small portion of the axon would produce catastrophic degeneration of the whole axon, it is possible that the local signaling interactions are key. It is possible that local loss of the myelin leads to alterations in the cytoskeleton that alter axon transport in subtle ways. These changes in axon homeostasis may eventually lead to axon degeneration or make the axon susceptible to previously relatively benign inflammatory mediators.

C. Molecular Immune Components

In the same manner that the cellular components leading to axon degeneration reflect both the different inflammatory cells and also the properties of the target axons, so the molecular mechanisms involved in axon injury reflect both the secretory products of the inflammatory cells, "the molecules of destruction," and the response of molecular components of the axon. At the present time little is known about the spectrum of molecules secreted by inflammatory cells that are involved in axon injury in MS. Even less is known about the molecular targets of these "molecular scissors" on, or within, axons of the CNS.

1. Antibodies and Complement

Immunologically specific injury to the axon may come about by the action of antibodies binding to axon antigens. A precedent comes from studies of the PNS where it has been shown that antibodies against axon antigens play a critical role in acute motor axon neuropathy (Hafer-Macko et al., 1996) (see Chapter 25). Antibodies to the ganglioside GD1a bind preferentially to motor axons; GD1b antibodies bind to dorsal root ganglion cell axons (Gong et al., 2002). If the antibodies activate the complement cascade, this provides a mechanism by which selected classes of axons may be injured. Recent evidence shows, however, that antibody-dependent activation of complement plays a role in axon damage even when the antibodies are not directed against the axon, as in MOG-induced EAE (Mead et al., 2002, 2004). In rats in which activation of the membrane attack complex is prevented by the deletion of C6, there is neither demyelination

nor axon injury, despite the invasion of the CNS by mononuclear cells (Mead et al., 2002). In contrast, deletion of CD59a, a key regulator of membrane attack complex assembly, led to enhanced axon injury in MOG EAE (Mead et al., 2004).

2. Cytotoxic T-Cell Products

There is at present no evidence that in patients with MS there exist specific T-cell populations directed specifically against axon antigens, but if such cells exist, this would add a new dimension to our understanding of the pathogenesis of MS. There is indirect evidence to suggest that CD8 T-cells may be involved in axon injury in the MS brain (Bitsch et al., 2000). There is evidence from *in vitro* studies that granules contained in CD8 T-cells are directed toward neurites, which may be damaged by soluble mediators contained in the granules (Neumann et al., 2002). There is little direct evidence to implicate either perforin or granzyme but the cytotoxic mechanism may vary with cell type and conditions.

3. Free Radicals

Macrophages activated by Th1 cytokines express inducible nitric oxide, and the macrophages and microglia associated with MS lesions are no exception (De Groot et al.,1997; Bitsch et al., 2000). The studies of Smith and colleagues have identified nitric oxide as a potential mediator of axon injury in MS (Smith et al., 2001) (see Chapter 18). Their studies show that when axons are exposed to nitric oxide (NO), at concentrations believed to represent physiological concentrations *in vivo*, the axons are not injured but when the axon is exposed to the same levels of NO and stimulated to conduct a high frequency train of impulses, this may lead to axon degeneration. The precise mechanism by which the NO damages axons is unclear, but it is possible that the mitochondria are the primary target, as it has been demonstrated that NO can inhibit neuronal energy production (Brorson et al., 1999). It would be of considerable interest to know whether there is significant mitochondrial damage in axons in an inflammatory milieu and whether this leads to activation of other potentially cytotoxic cascades (Mattson, 2000).

4. Matrix Metalloproteases

There has been much interest in the possible role of matrix metalloproteases (MMPs) in MS. Although this family of molecules derive their name from their role in modeling components of the extracellular matrix, it is clear that they have diverse other roles, and this is nowhere more true than in the CNS (Yong et al., 2001). MMPs, in particular MMP-9 and MMP-2, have been implicated in the migration of T-cells across the blood-brain barrier and also in the degradation of myelin proteins (Hartung and Kieseier, 2000). When MMP-2, -9, or -7, which are known to be expressed in mononuclear cells in both MS and EAE lesions, are microinjected into fiber tracts of the rodent

CNS, they produce rapid and extensive transection of axons (Newman et al., 2001). It is not known how these molecules mediate their effects on the axon, whether it is a consequence of their direct action on molecules on the axon plasma membrane, or a consequence of local destruction of the surrounding matrix. The degradation of the matrix surrounding the axon may be of import and may lead to an anoikis-like axon degeneration (Grossmann, 2002).

5. Cytokines

A number of schemas of axon degeneration in MS have suggested that cytokines may play a role in axon degeneration (Bjartmar et al., 2003; Medana and Esiri, 2003). At the present time, there is little evidence to implicate cytokines *per se* in axon degeneration. Studies on neuronal cell degeneration in models of acute brain injury show that the cytokines interleukin-1β and tumor necrosis factor-α exert their effects on neurons that are in some manner already compromised (Allan and Rothwell, 2001), and a similar situation may apply to compromised axons. In mice with the gene for tumor necrosis factor-α, deleted injured PNS axons persist slightly longer than in wild-type mice, suggesting that this cytokine may play a part in the degeneration cascade of already-injured axons (Siebert and Bruck, 2003).

D. Molecular Axon Components

Although a number of molecules, or classes of molecules, secreted by activated immune cells have been implicated in axon injury in MS, the early events leading to transection of the axon have not been studied in any depth. The appearance of the axon end-bulb already indicates that axon injury has proceeded to an irreversible state. The sealing of the ends of an injured axon involves calcium-dependent processes including activation of calpain and phospholipase A2 (Howard et al., 1999; Geddis and Rehder, 2003), but we know little of the molecular events that precede this catastrophic event.

1. Active Axon Degeneration

Axon degeneration accompanies an extraordinary diversity of injury to, and diseases of, the nervous system, and a favored model to study the mechanisms that underlie axon degeneration has been the study of degeneration of the distal segment of a transected axon, wallerian degeneration. The morphological events that appear in wallerian degeneration are found at the end stage of almost every form of axon degeneration, suggesting that there is a final common pathway in the degeneration process (Griffin et al., 1996). It was long thought that the axon degenerated as a consequence of separation from the cell body leading to a withering of the distal process, an essentially passive process (Finn et al., 2000). The degeneration of the axon was also linked in acute transection to an influx of calcium that activated calcium-

activated proteases within the axoplasm, which in turn degraded the axon cytoskeletal elements (Schlaepfer and Hasler, 1979).

The serendipitous discovery of a strain of mouse carrying a mutation that dramatically slows wallerian degeneration (Lunn et al., 1989) has radically changed our views of how axons degenerate (Finn et al., 2000; Coleman and Perry, 2002). In wild-type mice, and indeed all mammals, the axon segment distal to an injury normally undergoes wallerian degeneration within a few days of transection. In the mutant Wld^s mice the axons of both CNS and PNS neurons may survive for several weeks separated from the cell body (Fig. 3). This simple observation tells us that axon degeneration in wild-type axons must be an active autodestructive process akin to programmed-cell-death or apoptosis of the cell body of neurons and other cells. The mutation in these mice has now been identified, and the Wld^s gene was found to be a chimeric protein formed from UbE4b, an ubiquitin ligase, and nicotinamide mononucleotide adenylyltransferase (Nmnat), an NAD synthesizing enzyme (Mack et al., 2001). The mechanism of action of this gene is not known, but it clearly implicates the ubiquitin-proteasome pathway in axon degeneration (see later).

The programmed-cell-death-like process in axons shares some similarities with the apoptotic cascades described at the neuronal cell soma, but there are also notable differences. Transected neurites undergoing wallerian degeneration *in vitro* express phosphatidylserine residues on the plasma membrane as detected by Annexin V, undergo blebbing, and lose their mitochondrial potential before degeneration (Sievers et al., 2003). Manipulations that protect the cell bodies of some neurons from apoptosis, such as raising extracellular potassium or intracellular cyclic adenosine monophosphate, also protect transected neurites *in vitro* (Buckmaster et al, 1995). However, the degeneration of neurites *in vitro* is not protected by caspase inhibitors (Finn et al., 2000; Sievers et al, 2003), and axons *in vivo* are not protected by overexpression of Bcl-2 (Burne et al., 1996), although they are protected in Bax deficient mice (Dong et al 2003; J.W. McDonald, personal communication).

Thus, the "molecules of destruction" secreted by inflammatory cells in the MS lesion act on axons that contain the biochemical machinery that maintains the balance between life and death of the axon. These pathways act in an analogous fashion to, but distinct from, the pro-apoptic and anti-apoptotic pathways maintaining the balance between life and death of the cell soma. It is important to note that the protection of the axon in wallerian degeneration by the Wld^s gene has now been shown to extend to protection of axons subjected to taxol toxicity (Wang et al. 2003), to protection of axons in a mouse model of motorneuron disease (Ferri et al., 2003), and protection of axons from the axon degeneration present in a dysmyelinating mutant, the Po knockout mouse (Samsam et al., 2003). A simple hypothesis is that secretory

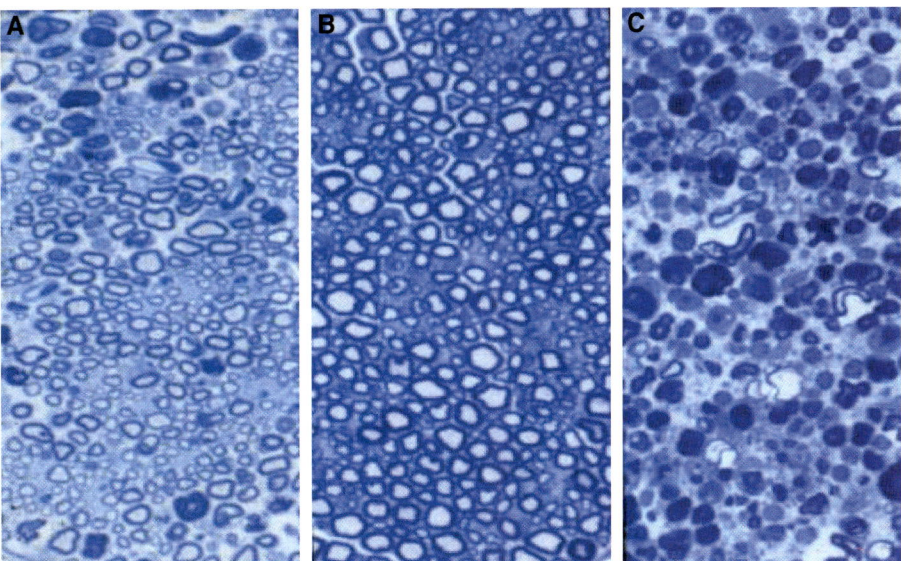

Figure 3 The remarkable phenotype of the Wld[s] mouse (Lunn et al., 1989). Central panel (**B**) illustrates the appearance of the normal sciatic nerve in a 1-μm semithin section stained with toluidine blue. Panel (**C**) illustrates the appearance of the distal nerve of a wild-type mouse nerve undergoing wallerian degeneration 7 days after transection. Panel (**A**) shows the remarkable preservation of the distal axon segment 7 days after sciatic nerve transection in the Wld[s] mouse.

products of inflammatory cells, or contact with inflammatory cells, leads to local activation of these autodestruction pathways in the axon, and thus, a local axon transection.

2. Axon Calcium Levels

The loss of Ca^{2+} homeostasis in the axon has long been proposed as an early event in axon degeneration (Schlaepfer and Hasler, 1979). Alterations in ion homeostasis leading to increased permeability of the axolemma allows intra-axonal Ca^{2+} to rise, and reversal of the Na^+-Ca^{2+} transporter has also been implicated in axon injury in ischemia (Stys, 1998) (Chapter 19). A rise in intra-axonal Ca^{2+} can activate proteases, in particular calpains (see Chapter 20), which in turn play a role in the degradation of the axon cytoskeleton. Although it is possible that changes in intra-axonal Ca^{2+} levels are critical in axon injury in MS lesions, there is no direct information on the link between inflammation and Ca^{2+} homeostasis in axons.

3. Caspases

The caspases are key players in the apoptotic execution of many different types of cells including neurons (Friedlander, 2003); however, the role of the caspases in axon degeneration is unclear. Caspase activation and the release of cytochrome-c have been described in axons after traumatic injury (Buki et al., 2000) and in the spinal cord of animals with EAE (Ahmed et al., 2002). It has been suggested that the caspases could play a role in degradation of the cytoskeleton. On the other hand, it has been shown that caspase inhibitors do not prevent axon or neurite degeneration in studies of wallerian degeneration *in vitro* (Finn et al., 2000; Sievers et al., 2003). However, there are a number of

routes to programmed cell death that are caspase-independent (Jaattela and Tschopp, 2003), and these pathways have yet to be explored in axon degeneration.

4. Ubiquitin-Proteasome Pathway

The role of the ubiquitin proteasome pathway (UPP) in axon degeneration has been brought to the fore by the discovery of two spontaneously occurring mutant strains of mice. The phenotype of the gracile axon dystrophy mouse (gad) is spontaneous axon degeneration in the gracile nucleus of the midbrain (Mukoyama et al., 1989), which leads to a progressive degeneration of the sensory neurons. The mutation was found to be in a gene encoding the ubiquitin hydrolase, UCH-L1, an enzyme involved in the release of ubiquitin from its substrate (Saigoh et al., 1999). This enzyme is one of the most abundant cytoplasmic enzymes in neurons, but it is not known how loss of this enzyme activity results in axon degeneration. In contrast, the Wld[s] mouse was found to have a phenotype in which axons and synapses of both the CNS and PNS exhibited very slow wallerian degeneration (see Coleman and Perry, 2002, for review). The Wld[s] gene was found to be a chimeric gene affecting the function of the ubiquitin ligase UbE4b (Mack et al., 2001). This ligase is normally involved in the selection of substrates for ubiquitination before processing in the proteasome. The vertebrate-specific 300 amino acid N-terminal domain is essential for ubiquitin chain extension of the substrate by the ligase (Mahoney et al., 2002). The active site of the ligase U-box region has been replaced in the chimeric protein by the enzyme Nmnat. It seems possible that the fusion between the first 70 amino acids of UbE4b and the entire open-reading frame of Nmnat acts as a dominant negative inhibitor of normal UbE4b activity. Transgenic mice expressing the chimeric Wld^s gene show a dose-dependent delay in wallerian degeneration (Mack et al., 2001), whereas transgenic mice expressing only the Nmnat portion of the chimeric gene do not show this phenotype (Coleman and Perry, 2002). The role of UbE4b in the axon is not known, and indeed in Wld^s mice the Wld^s protein is only detectable in the neuronal nucleus and not in the axon (Feng, Coleman, and Perry, unpublished observations).

Further evidence to support the role of the UPP in axon degeneration comes from *in vitro* studies using proteasome inhibitors (Zhai et al., 2003). These authors showed that axon and neurite degeneration could be delayed by application of proteasome inhibitors *in vivo* and *in vitro*. It should be noted, however, that the delay in degeneration was hours rather than the delay of several days induced by the Wld^s gene *in vitro* (Buckmaster et al., 1995) or weeks *in vivo* (Perry et al., 1991). The role of the proteasome in neuronal survival is complex, as inhibitors of the proteasome may also induce neuronal apoptosis (Qiu et al., 2000).

5. Axonal Transport

The axon and its terminals are maintained in a state of homeostasis by transport systems that move materials in an anterograde and retrograde direction. The family of molecules responsible for anterograde movement of organelles and proteins are the kinesins, and some 38 members of this family have been detected in the brain (Miki et al., 2001). How inflammatory molecules might affect these transport systems has not been studied, and this potentially interesting and important area of research has been largely neglected. In a guinea pig model of EAE, despite a loss of only 25% of the axons, there is a 75% decrement in the amount of material transported along the optic nerve (Guy et al., 1989). Evidence also suggests that raised levels of glutamate may interfere with fast axonal transport (Ackerley et al., 2000), and treatment of mice with riluzole in MOG-induced EAE was found to reduce axon damage (Gilgun-Sherki et al., 2003). If axon transport processes can be affected by inflammatory mediators or glutamate, the consequences may not be immediate. In patients with Charcot-Marie-Tooth type 2a, patients develop a progressive late-onset peripheral neuropathy. The mutation underlying this disease is a mutation in one of the genes of the kinesin family, KIF-1B, a transporter involved in the movement of mitochondria (Zhao et al., 2001).

III. Secondary Consequences of Axon Injury: Beyond the Plaque

The focus of investigations into the neuropathology of MS has been on the plaques within the white matter tracts. White matter distal to the plaques is commonly referred to as normal-appearing white matter (NAWM). Once we accept that axon injury is a major part of MS pathology, the term NAWM is clearly a misnomer and reflects a somewhat limited level of analysis of the pathology. Axon injury results in wallerian degeneration of the segment of axon distal to the lesion and a retrograde reaction in the cell body. Both of these components of the neuropathology resulting from axon injury have received little attention in MS, yet both lead to activation of the resident microglia, which may in turn influence immune reactions within the CNS, and impact on neighboring axons and neurons.

A. Wallerian Degeneration

After transection of an axon in the CNS, the cut ends rapidly seal and the distal axon may survive for several days before it begins to undergo wallerian degeneration, the larger axons degenerating before finer caliber axons. After the axon has degenerated, the myelin sheath begins to degenerate; but in marked contrast to the rapid removal of axon and myelin debris from the PNS, the debris in the CNS is slowly cleared over a period of months (Bignami and Eng, 1973). In the human brain and spinal cord, the debris in fiber tracts undergoing wallerian degeneration may persist for years, as it is very slowly removed by mononuclear phagocytes (Miklossy and Van der Loos, 1991; Buss et al., 2004). For reasons that are not well understood, the myelin sheath may persist in a remarkably intact state despite the loss of the axon (Fig. 4).

Wallerian degeneration in the CNS results in the activation of the microglia along the degenerating tract (Fig. 5) (Lawson et al., 1994). These activated microglia are largely composed of proliferating resident microglia, although some monocytes may be recruited at later stages. Activated microglia have been demonstrated in so-called NAWM of the MS brain, in both postmortem material (Allen et al., 2001) and *in vivo* (Banati et al., 2000). Activated microglia are often attributed with a pro-inflammatory phenotype synthesizing inflammatory cytokines, such as interleukin-1β and tumor necrosis factor-α, but it is now clear that morphological activation of microglia is not synonymous with pro-inflammatory cytokine production (Perry et al., 2002). Indeed the profile of cytokines, or other inflammatory mediators, secreted by a phagocytic macrophage critically depends on the nature of the phagocytosed material and the receptor repertoire used by the macrophage to ingest the debris. It has been shown that macrophages that have ingested apoptotic cells have an anti-inflammatory profile (Henson et al., 2001). A key receptor involved in the generation of this anti-inflammatory profile is the phosphatidylserine receptor that recognizes phosphatidylserine residues expressed on the external leaflet of the plasma membrane of apoptotic cells. Given the evidence that axons degenerate by an active programmed-cell-death-like process

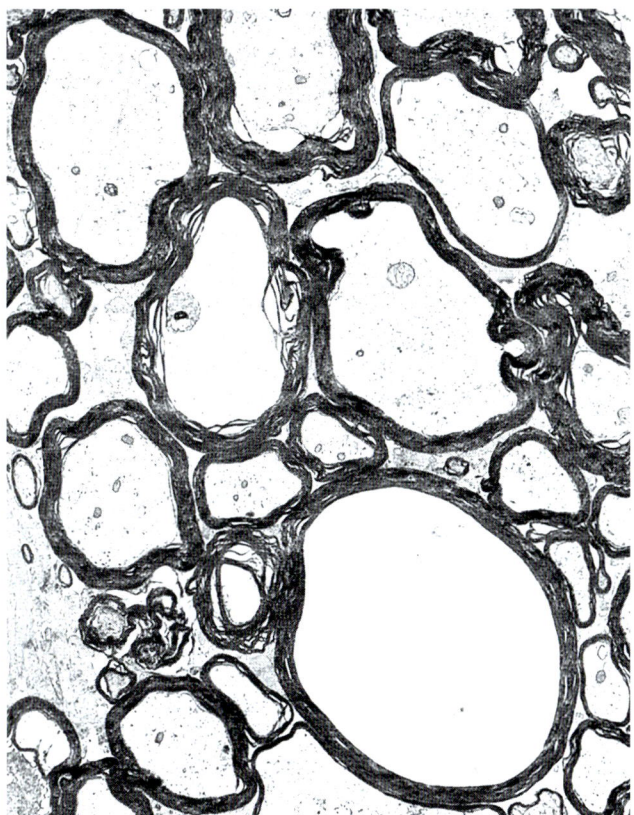

Figure 4 Preservation of CNS myelin during wallerian degeneration in the spinal cord, although some of the axons have degenerated 3 days previously (× 3000).

and that neurites undergoing wallerian degeneration *in vitro* express phosphatidylserine residues on the external axolemma (Sievers et al., 2003), it is of interest to study the

cytokine profile associated with the activation of microglia in CNS wallerian degeneration. In contrast to that found in peripheral nerves undergoing wallerian degeneration, it has been found that wallerian degeneration of optic nerve is associated with inflammatory profile with increased expression of transforming growth factor-β1 (TGF-β1) and cyclo-oxygenase-2 consistent with their having phagocytosed apoptotic cells or cellular material undergoing an apoptotic-like process (Palin, Cunningham, Perry, unpublished). These activated microglia, however, are "primed" and after a systemic challenge with endotoxin, to mimic a systemic infection, the cytokine profile is switched to the expression of significant levels of pro-inflammatory cytokines. A recent microarray analysis of white matter taken from distal to plaques in MS postmortem material also failed to find a typical pro-inflammatory profile despite the large numbers of activated microglia present (Graumann et al., 2003). These authors found upregulation of genes involved in pathways related to the response to oxidative stress and ischemic pre-conditioning.

The presence of activated microglia distal to plaques may have two obvious consequences. First, it has been shown in experimental models of EAE that degenerating fiber tracts and the presence of activated microglia may act as a target for the entry of activated T-cells and the initiation of an inflammatory lesion (Konno et al., 1990). The mechanisms underlying the targeting of inflammation to the degenerating fiber tracts are not known, and it is unclear to what extent this also happens in the human CNS. Second, the phagocytosis of material from degenerating axons and myelin may act to prime the microglia so that a secondary stimulus, such as that evoked by a systemic infection, may further activate the microglia (Perry et al., 2003). A significant proportion of clinical relapses are triggered by systemic infections (Buljevac et al., 2002).

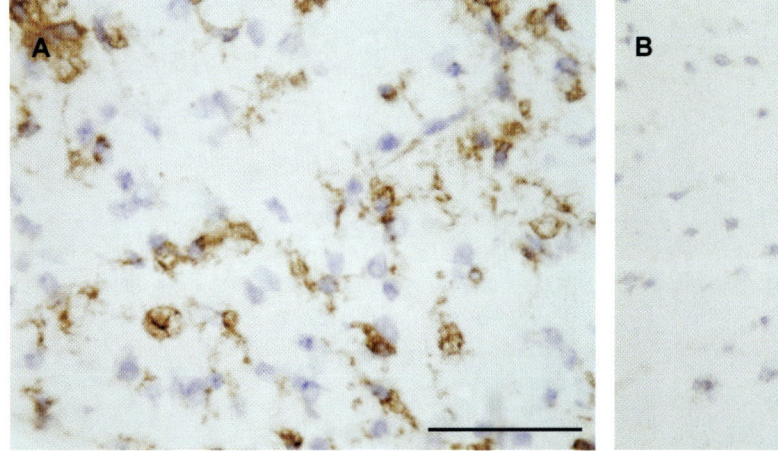
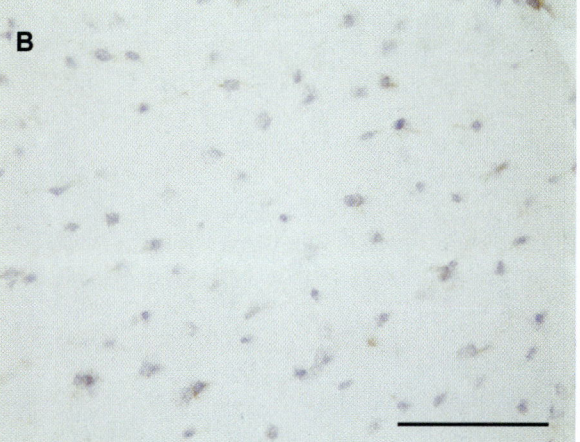

Figure 5 Activated microglia in the murine optic nerve undergoing wallerian degeneration 28 days postinjury. The activated microglia as revealed by CD68 (**A**) are readily visible, whereas those in the normal optic nerve (**B**) are fewer, and express low levels of CD68. Scale bar = 80 μm.

B. Retrograde Degeneration

In the CNS the retrograde response to axon transection is dependent on a number of variables including the particular neuron population, the proximity of the transection to the cell body, and the number of axon collaterals the cell may possess (Lieberman, 1971). A well-described model for the study of inflammation in the vicinity of neurons undergoing the retrograde reaction is the facial nucleus after injury of the facial nerve (Streit and Graeber, 1993). After nerve injury there is rapid activation of the microglia around the cell bodies of the injured cells, and it has been suggested that the proliferation and activation of the microglia may be neuroprotective (Kreutzberg, 1996). Studies in mice lacking the cytokine macrophage-colony stimulating factor, however, reveal that even in the absence of microglia proliferation and reduced microglia activation, neuron survival and nerve regeneration are not affected (Kalla et al., 2001). The cytokine profile associated with the microglia activated in this retrograde reaction show some important species differences. In the rat the cytokine TGF-β1 is upregulated but the pro-inflammatory cytokines interleukin-1β, tumor necrosis factor-α, and interferon-γ are not detectable (Kiefer et al., 1993). In contrast in the mouse, some loss of neurons occurs after the lesion, T-cells invade the facial nucleus and pro-inflammatory cytokines are detected (Raivich et al., 1998). Recent studies show that the microglia response, cytokine expression, and neuronal viability after nerve root evulsion is under genetic control and varies between rat strains in a largely independent manner (Olsson et al., 2000). The genes that regulate these components of the innate response to CNS injury are likely to be of particular importance in the pathology distal to the plaque in MS. Given the diverse retrograde responses of neurons to axon injury and the species and genetic differences, it is unclear whether findings from the facial nucleus can be extrapolated to other populations of neurons such as thalamic neurons, or neurons of the cerebral cortex.

It is important to investigate whether the innate inflammatory response can contribute to the progression of MS. Evidence to suggest that it does comes from long-term observations of patients in which the majority of T-cells have been depleted by the humanized antileukocyte (CD25) monoclonal antibody Campath-1H (Coles et al., 1999). Despite the suppression of T-cell-mediated inflammation, about half of the patients experienced progressive disability and continuing brain atrophy.

IV. Conclusion

Axon injury is a significant part of MS pathology. Postmortem analysis shows that axon injury occurs early in the evolution of the plaque, and the degree of axon injury correlates with the intensity of the inflammatory response. Quantitative analysis reveals that a significant percentage of axons degenerate in major fiber tracts. Studies in animal models of MS show that axon injury also occurs in a number of these models. The transection of an axon by inflammatory cells and their products is an irreversible lesion and insights into the early stages of this process are needed.

A spectrum of molecules secreted by inflammatory cells including T-cells, B-cells, and macrophages in an immunologically nonspecific manner may precipitate axon transection. These "molecular scissors" may act on the axon in a number of different ways. They may activate biochemical pathways, intrinsic to the axon, that lead to local autodestruction akin to programmed-cell-death, or apoptosis, of the cell body.

The myelin sheath may protect the axon from some of the potentially destructive molecules, but exposed parts of the axon, such as the node of Ranvier and axon terminal, remain sites susceptible to injury. Demyelination may compromise axon homeostasis and axonal transport and thus predispose these axons to injury by inflammatory mediators. Changes in axon transport or other aspects of axon homeostasis may have subtle effects on synaptic signaling, particularly over a long period of time.

Axon transection in plaques within the fiber tracts leads to wallerian degeneration of the distal axon segment and a retrograde reaction at the cell body. These processes are associated with the activation of microglia distal to the plaque. The possible role of this innate immune response on adjacent intact axons and neuronal function and integrity has not been explored. Comparison of the innate inflammatory response in MS with the innate response in acute brain injury and the consequences of this inflammation may provide useful insights.

Strategies to prevent axon injury by inflammatory cells or demyelination are much needed. Current anti-inflammatory therapies do not appear to affect long-term outcome, suggesting that the mechanisms of axon injury and the innate inflammatory response as a consequence of this axon injury are not being targeted. Therapeutic interventions to target the molecules of destruction that are secreted by inflammatory cells that act as molecular scissors to precipitate axon transection are much needed.

Acknowledgments

Supported by The Multiple Sclerosis Society (UK), the Wellcome Trust, and MRC (UK).

I thank my colleagues who have contributed to many fruitful discussions on the topic of this chapter.

References

Ackerley, S., Grierson, A. J., Brownlees, J., Thornhill, P., Anderton, B. H., Leigh, P. N., Shaw, C. E., and Miller, C. C. (2000). Glutamate slows axonal transport of neurofilaments in transfected neurons. *J. Cell Biol.* **150,** 165–176.

Ahmed, Z., Doward, A. I., Pryce, G., Taylor, D. L., Pocock, J. M., Leonard, J. P., Baker, D., and Cuzner, M. L. (2002). A role for caspase-1 and -3 in the pathology of experimental allergic encephalomyelitis : Inflammation versus degeneration. *Am. J. Pathol.* **161,** 1577–1586.

Allan, S. M., and Rothwell, N. J. (2001). Cytokines and acute neurodegeneration. *Nat. Rev. Neurosci.* **2,** 734–744.

Allen, I. V., McQuaid, S., Mirakhur, M., and Nevin, G. (2001). Pathological abnormalities in the normal-appearing white matter in multiple sclerosis. *Neurol. Sci.* **22,** 141–144.

Banati, R. B., Newcombe, J., Gunn, R. N., Cagnin, A., Turkheimer, F., Heppner, F., Price, G., Wegner, F., Giovannoni, G., Miller, D. H., Perkin, G. D., Smith, T., Hewson, A. K., Bydder, G., Kreutzberg, G. W., Jones, T., Cuzner, M. L., and Myers, R. (2000). The peripheral benzodiazepine binding site in the brain in multiple sclerosis: quantitative *in vivo* imaging of microglia as a measure of disease activity. *Brain* **123,** 2321–2337.

Bignami, A., and Eng, L. F. (1973). Biochemical studies of myelin in Wallerian degeneration of rat optic nerve. *J. Neurochem.* **20,** 165–173.

Bitsch, A., Schuchardt, J., Bunkowski, S., Kuhlmann, T., and Bruck, W. (2000). Acute axonal injury in multiple sclerosis. Correlation with demyelination and inflammation. *Brain* **12,** 1174–1183.

Bjartmar, C., Wujek, J. R., and Trapp, B. D. (2003). Axonal loss in the pathology of MS: Consequences for understanding the progressive phase of the disease. *J. Neurol. Sci.* **206,** 165–171.

Brex, P. A., Ciccarelli, O., O'Riordan, J. I., Sailer, M., Thompson, A. J., and Miller, D. H. (2002). A longitudinal study of abnormalities on MRI and disability from multiple sclerosis. *N. Engl. J. Med.* **17,** 158–164.

Brorson, J. R., Schumacker, P. T., and Zhang, H. (1999). Nitric oxide acutely inhibits neuronal energy production. The Committees on Neurobiology and Cell Physiology. *J. Neurosci.* **19,** 147–158.

Buckmaster, E. A., Perry, V. H., and Brown, M. C. (1995). The rate of Wallerian degeneration in cultured neurons from wild type and C57BL/WldS mice depends on time in culture and may be extended in the presence of elevated K+ levels. *Eur. J. Neurosci.* **7,** 1596–1602.

Buki, A., Okonkwo, D. O., Wang, K. K., and Povlishock, J. T. (2000). Cytochrome c release and caspase activation in traumatic axonal injury. *J. Neurosci.* **20,** 2825–2834.

Buljevac, D., Flach, H. Z., Hop, W. C., Hijdra, D., Laman, J. D., Savelkoul, H. F., van Der Meche, F. G., van Doorn, P. A., and Hintzen, R. Q. (2002). Prospective study on the relationship between infections and multiple sclerosis exacerbations. *Brain* **125,** 952–960.

Burne, J. F., Staple, J. K., and Raff, M. C. (1996). Glial cells are increased proportionally in transgenic optic nerves with increased numbers of axons. *J. Neurosci.* **16,** 2064–2073.

Buss, A., Brook, G. A., Kakulas, B., Martin, D., Franzen, R., Schoenen, J., Noth, J., and Schmitt, A. B. (2004). Gradual loss of myelin and formation of an astrocytic scar during Wallerian degeneration in the human spinal cord. *Brain* **127,** 34–44.

Coleman, M. P., and Perry, V. H. (2002). Axon pathology in neurological disease: A neglected therapeutic target. *Trends Neurosci.* **25,** 532–537.

Coles A. J., Wing, M. G., Molyneux, P., Paolillo, A., Davie, C. M., Hale, G., Miller, D., Waldmann, H., and Compston, A. (1999). Monoclonal antibody treatment exposes three mechanisms underlying the clinical course of multiple sclerosis. *Ann. Neurol.* **46,** 296–304.

Compston, A., and Coles, A. (2002). Multiple sclerosis. *Lancet* **359(9313),** 1221–1231.

Davie, C. A., Hawkins, C. P., Barker, G. J., Brennan, A., Tofts, P. S., and Miller, D. H., and McDonald, W. I. (1994). Serial proton magnetic resonance spectroscopy in acute multiple sclerosis lesions. *Brain* **117,** 49–58.

De Groot, C. J., Ruuls, S. R., Theeuwes, J. W., Dijkstra, C. D., and Van der Valk, P. (1997). Immunocytochemical characterization of the expression of inducible and constitutive isoforms of nitric oxide synthase in demyelinating multiple sclerosis lesions. *J. Neuropathol. Exp. Neurol.* **56,** 10–20.

Dewar, D., Yam, P., and McCulloch, J. (1999). Drug development for stroke: Importance of protecting cerebral white matter. *Eur. J. Pharmacol.* **375,** 41–50.

Dong, H., Fazzaro, A., Xiang, C., Korsmeyer, S. J., Jacquin, M. F., and McDonald J. W. (2003). Enhanced oligodendrocyte survival after spinal cord injury in Bax-deficient mice and mice with delayed Wallerian degeneration. *J. Neurosci.* **25,** 6882–6891.

Eikelenboom, M. J., Petzold, A., Lazeron, R. H., Silber, E., Sharief, M., Thompson, E. J., Barkof, F., Giovannoni, G., Polman, C. H., and Uitdehaag, E. M. (2003). Multiple sclerosis: Neurofilament light chain antibodies are correlated to cerebral atrophy. *Neurology* **60,** 219–223.

Evangelou, N., Konz, D., Esiri, M. M., Smith, S., Palace, J., and Matthews, P. M. (2000). Regional axonal loss in the corpus callosum correlates with cerebral white matter lesion volume and distribution in multiple sclerosis. *Brain* **123,** 1845–1849.

Ferguson, B., Matyszak, M. K., Esiri, M. M., and Perry, V. H. (1997). Axonal damage in acute multiple sclerosis lesions. *Brain* **120,** 393–399.

Ferri, A., Sanes, J. R., Coleman, M. P., Cunningham, J. M., and Kato, A. (2003). Inhibiting axon degeneration and synapse loss attenuates apoptosis and disease progression in a mouse model of motoneuron disease. *Curr. Biol.* **13,** 669–673.

Filippi, M. (2003). MRI-clinical correlations in the primary progressive course of MS: New insights into the disease pathophysiology from the application of magnetization transfer, diffusion tensor, and functional MRI. *J. Neurol. Sci.* **206,** 157–164.

Finn, J. T., Weil, M., Archer, F., Siman, R., Srinivasan, A., and Raff, M. C. (2000). Evidence that Wallerian degeneration and localized axon degeneration induced by local neurotrophin deprivation do not involve caspases. *J. Neurosci.* **20,** 1333–1341.

Franklin R. J. (2002). Why does remyelination fail in multiple sclerosis? *Nat. Rev. Neurosci.* **3,** 705–714.

Friedlander, R. M. (2003). Apoptosis and caspases in neurodegenerative diseases. *N. Engl. J. Med.* **348,** 1365–1375.

Geddis, M. S., and Rehder, V. (2003). Initial stages of neural regeneration in *Helisoma trivolvis* are dependent upon PLA2 activity. *J. Neurobiol.* **54,** 555–565.

Genain, C. P., Nguyen, M. H., Letvin, N. L., Pearl, R., Davis, R. L., Adelman, M., Lees, M. B., Linington, C., and Hauser, S. L. (1995). Antibody facilitation of multiple sclerosis-like lesions in a nonhuman primate. *J. Clin. Invest.* **96,** 2966–2974.

Gilgun-Sherki, Y., Panet, H,. Melamed, E., and Offen, D. (2003). Riluzole suppresses experimental autoimmune encephalomyelitis: Implications for the treatment of multiple sclerosis. *Brain Res.* **989,** 196–204.

Giovannoni, G., Silver, N. C., Good, C. D., Miller, D. H., and Thompson, E. J. (2000). Immunological time-course of gadolinium-enhancing MRI lesions in patients with multiple sclerosis. *Eur. Neurol.* **44,** 222–228.

Gong, Y., Tagawa, Y., Lunn, M. P., Laroy, W., Heffer-Lauc, M., Li, C. Y., Griffin, J. W., Schnaar, R. L., and Sheikh, K. A. (2002). Localization of major gangliosides in the PNS: Implications for immune neuropathies. *Brain* **125,** 2491–2506.

Gordon, S. (2003). Alternative activation of macrophages. *Nat. Rev. Immunol.* **3,** 23–35.

Graumann, U., Reynolds, R., Steck, A. J., and Sand Schaeren-Wiemers, N. (2003). Molecular changes in normal appearing white matter in multiple sclerosis are characteristic of neuroprotective mechanisms against hypoxic insult. *Brain Pathol.* **13(4):554–573.**

Griffin, J. W., Li, C. Y., Macko, C., Ho, T. W., Hsieh, S. T., Xe, P., Wang, F. A., Comblath, D. R., McKhann, G. M., and Asbury, A. K. (1996). Early nodal changes in the acute motor axonal neuropathy pattern of the Guillain-Barre syndrome. *J. Neurocytol.* **25,** 33–51.

Grossmann, J. (2002). Molecular mechanisms of "detachment-induced apoptosis—Anoikis." *Apoptosis* **7,** 247–260.

Guy, J., Ellis, E. A., Tark, E. F. 3rd, Hope G. M., and Rao, N. M. (1989). Axonal transport reductions in acute experimental allergic encephalomyelitis: qualitative analysis of the optic nerve. *Curr. Eye Res.* **8**, 261–269.

Hafer-Macko, C., Hsieh, S. T., Li, C. Y., Ho, T. W., Sheikh, K., Cornblath, D. R., McKhann, G. M., Asbury, A. K., and Griffin, J. W. (1996). Acute motor axonal neuropathy: an antibody-mediated attack on axolemma. *Ann. Neurol.* **40**, 635–644 .

Hartung, H. P., and Kieseier, B. C. (2000).The role of matrix metalloproteinases in autoimmune damage to the central and peripheral nervous system. *J. Neuroimmunol.* **107**, 140–147.

Henson, P. M., Bratton, D. L., and Fadok, V. A. (2001). The phosphatidylserine receptor: a crucial molecular switch? *Nat. Rev. Mol. Cell Biol.* **2**, 627–633.

Herrera, A. J., Castano, A., Venero, J. L., Cano, J., and Machado, A. (2000). The single intranigral injection of LPS as a new model for studying the selective effects of inflammatory reactions on dopaminergic system. *Neurobiol. Dis.* **7**, 429–447.

Hirano, A., and Llena, J. F. (1995). Morphology of central nervous system axons. *In:* "The Axon: Structure, Function and Pathophysiology" (S. G. Waxman, J. D. Koscis, and P. K. Stys., eds.). OUP, Oxford.

Howard, M. J., David, G., and Barrett, J. N. (1999). Resealing of transected myelinated mammalian axons in vivo: evidence for involvement of calpain. *Neuroscience* **93**, 807–815.

Jaattela, M., and Tschopp, J. (2003). Caspase-independent cell death in T lymphocytes. *Nat. Immunol.* **4**, 416–423.

Kalla, R., Liu, Z., Xu, S., Koppius, A., Imai, Y., Kloss, C. U., Kohsaka, S., Gschwendtner, A., Moller, J. C., Werner, A., and Raivich, G. (2001). Microglia and the early phase of immune surveillance in the axotomized facial motor nucleus: impaired microglial activation and lymphocyte recruitment but no effect on neuronal survival or axonal regeneration in macrophage-colony stimulating factor-deficient mice. *J. Comp. Neurol.* **436**, 182–201.

Kiefer, R., Lindholm, D., and Kreutzberg, G. W. (1993). Interleukin-6 and transforming growth factor-beta 1 mRNAs are induced in rat facial nucleus following motoneuron axotomy. *Eur. J. Neurosci.* **5**, 775–781.

Konno, H., Yamamoto, T., Suzuki, H., Yamamoto, H., Iwasaki, Y., Ohara, Y., Terunuma, H., and Harata, N. (1990). Targeting of adoptively transferred experimental allergic encephalitis lesion at the sites of wallerian degeneration. *Acta Neuropathol. (Berl)* **80**, 521–526.

Kornek, B., and Lassmann, H. (1999). Axonal pathology in multiple sclerosis. A historical note. *Brain Pathol.* **9**, 651–656.

Kornek, B., Storch, M. K., Weissert, R., Wallstroem, E., Stefferl, A., Olsson, T., Linington, C., Schmidbauer, M., and Lassmann, H. (2000). Multiple sclerosis and chronic autoimmune encephalomyelitis: A comparative quantitative study of axonal injury in active, inactive, and remyelinated lesions. *Am. J. Pathol.* **157**, 267–276.

Kreutz, M., Fritsche, J., and Andreesen, R (2002). Macrophages in tumor biology. *In:* "The Macrophage" (B. Burke and C. E. Lewis, eds.). OUP, Oxford.

Kreutzberg, G. W. (1996). Microglia: a sensor for pathological events in the CNS. *Trends Neurosci.* **19**, 312–318.

Lawson, L. J., Frost, L., Risbridger, J., Fearn, S., and Perry V. H. (1994). Quantification of the mononuclear phagocyte response to Wallerian degeneration of the optic nerve. *J. Neurocytol.* **23**, 729–744.

Lieberman, A. R. (1971). The axon reaction: a review of the principal features of perikaryal responses to axon injury. *Int. Rev. Neurobiol.* **14**, 49–124.

Linington, C., Bradl, M., Lassmann, H., Brunner, C., and Vass, K. (1988). Augmentation of demyelination in rat acute allergic encephalomyelitis by circulating mouse monoclonal antibodies directed against a myelin/oligodendrocyte glycoprotein. *Am. J. Pathol.* **130**, 443–454.

Losseff, N. A., Webb, S. L., O'Riordan, J. I., Page, R., Wang, L., Barker, G. J., Tofts, P. S., McDonald, W. I., Miller, D. H., and Thompson, A. J. (1996). Spinal cord atrophy and disability in multiple sclerosis. A new reproducible and sensitive MRI method with potential to monitor disease progression. *Brain* **119**, 701–708.

Lunn, E. R., Perry, V. H., Brown, M. C., Rosen, H., and Gordon, S. (1989). Absence of wallerian degeneration does not hinder regeneration in peripheral nerve. *Eur. J. Neurosci.* **1**, 27–33.

Mack, T. G., Reiner, M., Beirowski, B., Mi, W., Emanuelli, M., Wagner, D., Thomson, D., Gillingwater, T., Court, F., Conforti, L., Fernando, F. S., Tarlton, A., Andressen, C., Addicks, K., Magni, G., Ribchester, R. R., Perry, V. H., and Coleman, M. P. (2001).Wallerian degeneration of injured axons and synapses is delayed by a Ube4b/Nmnat chimeric gene. *Nat. Neurosci.* **4**, 1199–1206.

Mahoney, J. A., Odin, J. A., White S. M., Shaffer, D., Koff, A., Casciolarosen, L., and Rosen, A. (2002). The human homologue of the yeast polyubiquitination factor Ufd2p is cleaved by caspase 6 and granzyme B during apoptosis. *Biochem. J.* **361**, 587–595.

Mattson, M. P. (2000). Apoptosis in neurodegenerative disorders. *Nat. Rev. Mol. Cell Biol.* **1**, 120–129.

Matyszak, M. K., Townsend, M. J., and Perry, V. H. (1997). Ultrastructural studies of an immune-mediated inflammatory response in the CNS parenchyma directed against a non-CNS antigen. *Neuroscience* **78**, 549–560.

Matyszak, M. K., and Perry, V. H. (1996). The potential role of dendritic cells in immune-mediated inflammatory diseases in the central nervous system. *Neuroscience* **74**, 599–608.

Matyszak, M. K., and Perry, V. H. (1995). Demyelination in the central nervous system following a delayed-type hypersensitivity response to bacillus Calmette-Guerin. *Neuroscience* **64**, 967–977.

Maxwell, W. L., and Graham, D. I. (1997). Loss of axonal microtubules and neurofilaments after stretch-injury to guinea pig optic nerve fibers. *J. Neurotrauma* **14**, 603–614.

Mead, R. J., Singhrao, S. K., Neal, J. W., Lassmann, H., and Morgan, B. P. (2002). The membrane attack complex of complement causes severe demyelination associated with acute axonal injury. *J. Immunol.* **168**, 458–465.

Mead, R. J., Neal, J. W., Griffiths, M. R., Linington, C., Botto, M., Lassmann, H., and Morgan, B. P. (2004). Deficiency of the complement regulator CD59a enhances disease severity, demyelination and axonal injury in murine acute experimental allergic encephalomyelitis. *Lab. Invest.* **84**, 21–28.

Medana, I. M., and Esiri, M. M. (2003). Axonal damage: a key predictor of outcome in human CNS diseases. *Brain* **126**, 515–530.

Miki, H., Setou, M., Kaneshior, K., and Hirokawa, N. (2001). All kinesin superfamily protein, KIF, genes in mouse and human. *Proc. Natl. Acad. Sci. U.S.A.* **98**, 7004–7011.

Miklossy, J., and Van der Loos, H. (1991). The long-distance effects of brain lesions: Visualization of myelinated pathways in the human brain using polarizing and fluorescence microscopy. *J. Neuropathol. Exp. Neurol.* **50**, 1–15.

Mukoyama, M., Yamazaki, K., Kikuchi, T., and Tomita, T. (1989). Neuropathology of gracile axonal dystrophy (GAD) mouse. An animal model of central distal axonopathy in primary sensory neurons. *Acta Neuropathol.* **79**, 294–299

Neumann, H., Medana, I. M., Bauer, J., and Lassmann, H. (2002). Cytotoxic T lymphocytes in autoimmune and degenerative CNS diseases. *Trends Neurosci.* **25**, 313–319.

Newman, T. A., Woolley, S. T., Hughes, P. M., Sibson, N. R., Anthony, D. C., and Perry, V. H. (2001). T-cell- and macrophage-mediated axon damage in the absence of a CNS-specific immune response: involvement of metalloproteinases. *Brain* **124**, 2203–2214.

Olsson, T., Lundberg, C., Lidman, O., and Piehl, F. (2000). Genetic regulation of nerve avulsion-induced spinal cord inflammation. *Ann. N. Y. Acad. Sci.* **917**, 186–196.

Perry, V. H. (1998). A revised view of the central nervous system microenvironment and major histocompatibility complex class II antigen presentation. *J. Neuroimmunol.* **90**, 113–121.

Perry, V. H., Brown, M. C., and Lunn E. R. (1991). Very slow retrograde and Wallerian degeneration in the CNS of C57BL/Ola mice. *Eur. J. Neurosci.* **3**, 102–101.

Perry, V. H., Cunningham, C., and Boche, D. (2002). Atypical inflammation in the central nervous system in prion disease. *Curr. Opin. Neurol.* **15**, 349–354.

Perry, V. H., Newman, T. A., and Cunningham, C. (2003). The impact of systemic infection on the progression of neurodegenerative disease. *Nat. Rev. Neurosci.* **4**, 103–112.

Peterson, J. W., Bo, L., Mork, S., Chang, A., and Trapp, B. D. (2001). Transected neurites, apoptotic neurons, and reduced inflammation in cortical multiple sclerosis lesions. *Ann. Neurol.* **50**, 389–400.

Plumb, J., Armstrong, M. A., Duddy, M., Mirakhur, M., and McQuaid, S. (2003). CD83-positive dendritic cells are present in occasional perivascular cuffs in multiple sclerosis lesions. *Multiple Sclerosis* **9**, 142–147.

Qiu, J. H., Asai, A., Chi, S., Saito, N., Hamada, H., and Kirino, T. (2000). Proteasome inhibitors induce cytochrome c-caspase-3-like protease-mediated apoptosis in cultured cortical neurons. *J. Neurosci.* **20**, 259–265.

Raivich, G., Jones, L. L., Kloss, C. U., Werner, A., Neumann, H., and Kreutzberg, G. W. (1998). Immune surveillance in the injured nervous system: T-lymphocytes invade the axotomized mouse facial motor nucleus and aggregate around sites of neuronal degeneration. *J. Neurosci.* **18**, 5804–5816.

Saigoh, K., Wang, Y. L., Suh, J. G., Yamanishi, T., Sakai, Y., Kiyosawa, H., Harada, T., Ichihara, N., Wakana, S., Kikuchi, T., and Wada, K. (1999). Intragenic deletion in the gene encoding ubiquitin carboxy-terminal hydrolase in gad mice. *Nat. Genet.* **23**, 47–51.

Salzer, J. L. (1995). Mechanisms of adhesion between axons and glial cells. In: "The Axon: Structure, Function and Pathophysiology." (S. G. Waxman, J. D. Koscis, and P. K. Stys., eds.). OUP, Oxford.

Samsam, M., Mi, W., Wessig, C., Zielasek, J., Toyka, K. V., Coleman, M. P., and Martini, R. (2003). The Wlds mutation delays robust loss of motor and sensory axons in a genetic model for myelin-related axonopathy. *J. Neurosci.* **23**, 2833–2839.

Schlaepfer, W. W., and Hasler, M. B. (1979). Characterization of the calcium-induced disruption of neurofilaments in rat peripheral nerve. *Brain Res.* **168**, 299–309.

Schroeter, M., Stoll, G., Weissert, R., Hartung, H. P., Lassmann, H., and Jander, S. (2003). CD8+ phagocyte recruitment in rat experimental autoimmune encephalomyelitis: Association with inflammatory tissue destruction. *Am. J. Pathol.* **163**, 1517–1524.

Siebert, H., and Bruck, W. (2003). The role of cytokines and adhesion molecules in axon degeneration after peripheral nerve axotomy: a study in different knockout mice. *Brain Res.* **960**, 152–156.

Sievers, C., Platt, N., Perry, V. H., Coleman, M. P., and Conforti, L. (2003). Neurites undergoing Wallerian degeneration show an apoptotic-like process with Annexin V positive staining and loss of mitochondrial membrane potential. *Neurosci. Res.* **46**, 161–169.

Smith, K. J., Kapoor, R., Hall, S. M., and Davies, M. (2001). Electrically active axons degenerate when exposed to nitric oxide. *Ann. Neurol.* **49**, 470–476.

Storch, M. K., Weissert, R., Steffer, A., Birnbacher, R., Wallstrom, E., Dahlman, I., Ostensson, C. G., Linington, C., Olsson, T., and Lassmann, H. (2002). MHC gene related effects on microglia and macrophages in experimental autoimmune encephalomyelitis determine the extent of axonal injury. *Brain Pathol.* **12**, 287–299.

Streit, W. J., and Graeber, M. B. (1993). Heterogeneity of microglial and perivascular cell populations: Insights gained from the facial nucleus paradigm. *Glia* **7**, 68–74.

Stys, P. K. (1998). Anoxic and ischemic injury of myelinated axons in CNS white matter: From mechanistic concepts to therapeutics. *J. Cereb. Blood. Flow Metab.* **18**, 2–25.

Trapp, B. D., Peterson, J., Ransohoff, R. M., Rudick, R., Mork, S., and Bo, L. (1998). Axonal transection in the lesions of multiple sclerosis. *N. Engl. J. Med.* **338**, 278–285.

Trebst, C., and Ransohoff, R. M. (2001). Investigating chemokines and chemokine receptors in patients with multiple sclerosis: Opportunities and challenges. *Arch. Neurol.* **58**, 1975–1980.

Tuohy, V. K., Yu, M., Yin, L., Kawczak, J. A., Johnson, J. M., Mathisen, P. M., Weinstock-Guttman, B., and Kinkel, R. P. (1998). The epitope spreading cascade during progression of experimental autoimmune encephalomyelitis and multiple sclerosis. *Immunol. Rev.* **164**, 93–100.

Wang, M. S., Davis, A. A., Culver, D. G., and Glass, J. D. (2002). WldS mice are resistant to paclitaxel (taxol) neuropathy. *Ann. Neurol.* **52**, 442–447.

Wekerle, H., Kojima, K., Lannes-Vieira, J., Lassmann, H., and Linington, C. (1994). Animal models. *Ann. Neurol.* **36 Suppl**, S47–53.

Yong, V. W., Power, C., Forsyth, P., and Edwards D. R. (2001). Metalloproteinases in biology and pathology of the nervous system. *Nat. Rev. Neurosci.* **2**, 502–511.

Zhai, Q., Wang, J., Kim, A., Liu, Q., Watts, R., Hoopfer, E., Mitchison, T., Luo, L., and He, Z. (2003). Involvement of the ubiquitin-proteasome system in the early stages of wallerian degeneration. *Neuron* **39**, 217–225.

Zhao, C., Takita, J., Tanaka, Y., Setou, M., Nakagawa, T., Takeda, S., Yang, H. W., Tereda, S., Nakata, T., Takei, Y., Saito, M., Tsuji, S., Hayashi, Y., and Hirokawa, N. (2001). Charcot-Marie-Tooth disease type 2A caused by mutation in a microtubule motor KIF1Bbeta. *Cell* **105**, 587–597.

18

Nitric Oxide and Axonal Pathophysiology

Kenneth J. Smith, Ph.D.

I. Introduction

Evidence that nitric oxide (NO) plays an important role in MS is accumulating rapidly. Certainly NO is produced within the inflammatory lesions of MS, seemingly in relatively high concentrations, and it has potent effects on immune and excitable cells. Indeed, NO appears to play a myriad of roles in MS as a whole (Santiago et al., 1998; Smith and Lassmann, 2002). This chapter is focused specifically on the effects of NO on axons because, on histological evidence, NO formation is likely to be particularly prominent in the white matter in MS. Thus this chapter is not concerned with the important roles of NO in immune modulation or the regulation of cerebral blood flow, nor is it concerned with the likely effects of NO in the gray matter, where it probably disturbs the function of neuronal and glial cell bodies, including the likely disruption of both normal synaptic function and signaling via glutamate receptors.

In the normal nervous system, axons in white matter tracts experience only very low concentrations of nitric oxide, but, in contrast, axons within inflammatory multiple sclerosis (MS) lesions may be surrounded by groups of inflammatory cells that are liberating nitric oxide (NO) in sustained, relatively high concentrations. These latter concentrations are likely to swamp any physiological signaling, and to have a range of potentially deleterious effects on the axons, some of which will be reversible, but some of which may be persistent or permanent. This chapter is concerned with these effects, as it seems likely (although unproven) that the effects of NO exposure may become manifest in the expression of temporary and permanent neurological deficits.

II. Basic Chemistry and Biology of Nitric Oxide

Although NO is one of the smallest molecules in biology, it has a remarkably rich chemistry and participates in a wide variety of biological events. The chemistry is complex and incompletely understood, even when studied in controlled conditions aside from biological systems. Within biological systems, the complexities are magnified, as tissues, especially inflamed tissues, are inherently complex and contain a myriad of microcompartments characterized by different pH, redox potential, NO, and oxygen concentrations etc., which can affect the form taken by "NO", and thus the consequences of NO production.

In tissues, NO behaves as a freely diffusible, reasonably reactive soluble gas, which, like oxygen, diffuses through the tissue with little restriction imposed by cell membranes. NO is produced from the amino acid L-arginine by the enzyme nitric oxide synthase (NOS), which predominantly exists in three forms, nNOS, inducible NOS (iNOS), and eNOS, indicating the neuronal, immunological/inflammatory, and endothelial cells in which the forms were first identified (Alderton et al., 2001; Stuehr, 1999). nNOS and eNOS are constitutively expressed (cNOS) (although they can also be induced by appropriate stimuli) and are concerned with signaling in the brain and vasculature primarily regarding, respectively, the modulation of neural processes and the regulation of blood flow. Thus under physiological conditions, the cNOS isoforms make small quantities of NO in response to (usually briefly) raised concentrations of intracellular calcium ions, and the NO functions as a signaling molecule by binding to its main receptor, soluble guanylate cyclase (sGC), resulting in the synthesis of cyclic guanosine 3,5'-monophosphate (cGMP) (Krumenacker et al., 2004; Ignarro, 1991; Bellamy and Garthwaite, 2001; Esplugues, 2002). This signaling occurs at concentrations of NO in the low nanomolar range, and one recent estimate based on the effect of NO on this enzyme suggests that the physiological concentration of NO may be as low as 1 nM (Griffiths et al., 2003).

In contrast, iNOS is not present in the normal central nervous system (CNS), but it is induced in some types of CNS cell (including microglia and astrocytes) in response to inflammation; it is also expressed by some inflammatory cells recruited into the CNS. iNOS makes NO continuously,

in high concentration (Aktan, 2004), and under these circumstances, NO can be toxic. Indeed, such production of NO is important in nonspecific defense against pathogens and tumor cells.

Although NO may be formed continuously by iNOS, this does not mean that NO concentrations will rise continuously, or that NO will diffuse further and further from its site of formation over time (Ledo et al., 2004). NO concentrations are limited by the presence of two major "sinks" in the form of oxyhemoglobin in blood vessels, and an as yet unidentified cellular sink (Griffiths and Garthwaite, 2001). Oxyhemoglobin will effectively provide a permanent sink while blood flow continues, but the cellular sink is saturable, and, once saturated, the NO concentration in tissue samples *in vitro* can rise to levels at which respiration is inhibited (see later) (Griffiths and Garthwaite, 2001). The half-life of NO within lesions, therefore, will not be a constant, and it may vary substantially in different microdomains, but as a guide it has been estimated to vary from approximately 90 ms to >2 seconds (Griffiths and Garthwaite, 2001; Thomas et al., 2001), and these values will be affected by the conditions prevailing within the tissue, including the NO and oxygen concentrations. The short half-life limits the effective diffusion radius of NO, which has been estimated to be approximately 100–200 μm from the NO-producing cell (Lancaster Jr., 1997).

Knowledge of the NO concentration in a lesion would be useful, but it would give a poor guide to the consequences of its presence, because these are strongly influenced by which reactive nitrogen species are formed under the prevailing conditions. As NO is a reactive molecule, it does not exist in tissues only as the free radical NO$^{\bullet}$, but it also gives rise, sometimes reversibly, to a number of related reactive nitrogen species (RNS), several of which are also reactive and which therefore have their own chemistries and biological activities (reviewed in Beckman and Koppenol, 1996; Smith et al., 1999; Crow and Beckman, 1996; Hogg, 2002; Feelisch, 1998; Espey et al., 2002). The details of these reactions need not concern us here (and are not understood in inflamed tissues), except to distinguish the agent peroxynitrite (ONOO$^-$) and a large group of molecules (including many ion channels) that contain a free thiol group that can be nitrosated to form nitrosothiols. Peroxynitrite is a strongly oxidizing, toxic agent formed by the combination of NO with superoxide (O$_2^-$). In fact, NO can out-compete superoxide dismutase for superoxide, which is produced as a byproduct of mitochondrial metabolism (Duchen, 2004). The formation of peroxynitrite is an important reaction of NO, and many of the toxic reactions attributed to NO may in fact be due to peroxynitrite (Crow and Beckman, 1996; Szabo, 2003).

Another important reaction of NO (more strictly, of RNS, especially N$_2$O$_3$) is a reaction with thiol groups to form nitrosothiols (Hogg, 2002; Ahern et al., 2002). Nitrosation can modify the function of proteins such as enzymes and ion channels (Mannick and Schonhoff, 2004; Martinez-Ruiz and Lamas, 2004). Conditions that favor the formation of the RNS responsible for nitrosation are present in cell membranes (where NO and oxygen can concentrate) and so such agents may be particularly prevalent in white matter, where myelin is plentiful. Once formed, nitrosothiols can modify other thiol groups by transnitrosation reactions, and they are often more effective in this than NO (RNS) itself. Furthermore, nitrosothiols can functionally stabilize NO, effectively prolonging its half-life, whereas the half-life of NO in tissues is approximately 1 second (see previously), and the half-life of nitrosated albumin (SNO-albumin) is closer to 1 day. This consideration may allow the effects of NO to be spread to more distant cells by prolonging the available time for diffusion.

Although the production of NO within MS lesions is known to be substantially higher than normal, the actual NO concentration achieved is not known, nor is much guidance obtained by reference to other inflammatory lesions. Estimates of NO concentration resulting from *in vitro* preparation are interesting, but are unlikely to faithfully model the concentration achieved *in vivo*. Over the years, estimates of maximal NO concentrations have tended to fall, but so too have the estimated thresholds for several of the effects of NO on other molecules (e.g., Bellamy et al., 2002). Factors that affect NO concentrations include the overall concentration of NOS enzyme in cells throughout the lesion (most particularly the amount of the iNOS form), the availability of substrate and co-factors, the proximity to sinks such as hemoglobin in blood vessels, the capacity of the local cellular sink (Griffiths and Garthwaite, 2001; Griffiths et al., 2002), and the quantity of other scavengers such as superoxide.

The uncertainty regarding the identity of the RNS present at sites of inflammation is established right from the time of "NO" synthesis, as there is discussion over whether the NOS enzyme actually produces NO, or related species such as the nitroxyl anion (NO$^-$) (Alderton et al., 2001). Depending on conditions, NOS may effectively form NO (i.e., the free radical), NO$^-$, nitrosothiols, and probably small amounts of peroxynitrite (Stamler, 1999). As the precise form of NO involved in different aspects of axonal pathophysiology is typically not known, in this chapter the term NO is used to include the possibility that other RNS are actually the effector molecules.

III. Evidence for the Production of NO in MS

Many lines of evidence show that the production of NO is significantly raised in MS, and within MS lesions in particular. For example, the nitrite/nitrate concentration in the urine and blood (the ultimate fate of most of the NO pro-

duced within the body is in the form of nitrite and nitrate) is significantly increased in patients with demyelinating disease (Giovannoni, 1998; Giovannoni et al., 1997, 1999). Furthermore, nitrotyrosine, regarded as a relatively stable marker of peroxynitrite production, is very significantly raised (approximately sixfold, $P < 0.0001$) in the serum of patients with MS compared with controls, particularly in patients with chronic progressive disease (Zabaleta et al., 1998). More particular to the CNS are studies that have examined nitrite and nitrate concentrations within the cerebrospinal fluid. Although two early studies involving only a small number of patients did not find raised NOx in the cerebrospinal fluid (Ikeda et al., 1995; De Bustos et al., 1999), most studies have found significant increases (Cross et al., 1998; Brundin et al., 1999; Drulovic et al., 2001; Giovannoni, 1998; Johnson et al., 1995; Peltola et al., 2001; Yamashita et al., 1997; Ali et al., 1996; Svenningsson et al., 1999; Speciale et al., 2000), and some concentrations that correlated with clinical disease activity (e.g., Danilov et al., 2003).

The evidence for the local production of NO in MS lesions is compelling, in that there is prominent expression of the inducible form of NOS. iNOS is not normally present within the CNS, but iNOS mRNA was "abundantly expressed" in a biopsy taken from a patient with Marburg's-type MS within 33 days of the onset of disseminated symptoms (Bitsch et al., 1999), indicating that NO production is likely to be present from very early in the disease process. iNOS mRNA was also found in all seven MS brains examined in another study (Bagasra et al., 1995), and it was the dominant isoform of NOS found in another (Broholm et al., 2004) (see also Bo et al., 1994). Expression of the iNOS protein has been demonstrated in acute lesions using immunohistochemical techniques (Oleszak et al., 1998; Liu et al., 2001; Broholm et al., 2004), but expression diminishes or is absent in chronic (noninflammatory) lesions (De Groot et al., 1997; Liu et al., 2001; Oleszak et al., 1998; Broholm et al., 2004). Expression has been described in cells of the macrophage/microglial lineage (De Groot et al., 1997; Oleszak et al., 1998; Hooper et al., 1997; Broholm et al., 2004) and in reactive astrocytes (Liu et al., 2001; Broholm et al., 2004). iNOS is prominently and widely expressed in white and gray matter that appears normal macroscopically, and expression was moderate to high in 67% of samples lacking the histological characteristics of MS plaques (Broholm et al., 2004). iNOS mRNA (Koprowski et al., 1993) and protein (van Dam et al., 1995; Cross et al., 1997) are also expressed within the inflammatory lesions of animals with experimental autoimmune encephalomyelitis (EAE), where the level of expression coincides temporally and quantitatively with the severity of the neurological deficit (Koprowski et al., 1993; Okuda et al., 1995). The eNOS isoform is also highly expressed in intraparenchymal vascular endothelial cells in MS tissue, unlike the normal brain (Broholm et al., 2004). At the pathological concentrations of NO likely to be present in MS lesions, the enzyme sGC is likely to be near maximally activated, in which case the advantages of being able to use this enzyme pathway to exert subtle effects on cellular metabolism will be denied.

Peroxynitrite has a half-life in tissue measured in milliseconds, so it cannot be directly detected histologically, but persistent evidence of its ephemeral presence is provided by the finding of nitrotyrosine in many active MS lesions, and labeling can be intense (Liu et al., 2001), with labeling of hypertrophic astrocytes (Cross et al., 1998; Oleszak et al., 1998), and, especially, iNOS positive macrophages/microglial cells (Cross et al., 1998; Oleszak et al., 1998; Bagasra et al., 1995; Hooper et al., 1997).

Of particular interest is the observation that iNOS-positive astrocytes and, to a lesser extent, macrophage/microglial cells were diffusely scattered throughout the cerebral white matter in a patient with a rapid primary progressive course (Broholm et al., 2004), and strongly nNOS-positive astrocytes were also present. Furthermore, labeling was prominent and widespread in microglia in patients with primary progressive MS (Hans Lassmann, personal communication). These findings may be relevant to understanding the cause of the "smoldering" level of axonal degeneration that appears to be responsible for the progressive accumula-

tion of neurological deficit in this form of the disease. The role of NO in MS has been reviewed in more detail elsewhere (Smith et al., 1999; Santiago et al., 1998; Smith and Lassmann, 2002).

IV. NO Impairs Axonal Conduction

The first electrophysiological effect of NO on axons to be described was the block of conduction, and NO is very effective in this respect (Fig. 1) (Redford et al., 1997; Shrager et al.,1998; Garthwaite et al., 2002; Kapoor et al., 2003). The block is imposed within a few minutes of exposure, maintained for the duration of exposure (at least for several hours) and relieved within minutes of washing (Redford et al., 1997; Kapoor et al., 2003). The effects of NO appear to be fully reversible, and no apparent lasting consequences are revealed during at least 10 hours after exposure (Kapoor et al., 2003). In this sense, NO appears to act like a local anesthetic.

There is not yet any proof that NO is involved in causing neurological deficits in patients, but several observations are consistent with this possibility. Perhaps the clearest has arisen from some surprising observations in patients treated with an experimental MS therapy, the administration of the antibody CAMPATH-1H (Moreau et al., 1996). Indeed, it

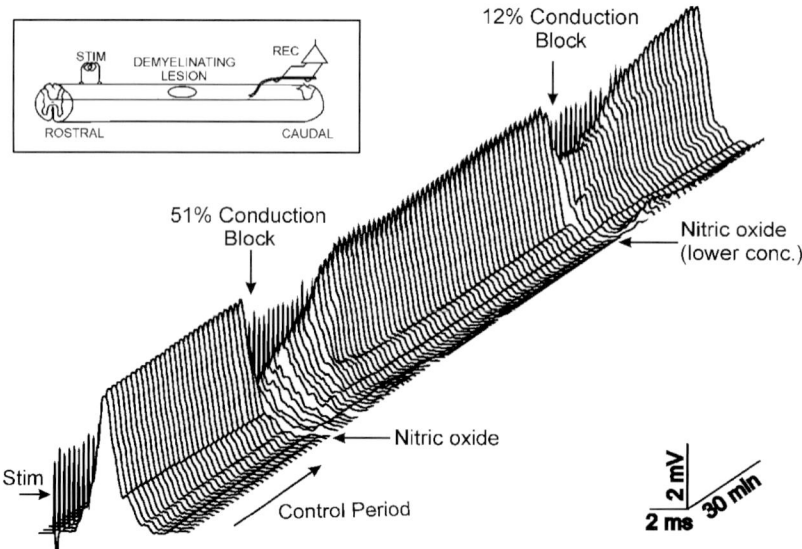

Figure 1 A series of records showing that NO causes a reversible block of conduction in central demyelinated axons when injected into an experimental lesion situated in the rat dorsal columns (*inset*). The records are plotted with three-dimensional perspective, with the earliest records shown at the front; the records were taken every 2 minutes and show about 5 hours of recording time. All the axons contributing to the compound action potentials were known to be affected by the demyelinating lesion on the basis of other recordings (not shown) and confirmed by histological examination. Conduction along the axons was stable until NO was applied by the injection of the NO donor spermine NONOate, when conduction in approximately half the axons was promptly blocked. The block reversed gradually over the next 30 minutes as the production of NO diminished. A second injection of a lower concentration of donor reinstated the block, in a smaller number of axons. (Modified from Redford et al., 1997.)

was a search for a mechanism to explain these observations that prompted the initial experiments with NO in the author's laboratory. The CAMPATH-1H antibody is directed against the CD52 antigen expressed on all lymphocytes, and its administration was intended to deplete patients of these lymphocytes as they are believed to be responsible for disease activity. Although the therapy had been administered with no ill effects to individuals without MS, when administered to patients with MS, the antibody quite promptly (2 to 4 hours) elicited a surprising reappearance of signs and symptoms that had previously been expressed, but from which recovery had occurred. New symptoms did not appear, indicating that the antibody administration had somehow reimposed conduction block in axons that had previously been damaged by the disease process. The reenactment of the symptoms occurred in conjunction with a surge in the level of circulating pro-inflammatory cytokines, but the initial suspicion that these were responsible for the exacerbation was not confirmed by experimentation (unpublished observations). Realization that the pro-inflammatory cytokines would result in the appearance of iNOS, however, directed attention to the potential role of NO and the findings described previously. In this regard, it is notable that demyelinated axons are particularly vulnerable to the effects of NO (Redford et al., 1997), providing a plausible explanation for the observations upon CAMPATH-1H administration.

Apart from the CAMPATH observations, other findings also indicate that inflammation may be capable of imposing severe conduction and neurological deficits in patients with inflammatory demyelinating disease (Youl et al., 1991; Coles et al., 1999), even in the absence of demyelination (Bitsch et al., 1999). Whether NO is involved in causing the deficits remains unproven, although it may be worth noting that iNOS was abundantly expressed in the inflammatory lesions believed to cause neurological deficits (Bitsch et al., 1999).

The mechanisms underlying NO-mediated conduction block are not known. However, the discoveries that NO can impair mitochondrial respiration, affect sodium channel properties, and cause axonal depolarization have provided several reasonable candidates to explain the block of conduction. These effects of NO are discussed later.

It is interesting to speculate on whether NO may play a role in Uhthoff's phenomenon (Smith and McDonald, 1999) (see Chapter 6), namely the tendency for the expression of some symptoms to be modulated by changes in body temperature. Body warming is deleterious, and cooling beneficial, such that in extreme cases a patient might experience an improvement in vision upon drinking a glass of cold water (Hopper et al., 1972; McDonald, 1986). Such effects arise from the modulation of axonal conduction block in affected pathways, and although the effect is conventionally explained by reference to the effects of temperature on action potential duration (Smith and McDonald, 1999) (see

Chapter 6), NO might play a role (Beenakker et al., 2001). Patients with MS who are temperature-sensitive and who wore a cooling garment achieved a clinical improvement, as expected, but the effect was associated in this study with a substantial reduction in leukocytic NO production. Thus, although changes in action potential duration *can* explain the clinical observations, changes in the rate of NO production may also play a role.

V. NO and Axonal Depolarization

One effect of NO that could contribute to the conduction abnormalities described previously is that it causes a prompt depolarization of axons and neurons, respectively, when applied to rat optic nerve (Garthwaite et al., 2002) and neurons in the hypothalamic paraventricular region (Bains and Ferguson, 1997). In the neurons at least, the depolarization could be reproduced by a cGMP analog (Bains and Ferguson, 1997). In the optic nerve, the depolarization commenced almost immediately on exposure to NO and consisted of two stages (Fig. 2). The initial stage resulted in only

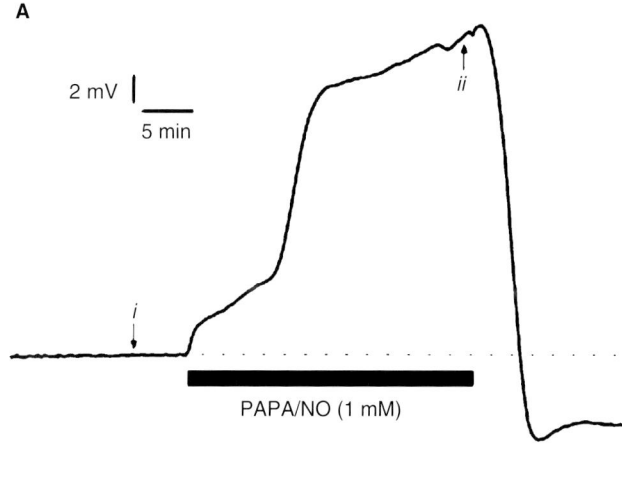

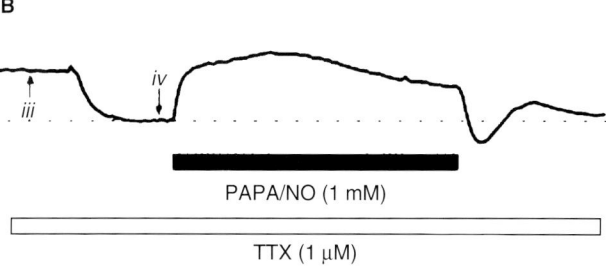

Figure 2 Depolarization of optic nerve axons in response to exposure to the NO donor PAPA NONOate (*solid bar*). (**A**) A small, prompt depolarization was followed by a larger depolarization that reversed rapidly on washout. (**B**) The sodium channel blocking agent tetrodotoxin (TTX) (*open bar*) caused a small hyperpolarization and abolished the delayed depolarization. (Reproduced from Garthwaite et al., 2002.)

a few millivolts of depolarization, but it progressed to a second, larger depolarization after 7 to 10 minutes. Depolarization was reversed on washing and was followed by a period of hyperpolarization. Although conduction persisted during the first stage of depolarization, it was blocked during the second. The cause of the first stage of depolarization is not certain, but the second stage appears to involve sodium entry via axolemmal sodium channels in conjunction with a reduction in adenosine triphosphate (ATP). The concentration of ATP fell by 44% after 10 minutes of NO exposure (Garthwaite et al., 2002). A potential cause of the reduction in ATP is described in the next section.

VI. Mitochondrial Dysfunction

Perhaps one of the most important consequences of NO production in MS lesions will prove to be an inhibition of mitochondrial respiration, leading to a reduced, and perhaps insufficient, production of ATP. At present it is not certain that NO has these effects in MS lesions, but there is a weight of circumstantial evidence suggesting this may be so.

The effects of NO on mitochondria have been the subject of several recent reviews (Brown and Bal-Price, 2003; Brown and Borutaite, 2002; Duchen, 2000, 2004; Brorson et al., 1999; Beltran et al., 2000a). In brief, there is good evidence that NO and its related molecules are potent in inhibiting enzymes of the respiratory chain. In particular, NO exerts an acute, potent, and reversible inhibition of cytochrome c oxidase (complex IV, the terminal component of the mitochondrial respiratory chain) in competition with oxygen (Brown and Cooper, 1994; Cleeter et al., 1994; Sarti et al., 2003), and reactive nitrogen species, such as peroxynitrite, can also irreversibly inhibit the respiratory pathway at several additional stages, including complexes I, II, and V (reviewed in Brown and Borutaite, 2002; Radi et al., 2002). The inhibition of these key components of mitochondrial respiration understandably reduces ATP production (Brookes et al., 1999; Brorson et al., 1999), and this can be expected to have prompt and marked deleterious consequences in axons because they have high energy demands. For example, a reduction in ATP could easily be sufficient to result in a failure to maintain the axonal ion gradients upon which conduction and normal axonal physiology depend (Ames III, 2000). Some potential consequences of this failure are discussed in the section NO and Axonal Degeneration.

There is an ongoing debate regarding whether NO may affect mitochondrial metabolism at *physiological* concentrations (e.g., Brown et al., 1995; Brown, 2000; Bellamy et al., 2002; Moncada and Erusalimsky, 2002; Keynes and Garthwaite, 2004; Brookes et al., 2003); that is, whether NO exists at a sufficient concentration in the normal nervous system to achieve a significant inhibition of cytochrome c oxidase. However, NO-mediated mitochondrial inhibition is less controversial when pathological concentrations of NO are concerned. Thus at tissue oxygen concentrations (e.g., 5-30μM oxygen), NO at only 100 nM concentration achieves an approximately 60% inhibition of mitochondrial respiration, at least *in vitro*, with a K_i reported to be as low as 27 or 60 nM (Fig. 3) (Brown, 2000; Brown and Cooper, 1994; Koivisto et al., 1997; Brookes et al., 2003). Although the NO concentration within MS lesions is not known, it seems likely that it will reach or exceed these levels, especially in the more intensely inflammatory lesions where iNOS-positive cells are plentiful. Furthermore, the effects of NO are significantly augmented by hypoxia, and there is recent evidence that hypoxia-like conditions exist within some MS lesions (Aboul-Enein et al., 2003). Moreover, the likelihood of irreversible damage to mitochondrial function increases not only with exposure to higher NO concentrations, but also with prolonged exposure to NO (Brookes et al., 1999; Beltran et al., 2000b; Stewart et al., 2000; Clementi et al., 1998), and such exposure will certainly occur in inflammatory MS lesions. On the basis of magnetic resonance imaging (MRI) observations, inflammation can persist within lesions for weeks or months.

NO can also open the mitochondrial permeability transition pore (Horn et al., 2002), a large conductance pore that, when open, can cause a collapse of the mitochondrial membrane potential, leading to ATP depletion (reviewed in Duchen, 2004). There is also evidence that the overall reduction in ATP synthesis can be sufficiently profound in neurons so that NO probably also inhibits glycolysis (Brorson et al., 1999), such as by the inhibition of glyceraldehyde-3-phosphate dehydrogenase (Brune and Mohr, 2001).

Apart from compromising ATP production, inhibition of complex IV can result in the increased production of super-

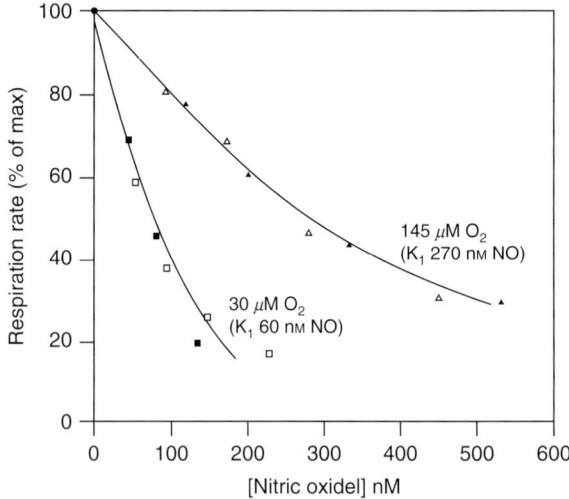

Figure 3 Curves showing the effect of different concentrations of NO on mitochondrial metabolism at two concentrations of oxygen. The potency of NO is enhanced at tissue concentrations of oxygen (~30μM). (Reproduced from Brown, 2000.)

oxide and other reactive oxygen species by mitochondria, with the likely consequence of an increased damaging production of peroxynitrite (Moncada and Erusalimsky, 2002; Brown and Borutaite, 2001). Beyond inhibiting several key molecules within mitochondria, this strong oxidizing agent will have additional deleterious effects on proteins, lipids, and other targets within MS lesions.

Several lines of evidence suggest that mitochondrial function is indeed impaired in MS and EAE, in line with expectations based on the previous observations, although whether NO is responsible for the impairment is not yet clear. However, oxidative damage to mitochondrial DNA has been reported in active MS plaques (Vladimirova et al., 1998; Lu et al., 2000) associated with an impaired NADH dehydrogenase activity (Lu et al., 2000). A pronounced reduction in the axonal density of ATPase-positive mitochondria has been described in a subset of acutely demyelinating plaques (reported in Smith and Lassmann, 2002). Microarray analysis of MS normal-appearing white matter has also revealed the upregulation of genes that reflect a higher energy metabolism (Graumann et al., 2003). The cause for this upregulation is not yet clear, but it is arguably in compensation for a diminished energy production from the existing mitochondria. The same study reported evidence suggesting a global defense against oxidative and perhaps nitrosative stress. In EAE, an inhibition of respiratory chain function has been reported in brain macrophage/microglial cells (Zielasek et al., 1995), and a lactic acidosis has also been noted during the onset of clinical signs (Simmons et al., 1982).

Demyelinated regions of axons might be especially vulnerable to an inhibition of mitochondrial respiration on the basis of the observation that they possess greater numbers of mitochondria than normal (Mutsaers and Carroll, 1998). This finding suggests that energy demand is higher in demyelinated than in normal axons, and it is easy to imagine many reasons why this should be so. For example, although unproven, it seems certain that the sodium load incurred per conducted action potential will be much greater along demyelinated membranes in comparison with the normally myelinated portions of the same axon (see Chapter 6).

Finally, it has recently been reported that NO can trigger the biogenesis of mitochondria in some cell types, by a cGMP-dependent mechanism (Nisoli et al., 2003). Whether such an event occurs within the CNS in MS has not been examined, but, if it occurs, it could tend to diminish the deleterious consequences of some of the phenomena described previously.

VII. NO and Ion Channels

A. NO and Sodium Channels

Sodium channels are perhaps the single-most important ion channel in axons (see Chapter 7, this volume), so it is sig-nificant that many reports describe potent effects of NO on sodium channel physiology. No single effect of NO emerges from the different reports, and this likely reflects the use in the different studies of different concentrations of NO (some of which may be supra-pathophysiological) and the examination of different NO species, studied in different ways on different subtypes of channel within different cell types (where different accessory proteins/factors may be present). It is also clear, however, that sodium channel properties are modified in whole cell preparations by the relatively low concentrations of NO produced by the cells themselves. Both cGMP-mediated (e.g. Smith and Otis, 2003) and cGMP-independent (e.g., thiol modification; Renganathan et al., 2002b; Ahern et al., 2000) actions of NO on sodium channels have been reported.

NO can both substantially potentiate the persistent sodium current (Ahern et al., 2000), or block both this current and the fast and slow sodium currents (Li et al., 1998; Renganathan et al., 2000, 2002a, 2002b; Bielefeldt et al., 1999). The persistent sodium current is normally a small fraction (~1%) of the transient sodium current associated with the formation of an action potential, but because it is persistent, it can significantly affect the physiological properties of axons by biasing axonal excitability. In one study, bath application of NO to pituitary nerve terminals increased the channel activity in excised outside-out patches from almost nothing >20 ms after the start of a depolarizing pulse, to high activity throughout the duration of a 50 ms pulse (Fig. 4) (Ahern et al., 2000). Similar findings regarding the persistent current, with little effect on the transient current, have also been reported in excised patches from hippocampal neurons (Hammarstrom and Gage, 1999) (see also Sawada et al., 1995).

In another preparation (cardiac myocytes), an increase in persistent sodium current resulted from ionomycin treatment to stimulate the endogenous production of NO (Ahern et al., 2000). Thus even relatively low concentrations of NO can produce an increase in channel open probability. Such changes would be expected to increase axonal excitability, and it is interesting to speculate on whether the changes may contribute to the hyperexcitability expressed by demyelinated axons (Smith et al., 1997; Baker, 2000). Indeed, there is evidence that the generation of ectopic impulses at sites of demyelination along central axons can be due to a persistent sodium current that develops at these sites (Rizzo et al., 1996b; Kapoor et al., 1997; Smith et al., 1997; Baker, 2000; Baker and Bostock, 1992; see Chapter 9). The potential effects of NO on axons may be expected to be diversified in MS because of the appearance along some demyelinated axons of atypical sodium channels for the site of expression. Thus although the dominant subtype of sodium channels at nodes of Ranvier in the adult is $Na_v1.6$, there is a switch to include $Na_v1.2$ along some demyelinated axons in animals with EAE

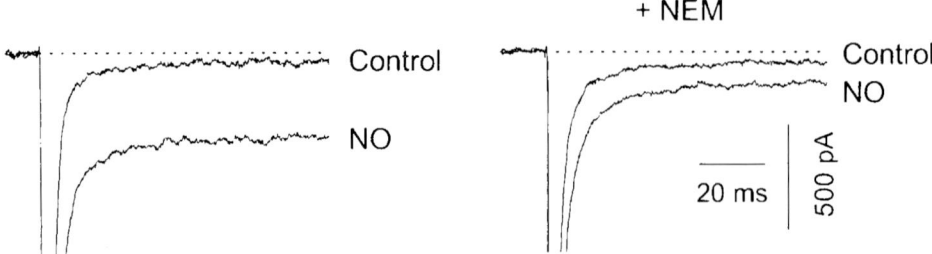

Figure 4 Records showing the effect of NO applied to myocytes on the flash photolysis of sodium nitroprusside. Note that the persistent sodium current following the spike (which goes off scale) is increased many fold. The increase was reversed by the sulphydryl alkylating agent *N*-ethylmaleimide (NEM). (Reproduced from Ahern et al., 2000.)

(Craner et al., 2003) and patients with MS (Craner et al., 2004b).

Unmyelinated axons from dorsal root ganglion cells enter the spinal cord and also, therefore, are affected by spinal inflammatory lesions in MS. Sodium channels in the neurons of such axons are prominently affected by NO, and NO donors block the fast, slow, and persistent sodium currents of such neurons by S-nitrosation (Renganathan et al., 2002b). Indeed, there is evidence that NO can act as an autocrine regulator of sodium currents in these cells (Renganathan et al., 2000).

Unsurprisingly, given its wide range of effects, exposure to NO can change the electrophysiological properties of whole neurons, and it has been found to excite or inhibit spontaneous firing in different neurons when applied to the whole spinal cord (Pehl and Schmid, 1997). Sustained (> 40 minute) increases in the spontaneous firing rate of Purkinje neurons has been observed in response to activation of the NO-cGMP signaling pathway using NO donors (Smith and Otis, 2003). Similar effects can result from NO generated by parallel fiber activity (Smith and Otis, 2003).

B. NO and Potassium Channels

The voltage-gated potassium channels expressed by central myelinated axons are predominantly of the Kv1.1, Kv1.2, and Kv3.1 subtypes (Devaux et al., 2003; Scherer and Arroyo, 2002); but in contrast to the several reports of effects of NO on sodium and calcium channels, few studies have examined the effects of NO specifically on these subtypes of potassium channels. The NO donor S-nitrosocysteine had few effects on Kv1.1 currents (Busch et al., 1996), but NO donors were found to suppress Kv3.1 currents by a cGMP-mediated pathway (Moreno et al., 2001).

C. NO and Calcium Channels

Functional calcium channels are not plentiful along axons, but there is immunohistochemical and pharmacological evidence that L-type calcium channels are present in normal mammalian CNS axons (Ouardouz et al., 2003;

Brown et al., 2001), and that N-type calcium channels can appear along demyelinated axons (Kornek et al., 2001). The effects of NO on calcium channels are complex. NO is reported to inhibit L-type calcium currents in rabbit glomus (carotid body) cells via a cGMP independent mechanism (Summers et al., 1999), whereas NO inhibited calcium currents in dorsal root ganglion cells by a cGMP-dependent mechanism (Kim et al., 2000). In contrast, but also in peripheral neurons, NO donors were found to enhance calcium currents, in superior cervical ganglion neurons after intracellular or extracellular application, by a cGMP-dependent mechanism (Chen and Schofield, 1995). However, most examinations have used muscle tissue, and here both a stimulation (Kirstein et al., 1995; Abi-Gerges et al., 2002) and an inhibition (Hu et al., 1997; Gallo et al., 2001; Dittrich et al., 2001) of L-type calcium current have been reported, apparently mediated by direct nitrosation of the channel and by cGMP in different preparations. Thus nitrosothiols and NO can have different effects. One study found that L-type calcium channels in ferret ventricular myocytes were stimulated by nitrosation of the channel and inhibited by cGMP, suggesting that sarcolemmal thiol redox state may be an important determinant of channel activity (Campbell et al., 1996). Some of the effects of NO appear to be biphasic, seemingly depending on the interplay between different biochemical pathways.

In whole-cell and single-channel studies of L-type calcium channels expressed in kidney cells, some data suggest that nitrosation of an intracellularly located channel thiol is important in determining channel gating and conductance (Poteser et al., 2001).

D. NO and Ryanodine Receptors

It has been reported that ryanodine receptors are present in axons (Ouardouz et al., 2003), which raises the interesting possibility that NO might affect axonal physiology via this route. There are so far no studies of the effects of NO on axonal ryanodine receptors, but guidance might be taken from studies in muscle. Here, NO is believed to play a role in the normal physiological function of muscle cells (i.e., contraction), where ryanodine receptors play a key role (Stamler and Meissner, 2001; Salama et al., 2000; Hare, 2003). In muscle, ryanodine receptors are well-established components in the calcium-induced calcium release mechanism, whereby calcium ions entering a muscle cell via its voltage-dependent, L-type calcium channels triggers the release of calcium ions from the sarcoplasmic reticulum (SR). The release is achieved by opening the high conductance SR calcium release channel, the ryanodine receptor. These receptors are exceptionally rich in free thiol groups, and certain of these have a high sensitivity to oxidation/ nitrosation, resulting in channel opening (Fig. 5) (Xu et al., 1998; Stoyanovsky et al., 1997; Eu et al., 1999). Indeed, S-nitrosation of up to 12 sites on the receptor can lead to the progressive activation of the channel, which is reversed by denitrosation (Xu et al., 1998), although nitrosation of a single cysteine may occur physiologically (Eu et al., 2000). In the initial studies, rather high, seemingly nonphysiological concentrations of exogenous nitric oxide were used to study these effects, but it is now emerging that within the normal

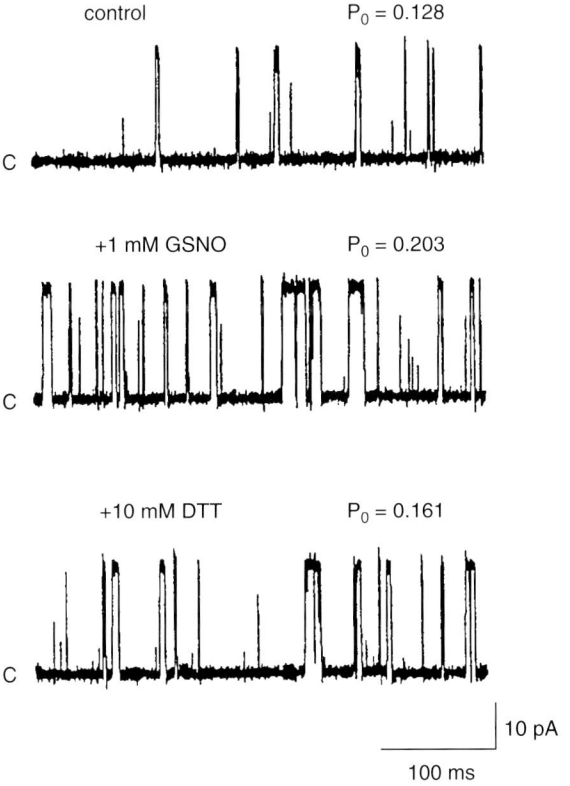

Figure 5 Records showing the effects of NO (in the form of the donor GSNO) on the cardiac ryanodine receptor located in a planar lipid bilayer. Single-channel currents are shown as upward deflections from the closed levels, before (top record) and 1 minute after 1 mM GSNO (middle record) and then 1 minute after 10 mM dithiothreitol (DTT) (bottom record). Exposure to NO increased the frequency of channel opening, which was reversed by DTT. (Modified from Xu et al., 1998.)

muscle cell NO formation can occur in distinct microdomains where nNOS (NOS1) and eNOS (NOS3) isoforms occur in close proximity with ryanodine receptors and SR calcium ATPase, and with L-type calcium channels, respectively (reviewed in Hare, 2003). In this way, NO is delivered as required in the immediate vicinity of its intended targets.

In muscle cells, NO can nitrosate critical thiols on the ryanodine receptor to effect activation and/or inhibition of the receptor, and these actions appear to play a role in normal muscle contraction. Indeed, NO cycles in the beating heart on millisecond time scales, and in canine heart cells, the ryanodine receptor is reported to be endogenously nitrosated (Xu et al., 1998; Eu et al., 2000). By analogy with the observations in muscle, it seems reasonable to propose on the basis of the observations by Ouardouz et al. (2003) that NO may promote calcium release in axons from intra-axonal stores. This may be especially prominent in inflammatory MS lesions, with sustained high concentrations of NO and axons unadapted for such NO exposure. When considered in conjunction with the fact that calcium concentrations within neuronal endoplasmic reticulum can be substantial, especially after electrical activity (Pozzo-Miller et al., 1999), it is clear that axons could become flooded with damaging concentrations of calcium. Indeed, whereas muscle cells contain high concentrations of the NO-scavenger myoglobin, this is not the case in axons, which may therefore be more sensitive to NO.

Apart from affecting the function of ryanodine receptors by the direct nitrosation of critical thiols, there is also evidence that NO may affect their function by phosphorylation via cGMP-dependent protein kinase (Suko et al., 1993). Also, apart from calcium release via ryanodine receptors, it is possible that inositol-1,4,5-triphosphate (IP3) receptors could be involved, although the effects of NO on IP3 receptors have not been extensively studied.

VIII. NO and the Na$^+$/K$^+$ ATPase (Sodium Pump)

Na$^+$/K$^+$ ATPase plays a key role in axonal physiology, being responsible for sodium extrusion after impulse activity, and contributing to the maintenance of resting potential. Indeed, Na$^+$/K$^+$ ATPase consumes approximately 50% of the energy supply in the CNS. It is significant, therefore, that NO is quite potent in impairing the function of the enzyme, both *in vitro* (Guzman et al., 1995; Sato et al., 1995; Muriel and Sandoval, 2000) and *in vivo* (Liu and Sheu, 1997) when NO production is raised by iNOS formation. Indeed, there is now evidence that the Na$^+$/K$^+$ ATPase is nitrosated under physiological conditions *in vivo* as a result of nNOS activity, even without the additional contribution from iNOS (Jaffrey et al., 2001). The inhibition appears to be due to an interaction between NO or a related reactive nitrogen species and a thiol group at the active site of the enzyme (Sato et al., 1997; Boldyrev et al., 1997), although other evidence also supports an action mediated via cGMP (McKee et al., 1994). Brain Na$^+$/K$^+$ ATPase is more vulnerable to inhibition than that from kidney (Boldyrev et al., 1997). If, as seems likely, function of the Na$^+$/K$^+$ ATPase is impaired in axons affected by inflammatory lesions in MS, the axons may become depolarized, and also prone to sodium loading, thereby becoming predisposed to degeneration (see later).

IX. NO and the Sodium-Calcium Exchanger

The axolemmal sodium-calcium exchanger is a non-ATP-dependent antiporter that normally functions to export calcium ions from the axon at the expense of importing sodium ions. There is evidence that under pathological circumstances, the exchanger can sometimes operate in reverse (see Chapter 19) (Stys et al., 1992), and then it can play a role in promoting deleterious calcium entry into axons when axons are exposed to NO (see later) (Kapoor et al., 2003). These observations become even more interesting when considered with evidence that the activity of the sodium-calcium exchanger can be modulated by NO in neuronal preparations in a cGMP-dependent mechanism (Asano et al., 1995) and in T-cells by an intimate association with constitutive NOS (cNOS) (Kiang et al., 2003). In T-cells it seems that it is the phosphorylation of the NOS enzyme that decreases the kinetic activity of the exchanger. The consequences of any modulation of this exchanger by NO would be different depending on the prevailing direction of transport at the time of NO exposure.

X. NO and Glial Cells

Apart from affecting axons directly, it is likely that NO will also affect them indirectly by effects on glial cells. Whereas astrocytes and microglia are likely to be relatively resistant to the effects of NO, as these cells can become iNOS positive themselves, there is evidence that oligodendrocytes are much more sensitive to NO-mediated toxicity (Mitrovic et al., 1994, 1996; Merrill et al., 1993). Indeed, depending on the concentration and duration of exposure, NO can kill oligodendrocytes by necrosis (Mitrovic et al., 1995; Boullerne et al., 1999; Garthwaite et al., 2002) or apoptosis (Molina-Holgado et al., 2001; Boullerne et al., 1999), and perhaps by inducing DNA strand breaks, with the subsequent energy-consuming action of poly(ADP-ribose) synthetase (Zhang et al., 1994). Reactive nitrogen species, especially peroxynitrite, may also damage oligodendrocytes and their myelin by inducing lipid peroxidation (Radi et al.,

1991; van der Veen and Roberts, 1999). If NO exposure in MS lesions does kill oligodendrocytes, demyelination will ensue, and this will have severe effects on axonal pathophysiology, as described by Smith and Waxman (see Chapter 6).

XI. NO-Preconditioning?

Axons within MS lesions may be exposed to NO for prolonged periods (weeks) and on repeated occasions if inflammation at a lesion is reactivated. Under these circumstances, it is not unreasonable to ask whether the affected axons may become partly tolerant to NO via mechanisms similar to those operating in ischemic preconditioning (Gonzalez-Zulueta et al., 2000). Indeed, microarray analysis of MS brain tissue has revealed the upregulation of neuroprotective genes known to be induced by ischemic preconditioning (and also genes suggesting a neuroprotective reaction against oxidative stress) (Graumann et al., 2003). Such preconditioning can be induced by sublethal exposure to NO, among other factors. Whether exposure of axons (rather than their cell bodies) to NO results in preconditioning is not yet clear.

XII. Other Effects of NO

There are reports that NO, acting either directly or indirectly, can affect Na$^+$/H$^+$ exchange (Chen and Guo, 1999; Gill et al., 2002) and that peroxynitrite can affect several types of glutamate transporters (Trotti et al., 1996). However, although this may be potentially important, it may be premature to speculate on the consequences to axonal pathophysiology of such effects beyond mentioning the possibility of demyelination resulting from injury to oligodendrocytes. These myelinating cells are particularly sensitive to glutamate (at least *in vitro*) (Oka et al., 1993). The role of glutamate in white matter injury is discussed by Stys (2004) and in Chapter 19.

There is also evidence that the calcium ATPase (calcium pump) can be nitrated, and probably inactivated, by peroxynitrite (Klebl et al., 1998; Viner et al., 1999). It is reasonable to suppose that this will be deleterious for axonal function.

XIII. Beneficial Effects of NO

This chapter has focused on the deleterious effects of NO, as NO is likely to be largely deleterious to axons when produced at the relatively high concentrations associated with iNOS production. However, NO can also have antioxidant properties by, for example, reacting with peroxyl and hydroxyl radicals (Halliwell et al., 1999; Kagan et al., 2001; Wink et al., 2001), and it can also break lipid peroxidation chain reactions (Hogg and Kalyanaraman, 1999; O'Donnell and Freeman, 2001), which may be important in the lipid-rich environment of the myelin sheath.

Beyond the margins of inflammatory lesions, NO will diminish in concentration, perhaps sharply, and at low concentrations the effects of the agent may be largely beneficial, as occurs at the margins of ischemic lesions (Keynes and Garthwaite, 2004). The majority of the beneficial effects of NO, however, probably occur outside of the brain parenchyma, where NO can suppress lymphocyte proliferation and inhibit their infiltration into the brain. Such events are beyond the subject of this review.

XIV. NO and Axonal Degeneration

Given the range of largely deleterious effects of NO outlined previously, it is perhaps not surprising that NO has been implicated in axonal degeneration. Interest in this phenomenon has been spurred in recent years by the realization that axonal degeneration is substantial in MS, and that it is an important cause of permanent neurological deficits. A consistent finding from several studies is that the degeneration occurs from early in the disease, that axons are transected within the inflammatory lesions, and that the number of axons affected is proportional to the intensity of the inflammation (Trapp et al., 1998; Ferguson et al., 1997). In fact, the extent of axonal destruction in MS lesions especially correlates with the number of activated (presumably iNOS positive) macrophages (Ferguson et al., 1997), which can be found in close apposition with injured axons (Trapp et al., 1998). There has been suspicion that factor(s) associated with inflammation are responsible, and NO is one of the factors for which evidence has accumulated.

Two patterns of axonal degeneration can be distinguished in MS. One pattern is that described previously, which is clearly related to inflammation, but there is also a "slow burning" axonal degeneration in chronic demyelinated plaques (Kornek et al., 2000), which may be responsible for the gradual accumulation of permanent neurological deficit in progressive disease. It has been argued that these latter lesions are noninflammatory as they do not enhance on MRI examination, in which case NO is unlikely to be involved. In contrast, we believe that NO may be involved in both patterns of degeneration, perhaps acting by similar mechanisms, as even in progressive disease axonal degeneration occurs on a background of residual inflammation (Guseo and Jellinger, 1975; Prineas and Wright, 1978) in an environment where many microglial cells are intensely iNOS-positive.

It is clear that simple exposure to a sufficiently high concentration of NO (low micromolar) can kill axons (Kapoor et al., 1999, 2003; Garthwaite et al., 2002) and that pro-

longed exposure to moderate concentrations (as may occur in MS lesions) is much more damaging than brief exposure to much higher concentrations. In fact, axons are much more sensitive to the deleterious effects of NO than are Schwann cells, oligodendrocytes, and astrocytes. Nonetheless, the extent to which NO kills axons in this way in MS lesions is not yet clear, nor is it clear whether such directly NO-mediated degeneration happens at all. Apart from such seemingly direct damage to axons, however, there is evidence to support a less directly toxic role for NO, in which several of its effects described previously may conspire together to effect axonal degeneration. In this mechanism another, usually innocuous, factor plays an important, indeed decisive, role, namely physiological levels of axonal impulse activity (Smith et al., 2001a). The mechanism involves a raised intra-axonal sodium ion concentration, which leads in turn to a lethally high intra-axonal calcium ion concentration mediated via reverse operation of the sodium-calcium exchanger.

The entry of sodium ions into axons is an inherent part of normal physiology, but several events theoretically exacerbate entry in MS lesions. Apart from the sodium entry inherent to the normal physiological impulse traffic, sodium entry is increased, probably dramatically, in demyelinated axons as a result of changes in the sodium channel distribution along the demyelinated axolemma (Smith et al., 1982; Bostock and Sears, 1976) (see Chapters 6 and 8), perhaps augmented by changes in the types of sodium channels expressed (Craner et al., 2003, 2004a) (see Chapter 7). Indeed, there is indirect evidence (Rizzo et al., 1996b; Kapoor et al., 1997; Smith et al., 1997; Baker, 2000; Baker and Bostock, 1992) that demyelinated axolemma can acquire properties that result in a persistent sodium current, namely a continuous drain of sodium ions into the axon. This entry will be markedly exacerbated if the axons become hyperexcitable (see Chapter 6) (Kapoor et al., 1997; Smith and McDonald, 1980, 1982; Baker and Bostock, 1992; Rizzo et al., 1996a). Demyelinated axons can generate ectopic activity continuously at frequencies of up to 50 Hz, which amounts to an additional 180,000 action potentials per hour. These causes of sodium entry will certainly put axons under more strain than normal, but, nonetheless, there is evidence that they can cope with the sodium load quite adequately, given that axons can generate ectopic activity continuously for at least 10 hours (Smith and McDonald, 1982) and probably indefinitely. The problem appears to be imposed by the presence of NO, acting in several of the different ways described previously.

First, NO can affect sodium channels in such a way that they have a much greater probability of being in the open configuration (Ahern et al., 2000; Hammarstrom and Gage, 1999), resulting in a marked increase in the persistent sodium current. This effect results in a substantial additional drain of sodium ions into the axon. Second, NO can inhibit mitochondrial metabolism (see previously) (Brown and

Cooper, 1994; Cleeter et al., 1994; Sarti et al., 2003), depriving the axon of the ATP required to extrude the sodium ions via the Na$^+$/K$^+$ ATPase. This failure may be augmented by a direct inhibition of the enzyme by NO (Guzman et al., 1995; Sato et al., 1995). If the pump does not function adequately, the internal concentration of sodium ions will start to increase inexorably. The increase may well be exacerbated by a separate increase in the persistent sodium current as a result of an effective hypoxia (Aboul-Enein et al., 2003; Hammarstrom and Gage, 1998), perhaps simulated in this case by the NO-mediated inhibition of mitochondrial activity. Although sodium ions are not particularly toxic, we know, from the elegant studies of Stys and Waxman and colleagues into the consequences of severe energy deprivation resulting from ischemia (Stys and LoPachin, 1997; Stys et al., 1991; Waxman et al., 1994) (see Chapter 19), that if the internal concentration of sodium ions rises to a sufficient level, the axolemmal sodium-calcium exchanger can start to operate in reverse (Stys and LoPachin, 1998; Waxman et al., 1994; Ransom et al., 1993), importing calcium into the axon instead of exporting it. Indeed, Na$_v$1.6 sodium channels (which produce a substantial persistent current (Herzog et al., 2003)) co-localize with the exchanger, and axons in MS lesions show evidence of damage at sites expressing the Na$_v$1.6 and the sodium-calcium exchanger (Craner et al., 2004a, 2004b). Calcium will be imported into an axon that is already deprived of ATP, so it will not be able to maintain calcium homeostasis by the normal energy-dependent mechanisms involving the calcium ATPase, or sequestration into mitochondria or the endoplasmic reticulum. This problem may be exacerbated by an NO-mediated opening of the axonal ryanodine receptors (Eu et al., 2000) discovered in axons (Ouardouz et al., 2003), and by calcium-mediated proteolysis of sodium channels adding to the persistent sodium current (Iwata et al., 2004). In these events the intra-axonal calcium ion concentration rises uncontrollably, eventually causing axonal degeneration by the activation of degradative enzymes. These enzymes cause the dissolution of the axoplasm, and this is observed histologically in experimental preparations (Smith et al., 2001a). This proposed mechanism is discussed in more detail by Bechtold and Smith (2004).

Although we hypothesize that this sequence of events can cause axonal degeneration if the NO concentration is sufficiently high (Smith et al., 2001a), there is also evidence that at more marginal NO concentrations, there is a window where the fate of axons depends on their level of impulse activity. Within this window, the decisive factor determining whether axons will degenerate or survive is the level of ongoing impulse activity (Smith et al., 2001a). Impulse formation is not an energy-dependent process; as long as there is a sufficient membrane potential and sufficient sodium current, even a metabolically poisoned axon will continue to make action potentials, adding to the sodium load.

Experimental evidence shows that this additional load can be fatal for the axon, such that axons in two spinal roots exposed to seemingly identical conditions, including vascular perfusion and NO concentration, can either all survive or all degenerate, depending simply on their frequency of impulse conduction (Fig. 6) (Smith et al., 2001a). Frequencies in the physiological range are sufficient in this respect, and it follows that physiological levels of impulse activity in patients may be sufficient to precipitate axonal degeneration at sites of inflammation where the axons will be exposed to NO.

XV. Implications for Therapy

Consideration of the preceding mechanism reveals several potential avenues by which axons might be protected from degeneration in inflammatory disorders such as MS. First, NO could be scavenged, or inflammatory NO production could be suppressed. These are attractive goals, but they are not only difficult to achieve in patients with currently available drugs; they are also potentially dangerous. Effective NO scavenging would lead to unacceptable increases in blood pressure, and experiments with iNOS inhibitors in EAE have revealed that such therapies can have lethal results (Willenborg et al., 1999), probably as a result of the release from NO-mediated suppression of peripheral immune events. Second, the sodium-calcium exchanger could be suppressed to avoid the damaging entry of calcium ions. The potential value of this avenue has already been demonstrated in a laboratory model of NO-induced axonal injury (Smith et al., 2001b; Kapoor et al., 2003), and we are currently examining its utility in animals with EAE. However, there are significant questions with regard to whether this will ever be an acceptable therapy for chronic use in patients. Finally, it should be possible to protect axons from degeneration by limiting the rise in intra-axonal sodium by partial blockade of their sodium channels. Such drugs are commonly used in neurological practice as anticonvulsants, and they are acceptable and safe for chronic administration. The potential efficacy in MS of this approach is suggested by the successful axonal protection that has recently been achieved using sodium channel-blocking agents in some simplified laboratory models (Kapoor et al., 1998, 2003; Smith et al., 2001b; Garthwaite et al., 2002) and in animal models of MS, namely phenytoin in progressive EAE (Lo et al., 2002, 2003) and flecainide in chronic relapsing EAE (Fig. 7) (Bechtold et al., 2004). The good results with flecainide have now been reproduced with lamotrigine, and to a lesser extent with phenytoin, in chronic relapsing EAE (DA Bechtold, KJ Smith, unpublished observations). Carbamazepine was not found to be effective in axonal protection in this study, but this result, and the limited protection produced by phenytoin, are

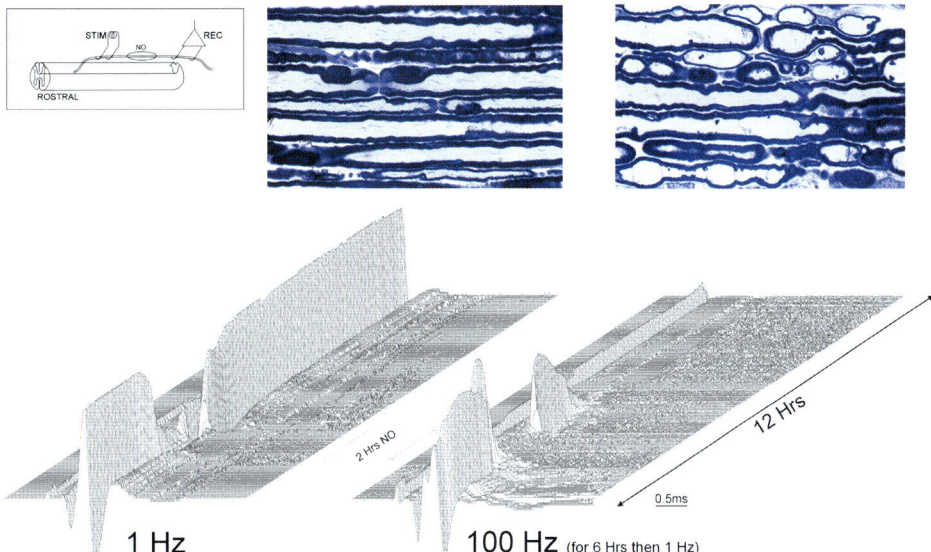

Figure 6 Two series of averaged compound action potentials recorded in parallel, in an anesthetized rat, over a 12-hour period from two separate dorsal roots using the arrangement indicated (*inset*). The data are shown in three-dimensional perspective, as in Figure 1. In the left plot, the root was stimulated at 1 Hz throughout, but in the right the stimulation was a 100 Hz for the first 6 hours, followed by 1 Hz for the remaining 6 hours. On both sides the records were relatively stable for the first 2.5 hours, but conduction block was imposed on nearly all the axons by a 2-hour exposure to NO. This block was released upon removal of the NO. In the left plot all the axons continued to conduct for the remaining 7.5 hours of the experiment. In contrast, in the right plot it is clear that exposure to the same concentration of NO, but experienced in conjunction with 100 Hz impulse activity, resulted in only a transient recovery of function, followed by persistent conduction block, despite the later reduction of the stimulus frequency to only 1 Hz. Histological examination of the roots at the end of the experiment revealed that whereas the root stimulated at only 1 Hz during the period of NO exposure was quite normal in appearance, all the axons exposed to NO in conjunction with stimulation of 100 Hz had undergone degeneration. (Redrawn from Smith et al., 2001a.)

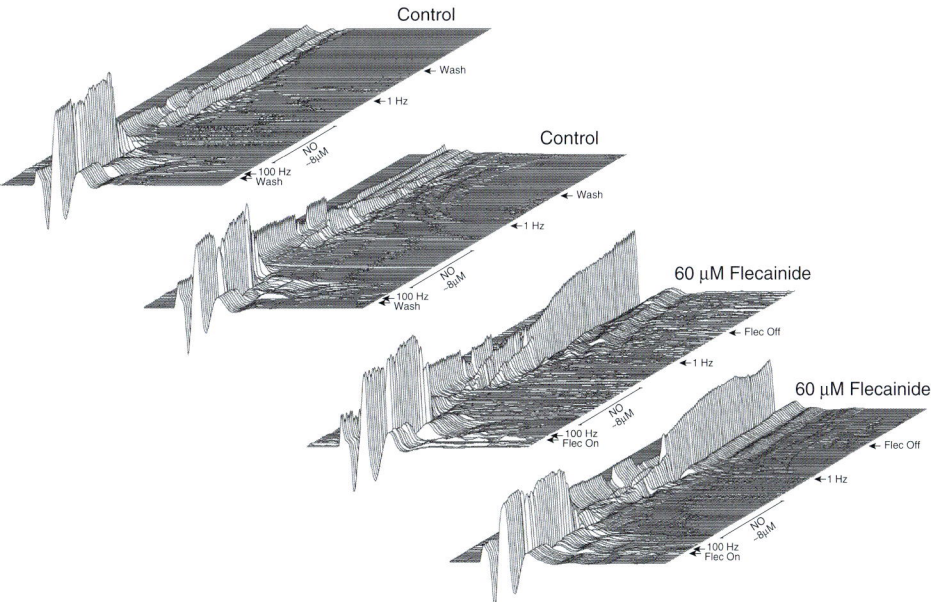

Figure 7 Four series of records obtained using the same protocol as in Figure 6. In the upper two plots the combination of impulse activity and NO exposure resulted in persistent conduction block in almost all of the axons, as in Figure 6. Despite experiencing exactly the same protocol, however, conduction in the adjacent roots (*lower two plots*) was restored, showing that almost all the axons survived. In these roots, the sodium channel-blocking agent flecainide was included with the NO donor, although in a sufficiently low dose that conduction persisted despite the presence of the drug. The inclusion of flecainide protected the axons from degeneration. (Modified from Kapoor et al., 2003.)

likely due to the short plasma half-life of these drugs in the rat, as monitoring of circulating levels revealed the presence of only subclinical concentrations during part of the day. In view of these findings, clinical trials are planned to examine the value of lamotrigine and phenytoin in patients with MS.

References

Abi-Gerges, N., Szabo, G., Otero, A. S., Fischmeister, R., and Mery, P. F. (2002). NO donors potentiate the beta-adrenergic stimulation of I(Ca,L) and the muscarinic activation of I(K,ACh) in rat cardiac myocytes. J. Physiol **540**, 411–424.

Aboul-Enein, F., Rauschka, H., Kornek, B., Stadelmann, C., Stefferl, A., Bruck, W., Lucchinetti, C., Schmidbauer, M., Jellinger, K., and Lassmann, H. (2003). Preferential loss of myelin-associated glycoprotein reflects hypoxia-like white matter damage in stroke and inflammatory brain diseases. J. Neuropathol. Exp. Neurol **62**, 25–33.

Ahern, G. P., Hsu, S.-F., Klyachko, V. A., and Jackson, M. B. (2000). Induction of persistent sodium current by exogenous and endogenous nitric oxide. J. Biol. Chem. **275**, 28810–28815.

Ahern, G. P., Klyachko, V. A., and Jackson, M. B. (2002). cGMP and S-nitrosylation: Two routes for modulation of neuronal excitability by NO. Trends Neurosci. **25**, 510–517.

Aktan, F. (2004). iNOS-mediated nitric oxide production and its regulation. Life Sci. **75**, 639–653.

Alderton, W. K., Cooper, C. E., and Knowles, R. G. (2001). Nitric oxide synthases: Structure, function and inhibition. Biochem. J. **357**, 593–615.

Ali, Q. G., Halawa, A., Baig, S., and Siden, A. (1996). Multiple sclerosis and neurotransmission. Biogenic Amines **12**, 353–376.

Ames, A., III (2000). CNS energy metabolism as related to function. Brain Res. Brain Res. Rev. **34**, 42–68.

Asano, S., Matsuda, T., Takuma, K., Kim, H. S., Sato, T., Nishikawa, T., and Baba, A. (1995). Nitroprusside and cyclic GMP stimulate Na$^+$-Ca^{2+} exchange activity in neuronal preparations and cultured rat astrocytes. J. Neurochem. **64**, 2437–2441.

Bagasra, O., Michaels, F. H., Zheng, Y. M., Bobroski, L. E., Spitsin, S. V., Fu, Z. F., Tawadros, R., and Koprowski, H. (1995). Activation of the inducible form of nitric oxide synthase in the brains of patients with multiple sclerosis. Proc. Natl. Acad. Sci. U.S.A. **92**, 12041–12045.

Bains, J. S., and Ferguson, A. V. (1997). Nitric oxide depolarizes type II paraventricular nucleus neurons in vitro. Neuroscience **79**, 149–159.

Baker, M., and Bostock, H. (1992). Ectopic activity in demyelinated spinal root axons of the rat. J. Physiol. London **451**, 539–552.

Baker, M. D. (2000). Axonal flip-flops and oscillators. Trends Neurosci. **23**, 514–519.

Bechtold, D. A., Kapoor, R., and Smith, K. J. (2004). Axonal protection using flecainide in experimental autoimmune encephalomyelitis. Ann. Neurol. **55**, 607–616.

Bechtold, D. A., and Smith, K. J. (2004). Sodium-mediated axonal degeneration in inflammatory demyelinating disease. J. Neurol. Sci.

Beckman, J. S., and Koppenol, W. H. (1996). Nitric oxide, superoxide, and peroxynitrite: the good, the bad, and the ugly. Am. J. Physiol. **271**, C1424-C1437.

Beenakker, E. A., Oparina, T. I., Hartgring, A., Teelken, A., Arutjunyan, A. V., and De Keyser, J. (2001). Cooling garment treatment in MS: Clinical improvement and decrease in leukocyte NO production. Neurology **57**, 892–894.

Bellamy, T. C., and Garthwaite, J. (2001). Sub-second kinetics of the nitric oxide receptor, soluble guanylyl cyclase, in intact cerebellar cells. J. Biol. Chem. **276**, 4287–4292.

Bellamy, T. C., Griffiths, C., and Garthwaite, J. (2002). Differential sensitivity of guanylyl cyclase and mitochondrial respiration to nitric oxide measured using clamped concentrations. J. Biol. Chem. **277**, 31801–31807.

Beltran, B., Mathur, A., Duchen, M. R., Erusalimsky, J. D., and Moncada, S. (2000a). The effect of nitric oxide on cell respiration: A key to understanding its role in cell survival or death. Proc. Natl. Acad. Sci. U.S.A. **97**, 14602–14607.

Beltran, B., Orsi, A., Clementi, E., and Moncada, S. (2000b). Oxidative stress and S-nitrosylation of proteins in cells. Br. J. Pharmacol. **129**, 953–960.

Bielefeldt, K., Whiteis, C. A., Chapleau, M. W., and Abboud, F. M. (1999). Nitric oxide enhances slow inactivation of voltage-dependent sodium currents in rat nodose neurons. Neurosci. Lett. **271**, 159–162.

Bitsch, A., Wegener, C., Da Costa, C., Bunkowski, S., Reimers, C. D., Prange, H. W., and Bruck, W. (1999). Lesion development in Marburg's type of acute multiple sclerosis: From inflammation to demyelination. Multiple Sclerosis **5**, 138–146.

Bo, L., Dawson, T. M., Wesselingh, S., Mork, S., Choi, S., Kong, P. A., Hanley, D., and Trapp, B. D. (1994). Induction of nitric oxide synthase in demyelinating regions of multiple sclerosis brains. Ann. Neurol. **36**, 778–786.

Boldyrev, A. A., Bulygina, E. R., Kramarenko, G. G., and Vanin, A. F. (1997). Effect of nitroso compounds on Na/K-ATPase. Biochim. Biophys. Acta **1321**, 243–251.

Bostock, H., and Sears, T. A. (1976). Continuous conduction in demyelinated mammalian nerve fibers. Nature **263**, 786–787.

Boullerne, A. I., Nedelkoska, L., and Benjamins, J. A. (1999). Synergism of nitric oxide and iron in killing the transformed murine oligodendrocyte cell line N20.1. J. Neurochem. **72**, 1050–1060.

Broholm, H., Andersen, B., Wanscher, B., Frederiksen, J. L., Rubin, I., Pakkenberg, B., Larsson, H. B., and Lauritzen, M. (2004). Nitric oxide synthase expression and enzymatic activity in multiple sclerosis. Acta Neurol. Scand. **109**, 261–269.

Brookes, P. S., Bolanos, J. P., and Heales, S. J. R. (1999). The assumption that nitric oxide inhibits mitochondrial ATP synthesis is correct. FEBS Lett. **446**, 261–263.

Brookes, P. S., Kraus, D. W., Shiva, S., Doeller, J. E., Barone, M. C., Patel, R. P., Lancaster, J. R., Jr., and Darley-Usmar, V. (2003). Control of mitochondrial respiration by NO, effects of low oxygen and respiratory state. J. Biol. Chem. **278**, 31603–31609.

Brorson, J. R., Schumacker, P. T., and Zhang, H. (1999). Nitric oxide acutely inhibits neuronal energy production. J. Neurosci. **19**, 147–158.

Brown, A. M., Westenbroek, R. E., Catterall, W. A., and Ransom, B. R. (2001). Axonal L-type Ca^{2+} channels and anoxic injury in rat CNS white matter. J. Neurophysiol. **85**, 900–911.

Brown, G. C. (2000). Nitric oxide as a competitive inhibitor of oxygen consumption in the mitochondrial respiratory chain. Acta Physiol. Scand. **168**, 667–674.

Brown, G. C., and Bal-Price, A. (2003). Inflammatory neurodegeneration mediated by nitric oxide, glutamate, and mitochondria. Mol. Neurobiol. **27**, 325–355.

Brown, G. C., Bolanos, J. P., Heales, S. J., and Clark, J. B. (1995). Nitric oxide produced by activated astrocytes rapidly and reversibly inhibits cellular respiration. Neurosci. Letters **193**, 201–204.

Brown, G. C., and Borutaite, V. (2001). Nitric oxide, mitochondria, and cell death. IUBMB. Life **52**, 189–195.

Brown, G. C., and Borutaite, V. (2002). Nitric oxide inhibition of mitochondrial respiration and its role in cell death. Free Rad. Biol. and Med. **33**, 1440–1450.

Brown, G. C., and Cooper, C. E. (1994). Nanomolar concentrations of nitric oxide reversibly inhibit synaptosomal respiration by competing with oxygen at cytochrome oxidase. FEBS Lett. **356**, 295–298.

Brundin, L., Morcos, E., Olsson, T., Wiklund, N. P., and Andersson, M. (1999). Increased intrathecal nitric oxide formation in multiple sclerosis: Cerebrospinal fluid nitrite as activity marker. *Eur. J. Neurol.* **6**, 585–590.

Brune, B., and Mohr, S. (2001). Protein thiol modification of glyceraldehyde-3-phosphate dehydrogenase and caspase-3 by nitric oxide. *Curr. Protein Pept. Sci.* **2**, 61–72.

Busch, A. E., Kopp, H. G., Waldegger, S., Samarzija, I., Sussbrich, H., Raber, G., Kunzelmann, K., Ruppersberg, J. P., and Lang, F. (1996). Effect of isosorbiddinitrate on exogenously expressed slowly activating K^+ channels and endogenous K^{+2} channels in Xenopus oocytes. *J. Physiol* **491 (Pt 3)**, 735–741.

Campbell, D. L., Stamler, J. S., and Strauss, H. C. (1996). Redox modulation of L-type calcium channels in ferret ventricular myocytes. Dual mechanism regulation by nitric oxide and S-nitrosothiols. *J. Gen. Physiol.* **108**, 277–293.

Chen, C., and Schofield, G. G. (1995). Nitric oxide donors enhanced Ca^{2+} currents and blocked noradrenaline-induced Ca^{2+} current inhibition in rat sympathetic neurons. *J. Physiol. (London)* **482**, 521–531.

Chen, H., and Guo, Z. G. (1999). Nitric oxide derived from endothelial cells inhibits Na^+/H^+ exchange in rabbit platelets activated by thrombin. *Zhongguo Yao Li Xue. Bao.* **20**, 333–337.

Cleeter, M. W. J., Cooper, A. M., Darley-Usmar, B. M., Moncada, D., and Schapira, A. H. V. (1994). Reversible inhibition of cytochrome c oxidase, the terminal enzyme of the mitochondrial respiratory chain, by nitric oxide. *FEBS Lett.* **345**, 50–54.

Clementi, E., Brown, G. C., Feelisch, M., and Moncada, S. (1998). Persistent inhibition of cell respiration by nitric oxide: Crucial role of S-nitrosylation of mitochondrial complex I and protective action of glutathione. *Proc. Natl. Acad. Sci. USA* **95**, 7631–7636.

Coles, A. J., Wing, M. G., Molyneux, P., Paolillo, A., Davie, C. M., Hale, G., Miller, D, Waldmann, H., and Compston, A. (1999). Monoclonal antibody treatment exposes three mechanisms underlying the clinical course of multiple sclerosis. *Ann. Neurol.* **46**, 296–304.

Craner, M. J., Hains, B. C., Lo, A. C., Black, J. A., and Waxman, S. G. (2004a). Co-localization of sodium channel Nav1.6 and the sodium-calcium exchanger at sites of axonal injury in the spinal cord in EAE. *Brain* **127**, 294–303.

Craner, M. J., Lo, A. C., Black, J. A., and Waxman, S. G. (2003). Abnormal sodium channel distribution in optic nerve axons in a model of inflammatory demyelination. *Brain* **126**, 1552–1561.

Craner, M. J., Newcombe, J., Black, J. A., Hartle, C., Cuzner, M. L., and Waxman, S. G. (2004b). Molecular changes in neurons in multiple sclerosis: altered axonal expression of Nav1.2 and Nav1.6 sodium channels and Na^+/Ca^{2+} exchanger. *Proc. Natl. Acad. Sci. U.S.A.* **101**, 8168–8173.

Cross, A. H., Manning, P. T., Keeling, R. M., Schmidt, R. E., and Misko, T. P. (1998). Peroxynitrite formation within the central nervous system in active multiple sclerosis. *J. Neuroimmunol.* **88**, 45–56.

Cross, A. H., Manning, P. T., Stern, M. K., and Misko, T. P. (1997). Evidence for the production of peroxynitrite in inflammatory CNS demyelination. *J. Neuroimmunol.* **80**, 121–130.

Crow, J. P., and Beckman, J. S. (1996). The importance of superoxide in nitric oxide-dependent toxicity: evidence for peroxynitrite-mediated injury. *Adv. Exp. Med.and Biol.* **387**, 147–161.

Danilov, A. I., Andersson, M., Bavand, N., Wiklund, N. P., Olsson, T., and Brundin, L. (2003). Nitric oxide metabolite determinations reveal continuous inflammation in multiple sclerosis. *J. Neuroimmunol.* **136**, 112–118.

De Bustos, F., Navarro, J. A., de Andres, C., Molina, J. A., Jimenez-Jimenez, F. J., Orti-Pareja, M., Gasalla, T., Tallon-Barranco, A., Martinez-Salio, A., and Arenas, J. (1999). Cerebrospinal fluid nitrate levels in patients with multiple sclerosis. *Eur. Neurol.* **41**, 44–47.

De Groot, C. J., Ruuls, S. R., Theeuwes, J. W., Dijkstra, C. D., and van der Valk, P. (1997). Immunocytochemical characterization of the expression of inducible and constitutive isoforms of nitric oxide synthase in demyelinating multiple sclerosis lesions. *J. Neuropathol. Exp. Neurol.* **56**, 10–20.

Devaux, J., Alcaraz, G., Grinspan, J., Bennett, V., Joho, R., Crest, M., and Scherer, S. S. (2003). Kv3.1b is a novel component of CNS nodes. *J. Neurosci.* **23**, 4509–4518.

Dittrich, M., Jurevicius, J., Georget, M., Rochais, F., Fleischmann, B., Hescheler, J., and Fischmeister, R. (2001). Local response of L-type Ca(2+) current to nitric oxide in frog ventricular myocytes. *J. Physiol.* **534**, 109–121.

Drulovic, J., Drulovic, J., Mesaros, S., Samard, I. T., Maksimovic, D., Stojsavljevic, N., Levic, Z., and Stojkovic, M. M. (2001). Raised cerebrospinal fluid nitrite and nitrate levels in patients with multiple sclerosis: no correlation with disease activity. *Multiple Sclerosis* **7**, 19–22.

Duchen, M. R. (2000). Mitochondria and calcium: From cell signalling to cell death. *J. Physiol.* **529**, 57–68.

Duchen, M. R. (2004). Roles of mitochondria in health and disease. *Diabetes* **53 Suppl 1**, S96–102.

Espey, M. G., Miranda, K. M., Thomas, D. D., Xavier, S., Citrin, D., Vitek, M. P., and Wink, D. A. (2002). A chemical perspective on the interplay between NO, reactive oxygen species, and reactive nitrogen oxide species. *Ann. N. Y. Acad. Sci.* **962**, 195–206.

Esplugues, J. V. (2002). NO as a signalling molecule in the nervous system. *Br. J. Pharmacol.* **135**, 1079–1095.

Eu, J. P., Sun, J., Xu, L., Stamler, J. S., and Meissner, G. (2000). The skeletal muscle calcium release channel: coupled O_2 sensor and NO signaling functions. *Cell* **102**, 499–509.

Eu, J. P., Xu, L., Stamler, J. S., and Meissner, G. (1999). Regulation of ryanodine receptors by reactive nitrogen species. *Biochem. Pharmacol.* **57**, 1079–1084.

Feelisch, M. (1998). The use of nitric oxide donors in pharmacological studies. *Naunyn-Schmiedebergs Arch. Pharmacol.* **358**, 113–122.

Ferguson, B., Matyszak, M. K., Esiri, M. M., and Perry, V. H. (1997). Axonal damage in acute multiple sclerosis lesions. *Brain* **120**, 393–399.

Gallo, M. P., Malan, D., Bedendi, I., Biasin, C., Alloatti, G., and Levi, R. C. (2001). Regulation of cardiac calcium current by NO and cGMP-modulating agents. *Pflugers Arch. Eur. J. Physiol.* **441**, 621–628.

Garthwaite, G., Goodwin, D. A., Batchelor, A. M., Leeming, K., and Garthwaite, J. (2002). Nitric oxide toxicity in CNS white matter: An in vitro study using rat optic nerve. *Neuroscience* **109**, 145–155.

Gill, R. K., Saksena, S., Syed, I. A., Tyagi, S., Alrefai, W. A., Malakooti, J., Ramaswamy, K., and Dudeja, P. K. (2002). Regulation of NHE3 by nitric oxide in Caco-2 cells. *Am. J. Physiol. Gastrointest. Liver Physiol.* **283**, G747–G756.

Giovannoni, G. (1998). Cerebrospinal fluid and serum nitric oxide metabolites in patients with multiple sclerosis. *Multiple Sclerosis* **4**, 27–30.

Giovannoni, G., Heales, S. J., Silver, N. C., O'Riordan, J., Miller, R. F., Land, J. M., Clark, J. B., and Thompson, E. J. (1997). Raised serum nitrate and nitrite levels in patients with multiple sclerosis. *J. Neurol. Sci.* **145**, 77–81.

Giovannoni, G., Silver, N. C., O'Riordan, J., Miller, R. F., Heales, S. J. R., Land, J. M., Elliot, M., Feldmann, M., Miller, D. H., and Thompson, E. J. (1999). Increased urinary nitric oxide metabolites in patients with multiple sclerosis correlates with early and relapsing disease. *Multiple Sclerosis* **5**, 335–341.

Gonzalez-Zulueta, M., Feldman, A. B., Klesse, L. J., Kalb, R. G., Dillman, J. F., Parada, L. F., Dawson, T. M., and Dawson, V. L. (2000). Requirement for nitric oxide activation of p21(ras)/extracellular regulated kinase in neuronal ischemic preconditioning. *Proc. Natl. Acad. Sci. U. S. A.* **97**, 436–441.

Graumann, U., Reynolds, R., Steck, A. J., and Schaeren-Wiemers, N. (2003). Molecular changes in normal appearing white matter in multiple sclerosis are characteristic of neuroprotective mechanisms against hypoxic insult. *Brain Pathol.* **13**, 554–573.

Griffiths, C., and Garthwaite, J. (2001). The shaping of nitric oxide signals by a cellular sink. *J. Physiol* **536**, 855–862.

Griffiths, C., Wykes, V., Bellamy, T. C., and Garthwaite, J. (2003). A new and simple method for delivering clamped nitric oxide concentrations in the physiological range: Application to activation of guanylyl cyclase-coupled nitric oxide receptors. *Mol. Pharmacol.* **64,** 1349–1356.

Griffiths, C., Yamini, B., Hall, C., and Garthwaite, J. (2002). Nitric oxide inactivation in brain by a novel O_2-dependent mechanism resulting in the formation of nitrate ions. *Biochem. J.* **362,** 459–464.

Guseo, A., and Jellinger, K. (1975). The significance of perivascular infiltrations in multiple sclerosis. *J. Neurol.* **211,** 51–60.

Guzman, N. J., Fang, M. Z., Tang, S. S., Ingelfinger, J. R., and Garg, L. C. (1995). Autocrine inhibition of Na^+/K^+-ATPase by nitric oxide in mouse proximal tubule epithelial cells. *J. Clin. Invest.* **95,** 2083–2088.

Halliwell, B., Zhao, K., and Whiteman, M. (1999). Nitric oxide and peroxynitrite. The ugly, the uglier and the not so good: a personal view of recent controversies. *Free Radic. Res.* **31,** 651–669.

Hammarstrom, A. K., and Gage, P. W. (1998). Inhibition of oxidative metabolism increases persistent sodium current in rat CA1 hippocampal neurons. *J. Physiol* **510 (Pt 3),** 735–741.

Hammarstrom, A. K. M., and Gage, P. W. (1999). Nitric oxide increases persistent sodium current in rat hippocampal neurons. *J. Physiol.* **520,** 451–461.

Hare, J. M. (2003). Nitric oxide and excitation-contraction coupling. *J. Mol. Cell Cardiol.* **35,** 719–729.

Herzog, R. I., Cummins, T. R., Ghassemi, F., Dib-Hajj, S., and Waxman, S. G. (2003). Distinct repriming and closed-state inactivation kinetics of Nav1.6 and Nav1.7 sodium channels in spinal sensory neurons. *J. Physiol. (Lond.)* **551.3,** 741–751.

Hogg, N., (2002). The biochemistry and physiology of s-nitrosothiols. *Annu. Rev. Pharmacol.and Toxicol.* **42,** 585–600.

Hogg, N., and Kalyanaraman, B. (1999). Nitric oxide and lipid peroxidation. *Biochim. Biophys. Acta* **1411,** 378–384.

Hooper, D. C., Bagasra, O., Marini, J. C., Zborek, A., Ohnishi, S. T., Kean, R., Champion, J. M., Sarker, A. B., Bobroski, L., Farber, J. L., Akaike, T., Maeda, H., and Koprowski, H. (1997). Prevention of experimental allergic encephalomyelitis by targeting nitric oxide and peroxynitrite: implications for the treatment of multiple sclerosis. *Proc. Natl. Acad. Sci. U. S. A.* **94,** 2528–2533.

Hopper, C. L., Matthews, C. G., and Cleeland, C. S. (1972). Symptom instability and thermoregulation in multiple sclerosis. *Neurology* **22,** 142–148.

Horn, T. F., Wolf, G., Duffy, S., Weiss, S., Keilhoff, G., and MacVicar, B. A. (2002). Nitric oxide promotes intracellular calcium release from mitochondria in striatal neurons. *FASEB J.* **16,** 1611–1622.

Hu, H., Chiamvimonvat, N., Yamagishi, T., and Marban, E. (1997). Direct inhibition of expressed cardiac L-type Ca^{2+} channels by S-nitrosothiol nitric oxide donors. *Circ. Res.* **81,** 742–752.

Ignarro, L. J. (1991). Signal transduction mechanisms involving nitric oxide. *Biochem. Pharmacol.* **41,** 485–490.

Ikeda, M., Sato, I., Matsunaga, T., Takahashi, M., Yuasa, T., and Murota, S. (1995). Cyclic guanosine monophosphate (cGMP), nitrite and nitrate in the cerebrospinal fluid in meningitis, multiple sclerosis and Guillain-Barre syndrome. *Intern. Med.* **34,** 734–737.

Iwata, A., Stys, P. K., Wolf, J. A., Chen, X. H., Taylor, A. G., Meaney, D. F., and Smith, D. H. (2004). Traumatic axonal injury induces proteolytic cleavage of the voltage-gated sodium channels modulated by tetrodotoxin and protease inhibitors. *J. Neurosci.* **24,** 4605–4613.

Jaffrey, S. R., Erdjument-Bromage, H., Ferris, C. D., Tempst, P., and Snyder, S. H. (2001). Protein S-nitrosylation: a physiological signal for neuronal nitric oxide. *Nat. Cell Biol.* **3,** 193–197.

Johnson, A. W., Land, J. M., Thompson, E. J., Bolanos, J. P., Clark, J. B., and Heales, S. J. (1995). Evidence for increased nitric oxide production in multiple sclerosis. *J. Neurol. Neurosurg and Psychiatry* **58,** 107.

Kagan, V. E., Kozlov, A. V., Tyurina, Y. Y., Shvedova, A. A., and Yalowich, J. C. (2001). Antioxidant mechanisms of nitric oxide against iron-catalyzed oxidative stress in cells. *Antioxid. Redox. Signal.* **3,** 189–202.

Kapoor, R., Davies, M., Blaker, P. A., Hall, S. M., and Smith, K. J. (2003). Blockers of sodium and calcium entry protect axons from nitric oxide-mediated degeneration. *Ann. Neurol.* **53,** 174–180.

Kapoor, R., Davies, M., Hall, S. M., and Smith, K. J. (1998). Nitric oxide causes axonal degeneration which is exacerbated by impulse activity. *J. Neurol. Neurosurg. Psychiatry* **65,** 415.

Kapoor, R., Davies, M., and Smith, K. J. (1999). Temporary axonal conduction block and axonal loss in inflammatory neurological disease: a potential role for nitric oxide? *Ann. NY Acad. Sci.* **893,** 304–308.

Kapoor, R., Li, Y. G., and Smith, K. J. (1997). Slow sodium-dependent potential oscillations contribute to ectopic firing in mammalian demyelinated axons. *Brain* **120,** 647–652.

Keynes, R. G., and Garthwaite, J. (2004). Nitric oxide and its role in ischaemic brain injury. *Curr. Mol. Med.* **4,** 179–191.

Kiang, J. G., McClain, D. E., Warke, V. G., Krishnan, S., and Tsokos, G. C. (2003). Constitutive NO synthase regulates the Na^+/Ca^{2+} exchanger in human T cells: Role of $[Ca^{2+}]_i$ and tyrosine phosphorylation. *J. Cell Biochem.* **89,** 1030–1043.

Kim, S. J., Song, S. K., and Kim, J. (2000). Inhibitory effect of nitric oxide on voltage-dependent calcium currents in rat dorsal root ganglion cells. *Biochem. Biophys. Res. Comm.* **271,** 509–514.

Kirstein, M., Rivet-Bastide, M., Hatem, S., Benardeau, A., Mercadier, J. J., and Fischmeister, R. (1995). Nitric oxide regulates the calcium current in isolated human atrial myocytes. *J. Clin. Invest* **95,** 794–802.

Klebl, B. M., Ayoub, A. T., and Pette, D. (1998). Protein oxidation, tyrosine nitration, and inactivation of sarcoplasmic reticulum Ca^{2+}-ATPase in low-frequency stimulated rabbit muscle. *FEBS Lett.* **422,** 381–384.

Koivisto, A., Matthias, A., Bronnikov, G., and Nedergaard, J. (1997). Kinetics of the inhibition of mitochondrial respiration by NO. *FEBS Lett.* **417,** 75–80.

Koprowski, H., Zheng, Y. M., Heber-Katz, E., Fraser, N., Rorke, L., Fu, Z. F., and Dietzschold, B. (1993). In vivo expression of inducible nitric oxide synthase in experimentally induced neurologic diseases. *Proc. Natl. Acad. Sci. U. S. A.* **90,** 3024–3027.

Kornek, B., Storch, M. K., Bauer, J., Djamshidian, A., Weissert, R., Wallstroem, E., Stefferl, A., Zimprich, F., Olsson, T., Linington, C., Schmidbauer, M., and Lassmann, H. (2001). Distribution of a calcium channel subunit in dystrophic axons in multiple sclerosis and experimental autoimmune encephalomyelitis. *Brain* **124,** 1114–1124.

Kornek, B., Storch, M. K., Weissert, R., Wallstroem, E., Stefferl, A., Olsson, T., Linington, C., Schmidbauer, M., and Lassmann, H. (2000). Multiple sclerosis and chronic autoimmune encephalomyelitis: A comparative quantitative study of axonal injury in active, inactive, and remyelinated lesions. *Am. J. Pathol.* **157,** 267–276.

Krumenacker, J. S., Hanafy, K. A., and Murad, F. (2004). Regulation of nitric oxide and soluble guanylyl cyclase. *Brain Res. Bull.* **62,** 505–515.

Lancaster, J. R., Jr. (1997). A tutorial on the diffusibility and reactivity of free nitric oxide. *Nitric Oxide* **1,** 18–30.

Ledo, A., Frade, J., Barbosa, R. M., and Laranjinha, J. (2004). Nitric oxide in brain: Diffusion, targets and concentration dynamics in hippocampal subregions. *Mol. Aspects Med.* **25,** 75–89.

Li, Z., Chapleau, M. W., Bates, J. N., Bielefeldt, K., Lee, H.-C., and Abboud, F. M. (1998). Nitric oxide as an autocrine regulator of sodium currents in baroreceptor neurons. *Neuron* **20,** 1039–1049.

Liu, J. S., Zhao, M. L., Brosnan, C. F., and Lee, S. C. (2001). Expression of inducible nitric oxide synthase and nitrotyrosine in multiple sclerosis lesions. *Am. J. Pathol.* **158,** 2057–2066.

Liu, S. H. and Sheu, T. J. (1997). The in vivo effect of lipopolysaccharide on Na^+,K^+-ATPase catalytic (alpha) subunit isoforms in rat sciatic nerve. *Neurosci. Lett.* **234,** 166–168.

Lo, A. C., Black, J. A., and Waxman, S. G. (2002). Neuroprotection of axons with phenytoin in experimental allergic encephalomyelitis. *Neuroreport* **13,** 1909–1912.

Lo, A. C., Saab, C. Y., Black, J. A., and Waxman, S. G. (2003). Phenytoin protects spinal cord axons and preserves axonal conduction and neurological function in a model of neuroinflammation in vivo. *J. Neurophysiol.* **90,** 3566–3571.

Lu, F., Selak, M., O'Connor, J., Croul, S., Lorenzana, C., Butunoi, C., and Kalman, B. (2000). Oxidative damage to mitochondrial DNA and activity of mitochondrial enzymes in chronic active lesions of multiple sclerosis. *J. Neurol. Sci.* **177,** 95–103.

Mannick, J. B., and Schonhoff, C. M. (2004). NO means no and yes: regulation of cell signaling by protein nitrosylation. *Free Radic. Res.* **38,** 1–7.

Martinez-Ruiz, A., and Lamas, S. (2004). S-nitrosylation: a potential new paradigm in signal transduction. *Cardiovasc. Res.* **62,** 43–52.

McDonald, W. I. (1986). The pathophysiology of multiple sclerosis. *In:* "Multiple Sclerosis" (W. I. McDonald, and D. H. Silberberg, D. H., Eds.). pp. 112–133. Butterworth, London.

McKee, M., Scavone, C., and Nathanson, J. A. (1994). Nitric oxide, cGMP, and hormone regulation of active sodium transport. *Proc. Natl. Acad. Sci. U. S. A.* **91,** 12056–12060.

Merrill, J. E., Ignarro, L. J., Sherman, M. P., Melinek, J., and Lane, T. E. (1993). Microglial cell cytotoxicity of oligodendrocytes is mediated through nitric oxide. *J. Immunol.* **151,** 2132–2141.

Mitrovic, B., Ignarro, L. J., Montestruque, S., Smoll, A., and Merrill, J. E. (1994). Nitric oxide as a potential pathological mechanism in demyelination: its differential effects on primary glial cells in vitro. *Neuroscience* **61,** 575–585.

Mitrovic, B., Ignarro, L. J., Vinters, H. V., Akers, M.-A., Schmid, I., Uittenbogaart, C., and Merrill, J. E. (1995). Nitric oxide induces necrotic but not apoptotic cell death in oligodendrocytes. *Neuroscience* **65,** 531–539.

Mitrovic, B., Parkinson, J., and Merrill, J. E. (1996). An in vitro model of oligodendrocyte destruction by nitric oxide and its relevance to multiple sclerosis. *Methods (Duluth)* **10,** 501–513.

Molina-Holgado, E., Vela, J. M., Arevalo-Martin, A., and Guaza, C. (2001). LPS/IFN-gamma cytotoxicity in oligodendroglial cells: Role of nitric oxide and protection by the anti-inflammatory cytokine IL-10. *Eur. J. Neurosci.* **13,** 493–502.

Moncada, S., and Erusalimsky, J. D. (2002). Does nitric oxide modulate mitochondrial energy generation and apoptosis? *Nat. Rev. Mol. Cell Biol.* **3,** 214–220.

Moreau, T., Coles, A., Wing, M., Isaacs, J., Hale, G., Waldmann, H., and Compston, A. (1996). Transient increase in symptoms associated with cytokine release in patients with multiple sclerosis. *Brain* **119,** 225–237.

Moreno, H., Vega-Saenz, d. M., Nadal, M. S., Amarillo, Y., and Rudy, B. (2001). Modulation of Kv3 potassium channels expressed in CHO cells by a nitric oxide-activated phosphatase. *J. Physiol.* **530,** 345–358.

Muriel, P., and Sandoval, G. (2000). Nitric oxide and peroxynitrite anion modulate liver plasma membrane fluidity and Na$^+$/K$^+$-ATPase activity. *Nitric Oxide* **4,** 333–342.

Mutsaers, S. E., and Carroll, W. M. (1998). Focal accumulation of intra-axonal mitochondria in demyelination of the cat optic nerve. *Acta Neuropathol. (Berl.)* **96,** 139–143.

Nisoli, E., Clementi, E., Paolucci, C., Cozzi, V., Tonello, C., Sciorati, C., Bracale, R., Valerio, A., Francolini, M., Moncada, S., and Carruba, M. O. (2003). Mitochondrial biogenesis in mammals: the role of endogenous nitric oxide. *Science* **299,** 896–899.

O'Donnell, V. B., and Freeman, B. A. (2001). Interactions between nitric oxide and lipid oxidation pathways: Implications for vascular disease. *Circ. Res.* **88,** 12–21.

Oka, A., Belliveau, M. J., Rosenberg, P. A., and Volpe, J. J. (1993). Vulnerability of oligodendroglia to glutamate: Pharmacology, mechanisms, and prevention. *J. Neurosci.* **13,** 1441–1453.

Okuda, Y., Nakatsuji, Y., Fujimura, H., Esumi, H., Ogura, T., Yanagihara, T., and Sakoda, S. (1995). Expression of the inducible isoform of nitric oxide synthase in the central nervous system of mice correlates with the severity of actively induced experimental allergic encephalomyelitis. *J. Neuroimmunol.* **62,** 103–112.

Oleszak, E. L., Zaczynska, E., Bhattacharjee, M., Butunoi, C., Legido, A., and Katsetos, C. D. (1998). Inducible nitric oxide synthase and nitrotyrosine are found in monocytes/macrophages and/or astrocytes in acute, but not in chronic, multiple sclerosis. *Clin. Diagn. Lab. Immunol.* **5,** 438–445.

Ouardouz, M., Nikolaeva, M. A., Coderre, E., Zamponi, G. W., McRory, J. E., Trapp, B. D., Yin, X., Wang, W., Woulfe, J., and Stys, P. K. (2003). Depolarization-induced Ca^{2+} release in ischemic spinal cord white matter involves L-type Ca^{2+} channel activation of ryanodine receptors. *Neuron* **40,** 53–63.

Pehl, U., and Schmid, H. A. (1997). Electrophysiological response of neurons in the rat spinal cord to nitric oxide. *Neuroscience* **77,** 563–573.

Peltola, J., Ukkonen, M., Moilanen, E., and Elovaara, I. (2001). Increased nitric oxide products in CSF in primary progressive MS may reflect brain atrophy. *Neurology* **57,** 895–896.

Poteser, M., Romanin, C., Schreibmayer, W., Mayer, B., and Groschner, K. (2001). S-nitrosation controls gating and conductance of the alpha 1 subunit of class C L-type Ca^{2+} channels. *J. Biol. Chem.* **276,** 14797–14803.

Pozzo-Miller, L. D., Pivovarova, N. B., Connor, J. A., Reese, T. S., and Andrews, S. B. (1999). Correlated measurements of free and total intracellular calcium concentration in central nervous system neurons. *Microsc. Res. Tech.* **46,** 370–379.

Prineas, J. W., and Wright, R. G. (1978). Macrophages, lymphocytes, and plasma cells in the perivascular compartment in chronic multiple sclerosis. *Lab. Invest.* **38,** 409–421.

Radi, R., Beckman, J. S., Bush, K. M., and Freeman, B. A. (1991). Peroxynitrite-induced membrane lipid peroxidation: the cytotoxic potential of superoxide and nitric oxide. *Arch. Biochem. Biophys.* **288,** 481–487.

Radi, R., Cassina, A., and Hodara, R. (2002). Nitric oxide and peroxynitrite interactions with mitochondria. *Biol. Chem.* **383,** 401–409.

Ransom, B. R., Waxman, S. G., and Stys, P. K. (1993). Anoxic injury of central myelinated axons: ionic mechanisms and pharmacology. *Research Publications - Association For Research In Nervous and Mental Disease* **71,** 121–151.

Redford, E. J., Kapoor, R., and Smith, K. J. (1997). Nitric oxide donors reversibly block axonal conduction: demyelinated axons are especially susceptible. *Brain* **120,** 2149–2157.

Renganathan, M., Cummins, T. R., Hormuzdiar, W. N., Black, J. A., and Waxman, S. G. (2000). Nitric oxide is an autocrine regulator of Na$^+$ currents in axotomized C-type DRG neurons. *J. Neurophysiol.* **83,** 2431–2442.

Renganathan, M., Cummins, T. R., and Waxman, S. G. (2002a). Nitric oxide blocks fast, slow and persistent sodium currents in C-type DRG neurons by a cGMP-independent mechanism. *J. Neurophysiol.* **87,** 761–775.

Renganathan, M., Cummins, T. R., and Waxman, S. G. (2002b). Nitric oxide blocks fast, slow, and persistent Na$^+$ channels in C-type DRG neurons by S-nitrosylation. *J. Neurophysiol.* **87,** 761–775.

Rizzo, M. A., Kocsis, J. D., and Waxman, S. G. (1996a). Mechanisms of paresthesiae, dysesthesiae, and hyperesthesiae: role of Na channel heterogeneity. *Eur. Neurol.* **36,** 3–12.

Rizzo, M. A., Kocsis, J. D., and Waxman, S. G. (1996b). Mechanisms of paresthesiae, dysesthesiae, and hyperesthesiae: role of Na+ channel heterogeneity. *Eur. Neurol.* **36,** 3–12.

Salama, G., Menshikova, E. V., and Abramson, J. J. (2000). Molecular interaction between nitric oxide and ryanodine receptors of skeletal and cardiac sarcoplasmic reticulum. *Antioxid. Redox. Signal* **2,** 5–16.

Santiago, E., Perez-Mediavilla, L. A., and Lopez-Moratalla, N. (1998). The role of nitric oxide in the pathogenesis of multiple sclerosis. *J. Physiol. Biochem.* **54,** 229–237.

Sarti, P., Arese, M., and Giuffre, A. (2003). The molecular mechanisms by which nitric oxide controls mitochondrial complex IV. *Ital. J. Biochem.* **52**, 37–42.

Sato, T., Kamata, Y., Irifune, M., and Nishikawa, T. (1995). Inhibition of purified (Na$^+$,K$^+$)-ATPase activity from porcine cerebral cortex by NO generating drugs. *Brain Res.* **704**, 117–120.

Sato, T., Kamata, Y., Irifune, M., and Nishikawa, T. (1997). Inhibitory effect of several nitric oxide-generating compounds on purified Na$^+$,K$^+$-ATPase activity from porcine cerebral cortex. *J. Neurochem.* **68**, 1312–1318.

Sawada, M., Ichinose, M., and Hara, N. (1995). Nitric oxide induces an increased Na$^+$ conductance in identified neurons of Aplysia. *Brain Res.* **670**, 248–256.

Scherer, S. S., and Arroyo, E. J. (2002). Recent progress on the molecular organization of myelinated axons. *J. Peripher. Nerv. Syst.* **7**, 1–12.

Shrager, P., Custer, A. W., Kazarinova, K., Rasband, M. N., and Mattson, D. (1998). Nerve conduction block by nitric oxide that is mediated by the axonal environment. *J. Neurophysiol.* **79**, 529–536.

Simmons, R. D., Bernard, C. C., Singer, G., and Carnegie, P. R. (1982). Experimental autoimmune encephalomyelitis. An anatomically-based explanation of clinical progression in rodents. *J. Neuroimmunol.* **3**, 307–318.

Smith, K. J., Bostock, H., and Hall, S. M. (1982). Saltatory conduction precedes remyelination in axons demyelinated with lysophosphatidyl choline. *J. Neurol. Sci.* **54**, 13–31.

Smith, K. J., Felts, P. A., and Kapoor, R. (1997). Axonal hyperexcitability: mechanisms and role in symptom production in demyelinating diseases. *The Neuroscientist* **3**, 237–246.

Smith, K. J., Kapoor, R., and Felts, P. A. (1999). Demyelination: the role of reactive oxygen and nitrogen species. *Brain Pathol.* **9**, 69–92.

Smith, K. J., Kapoor, R., Hall, S. M., and Davies, M. (2001a). Electrically active axons degenerate when exposed to nitric oxide. *Ann. Neurol.* **49**, 470–476.

Smith, K. J., Kapoor, R., Hall, S. M., and Davies, M. (2001b). Partial sodium channel blockade protects axons from degeneration caused by the combination of impulse activity and exposure to nitric oxide. *Society for Neuroscience Meeting Abstracts* 103.12.

Smith, K. J., and Lassmann, H. (2002). The role of nitric oxide in multiple sclerosis. *Lancet Neurol.* **1**, 232–241.

Smith, K. J., and McDonald, W. I. (1980). Spontaneous and mechanically evoked activity due to central demyelinating lesion. *Nature* **286**, 154–155.

Smith, K. J., and McDonald, W. I. (1982). Spontaneous and evoked electrical discharges from a central demyelinating lesion. *J. Neurol. Sci.* **55**, 39–47.

Smith, K. J., and McDonald, W. I. (1999). The pathophysiology of multiple sclerosis: The mechanisms underlying the production of symptoms and the natural history of the disease. *Phil. Trans. R. Soc. Lond. B* **354**, 1649–1673.

Smith, S. L., and Otis, T. S. (2003). Persistent changes in spontaneous firing of Purkinje neurons triggered by the nitric oxide signaling cascade. *J. Neurosci.* **23**, 367–372.

Speciale, L., Sarasella, M., Ruzzante, S., Caputo, D., Mancuso, R., Calvo, M. G., Guerini, F. R., and Ferrante, P. (2000). Endothelin and nitric oxide levels in cerebrospinal fluid of patients with multiple sclerosis. *J. Neurovirol.* **6**, S62–S66.

Stamler, J. (1999). Nitric oxide in the cardiovascular system. Review in depth. *In:* "Nitric Oxide in the Cardiovascular System" p. 273. Williams and Wilkins, Baltimore.

Stamler, J. S., and Meissner, G. (2001). Physiology of nitric oxide in skeletal muscle. *Physiol. Rev.* **81**, 209–237.

Stewart, V. C., Sharpe, M. A., Clark, J. B., and Heales, S. J. R. (2000). Astrocyte-derived nitric oxide causes both reversible and irreversible damage to the neuronal mitochondrial respiratory chain. *J. Neurochem.* **75**, 694–700.

Stoyanovsky, D., Murphy, T., Anno, P. R., Kim, Y. M., and Salama, G. (1997). Nitric oxide activates skeletal and cardiac ryanodine receptors. *Cell Calcium* **21**, 19–29.

Stuehr, D. J. (1999). Mammalian nitric oxide synthases. *Biochim. Biophys. Acta* **1411**, 217–230.

Stys, P. K. (2004). White matter injury mechanisms. *Curr. Mol. Med.* **4**, 113–130.

Stys, P. K., and LoPachin, R. M. (1997). Mechanisms of calcium and sodium fluxes in anoxic myelinated central nervous system axons. *Neuroscience* **82**, 21–32.

Stys, P. K., and LoPachin, R. M. (1998). Mechanisms of calcium and sodium fluxes in anoxic myelinated central nervous system axons. *Neuroscience* **82**, 21–32.

Stys, P. K., Waxman, S. G., and Ransom, B. R. (1991). Na(+)-Ca2+ exchanger mediates Ca^{2+} influx during anoxia in mammalian central nervous system white matter. *Ann. Neurol.* **30**, 375–380.

Stys, P. K., Waxman, S. G., and Ransom, B. R. (1992). Ionic mechanisms of anoxic injury in mammalian CNS white matter: role of Na+ channels and Na$^+$-Ca^{2+} exchanger. *J. Neurosci.* **12**, 430–439.

Suko, J., Maurer-Fogy, I., Plank, B., Bertel, O., Wyskovsky, W., Hohenegger, M., and Hellmann, G. (1993). Phosphorylation of serine 2843 in ryanodine receptor-calcium release channel of skeletal muscle by cAMP-, cGMP- and CaM-dependent protein kinase. *Biochim. Biophys. Acta* **1175**, 193–206.

Summers, B. A., Overholt, J. L., and Prabhakar, N. R. (1999). Nitric oxide inhibits L-type Ca^{2+} current in glomus cells of the rabbit carotid body via a cGMP-independent mechanism. *J. Neurophysiol.* **81**, 1449–1457.

Svenningsson, A., Petersson, A.-S., Andersen, O., and Hansson, G. K. (1999). Nitric oxide metabolites in CSF of patients with MS are related to clinical disease course. *Neurology* **53**, 1880–1882.

Szabo, C. (2003). Multiple pathways of peroxynitrite cytotoxicity. *Toxicol. Lett.* **140-141**, 105–112.

Thomas, D. D., Liu, X., Kantrow, S. P., and Lancaster, J. R., Jr. (2001). The biological lifetime of nitric oxide: implications for the perivascular dynamics of NO and O$_2$. *Proc. Natl. Acad. Sci. U. S. A.* **98**, 355–360.

Trapp, B. D., Peterson, J., Ransohoff, R. M., Rudick, R., Mork, S., and Bo, L. (1998). Axonal transection in the lesions of multiple sclerosis. *N. Engl. J. Med.* **338**, 278–285.

Trotti, D., Rossi, D., Gjesdal, O., Levy, L. M., Racagni, G., Danbolt, N. C., and Volterra, A. (1996). Peroxynitrite inhibits glutamate transporter subtypes. *J. Biol. Chem.* **271**, 5976–5979.

van Dam, A. M., Bauer, J., Man-A-Hing, W. K., Marquette, C., and Tilders, F. J. B. F. (1995). Appearance of inducible nitric oxide synthase in the rat central nervous system after rabies virus infection and during experimental allergic encephalomyelitis but not after peripheral administration of endotoxin. *J. Neurosci. Res.* **40**, 251–260.

van der Veen, R. C., and Roberts, L. J. (1999). Contrasting roles for nitric oxide and peroxynitrite in the peroxidation of myelin lipids. *J. Neuroimmunol.* **95**, 1–7.

Viner, R. I., Ferrington, D. A., Williams, T. D., Bigelow, D. J., and Schoneich, C. (1999). Protein modification during biological aging: selective tyrosine nitration of the SERCA2a isoform of the sarcoplasmic reticulum Ca^{2+}-ATPase in skeletal muscle. *Biochem. J.* **340 (Pt 3)**, 657–669.

Vladimirova, O., O'Connor, J., Cahill, A., Alder, H., Butunoi, C., and Kalman, B. (1998). Oxidative damage to DNA in plaques of MS brains. *Multiple Sclerosis* **4**, 413–418.

Waxman, S. G., Black, J. A., Ransom, B. R., and Stys, P. K. (1994). Anoxic injury of rat optic nerve: ultrastructural evidence for coupling between Na$^+$ influx and Ca^{2+}-mediated injury in myelinated CNS axons. *Brain Res.* **644**, 197–204.

Willenborg, D. O., Staykova, M. A., and Cowden, W. B. (1999). Our shifting understanding of the role of nitric oxide in autoimmune encephalomyelitis: A review. *J. Neuroimmunol.* **100**, 21–35.

Wink, D. A., Miranda, K. M., Espey, M. G., Pluta, R. M., Hewett, S. J., Colton, C., Vitek, M., Feelisch, M., and Grisham, M. B. (2001). Mechanisms of the antioxidant effects of nitric oxide. *Antioxid. Redox. Signal.* **3,** 203–213.

Xu, L., Eu, J. P., Meissner, G., and Stamler, J. S. (1998). Activation of the cardiac calcium release channel (Ryanodoine receptor) by poly-S-nitrosylation. *Science* **279,** 234–237.

Yamashita, T., Ando, Y., Obayashi, K., Uchino, M., and Ando, M. (1997). Changes in nitrite and nitrate (NO^{2-}/NO^{3-}) levels in cerebrospinal fluid of patients with multiple sclerosis. *J. Neurol. Sci.* **153,** 32–34.

Youl, B. D., Turano, G., Miller, D. H., Towell, A. D., Macmanus, D. G., Moore, S. G., Barrett, G., Kendall, B. E., Moseley, I. F., Tofts, P. S., Halliday, A. M., and McDonald, W. I. (1991). The pathophysiology of acute optic neuritis. An association of gadolinium leakage with clinical and electrophysiological deficits. *Brain* **114,** 2437–2450.

Zabaleta, M. E., Bianco, N. E., and De Sanctis, J. B. (1998). Serum nitrotyrosine levels in patients with multiple sclerosis: Relationship with clinical activity. *Med. Sci. Res.* **26,** 407–408.

Zhang, J., Dawson, V. L., Dawson, T. M., and Snyder, S. H. (1994). Nitric oxide activation of poly(ADP-ribose) synthetase in neurotoxicity. *Science* **263,** 687–689.

Zielasek, J., Reichmann, H., Kunzig, H., Jung, S., Hartung, H.-P., and Toyka, K. V. (1995). Inhibition of brain macrophage/microgial respiratory chain enzyme activity in experimental autoimmune encephalomyelitis of the Lewis rat. *Neurosci. Lett.* **184,** 129–132.

19

Molecular Mechanisms of Calcium Influx in Axonal Degeneration

Peter K. Stys, M.D.

Stephen G. Waxman, M.D., Ph.D.

I. Introduction

Axonal degeneration is a key feature in multiple sclerosis (MS) and other central nervous system (CNS) disorders, accounting for much of the irreversible clinical disability. The precise mechanisms are poorly understood, but likely involve axonal overload of calcium (Ca) ions. Under normal conditions, adenosine triphosphate (ATP)-dependent pumps maintain rigid control over sodium (Na), potassium (K), and Ca gradients. When energy supply is limited, either because of inadequate delivery (e.g., ischemia, mitochondrial dysfunction) and/or excessive utilization (e.g., inefficient conduction in demyelinated axons), ion gradients collapse leading in turn to inappropriate and excessive gating of channels, aberrant operation of coupled ion and chemical transporters, and Ca overload. During Na-K-ATPase compromise, Na can enter axons through noninactivating Na channels, promoting axonal Na overload and depolarization by allowing K egress. This will gate voltage-sensitive Ca channels and stimulate reverse Na Ca exchange, leading to further Ca entry. ATP depletion will also promote Ca release from intracellular stores. Neurotransmitters such as glutamate will also be released by reverse operation of Na-dependent transporters. This excitotoxin will then overactivate a variety of ionotropic and metabotropic glutamate receptors, leading to further Ca overload in glia, and possibly axons and myelin as well, in addition to releasing Ca from inositol 1, 4, 5-triphosphate (IP3)-dependent stores. Together, this Ca overload will overactivate a variety of Ca-dependent enzyme systems (e.g., calpains, phospholipases) leading to structural and functional axonal injury.

MS has traditionally been considered a chronic neurological disorder characterized by multifocal inflammatory demyelination of central white matter tracts and degeneration of axons (Bjartmar et al., 2003; Lazzarini et al., 2004). The human CNS has a capacity to partially compensate for demyelination by establishing increased densities of Na channels along demyelinated domains of axons (see Chapters 7 and 8) and by recruiting glial cells that can remyelinate denuded axons to some degree (Prineas et al., 1993; Lassmann et al., 1997). These mechanisms contribute to remission and to the subclinical (functionally silent) nature of some lesions in patients with MS. However, degeneration of axons also occurs in MS and is of great clinical importance because it is thought to underlie permanent, irreversible clinical disability (De Stefano et al., 1998; Bjartmar et al., 2003). Although pathological features of axonopathy in MS were observed more than a century ago (Charcot, 1868; Kornek and Lassmann, 1999), virtually nothing is known about the molecular mechanisms of axonal injury in this disease. This chapter summarizes the pathophysiological mechanisms of white matter injury studied in other pathological states such as ischemia and trauma, with an emphasis on the routes of cellular Ca overload, which appears to be a cardinal event in axonal damage. Emerging evidence suggests that these mechanisms may contribute in important ways to axonal injury in inflammatory CNS disorders such as experimental autoimmune encephalomyelitis (EAE) and MS.

II. Molecular Architecture of Myelinated Axons: A Brief Overview

Myelinated fibers are uniquely constructed to transmit electrical signals reliably and efficiently. A detailed description of the structure and physiology of myelinated axons can be found elsewhere in this volume (see Chapters 1, 5, and 6). Axons have evolved into cablelike structures to support transmission of information within ever larger organisms. Insertion of Na and K channels in a homogeneous manner into the axolemma supports continuous conduction in unmyelinated fibers well, although velocities are modest ($\approx$20 m/s for a 500-μm diameter squid axon; 2 m/s for a 1-μm mammalian C-fiber; 1 m/s or slower in a mammalian CNS nonmyelinated axon [Waxman and Bennett, 1972]). As nervous systems became larger and more complex, and more "transmission lines" were needed to be packed into finite volumes, the requirement for more rapid conduction velocities led to a radical design shift (i.e., the evolution of the myelinated axon). Here the axolemmal channel distributions are highly inhomogenous, with extremely high densities (>1000 μm^{-2}) of voltage-gated Na channels (mainly Na$_v$1.6 in mature mammalian fibers [Caldwell et al., 2000; Poliak and Peles, 2003]) secured at nodes of Ranvier by ankyrin$_G$, and with a far lower density in the paranodal and

internodal axolemma, which is wrapped by myelin (Ritchie and Rogart, 1977; Waxman, 1977). Myelination greatly reduces internodal current losses mainly by decreasing capacitance, rather than increasing resistance, of the internodal axon (Funch and Faber, 1984). Delayed rectifier K channels (K$_v$1.1 and 1.2) are located at the juxtaparanodal axolemma and may serve to reduce nodal re-excitation (Poliak and Peles, 2003) (see Chapters 4 and 5). Also, other K channels have been found on axons such as the mixed permeability inward rectifier, slow and voltage-independent "flicker" K channels, and K channels modulated by axoplasmic Ca and ATP concentrations (Vogel and Schwarz, 1995). Cl channels have also been detected electrophysiologically. Although the presence of voltage-gated Ca channels on axons has been controversial, recent evidence shows that Ca$_v$ 1.2 and 1.3 (L-type, dihydropyridine-sensitive) are present in discrete clusters in the internodal axolemma of central fibers (Ouardouz et al., 2003) (see later in this chapter and Chapter 5). Together, the highly segregated distribution of voltage-gated ion channels and overlying myelin sheath support saltatory conduction from node to node, with a high safety factor and with minimal delays along the internodal regions. This elegant design solution allows rapid conduction ($\approx$120 m/s for larger myelinated peripheral nervous system fibers) along myelinated axons.

Although saltatory conduction is efficient in terms of ionic translocation and energy consumption, resting membrane potentials must be maintained, and action currents balanced by pumping of ions back across the axolemma. Axons therefore are also endowed with pumps and transporters to maintain electrochemical homeostasis. The workhorse of ATP-dependent ion transport is the Na-K-ATPase, which functions as an Na and K pump; the Ca-ATPase plays an important role in direct transport of Ca across the plasmalemma and intracellular membranes. Abundant immunohistochemical and electrophysiological evidence exists for the presence of the Na pump in both myelinated and unmyelinated fibers. In the former, the pump has been shown to be localized to the nodal (Wood et al., 1977; Schwartz et al., 1981; Ariyasu and Ellisman, 1987; Kanoh et al., 1994, 1997) or internodal (Bostock et al., 1991; Mata et al., 1991; Kanoh, 1997) axolemma, depending on the preparation. The Na-K-ATPase is a central mechanism responsible for electrochemical homeostasis in excitable cells, and accounts for roughly 50% of their resting ATP consumption (Erecinska and Silver, 1989; Erecinska and Dagani, 1990). In addition to supporting electrogenesis, the energy stored in the Na gradient is used by many Na-coupled passive co-transporters and counter-transporters to regulate concentrations of other ions, transmitters, amino acids, and other substances. Examples include the Na-Ca, Na-H, Na-Mg, and Na-dependent Cl-HCO$_3$ exchangers; Na-K-Cl and Na-HCO$_3$ co-transporters; Na-dependent glutamate, GABA, and glycine transport; glucose, ascorbate, taurine, and many other small organic molecules. It is apparent, therefore, that compromise of the Na-K-ATPase, such as occurs during acute or chronic hypoxia/ischemia, will directly and indirectly disrupt a large number of critical cellular regulatory systems, which may lead to functional failure and ultimately degeneration.

III. Ca Homeostasis in Excitable Cells

Calcium is a key ion that contributes to excitation and links cellular activity to metabolism. This ion affects a wide variety of neuronal functions including synaptic transmission and plasticity, axoplasmic transport, gene expression, growth, apoptosis, and energy metabolism (Bootman et al., 2001 a, 2001b; Spira et al., 2001; West et al., 2001). Therefore its concentration and spatiotemporal distribution in excitable cells are tightly controlled (Bootman et al., 2001a; Petersen, 2002). Cells possess a number of powerful homeostatic systems charged with maintaining control over Ca concentrations in the cytosol (Carafoli, 2002). The components include plasmalemmal Ca extrusion systems (Ca-ATPase, Na-Ca and Na-K-Ca exchangers) (Blaustein and Lederer, 1999; Lytton et al., 2002; Shull et al., 2003), cytosolic Ca-binding proteins (parvalbumin, calbindin-D28K, calmodulin and others) (Heizmann and Hunziker, 1991; Schwaller et al., 2002), mitochondrial Ca uptake and release, and the SR/ER Ca-ATPase (or SERCA) on organelles such as the endoplasmic reticulum and nuclear envelope (Wuytack et al., 2002). Together, these Ca buffering systems restore Ca gradients dissipated during normal cellular signaling mediated by a variety of Ca-permeable channels activated by voltage, ligands, or by the emptying of internal Ca stores ("I_{CRAC}"). These in turn can be found on the plasma membrane (e.g., Ca_v family; channels gated by transmitters such as glutamate, acetylcholine, serotonin, ATP; transient receptor potential [TRP] channels [Clapham, 2003]) or on membranes of intracellular organelles, particularly the endoplasmic reticulum (e.g., receptors activated by ryanodine, IP3, nicotinic acid adenine dinucleotide phosphate [NAADP], and "sphingolipid Ca release-mediating protein of the ER" [SCaMPER] [Pozzan et al., 1994; Berridge et al., 2000; Fill and Copello, 2002; Rutter, 2003]). Taken together, these Ca sourcing and buffering systems support a highly complex spatially and temporally organized fluctuation of [Ca] in excitable cells that is critical for normal function. It follows that disturbing this finely tuned Ca handling arrangement can quickly lead to aberrant function and cell damage. Such a disturbance can result from excessive sourcing of this cation and/or impairment of the buffering systems, usually as a result of a deficit in cellular energy supply. Many of these Ca transport systems have been identified in axons, and their alteration by pathological states plays a pivotal role in the degeneration of these structures. Most of the work in this area has been carried out using hypoxia/ischemia as the

injury paradigm, and the following sections summarize our current knowledge obtained from such experimental models. It is becoming apparent, however, that injury mechanisms related to energy failure are also recruited in other pathological states that include MS and its animal models (Lassmann, 2003; Waxman, 2003); therefore these cascades may reflect a stereotyped sequence leading to axonal injury regardless of the initial insult.

IV. Acute Axonal Injury: Depolarization and Ionic Deregulation

Central mammalian axons are critically dependent on a continuous supply of oxygen and glucose for survival. Interruption of the supply of these substrates rapidly leads to failure of excitability (although some central tracts such as mouse optic nerve can maintain excitability for longer periods *in vitro* [Tekkok et al., 2003]), depolarization and ionic deregulation (Utzschneider et al., 1991; Ransom et al., 1992; LoPachin and Stys, 1995; Leppanen and Stys, 1997; Fern et al., 1998; Stys, 1998; Stys et al., 1998; Brown et al., 2001a). Figure 1 shows an example of the acute effects of anoxia on rat optic nerve *in vitro*. Within minutes, rat optic nerves lose the capacity to conduct action potentials (Fig. 1A) in parallel with a rapid and robust depolarization (Fig. 1B). Glycolysis is able to sustain a small residual resting membrane potential during anoxia as shown by the modest additional depolarization after application of ouabain, an Na pump inhibitor. This experiment shows that Na-K-ATPase activity was only minimally supported during anoxia. This does not imply that glycolysis plays only a minor role in the overall energy supply of central axons. During anoxic conditions, mitochondria are known to consume ATP by reverse operation of the ATP-synthase (Nicholls and Budd, 2000). Therefore it is likely that the inability of glycolysis to support the required energy demands is also due to paradoxical consumption of ATP by dysfunctional mitochondria. Aglycemia (without anoxia) shows a longer delay before depolarization and action potential failure become apparent (Stys, 1998; Stys et al., 1998; Brown et al., 2001a), likely caused by additional supply by glycogen stores from supporting astrocytes, with shuttling of lactate to axons by specific monocarboxylate transporters (Wender et al., 2000; Brown et al., 2003).

A more detailed study of the ionic deregulation that occurs in the acute phases of anoxia/ischemia showed that extracellular [K] rises to ≈ 15 mM, along with an acidification of the extracellular space by 0.3 pH units (Ransom et al., 1992). The rise in $[K]_o$ closely parallels the rapid anoxic depolarization and loss of excitability. Studies using electron probe microanalysis have revealed that it is largely axons that source the observed increase in $[K]_o$, with axoplasmic [K] falling to 10% of normal, together with a parallel increase in $[Na]_i$ from approximately 20 to approximately

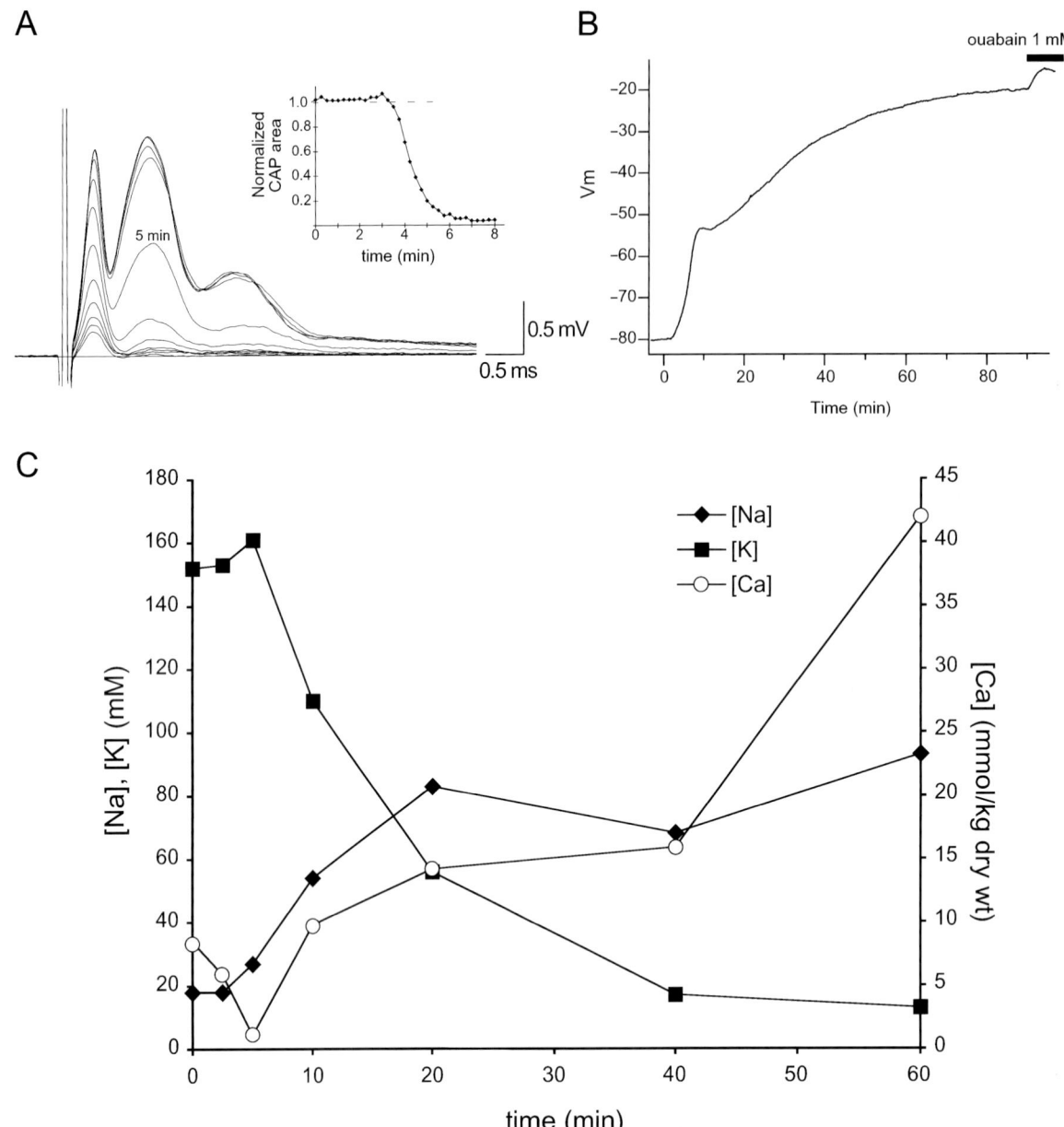

Figure 1 Representative traces of compound action potential (**A**) and resting membrane potential (**B**) from rat optic nerve recorded *in vitro* and exposed to anoxia (beginning at time 0). In the rat, optic nerve action potential conduction is abolished within minutes of anoxia onset, paralleling the rapid phase of depolarization. Blocking the Na-K-ATPase with ouabain (**B**) after the resting potential has plateaued in anoxia reveals that a small component is supported by glycolysis. (**C**) Time course of changes in axoplasmic [Na], [K], and [Ca] in anoxic optic nerve axons measured by electron probe microanalysis (LoPachin and Stys, 1995). [Na] and [K] are shown as calculated free concentrations in mM, whereas Ca, which exists largely in the bound state in cells, is shown as mmol/kg dry weight. Axoplasmic Na increases from a resting level of approximately 20 mM, with a parallel severe loss of axoplasmic K. Total axonal Ca content increases gradually during the hour of anoxic exposure to about five times normal. (**A, B**: Reproduced from Stys, P. K. [1998]. *J. Cereb. Blood Flow Metab.*, 18:2–25, with permission from Lippincott, Williams and Wilkins. **C**: Reproduced from Stys, P. K., and Waxman, S. G. [2003]. Ischemic white matter damage. *In:* "Myelin Biology and Disorders," R. Lazzarini, J. Griffin, H. Lassmann, K.-A. Nave, R. J. Miller, and B. D. Trapp, eds. Copyright 2003, with permission from Elsevier.)

100 mM (Fig. 1C). A gradual but substantial increase in *total* axonal [Ca] was also observed during the 60-minute anoxic exposure, which worsens in large axons after reoxygenation (LoPachin and Stys, 1995; Stys and LoPachin, 1996). As expected, the observed rise in total axonal Ca is paralleled by a reduction in extracellular [Ca] as measured

by ion-sensitive microelectrodes (Brown et al., 1998), reflecting the translocation of this ion across the axolemma. *Free* [Ca] (that sensed by Ca-sensitive dyes) also increases substantially during anoxia/ischemia in central axons, with estimates exceeding 10 μM after 20 to 30 minutes of *in vitro* ischemia (Ren et al., 2000; Nikolaeva and Stys, 2003). Of interest, although as expected total axoplasmic [Ca] (as measured by electron probe microanalysis) does not increase during anoxia in Ca-free perfusate, both optic nerve and dorsal column axons exhibit substantial *free* [Ca] increases, even in Ca-free bath. In dorsal column axons, this internally sourced Ca rise is sufficient to severely damage the axons (Ouardouz et al., 2003). Reoxygenation appears particularly harmful to mitochondria, which suffer a greater than 100-fold increase in total matrix Ca, occurring largely after oxygen is restored (LoPachin and Stys, 1995; Stys and LoPachin, 1996). This is not unexpected as these organelles accumulate Ca electrophoretically via a Ca uniporter, which relies on the negative matrix potential (Crompton, 1985; Nicholls, 1985). This potential is rapidly dissipated when electron transport fails during anoxia/ischemia, limiting the amount of Ca entry into the matrix. During reoxygenation, however, with a high axoplasmic free [Ca] (see previously), re-energized mitochondria paradoxically accumulate large quantities of this ion, which will in turn short-circuit the newly re-established flux of protons pumped by the respiratory chain complexes, and overload the matrix with Ca, causing further damage to these organelles. Similar Ca changes are seen in CNS axons injured by mechanical trauma (LoPachin et al., 1999).

Axonal Ca overload is not merely an epiphenomenon but appears central in the pathogenesis of structural and functional injury. Removal of Ca from the perfusate during *in vitro* anoxia or ischemia prevents net accumulation of Ca and reduces free [Ca] increases and is also highly neuroprotective under many conditions (Stys et al., 1990; Imaizumi et al., 1997; Tekkok and Goldberg, 2001). One notable exception is ischemic injury of spinal dorsal columns, where in addition to control of extracellular Ca influx, release from intracellular stores must also be reduced for functional improvement (Ouardouz et al., 2003). Regardless of the source, however, in central white matter an increased concentration of Ca appears to be the "final common pathway" of cell death, as proposed for other cell types by Schanne and colleagues 25 years ago (Schanne et al., 1979; Orrenius and Nicotera, 1996). For this reason, deciphering the various modes of cellular Ca overload, whether sourced from outside or inside the cell, is of great importance.

An initial series of *in vitro* experiments on mature rat optic nerve in the early 1990s showed that acute anoxic injury to this structure is almost entirely dependent on influx of extracellular Ca. Removal of this cation from the perfusate allowed virtually complete functional (Stys et al., 1990) and ultrastructural (Waxman et al., 1993) recovery. Follow-up studies uncovered a Na-dependence of the Ca entry. Removal of bath Ca *or* Na strongly protects optic nerves against *in vitro* anoxia (Fig. 2A). Similarly, preventing Na influx through voltage-gated Na channels by applying TTX is highly protective, indicating that Na loading (later directly shown to be axonal [Stys and LoPachin, 1998]), not merely depolarization, secondarily leads to

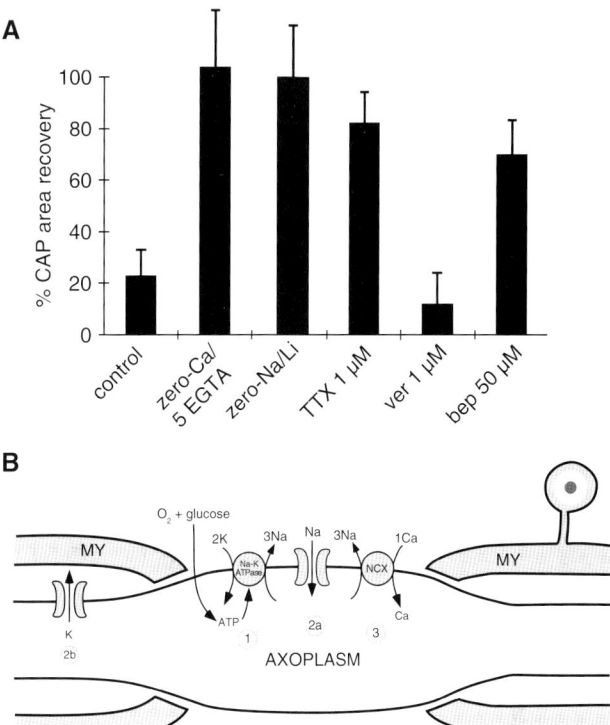

Figure 2 (**A**) Bar graph summarizing the degree of compound action potential recovery recorded electrophysiologically after exposure of adult rat optic nerves to *in vitro* anoxia. In normal artificial CSF containing 2 mM Ca, CAP magnitude recovers to approximately 20% of control after 1 hour of anoxia. Removing Ca from the perfusate (with the addition of the Ca chelator EGTA) allows virtually complete recovery, as does removal of Na ions from the bath. Blocking voltage-gated Na channels with TTX is also highly protective, whereas increasing Na permeability with the Na channel inactivation blocker veratridine worsens anoxic injury. The Na-Ca exchange inhibitor bepridil is also very protective. (**B**) Taken together, these results suggest a Ca- and Na-dependent mechanism of anoxic optic nerve injury summarized in the diagram. Energy failure (1) causes Na influx through non-inactivating Na channels (2a) and K loss through K channels (2b). The Na accumulation and depolarization together drive the Na-Ca exchanger to admit damaging amounts of axoplasmic Ca from the extracellular space. (**A**: data from Stys et al., 1992a; **B**: Modified from Stys et al., 1992a.)

axoplasmic Ca accumulation. Reverse operation of the Na-Ca exchanger and resultant Ca influx would be recruited by these steps, which was directly shown by the protective effects of Na-Ca exchange inhibitors (Fig. 2A) (Stys et al., 1992a; Imaizumi et al., 1997; Li et al., 2000; Tekkok et al., 2000; Brown et al., 2001a). This preliminary model of axonal Ca overload is illustrated in Fig. 2B. According to this model, energy depletion leads to Na pump failure, influx of Na through noninactivating Na channels (Stys et al., 1993; Taylor, 1993), and stimulation of the Na-efflux, Ca-import mode of the Na-Ca exchanger, shown to be present on central axons (Steffensen et al., 1997; Craner et al., 2004a) (see also Chapter 7). (More recently, a K-coupled Na-K-Ca exchanger has been found in the CNS outside of its traditional territory in the retina [Dong et al., 2001; Kiedrowski et al., 2002]. [For a review, see Lytton, 2002]). Its contribution to Ca loading cannot be ruled out, if it were proven to be present in axons. Indeed, given the K dependence of this transporter and the known collapse of the K gradient and K accumulation in the extracellular space, the Na-K-Ca exchanger would be even more strongly driven than the K-independent Na-Ca exchanger to import Ca into cells).

The proximal role played by voltage-gated Na channels appears to extend to other modes of white matter injury, such as inflammatory demyelination. Two recent studies indicate that use-dependent Na channel blockers, such as phenytoin (Lo et al., 2003) and flecainide (Bechtold et al., 2004), significantly improve the survival of CNS axons, their ability to conduct impulses, and clinical scores in rats with EAE, an animal model of MS (see Chapter 29). Taken together, it is becoming apparent that the fundamental steps illustrated in Fig. 2B may represent a ubiquitous cascade of events unleashed in injured white matter, regardless of initial insult. This raises important therapeutic opportunities for a variety of white matter disorders.

V. Ca Channels May Promote Influx and Trigger Release from Internal Stores

Other Ca influx pathways also likely contribute to Ca accumulation. Experiments in rat optic nerve (Fern et al., 1995a; Brown et al., 2001b) and spinal dorsal columns (Imaizumi et al., 1999) indicate that L- and N-type Ca channels contribute to anoxic injury in these preparations. Although it is likely that these channels allow flux of Ca across plasma membranes, L-type channels may contribute in another role by sensing axonal depolarization and activating Ca release from ryanodine receptors (Ouardouz et al., 2003). Indeed, electron probe studies failed to show a reduction of *net* Ca accumulation in anoxic optic axons exposed to L-type Ca channel blockers such as nifedipine or nimodipine (Stys and LoPachin, 1998). It is possible that an important role of L-type channels in ischemic axons is activation of ryanodine receptors and release of internal Ca stores, rather than flux of extracellular Ca across the axolemma. Recent experiments in ischemic rat dorsal column (Ouardouz et al., 2003) have shown that unlike anoxia, more prolonged exposure to *in vitro* ischemia (oxygen-glucose deprivation) results in severe functional injury that cannot be rescued by removal of extracellular Ca. Yet robust protection is afforded by pretreatment with the high affinity Ca chelator BAPTA as the acetoxymethyl ester to allow penetration across cell membranes. These findings strongly suggest that deleterious Ca is released from an intracellular source, such as endoplasmic reticulum or mitochondria. Of interest, adding the

L-type Ca channel blocker nimodipine to ischemic dorsal columns already perfused with zero-Ca/EGTA solution increased postischemic recovery of compound action potential amplitudes from 2% in zero-Ca/EGTA alone to 62% with the addition of nimodipine. Clearly, this agent was not neuroprotective as a result of reduction of Ca *influx* through L-type channels. Instead, it was hypothesized that its interference with voltage sensing by these channels inhibited depolarization-induced release of Ca from endoplasmic reticulum, which proceeded through ryanodine receptors, analogous to Ca-independent "excitation-contraction coupling" in skeletal muscle (Franzini-Armstrong and Protasi, 1997). This mechanism is further supported by protective effects of thapsigargin, which depletes Ca stores; ryanodine, which partially blocks release of Ca from endoplasmic reticulum; and either zero-Na perfustate or TTX, which will reduce ischemic depolarization, thereby dampening the change in membrane potential sensed by the Ca channels. Ryanodine receptors (RyR1 and RyR2) and Ca channels ($Ca_v1.2$ and $Ca_v1.3$) were shown to co-immunoprecipitate (respectively) and be spatially co-localized at the axolemma of dorsal column axons (Fig. 3), further supporting an "excitation-contraction coupling"-like Ca release in these fibers (Ouardouz et al., 2003). Indeed, ryanodine receptor-dependent Ca release may not be the only source of intracellular Ca in ischemic central axons. Inhibition of group I metabotropic glutamate receptors, in addition to external Ca removal and application of nimodipine to block the aforementioned mode of release, allows virtually complete functional recovery of dorsal columns after an hour of severe ischemia (Stys and Ouardouz, 2002). We interpret this additional protection as inhibition of Ca release from IP3 receptors, stimulated by IP3 generated by phospholipase C through mGluR1 activation. These mechanisms may be of great importance because they underscore the argument that control of extracellular Ca influx is necessary, but not sufficient, to protect central axons from more severe ischemic injury.

Pathological states such as inflammatory demyelination may promote inappropriate ectopic insertion of channels into the axon membrane. Lassmann and co-workers showed an excess of N-type Ca channel subunit accumulation at the axolemma in areas of spheroid formation within actively demyelinating lesions in both human brain and EAE animals (Kornek et al., 2001). This raises the interesting possibility that normal axons (at least those not previously exposed to a chronic insult such and inflammatory demyelination) may have very low densities of Ca channels, but chronic pathological states may increase channel densities, thus promoting Ca influx and Ca-dependent injury. What is not yet clear is whether these accumulated channels are functionally inserted into the axolemma of pathological axons where they can impart an increased Ca permeability.

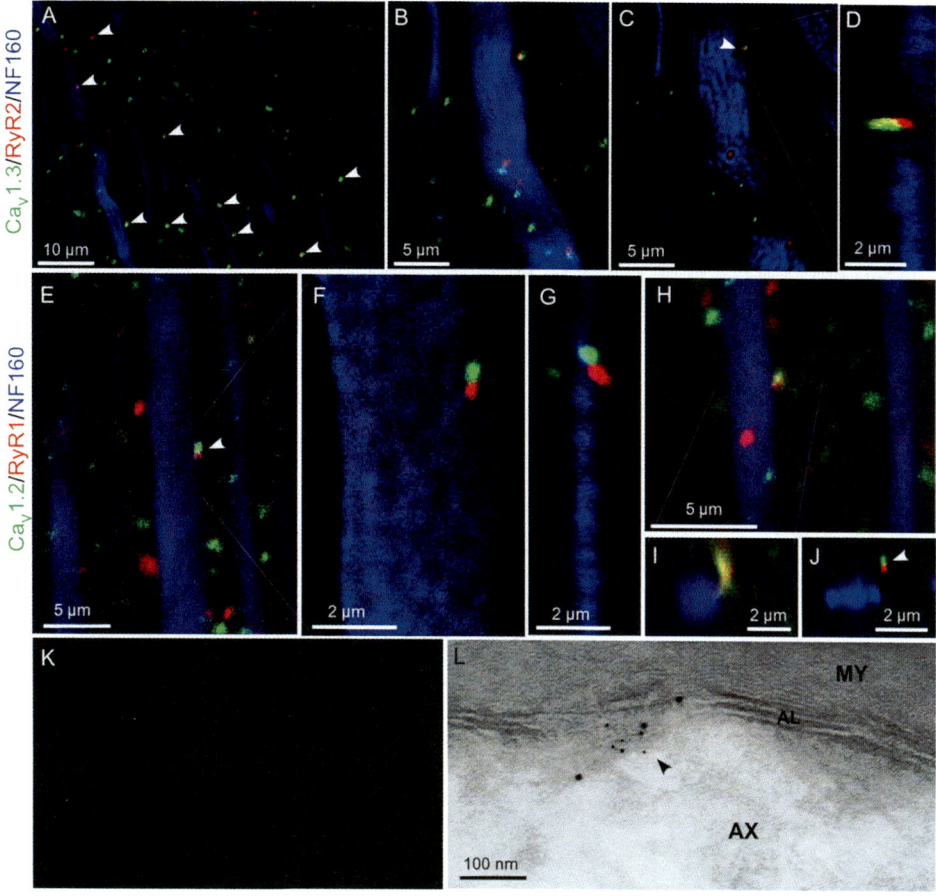

Figure 3 Immunolocalization of Ca$_v$ and RyR in spinal dorsal columns. (**A–D**) Triple labeled sections (Ca$_v$1.3/RyR2/neurofilament) show many Ca$_v$ and RyR clusters, which are occasionally co-localized. Clusters were found near the surfaces of axon cylinders and within glial structures. Deconvolution (**C, D**) reveals a more accurate localization of cluster pairs at the surface of an axon cylinder, overlying a neurofilament-poor area, possibly representing an ER cistern. YZ projection (**D**) shows elongated "fingers" of associated Ca$_v$/RyR complexes. Similar distributions of Ca$_v$1.2/RyR1 profiles are shown in panels **E–J**, also associated with axon cylinders and glial regions (**I**; deconvolved: **J**). Control sections with primary antibodies omitted showed no signal (**K**). Double immuno-gold staining (**L**) using pan-RyR (small grains) and Ca$_v$1.3 (large grains) shows close association of both proteins at the axolemma. (Reproduced from Ouardouz et al., 2003, with permission.)

VI. Glutamate Release from Axons as a Trigger of Ca Overload

Another consequence of axonal Na loading and depolarization, regardless of initial insult, is the aberrant ion-coupled transport of small organic molecules, such as neurotransmitters, in particular, the excitatory transmitter glutamate. Under normal conditions in the CNS, glutamate is taken back up into cells by a series of Na-dependent glutamate transporters. These molecules support electrogenic transport and are also coupled to K (and protons) (Zerangue and Kavanaugh, 1996; Levy et al., 1998), therefore depolarization, Na influx, and/or K loss (all of which occur in damaged axons) will drive these transporters in the Na and glutamate efflux mode. In support of this contention, experiments on anoxic dorsal columns have shown that reverse Na-dependent glutamate transport contributes to a significant degree to anoxic glutamate release in this tissue (Fig. 4B), with most of the transmitter released from axon trunks (Li, 1999). This does not preclude additional non-vesicular modes of glutamate release of which there are several, including flux through volume-sensitive anion channels (Kimelberg et al., 1990; Rutledge et al., 1998), exocytosis from astrocytes (Pasti et al., 2001), or release from astrocytes through gap junction hemichannels (Ye et al., 2003). Volume changes and early cytosolic Ca dysregulation promote these modes of glutamate release, so it is quite plausible that these systems contribute as well; however no firm evidence has yet been provided in injured CNS white matter tracts.

The search for glutamate-release mechanisms in damaged white matter was prompted by prior studies from several laboratories indicating a prominent role of ionotropic glutamate receptors in the pathogenesis of white matter ischemia and trauma (Agrawal and Fehlings, 1997; Wrathall et al., 1997; Li et al., 1999; Rosenberg et al., 1999a; Tekkok and Goldberg, 2001). Some studies have even shown that excitotoxic mechanisms play a role in immune-mediated demyelinating disease in rodents (Pitt et al., 2000; Smith et al., 2000), again emphasizing a stereotyped response of CNS white matter to injury (see previously). Glial cells express a variety of glutamate receptors and thus represent a major target of glutamate-triggered Ca overload. AMPA and kainate receptors are found on mature oligodendrocytes and astrocytes (Jensen and Chiu, 1993; Garcia-Barcina and Matute, 1996; Agrawal and Fehlings, 1997; Matute et al., 1997) (for reviews see Steinhauser and Gallo, 1996; Matute et al., 2002; and Dewar et al., 2003), whereas NMDA receptor-mediated currents only appear transiently on both glial cell types until approximately 2 weeks of age (Ziak et al., 1998). White matter astrocytes express all AMPA and kainate receptor subunits except GluR4, whereas oligodendrocytes express only GluR3 and GluR4 AMPA receptor subunits (notably lacking GluR2), as well as all kainate subunits except GluR5 (Garcia-Barcina and Matute, 1996, 1998; Matute et al., 2002). Persistent activation of these non-NMDA ionotropic receptors injures oligodendrocytes, both in cell culture and *in vivo* (Yoshioka et al., 1995, 1996; Matute et al., 1997; Matute, 1998; McDonald et al., 1998; Liu et al., 2002). The absence of GluR2 imparts significant Ca permeability and may render oligodendrocytes particularly susceptible to Ca flux through these receptors. AMPA and kainate receptor expression is particularly robust in oligodendrocyte progenitors (Barres et al., 1990; Kastritsis and McCarthy, 1993; Holzwarth et al., 1994), which may contribute to the exquisite sensitivity of these cells to ischemia (Fern and Moller, 2000; Follett et al., 2000). Astrocytes can also be injured when exposed to AMPA receptor agonists (Li and Stys, 2000), particularly when desensitization is blocked (David et al., 1996).

The question of whether myelinated axons *per se* possess glutamate receptor subunits has not been resolved. Axonal protection by the AMPA/kainate receptor blocker NBQX has been demonstrated in an animal model of EAE (Pitt et al., 2000; Smith et al., 2000). More recently, Tekkök and Goldberg (2001) presented evidence of axonal protection by NBQX in an *in vitro* model of central white matter ischemic injury. However, more recent data from this group indicate that the axonal protection by glutamate antagonists may be secondary to sparing of oligodendroglia, thereby reducing the generation of free radicals that could be toxic to neighboring axons (Underhill and Goldberg, 2002). Irrespective of whether they are present on axons or glial cells, AMPA/kainate receptors appear to play a prominent role in various modes of white mat-

ter injury, including hypoxia/ischemia (Li et al., 1999; Follett et al., 2000; Kanellopoulos et al., 2000; Tekkok and Goldberg, 2001; McCracken et al., 2002), trauma (Agrawal and Fehlings, 1997; Wrathall et al., 1997; Rosenberg et al., 1999a), and inflammatory demyelination (Pitt et al., 2000; Smith et al., 2000; Werner et al., 2000; Groom et al., 2003). Representative results from anoxic dorsal columns in the adult rat are shown in Fig. 4. Under normoxic conditions, application of either glutamate or kainate (the latter to activate AMPA and kainate receptors) causes functional injury to dorsal columns, whereas NMDA has no effect, as measured by the propagated compound action potential. Moreover, the broad-spectrum ionotropic glutamate receptor antagonist kynurenic acid, or the more selective AMPA receptor blocker GYKI52466, display robust neuroprotective activity against dorsal column anoxia. Similarly, blocking glutamate release via Na-dependent transporters with dihydrokainate or L-trans-pyrrolidine-2,4-dicarboxylic acid (Arriza et al., 1994; Griffiths et al., 1994) is also protective against anoxic damage in this tissue. These results do not distinguish between axonal and glial targets of glutamate-triggered injury, but taken together, they indicate that not only is dorsal column white matter injured by glutamate exposure, but that endogenous glutamate is released in sufficient quantities during anoxia to trigger substantial excitotoxicity.

The mechanisms of excitotoxic damage in white matter may be more complex than simple activation of Ca-permeable receptors. For instance, preliminary data indicate that selective AMPA receptor blockade (using GYKI52466 or SYM2206) is far more protective against white matter anoxia/ischemia using the optic nerve model (in contrast to spinal cord white matter) than combined inhibition of AMPA and kainate receptors using a less selective agent such as NBQX (Jiang and Stys, 2003) or kynurenic acid. Although these observations have yet to be confirmed and mechanisms elucidated, they raise the intriguing, if not counterintuitive, possibility that kainate-receptor activation may in fact be partially protective in some central white matter tracts. Complicating matters further is the possibility that metabotropic glutamate receptors may also contribute to the injury cascade in ischemia and trauma, by coupling back to the potentially important mechanism of release from internal Ca stores, via a phospholipase C-dependent mechanism acting on IP3 receptors (Agrawal et al., 1998; Stys and Ouardouz, 2002). On the basis of immunocytochemical findings, one study suggests the presence of metabotropic glutamate receptors along axons in MS (Geurts et al., 2003).

It is generally accepted that NMDA receptors do not play a significant role in the pathophysiology of mature white matter injury, as these receptors appear absent in adult tissue (Wyllie et al., 1991; Ziak et al., 1998), although they are transiently expressed on glia of immature spinal cord (Ziak et al., 1998), and neither NMDA receptor activation nor antagonism

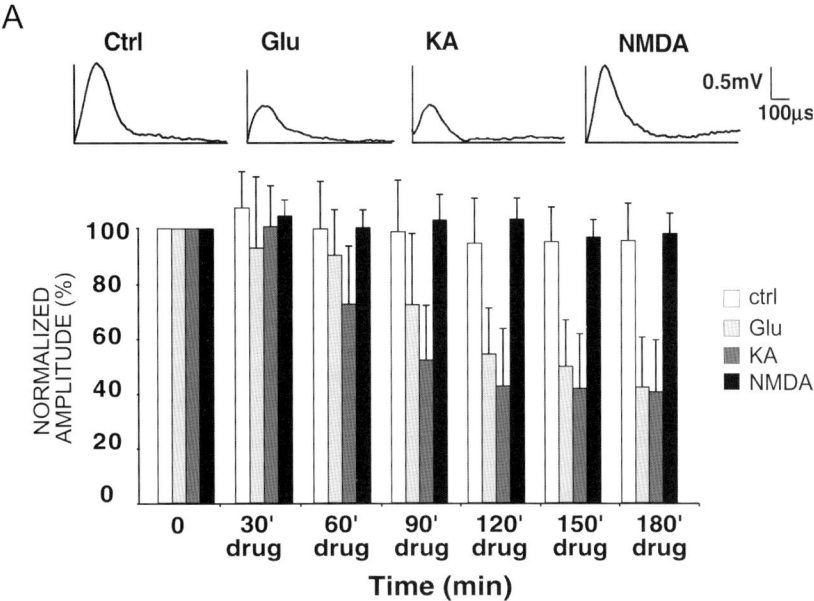

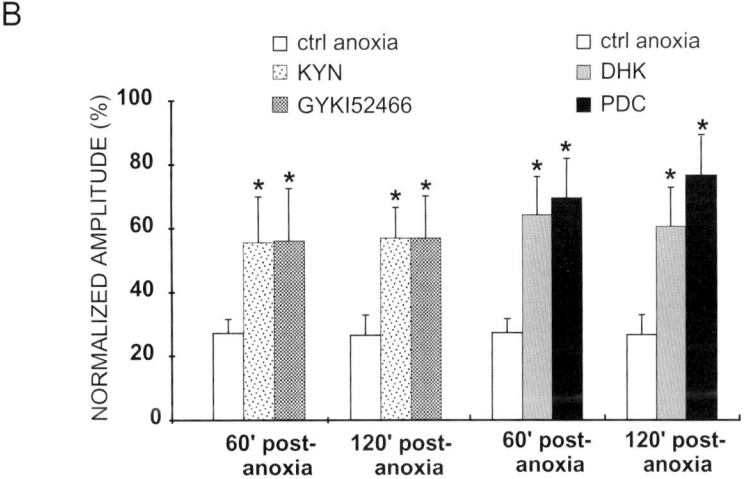

Figure 4 (**A**) Effect of glutamate (Glu), kainate (KA), or NMDA on *in vitro* dorsal columns. Representative CAP tracings after 180 minutes of exposure and bar graph show controls to be stable for 180 minutes, whereas glutamate (1 mM) or kainate (500 μM) irreversibly reduced CAP amplitude to approximately 40% of control. In contrast, NMDA (500 μM, with 20 μM glycine and in the absence of Mg^{2+}) had no effect on propagated CAP. (**B**) Protective effects of ionotropic glutamate receptor antagonists or glutamate transport blockers against dorsal column anoxic injury. The broad spectrum (NMDA, AMPA, kainate receptor) blocker kynurenic acid (1 mM) and the more selective AMPA receptor antagonist GYKI52466 (30 μM) are both protective against anoxic injury. Similarly, the Na-dependent glutamate transport blockers dihydrokainate (DHK) or L-trans-pyrrolidine-2,4-dicarboxylic acid (PDC; 1 mM each) were also protective. Taken together, these data indicate that endogenous glutamate is released from dorsal columns during anoxia/ischemia via reverse transport due to Na influx and depolarization, causing damage by activation of AMPA-preferring ionotropic receptors. (**A**: Modified from Li and Stys, 2000, with permission. Copyright 2000 by the Society for Neuroscience; **B**: Modified from Li et al., 1999, with permission. Copyright 1999 by the Society for Neuroscience.)

exerts any obvious deleterious or protective effects (respectively) in central white matter tracts (Fig. 4) (Agrawal and Fehlings, 1997; Li and Stys, 2000; Yam et al., 2000). This receptor has not been studied in great detail in this context, so its role in white matter pathophysiology cannot be ruled out.

VII. Adenosine and GABA as Modulators of Ca Influx

Experiments on rat optic nerve *in vitro* have provided evidence suggesting that release of two other neurotransmitters/neuromodulators, GABA and adenosine, from endogenous stores within white matter may provide a mechanism that modulates calcium influx into axons (Fig. 5). Fern et al. (1994, 1995b, 1996) showed that anoxia triggers the release of GABA and adenosine from endogenous stores within the optic nerve. These act on GABA-B and adenosine receptors, respectively, and increase resistance to anoxia, thus playing an autoprotective role. This autoprotection appears to involve a G-protein/protein kinase C (PKC) pathway that is activated as a result of binding of GABA or adenosine to their receptors. Although the target of PKC activity is not known, these experiments indicate that there are endogenous mechanisms that can modulate at least some of the pathways for calcium influx into axons. Thus, the response of CNS white matter to injury displays a surprisingly rich dependence on a spectrum of traditional neurotransmitters.

VIII. Nitric Oxide and Free Radicals

Nitric oxide (NO) is synthesized from L-arginine by three isoforms of NO synthase, the constitutively expressed eNOS and nNOS, and a third (iNOS), which is induced during inflammation (for a review see Brown and Borutaite, 2002). The biological chemistry of NO and its reaction pathways are complex (for reviews see Brown and Borutaite, 2002 and Chapter 18). However, this molecule may be converted to a number of more active derivatives, known collectively as reactive nitrogen species, which in turn can react with and chemically modify a large number of key cellular proteins, lipids, and nucleic acids. In the present context, perhaps one of the most important structures adversely influenced by NO are mitochondria. This gas inhibits cytochrome oxidase (complex IV) competitively with O_2, and certain NO derivatives such as peroxynitrite ($ONOO^-$) may inactivate all respiratory complexes (I-IV) and the ATP synthase. To make matters worse, peroxynitrite stimulates proton leak across the inner mitochondrial membrane (Gadelha et al., 1997), which, together with impaired complex activity, can effectively render a cell hypoxic or at a minimum exacerbate an existing injury.

The effects of NO may have profound effects on central white matter tracts. Smith and colleagues (Redford et al., 1997) (see also Chapter 18) showed that exposure of demyelinated spinal axons to NO induced reversible conduction block, whereas myelinated axons in the same tract were affected only at higher concentrations (Fig. 6). Subsequent studies confirmed and extended this observation, suggesting that active axons are particularly sensitive to NO exposure (Smith et al., 2001). Although the precise mechanisms of NO toxicity are not fully understood, direct nitration of key proteins, such as Na channels (Hammarstrom and Gage, 1999; Renganathan et al., 2002) and mito-

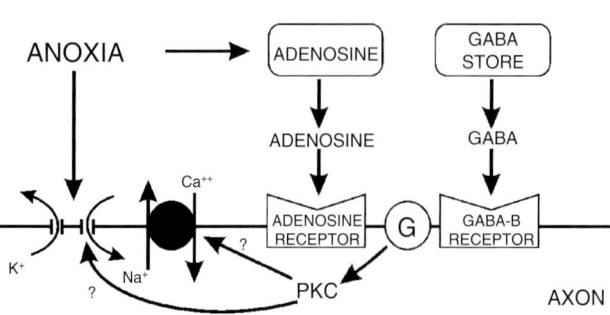

Figure 5 Proposed model for protective effect of adenosine and GABA in the anoxic optic nerve. According to this model, anoxia triggers K efflux and Na influx which lead to reverse operation of the Na-Ca exchanger and influx of calcium into axons. Anoxia also induces release of GABA and adenosine from endogenous stores within white matter with a resultant activation of GABA-B and adenosine receptors, initiating a G-protein/PKC cascade, which increases the tolerance of axons to anoxia. The target of PKC phosphorylation is not known, but could be the Na-Ca exchanger or Na channels. (From Fern et al., 1996, with permission.)

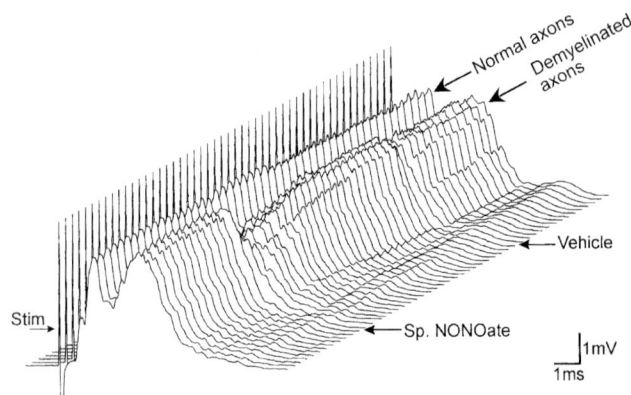

Figure 6 CAPs recorded from a demyelinated lesion induced in the rat dorsal column by a previous intraspinal injection of ethidium bromide. Records are plotted at 2-minute intervals. Application of the NO donor spermine NONOate (NO concentration aapproximately 3 μM) resulted in conduction block in many of the demyelinated axons, whereas normal fibers remained largely unaffected. This study underscores the increased susceptibility of demyelinated fibers to NO that may exert its effects by partial mitochondrial inhibition and/or Na channel nitrosylation (see text). (Modified from Redford et al., 1997, with permission.)

chondrial impairment, are highly likely. Indeed, it appears that the steps set in motion by NO may overlap to a significant extent with those during hypoxia/ischemia. Blockade of voltage-gated Na channels or reduction of axonal Ca load with pharmacological block of the Na-Ca exchanger protect against NO exposure (Garthwaite et al., 2002; Kapoor et al., 2003). Thus, the major effect of NO production under pathological conditions such as inflammatory demyelination may be to further exacerbate the cellular hypoxic state, driving the anoxic/ischemic injury cascade (Fig. 7) even more strongly. If so, neuroprotective strategies (see next section)

may simultaneously mitigate at least some of the damaging effects of NO in CNS white matter.

IX. Potential Neuroprotective Strategies

The last 15 years have generated substantial advances in our understanding of CNS white matter injury mechanisms, from the simple three-step model illustrated in Fig. 2B to a much more complex network of inter-related events summarized in Fig. 7. A more thorough understanding of these

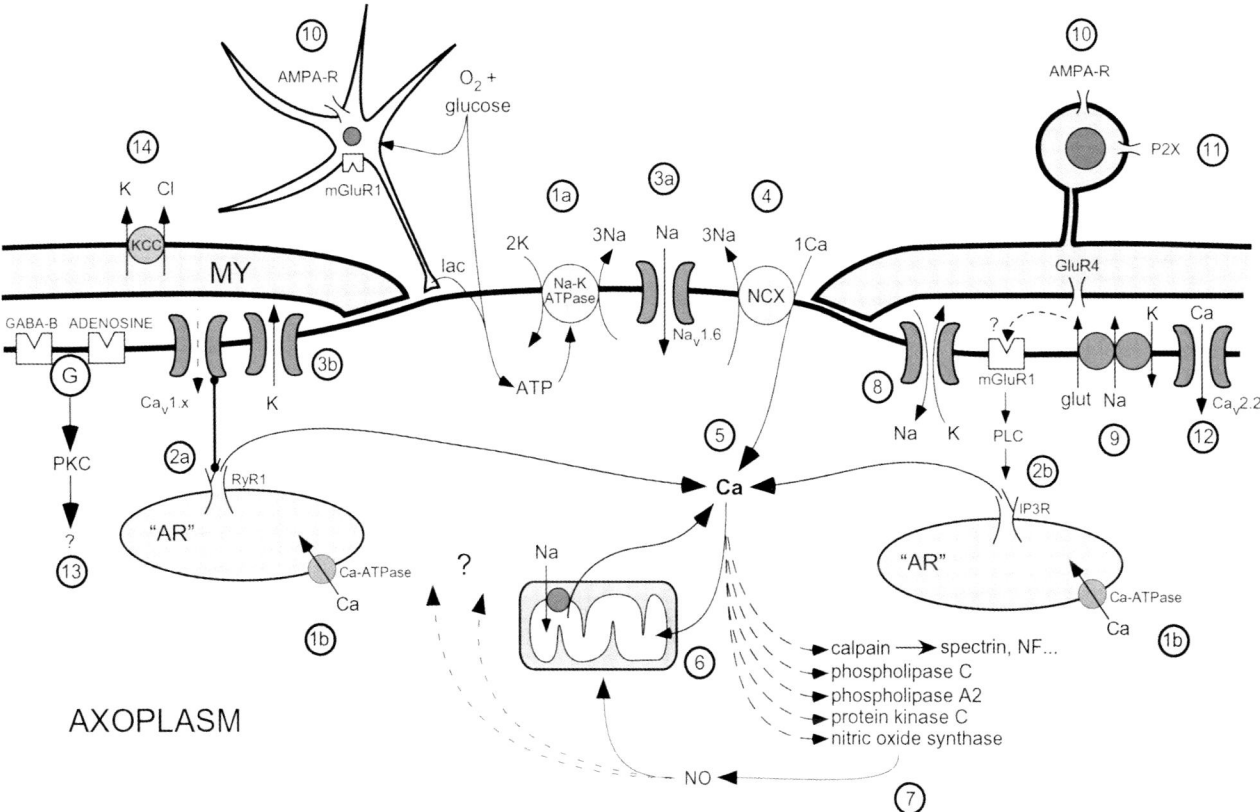

Figure 7 **Diagram summarizing events of the acute phase of CNS white matter injury.** White matter is critically dependent on a continuous supply of O_2 and either glucose or lactate supplied by astrocytes and then shuttled to axons through monocarboxylate transporters (Wender et al., 2000). An energy deficit and/or excess demand lead to impairment of ATP-dependent pumps such as the Na-K-ATPase (**1a**) and Ca-ATPase (**1b**), including those located on the "axoplasmic reticulum." Axonal Ca accumulation may begin due to release from internal stores, triggered by depolarization via L-type Ca channels (**2a**), and generation of IP3 (**2b**). The rise in $[Na]_i$ by flux through non-inactivating Na channels (**3a**) coupled with depolarization caused by K efflux through a variety of K channels (**3b**) stimulates the Na-Ca exchanger to operate in the reverse, Ca import mode (**4**). This Ca accumulation (**5**) triggers a variety of destructive events including mitochondrial Ca overload (especially during reoxygenation) (**6**), and over-activation of a number of Ca-dependent enzyme systems (**7**). NO generated by NO-synthase may inhibit mitochondrial respiration and alter other cellular proteins. Some Na influx may occur through Na/K permeable inward rectifier channels (**8**) (Eng et al., 1990; Stys et al., 1998). Na overload and depolarization also stimulate glutamate release through reversal of Na-dependent glutamate transport (**9**), leading to glial injury from activation of ionotropic glutamate receptors (**10**). Very recently, ATP-activated P2X purinergic receptors were shown to cause Ca-dependent oligodendroglial injury (**11**) (Matute et al., 2003). A component of Ca influx into damaged axons directly through voltage-gated Ca channels is also likely (**12**). Endogenously released transmitters such as GABA and adenosine may play an "autoprotective" role (**13**). Anion transporters such as the K-Cl co-transporter participate in volume dysregulation in glia and the myelin sheath, contributing to conduction abnormalities (**14**). The locations of the various channels and transporters are drawn for clarity and do not necessarily reflect their real distributions in myelinated axons. Modified from reference Stys, 2004a with permission from Bentham Science Publishers Ltd.

events may allow a more rational and, it is hoped, more effective design of therapeutic intervention. "Energy deficit," whether due to inadequate supply such as ischemia, impaired energy producing machinery such as mitochondria altered by NO, or excess energy utilization as would occur in a demyelinated axon (see Fig. 8), will inhibit ATP-dependent pumps such as the Na-K- and Ca-ATPases, resulting in flux of ions down their electrochemical gradients. Ca leak from internal stores plays a major role in some white matter tracts, whereas Na influx through noninactivating channels is a proximal event, which in turn triggers a variety of deleterious cascades including the following: (a) Na loading; (b) depolarization; (c) reverse Na-Ca exchange and Ca overload; (d) glutamate efflux from axons as well as glia through reversal of electrogenic Na-dependent glutamate transporters, with subsequent activation of ionotropic and metabotropic glutamate receptors on glial cells and possibly on axons; (e) activation of voltage-gated Ca channels, which may flux Ca directly or further exacerbate release from internal stores; and other steps illustrated in Fig. 7.

From such an "injury map," one can now select targets that will most likely be beneficial. On the one hand, blocking one or several of the Ca-dependent enzymes (e.g., calpain) may confer modest protection, because the accumulated Ca ions will go on to stimulate other deleterious Ca-sensitive pathways, a prediction borne out experimentally (Jiang and Stys, 2000) (see also Chapter 20). On the other hand, addressing a proximal step on which several downstream events are dependent appears most attractive. One obvious candidate is the voltage-dependent Na channel, and in particular, the noninactivating component of the $Na_v 1.6$ channel (Smith et al., 1998; Herzog et al., 2003b). This channel has been shown to be the predominant Na channel subtype at nodes of mature myelinated axons (Caldwell et al., 2000) and along demyelinated axons in EAE (Craner et al., 2004a) and in MS (Craner et al., 2004b). This channel presumably contributes a substantial fraction of the resting axon membrane Na permeability that is known to be present in axons of the optic nerve (Stys et al., 1993). Interestingly, the inactivation properties of the

$Na_v 1.6$ channel have been shown to be Ca-dependent. Increased intracellular Ca leads to slower inactivation and thus an increased Na flux through the channel (Herzog et al., 2003a). This raises the possibility that, as a result of increased levels of intracellular Ca, there is an increased Na influx that could, in turn, have a positive feedback effect, further increasing Na-dependent Ca entry mechanisms such as reverse Na-Ca exchange. Such a mechanism is quite plausible because Ca imaging experiments in optic axons have shown that slowing Na channel inactivation pharmacologically with veratridine greatly increases the amount of Ca influx, even after a single action potential (Verbny et al., 2002). Therefore, active fibers may be particularly vulnerable to such a runaway positive feedback cycle of increased Ca, slowed Na channel inactivation, further activity-dependent increase in Na loads leading to greater Ca entry, and so on, finally culminating in degeneration of the fiber.

In fact a selective block of the persistent component of sodium current may be essential to avoid interfering with normal excitability. For example, TTX, a state-independent Na channel blocker (Catterall, 1980), is protective in many white matter injury models (Stys et al., 1992a; Imaizumi et al., 1997; Teng and Wrathall, 1997; Rosenberg et al., 1999b; Tekkok and Goldberg, 2001). However, this agent is unlikely to be clinically useful because it potently blocks normal neural excitability. There are several classes of Na channel blockers (e.g., local anesthetic, antiarrhythmic, anticonvulsant) that display "use-dependence," that is, potency of block that varies with the rate of activation of the channels and are more selective for the open state of the Na channel. These state-dependent Na channel blockers have the potential of allowing normal signaling to proceed unhindered along axons, yet effectively blocking a persistently open state that would leak excessive Na ions during pathological conditions. This proposition has been tested in the *in vitro* anoxic optic nerve model using analogs of local anesthetics and antiarrhythmic agents known to preferentially block open, noninactivating Na channels (Stys et al., 1992b, 1995). The permanently charged quaternary lido-

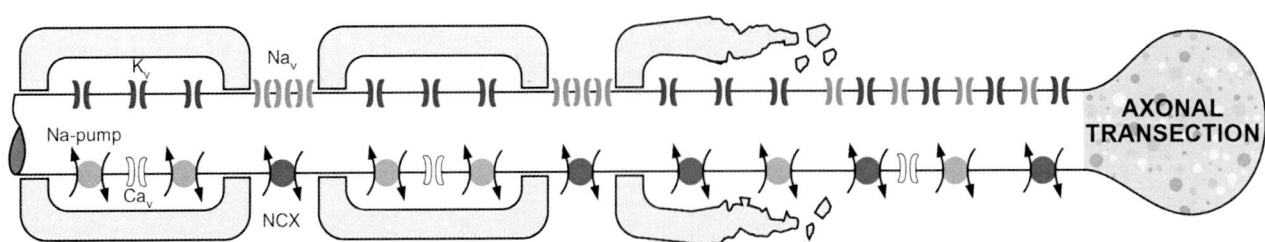

Figure 8 Architectural changes occurring in demyelinated axons, and the hypothesis of an unbalanced energy supply-demand equation. Normal axons (*left*) are only vulnerable when energy supply is interrupted (e.g., during ischemia). In a demyelinated fiber (*right*), the increased energy demand, particularly in active axons, coupled with a reduced ATP-producing capacity by altered mitochondria, may create a state of "virtual hypoxia" promoting a loss of Ca homeostasis and ultimately structural failure of the fiber, manifested as spheroid formation and finally transection. Na_v, K_v, Ca_v: voltage-gated ion channels; NCX: Na-Ca exchanger. (Reproduced from Stys, 2004b, with permission.)

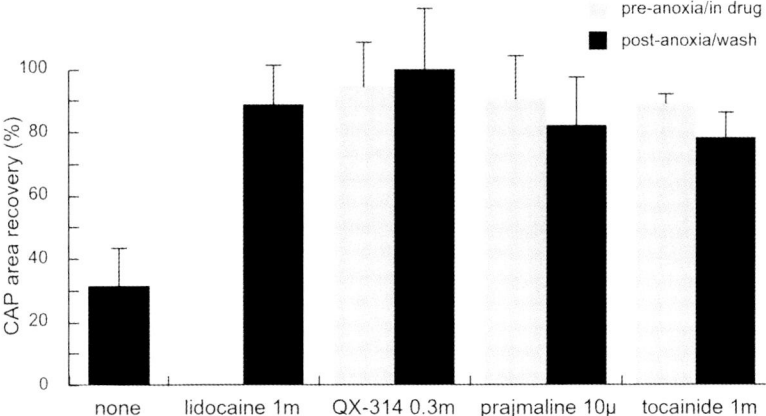

Figure 9 Bar graph showing effects of selected Na channel blockers on pre-anoxic and post-anoxic optic nerve compound action potential (CAP). Gray bars show depression of excitability before anoxia is applied, reflecting the drug's anesthetic properties. Black bars show CAP recovery after anoxia and wash of drug. Control recovery without blockers is ≈20–30% of control. Lidocaine (1 mM) is an effective neuroprotectant but at anesthetic concentrations. In contrast, charged compounds such as QX-314 and prajmaline that are thought to be more selective for the open conformation of the Na channel, are highly neuroprotective with minimal CAP depression. Prajmaline and tocainide are anti-arrhythmic drugs in clinical use. (Reproduced from Stys, P. K., and Waxman, S. G. [2004]. Ischemic white matter damage. In: "Myelin Biology and Disorders," R. Lazzarini, J. Griffin, H. Lassmann, K.-A. Nave, R. J. Miller and B. D. Trapp, eds. Copyright 2004, with permission from Elsevier. Data from Stys, 1995.)

caine analog QX-314 (known to be more selective for the open conformation of Na channels) (Yeh and Tanguy, 1985; Wang et al., 1987; Khodorov, 1991) was very effective at a concentration that showed little inhibition of normal electrogenesis. A sampling of effective compounds against *in vitro* white matter anoxic injury is shown in Fig. 9. The prototypical local anesthetic lidocaine was a potent neuroprotectant, but at concentrations that severely impaired conduction. Charged quaternary amines such as QX-314 and prajmaline were also effective, but at concentrations that exhibited little suppression of excitability.

Unfortunately such charged molecules are unlikely to be effective *in vivo* because of poor penetration of the blood-brain barrier and cell membranes, which is required for access to the local anesthetic binding site on the cytoplasmic face of the Na channel (Hille, 1977; Ragsdale et al., 1996; Salazar et al., 1996). However, certain anticonvulsants and antiarrhythmic agents can penetrate into the brain and have been shown to be effective against brain ischemia (e.g., mexiletine) (Lee et al., 1999; Hewitt et al., 2001). Even more intriguing is the ability of some of these agents to improve outcome in EAE after systemic administration. Lo et al. (2002, 2003) showed a substantial protective effect of the Na-channel blocking anticonvulsant phenytoin, which substantially lessened the incidence of degeneration of optic nerve and spinal cord axons, maintained conduction in these axons, and improved clinical outcome in progressive EAE. Phenytoin also protected against the reduction in conduction velocity seen in untreated EAE, leading these investigators

to suggest that it protected against demyelination (Lo et al., 2003). Another study using flecainide (a use-dependent Na channel blocking antiarrhythmic agent) in a chronic relapsing EAE model also showed a substantial protective effect against axonal degeneration, improvement in electrophysiological conduction parameters in the cord, clinical scores, and a sparing of myelin loss (Bechtold et al., 2004). Together, these studies unite at least part of the injury model proposed for anoxia/ischemia, with the still-unresolved sequence of events responsible for white matter injury in neuroinflammatory disorders. Indeed, even the myelin-sparing effect of phenytoin and flecainide can be explained by a reduction of glutamate release (by reverse transport, or later because of axonal degeneration), which is thought to target glial elements, potentially including myelin.

It is of course possible that the positive results discussed in the previous paragraph may not be achievable clinically in humans. The concentrations of a Na channel blocker required to adequately block Na influx may not be tolerated *in vivo*, or other pathways (e.g., poorly selective cation channels such as the inward rectifier, or AMPA/kainate receptors activated by glutamate from other sources such as inflammatory cells) may also contribute to Na influx. Although the primary site of action (on glial cells? on axons?) is not known at this time, a number of studies have confirmed the efficacy of AMPA receptor antagonists such as NBQX and GYKI52466 in *in vitro* anoxic, ischemic, and traumatic white matter injury models (Agrawal and Fehlings, 1997; Li et al., 1999; Stys and Ouardouz, 2002), as well as in *in vivo* models of ischemia, spinal cord injury, and EAE (Wrathall et al., 1994, 1997; Rosenberg et al., 1999a; Kanellopoulos et al., 2000; Pitt et al., 2000; Smith et al., 2000; McCracken et al., 2002; Groom et al., 2003). Together with the known neuroprotective actions of these agents in gray matter (Akins and Atkinson, 2002), this class of drug represents an attractive option, perhaps for use in combination with Na channel blockers, and deserves further study.

X. Conclusions

Our understanding of multiple sclerosis has evolved from its being considered an inflammatory disorder that results in immune-mediated demyelination to one where degeneration of the neuronal elements (in particular axons) is recognized as a critically important event. Axonopathy begins early in the course of MS and likely underlies the irreversible clinical deficits that patients accumulate over the years. Our understanding of this key component of the disease is still rudimentary, but studies on injury mechanisms in white matter have shed light on the molecular events that may be triggered to cause axonal transection and degeneration in MS and related disorders. Thus the time has come to seriously consider MS as a disorder that requires coordinated therapeutic efforts aimed at both (1) halting or slowing the initiating immunological aberration, and (2) providing neuroprotection that reduces the damage to glia and particularly axons. Practical and partially effective treatment options have been devised for the immune component, and a challenge for the future will be to devise, test, and bring into clinical use a safe and effective adjunctive neuroprotective treatment. Ironically, MS may present an ideal scenario for such an approach. Unlike acute CNS injuries such as stroke and trauma, where minutes count and posttreatment is largely ineffective, the chronic nature of MS creates the opportunity to pretreat patients before much irreversible damage is done.

Acknowledgments

Work in the laboratory of PKS is supported by grants from the Heart and Stroke Foundation of Ontario, National Institute of Neurological Disorders and Stroke, Canadian Institutes of Health Research, Ontario Neurotrauma Foundation, Canadian Stroke Network, Premier's Research Excellence Award from the Province of Ontario, National Multiple Sclerosis Society, Canadian Multiple Sclerosis Society, and the generosity of private donors.

Research in the laboratory of SGW has been supported in part by the Medical Research Service and Rehabilitation Research Service, Department of Veterans Affairs, and by grants from the National Multiple Sclerosis Society, the Paralyzed Veterans of America, the United Spinal Association, and the Nancy Davis Foundation.

We thank our many co-workers whose research is described in this chapter.

References

Agrawal, S. K., and Fehlings, M. G. (1997). Role of NMDA and non-NMDA ionotropic glutamate receptors in traumatic spinal cord axonal injury. *J. Neurosci.* **17**, 1055–1063.

Agrawal, S. K., Theriault, E., and Fehlings, M. G. (1998). Role of group I metabotropic glutamate receptors in traumatic spinal cord white matter injury. *J. Neurotrauma* **15**, 929–941.

Akins, P. T., and Atkinson, R. P. (2002). Glutamate AMPA receptor antagonist treatment for ischaemic stroke. *Curr. Med. Res. Opin.* **18 (Suppl 2)**, s9–13.

Ariyasu, R. G., and Ellisman, M. H. (1987). The distribution of (Na+ − K+)ATPase is continuous along the axolemma of unensheathed axons from spinal roots of "dystrophic" mice. *J. Neurocytol.* 16, 239–248.

Arriza, J. L., Fairman, W. A., Wadiche, J. I., Murdoch, G. H., Kavanaugh, M. P., and Amara, S. G. (1994). Functional comparisons of three glutamate transporter subtypes cloned from human motor cortex. *J. Neurosci.* **14**, 5559–5569.

Barres, B. A., Chun, L. L., and Corey, D. P. (1990). Ion channels in vertebrate glia. *Annu. Rev. Neurosci.* **13**, 441–474.

Bechtold, D. A., Kapoor, R., and Smith, K. J. (2004). Axonal protection using flecainide in experimental autoimmune encephalomyelitis. *Ann. Neurol.* 55:607–616.

Berridge, M. J., Lipp, P., and Bootman, M. D. (2000). The versatility and universality of calcium signalling. *Nat. Rev. Mol. Cell Biol.* **1**, 11–21.

Bjartmar, C., Wujek, J. R., and Trapp, B. D. (2003). Axonal loss in the pathology of MS: consequences for understanding the progressive phase of the disease. *J. Neurol. Sci.* **206**, 165–171.

Blaustein, M. P., and Lederer, W. J. (1999). Sodium/calcium exchange: its physiological implications. *Physiol. Rev.* **79**, 763–854.

Bootman, M. D., Lipp, P., and Berridge, M. J. (2001a). The organisation and functions of local Ca(2+) signals. *J. Cell Sci.* **114**, 2213–2222.

Bootman, M. D., Collins, T. J., Peppiatt, C. M., Prothero, L. S., MacKenzie, L., De Smet, P., Travers, M., Tovey, S. C., Seo, J. T., Berridge, M. J., Ciccolini, F., and Lipp, P. (2001b). Calcium signalling: an overview. *Semin. Cell Dev. Biol.* **12**, 3–10.

Bostock, H., Baker, M., and Reid, G. (1991). Changes in excitability of human motor axons underlying post-ischaemic fasciculations: Evidence for two stable states. *J. Physiol. (Lond.)* **441**, 537–557.

Brown, A. M., Wender, R., and Ransom, B. R. (2001a). Ionic mechanisms of aglycemic axon injury in mammalian central white matter. *J. Cereb. Blood Flow Metab.* **21**, 385–395.

Brown, A. M., Tekkok, S. B., and Ransom, B. R. (2003). Glycogen regulation and functional role in mouse white matter. *J. Physiol.* **549**, 501–512.

Brown, A. M., Westenbroek, R. E., Catterall, W. A., and Ransom, B. R. (2001b) Axonal L-type Ca(2+) channels and anoxic injury in rat CNS white matter. *J. Neurophysiol.* **85**, 900–911.

Brown, A. M., Fern, R., Jarvinen, J. P., Kaila, K., and Ransom, B. R. (1998). Changes in [Ca^{2+}] during anoxia in CNS white matter. *Neuroreport* **9**, 1997–2000.

Brown, G. C., and Borutaite, V. (2002). Nitric oxide inhibition of mitochondrial respiration and its role in cell death. *Free Radic. Biol. Med.* **33**, 1440–1450.

Caldwell, J. H., Schaller, K. L., Lasher, R. S., Peles, E., and Levinson, S. R. (2000). Sodium channel Nav1.6 is localized at nodes of Ranvier, dendrites, and synapses. *Proc. Natl. Acad. Sci. U. S. A.* 97:5616–5620.

Carafoli, E. (2002). Calcium signaling: a tale for all seasons. *Proc Natl Acad Sci U. S. A.* **99**, 1115–1122.

Catterall, W. A. (1980). Neurotoxins that act on voltage-sensitive sodium channels in excitable membranes. *Annu. Rev. Pharmacol. Toxicol.* **20**, 15–43.

Charcot, M. (1868). Histologie de la sclerose en plaques. *Gaz. Hop.* **141**, 554–558.

Clapham, D. E. (2003). TRP channels as cellular sensors. *Nature* **426**, 517–524.

Craner, M. J., Hains, B. C., Lo, A. C., Black, J. A., and Waxman, S. G. (2004a). Co-localization of sodium channel Nav1.6 and the sodium-calcium exchanger at sites of axonal injury in the spinal cord in EAE. *Brain* **127**, 294–303.

Craner, M. J., Newcombe, J., Black, J. A., Hartle, C., Cuzner, M. L., and Waxman, S. G. (2004b). Molecular changes in neurons in MS: Altered axonal expression of Nav1.2 and Nav1.6 sodium channels and Na/Ca exchanger. *Proc. Natl. Acad. Sci. U. S. A.* 101:8168–8173.

Crompton, M. (1985). The regulation of mitochondrial calcium transport in heart. *Curr. Top. Membr. Trans.* **25**, 231–275.

David, J. C., Yamada, K. A., Bagwe, M. R., and Goldberg, M. P. (1996). AMPA receptor activation is rapidly toxic to cortical astrocytes when desensitization is blocked. *J. Neurosci.* **16**, 200–209.

De Stefano, N., Matthews, P. M., Fu, L., Narayanan, S., Stanley, J., Francis, G. S., Antel, J. P., and Arnold, D. L. (1998). Axonal damage correlates with disability in patients with relapsing-remitting multiple sclerosis. Results of a longitudinal magnetic resonance spectroscopy study. *Brain* **121 (Pt 8)**, 1469–1477.

Dewar, D., Underhill, S. M., and Goldberg, M. P. (2003). Oligodendrocytes and ischemic brain injury. *J. Cereb. Blood Flow Metab.* **23**, 263–274.

Dong, H., Light, P. E., French, R. J., and Lytton, J. (2001). Electrophysiological characterization and ionic stoichiometry of the rat brain K(+)-dependent NA(+)/CA(2+) exchanger, NCKX2. *J. Biol. Chem.* **276**, 25919–25928.

Eng, D. L., Gordon, T. R., Kocsis, J. D., and Waxman, S. G. (1990). Current-clamp analysis of a time-dependent rectification in rat optic nerve. *J. Physiol. (Lond.)* **421**, 185–202.

Erecinska, M., and Silver, I. A. (1989). ATP and brain function. *J. Cereb. Blood Flow Metab.* **9**, 2–19.

Erecinska, M., and Dagani, F. (1990). Relationships between the neuronal sodium/potassium pump and energy metabolism. Effects of K+, Na+, and adenosine triphosphate in isolated brain synaptosomes. *J. Gen. Physiol.* 95, 591–616.

Fern, R., and Moller, T. (2000). Rapid ischemic cell death in immature oligodendrocytes: A fatal glutamate release feedback loop. *J. Neurosci.* **20**, 34–42.

Fern, R., Waxman, S. G., and Ransom, B. R. (1994). Modulation of anoxic injury in CNS white matter by adenosine and interaction between adenosine and GABA. *J. Neurophysiol.* **72**, 2609–2616.

Fern, R., Ransom, B. R., and Waxman, S. G. (1995a). Voltage-gated calcium channels in CNS white matter: role in anoxic injury. *J. Neurophysiol.* **74**, 369–377.

Fern, R., Waxman, S. G., and Ransom, B. R. (1995b). Endogenous GABA attenuates CNS white matter dysfunction following anoxia. *J. Neurosci.* **15**, 699–708.

Fern, R., Ransom, B. R., and Waxman, S. G. (1996). White matter stroke: Autoprotective mechanisms with therapeutic implications. *Cerebrovasc. Dis.* 6, 59–65.

Fern, R., Davis, P., Waxman, S. G., and Ransom, B. R. (1998). Axon conduction and survival in CNS white matter during energy deprivation: A developmental study. *J. Neurophysiol.* **79**, 95–105.

Fill, M., and Copello, J. A. (2002). Ryanodine receptor calcium release channels. *Physiol. Rev.* **82**, 893–922.

Follett, P. L., Rosenberg, P. A., Volpe, J. J., and Jensen, F. E. (2000). NBQX attenuates excitotoxic injury in developing white matter. *J. Neurosci.* **20**, 9235–9241.

Franzini-Armstrong, C., and Protasi, F. (1997). Ryanodine receptors of striated muscles: a complex channel capable of multiple interactions. *Physiol. Rev.* **77**, 699–729.

Funch, P. G., and Faber, D. S. (1984). Measurement of myelin sheath resistances: implications for axonal conduction and pathophysiology. *Science* **225**, 538–540.

Gadelha, F. R., Thomson, L., Fagian, M. M., Costa, A. D., Radi, R., and Vercesi, A. E. (1997). Ca2+-independent permeabilization of the inner mitochondrial membrane by peroxynitrite is mediated by membrane protein thiol cross-linking and lipid peroxidation. *Arch. Biochem. Biophys.* **345**, 243–250.

Garcia-Barcina, J. M., and Matute, C. (1996). Expression of kainate-selective glutamate receptor subunits in glial cells of the adult bovine white matter. *Eur. J. Neurosci.* **8**, 2379–2387.

Garcia-Barcina, J. M., and Matute, C. (1998). AMPA-selective glutamate receptor subunits in glial cells of the adult bovine white matter. *Brain Res. Mol. Brain Res.* **53**, 270–276.

Garthwaite, G., Goodwin, D. A., Batchelor, A. M., Leeming, K., and Garthwaite, J. (2002). Nitric oxide toxicity in CNS white matter: An in vitro study using rat optic nerve. *Neuroscience* **109**, 145–155.

Geurts, J. J., Wolswijk, G., Bo, L., van der Valk, P., Polman, C. H., Troost, D., and Aronica, E. (2003). Altered expression patterns of group I and II metabotropic glutamate receptors in multiple sclerosis. *Brain* **126**, 1755–1766.

Griffiths, R., Dunlop, J., Gorman, A., Senior, J., and Grieve, A.(1994). L-trans-pyrrolidine-2,4-dicarboxylate and cis-1-aminocyclobutane-1,3-dicarboxylate behave as transportable, competitive inhibitors of the high-affinity glutamate transporters. *Biochem. Pharmacol.* **47**, 267–274.

Groom, A. J., Smith, T., and Turski, L. (2003). Multiple sclerosis and glutamate. *Ann. N. Y. Acad. Sci.* **993**, 229–275.

Hammarstrom, A. K., and Gage, P. W. (1999). Nitric oxide increases persistent sodium current in rat hippocampal neurons. *J. Physiol. (Lond.)* **520 Pt 2**, 451–461.

Heizmann, C. W., and Hunziker, W. (1991). Intracellular calcium-binding proteins: More sites than insights. *Trends Biochem. Sci.* 16, 98–103.

Herzog, R. I., Liu, C., Waxman, S. G., and Cummins, T. R. (2003a). Calmodulin binds to the C terminus of sodium channels Nav1.4 and Nav1.6 and differentially modulates their functional properties. *J. Neurosci.* **23**, 8261–8270.

Herzog, R. I., Cummins, T. R., Ghassemi, F., Dib-Hajj, S. D., and Waxman, S. G. (2003b). Distinct repriming and closed-state inactivation kinetics of Nav1.6 and Nav1.7 sodium channels in mouse spinal sensory neurons. *J. Physiol.* **551**, 741–750.

Hewitt, K. E., Stys, P. K., and Lesiuk, H. J. (2001). The use-dependent sodium channel blocker mexiletine is neuroprotective against global ischemic injury. *Brain Res.* **898**, 281–287.

Hille, B. (1977). Local anesthetics: hydrophilic and hydrophobic pathways for the drug-receptor reaction. *J. Gen. Physiol.* **69**, 497–515.

Holzwarth, J. A., Gibbons, S. J., Brorson, J. R., Philipson, L. H., and Miller, R. J. (1994). Glutamate receptor agonists stimulate diverse calcium responses in different types of cultured rat cortical glial cells. *J. Neurosci.* **14**, 1879–1891.

Imaizumi, T., Kocsis, J. D., and Waxman, S. G. (1997). Anoxic injury in the rat spinal cord: Pharmacological evidence for multiple steps in Ca2+-dependent injury of the dorsal columns. *J. Neurotrauma* **14**, 299–311.

Imaizumi, T., Kocsis, J. D., and Waxman, S. G. (1999). The role of voltage-gated Ca2+ channels in anoxic injury of spinal cord white matter. *Brain Res.* **817**, 84–92.

Jensen, A. M., and Chiu, S. Y. (1993). Expression of glutamate receptor genes in white matter: developing and adult rat optic nerve. *J. Neurosci.* **13**, 1664–1675.

Jiang, Q., and Stys, P. K. (2000). Calpain inhibitors confer biochemical, but not electrophysiological, protection against anoxia in rat optic nerves. *J. Neurochem.* **74**, 2101–2107.

Jiang, Q., and Stys, P. K. (2003). Inhibition of AMPA receptors alone is more protective than combined AMPA/kainate receptor antagonism in white matter anoxia. *Soc. Neurosci.* Abstr:951.915.

Kanellopoulos, G. K., Xu, X. M., Hsu, C. Y., Lu, X., Sundt, T. M., and Kouchoukos, N. T. (2000). White matter injury in spinal cord ischemia: protection by AMPA/kainate glutamate receptor antagonism. *Stroke* **31**, 1945–1952.

Kanoh, N. (1997). Cytochemical localization of ouabain-sensitive, K(+)-dependent p-nitrophenylphosphatase activity in the facial nerve of reserpinized guinea pigs. *J. Histochem. Cytochem.* **45**, 1129–1135.

Kanoh, N., Kobayashi, T., Okada, T., and Seguchi, H. (1994). Ultracytochemical demonstration of ouabain-sensitive, K(+)-dependent, p-nitrophenylphosphatase (Na-K ATPase) activity in cat facial nerve. *Eur. Arch. Otorhinolaryngol.* **251**, 238–240.

Kapoor, R., Davies, M., Blaker, P. A., Hall, S. M., and Smith, K. J. (2003). Blockers of sodium and calcium entry protect axons from nitric oxide-mediated degeneration. *Ann. Neurol.* **53**, 174–180.

Kastritsis, C. H., and McCarthy, K. D. (1993). Oligodendroglial lineage cells express neuroligand receptors. *Glia* **8**, 106–113.

Khodorov, B. I. (1991). Role of inactivation in local anesthetic action. *Ann. N. Y. Acad. Sci.* **625**, 224–248.

Kiedrowski, L., Czyz, A., Li, X. F., and Lytton, J. (2002). Preferential expression of plasmalemmal K-dependent Na+/Ca2+ exchangers in neurons versus astrocytes. *Neuroreport* **13**, 1529–1532.

Kimelberg, H. K., Goderie, S. K., Higman, S., Pang, S., and Waniewski, R. A. (1990). Swelling-induced release of glutamate, aspartate, and taurine from astrocyte cultures. *J. Neurosci.* **10**, 1583–1591.

Kornek, B., and Lassmann, H. (1999). Axonal pathology in multiple sclerosis. A historical note. *Brain Pathol.* **9**, 651–656.

Kornek, B., Storch, M. K., Bauer, J., Djamshidian, A., Weissert, R., Wallstroem, E., Stefferl, A., Zimprich, F., Olsson, T., Linington, C., Schmidbauer, M., and Lassmann, H. (2001). Distribution of a calcium channel subunit in dystrophic axons in multiple sclerosis and experimental autoimmune encephalomyelitis. *Brain* **124**, 1114–1124.

Lassmann, H. (2003). Hypoxia-like tissue injury as a component of multiple sclerosis lesions. *J. Neurol. Sci.* **206**, 187–191.

Lassmann, H., Bruck, W., Lucchinetti, C., and Rodriguez, M. (1997). Remyelination in multiple sclerosis. *Multiple Sclerosis* **3**, 133–136.

Lazzarini, R. A., Griffin, J. W., Lassmann, H., Nave, K.-A., Miller, R. H., and Trapp, B. D., eds (2004). *Myelin Biology and Disorders.* Elsevier Academic Press, Amsterdam.

Lee, E. J., Ayoub, I. A., Harris, F. B., Hassan, M., Ogilvy, C. S., and Maynard, K. I. (1999). Mexiletine and magnesium independently, but not combined, protect against permanent focal cerebral ischemia in Wistar rats. *J. Neurosci. Res.* **58**, 442–448.

Leppanen, L. L., and Stys, P. K. (1997). Ion transport and membrane potential in CNS myelinated axons. II: Effects of metabolic inhibition. *J. Neurophysiol.* **78**, 2095–2107.

Levy, L. M., Warr, O., and Attwell, D. (1998). Stoichiometry of the glial glutamate transporter GLT-1 expressed inducibly in a Chinese hamster ovary cell line selected for low endogenous Na+-dependent glutamate uptake. *J. Neurosci.* **18**, 9620–9628.

Li, S., and Stys, P. K. (2000). Mechanisms of ionotropic glutamate receptor-mediated excitotoxicity in isolated spinal cord white matter. *J. Neurosci.* **20**, 1190–1198.

Li, S., Jiang, Q., and Stys, P. K. (2000). Important role of reverse Na(+)-Ca(2+) exchange in spinal cord white matter injury at physiological temperature. *J. Neurophysiol.* **84**, 1116–1119.

Li S., Mealing G. A., Morley, P., and Stys, P. K. (1999). Novel injury mechanism in anoxia and trauma of spinal cord white matter: Glutamate release via reverse Na+-dependent glutamate transport. *J. Neurosci.* **19**, RC16.

Liu, H. N., Giasson, B. I., Mushynski, W. E., and Almazan, G. (2002). AMPA receptor-mediated toxicity in oligodendrocyte progenitors involves free radical generation and activation of JNK, calpain and caspase 3. *J. Neurochem.* **82**, 398–409.

Lo, A. C., Black, J. A., and Waxman, S. G. (2002). Neuroprotection of axons with phenytoin in experimental allergic encephalomyelitis. *Neuroreport* **13**, 1909–1912.

Lo, A. C., Saab, C. Y., Black, J. A., and Waxman, S. G. (2003). Phenytoin protects spinal cord axons and preserves axonal conduction and neurological function in a model of neuroinflammation *in vivo*. *J. Neurophysiol.* **90**, 3566–3571.

LoPachin, R. M., and Stys, P. K. (1995). Elemental composition and water content of rat optic nerve myelinated axons and glial cells: effects of in vitro anoxia and reoxygenation. *J. Neurosci.* **15**, 6735–6746.

LoPachin, R. M., Gaughan, C L., Lehning, E. J., Kaneko, Y., Kelly, T. M., and Blight, A. (1999). Experimental spinal cord injury: spatiotemporal characterization of elemental concentrations and water contents in axons and neuroglia. *J. Neurophysiol.* **82**, 2143–2153.

Lytton, J., Li, X. F., Dong, H., and Kraev, A. (2002). K+-dependent Na+/Ca2+ exchangers in the brain. *Ann. N. Y. Acad. Sci.* **976**, 382–393.

Mata, M., Fink, D. J., Ernst, S. A., and Siegel, G. J. (1991). Immunocytochemical demonstration of Na(+),K(+)-ATPase in internodal axolemma of myelinated fibers of rat sciatic and optic nerves. *J. Neurochem.* **57**, 184–192.

Matute, C. (1998). Characteristics of acute and chronic kainate excitotoxic damage to the optic nerve. *Proc. Natl. Acad. Sci. U. S. A.* **95**, 10229–10234.

Matute, C., Sanchez-Gomez, M. V., Martinez-Millan, L., and Miledi, R. (1997). Glutamate receptor-mediated toxicity in optic nerve oligodendrocytes. *Proc. Natl. Acad. Sci. U. S. A.* **94**, 8830–8835.

Matute, C., Alberdi, E., Ibarretxe, G., and Sanchez-Gomez, M. V. (2002). Excitotoxicity in glial cells. *Eur. J. Pharmacol.* **447**, 239–246.

Matute, C. J., Domercq, M., Alberdi, M. E., Sanchez-Gomez, M. V., Perez-Samartin, A., Perez-Cerda, F., Torre, I., and Etxebarria, E. (2003). ATP excitotoxicity in oligodendrocytes. *Soc. Neurosci. Abstr.* 213.213.

McCracken, E., Fowler, J. H., Dewar, D., Morrison, S., and McCulloch, J. (2002). Grey matter and white matter ischemic damage is reduced by the competitive AMPA receptor antagonist, SPD 502. *J. Cereb. Blood Flow Metab.* **22**, 1090–1097.

McDonald, J. W., Althomsons, S. P., Hyrc, K. L., Choi, D. W., and Goldberg, M. P. (1998). Oligodendrocytes from forebrain are highly vulnerable to AMPA/kainate receptor-mediated excitotoxicity. *Nat. Med.* **4**, 291–297.

Nicholls, D. G. (1985). A role for the mitochondrion in the protection of cells against calcium overload? *In:* "Progress in Brain Research" (K, Kogure K.-A. Hossmann, B. K. Siesjo, and F. A. Welsh, eds), pp. 97–106, Elsevier, St. Louis.

Nicholls, D. G., and Budd, S. L. (2000). Mitochondria and neuronal survival. *Physiol. Rev.* **80**, 315–360.

Nikolaeva, M., and Stys, P. K. (2003). Sources of ischemia-induced Ca increase in rat optic nerve axons. *Sixth IBRO World Congress of Neuroscience*, Prague, Czech Republic.

Orrenius, S., and Nicotera, P. (1996). Mechanisms of calcium-related cell death. *In:* "Cellular and Molecular Mechanisms of Ischemic Brain Damage" (B. K. Siesjo, and T. Wieloch, eds.), pp. 137–152. Raven Press, New York.

Ouardouz, M., Nikolaeva, M., Coderre, E., Zamponi, G. W., McRory, J. E., Trapp, B. D., Yin, X., Wang, W., Woulfe, J., and Stys, P. K. (2003). Depolarization-induced Ca2+ release in ischemic spinal cord white matter involves L-type Ca2+ channel activation of ryanodine receptors. *Neuron* **40**, 53–63.

Pasti, L., Zonta, M., Pozzan, T., Vicini, S., and Carmignoto, G. (2001). Cytosolic calcium oscillations in astrocytes may regulate exocytotic release of glutamate. *J. Neurosci.* **21**, 477–484.

Petersen, O. H. (2002). Calcium signal compartmentalization. *Biol. Res.* **35**, 177–182.

Pitt, D., Werner, P., and Raine, C. S. (2000). Glutamate excitotoxicity in a model of multiple sclerosis. *Nat. Med.* **6**, 67–70.

Poliak, S., and Peles, E. (2003). The local differentiation of myelinated axons at nodes of Ranvier. *Nat. Rev. Neurosci.* **4**, 968–980.

Pozzan, T., Rizzuto, R., Volpe, P., and Meldolesi, J. (1994). Molecular and cellular physiology of intracellular calcium stores. *Physiol. Rev.* **74**, 595–636.

Prineas, J. W., Barnard, R. O., Kwon, E. E., Sharer, L. R., and Cho, E. S. (1993). Multiple sclerosis: Remyelination of nascent lesions. *Ann. Neurol.* **33**, 137–151.

Ragsdale, D. S., McPhee, J. C., Scheuer, T., and Catterall, W. A. (1996). Common molecular determinants of local anesthetic, antiarrhythmic, and anticonvulsant block of voltage-gated Na+ channels. *Proc. Natl. Acad. Sci. U. S. A.* **93**, 9270–9275.

Ransom, B. R., Walz, W., Davis, P. K., and Carlini, W. G. (1992). Anoxia-induced changes in extracellular K+ and pH in mammalian central white matter. *J. Cereb. Blood Flow Metab.* **12,** 593–602.

Redford, E. J., Kapoor, R., and Smith, K. J. (1997). Nitric oxide donors reversibly block axonal conduction: Demyelinated axons are especially susceptible. *Brain* **120,** 2149–2157.

Ren, Y., Ridsdale, A., Coderre, E., and Stys, P. K. (2000). Calcium imaging in live rat optic nerve myelinated axons in vitro using confocal laser microscopy. *J. Neurosci. Methods* **102,** 165–176.

Renganathan, M., Cummins, T. R., and Waxman, S. G. (2002). Nitric oxide blocks fast, slow, and persistent Na+ channels in C-type DRG neurons by S-nitrosylation. *J. Neurophysiol.* **87,** 761–775.

Ritchie, J. M., and Rogart, R. B. (1977). Density of sodium channels in mammalian myelinated nerve fibers and nature of the axonal membrane under the myelin sheath. *Proc. Natl. Acad. Sci. U. S. A.* **74,** 211–215.

Rosenberg, L. J., Teng, Y. D., and Wrathall, J. R. (1999a). 2,3-dihydroxy-6-nitro-7-sulfamoyl-benzo(*f*)quinoxaline reduces glial loss and acute white matter pathology after experimental spinal cord contusion. *J. Neurosci.* **19,** 464–475.

Rosenberg, L. J., Teng, Y. D., and Wrathall, J. R. (1999b). Effects of the sodium channel blocker tetrodotoxin on acute white matter pathology after experimental contusive spinal cord injury. *J. Neurosci.* **19,** 6122–6133.

Rutledge, E. M., Aschner, M., and Kimelberg, H. K. (1998). Pharmacological characterization of swelling-induced D-[3H]aspartate release from primary astrocyte cultures. *Am. J. Physiol.* **274,** C1511–1520.

Rutter, G. A. (2003). Calcium signalling: NAADP comes out of the shadows. *Biochem. J.* **373,** e3–4.

Salazar, B. C., Castillo, C., Diaz, M. E., and Recio-Pinto, E. (1996). Multiple open channel states revealed by lidocaine and QX-314 on rat brain voltage-dependent sodium channels. *J. Gen. Physiol.* **107,** 743–754.

Schanne, F. A., Kane, A. B., Young, E. E., and Farber, J. L. (1979). Calcium-dependence of toxic cell death: A final common pathway. *Science* **206,** 700–702.

Schwaller, B., Meyer, M., and Schiffmann, S. (2002). "New" functions for "old" proteins: The role of the calcium-binding proteins calbindin D-28k, calretinin and parvalbumin, in cerebellar physiology. Studies with knockout mice. *Cerebellum* **1,** 241–258.

Schwartz, M., Ernst, S. A., Siegel, G. J., and Agranoff, B. W. (1981). Immunocytochemical localization of (Na+, K+)-ATPase in the goldfish optic nerve. *J. Neurochem.* **36,** 107–115.

Shull, G. E., Okunade, G., Liu, L. H., Kozel, P., Periasamy, M., Lorenz, J. N., and Prasad, V. (2003). Physiological functions of plasma membrane and intracellular Ca2+ pumps revealed by analysis of null mutants. *Ann. N. Y. Acad. Sci.* **986,** 453–460.

Smith, K. J., Kapoor, R., Hall, S. M., and Davies, M. (2001). Electrically active axons degenerate when exposed to nitric oxide. *Ann. Neurol.* **49,** 470–476.

Smith, M. R., Smith, R. D., Plummer, N. W., Meisler, M. H., and Goldin, A. L. (1998). Functional analysis of the mouse Scn8a sodium channel. *J. Neurosci.* **18,** 6093–6102.

Smith, T., Groom, A., Zhu, B., and Turski, L. (2000). Autoimmune encephalomyelitis ameliorated by AMPA antagonists. *Nat. Med.* **6,** 62–66.

Spira, M. E., Oren, R., Dormann, A., Ilouz, N., and Lev, S. (2001). Calcium, protease activation, and cytoskeleton remodeling underlie growth cone formation and neuronal regeneration. *Cell Mol. Neurobiol.* **21,** 591–604.

Steffensen, I., Waxman, S. G., Mills, L., and Stys, P. K. (1997). Immunohistochemical localization of the Na+-Ca2+ exchanger in rat central and peripheral myelinated axons. *Brain Res.* **776,** 1–9.

Steinhauser, C., and Gallo, V. (1996). News on glutamate receptors in glial cells. *Trends Neurosci.* **19,** 339–345.

Stys, P. K. (1995). Protective effects of antiarrhythmic agents against anoxic injury in CNS white matter. *J. Cereb. Blood Flow Metab.* **15,** 425–432.

Stys, P. K. (1998). Anoxic and ischemic injury of myelinated axons in CNS white matter: from mechanistic concepts to therapeutics. *J. Cereb. Blood Flow Metab.* **18,** 2–25.

Stys, P. K. (2004a). White matter injury mechanisms. *Curr. Mol. Med.* **4,** 109–126.

Stys, P. K. (2004b). Axonal degeneration in MS: Is it time for neuroprotective strategies? *Ann. Neurol.* **55,** 601–603.

Stys, P. K., and LoPachin, R. M. (1996). Elemental composition and water content of rat optic nerve myelinated axons during in vitro post-anoxia reoxygenation. *Neuroscience* **73,** 1081–1090.

Stys, P. K., and LoPachin, R. M. (1998). Mechanisms of ion flux in anoxic myelinated CNS axons. *Neuroscience* **82,** 21–32.

Stys, P. K., and Ouardouz, M. (2002). Role of glutamate receptors in spinal cord dorsal column ischemia. *Soc. Neurosci. Abstr.* 298.

Stys, P. K., Waxman, S. G., and Ransom, B. R. (1992a). Ionic mechanisms of anoxic injury in mammalian CNS white matter: role of Na+ channels and Na+-Ca2+ exchanger. *J. Neurosci.* **12,** 430–439.

Stys, P. K., Ransom, B. R., and Waxman, S. G. (1992b). Tertiary and quaternary local anesthetics protect CNS white matter from anoxic injury at concentrations that do not block excitability. *J. Neurophysiol.* **67,** 236–240.

Stys, P. K., Hubatsch, D. A., and Leppanen, L. L. (1998). Effects of K+ channel blockers on the anoxic response of central myelinated axons. *NeuroReport* **9,** 447–453.

Stys, P. K., Ransom, B. R., Waxman, S. G., and Davis, P. K. (1990). Role of extracellular calcium in anoxic injury of mammalian central white matter. *Proc. Natl. Acad. Sci. U. S. A.* **87,** 4212–4216.

Stys, P. K., Sontheimer, H., Ransom B. R., and Waxman, S. G. (1993). Non-inactivating, TTX-sensitive Na+ conductance in rat optic nerve axons. *Proc. Natl. Acad. Sci. U. S. A.* **90,** 6976–6980.

Taylor, C. P. (1993). Na+ currents that fail to inactivate. *Trends Neurosci.* **16,** 455–460.

Tekkok, S. B., and Goldberg, M. P. (2001). AMPA/kainate receptor activation mediates hypoxic oligodendrocyte death and axonal injury in cerebral white matter. *J. Neurosci.* **21,** 4237–4248.

Tekkok, S. B., Brown, A. M., and Ransom, B. R. (2003). Axon function persists during anoxia in mammalian white matter. *J. Cereb. Blood Flow Metab.* **23,** 1340–1347.

Tekkok, S. B., Hyrc, K L., Underhill, S. M., and Goldberg, M. P. (2000). Na+/Ca2+ exchange blocker KB-R7943 protects axons and oligodendrocytes during oxygen glucose deprivation. *Soc. Neurosci. Abstr.* **26,** 2065.

Teng, Y. D., and Wrathall, J. R. (1997). Local blockade of sodium channels by tetrodotoxin ameliorates tissue loss and long-term functional deficits resulting from experimental spinal cord injury. *J. Neurosci.* **17,** 4359–4366.

Underhill, S. M., and Goldberg, M. P. (2002). Axons potentiate oligodendrocyte vulnerability to excitotoxicity. *Soc. Neurosci. Abstr.* 299.7.

Utzschneider, D. A., Kocsis, J. D., and Waxman, S. G. (1991). Differential sensitivity to hypoxia of the peripheral versus central trajectory of primary afferent axons. *Brain Res.* **551,** 136–141.

Verbny, Y., Zhang, C. L., and Chiu, S. Y. (2002). Coupling of calcium homeostasis to axonal sodium in axons of mouse optic nerve. *J. Neurophysiol.* **88,** 802–816.

Vogel, W., and Schwarz, J. R. (1995). Voltage-clamp studies in axons: macroscopic and single channel currents. *In:* "The Axon: Structure, Function and Pathophysiology" (S. G. Waxman, J. D. Kocsis, and P. K. Stys, eds.), pp. 257–280. Oxford University Press, New York.

Wang, G. K., Brodwick, M. S., Eaton, D. C., and Strichartz, G. R. (1987). Inhibition of sodium currents by local anesthetics in chloramine-T-treated squid axons. The role of channel activation. *J. Gen. Physiol.* **89,** 645–667.

Waxman, S. G. (1977). Conduction in myelinated, unmyelinated, and demyelinated fibers. *Arch. Neurol.* **34,** 585–599.

Waxman, S. G. (2003). Nitric oxide and the axonal death cascade. *Ann. Neurol.* **53,** 150–153.

Waxman, S. G., and Bennett. M. V. (1972). Relative conduction velocities of small myelinated and non-myelinated fibres in the central nervous system. *Nat. New Biol.* **238**, 217–219.

Waxman, S. G., Black, J. A., Ransom, B. R., and Stys, P. K. (1993). Protection of the axonal cytoskeleton in anoxic optic nerve by decreased extracellular calcium. *Brain Res.* **614**, 137–145.

Wender, R., Brown, A. M., Fern, R., Swanson, R. A., Farrell, K., and Ransom, B. R. (2000). Astrocytic glycogen influences axon function and survival during glucose deprivation in central white matter. *J. Neurosci.* **20**, 6804–6810.

Werner, P., Pitt, D., and Raine, C. S. (2000). Glutamate excitotoxicity: A mechanism for axonal damage and oligodendrocyte death in multiple sclerosis? *J. Neural. Transm. Suppl.* 60:375–385.

West, A. E., Chen, W. G., Dalva, M B., Dolmetsch, R. E., Kornhauser, J. M., Shaywitz, A. J., Takasu, M A., Tao, X., and Greenberg, M. E. (2001). Calcium regulation of neuronal gene expression. *Proc. Natl. Acad. Sci. U. S. A.* **98**, 11024–11031.

Wood, J. G., Jean, D. H., Whitaker, J. N., McLaughlin, B. J., and Albers, R. W. (1977). Immunocytochemical localization of the sodium, potassium activated ATPase in knifefish brain. *J. Neurocytol.* **6**, 571–581.

Wrathall, J. R., Choiniere, D., and Teng, Y. D. (1994). Dose-dependent reduction of tissue loss and functional impairment after spinal cord trauma with the AMPA/kainate antagonist NBQX. *J. Neurosci.* **14**, 6598–6607.

Wrathall, J. R., Teng, Y. D., and Marriott, R. (1997). Delayed antagonism of AMPA/kainate receptors reduces long-term functional deficits resulting from spinal cord trauma. *Exp. Neurol.* **145**, 565–573.

Wuytack, F., Raeymaekers, L., and Missiaen, L. (2002). Molecular physiology of the SERCA and SPCA pumps. *Cell Calcium* **32**, 279–305.

Wyllie, D. J., Mathie, A., Symonds, C. J., and Cull-Candy, S. G. (1991). Activation of glutamate receptors and glutamate uptake in identified macroglial cells in rat cerebellar cultures. *J. Physiol.* **432**, 235–258.

Yam, P. S., Dunn, L. T., Graham, D. I., Dewar, D., and McCulloch, J. (2000). NMDA receptor blockade fails to alter axonal injury in focal cerebral ischemia. *J. Cereb. Blood Flow Metab.* **20**, 772–779.

Ye, Z. C., Wyeth, M. S., Baltan-Tekkok, S., and Ransom, B. R. (2003). Functional hemichannels in astrocytes: A novel mechanism of glutamate release. *J. Neurosci.* **23**, 3588–3596.

Yeh, J. Z., and Tanguy, J. (1985). Na channel activation gate modulates slow recovery from use-dependent block by local anesthetics in squid giant axons. *Biophys. J.* **47**, 685–694.

Yoshioka, A., Bacskai, B., and Pleasure, D. (1996). Pathophysiology of oligodendroglial excitotoxicity. *J. Neurosci. Res.* **46**, 427–437.

Yoshioka, A., Hardy, M., Younkin, D P., Grinspan, J. B., Stern, J. L., and Pleasure, D. (1995). Alpha-amino-3-hydroxy-5-methyl-4-isoxazolepropionate (AMPA) receptors mediate excitotoxicity in the oligodendroglial lineage. *J. Neurochem.* **64**, 2442–2448.

Zerangue, N., and Kavanaugh, M. P. (1996). Flux coupling in a neuronal glutamate transporter. *Nature* **383**, 634–637.

Ziak, D., Chvatal, A., and Sykova, E. (1998).Glutamate-, kainate- and NMDA-evoked membrane currents in identified glial cells in rat spinal cord slice. *Physiol. Res.* **47**, 365–375.

20

Axonal Damage and Neuronal Death in Multiple Sclerosis and Experimental Autoimmune Encephalomyelitis: The Role of Calpain

M. K. Guyton, M.S.

E. A. Sribnick, B.A., B.S.

J. M. Wingrave, M.S.

S. K. Ray, Ph.D.

N. L. Banik, Ph.D.

I. Introduction

The inflammatory response of autoreactive T-cells and other immune cells in multiple sclerosis (MS) and its widely used animal model, experimental autoimmune encephalomyelitis (EAE), is well established; however, it is now thought that remitting neurological deficits of MS and EAE occur primarily through demyelination of axons (Ray and Banik, 2003; Shields and Banik, 2001). In addition, current knowledge indicates that neuronal injury and axonal damage, particularly in the progressive phase of the disease, are important neurodegenerative components responsible for nonremitting functional loss in MS (Trapp et al., 1999). The various mechanisms of myelin breakdown, axonal damage, and neuronal cell death in MS and EAE are not clearly established, although roles for proteases are strongly indicated.

One such protease is the calcium-(Ca^{2+}) activated neutral protease, calpain, which requires Ca^{2+} for activation. Ca^{2+} influx and calpain activation have been implicated in the neurodegenerative effects of many disorders of the central nervous system (CNS), including spinal cord injury (SCI), traumatic brain injury (TBI), Parkinson's disease, Alzheimer's disease, and ischemia (Ray and Banik, 2003; Shields and Banik, 2001). Also, studies in our laboratory demonstrate increased calpain expression and activity in EAE

293

spinal cord (Shields et al., 1998b) and optic nerve tissue (Shields et al., 1998a), as well as in MS brain lesions (Shields et al., 1999b). Furthermore, the use of calpain inhibitors as a neuroprotectant has been established in several animal models of these diseases (Banik et al., 1998; Bartus et al., 1994), suggesting that calpain is directly involved in axonal damage and neuronal death. The molecular basis for the importance of calpain in neurodegeneration in MS and EAE is twofold: calpain mediates axonal degeneration (Shields and Banik, 2001) and calpain serves a pivotal role in several apoptotic cascades (Neumar et al., 2003) in various neurological disorders. After axonal injury, degradation and dephosporylation of neurofilament proteins (NFPs) and other proteins in axons can occur, and our laboratory (Ray et al., 2001; Shields and Banik, 1998b) and others (Stys and Jiang, 2002) have shown that (1) calpain activity is associated with NFP degradation and (2) treatment with calpain inhibitors can decrease NFP degradation. Furthermore, although calpain activation has been reported to be necessary for axonal regeneration (Godell et al., 1997), calpain activity may also inhibit axonal development (Robles et al., 2003), potentially leading to neuronal cell death.

Calpain plays a role in cell death through modifications in apoptotic signaling. Many calpain substrates are key proteins in apoptotic pathways. After the posttraumatic influx of Ca^{2+} into cells, calpain is activated, and has been demonstrated to cleave Bid to its truncated form, tBid (Chen et al., 2001), which leads to the activation of the pro-apoptotic protein Bax (Daniel, 2000). Bax is also a calpain substrate and can be directly activated by calpain-induced cleavage (Choi et al., 2001). Calpain activation can lead to the downregulation of the antiapoptotic protein Bcl-2 through cleavage of the Bcl-2 transcription upregulator cAMP-responsive element-binding protein (See and Loeffler, 2001). Calpain has been shown to degrade calcium/calmodulin-dependent protein kinase IV (McGinnis et al., 1998), whose activity blocks apoptosis. Furthermore, calpain also cleaves cain/cabin1, the endogenous inhibitor of calcineurin, thereby leading to calcineurin activation and subsequent Ca^{2+}-induced cell death (Kim et al., 2002). Calpain-like protease activity has also been demonstrated in the formation of the mitochondrial permeability transition pore (Gores et al., 1998), which leads to necrosis. Treatment with calpain inhibitors blocked the formation of the mitochondrial permeability transition pore, suggesting that calpain also plays a role in necrotic cell death (Gores et al., 1998).

Cross-talk between the calpain and caspase families complicates the role of calpain in apoptosis. For instance, although calpain inhibition has been shown to restore caspase-3 and -9 activity (Neumar et al., 2003), other studies have demonstrated that calpain inhibition decreases caspase-3 activity and cleavage of procaspase-3 to the activated form (Blomgren et al., 2001; Varghese et al., 2001). To further complicate the story, calpain activity has been shown to

facilitate the cleavage of the endogenous calpain inhibitor calpastatin by caspases (Neumar et al., 2003). In addition, caspase-12 is activated by increased levels of CA^{2+} in the endoplasmic reticulum, and caspase-12 activity is decreased following calpain inhibition, indicating that Ca^{2+} influx, leading to calpain activation, is involved in caspase-12-induced apoptosis (Nakagawa and Yuan, 2000).

The purpose of this article is to analyze the current literature pertaining to the roles of calpain in the neurodegenerative events in MS and EAE. First, a brief synopsis of the roles of Ca^{2+}-independent proteases is discussed. We also examine studies suggesting that altered Ca^{2+} influx via alterations in Ca^{2+} channels and glutamate excitotoxicity play a role in pathogenesis. The role of calpain in the inflammatory events and in the CNS is summarized and followed by a discussion of the current literature. Studies in our laboratory suggesting that calpain is involved in axonal damage and neuronal death are described, and the potential therapeutic effects that treatment with calpain inhibitors may have in MS and EAE are discussed.

II. Participation of Proteases in Demyelination in MS and EAE

The roles of acidic and neutral proteases have long been established in demyelination and demyelinating diseases (Banik, 1979), and both Ca^{2+}-independent and Ca^{2+}-dependent proteases are thought to participate in this process. There are a large number of Ca^{+2}-independent proteases such as caspases, lysosomal enzymes (e.g., cathepsins), and matrix metalloproteases (MMPs) (e.g., gelatinases) that have been suggested to contribute to myelinolysis in MS and EAE. Many of these proteases have been identified. In addition, Ca^{2+} is involved in many aspects of cellular function, one of which is the activation of proteases, including calpain. Ca^{2+} influx after injury has been associated with various neurodegenerative diseases, including ischemia, Alzheimer's disease, amylotrophic lateral sclerosis, and EAE (Ray et al., 2003). While the mechanisms of Ca^{2+} influx are unclear, it is speculated that alterations in Ca^{2+}-gated channels and glutamate excitotoxicity play a role in the pathophysiology of EAE and MS. The increase in intracellular Ca^{2+} levels is thought to lead to the induction of Ca^{2+}-dependent events including calpain-mediated axonal damage and neuronal death.

A. Ca^{2+}-Independent Proteases

1. Caspases

The cysteine protease caspase-1 plays a crucial part in the inflammatory process due to its ability to proteolitically activate pro-inflammatory cytokine precursors such as interleukin (IL)-1β and IL-18 (Fantuzzi and Dinarello, 1999).

In patients with MS, a twofold to threefold increase of caspase-1 mRNA level was found in the week preceding an acute attack (Furlan et al., 1999). Although caspase-1 expression was evident in the spinal cord during the first two episodes in an IL-12-induced mouse model of EAE, caspase-3 expression was not immunolocalized in axons and apoptotic neurons until episode 3, which also correlated with the increased axonal degeneration at the later episode (Ahmed et al., 2002). Also, oligodendrocytes (the cells that myelinate axons) from caspase-11-deficient mice were highly resistant to cell death induced by cytotoxic cytokines, suggesting that oligodendrocyte death was mediated by a pathway involving caspase-11 activation (Hisahara et al., 2001). In one study, apoptosis of neurons was induced by the cerebrospinal fluid (CSF) from patients with MS. The treatment of MS CSF-induced neuron damage with caspase inhibitors completely preserved neuronal survival and largely attenuated DNA fragmentation, suggesting that caspase inhibitors could be neuroprotective in patients with MS (Cid et al., 2003).

2. Cathepsins

Lysosomal enzymes are also involved in the pathogenesis of demyelinating diseases. A significant increase in activities of the lysosomal enzymes in spinal cords of rats during the course of EAE correlated with the intensity of the disease (Massacesi et al., 1988). Two lysosomal proteases, cathepsin B (CB) and cathepsin D (CD), which are implicated in the proteolysis of myelin basic protein (MBP), have been examined in peripheral blood mononuclear cells (PBMCs) of 20 stable patients with relapsing-remitting MS (Bever et al., 1994). CB activity in PBMCs was significantly increased in all patients with MS, although CD levels were not significantly altered. It was suggested that an increase in CB levels in monocytes and macrophages of patients with MS could act as a modulator of demyelination (Bever et al., 1994).

3. Matrix Metalloproteinases

Matrix metalloproteinases (MMPs) are a group of enzymes (e.g., collagenases, gelatinases, stromelysin-1, matrilysin) responsible for the degradation of interstitial connective tissue and basement membrane (Kieseier et al., 1999). In one study, a substrate conversion assay was used to detect gelatinase activity in the CSF of patients with various neurological disorders including MS (Gijbels et al., 1992), and two main forms of gelatinase with molecular masses of 65 kD (gelatinase A) and 85 kD (gelatinase B) could be discerned. The high molecular mass gelatinase (i.e., gelatinase B) was significantly elevated only in samples of patients with MS or other inflammatory neurological disorders. Subsequently, high levels of gelatinase B were also detected in the CSF of EAE animals (Gijbels et al., 1993). It was suggested that gelatinase production within the CNS might constitute an important pathogenic mechanism for both the disruption of the blood-brain barrier and the destruction of myelin, as observed in several neuroinflammatory disorders. Also, treatment of EAE animals with a single intraperitoneal dose of GM 6001, a hydroxamate inhibitor of MMPs, was sufficient to induce at least a partial inhibition of the gelatinase activity in the CSF of EAE animals (Gijbels et al., 1994). When administered daily, either from the time of disease induction or from the onset of clinical signs, GM 6001 suppressed the development or reversed clinical symptoms of EAE in a dose-dependent manner, respectively. These results indicated that MMP inhibition could reverse ongoing EAE, mainly through restoration of the damaged blood-brain barrier in the inflammatory phase of the disease, as the degree of demyelination and inflammation did not differ between treatment groups (Gijbels et al., 1994).

In other studies, various MMPs were shown to digest MBP, the major extrinsic membrane protein of CNS myelin (Chandler et al., 1995). Production of these enzymes by glia or infiltrating inflammatory cells, therefore, could contribute to demyelination in neuroinflammatory diseases. Studies have shown that upregulation of MMP-3 in a spontaneously demyelinating transgenic mouse precedes onset of the disease (D'Souza et al., 2002) and that MMP-9 (gelatinase B) was selectively elevated in CSF during relapses and stable phases of MS (Leppert et al., 1998). The use of interferon-β1b (IFN-β1b) as a therapeutic agent has substantial clinical benefit in treating MS, yet the mechanism of its action in the disease remains largely unknown; however, a study showing that IFN-β1b inhibits gelatinase secretion and *in vitro* migration of human T-cells suggests a possible mechanism of action (Leppert et al., 1996; Yong et al., 1998).

B. The Role of Ca²⁺ Influx and the Ca²⁺-Dependent Protease Calpain

1. Ca²⁺ Influx

Recent studies have implicated increases in intracellular Ca^{2+} levels by alterations in Ca^{2+} channels in the development of EAE. For instance, the pore-forming subunit of neuronal-type voltage-gated Ca^{2+} channels was upregulated in activated and inactivated lesions with active demyelination in both MS and EAE, suggesting that Ca^{2+} influx in EAE may be facilitated by this increase (Kornek et al., 2001). Studies have also demonstrated that upregulation of the sodium (Na^+) channel $Na_v1.6$ in EAE spinal cord, which results in the intracellular flow of Na^+ and reversal of the Na^+/Ca^{2+} exchanger, might allow damaging concentrations of Ca^{2+} into the demyelinated axon (Craner et al., 2004).

Ca^{2+} influx may also be increased in EAE as a result of glutamate neurotoxicity, which alters intracellular Ca^{2+} homeostasis (Pitt et al., 2000; Smith et al., 2000). Since glutamate AMPA receptor antagonists ameliorated disease severity (Pitt et al., 2000; Smith et al., 2000), restored density of motor neurons (Smith et al., 2000), increased oligodendrocytes survival (Pitt et al., 2000), and reduced dephosphorylation of NFP (Pitt et al., 2000) in EAE animals.

The true intracellular Ca^{2+} concentration in the EAE lesion is currently unknown, and as activation of calpain is absolutely dependent on Ca^{2+}, it is essential to determine the intracellular Ca^{2+} level in tissues from EAE and MS. Increased Ca^{2+} influx may promote calpain activation and expression, axonal damage, and cell death. In support of this, studies in our laboratory indicate that the intracellular Ca^{2+} levels are substantially increased in EAE lumbar spinal cord (Guyton et al., 2004b) and in optic nerve (Guyton et al., 2002) compared to controls. In addition, increased intracellular Ca^{2+} concentrations in cultured glioblastoma (Sur et al., 2003) and neuronal PC12 (Ray et al., 2000) cells treated with glutamate or oxidants have been found to activate calpain, leading to cell death, further supporting the hypothesis that calpain activation may be neurodegenerative in EAE.

2. Calpain Expression and Activity

Among the Ca^{2+}-dependent proteases, calpain has been widely recognized as a prominent player in the pathogenesis of demyelinating diseases (Ray et al., 2003). Calpains exist as ubiquitous forms, microcalpain and millicalpain, requiring μM and mM calcium concentrations for activation, respectively (Saido et al., 1994; Shields and Banik, 1998a). The endogenous inhibitor, calpastatin, also is endogenously expressed and is specific only for calpain, suggesting the importance of calpain regulation in cell homeostasis. Generally, calpain exists as a proenzyme in an inactive form in the cytosol, where the normal Ca^{2+} levels are below concentrations needed for activation. During pathophysiological conditions, however, increased intracellular Ca^{2+} influx could potentially activate calpain (Ray and Banik, 2003; Saido et al., 1994). Calpain degrades myelin proteins (myelin-associated glycoproteins, proteolipid protein, MBP), NFP, cytoskeletal proteins (spectrin, talin, actin), and nuclear laminins on axons and cell membranes (Ray et al., 2003; Shields and Banik, 2001).

Calpain expression and activity has been demonstrated before disease onset in splenic cells (Shields et al., 1999a) and after disease onset in the spinal cord (Shields and Banik, 1998b) and optic nerve (Shields and Banik, 1998a), as well as in active brain lesions from patients with MS (Shields et al., 1999b). Studies have demonstrated that calpain is involved in the activation of T-cells, myelin degradation, axonal damage, and cell death mechanisms leading to apoptosis (Ray and Banik, 2003; Schaecher et al., 2001).

a. The Role of Calpain in Immune Cells. About 28 years ago, detection of a neutral protease in inguinal and popliteal lymph nodes of rats with EAE which degraded MBP suggested a possible role for this enzyme in demyelination (Smith, 1976). Further support was demonstrated in studies showing that stimulated macrophages secreted several neutral proteases, which selectively degraded MBP (Norton et al., 1978). Increased neutral protease activity was found in leukocytes of patients with MS during relapse as compared to remission and controls (Cuzner et al., 1975). Later, neutral protease activity was also identified in lymphocytes and in serum of Lewis rats with EAE (Banik, 1979; Smith, 1979). It is now well known that this neutral protease is calpain. Activated lymphoid cells are readily recognized in patients with MS. *In vitro* studies showed that calpain expression, both at the mRNA and protein levels, was increased in activated lymphoid cells, and calpain secreted from activated human lymphoid cells could degrade MBP (Deshpande et al., 1995b).

Previous studies in our laboratory have demonstrated increased calpain expression in splenic inflammatory cells before disease onset in EAE. Calpain inhibition blocked T-cell activation *in vitro*, suggesting that calpain may play a role in the production by autoreactive T-cells of factors that are involved in myelin destruction in EAE (Schaecher et al., 2001). Subsequent work demonstrated that calpain expression and activity were also increased in activated T-cells and in macrophages that infiltrated into the spinal cord of EAE animals, beginning with disease onset (Schaecher et al., 2002). This suggested that calpain expression and activity in peripheral immune cells occurs early after disease induction but is not detected in the CNS until after clinical symptoms develop.

b. The Role of Calpain in the CNS. In addition to increased calpain expression in inflammatory cell infiltrates such as OX42[+] mononuclear phagocytes and activated CD25[+] T-cells, calpain was also intensely increased in astrocytes in EAE spinal cord and optic nerve. Calpain-induced degradation of 68 kD NFP and spectrin demonstrated increased calpain activity in EAE (Shields and Banik, 2001). Studies from our laboratory have demonstrated increased calpain activity and expression with degradation of myelin and axonal proteins, such as NFP, occurring in EAE spinal cord, as compared to control (Shields and Banik, 2001). Increased calpain expression in activated GFAP[+] astrocytes and infiltrating IFNγ[+] inflammatory cells (Fig. 1) coincided with increased calpain activity and the appearance of clinical symptoms. These activated inflammatory cells (T-cells, macrophages) and reactive cells (astrocytes and microglia), which express more calpain, are the major source of calpain activity, confirming our earlier finding(s) that calpain activity is upregulated in EAE spinal cord and optic nerve, thus leading to degradation of NFP and other cytoskeletal proteins.

Subsequent studies in postmortem tissue from patients with MS revealed increased calpain activity as measured by

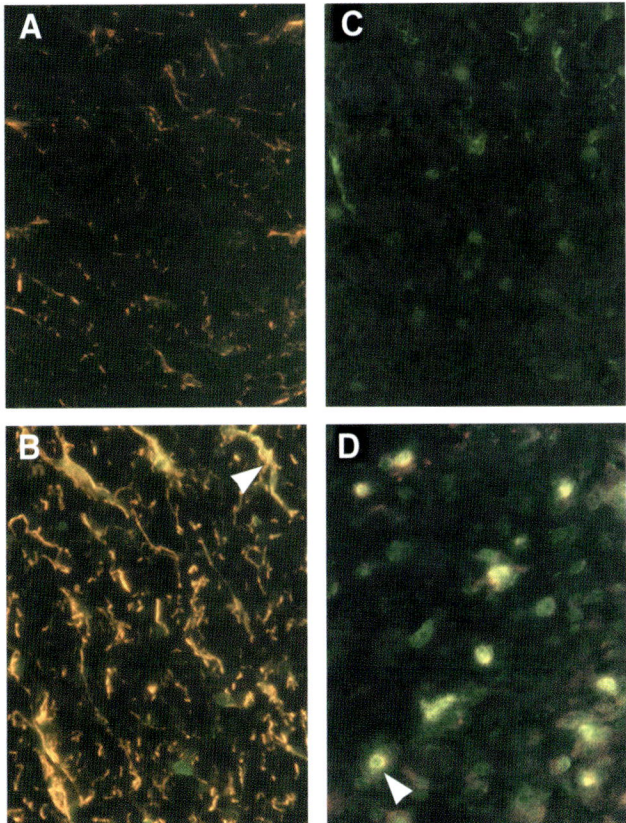

Figure 1 Double immunofluorescent labeling using antibodies for calpain (*green*) and cell-specific markers (*red*). (**A–B**) Antibodies specific for astrocytes (GFAP). (**C–D**) Antibodies specific for IFN-γ in control (**A, C**) and EAE (**B, D**) spinal cord white matter from Lewis rats. Arrows indicate co-localization shown in yellow (× 200). (Reproduced with permission from Shields et al., *Proc. Natl. Acad. Sci. U. S. A.* **95**, 5768–5772, 1998.)

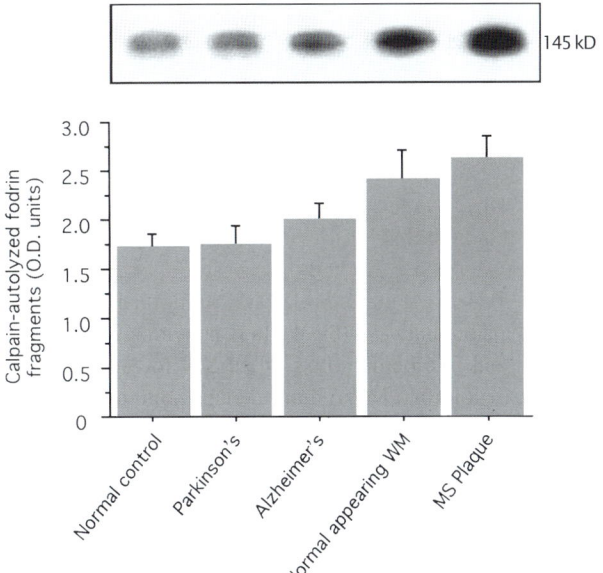

Figure 2 Calpain activity as measured by Western blot detection of the 145 kD calpain-dependent fodrin breakdown product in CNS white matter from normal control, Parkinson's, Alzheimer's, normal-appearing white matter (NAWM), and MS plaque samples (n = 8–10). Western blots were quantified via densitometry and analyzed by one-way ANOVA (±SEM). (Reproduced with permission from Shields et al., *Proc. Natl. Acad. Sci. U. S. A.* **96**,11486-11491, 1999.)

antibody specific for the calpain-cleaved fodrin fragment in MS white matter, compared to white matter tissue from controls and patients with Alzheimer's disease or Parkinson's disease (Fig. 2). Double immunofluorescent labeling, using calpain antibody and cell-specific marker antibodies, demonstrated substantial increases in calpain expression in MHC-II⁺ cells and mononuclear phagocytes (Fig. 3) in MS lesions. Similarly, calpain expression was also upregulated in reactive astrocytes and CD4⁺ T-cells from MS plaque and normal appearing white matter, as compared to tissue from patients with other neurological disorders, and control white matter (Shields et al., 1999b). In the lesion, there was extensive upregulation of calpain expression in CD4⁺ cells. It is important to note that in Alzheimer's disease and Parkinson's disease, gray matter is affected, and this is where calpain activation would potentially be involved in the neurodegeneration of these diseases. These findings, that calpain expression and activity are upregulated in EAE and MS, provide support for calpain's role in axonal damage and neuronal cell death in the pathology of these diseases.

III. Axonal Damage and Cell Death Result in Loss of Function in EAE and MS

Demyelination and the subsequent impairment of impulse conduction are thought to contribute to disabilities associated with MS and EAE (Raine, 1997). However, there is not only a loss of myelin, but also axonal damage and a loss of neurons and glial cells, indicating that the disease is more complex than originally presumed (Peterson et al., 2001; Pitt et al., 2000; Smith et al., 2000; Trapp et al., 1999). Magnetic resonance imaging studies consistently fail to correlate demyelinating lesions with significant clinical deficits (Antel, 1999; Hickey, 1999), but these studies do indicate possible damage to axons, as well as abnormalities in gray matter, contributing to dysfunction. Also, recent magnetic resonance spectroscopy studies demonstrated axonal damage with functional deficit in MS in the early phase, as well as in the progressive phase of the disease (Bozzali et al., 2002; Kuhlmann et al., 2002). The neurodegenerative component (neuronal death) is thought to be present at the later stage or in progressive phases of the disease.

A. Mechanisms of Axonal Damage

Activated calpain, released from activated mononuclear phagocytes and T-cells, participates in myelin protein degradation for antigen presentation (contributing to epitope

Normal Control   **MS Lesion**   **NAWM**

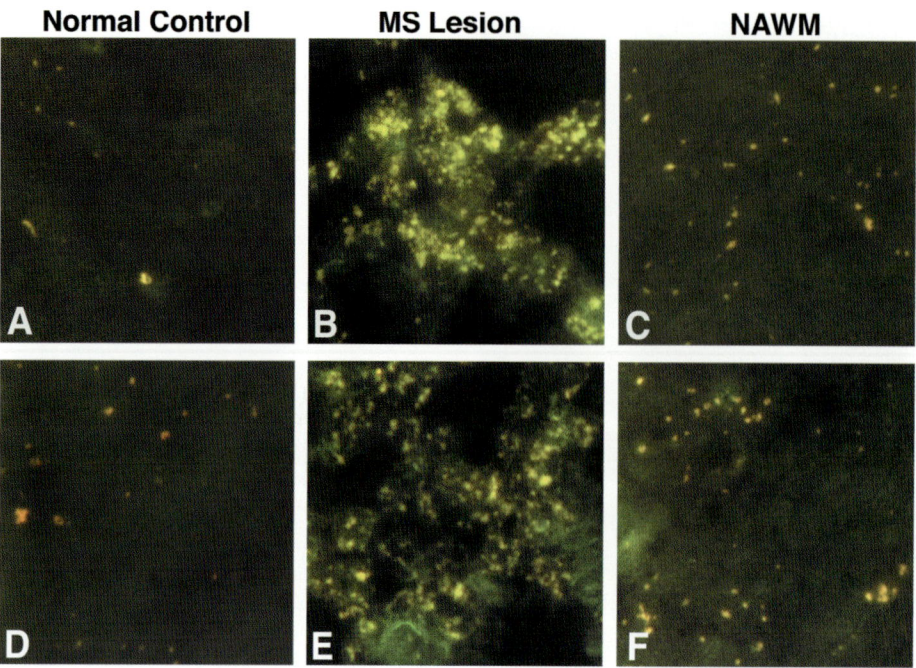

Figure 3 Double immunofluorescent labeling using antibodies for calpain (*green*) and cell-specific marker (*red*) in normal control white matter, normal appearing white matter, and MS lesion. (**A–C**) Antibodies specific for cells expression MHC class II (L243). (**D–F**) Mononuclear phagocytes (EBM-11). Co-localization appears yellow (× 400). (Reproduced with permission from Shields et al., *Proc. Natl. Acad. Sci. U. S. A.* **96,**11486-11491, 1999.)

spreading) (Shields and Banik, 1998a). In support of this hypothesis, we have recently demonstrated increased calpain expression (transcriptional, translational) in activated human lymphoid cell lines, which also secreted the enzyme (Deshpande et al., 1995a, 1995b). Furthermore, it is relevant to suggest that activated calpain secreted from MBP-specific T-cells may be detrimental to neuronal, oligodendroglial, and axonal preservation.

The degradation of 3P, NFP, and spectrin integrity, all of which maintain the architecture of axon and cell membrane, will lead to axonal degeneration and cell death in demyelinating diseases, as previously suspected (Newcombe et al., 1982), and axonal damage can be assessed by measuring increases in dephosphorylation of high molecular weight NFPs, which precede actual loss of NFP protein (Trapp et al., 1998), or by measuring changes in amyloid precursor protein transport (Kornek et al., 2000). Although our previous studies indicated that calpain activation, infiltration of cells, and upregulation of calpain expression in EAE spinal cord occurred after the appearance of clinical symptoms, they did not precisely determine at which point and in which cells calpain is detected first. Subsequent studies (Schaecher et al., 2002) demonstrated that calpain expression was increased in microglia/macrophages in EAE spinal cord at day 9 after induction of EAE (first day

after disease onset); however, although there was a substantial increase in the number of activated T-cells. T-cells did not express calpain until day 10 (Fig. 4). In addition, degradation of MBP and NFP was increased, indicating that axonal damage was occurring after disease onset and suggesting that calpain production from infiltrating immune cells may contribute to axonal damage and neurodegeneration.

To better understand the timing of calpain-induced damage in EAE, we also examined calpain expression in neurons in spinal cord gray matter via immunohistochemical staining of control and EAE spinal cord using an antibody specific for m-calpain and a neuron-specific anti-NeuN antibody (Fig. 5). Calpain expression was negligible in neurons from control spinal cord tissue; however, a large number of neurons, as well as other cells, stained positive for calpain after onset of disease, indicating that EAE neurons do express calpain at an elevated level after onset of disease. Current preliminary studies conducted in our laboratory indicate that axonal damage and neuronal death correlate with increased calpain expression and activity in EAE spinal cord after onset of disease (Figs. 5 and 6).

Because optic neuritis (which results in impairment of vision) can be an early clinical manifestation of MS and because the majority of patients with optic neuritis develop

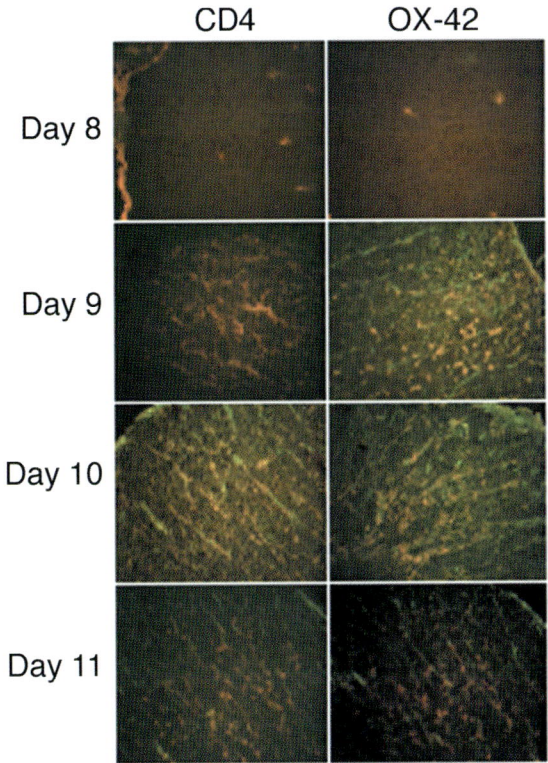

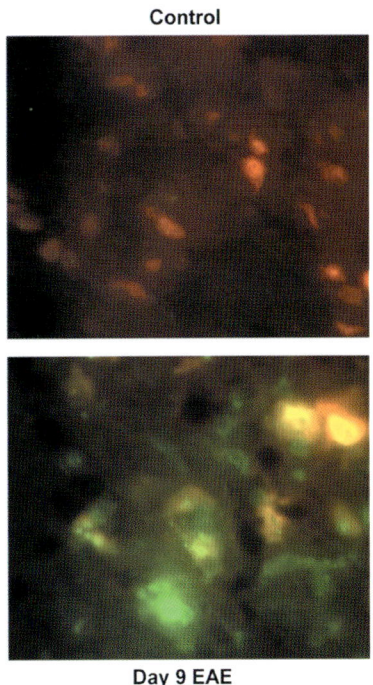

Figure 5 Double immunofluorescent staining using antibodies for calpain (*green*) and neuron specific marker (NeuN) in control EAE spinal cord. Co-localization appears yellow (× 400).

Figure 4 Double immunofluorescent labeling using antibodies for calpain (*green*) and cell-specific markers (*red*) over time. Control and EAE spinal cord were stained with T-cell (CD4) or macrophage/microglia (OX-42) antibodies at days 8–11. Co-localization appears yellow (×400). (Reproduced with permission from Schaecher et al., *J. Neuroimmunol.* 129:1-9, 2002.)

MS (Compston et al., 1991), it is likely that glial cells (oligodendrocytes) and axons in the optic nerve are damaged early in EAE, which is also used as an animal model for optic neuritis (Raine et al., 1980). As previously mentioned, calpain expression and activity are upregulated in EAE after onset of disease. Damage to retinal ganglion cells and visual impairment, as assayed by electroretinograms and visual-evoked potentials, have been demonstrated in EAE (Meyer et al., 2001). This suggested that increased calpain might damage cells and axons in the optic nerve, leading to visual dysfunction. We have found that axons are damaged, as assessed by measuring increases in dephosphorylated NFP, before onset of clinical symptoms (Fig. 6). Increased calpain expression and apoptotic/necrotic glial cells also occurred before disease onset (Guyton et al., 2004a), suggesting that the optic nerve is affected early with loss of

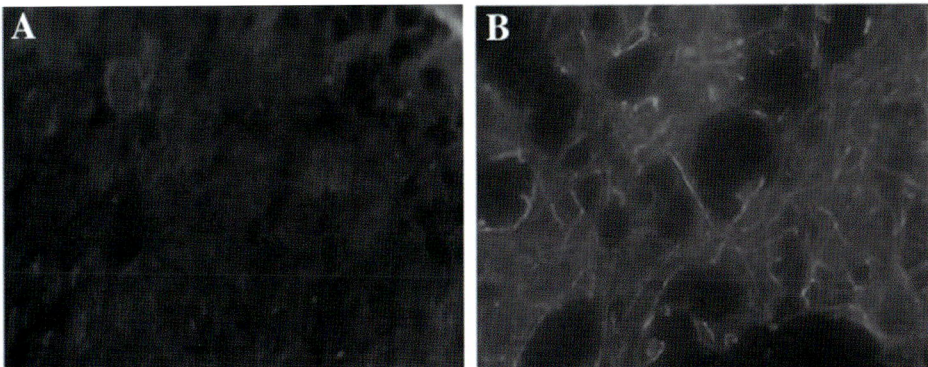

Figure 6 Degeneration of axons in EAE optic nerve Day 8 as assessed by production of dNFP. Immunohistochemical staining of dNFP using the SMI-32 antibody in control and EAE spinal cord.

function before clinical symptoms appear and treatment of EAE animals with calpain inhibitors may prevent cell and axon damage and help restore visual function.

B. Mechanisms of Neuronal Death

Apoptosis or programmed cell death is normal also in tissue development, including the CNS. In CNS, cells may die of traumatic apoptosis and necrosis, augmented by secondary injury factors. This is true in a number of CNS disorders, and treatment with calpain inhibitors blocks apoptosis in several of these diseases (Ray et al., 2003; Shields and Banik, 2001). Specific cell types, including T-cells and macrophages, are known to undergo programmed cell death in EAE (Sarin et al., 1994; Smith et al., 1996). In apoptosis, many mediators participate, including Ca^{2+}, free radicals, cytokines, and proteases. The increased calpain activity and expression in EAE optic nerve and spinal cord suggest that calpain is one of the cysteine proteases responsible for cell death in EAE. This is supported by many *in vitro* studies using various cell types, including lymphocytes, cardiomyocytes, neurons, and glial cells (Ray et al., 2000; Saido et al., 1994; Sarin et al., 1994). Calpains can also cleave many signaling proteins that are related to apoptosis (Ray et al., 2003). Although the role of activated calpain is potentially important in apoptosis, this has not yet been investigated in MS and EAE. Therefore, studies on calpain-mediated apoptotic death of neuronal/glial cells in culture will provide important information on the mechanism of cell death in EAE/MS. IFN-γ has been found to induce apoptosis in cultured oligodendrocytes (Vartanian et al., 1995), and apoptosis in glial cells has been demonstrated in MS plaques, injured spinal cord (Dowling et al., 1997; Li et al., 1996; Squier and Cohen, 1997), and EAE spinal cord (Pitt et al., 2000; Smith and Hall, 2001).

C. Excitotoxic Injury and Neuronal Death in Culture

We, and others, have recently demonstrated that neurons and glial cells in culture under oxidative stress, glutamate exitotoxicity, and/or in the presence of cytokines such as IFN-γ die of apoptotic or necrotic death after calpain activation, and that cell death can be prevented by treatment with calpain inhibitors (Ray et al., 2000; Squier et al., 1994). However, these studies did not indicate the concentration of intracellular-free Ca^{2+} involved in calpain activation, if mitochondria were damaged, or whether the protected cells were functional. Our studies on glial and primary cortical neurons after glutamate toxicity and oxidative stress resulted in increased Ca^{2+} influx, calpain and caspase activation, free radical production, and mitochondrial damage leading to cell death. Pretreatment of these cells with either calpain inhibitor calpeptin, caspase-3 inhibitor z-DEVD-fmk, or

with estrogen provided neuroprotection with restoration of function, as determined by electrophysiological recording of membrane potential (Sribnick et al., 2003). These *in vitro* findings support the hypothesis that calpain is associated with cell death in demyelinating diseases such as MS and EAE and that treatment with calpain inhibitors may ameliorate neurodegenerative effects.

IV. The Effects of Calpain Inhibition in MS and EAE

Information obtained on the involvement of calpain in various neurological diseases suggests that calpain may be a therapeutic target in MS and EAE. Calpastatin is the endogenous inhibitor of calpain but will not cross the blood-brain barrier because of its large size; however, cell-permeable synthetic calpain inhibitors might provide therapies for MS and EAE.

A. The Role of the Endogenous Calpain Inhibitor Calpastatin

The critical regulator of calpain is calpastatin, an endogenous calpain-specific inhibitor with no inhibitory effect on other proteases (Crawford, 1990). Normally, the calpastatin/calpain ratio determines calpain activity and calpastatin becomes a suicide substrate when the ratio increases (Takano and Maki, 1999). Previous studies in our laboratory have demonstrated that calpastatin translational expression is upregulated in EAE splenic inflammatory cells (Shields et al., 1999a) and in EAE spinal cord (Shields and Banik, 1998b), as compared to controls, suggesting that cells are trying to compensate for the increased calpain expression.

The role of calpastatin in CNS disease and injury has been largely ignored, although changes in calpain/calpastatin ratios have been reported in animal models of other neurological diseases including muscular dystrophy, ischemia, SCI, and TBI (Ray et al., 2003; Shields and Banik, 2001). It is particularly noteworthy that calpastatin is degraded by caspase-3 and that caspase activity in increased in the SCI lesion (Springer et al., 1999). The finding that increased caspase activity resulting from mitochondrial damage degrades calpastatin in SCI adds a new dimension because degradation of calpastatin eliminates its regulatory role and fosters cell damage by the calpain release (Shields et al., 2000).

B. The Effects of Calpain Inhibitors

Involvement of calpain in the destruction of myelin, cell death, and axonal damage in MS and EAE warrants examination of the effects of cell-penetrating, calpain-specific inhibitors such as calpeptin and SJA6017, which have been found to be neuroprotective in cataract formation (Fukiage et al., 1997; Tamada et al., 2001) and brain injury (Kupina et al., 2001). Proteinase inhibitors (AMCA, pepstatin) suppress clinical symptoms and reduce the number of CNS lesions in EAE and experimental allergic neuritis (Schabet et al., 1991); however, results using these nonspecific protease inhibitors offer few clues as to which proteases are involved.

The finding of an early increase in calpain expression in activated T-lymphocytes and subsequent increase in the CNS after disease onset suggests a pivotal role for calpain in the pathogenesis of EAE. Studies have shown that cell migration depends on calpain activation, as calpain-specific inhibitors block integrin-mediated cell detachment (Huttenlocher et al., 1997). Thus, calpain activation may also affect T-cell migration from the spleen/lymph nodes during the early stages of EAE. The immunocytochemical distribution of calpain in peripheral lymphatic tissue at different times after challenge demonstrated the source and progression (T-lymphocytes) of the developmental phases of this disease (Shields et al., 1999a).

Current information indicates that calpain activation occurs in the spinal cord after clinical symptoms are apparent, but may be upregulated in the optic nerve before disease onset. This will have important implications in the timing of treatment of EAE animals with calpain inhibitors as therapeutic agents. Drugs may be administered before the clinical symptoms appear to block activation of autoreactive T-cells and/or during the disease phase, so that the disease development may be delayed or severity of the disease may be reduced. Thus, the use of effective cell-permeable, calpain-specific inhibitors (calpeptin, SJA6017) would be expected to promote attenuation of cell death, prevention of axonal damage, migration of activated T-cells, reduction of inflammation by preventing NFκB translocation, and inhibition of MBP-peptide formation. If calpain inhibitors can change the clinical course of EAE and restore/preserve function, treatment for the human disease may be possible.

V. Conclusion

Increased calpain expression and activation in immune cells, glial cells, and neurons, correlating with increases in axonal degeneration and neuronal cell death, suggest that calpain plays a pivotal role not only in demyelination but also in neurodegeneration in MS and EAE. Results from these studies offer some clues suggesting that neuroprotective strategies that involve cell-permeable calpain inhibitors may be beneficial for treatment of EAE and MS.

Acknowledgments

Supported, in part, by grants from NIH-NINDS NS-31622, NS-38146, NS-41088, NS-45967, and CA-91460, as well as from the National Multiple Sclerosis Society and American Health Assistance Foundation. The authors also thank Denise Matzelle and Gloria Wilford for their assistance.

References

Ahmed, Z., Doward, A. I., Pryce, G., Taylor, D. L., Pocock, J. M., Leonard, J. P., Baker, D., and Cuzner, M. L. (2002). A role for caspase-1 and -3 in the pathology of experimental allergic encephalomyelitis: inflammation versus degeneration. *Am. J. Pathol.* **161**, 1577–1586.

Antel, J. (1999). Multiple sclerosis: Emerging concepts of disease pathogenesis. *J. Neuroimmunol.* **98**, 45–48.

Banik, N. L. (1979). The degradation of myelin basic protein by serum proteinase in experimental allergic encephalomyelitis and control rats. *Neurosci. Lett.* **11**, 307–312.

Banik, N. L., Shields, D. C., Ray, S., Davis, B., Matzelle, D., Wilford, G., and Hogan, E.L. (1998). Role of calpain in spinal cord injury: effects of calpain and free radical inhibitors. *Ann. N. Y. Acad. Sci.* **844**, 131–137.

Bartus, R. T., Hayward, N. J., Elliott, P. J., Sawyer, S. D., Baker, K. L., Dean, R. L., Akiyama, A., Straub, J. A., Harbeson, S. L., Li, Z., et al., (1994). Calpain inhibitor AK295 protects neurons from focal brain ischemia. Effects of postocclusion intra-arterial administration. *Stroke* **25**, 2265–2270.

Bever, C. T. Jr., Panitch, H. S., and Johnson, K. P. (1994). Increased cathepsin B activity in peripheral blood mononuclear cells of multiple sclerosis patients. *Neurology* **44**, 745–748.

Blomgren, K., Zhu, C., Wang, X., Karlsson, J. O., Leverin, A. L., Bahr, B. A., Mallard, C., and Hagberg, H. (2001). Synergistic activation of caspase-3 by m-calpain after neonatal hypoxia-ischemia: a mechanism of "pathological apoptosis"? *J. Biol. Chem.* **276**, 10191–10198.

Bozzali, M., Cercignani, M., Sormani, M. P., Comi, G., and Filippi, M. (2002). Quantification of brain gray matter damage in different MS phenotypes by use of diffusion tensor MR imaging. *AJNR Am. J. Neuroradiol.* **23**, 985–988.

Chandler, S., Coates, R., Gearing, A., Lury, J., Wells, G., and Bone, E. (1995). Matrix metalloproteinases degrade myelin basic protein. *Neurosci. Lett.* **201**, 223–226.

Chen, M., He, H. P., Zhan, S. X., Krajewski, S., Reed, J. C., and Gottlieb, R. A. (2001). Bid is cleaved by calpain to an active fragment in vitro and during myocardial ischemia/reperfusion. *J. Biol. Chem.* **276**, 30724–30728.

Choi, W. S., Lee, E. H., Chung, C. W., Jung, Y. K., Jin, B. K., Kim, S. U., Oh, T. H., Saido, T. C., and Oh, Y. J. (2001). Cleavage of Bax is mediated by caspase-dependent or independent calpain activation in dopaminergic neuronal cells: protective role of Bcl-2. *J. Neurochem.* **77**, 1531–1541.

Cid, C., Alvarez-Cermeno, J. C., Regidor, I., Plaza, J., Salinas, M., and Alcazar, A. (2003). Caspase inhibitors protect against neuronal apoptosis induced by cerebrospinal fluid from multiple sclerosis patients. *J. Neuroimmunol.* **136**, 119–124.

Compston, A., Scolding, N., Wren, D., and Noble, M. (1991). The pathogenesis of demyelinating disease: insights from cell biology. *Trends Neurosci.* **14**, 175–182.

Craner, M. J., Hains, B. C., Lo, A. C., Black, J. A., and Waxman, S. G., (2004). Co-localization of sodium channel Nav1.6 and the sodium-calcium exchanger at sites of axonal injury in the spinal cord in EAE. *Brain* **127**, 294–303.

Crawford, C. (1990). Protein and peptide inhibitors of calpains. *In:* "Intracellular Calcium-Dependent Proteolysis" (R. Mellgren and T. Murachi, Eds.). pp. 75–89. CRC Press, Boca Raton.

Cuzner, M. L., McDonald, W. I., Rudge, P., Smith, M., Borshell, N., and Davison, A. N. (1975). Leucocyte proteinase activity and acute multiple sclerosis. *J. Neurol. Sci.* **26**, 107–111.

D'Souza, C. A., Mak, B., and Moscarello, M. A. (2002). The up-regulation of stromelysin-1 (MMP-3) in a spontaneously demyelinating transgenic mouse precedes onset of disease. *J. Biol. Chem.* **277**, 13589–13596.

Daniel, P. T. (2000). Dissecting the pathways to death. *Leukemia* **14**, 2035–2044.

Deshpande, R. V., Goust, J. M., Chakrabarti, A. K., Barbosa, E., Hogan, E. L., and Banik, N. L. (1995a). Calpain expression in lymphoid cells. Increased mRNA and protein levels after cell activation. *J. Biol. Chem.* **270**, 2497–2505.

Deshpande, R. V., Goust, J. M., Hogan, E. L., and Banik, N. L. (1995b). Calpain secreted by activated human lymphoid cells degrades myelin. *J. Neurosci. Res.* **42**, 259–265.

Dowling, P., Husar, W., Menonna, J., Donnenfeld, H., Cook, S., and Sidhu, M. (1997). Cell death and birth in multiple sclerosis brain. *J. Neurol. Sci.* **149**, 1–11.

Fantuzzi, G., and Dinarello, C. A. (1999). Interleukin-18 and interleukin-1 beta: two cytokine substrates for ICE (caspase-1). *J. Clin. Immunol.* **19**, 1–11.

Fukiage, C., Azuma, M., Nakamura, Y., Tamada, Y., Nakamura, M., and Shearer, T. R. (1997). SJA6017, a newly synthesized peptide aldehyde inhibitor of calpain: amelioration of cataract in cultured rat lenses. *Biochim. Biophys. Acta* **1361**, 304–312.

Furlan, R., Filippi, M., Bergami, A., Rocca, M. A., Martinelli, V., Poliani, P. L., Grimaldi, L. M., Desina, G., Comi, G., and Martino, G. (1999). Peripheral levels of caspase-1 mRNA correlate with disease activity in patients with multiple sclerosis: a preliminary study. *J. Neurol. Neurosurg. Psychiatry* **67**, 785–788.

Gijbels, K., Galardy, R. E., and Steinman, L. (1994). Reversal of experimental autoimmune encephalomyelitis with a hydroxamate inhibitor of matrix metalloproteases. *J. Clin. Invest.* **94**, 2177–2182.

Gijbels, K., Masure, S., Carton, H., and Opdenakker, G. (1992). Gelatinase in the cerebrospinal fluid of patients with multiple sclerosis and other inflammatory neurological disorders. *J. Neuroimmunol.* **41**, 29–34.

Gijbels, K., Proost, P., Masure, S., Carton, H., Billiau, A., and Opdenakker, G. (1993). Gelatinase B is present in the cerebrospinal fluid during experimental autoimmune encephalomyelitis and cleaves myelin basic protein. *J. Neurosci. Res.* **36**, 432–440.

Godell, C. M., Smyers, M. E., Eddleman, C. S., Ballinger, M. L., Fishman, H. M., and Bittner, G. D. (1997). Calpain activity promotes the sealing of severed giant axons. *Proc. Natl. Acad. Sci. U. S. A.* **94**, 4751–4756.

Gores, G. J., Miyoshi, H., Botla, R., Aguilar, H. I., and Bronk, S. F. (1998). Induction of the mitochondrial permeability transition as a mechanism of liver injury during cholestasis: a potential role for mitochondrial proteases. *Biochim. Biophys. Acta* **1366**, 167–175.

Guyton, M., Banik, N., Crosson, C., and Rohrer, B. (2004a). Neurodegeneration of the optic nerve occurs in EAE: aan animal model of optic neuritis. Arvo Meeting, Fort Lauderdale, Florida.

Guyton, M., Sribnick, E. A., Wingrave, J. M., Ray, S., and Banik, N. L. (2004b). Axonal Damage and Neurodegeneration Correlate with Increased Calpain Activation in EAE. American Society for Neurochemistry Meeting, New York.

Guyton, M., Wingrave, M., Rocchini, A., Schaecher, K., George, M., Ray, S., and Banik, N. (2002). Apoptosis of neurons in rats with EAE. American Society for Neurochemistry, Palm Beach, FL.

Hickey, W. F. (1999). The pathology of multiple sclerosis: a historical perspective. *J. Neuroimmunol.* **98**, 37–44.

Hisahara, S., Yuan, J., Momoi, T., Okano, H., and Miura, M. (2001). Caspase-11 mediates oligodendrocyte cell death and pathogenesis of autoimmune-mediated demyelination. *J. Exp. Med.* **193**, 111–122.

Huttenlocher, A., Palecek, S. P., Lu, Q., Zhang, W., Mellgren, R. L., Lauffenburger, D. A., Ginsberg, M. H., and Horwitz, A. F. (1997). Regulation of cell migration by the calcium-dependent protease calpain. *J. Biol. Chem.* **272**, 32719–32722.

Kieseier, B. C., Seifert, T., Giovannoni, G., and Hartung, H. P. (1999). Matrix metalloproteinases in inflammatory demyelination: targets for treatment. *Neurology* **53**, 20–25.

Kim, M. J., Jo, D. G., Hong, G. S., Kim, B. J., Lai, M., Cho, D. H., Kim, K. W., Bandyopadhyay, A., Hong, Y. M., Kim do, H., Cho, C., Liu, J. O.,

Snyder, S. H., and Jung, Y. K. (2002). Calpain-dependent cleavage of cain/cabin1 activates calcineurin to mediate calcium-triggered cell death. *Proc. Natl. Acad. Sci. U. S. A.* **99**, 9870–9875.

Kornek, B., Storch, M. K., Bauer, J., Djamshidian, A., Weissert, R., Wallstroem, E., Stefferl, A., Zimprich, F., Olsson, T., Linington, C., Schmidbauer, M., and Lassmann, H. (2001). Distribution of a calcium channel subunit in dystrophic axons in multiple sclerosis and experimental autoimmune encephalomyelitis. *Brain* **124**, 1114–1124.

Kornek, B., Storch, M. K., Weissert, R., Wallstroem, E., Stefferl, A., Olsson, T., Linington, C., Schmidbauer, M., and Lassmann, H. (2000). Multiple sclerosis and chronic autoimmune encephalomyelitis: a comparative quantitative study of axonal injury in active, inactive, and remyelinated lesions. *Am. J. Pathol.* **157**, 267–276.

Kuhlmann, T., Lingfeld, G., Bitsch, A., Schuchardt, J., and Bruck, W. (2002). Acute axonal damage in multiple sclerosis is most extensive in early disease stages and decreases over time. *Brain* **125**, 2202–2212.

Kupina, N. C., Nath, R., Bernath, E. E., Inoue, J., Mitsuyoshi, A., Yuen, P. W., Wang, K. K., and Hall, E. D. (2001). The novel calpain inhibitor SJA6017 improves functional outcome after delayed administration in a mouse model of diffuse brain injury. *J. Neurotrauma* **18**, 1229–1240.

Leppert, D., Ford, J., Stabler, G., Grygar, C., Lienert, C., Huber, S., Miller, K. M., Hauser, S. L., and Kappos, L. (1998). Matrix metalloproteinase-9 (gelatinase B) is selectively elevated in CSF during relapses and stable phases of multiple sclerosis. *Brain* **121 (Pt 12)**, 2327–2334.

Leppert, D., Waubant, E., Burk, M. R., Oksenberg, J. R., and Hauser, S. L. (1996). Interferon beta-1b inhibits gelatinase secretion and in vitro migration of human T cells: a possible mechanism for treatment efficacy in multiple sclerosis. *Ann. Neurol.* **40**, 846–852.

Li, G. L., Brodin, G., Farooque, M., Funa, K., Holtz, A., Wang, W. L., and Olsson, Y. (1996). Apoptosis and expression of Bcl-2 after compression trauma to rat spinal cord. *J. Neuropathol. Exp. Neurol.* **55**, 280–289.

Massacesi, L., Abbamondi, A. L., Raimondi, L., Giorgi, C., and Amaducci, L. (1988). Lysosomal enzymes in experimental allergic encephalomyelitis: time course and evidence of the source. *Neurochem. Res.* **13**, 165–169.

McGinnis, K. M., Whitton, M. M., Gnegy, M. E., and Wang, K. K. (1998). Calcium/calmodulin-dependent protein kinase IV is cleaved by caspase-3 and calpain in SH-SY5Y human neuroblastoma cells undergoing apoptosis. *J. Biol. Chem.* **273**, 19993–20000.

Meyer, R., Weissert, R., Diem, R., Storch, M. K., de Graaf, K. L., Kramer, B., and Bahr, M. (2001). Acute neuronal apoptosis in a rat model of multiple sclerosis. *J. Neurosci.* **21**, 6214–6220.

Nakagawa, T., and Yuan, J. (2000). Cross-talk between two cysteine protease families. Activation of caspase-12 by calpain in apoptosis. *J. Cell Biol.* **150**, 887–894.

Neumar, R. W., Xu, Y. A., Gada, H., Guttmann, R. P., and Siman, R. (2003). Cross-talk between calpain and caspase proteolytic systems during neuronal apoptosis. *J. Biol. Chem.* **278**, 14162–14167.

Newcombe, J., Glynn, P., and Cuzner, M. L. (1982). The immunological identification of brain proteins on cellulose nitrate in human demyelinating disease. *J. Neurochem.* **38**, 267–274.

Norton, W. T., Cammer, W., Bloom, B. R., and Gordon, S. (1978). Neutral proteinases secreted by macrophages degrade basic protein: a possible mechanism of inflammatory demyelination. *Adv. Exp. Med. Biol.* **100**, 365–381.

Peterson, J. W., Bo, L., Mork, S., Chang, A., and Trapp, B. D. (2001). Transected neurites, apoptotic neurons, and reduced inflammation in cortical multiple sclerosis lesions. *Ann. Neurol.* **50**, 389–400.

Pitt, D., Werner, P., and Raine, C. S. (2000). Glutamate excitotoxicity in a model of multiple sclerosis. *Nat. Med.* **6**, 67–70.

Raine, C. (1997). Demyelinating diseases. *In:* "Textbook of Neuropathology" (R. Davis and D. Robertson, Eds.), pp. 627–714. Williams and Wilkins, New York.

Raine, C. S., Traugott, U., Nussenblatt, R. B., and Stone, S. H. (1980). Optic neuritis and chronic relapsing experimental allergic encephalomyelitis:

relationship to clinical course and comparison with multiple sclerosis. *Lab. Invest.* **42**, 327–335.

Ray, S., Fedan, M., Nowak, M., Wilford, G., Hogan, E., and Banik, N. (2000). Oxidative stress and Ca2+ influx upregulate calpain and induce apoptosis in PC12 cells. *Brain Res.* **852**, 326–334.

Ray, S. K., and Banik, N. L. (2003). Calpain and its involvement in the pathophysiology of CNS injuries and diseases: therapeutic potential of calpain inhibitors for prevention of neurodegeneration. *Curr. Drug Target CNS Neurol. Disord.* **2**, 173–189.

Ray, S. K., Matzelle, D. D., Sribnick, E. A., Guyton, M. K., Wingrave, J. M., and Banik, N. L. (2003). Calpain inhibitor prevented apoptosis and maintained transcription of proteolipid protein and myelin basic protein genes in rat spinal cord injury. *J. Chem. Neuroanat.* **26**, 119–124.

Ray, S. K., Matzelle, D. D., Wilford, G. G., Hogan, E. L., and Banik, N. L. (2001). Cell death in spinal cord injury (SCI) requires de novo protein synthesis. Calpain inhibitor E-64-d provides neuroprotection in SCI lesion and penumbra. *Ann. N. Y. Acad. Sci.* **939**, 436–449.

Robles, E., Huttenlocher, A., and Gomez, T. M. (2003). Filopodial calcium transients regulate growth cone motility and guidance through local activation of calpain. *Neuron* **38**, 597–609.

Saido, T., Sorimachi, H., and Suzuki, K. (1994). Calpain: new perspectives in molecular diversity and physiological-pathological involvement. *FASEB J.* **8**, 814–822.

Sarin, A., Cleirci, M., Blatt, A., Hendrix, C., Shearer, G., and Henkart, P. (1994). Inhibition of activation-induced programmed cell death and restoration of defective responses of HIV+ donors by cysteine protease inhibitors. *J. Immunol.* **153**, 862–872.

Schabet, M., Whitaker, J. N., Schott, K., Stevens, A., Zurn, A., Buhler, R., and Wietholter, H. (1991). The use of protease inhibitors in experimental allergic neuritis. *J. Neuroimmunol.* **31**, 265–272.

Schaecher, K., Rocchini, A., Dinkins, J., Matzelle, D. D., and Banik, N. L. (2002). Calpain expression and infiltration of activated T cells in experimental allergic encephalomyelitis over time: increased calpain activity begins with onset of disease. *J. Neuroimmunol.* **129**, 1–9.

Schaecher, K. E., Goust, J. M., and Banik, N. L. (2001). The effects of calpain inhibition upon IL-2 and CD25 expression in human peripheral blood mononuclear cells. *J. Neuroimmunol.* **119**, 333–342.

See, V., and Loeffler, J. P. (2001). Oxidative stress induces neuronal death by recruiting a protease and phosphatase-gated mechanism. *J. Biol. Chem.* **276**, 35049–35059.

Shields, D., and Banik, N. (2001). Calcium activated neutral proteinase in demyelinating diseases. *In:* "The Role of Proteolytic Enzymes in the Pathophysiology of Neurodegenerative Diseases" (N. Banik and A. Lajtha, Eds.), pp. 25–45. Plenum Press, New York.

Shields, D., Schaecher, K., Hogan, E., and Banik, N. (2000). Calpain expression increased in activated glial and inflammatory cells in the penumbra of spinal cord injury lesion. *J. Neurosci. Res.* **61**, 146–150.

Shields, D. C., and Banik, N. L. (1998a). Putative role of calpain in the pathophysiology of experimental optic neuritis. *Exp. Eye Res.* **67**, 403–410.

Shields, D. C., and Banik, N. L.(1998b). Upregulation of calpain activity and expression in experimental allergic encephalomyelitis: a putative role for calpain in demyelination. *Brain Res.* **794**, 68–74.

Shields, D. C., Schaecher, K. E., Goust, J. M., and Banik, N. L. (1999a). Calpain activity and expression are increased in splenic inflammatory cells associated with experimental allergic encephalomyelitis. *J. Neuroimmunol.* **99**, 1–12.

Shields, D. C., Schaecher, K. E., Saido, T. C., and Banik, N. L. (1999b). A putative mechanism of demyelination in multiple sclerosis by a proteolytic enzyme, calpain. *Proc. Natl. Acad. Sci. U. S. A.* **96**, 11486–11491.

Shields, D. C., Tyor, W. R., Deibler, G. E., and Banik, N. L. (1998a). Increased calpain expression in experimental demyelinating optic neuritis: an immunocytochemical study. *Brain Res.* **784**, 299–304.

Shields, D. C., Tyor, W. R., Deibler, G. E., Hogan, E. L., and Banik, N. L. (1998b). Increased calpain expression in activated glial and inflammatory cells in experimental allergic encephalomyelitis. *Proc. Natl. Acad. Sci. U. S. A.* **95**, 5768–5772.

Smith, K. J., and Hall, S. M. (2001). Factors directly affecting impulse transmission in inflammatory demyelinating disease: recent advances in our understanding. *Curr. Opin. Neurol.* **14**, 289–298.

Smith, M. E. (1976). A lymph node neutral proteinase acting on myelin basic protein. *J. Neurochem.* **27**, 1077–1082.

Smith, M. E. (1979). Neutral protease activity in lymphocytes of Lewis rats with acute experimental allergic encephalomyelitis. *Neurochem. Res.* **4**, 689–702.

Smith, T., Groom, A., Zhu, B., and Turski, L. (2000). Autoimmune encephalomyelitis ameliorated by AMPA antagonists. *Nat. Med.* **6**, 62–66.

Smith, T., Schmied, M., Hewson, A. K., Lassmann, H., and Cuzner, M. L. (1996). Apoptosis of T cells and macrophages in the central nervous system of intact and adrenalectomized Lewis rats during experimental allergic encephalomyelitis. *J. Autoimmun.* **9**, 167–174.

Springer, J., Azbill, R., and Knapp, P. (1999). Activation of the caspase-3 apoptotic cascade in traumatic spinal cord injury. *Nat. Med.* **5**, 943–046.

Squier, M., and Cohen, J. (1997). Calpain, an upstream regulator of thymocyte apoptosis. *J. Immunol.* **158**, 3690–3697.

Squier, M., Miller, A., Malkinson, A., and Cohen, J. (1994). Calpain activation in apoptosis. *J.Cell Physiol.* **159**, 229–237.

Sribnick, E. A., Wingrave, J. M., Matzelle, D. D., Ray, S. K., and Banik, N. L. (2003). Estrogen as a neuroprotective agent in the treatment of spinal cord injury. *Ann. N. Y. Acad. Sci.* **993**, 125–133; discussion 159–160.

Stys, P. K., and Jiang, Q. (2002). Calpain-dependent neurofilament breakdown in anoxic and ischemic rat central axons. *Neurosci. Lett.* **328**, 150–154.

Sur, P., Sribnick, E. A., Wingrave, J. M., Nowak, M. W., Ray, S. K., and Banik, N. L. (2003). Estrogen attenuates oxidative stress-induced apoptosis in C6 glial cells. *Brain Res.* **971**, 178–188.

Takano, E., and Maki, M. (1999). Structure of calpastatin and its inhibitory control of calpain. *In:* "Calpain: Pharmacology and Toxicology of Calcium-Dependent Protease" (K. Wang and P.-W. Yuen, Eds.), pp. 25–49. Francis and Taylor, Philadelphia.

Tamada, Y., Fukiage, C., Mizutani, K., Yamaguchi, M., Nakamura, Y., Azuma, M., and Shearer, T. R. (2001). Calpain inhibitor, SJA6017, reduces the rate of formation of selenite cataract in rats. *Curr. Eye Res.* **22**, 280–285.

Trapp, B. D., Peterson, J., Ransohoff, R. M., Rudick, R., Mork, S., and Bo, L. (1998). Axonal transection in the lesions of multiple sclerosis. *N. Engl. J. Med.* **338**, 278–285.

Trapp, B. D., Ransohoff, R., and Rudick, R, (1999). Axonal pathology in multiple sclerosis: Relationship to neurologic disability. *Curr. Opin. Neurol.* **12**, 295–302.

Varghese, J., Radhika, G., and Sarin, A. (2001). The role of calpain in caspase activation during etoposide induced apoptosis in T cells. *Eur. J. Immunol.* **31**, 2035–2041.

Vartanian, T., Li, Y., Zhao, M., and Stefansson, K. (1995). Interferon-gamma-induced oligodendrocyte cell death: implications for the pathogenesis of multiple sclerosis. *Mol. Med.* **1**, 732–743.

Yong, V. W., Chabot, S., Stuve, O., and Williams, G. (1998). Interferon beta in the treatment of multiple sclerosis: mechanisms of action. *Neurology* **51**, 682–689.

21

Mutations of Myelination-Associated Genes That Affect Axonal Integrity

Klaus-Armin Nave, Ph.D.
Hauke Werner, Ph.D.

I. Axon-Glia Interaction and Myelin Assembly

The principal function of oligodendrocytes is the ensheathment of axons with the subsequent assembly of myelin. Myelin sheaths, when viewed by electron microscopy in cross-section, are multilamellar stacks of spirally wrapped cell membrane, flanked by nodal and paranodal specializations. Myelin membranes provide the axon surface with a high radial membrane resistance and a low capacitance, both of which are required for rapid saltatory impulse conduction (Waxman, 1997).

Axonal caliber and the degree of myelination (i.e., myelin thickness and internodal length) are the major determinants of axonal conduction velocity in myelinated fiber tracts. Establishing optimal nerve conduction velocity is critical, as millisecond precision is required for many neural functions, including higher brain functions. By reaching the minimal size of about 1 μm in cross-section, a peripheral nervous system (PNS) axon can induce its myelination (Friede and Bischhausen, 1982; Voyvodic, 1989). Similarly, central nervous system (CNS) axons trigger myelination when they reach a diameter of about 0.2 μm (Waxman and Bennett, 1972). In turn, myelin itself is a positive modulator of axon caliber (de Waegh et al., 1992). Thus, active axoglial interactions play a major role in establishing the normal conduction properties within the nervous system.

Both Schwann cells and oligodendrocytes require axonal signals, not only in development but throughout adult life. Myelin sheaths remain in active metabolic contact to the glial cell soma, and may be considered an "external" glial organelle. When the axonal contact is lost, for example after an experimental lesion, myelin degenerates distal to the site of injury (Wallerian degeneration) (reviewed by Raff et al., 2002). Conversely, axons are lost as a consequence of glial dysfunction, as detailed in this chapter. Thus, there is a bidirectional dependency between axons and their ensheathing glial cells, and defects of this communication may cause severe neurological disability (see also Chapter 2).

Multiple sclerosis (MS) is a demyelinating disorder with immune-mediated attacks on the integrity of CNS myelin and myelin-forming oligodendrocytes. Charcot's early histopathological findings in 1868 pointed to a neuronal-axonal component of MS, confirmed in more recent studies by immunohistochemistry and laser confocal microscopy (Ferguson et al., 1997; Trapp et al., 1998).

It is now widely accepted that a progressive axonal loss is of major clinical relevance in MS. Acute axonal pathology could be the result of a bystander effect of CNS inflammation, as suggested by *in vitro* observation or animal models of experimental allergic encephalomyelitis (reviewed in Neumann, 2003; Bjartmar et al., 2003). Alternatively, the loss of functional oligodendrocytes or myelin itself may also underlie the loss of axonal integrity, specifically in the slowly progressive late phase of MS. Unfortunately, the relative contribution of inflammation and demyelination is difficult to estimate.

Thus, with respect to axonal integrity it is helpful to compare the histopathology of MS with that of inherited myelin diseases (i.e., in the absence of inflammation). Although this opportunity is rare in humans, several mouse models with mutations in myelin-specific genes have been developed that allow such a detailed histopathological analyses. These studies point to a critical function of oligodendrocytes in long-term axonal support. Schwann cells play an equally important role in the peripheral nervous system. The molecular nature of this supportive glial function remains to be defined.

II. Mouse Mutants as Human Myelin Disease Models

Inherited defects of myelin are generally rare disorders, although collectively they comprise a sizeable group of leukodystrophies and spastic paraplegias in the CNS, or peripheral neuropathies in the PNS. In all these diseases, there is growing evidence that a primary disorder of oligodendrocytes (or Schwann cells) results ultimately in axonal loss that contributes to a progressive clinical disability. This insight is derived in part from observations in homologous mouse mutants.

As early as 50 years ago, spontaneous neurological mutation in the mouse were described that exhibited abnormal myelin formation, providing the first rodent models of non-inflammatory myelin diseases (Falconer and Sierts-Roth, 1951; Phillips, 1954). In the last 20 years, the ability to generate transgenic mice and rats, with mutations of virtually any gene (in the mouse), has resulted in a rapid increase in the number of myelin mutants and myelin disease models (reviewed in Werner et al., 1998).

Following is a short overview of animal models that are genetically defined by mutations in myelin-specific genes, a variable degree of dysmyelination and demyelination, and progressive axonal defects. Collectively, these mutants show that myelin-forming glial cells are required to maintain long-term axonal integrity. With respect to nervous system evolution, the hypothesis is put forward that axonal support is the primary function of axon-ensheathing glial cells.

III. Axonal Defects in the Peripheral Nervous System

When comparing myelin of the central and peripheral nervous system, the principal relationship between axons and myelinating glia appears the same, although Schwann cells and oligodendrocytes are of different embryological origin. Many peripheral axons are derived from neurons within the CNS, where they are also myelinated, suggesting that the underlying axoglial interactions are related or even the same. Different from oligodendrocytes, Schwann cells ensheath axonal segments in a 1:1 ratio (reviewed in Hildebrand et al., 1993, 1994), and their differentiated phenotype is dependent on axonal signaling (Jessen et al., 1994). Also, non-myelin-forming Schwann cells are highly specialized cells in the PNS that interact with numerous small-caliber axons, by engulfing without enwrapping them. This non-myelin-forming Schwann cell has no obvious counterpart in the CNS.

Peripheral neuropathies in humans can be caused by a number of Schwann cell-intrinsic defects that have a common clinical phenotype of progressive muscle weakness. Because this results from a functional denervation of muscle fibers, a secondary loss of motor units demonstrates indirectly the extent to which Schwann cell dysfunction causes axonal degeneration.

A. Peripheral Myelin Protein 22-Associated Neuropathies

The peripheral myelin protein of 22 kDa (PMP22) is a small integral myelin membrane glycoprotein with a tetraspan topology. The *Pmp22* gene, located on mouse chromosome 11, is nearly exclusively expressed in Schwann cells and a few epithelial cell types outside the nervous system. Its primary cellular function is not well understood, and it has been suggested that PMP22 was "recruited" as a myelin protein from a primary function in cell growth control (Naef and Suter, 1998, Müller, 2000).

Two autosomal-dominant mouse mutants, Trembler (Tr) and Tr-J are defined by point mutations in the *Pmp22* gene and alter the primary structure of the protein (G150D and L16P, respectively) (Suter et al., 1992a, 1992b). Additional *Pmp22* mutant mice were described later, including an *in-frame* deletion of exon 4 (Suh et al., 1997) and two mutagen-induced point mutations (Isaacs et al., 2000).

The altered structure of PMP22 causes defects of intracellular protein trafficking in Schwann cells (Tobler et al., 1999) that are increased in number but fail to properly myelinate (Sancho et al., 2001). Trembler mice remain severely dysmyelinated in the PNS, whereas CNS myelin appears normal (Falconer & Sierts-Roth, 1951; Henry and Sidman, 1988). The clinical phenotype of Trembler (ataxia, tremors) can be largely explained by the absence of peripheral myelin, a Schwann-cell autonomous defect (Aguayo et al., 1977).

The primary Schwann cell defect in Trembler mice has a strong effect on the dysmyelinated peripheral axons (Sancho et al., 1999; Maier et al., 2002). It has been argued that muscular dystrophy in Trembler may not only be due to axonal damage (Gale et al., 1982), which is difficult to assess in the sciatic nerve, but significant axonal loss has been documented in the dorsal roots (Robertson et al., 1997).

In the absence of overt axonal loss, Trembler mice were the first to show that dysmyelination and demyelination alter the slow axonal transport rates in peripheral nerves (de Waegh and Brady, 1990, 1991). Of interest, in nerve graft experiments, Trembler Schwann cells reduced the diameter of the regenerated axons, but just locally. Reduced axonal transport rates and the reduced phosphorylation of cytoskeletal proteins were also strictly localized to the segment associated with mutant myelin. These data suggest that myelin, when contacting axons, modulates a kinase-phosphatase system (de Waegh et al. 1992; Starr et al., 1996) acting on neurofilaments and presumably other axonal proteins.

A bona-fide human disease model is provided by *Pmp22* overexpressing transgenic mice and rats that closely mimic Charcot-Marie-Tooth disease Type IA (CMT1A), also associated with progressive axonal loss (Sereda et al., 1996; Magyar et al, 1996; Huxley et al., 1996). The overall clinical phenotype of *Pmp22*-transgenic animals is correlated with the degree of PMP22 overexpression. Clinically, CMT1A and its rodent models are neuromuscular disorders with progressive muscle weakness and gait abnormalities. The phenotype is not directly caused by the lack of myelin or reduced nerve conduction velocity, but rather by the progressive loss of motor axons and, thus, a loss of the deafferented muscle fibers. For example, the *CMT rat* model overexpresses the PMP22 gene about 1.6-fold in Schwann cells (Sereda et al, 2003), thereby causing reduced nerve conduction velocities and, at the histological level, Schwann cell hypertrophy with prominent and abundant "onion bulbs." These features closely resemble the pathological findings of the human disease. Higher expression levels cause even more severe dysmyelination (Magyar et al, 1996; Niemann et al, 2000). The extent of axonal and muscular involvement has been demonstrated and quantified also in the rat CMT model, using electrophysiological and histological techniques (Sereda et al, 1996).

Mouse mutants that lack PMP22 expression (null mutation) have a slightly delayed onset of myelination and exhibit a severe neuropathy later (Adlkofer et al., 1995). Loss of PMP22 is associated with formation of "hypermyelinated" tomacula that are unstable and degenerate, again causing progressive demyelination and axonal degeneration (Sancho et al., 1999).

Taken together, altered expression of PMP22, a Schwann cell-specific myelin protein of unknown primary function, results in a variable degree of Schwann cell dysmyelination and demyelination. Whereas the effects of slowed nerve conduction are minimal, the progressive loss of peripheral myelin or another function of PMP-mutant Schwann cells causes axonal abnormalities and, ultimately axonal loss, the basis for muscle weakness and clinical symptoms. These observations indicate that myelin-forming Schwann cells are essential for the long-term survival of axons in the PNS. This function is certainly not specific to PMP22, as related phenotypes can be observed in other PNS myelin mutant mice.

B. Axonal Loss in Other PNS Myelin Mutants

Mice lacking expression of myelin protein zero (MPZ/P0), a major structural component of PNS myelin, exhibit defects of myelin compaction, predominantly at the intraperiod line (Giese et al., 1992). Later, P0-deficient myelin sheaths degenerate, again leading to a significant fraction of degenerating axons in older mutants (Frei et al, 1999). Mice with only 50% reduced P0 gene dosage appear normally myelinated at first but develop a late-onset progressive neuropathy (Martini et al., 1995), providing a bona-fide model for human CMT1B (Warner et al., 1996). As in other neuropathies, the histopathological features of CMT type I, including demyelinated axons, thinly remyelinated axons, and onion bulbs with supernumerary Schwann cells, are present but only indirectly related to the clinical phenotype. Human CMT1B patients suffer from progressive muscle weakness, suggesting that dysmyelination and demyelination underlie axonal loss. The latter is less obvious in P0 ± mice compared to other Schwann cell defects. Also, experimental overexpression of P0 in Schwann cells of transgenic mice causes, in addition to a dysmyelination, secondary axonal loss (Wrabetz et al., 2000). The mechanism of P0-dependent axonopathy is unknown but may have molecular features of pathogenesis in common with wallerian-type axon degeneration (Samsam et al., 2003).

Myelin-associated glycoprotein (MAG), an immunoglobulin-like Type I membrane protein, exhibits a very restricted localization at the adaxonal surface of myelin. It was a prime candidate for the axon-glial recognition underlying myelination (Schachner and Bartsch, 2000). However, Schwann cells in MAG-deficient mice are able to recognize axons and assemble normal amounts of myelin, without major abnormalities or developmental delays (Montag et al., 1994;

Li et al., 1994). Nevertheless, long-term observation of these mutants identified onion-bulb formations, paranodal myelin tomaculi, and degenerating axons, comprising a mild peripheral neuropathy (Fruttiger et al., 1995; Guenard et al., 1996; Weiss et al., 2001). In MAG*N-CAM double mutant mice, peripheral myelination was initially uncompromised, but secondary axonal degeneration was noted several months earlier than in MAG-deficient mice (Carenini et al., 1997).

An unexpected observation in MAG mutants was a reduced phosphorylation of axonal neurofilaments, at least in the PNS. This was associated with an increase of neurofilament density and a reduction of axon caliber (Yin et al., 1998; Dashiell et al., 2002). Thus, one direct or indirect function of MAG is the regulation of stuctural features in myelinated axons. MAG may mediate glia-to-axon signaling, as it can function as a glial ligand for axonal gangliosides and the p75/nogo receptor complex (reviewed by Sandvig et al., 2004). The mechanisms by which MAG binding causes phosphorylation of neurofilaments remain to be defined (Sanchez et al., 2000) (see Chapter 2). In the CNS of MAG-deficient mice, a late onset phenotype is a dying back axonopathy (Lassmann et al., 1997).

C. Axonal Support by Nonmyelinforming Schwann Cells

Support of axons is not restricted to the intimate relationship with myelinating Schwann cells. Some sensory and all postganglionic sympathetic axons have diameters below 1 μm and are unmyelinated (Type C fibers). These axons assemble in "Remak bundles" and are engulfed as groups of axons by nonmyelinating Schwann cells. In one study, axoglial signaling was specifically ablated for these nonmyelinating Schwann cells by transgenic overexpression of a dominant-negative ErbB4 receptor (Chen et al., 2003). Mutant mice develop a progressive neuropathy, including apoptosis and proliferation of nonmyelinating Schwann cells. Of importance, there was secondary degeneration of sensory C fibers and subsequent apoptosis of DRG neurons. These results indicate bidirectional interactions and signaling also between small-diameter axons and their associated (nonmyelinating) Schwann cells in the Remak bundle. The molecular mechanism of glial support was suggested to involve neurotrophic factors, as GDNF protein was reduced in the sciatic nerves (Chen et al., 2003). Neuregulin and ErbB receptor expression is induced in a model of wallerian degeneration (Carroll et al., 1997).

IV. Axonal Defects in CNS Myelin Mutants

Recognizing long-term interactions between oligodendrocytes and axons is more difficult in the CNS than in the PNS, because mutations that disrupt central myelination are usually associated with premature death. More recently, mouse mutants with quite subtle defects of CNS myelin have been described that allowed the identification of a role of oligodendrocytes in long-term axonal support in the absence of demyelination, dysmyelination, or gain-of-function mutations.

A. PLP-Associated Myelin Disorders

Mice with altered expression of the X-linked myelin proteolipid protein (PLP) gene were the first to show clear axonal involvement within a wide spectrum of phenotypic disease expression. Expression of the PLP gene is restricted to myelin-forming oligodendrocytes, although Schwann cells express PLP/DM20 at a low level. Natural and transgenic PLP mouse mutants are models for human Pelizaeus-Merzbacher disease (PMD), ranging in phenotype from severe leukodystrophy with premature death, to milder forms resembling spastic paraplegia type-2 (SPG2).

The PLP gene is linked to the X chromosome and encodes a myelin protein of 30 kDa, highly conserved in sequence and topology between mouse and human (Stoffel et al., 1984; Milner et al., 1985). PLP has four transmembrane domains, with the amino- and carboxyl-termini facing the cytoplasmic side of the myelin membrane (Popot et al., 1991; Wahle and Stoffel, 1998). By alternative RNA splicing, a smaller PLP isoform is generated (termed DM20) that lacks 35 residues from the cytoplasmic loop. This portion of PLP may harbor signals for the efficient sorting of PLP and possibly PLP-associated molecules into the myelin compartment (Anderson et al., 1997; Trapp et al., 1997). There is indirect evidence that PLP and DM20 assemble into homo-oligomeric complexes before reaching the myelin compartment (Jung et al., 1996; McLaughlin et al., 2002). Posttranslational palmitoylation and the binding of cholesterol to PLP and DM20 (Simons et al., 2000) explain the unusual overall hydrophobicity of proteolipids. For a detailed review on PLP structure and function, see Griffiths et al. (1998) and Greer and Lees (2002).

The natural mouse mutant *jimpy* (Phillips, 1954; Sidman et al., 1964) is defined by a point mutation of the X chromosome-linked PLP gene (Nave et al., 1986; Hudson et al., 1987) and is the prototype of a leukodystrophy model caused by aberrant PLP expression. The clinical signs of *jimpy* mice—ataxia, tremors, and seizures—begin in the second postnatal week, coinciding with the onset of CNS myelination in wild-type animals. *Jimpy* mice are bona-fide models for the connatal form of human PMD (Seitelberger et al., 1996; Koeppen and Robitaille, 2002). The histological phenotype is an almost complete lack of CNS myelin, associated with the absence of mature oligodendrocytes (Hirano et al., 1969; Meier and Bischoff, 1974, 1975; Meier et al., 1974). Increased oligodendrocyte cell death (Skoff, 1982, 1995) shows features of apoptotic (Vela et al., 1996; Knapp et al., 1999) and is likely caused by retention of abnormally folded PLP and ER stress (Gow and Lazzarini, 1996). A small percentage of *jimpy* oligodendrocytes survive, generating small patches of myelin. The abnormal ultrastructure of myelin at the intraperiod line (fused in *jimpy* to a single electron-dense structure, indistinguishable from the major dense line) suggests that PLP serves here as an adhesive strut stabilizing compacted myelin (Duncan et al., 1989; Schneider et al., 1995). *Jimpy* mice and other severe mutants of the PLP gene do not live long enough, however, to exhibit secondary effects on axonal integrity.

The allelic *rumpshaker* mice, with a mutation of the PLP gene, live considerably longer than *jimpy* but show no obvious axonal involvement. However, these mice have reduced oligodendrocyte death, and the mutant proteolipid (I186T) is only partially retained in the ER (Southwood et al., 2002). Instead, mutant PLP is incorporated into myelin that becomes less stably packaged (Schneider et al., 1992; Fanarraga et al., 1993; Karthigasan et al., 1996). When compared to PLP-null mutants (see later) this incorporation of PLP into myelin appears to protect axons from degeneration. Of interest, *rumpshaker* mice are good animal models for human SPG-2, with the index family of this disease carrying the same PLP point mutation (Kobayashi et al., 1994; Naidu et al., 1997).

The first hint of an axonal involvement came from transgenic mice that overexpress PLP and DM20 less than twofold at the transcriptional level (Readhead et al., 1994; Anderson et al., 1998). After a rather normal development, they showed progressive ataxia and behavioral abnormalities at age 2 months caused by a demyelination with substantial axonal loss in the long tracts of the spinal cord (Anderson et al., 1998). Although this axonal loss could be secondary to severe demyelination, PLP *null* mutants demonstrated significant axonal loss in the presence of nearly-normal amounts of myelin membrane.

Several laboratories have used gene targeting to completely ablate the expression of PLP/DM20 (Boison and Stoffel, 1994; Klugmann et al., 1997). Isoform-specific gene targeting addressed functional differences between PLP and DM20 (Stecca et al., 2000; Sporkel et al., 2002). Surprisingly, interpretation of these data is more difficult than anticipated. The mice have clearly demonstrated that PLP/DM20 physically stabilizes myelin (Rosenbluth et al., 1996; Klugmann et al., 1997), but neither protein isoform is required for myelin assembly. When compared to *jimpy* or PLP/DM20-overexpressing mice, it is the toxic gain-of-function effect that emerges as the major cause of dysmyelination and cell death.

Functionally, there is no motor deficit in young adult PLP-deficient mice (Klugmann et al.,1997) and the PNS is normal, at least in the short-lived model system mouse, a remarkable difference from human patients with the *PLP*

null mutation who develop a demyelinating peripheral neuropathy (Garbern et al., 1997).

A striking observation was that, in the absence of PLP/DM20, axonal swellings develop throughout the CNS, causing widespread neurodegeneration within several months (Griffiths et al., 1998). The associated motor defects differ from the phenotype of dysmyelinated mice. This fiber degeneration, predominantly affecting small-caliber axons, is probably secondary to impaired fast axonal transport (Edgar et al., 2004), originating at the paranodal region (Fig. 1). Length-dependent axonal degenerations of the CNS have also been found in human patients with PMD caused by a PLP null mutation (Garbern et al., 2002).

The principal cellular function of PLP/DM20 remains to be identified. It is likely that a PLP-related proteolipid, termed M6B, expressed in oligodendrocytes, is masking the full loss-of-function of PLP/DM20. This is suggested because both PLP-deficient and M6B-deficient single mutant mice are myelinated with few ultrastructural abnormalities, whereas PLP*M6B double deficient mice exhibit major developmental defects of CNS myelination, including severe axonal involvement (Werner et al., unpublished).

Female heterozygous mice of the X-linked PLP *null* allele are natural mosaics with respect to PLP gene expression, as a result of the random nature of X-chromosome inactivation. This allowed investigation in older females of whether the novel axon-supportive function of oligodendrocytes is long range and can be provided by only 50% of oligodendrocytes for significantly more than 50% of the axons. Alternatively, it might be a local support, predicting that 50% of the axons associated with mutant oligodendrocytes are abnormal. Indeed, by quantitative analysis, the latter was the case. The presence of roughly 50% of axonal swellings in the optic nerve suggested a rather localized support function (Griffiths et al., 1998).

Taken together, PLP mutant mice have demonstrated that the long-term integrity of myelinated axons requires local oligodendroglial support, and that oligodendrocytes require proteolipids to efficiently serve this function. However, axonal swellings and degeneration are not a feature of myelin mutants in general.

B. CNP-Deficient Mice

In the absence of PLP, the destabilization of the myelin sheath could be a primary cause of axon swellings and degeneration. It was important, therefore, to identify a protein that also contributes to axonal integrity, but was unrelated to the physical stability of myelin.

The enzyme 2′,3′-cyclic nucleotide 3′-phosphodiesterase (CNP) is a widely used marker protein of myelin-forming glial cells. In addition to the glial cell soma, CNP is associated with noncompacted regions of myelin such as the inner mesaxon, paranodal loops, and Schmidt-Lantermann

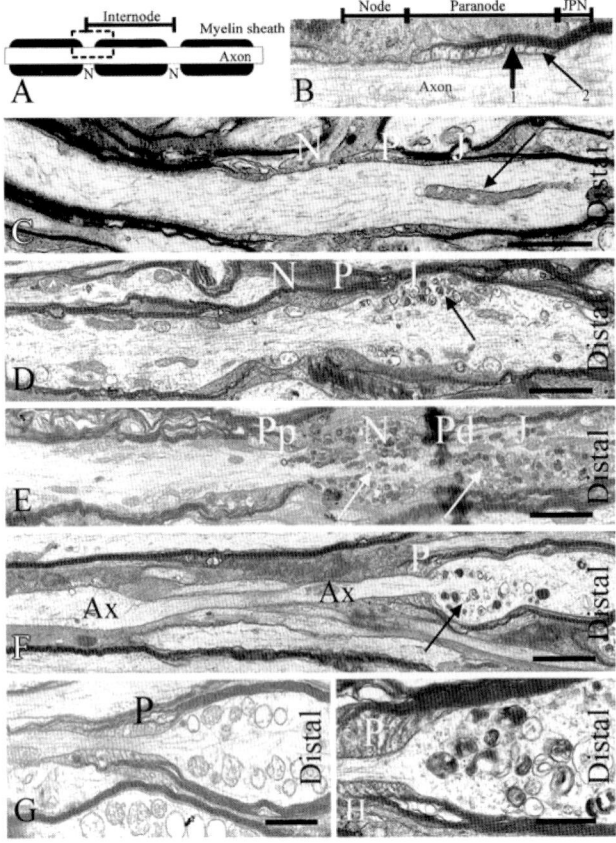

Figure 1 Axonal swelling and degeneration in mice lacking PLP/DM20. Membranous organelles accumulate preferentially distal to the nodal complex in optic nerve axons of PLP/DM20-deficient mice. (**A**) Schematic showing the axon and surrounding myelin sheath. The length of axon myelinated by a single oligodendrocyte process is termed the *internode* and terminates at the nodes of Ranvier (N). (**B**) The boxed area from **A** is shown in detail. The node of Ranvier is abutted by the paranode, the region at which the terminal loops of individual myelin lamellae (*arrow 1*) appose the axolemma in an orderly manner. The juxtaparanode (JPN) is the region between the paranode and the internode. The paranodal axoglial junction (*arrow 2*) is a highly specialized intercellular junction. (**C**) Wild-type axon showing a nodal complex. The node (N), paranode (P), and juxtaparanodal (J) regions are indicated, as is the distal (chiasmal) side. An axonal mitochondrion is evident (*arrow*). Bar 2 μm. (**D**) In this and subsequent images the axons are from PLP null mice. A small accumulation of dense bodies and mitochondria (*arrow*) are present at the distal juxtaparanode (J). The proximal juxtaparanode and internode contain several nonclustered mitochondria, which is slightly in excess of the maximum number observed in wild-type axons. However, there is a distinct difference between proximal and distal regions. Bar 2 μm. (**E**) In this example the accumulated dense bodies and mitochondria occupy the distal internode, juxtaparanode (J), and paranode (Pd), and have also extended into the nodal (N) region; the proximal paranode (Pp) remains unaffected. Bar 2 μm. (**F**) A proportion of optic nerve axons in PLP null mice have nonmyelinated regions interposed between myelinated internodes. In this example, the proximal axon (Ax) is unmyelinated, whereas the distal axon is myelinated. A heminode with its paranode (P) is present. A collection of organelles, predominantly dense bodies (*arrow*), is present distal to the paranode, whereas no accumulation is present proximally. Bar 2 μm. (**G**) The distal aspect of a nodal complex is shown with the paranode (P) marked. The distal axon contains a small accumulation of mitochondria. Bar, 1 μm. (**H**) Another axon shows accumulation of dense bodies distal to the paranode (P). Bar 1 μm. (Reproduced from Edgar et al., *The Journal of Cell Biology* 2004, **166**:121–131 by copyright permission of The Rockefeller University Press.)

incisures (Trapp et al., 1988), but it is absent from compact myelin. CNP is maintained in mature oligodendrocytes throughout life. By immunoelectron microscopy, the *CNP* gene is also expressed at a low level outside the nervous system, including a subset of immune cells, photoreceptor cells, and in testis (Giulian and Moore, 1980; Sprinkle et al., 1985; Scherer et al., 1994).

CNP transcripts encode two protein isoforms (46 kDa and 48 kDa) (Scherer et al., 1994; O'Neill et al., 1997) that are isoprenylated at the carboxyl-terminus for efficient association with cellular membranes (Agrawal et al., 1990; Braun et al., 1991). The CNP biochemical substrates (2′,3′-cyclic nucleotides) are not present in brain, leaving the enzyme activity puzzling, because they are known only as intermediates of RNA metabolism (Heaton and Eckstein, 1996). It has been suggested that CNP interacts with mitochondria and cytoskeletal proteins, and serves as a membrane anchor for tubulin (McFerran and Burgoyne, 1997; Laezza et al., 1997; Bifulco et al., 2002), although the normal cellular function of this protein remains unclear. Overexpression on CNP in transgenic mice causes myelin abormalities (Gravel et al., 1996; Yin et al., 1997). However, targeted disruption of CNP function by homologous recombination failed to unequivocally reveal the cellular function of CNP for myelination. Mutant animals show no major myelin abnormality during the first 4 months of age. The protein and lipid composition of purified myelin membranes reveal no difference, except for the lack of CNP. By electron microscopy and light microscopy, the amount and ultrastructure of CNS myelin are initially normal (Lappe-Siefke et al., 2003).

The lack of CNP from myelin, however, eventually manifests as a severe neurodegenerative disorder with premature death and similar features as described for PLP null mutants. Whereas 3-month-old CNP-deficient mice are indistinguishable in motor behavior from wild-type littermates, at about 4 months, many mutants develop ataxia and visible hind-limb impairments. At 6 months, many mutants are unable to grasp a horizontal bar and balance on top of it. Frequently, mice have convulsions, for example, when lifted at their tails. This late phenotype is associated with muscle weakness, weight loss, and kyphosis. Premature death occurs at 7 to 14 months (Lappe-Siefke et al., 2003).

On Nissl-stained sections, CNP-deficient mice reveal a reduction of overall brain size in combination with enlarged ventricles (hydrocephalus), indicating underlying neurodegenerative changes (Fig. 2). Indeed, myelinated axons are visibly lost in the upper layers of the mutant cortex. Antibodies against the amyloid precursor protein reveal axonal swellings in the corpus callosum and in the lumbar spinal cord (Lappe-Siefke et al., 2003). At the electron microscopic level, axonal swellings are filled with microtubules, dense bodies, multivesicular bodies, and mitochondria. Myelin sheaths are generally preserved over small axonal swellings, but become attenuated through slippage

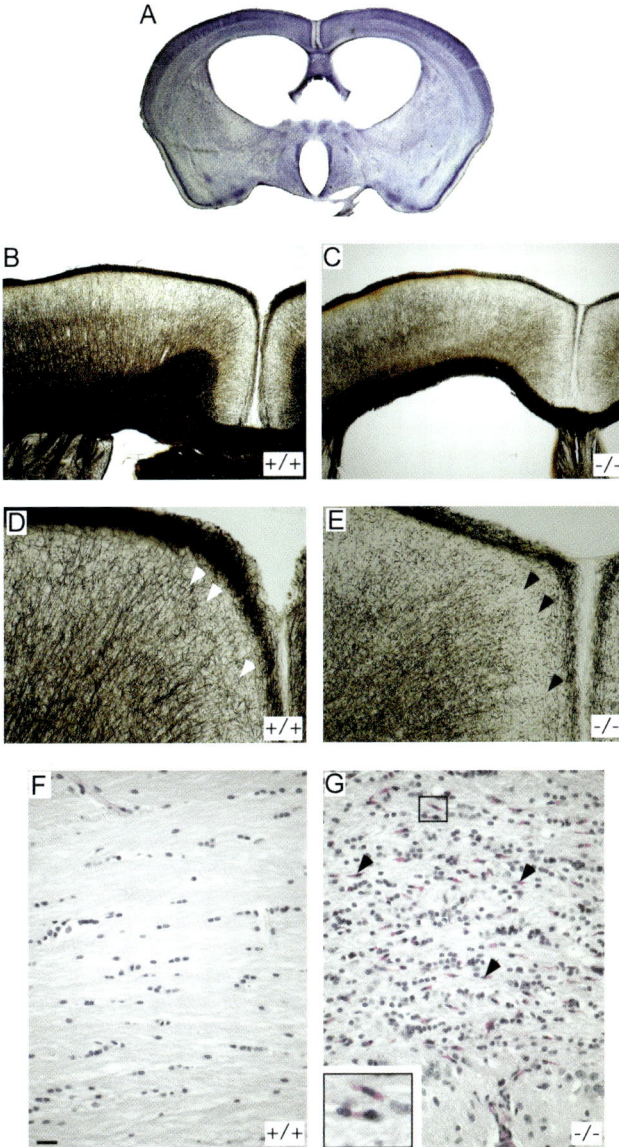

Figure 2 Neurodegeneration and hydrocephalus in mice lacking CNP. (A–E) Brain sections from CNP1 mutants and wild-type mice (age, 12 months), Nissl-stained (A) and Gallyas-impregnated to show myelin (B–E). The severely affected CNP1 mutant mouse brain (C, E) had enlarged ventricles and a reduced thickness in cortical gray and subcortical white matter (corpus callosum). Many myelinated fibers within the cortex seemed to have degenerated (*arrowheads*, E) compared with the equivalent layers of wild-type cortices (*arrowheads*, D). (F, G) PAS reaction on brain paraffin sections prepared from wild-type (F) and homozygous mutant (G) brains (corpus callosum; age, 14 mo). Many cells that accumulated PAS-positive material (*arrowheads*, G and *inset enlargement*) showed phagocytic activity, an indirect sign of neurodegeneration. Cell density was increased in this area, as the thickness of the corpus callosum was reduced. Bar 20 μm. (Reproduced from Lappe-Siefke et al., *Nature Genetics* 2003, **33**: 366–374 by copyright permission of Nature Publishing Group.)

when swellings enlarge at the nodal region, similar to the situation in PLP-null mutant mice. The periodicity of myelin itself is always maintained, and its physical stability appears

not to be compromised. The ultrastructure of paranodes, in which CNP is normally localized, is initially normal but may change as the animal ages. The inner adaxonal tongue is sometimes enlarged, but the relevance of this finding is unclear.

As expected, the axonal swellings are followed by wallerian degeneration and are accompanied by strong activation of microglial cells and reactive astrogliosis, but no inflammation. Astrogliosis is more prominent in the corpus callosum, whereas reactive microglia are increased most in cerebellum. Compared to the subcortical white matter, gliosis is less pronounced in the spinal cord. The reason for this regional heterogeneity is not known.

Taken together, CNP-mutant mice demonstrate more clearly than PLP mutants that two functions of oligodendrocytes, CNS myelin assembly and long-term axonal preservation, can be genetically uncoupled.

V. An Ancestral Glial Function in Axonal Support?

Mouse mutants with inherited defects of oligodendrocyte and Schwann cell function provide *in vivo* evidence that myelin-forming glial cells contribute to long-term axonal integrity. Loss of this supportive function in mice can occur even in the presence of intact myelin, as measured by rapid impulse propagation and the physical stability of myelin itself. Thus, glial support of myelinated axons emerges as a principal function of myelin-forming glial cells.

Oligodendroglial support of axonal integrity throughout adult life is relevant for any demyelinating disease. Axonal loss occurs in MS, but the causal relationship of acute inflammation, chronic demyelination, and axonal loss is difficult to solve. PLP or CNP-null mice show that progressive axonal loss can be caused by local dysfunction of oligodendrocytes in the absence of overt inflammation and demyelination. The molecular nature of this supportive function remains to be determined. Myelination itself appears to trigger this mutual dependency, as normally unmyelinated axons remain intact in the absence of glial support.

These considerations suggest that in human MS lesions, the widespread loss of myelin and functional oligodendrocytes contributes to the described axonal pathology, including wallerian degeneration and persistent clinical disabilities. At least at later stages of the disease, the axonal pathology described in chronic demyelinated lesions (Bitsch et al., 2000; Bjartmar and Trapp, 2003) may correspond to the neuropathology of mouse mutants with noninflammatory myelin defects.

In several vertebrate species, the ensheathment of axons that emanates from retinal ganglion cells is by loose myelin (Easter et al., 1984; Fujita et al., 2001). These sheaths are ultrastructurally similar to myelin in some of the mutants described here and may represent a link between ensheathments by myelinating and nonmyelinating glia.

If glial cells provide local axonal support independent of the elaboration of myelin, this interaction may reflect a primary function of glial cells in vertebrate evolution. Although it is possible that myelinating glial cells have adopted a secondary support function for axons, it seems more reasonable to assume that the evolution of myelin in early vertebrates (Witkovsky, 1971; Agrawal et al., 1971; Bullock et al., 1984) was a recruitment of glial cells already functionally associated with axons (similar to non-myelinforming Schwann cells), possibly to provide long-term axonal support.

References

Adlkofer, K., Martini, R., Aguzzi, A., Zielasek, J., Toyka, K. V., and Suter, U. (1995). Hypermyelination and demyelinating peripheral neuropathy in Pmp22-deficient mice. *Nat. Genet.* **11(3)**, 274–280.

Agrawal, H. C., Banik, N. L., Bone, A. H., Cuzner, M. L., Davison, A. N., and Mitchell, R. F. (1971). The chemical composition of dogfish myelin. *Biochem. J.* **124(5)**, 70P.

Agrawal, H. C., Sprinkle, T. J., and Agrawal, D. (1990). 2′,3′-cyclic nucleotide-3′-phosphodiesterase in the central nervous system is fatty-acylated by thioester linkage. *J. Biol. Chem.* **265(20)**, 11849–11853.

Aguayo, A. J., Attiwell, M., Trecarten, J., Perkins, S., and Bray, G. M. (1977). Abnormal myelination in transplanted Trembler mouse Schwann cells. *Nature* **265(5589)**, 73–75.

Anderson, T. J., Montague, P., Nadon, N., Nave, K. A., and Griffiths, I. R. (1997). Modification of Schwann cell phenotype with Plp transgenes: Evidence that the PLP and DM20 isoproteins are targeted to different cellular domains. *J. Neurosci. Res.* **50(1)**, 13–22.

Anderson, T. J., Schneider, A., Barrie, J. A., Klugmann, M., McCulloch, M. C., Kirkham, D., Kyriakides, E., Nave, K. A., and Griffiths, I. R. (1998). Late-onset neurodegeneration in mice with increased dosage of the proteolipid protein gene. *J. Comp. Neurol.* **394(4)**, 506–519.

Bifulco, M., Laezza, C., Stingo, S., and Wolff, J. (2002). 2′,3′-Cyclic nucleotide 3′-phosphodiesterase: a membrane-bound, microtubule-associated protein and membrane anchor for tubulin. *Proc. Natl. Acad. Sci. U. S. A.* **99(4)**, 1807–1812.

Bitsch, A., Schuchardt, J., Bunkowski, S., Kuhlmann, T., and Bruck, W. (2000). Axonal injury in multiple sclerosis. Correlation with demyelination and inflammation. *Brain* **123 (Pt 6)**, 1174–1183.

Bjartmar, C., and Trapp, B. D. (2003). Axonal degeneration and progressive neurologic disability in multiple sclerosis. *Neurotox. Res.* **5(1-2)**, 157–164.

Bjartmar, C., Wujek, J. R., and Trapp, B. D. (2003). Axonal loss in the pathology of MS: Consequences for understanding the progressive phase of the disease. Review. *J. Neurol. Sci.* **206(2)**, 165–171.

Boison, D., and Stoffel, W. (1994). Related Articles, Links Free in PMC Disruption of the compacted myelin sheath of axons of the central nervous system in proteolipid protein-deficient mice. *Proc. Natl. Acad. Sci. U. S. A.* **91(24)**, 11709–11713.

Braun, P. E., De Angelis, D., Shtybel, W. W., and Bernier, L. (1991). Isoprenoid modification permits 2′,3′-cyclic nucleotide 3′-phosphodiesterase to bind to membranes. *J. Neurosci. Res.* **30(3)**, 540–544.

Bullock, T. H., Moore, J. K., and Fields, R. D. (1984). Evolution of myelin sheaths: Both lamprey and hagfish lack myelin. *Neurosci. Lett.* **48(2)**, 145–148.

Carenini, S., Montag, D., Cremer, H., Schachner, M., and Martini, R. (1997). Absence of the myelin-associated glycoprotein (MAG) and the neural cell adhesion molecule (N-CAM) interferes with the mainte-

nance, but not with the formation of peripheral myelin. *Cell Tissue Res.* **287(1)**, 3–9.

Carroll, S. L., Miller, M. L., Frohnert, P. W., Kim, S. S., and Corbett, J. A. (1997). Expression of neuregulins and their putative receptors, ErbB2 and ErbB3, is induced during Wallerian degeneration. *J. Neurosci.* **17(5)**, 1642–1659.

Chen, S., Rio, C., Ji, R. R., Dikkes, P., Coggeshall, R. E., Woolf, C. J., and Corfas, G. (2003). Disruption of ErbB receptor signaling in adult non-myelinating Schwann cells causes progressive sensory loss. *Nat. Neurosci.* **6(11)**, 1186–1193.

Dashiell, S. M., Tanner, S. L., Pant, H. C., and Quarles, R. H. (2002). Myelin-associated glycoprotein modulates expression and phosphorylation of neuronal cytoskeletal elements and their associated kinases. *J. Neurochem.* **81(6)**, 1263–1272.

de Waegh, S., and Brady, S. T. (1990). Altered slow axonal transport and regeneration in a myelin-deficient mutant mouse: the trembler as an in vivo model for Schwann cell-axon interactions. *J. Neurosci.* **10(6)**, 1855–1865.

de Waegh, S. M., and Brady, S. T. (1991). Local control of axonal properties by Schwann cells: Neurofilaments and axonal transport in homologous and heterologous nerve grafts. *J. Neurosci. Res.* **30(1)**, 201–212.

de Waegh, S. M., Lee, V. M., and Brady, S. T. (1992). Local modulation of neurofilament phosphorylation, axonal caliber, and slow axonal transport by myelinating Schwann cells. *Cell* **68(3)**, 451–463.

Duncan, I. D., Hammang, J. P., Goda, S., and Quarles, R. H. (1989). Myelination in the jimpy mouse in the absence of proteolipid protein. *Glia* **2(3)**, 148–154.

Easter, S. S., Jr., Bratton, B., and Scherer, S. S. (1984). Growth-related order of the retinal fiber layer in goldfish. *J. Neurosci.* **4(8)**, 2173–2190.

Edgar, J. M., McLaughlin, M., Yool, D., Zhang, S. C., Fowler, J. H., Montague, P., Barrie, J. A., McCulloch, M. C., Duncan, I. D., Garbern, J., Nave, K. A., and Griffiths, I. R. (2004). Oligodendroglial modulation of fast axonal transport in a mouse model of hereditary spastic paraplegia. *J. Cell Biol.* **166(1)**, 121–131.

Falconer, D. S., and Sierts-Roth, U. (1951). Dreher, a new gene of the waltzer-shaker group in the house mouse. *Z. Indukt. Abstamm. Vererbungsl.* **84(2)**, 71–73.

Fanarraga, M. L., Sommer, I. U., Griffiths, I. R., Montague, P., Groome, N. P., Nave, K. A., Schneider, A., Brophy, P. J., and Kennedy, P. G. (1993). Oligodendrocyte development and differentiation in the rumpshaker mutation. *Glia* **9(2)**, 146–156.

Ferguson, B., Matyszak, M. K., Esiri, M. M., and Perry, V. H. (1997). Axonal damage in acute multiple sclerosis lesions. *Brain* **120 (Pt 3)**, 393–399.

Frei, R., Motzing, S., Kinkelin, I., Schachner, M., Koltzenburg, M., and Martini, R. (1999). Loss of distal axons and sensory Merkel cells and features indicative of muscle denervation in hindlimbs of P0-deficient mice. *J. Neurosci.* **19(14)**, 6058–6067

Friede, R. L., and Bischhausen, R. (1982). How are sheath dimensions affected by axon caliber and internode length? *Brain Res.* **235(2)**, 335–350.

Fruttiger, M., Montag, D., Schachner, M., and Martini, R. (1995). Crucial role for the myelin-associated glycoprotein in the maintenance of axon-myelin integrity. *Eur. J. Neurosci.* **7(3)**, 511–515.

Fujita, Y., Imagawa, T., and Uehara, M. (2001). Fine structure of the retino-optic nerve junction in the chicken. *Tissue Cell.* **33(2)**, 129–134.

Gale, A. N., Gomez, S., and Duchen, L. W. (1982). Changes produced by a hypomyelinating neuropathy in muscle and its innervation. Morphological and physiological studies in the Trembler mouse. *Brain* **105 (Pt 2)**, 373–393.

Garbern, J. Y., Cambi, F., Tang, X. M., Sima, A. A., Vallat, J. M., Bosch, E. P., Lewis, R., Shy, M., Sohi, J., Kraft, G., Chen, K. L., Joshi, I., Leonard, D. G., Johnson, W., Raskind, W., Dlouhy, S. R., Pratt, V., Hodes, M E., Bird, T., and Kamholz, J. (1997). Proteolipid protein is necessary in peripheral as well as central myelin. *Neuron* **19(1)**, 205–218.

Garbern, J. Y., Yool, D. A., Moore, G. J., Wilds, I. B., Faulk, M. W., Klugmann, M., Nave, K. A., Sistermans, E. A., van der Knaap, M. S., Bird, T. D., Shy, M. E., Kamholz, J. A., and Griffiths, I. R. (2002). Patients lacking the major CNS myelin protein, proteolipid protein 1, develop length-dependent axonal degeneration in the absence of demyelination and inflammation. *Brain* **125 (Pt 3)**, 551–561.

Giese, K. P., Martini, R., Lemke, G., Soriano, P., and Schachner, M. (1992). Mouse P0 gene disruption leads to hypomyelination, abnormal expression of recognition molecules, and degeneration of myelin and axons. *Cell* **71(4)**, 565–76.

Giulian, D., and Moore, S. (1980). Identification of 2′:3′-cyclic nucleotide 3′-phosphodiesterase in the vertebrate retina. *J. Biol. Chem.* **255(13)**, 5993–5995.

Gow, A., and Lazzarini, R. A. (1996). A cellular mechanism governing the severity of Pelizaeus-Merzbacher disease. *Nat. Genet.* **13(4)**, 422–428.

Gravel, M., Peterson, J., Yong, V. W., Kottis, V., Trapp, B., and Braun P. E. (1996). Overexpression of 2′,3′-cyclic nucleotide 3′-phosphodiesterase in transgenic mice alters oligodendrocyte development and produces aberrant myelination. *Mol. Cell Neurosci.* **7(6)**, 453–466.

Greer, J. M., and Lees, M. B. (2002). Myelin proteolipid protein: the first 50 years. Review. *Int. J. Biochem. Cell Biol.* **34(3)**, 211–215.

Griffiths, I., Klugmann, M., Anderson, T., Thomson, C., Vouyiouklis, D., and Nave, K. A. Current concepts of PLP and its role in the nervous system. Review. *Microsc. Res. Tech.* **41(5)**, 344–358.

Griffiths, I., Klugmann, M., Anderson, T., Yool, D., Thomson, C., Schwab, M. H., Schneider, A., Zimmermann, F., McCulloch, M., Nadon, N., and Nave, K. A. (1998). Swellings and degeneration in mice lacking the major proteolipid of myelin. *Science* **280(5369)**, 1610–1613.

Guenard, V., Montag, D., Schachner, M., and Martini, R. (1996). Onion bulb cells in mice deficient for myelin genes share molecular properties with immature, differentiated non-myelinating, and denervated Schwann cells. *Glia* **18(1)**, 27–38.

Heaton, P. A., and Eckstein, F. (1996). Diastereomeric specificity of 2′,3′-cyclic nucleotide 3′-phosphodiesterase. *Nucleic Acids Res.* **24(5)**, 850–853.

Henry, E. W., and Sidman, R. L. (1988). Long lives for homozygous trembler mutant mice despite virtual absence of peripheral nerve myelin. *Science* **241(4863)**, 344–346.

Hildebrand, C., Bowe, C. M., and Remahl, I. N. (1994). Myelination and myelin sheath remodelling in normal and pathological PNS nerve fibres. Review. *Prog. Neurobiol.* **43(2)**, 85–141.

Hildebrand, C., Remahl, S., Persson, H., and Bjartmar, C. (1993). Myelinated nerve fibres in the CNS. Review. *Prog. Neurobiol.* **40(3)**, 319–384.

Hirano, A., Sax, D. S., and Zimmerman, H. M. (1969). The fine structure of the cerebella of jimpy mice and their "normal" litter mates. *J. Neuropathol. Exp. Neurol.* **28(3)**, 388–400.

Hudson, L. D., Berndt, J. A., Puckett, C., Kozak, C. A., and Lazzarini, R. A. (1987). Aberrant splicing of proteolipid protein mRNA in the dysmyelinating jimpy mutant mouse. *Proc. Natl. Acad. Sci. U. S. A.* **84(5)**, 1454–1458

Huxley, C., Passage, E., Manson, A., Putzu, G., Figarella-Branger, D., Pellissier, J. F., and Fontes, M. (1996). Construction of a mouse model of Charcot-Marie-Tooth disease type 1A by pronuclear injection of human YAC DNA. *Hum. Mol. Genet.* **5(5)**, 563–9.

Isaacs, A. M., Davies, K. E., Hunter, A. J., Nolan, P. M., Vizor, L., Peters, J., Gale, D. G., Kelsell, D. P., Latham, I. D., Chase, J. M., Fisher, E. M., Bouzyk, M. M., Potter, A., Masih, M., Walsh, F. S., Sims, M. A., Doncaster, K. E., Parsons, C. A., Martin, J., Brown, S. D., Rastan, S., Spurr, N. K., and Gray, I. C. (2000). Identification of two new Pmp22 mouse mutants using large-scale mutagenesis and a novel rapid mapping strategy. *Hum. Mol. Genet.* **9(12)**, 1865–1871.

Jessen, K. R., Brennan, A., Morgan, L., Mirsky, R., Kent, A., Hashimoto, Y., and Gavrilovic, J. (1994). The Schwann cell precursor and its fate: a study of cell death and differentiation during gliogenesis in rat embryonic nerves. *Neuron* **12(3)**, 509–527.

Jung, M., Sommer, I., Schachner, M., and Nave, K. A. (1996). Monoclonal antibody O10 defines a conformationally sensitive cell-surface epitope of proteolipid protein (PLP): Evidence that PLP misfolding underlies dysmyelination in mutant mice. *J. Neurosci.* **16(24)**, 7920–7929.

Karthigasan, J., Evans, E. L., Vouyiouklis, D. A., Inouye, H., Borenshteyn, N., Ramamurthy, G. V., and Kirschner, D. A. (1996). Effects of rumpshaker mutation on CNS myelin composition and structure. *J. Neurochem.* **66(1)**, 338–345.

Klugmann, M., Schwab, M. H., Puhlhofer, A., Schneider, A., Zimmermann, F., Griffiths, I. R., and Nave, K. A. (1997). Assembly of CNS myelin in the absence of proteolipid protein. *Neuron* **18(1)**, 59–70.

Knapp, P. E., Bartlett, W. P., Williams, L A., Yamada, M., Ikenaka, K., and Skoff, R. P. (1999). Programmed cell death without DNA fragmentation in the jimpy mouse: secreted factors can enhance survival. *Cell Death Differ.* **6(2)**, 136–145.

Kobayashi, H., Hoffman, E. P., and Marks, H. G. (1994). The rumpshaker mutation in spastic paraplegia. *Nat. Genet.* **7(3)**, 351–352.

Koeppen, A. H., and Robitaille, Y. (2002). Pelizaeus-Merzbacher disease. Review. *J. Neuropathol. Exp. Neurol.* **61(9)**, 747–759.

Laezza, C., Wolff, J., and Bifulco, M. (1997). Identification of a 48-kDa prenylated protein that associates with microtubules as 2′,3′-cyclic nucleotide 3′-phosphodiesterase in FRTL-5 cells. *FEBS Lett.* **413(2)**, 260–4.

Lappe-Siefke, C., Goebbels, S., Gravel, M., Nicksch, E., Lee, J., Braun, P. E., Griffiths, I. R., and Nave, K. A. (2003). Disruption of Cnp1 uncouples oligodendroglial functions in axonal support and myelination. *Nat. Genet.* **33**, 366–374.

Lassmann, H., Bartsch, U., Montag, D., and Schachner, M. (1997). Dyingback oligodendrogliopathy: a late sequel of myelin-associated glycoprotein deficiency. *Glia* **19(2)**, 104–110.

Li, C., Tropak, M. B., Gerlai, R., Clapoff, S., Abramow-Newerly, W., Trapp, B., Peterson, A., and Roder, J. (1994). Myelination in the absence of myelin-associated glycoprotein. *Nature* **369(6483)**, 747–750.

Magyar, J. P., Martini, R., Ruelicke, T., Aguzzi, A., Adlkofer, K., Dembic, Z., Zielasek, J., Toyka, K. V., and Suter, U. (1996). Impaired differentiation of Schwann cells in transgenic mice with increased PMP22 gene dosage. *J. Neurosci.* **16(17)**, 5351–5360.

Maier, M., Berger, P., and Suter, U. (2002). Understanding Schwann cell-neurone interactions: The key to Charcot-Marie-Tooth disease? Review. *J. Anat.* **200(4)**, 357–366.

Martini, R., Zielasek, J., Toyka, K. V., Giese, K. P., and Schachner, M. (1995). Protein zero (P0)-deficient mice show myelin degeneration in peripheral nerves characteristic of inherited human neuropathies. *Nat. Genet.* **11(3)**, 281–286.

McFerran, B., and Burgoyne, R. (1997). 2′,3′-Cyclic nucleotide 3′-phosphodiesterase is associated with mitochondria in diverse adrenal cell types. *J. Cell Sci.* **110 (Pt 23)**, 2979–2985.

McLaughlin, M., Hunter, D. J., Thomson, C. E., Yool, D., Kirkham, D., Freer, A. A., and Griffiths, I. R. (2002). Evidence for possible interactions between PLP and DM20 within the myelin sheath. *Glia* **39(1)**, 31–36.

Meier, C., and Bischoff, A. (1974). Dysmyelination in "jimpy" mouse. Electron microscopic study. *J. Neuropathol. Exp. Neurol.* **33(3)**, 343–353.

Meier, C., and Bischoff, A. (1975). Oligodendroglial cell development in jimpy mice and controls. An electron-microscopic study in the optic nerve. *J. Neurol. Sci.* **26(4)**, 517–528.

Meier, C., Herschkowitz, N., and Bischoff, A. (1974). Morphological and biochemical observations in the Jimpy spinal cord. *Acta Neuropathol. (Berl.).* **27(4)**, 349–362.

Milner, R. J., Lai, C., Nave, K. A., Lenoir, D., Ogata, J., and Sutcliffe, J. G. (1985). Nucleotide sequences of two mRNAs for rat brain myelin proteolipid protein. *Cell* **42(3)**, 931–939.

Montag, D., Giese, K. P., Bartsch, U., Martini, R., Lang, Y., Bluthmann, H., Karthigasan, J., Kirschner, D. A., Wintergerst, E. S., Nave, K. A., et al. (1994). Mice deficient for the myelin-associated glycoprotein show subtle abnormalities in myelin. *Neuron* **13(1)**, 229–246.

Muller, H. W. (2000). Tetraspan myelin protein PMP22 and demyelinating peripheral neuropathies: New facts and hypotheses. Review. *Glia* **29(2)**, 182–185.

Naef, R., and Suter, U. (1998). Facets of the peripheral myelin protein PMP22 in myelination and disease. Review. *Microsc. Res. Tech.* **41(5)**, 359–371.

Naidu, S., Dlouhy, S. R., Geraghty, M. T., and Hodes, M. E. (1997). A male child with the rumpshaker mutation, X-linked spastic paraplegia/ Pelizaeus-Merzbacher disease and lysinuria. *J. Inherit. Metab. Dis.* **20(6)**, 811–816.

Nave, K. A, Lai, C., Bloom, F. E., and Milner, R. J. (1986). Jimpy mutant mouse: a 74-base deletion in the mRNA for myelin proteolipid protein and evidence for a primary defect in RNA splicing. *Proc. Natl. Acad. Sci. U. S. A.* **83(23)**, 9264–9268.

Neumann, H. (2003). Molecular mechanisms of axonal damage in inflammatory central nervous system diseases. *Curr. Opin. Neurol.* **16(3)**, 267–273.

Niemann, S., Sereda, M. W., Suter, U., Griffiths, I. R., and Nave, K. A. (2000). Uncoupling of myelin assembly and schwann cell differentiation by transgenic overexpression of peripheral myelin protein 22. *J. Neurosci.* **20(11)**, 4120–4128.

O'Neill, R. C., Minuk, J., Cox, M. E., Braun, P. E., and Gravel, M. (1997). CNP2 mRNA directs synthesis of both CNP1 and CNP2 polypeptides. *J. Neurosci. Res.* **50(2)**, 248–257.

Phillips, R. J. (1954). Jimpy, a new totally sexlinked gene in the house mouse. *Z. Indukt. Abstamm. Vererbungsl.* **86(3)**, 322–326.

Popot, J. L., Pham Dinh, D., and Dautigny, A. (1991). Major myelin proteolipid: The 4-alpha-helix topology. *J. Membr. Biol.* **120(3)**, 233–246.

Raff, M. C., Whitmore, A. V., and Finn, J. T. (2002). Axonal self-destruction and neurodegeneration. Review. *Science* **296(5569)**, 868–871.

Readhead, C., Schneider, A., Griffiths, I., and Nave, K. A. (1994). Premature arrest of myelin formation in transgenic mice with increased proteolipid protein gene dosage. *Neuron* **12(3)**, 583–595.

Robertson, A. M., King, R. H., Muddle, J. R., and Thomas, P. K. (1997). Abnormal Schwann cell/axon interactions in the Trembler-J mouse. *J. Anat.* **190 (Pt 3)**, 423–432

Rosenbluth, J., Stoffel, W., and Schiff. R. (1996). Myelin structure in proteolipid protein (PLP)-null mouse spinal cord. *J. Comp. Neurol.* **371(2)**, 336–344.

Samsam, M., Mi, W., Wessig, C., Zielasek, J., Toyka, K. V., Coleman, M. P., and Martini, R. (2003). The Wlds mutation delays robust loss of motor and sensory axons in a genetic model for myelin-related axonopathy. *J. Neurosci.* **23(7)**, 2833–2839.

Sanchez, I., Hassinger, L., Sihag, R. K., Cleveland, D. W., Mohan, P., and Nixon, R. A. (2000). Local control of neurofilament accumulation during radial growth of myelinating axons in vivo. Selective role of site-specific phosphorylation. *J. Cell Biol.* **151(5)**, 1013–1024.

Sancho, S., Magyar, J. P., Aguzzi, A., and Suter1, U. (1999). Distal axonopathy in peripheral nerves of PMP22-mutant mice. *Brain* **122 (Pt 8)**, 1563–1577.

Sancho, S., Young, P., and Suter, U. (2001). Regulation of Schwann cell proliferation and apoptosis in PMP22-deficient mice and mouse models of Charcot-Marie-Tooth disease type 1A. *Brain* **124 (Pt 11)**, 2177–2187.

Sandvig, A., Berry, M., Barrett, L. B., Butt, A., and Logan, A. (2004). Myelin-, reactive glia-, and scar-derived CNS axon growth inhibitors: expression, receptor signaling, and correlation with axon regeneration. Review. *Glia* **46(3)**, 225–251.

Schachner, M., and Bartsch, U. (2000). Multiple functions of the myelin-associated glycoprotein MAG (siglec-4a) in formation and maintenance of myelin. Review. *Glia* **29(2)**, 154–165.

Scherer, S. S., Braun, P. E., Grinspan, J., Collarini, E., Wang, D. Y., and Kamholz, J. (1994). Differential regulation of the 2′,3′-cyclic nucleotide 3′-phosphodiesterase gene during oligodendrocyte development. *Neuron* **12(6)**, 1363–1375.

Schneider, A., Montague, P., Griffiths, I., Fanarraga, M., Kennedy, P., Brophy, P., and Nave, K. A. (1992). Uncoupling of hypomyelination and glial cell death by a mutation in the proteolipid protein gene. *Nature* **358(6389)**, 758–761.

Schneider, A. M., Griffiths, I. R., Readhead, C., and Nave, K. A. (1995). Dominant-negative action of the jimpy mutation in mice complemented with an autosomal transgene for myelin proteolipid protein. *Proc. Natl. Acad. Sci. U. S. A.* **92(10)**, 4447–4451.

Seitelberger, F. , Urbanitz, I., and Nave, K.-A. (1996). Pelizaeus-Merzbacher disease. *In:* "Handbook of Clinical Neurology," Vol. 22 (P. J. Vinken and G. W. Bruyn, Eds.), pp. 559–579. Elsevier Science B.V., Amsterdam.

Sereda, M., Griffiths, I., Puhlhofer, A., Stewart, H., Rossner, M. J., Zimmerman, F., Magyar, J. P., Schneider, A., Hund, E., Meinck, H. M., Suter, U., and Nave, K. A. (1996). A transgenic rat model of Charcot-Marie-Tooth disease. *Neuron* **16(5)**, 1049–1060.

Sereda, M. W., Meyer zu Horste, G., Suter, U., Uzma, N., and Nave, K. A. (2003). Therapeutic administration of progesterone antagonist in a model of Charcot-Marie-Tooth disease (CMT-1A). *Nat. Med.* **9(12)**, 1533–1537.

Sidman, R. L., Dickie, M M., and Appel, S. H. (1964). Mutant mice (QUAKING and JIMPY) with deficient myelination in the central nervous system. *Science* **144**, 309–311.

Simons, M., Kramer, E. M., Thiele, C., Stoffel, W., and Trotter, J. (2000). Assembly of myelin by association of proteolipid protein with cholesterol- and galactosylceramide-rich membrane domains. *J. Cell Biol.* **151(1)**, 143–154.

Skoff, R. P. (1982). Increased proliferation of oligodendrocytes in the hypomyelinated mouse mutant-jimpy. *Brain Res.* **248(1)**, 19–31.

Skoff, R. P. (1995). Programmed cell death in the dysmyelinating mutants. *Brain Pathol.* **5(3)**, 283–288.

Southwood, C. M., Garbern, J., Jiang, W., and Gow, A. (2002). The unfolded protein response modulates disease severity in Pelizaeus-Merzbacher disease. *Neuron* **36(4)**, 585–96.

Sporkel, O., Uschkureit, T., Bussow, H., and Stoffel, W. (2002). Oligodendrocytes expressing exclusively the DM20 isoform of the proteolipid protein gene: myelination and development. *Glia* **37(1)**, 19–30.

Sprinkle, T. J., McMorris, F. A., Yoshino, J., and DeVries, G. H. (1985). Differential expression of 2′:3′-cyclic nucleotide 3′-phosphodiesterase in cultured central, peripheral, and extraneural cells. *Neurochem. Res.* **10(7)**, 919–931.

Starr, R., Attema, B., DeVries, G. H., and Monteiro, M. J. (1996). Neurofilament phosphorylation is modulated by myelination. *J. Neurosci. Res.* **44(4)**, 328–337.

Stecca, B., Southwood, C. M., Gragerov, A., Kelley, K. A., Friedrich, V. L., Jr., and Gow, A. (2000). The evolution of lipophilin genes from invertebrates to tetrapods: DM-20 cannot replace proteolipid protein in CNS myelin. *J. Neurosci.* **20(11)**, 4002–4010.

Stoffel, W., Hillen, H., and Giersiefen, H. (1984). Structure and molecular arrangement of proteolipid protein of central nervous system myelin. *Proc. Natl. Acad. Sci. U. S. A.* **81(16)**, 5012–5016.

Suh, J. G., Ichihara, N., Saigoh, K., Nakabayashi, O., Yamanishi, T., Tanaka, K., Wada, K., and Kikuchi, T. (1997). An in-frame deletion in peripheral myelin protein-22 gene causes hypomyelination and cell death of the Schwann cells in the new Trembler mutant mice. *Neuroscience* **79(3)**, 735–744.

Suter, U., Moskow, J. J., Welcher, A. A., Snipes, G. J., Kosaras, B., Sidman, R. L., Buchberg, A. M., and Shooter, E. M. (1992). A leucine-to-proline mutation in the putative first transmembrane domain of the 22-kDa peripheral myelin protein in the trembler-J mouse. *Proc. Natl. Acad. Sci. U. S. A.* **89(10)**, 4382–4386, 1992.

Suter, U., Welcher, A. A., Ozcelik, T., Snipes, G. J., Kosaras, B., Francke, U., Billings-Gagliardi, S., Sidman, R. L., and Shooter, E. M. (1992). Trembler mouse carries a point mutation in a myelin gene. *Nature* **356(6366),** 241–244.

Tobler, A. R., Notterpek, L., Naef, R., Taylor, V., Suter, U., and Shooter, E. M. (1999). Transport of Trembler-J mutant peripheral myelin protein 22 is blocked in the intermediate compartment and affects the transport of the wild-type protein by direct interaction. *J. Neurosci.* **19(6),** 2027–2036.

Trapp, B. D., Bernier, L., Andrews, S. B., and Colman, D. R. (1988). Cellular and subcellular distribution of 2′,3′-cyclic nucleotide 3′-phosphodiesterase and its mRNA in the rat central nervous system. *J. Neurochem.* **51(3),** 859–868.

Trapp, B. D., Nishiyama, A., Cheng, D., and Macklin, W. (1997). Differentiation and death of premyelinating oligodendrocytes in developing rodent brain. *J. Cell Biol.* **137(2),** 459–468.

Trapp, B. D., Peterson, J., Ransohoff, R. M., Rudick, R., Mork, S., and Bo, L. (1998). Axonal transection in the lesions of multiple sclerosis. *N. Engl. J. Med.* **338(5),** 278–285, 1998.

Vela, J. M., Dalmau, I., Gonzalez, B., and Castellano, B. (1996). The microglial reaction in spinal cords of jimpy mice is related to apoptotic oligodendrocytes. *Brain Res.* **712(1),** 134–142.

Voyvodic, J. T. (1989). Target size regulates calibre and myelination of sympathetic axons. *Nature* **342(6248),** 430–433.

Wahle, S., and Stoffel, W. (1998). Cotranslational integration of myelin proteolipid protein (PLP) into the membrane of endoplasmic reticulum: analysis of topology by glycosylation scanning and protease domain protection assay. *Glia* **24(2),** 226–235.

Warner, L. E., Hilz, M. J., Appel, S. H., Killian, J. M., Kolodry, E. H., Karpati, G., Carpenter, S., Watters, G. V., Wheeler, C., Witt, D., Bodell, A., Nelis, E., Van Broeckhoven, C., and Lupski, J. R. (1996). Clinical phenotypes of different MPZ (P0) mutations may include Charcot-Marie-Tooth type 1B, Dejerine-Sottas, and congenital hypomyelination. *Neuron* **17(3),** 451–460.

Waxman, S. G. (1997). Axon-glia interactions: building a smart nerve fiber. Review. *Curr. Biol.* **7(7),** R406–410.

Waxman, S. G., and Bennett, M. V. L: (1972). Relative conduction velocities of small myelinated and non-myelinated fibers in the central nervous system. *Nat. New Biol.* **238,** 217–219.

Weiss, M. D., Luciano, C. A., and Quarles, R. H. (2001). Nerve conduction abnormalities in aging mice deficient for myelin-associated glycoprotein. *Muscle Nerve* **24(10),** 1380–1387.

Werner, H., Jung, M., Klugmann, M., Sereda, M., Griffiths, I. R., and Nave, K. A. (1998). Mouse models of myelin diseases. Review. *Brain Pathol.* **8(4),** 771–793.

Witkovsky, P. (1971). Synapses made by myelinated fibers running to teleost and elasmobranch retinas. *J. Comp. Neurol.* **142(2),** 205–221.

Wrabetz, L., Feltri, M. L., Quattrini, A., Imperiale, D., Previtali, S., D'Antonio, M., Martini, R., Yin, X., Trapp, B. D., Zhou, L., Chiu, S. Y., and Messing, A. P. (2000). (0) glycoprotein overexpression causes congenital hypomyelination of peripheral nerves. *J. Cell Biol.* **48(5),** 1021–1034.

Yin, X., Crawford, T. O., Griffin, J. W., Tu, P., Lee, V. M., Li, C., Roder, J., and Trapp, B. D. (1998). Myelin-associated glycoprotein is a myelin signal that modulates the caliber of myelinated axons. *J. Neurosci.* **18(6),** 1953–1962.

Yin, X., Peterson, J., Gravel, M., Braun, P. E., and Trapp, B. D. (1997). CNP overexpression induces aberrant oligodendrocyte membranes and inhibits MBP accumulation and myelin compaction. *J. Neurosci. Res.* **50(2),** 238–247.

22

Neuronal Blocking Factors in Demyelinating Diseases

Theodore R. Cummins, Ph.D.
Stephen G. Waxman, M.D., Ph.D.

I. Introduction

It is well established that conduction block resulting from demyelination and axonal degeneration contribute to the production of clinical deficits in experimental models of demyelinating disease and in multiple sclerosis (MS), Guillain-Barré syndrome (GBS), and chronic inflammatory demyelinating polyneuropathy. Clinical observations, however, raise the possibility that other factors may also contribute to the waxing and waning of symptoms in MS and GBS. Rapid clinical fluctuations, in some cases unaccompanied by changes in metabolic status or temperature sufficient to interfere with axonal conduction, are commonly encountered by patients with MS. In patients with GBS, clinical recovery can occur over hours during plasma exchange, a time course that cannot be explained by remyelination. It has been speculated that these rapid changes in neurological status may involve blocking factors that interfere with axonal conduction. A variety of putative blocking factors have been proposed over the last four decades including antibodies, cytokines, small peptides, and nitric oxide. Many of the putative blocking factors that have been investigated are thought to target voltage-gated sodium channels. Although modulation of other channels or membrane proteins might also contribute to block of impulse transmission, most of the work on the role of blocking factors in inflammatory demyelinating diseases has focused on voltage-gated sodium channels; therefore sodium channels are also the main focus of this chapter.

II. Basic Properties of Voltage-Gated Sodium Channels

Voltage-gated sodium channels are transmembrane proteins (Fig. 1A) that are responsible for the rapid depolarization

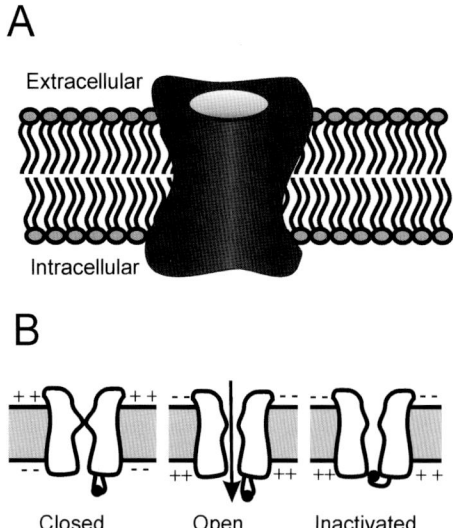

Figure 1 Voltage-gated sodium channels form a pore in the cell membrane of neurons and muscle (**A**). These channels are gated by changes in the membrane potential (**B**). At negative potentials, voltage-gated sodium channels are typically "closed" (*left*). Depolarization produces a conformational change that "opens" the channel and allows ions to traverse the pore (*center*). At depolarized potentials, however, the ionic conductance is rapidly shut down by the action of an intracellular loop that "inactivates" the channel (*right*).

that underlies the upstroke of action potentials in neurons and are thus crucial to nerve impulse conduction. Because of their crucial role in electrogenesis, factors that decrease the activity of voltage-gated sodium channels can have major effects on axonal conduction. Indeed, several different clinically useful drugs that inhibit neuronal excitability, such as local anesthetics and anticonvulsants, act by suppressing the activity of voltage-gated sodium channels. To understand how blocking factors might alter the activity of voltage-gated sodium channels, it is useful to consider that sodium channels are found in one of three basic states or configurations (Fig. 1B). Typically, sodium channels are in a resting or "closed" state in neurons or muscle cells that are at rest (with a membrane potential of approximately −60 to −80 mV). Closed sodium channels do not conduct sodium ions, but are ready to be activated or "opened" when stimulated by membrane depolarization. In the open state, voltage-gated sodium channels form a pore in the cytoplasmic membrane that allows sodium ions to flow into the cell, depolarizing the cell and generating the upstroke of the action potential; however, most sodium channels rapidly transit into the "inactivated" state at depolarized potentials. In the inactivated state, the sodium channel pore is occluded by an inactivation particle from the intracellular side of the channel, thus blocking the flow of sodium ions and contributing to the termination of the action potential.

Several mechanisms by which drugs and other factors can reduce the activity of voltage-gated sodium channels have been identified. Some biological toxins, such as

tetrodotoxin (the toxin found in the puffer fish Fugu), directly block sodium currents by binding in the pore of the channel and preventing the flow of sodium ions through the pore. Lidocaine and several other clinically relevant drugs primarily reduce sodium channel activity by enhancing the "inactivation" process of these channels (Fig. 2). This enhancement of sodium channel inactivation causes the channels to become inactivated at potentials where they would normally be in the closed or resting state, and can be measured by examining the voltage dependence of channel availability. The enhanced inactivation can also contribute to a use-dependent block, where channels that are rapidly and repeatedly activated are more susceptible to inactivation in the presence of the drug. Some of the blocking factors that may be important in inflammatory demyelinating diseases are thought to exert their effects via similar mechanisms. Blocking factors could affect axonal impulse transmission by directly blocking the sodium channel pore (like tetrodotoxin), by enhancing the inactivation process (like lidocaine), or by altering other gating properties of the sodium channels (perhaps preventing the closed-to-open gating transition).

Ten different voltage-gated sodium channel genes have been identified in humans (Nav1.1–Nav1.9 and Nax (Goldin et al., 2000)). Many of these different genes are known to

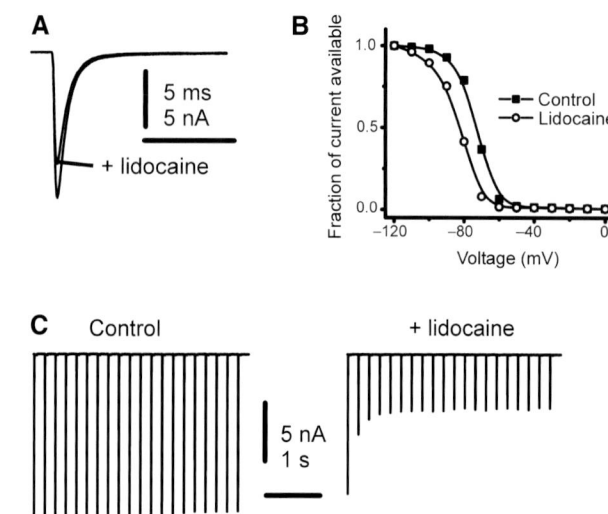

Figure 2 Voltage-gated sodium channels are inhibited by drugs such as lidocaine. (**A**) Lidocaine (500 μM) reduces the amplitude of the peak sodium current amplitude. (**B**) Lidocaine alters the voltage dependence of sodium channel steady-state inactivation and enhances inactivation. This is manifested as a reduction in the fraction of current available for activation at potentials near −80 mV after exposure to lidocaine (*unfilled circles*). (**C**) Lidocaine also induces use-dependent inhibition of sodium currents. Under control conditions (*left*) the peak sodium current amplitude is only slightly reduced during a 5-Hz train of stimulating depolarizations. By contrast, after exposure to lidocaine (*right*), the peak current amplitude substantially decreases during the same stimulation train.

produce voltage-gated sodium channels expressed in neurons; however, not all of these different channels are found in axons. Substantial evidence indicates that the specific isoforms that are present differ between peripheral and central nervous system axons, developing and mature axons, myelinated and unmyelinated axons, normal and injured axons, and myelinated and demyelinated axons. For example, Nav1.6 is the predominant isoform located at nodes of Ranvier in adult axons but Nav1.2 is found in unmyelinated axons and axons undergoing myelination (Kaplan et al., 2001). In an animal model of inflammatory demyelination (Craner et al., 2003) and in human MS (Craner et al., 2004), Nav1.6 protein levels in optic nerve axons decrease and Nav1.2 protein levels increase, indicating that disease processes can alter sodium channel expression and distribution in axons. Altered sodium channel isoform expression could be important in determining the sensitivity of axons to specific blocking factors. For example, Sakurai and colleagues (1992) reported that intravenously administered lidocaine elicited reversible subclinical symptoms in 23 out of 28 patients with MS, but had no effect on 19 control subjects. Demyelinated fibers, with a relatively low density of sodium channels in the demyelinated internodal membrane regions, have low safety factors and thus may be sensitive to conduction block at dosages of lidocaine that do not alter conduction in normal fibers. Alternatively, Nav1.2 and Nav1.6 channels might have differences in their sensitivity to lidocaine that could contribute to the differential block. Regardless of the mechanism that underlies the apparent higher sensitivity of demyelinated fibers to lidocaine, this study clearly demonstrates that endogenous blocking factors, if they indeed do exist, could play important roles in negative symptoms associated with demyelinating disease.

III. Antibodies as Neuroelectric Blocking Factors

Many studies have attempted to determine if factors in the serum or cerebrospinal fluid (CSF) from patients with demyelinating diseases can alter the electrical activity of neurons. During the last 40 years, a number of different studies have suggested that antibodies in serum may act as neuroelectric blocking factors in demyelinating disorders and thus contribute to the clinical symptoms. Although there is substantial evidence to support this idea, however, other studies have challenged the hypothesis that certain antibodies in patients with demyelinating disorders block the electrical activity of neurons; therefore this subject remains controversial. Perhaps the earliest study that proposed a role for antibodies as neuroelectric blocking factors was by Bornstein and Crain (1965). This study reported that serums from animals with experimental autoimmune encephalomyelitis (EAE) and humans with MS induced rapid, yet readily reversible, block

of synaptic activity in cultured mouse cerebral and spinal cord tissue. This block was determined to be heat-labile and complement-dependent, implicating antibodies in the process. Of importance, serum from control individuals did not produce block in this study. However, definitive evidence that antibodies in the serum of patients with demyelinating disorders play a crucial role in the rapid onset and/or recovery of negative symptoms that are often observed has been elusive. Seil et al. (1976) reported that serum from patients with MS and serum from controls showed neuroelectric blocking activity against mouse cortical cultures. Although the degree of block tended to be highly variable, it was concluded that this activity was a nonspecific property of serum that was not related to the pathogenesis of demyelinating disorders. By contrast Schauf et al. (1976, 1978) reported that factors in the serum from patients with MS (but not from controls) were able to inhibit electrical activity in an invertebrate spinal cord preparation and found that the degree of inhibition was closely correlated with the severity of clinical symptoms. The blocking activity of the factors in the MS serum were destroyed by heating and restored by the addition of normal serum and therefore appeared to be antibody mediated. The mechanism by which electrical activity was altered was investigated and, surprisingly, the serum factors blocked transmitter release but not axonal conduction, suggesting that the antibody might be synaptically directed. The specific antibodies and target molecules involved in this synaptic inhibition have not been identified.

Antibodies against GM1 gangliosides may alter axonal conduction by altering sodium channel activity. High titers of antibodies against GM1 ganglioside have been found in many patients with GBS, as well as in patients with lower motor neuron disease and motor neuropathy (Kornberg et al., 1994). Anti-GM1 antibodies exhibited a complement-dependent inhibition of sodium currents in rabbit sciatic nerve (Takigawa et al., 1995), identifying for the first time a specific antibody that inhibited a crucial component of axonal conduction. This result was especially intriguing because GM1 may be localized at the node of Ranvier where sodium channels are clustered along axons (Corbo et al., 1993), suggesting that anti-GM1 antibodies might bind at nodal membrane, where they could block sodium channels and disrupt axonal conduction. A study of conduction in rat ventral roots, however, failed to confirm that anti-GM1 antibody could block nerve conduction or sodium channels (Hirota et al., 1997), raising doubts about the role of this antibody in the conduction block observed in demyelinating diseases. A subsequent study by Arasaki et al. (1998) reported that although anti-GM1 IgG antibodies did not block conduction, anti-GM1 IgM antibodies did. This suggested that differences in the reactivities and complexes that are ultimately formed by IgG and IgM antibodies may underlie the conflicting results reported in the previous studies. Other studies have come down on different sides of the issue, with reports both supporting (Kuwabara et al., 1998; Weber et al., 2000) and arguing against (Benatar et al., 1999) the idea that anti-GM1 antibodies inhibit axonal conduction by blocking voltage-gated sodium channels. The strongest evidence for the role of blocking antibodies in GBS is presented in a study of neonatal GBS (Buchwald et al., 1999). This study showed that antibodies to GM1 were passed from a mother with ongoing GBS to her child. The child developed GBS 12 days postpartum, which, in conjunction with earlier studies implicating GM1 in blockage of neuromuscular transmission (Buchwald et al., 1998), led to speculation that GM1 antibodies were able to bind epitopes in the mature neuromuscular junction. Despite these studies relating to GM1 antibodies and GBS, the role of antibodies as neuroelectric blocking factors in demyelinating diseases remains controversial.

A number of experimental variables could contribute to the disparate findings regarding antibodies and neuroelectric blocking factors. For example, although Schauf and colleagues reported that CSF samples from patients with MS did not exhibit neuroelectric blocking activity in their frog spinal cord preparation, several studies suggested that factors in the CSF from patients with GBS (Brinkmeier et al., 1992b) and MS (Brinkmeier et al., 1993) were able to inhibit mammalian voltage-gated sodium channels. In these latter studies the CSF was tested on sodium currents in myoballs prepared from primary human skeletal muscle cultures. CSF from patients with GBS and MS, but not from control patients, enhanced the inactivation of the skeletal muscle sodium currents. It was proposed that this enhancement of inactivation might impair conduction and contribute to muscle weakness and other neurological abnormalities associated with these disorders.

Because of the tissue and species differences between the various studies, it is difficult to compare results. Subtle differences in the amino-acid sequences of sodium channels in human, rodent, and invertebrate preparations could underlie some of the conflicting results concerning the blocking activity of different factors.

IV. Cytokines as Neuroelectric Blocking Factors

Cytokines, a diverse group of soluble secreted proteins with molecular weights of approximately 8 to 25 kDa, are often found at increased levels in the sera and CSF of patients with demyelinating disorders (Hartung et al., 1991; Hauser et al., 1990) and have also been proposed to play roles in the impairment of axonal conduction in demyelinating disorders. These factors can be secreted by a variety of different cell types, but one important source of cytokines are leukocytes. Cytokines typically bind to specific receptors on the cell surface and induce the activation of second

messenger systems within the target cells. Second messenger systems can modulate the activity of sodium channels (Cantrell and Catterall, 2001) and other ion channels, and thus activation of second-messenger systems by cytokines could alter neuroelectric activity.

Alternatively, cytokines may also act directly on transmembrane proteins such as ion channels. Cytokines were implicated as contributing to adverse symptoms of MS in a study on the effect of CAMPATH-1H treatment (Moreau et al., 1996). In this study transient systemic and neurological adverse effects were observed in 12 of 14 MS patients treated with humanized monoclonal antibody CAMPATH-1H, which depletes lymphocytes. Typically, this was either a worsening of persistent symptoms or reactivation of previous clinical manifestations. Patients who exhibited the transient adverse symptoms exhibited substantial increases in the serum levels of the cytokines interleukin-6 (IL-6), tumor necrosis factor-α (TNF-α), and γ-interferon (IFN-γ). Two patients who received methylprednisolone treatment did not exhibit transient increases in neurological symptoms and did not have elevated cytokines, suggesting that soluble immune mediators might contribute to transient symptoms in MS. Moreau et al. (1996) noted that CAMPATH-1H used in the treatment of rheumatoid arthritis (Isaacs et al., 1992) did not induce adverse neurological effects but did increase TNF-α levels, leading these investigators to propose that circulating cytokines might directly impair conduction by acting on partially demyelinated axons (Smith suggests that pro-inflammatory cytokines may trigger the appearance of inducible nitric oxide synthase with a resultant production of nitric oxide, see Chapter 18). In a subsequent study of 27 patients with MS (Coles et al., 1999) selective blockade of TNF-α failed to prevent the increase or reactivation of transient adverse neurological symptoms induced by CAMPATH-1H, indicating that soluble inflammatory factors other than TNF-α are involved.

Several studies have tried to determine if cytokines might be able to alter sodium channel activity. A study on sodium currents in cultured embryonic rat cortical neurons demonstrated that CSF of patients with MS, but not the CSF of control patients, significantly enhanced the inactivation of the voltage-gated sodium channels in these neurons (Koller et al., 1996). This enhancement of inactivation would be expected to decrease neuronal excitability. To determine if cytokines might be responsible for this effect, Koller and colleagues tested the effects of IL-1β, IL-2, IL-6, and TNF-α on the cultured embryonic rat cortical neurons. None of these cytokines were able to mimic the effect of the CSF from patients with MS. The lack of effect of cytokines on the voltage-gated sodium currents suggests that cytokines do not directly contribute to the transient neurological symptoms seen in patients with MS. Other studies, however, have reported effects of cytokines on voltage-gated sodium currents. IL-2 has been reported to inhibit the voltage-gated sodium currents in cultured human skeletal muscle cells (Brinkmeier et al., 1992a). This effect was not blocked by an anti-IL-2-receptor antibody (Kaspar et al., 1994). This and other evidence indicated that IL-2 acted directly on the sodium channel. Muscle cells express a distinct sodium channel isoform, raising the possibility that only specific sodium channel isoforms might be sensitive to cytokines. A study of NH15-CA2 neuroblastoma x glioma hybrid cells (which express neuronal type sodium currents) indicated that both IL-2 and IL-1β could inhibit some neuronal sodium currents (Hamm et al., 1996). Because neurons can express many different voltage-gated sodium channels and, more important, because we now know that demyelinated axons often express different sodium channels than myelinated axons, it needs to be determined whether cytokines can inhibit sodium currents in demyelinated axons, or at least the specific sodium channel isoforms that are expressed in demyelinated axons. Until this is directly tested, the possibility that cytokines contribute to the block of axonal conduction in demyelinated axons remains an open issue.

V. Small Peptides as Neuroelectric Blocking Factors

For more than a decade, Brinkmeier and colleagues have investigated sodium channel blocking factors in the CSF of patients with MS and GBS (Brinkmeier et al. 1992b, 1993, 1996, 2000; Weber et al., 1999; Aulkmeyer et al., 2000). Their initial studies were interpreted as showing that CSF from patients with GBS and MS, but not control patients, could induce rapid (complete within 5 seconds) and reversible inhibition of voltage-gated sodium currents *in vitro*. The primary mechanism underlying this inhibition of sodium channels appeared to be an enhancement of inactivation, which can be measured as a shift in the steady-state inactivation voltage relationship (Fig. 3). Thus CSF from a patient with GBS reduced the fraction of current that is available for activation from a holding potential of −75 mV from approximately 75% to 20%. As mentioned previously, local anesthetics reduce sodium current amplitudes and cellular excitability by enhancing sodium channel inactivation and inducing negative shifts in the steady-state inactivation voltage relationship. High-performance liquid chromatography analysis of CSF from patients with GBS and MS indicated that the active factor has a molecular weight <1,000 Daltons. This finding was surprising because proteins such as antibodies and cytokines, implicated in previous studies, are much larger than this. One possibility was that a small-peptide molecule might be the active factor. This hypothesis was supported by data showing that the factor was degraded by acid hydrolysis and a carboxypeptidase (Aulkemeyer et al., 2000). Because the factor in the CSF of MS, GBS, and chronic inflammatory demyeli-

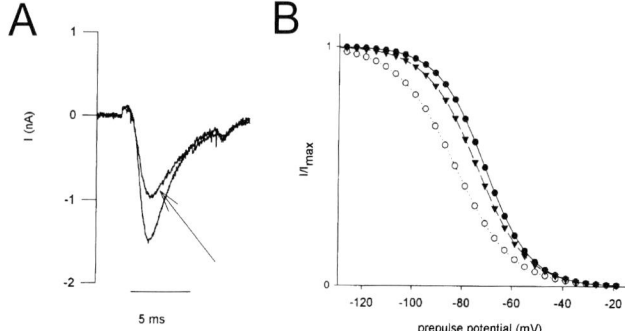

Figure 3 CSF from a patient with GBS inhibits voltage-gated sodium currents in NH15-CA2 cells. (**A**) Sodium currents recorded before and after (*arrow*) exposure to CSF are shown. (**B**) CSF alters the voltage dependence of sodium channel steady-state inactivation. The fraction of current available for activation is reduced at potentials near −80 mV after exposure to CSF (*unfilled circles*). The voltage dependence is similar before (*filled circles*) and after wash-out (*filled triangles*) of CSF. (Reprinted with permission from Weber et al., 1999.)

nating polyneuropathy patients seemed to be similar, Brinkmeier et al. (1996) proposed that demyelination or inflammation might induce production of a small oligopeptide that inhibits sodium channels.

Brinkmeier et al. (2000) reported that a previously unknown endogenous pentapeptide (Gln-Tyr-Asn-Ala-Asp; QYNAD) is present in human CSF. A QYNAD concentration of about 3 μM was measured in the CSF of healthy individuals, but concentrations of 300% to 1,400% higher were measured in the CSF of patients with MS and GBS. Substantial sodium channel blocking activity, associated with a hyperpolarizing shift in the voltage-dependence of inactivation without use dependence, was reported with 10 μM QYNAD, and it was suggested that, at the high concentrations present in the CSF of patients with MS and GBS, QYNAD might contribute to impaired conduction of action potentials along demyelinated axons. Because QYNAD and lidocaine have similar effects on the voltage-dependence of inactivation, it was suggested that QYNAD might be an endogenous lidocaine or endocaine. The initial experiments of Brinkmeier et al. (2000) investigated the effects of QYNAD on sodium currents in NH15-CA2 neuroblastoma x glioma cells. The same authors subsequently reported that QYNAD can block axonal conduction (Weber et al., 2002). These authors also reported that CSF filtration may be an effective treatment for GBS and suggested that reduction in QYNAD levels may contribute to the efficacy of CSF filtration (Wollinsky et al., 2001).

Because block of voltage-gated sodium channels by QYNAD could have important consequences in demyelinating disorders, Cummins et al. (2003) examined whether QYNAD blocked specific sodium channel isoforms. QYNAD was tested against several sodium channel isoforms expressed in mammalian cells, including the major isoforms found in myelinated (Na$_v$1.6) and abnormally myelinated (Na$_v$1.2) axons (Fig. 4A,B). In this study, 10 different batches of QYNAD prepared by four different facilities, including three separate batches from the facility that prepared QYNAD for the original report by Brinkmeier et al. (2000), were tested. QYNAD, tested at concentrations ranging from 10 to 500 μM, had no observable effect on Na$_v$1.2, Na$_v$1.4, Na$_v$1.6, or Na$_v$1.7 sodium channels. To address the possibility that QYNAD interacts with a sodium channel co-factor that is present in neurons but not other cell types, Cummins et al. also tested QYNAD on native sodium currents in acutely dissociated adult hippocampal neurons and in acutely cultured adult dorsal root ganglion neurons. QYNAD (100 μM) again had no effect on the native sodium currents recorded from either hippocampal CA1 neurons

(Fig. 4C) or dorsal root ganglion neurons. Finally, Cummins et al. tested QYNAD for any effects on axonal conduction in an intact central myelinated tract (rat optic nerve, a central tract that is commonly affected in MS). QYNAD failed to show any lidocaine-like effect on axonal conduction. Confirming this initial study, Quasthoff et al. (2003) also did not observe any sodium channel blocking activity with QYNAD. In their study, QYNAD was tested against two isoforms (Nav1.6 and Nav1.8) expressed in *Xenopus* oocytes and against isolated rat sural nerve; 5-minute exposures to QYNAD (10–100 μM) did not inhibit peak sodium currents or alter channel kinetics. Application of 100-μM QYNAD to isolated rat sural nerves *in vitro* for 45 minutes did not induce any detectable change in either A fiber or C fiber compound nerve action potentials in this study.

Although the studies by Cummins et al. (2003) and Quasthoff et al. (2003) raise serious concerns about the ability of QYNAD to block voltage-gated sodium channels, two other studies (Meuth et al., 2003; Padmashri et al., 2004) reported observations that support the hypothesis that QYNAD might modulate voltage-gated sodium currents; however, these studies raise additional questions. Padmashri et al. (2004) examined the effect of QYNAD on recombinant Nav1.2 currents expressed in Chinese hamster ovary cells. They found that prolonged exposure to QYNAD shifted the voltage dependence of inactivation in the negative direction, in a similar fashion to that reported by Brinkmeier et al. However, unlike Brinkmeier et al., they also found that QYNAD induced a major change in the voltage dependence of activation and showed a tendency to promote use-dependent inhibition, modulatory effects that are not consistent with those reported by Brinkmeier et al. Meuth et al. (2003) examined the effect of QYNAD on sodium currents in acutely isolated thalamic neurons *in vitro*. They did not find any effect of QYNAD on sodium channel activation, but reported that seven of nine batches of QYNAD were able to shift the steady-state inactivation of thalamic neuronal sodium currents in the negative direction, with a dose-response curve similar to that reported by Brinkmeier et al. (2000). However, Meuth et al. also reported that experiments carried out in rats with MOG-induced EAE, a model of relapsing and chronic MS, failed to demonstrate an *in vivo* effect of QYNAD. Thus, even if QYNAD is able to exhibit some sodium channel modulatory activity under specific *in vitro* conditions, it is unclear whether this is relevant to demyelinating disorders.

Brinkmeier et al. proposed that QYNAD is part of a larger protein and is generated by the action of an unknown protease. Of interest, Quasthoff et al. (2003) found that the QYNAD motif was conserved in a few mouse proteins, including some ankyrin-like proteins. This is intriguing because ankyrins may interact with voltage-gated sodium channels and play a role in anchoring channels at the nodes of Ranvier (Bennett and Lambert, 1999). Searches of human

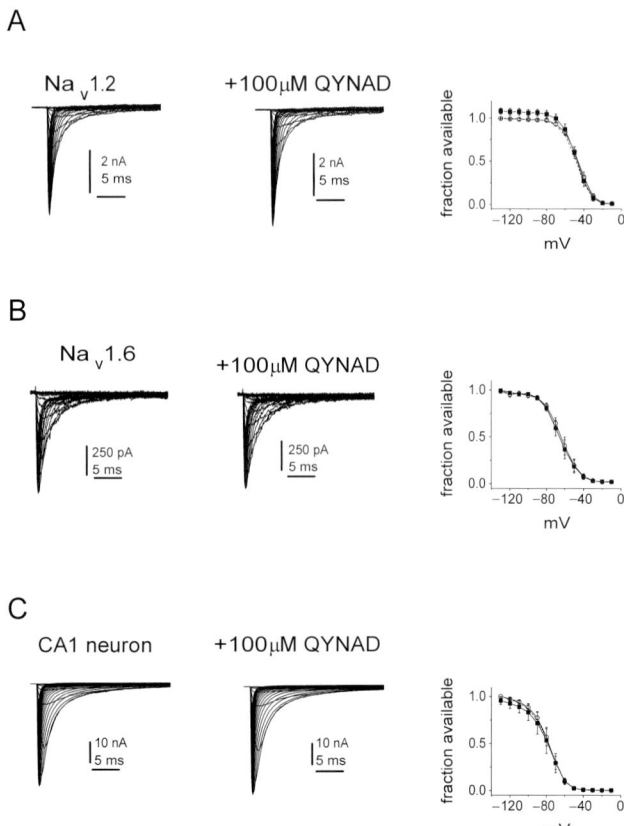

Figure 4 Sodium currents are not inhibited by QYNAD. (**A**) Representative Na$_v$1.2 sodium currents recorded before (*left*) and after 100 μM QYNAD (*center*). QYNAD (100 μM) did not alter the steady-state inactivation curve for Na$_v$1.2 sodium channels (*right*). (**B**) Representative Na$_v$1.6 sodium currents recorded before (*left*) and after 100 μM QYNAD (*center*). QYNAD (100 μM) did not alter the steady-state inactivation curve for Na$_v$1.6 sodium channels (*right*). (**C**) Representative sodium currents in acutely isolated rat hippocampal CA1 neuron currents recorded before (*left*) and after 100 μM QYNAD (*center*). QYNAD (100 μM) did not alter the steady-state inactivation curve for sodium currents in acutely isolated hippocampal CA1 neurons. (Reprinted with permission from Cummins et al., 2003.)

protein libraries, however, have not been successful in identifying the putative human precursor protein (Brinkmeier et al., 2000; Quasthoff et al., 2003; Cummins and Waxman, unpublished observations). Thus, it is also not clear how QYNAD might be generated *in vivo* and why the concentration of QYNAD is increased in the CSF of patients with MS and GBS. Another issue that should be examined is whether QYNAD concentrations in the CSF fluctuate and, if so, whether fluctuations are correlated with clinical status. Until some of these issues regarding the role of QYNAD in demyelinating disorders can be better addressed, the conclusion that QYNAD contributes to negative symptoms in MS and related disorders should be viewed with caution.

VI. Nitric Oxide as a Neuroelectric Blocking Factor

Nitric oxide has also been proposed as a factor that affects nerve conduction in demyelinating diseases (Redford et al., 1997) (see also Chapter 18). Nitric oxide production is significantly increased in inflamed tissue and in demyelinated MS lesions (Bo et al., 1994). The role of nitric oxide in demyelinating diseases is complex (Giovannoni et al., 1998; Parkinson et al., 1997). Nitric oxide can influence the immune response, the permeability of the blood-brain barrier, mitochondrial metabolism, and numerous other processes. Using nitric oxide donors, Redford et al. (1997) showed that nitric oxide could significantly block conduction in axons of the rat spinal cord dorsal column. Demyelinated and early remyelinated axons were much more susceptible to block than normal axons, presumably because conduction is more tenuous in demyelinated axons and more easily blocked. In this study, the mechanism of conduction block was not clear; however, the block was readily reversible.

To better understand how nitric oxide might alter neuronal function, Renganathan et al. (2000, 2001) examined the effects of nitric oxide on sodium currents in sensory neurons (Fig. 5A). These studies showed that nitric oxide donors could induce block of multiple types of voltage-gated sodium currents in sensory neurons. The inhibition was blocked by hemoglobin, a scavenger of nitric oxide, and was readily reversible. The inhibition was not affected by factors that modulate the guanyl cyclase, cGMP, or cGMP-dependent protein kinase, suggesting that the inhibition of sodium currents by nitric oxide was independent of guanyl cyclase and cGMP second-messenger signaling pathways. Alkylation of free thiols with *N*-ethylmaleimide was able to prevent the effect of nitric oxide, suggesting that S-nitrosylation of sodium channels by nitric oxide can block sodium currents in neurons and may contribute to impaired impulse conduction in pathological conditions.

Nitric oxide has also been implicated in degeneration of axons in inflammatory neurological diseases. Smith et al.

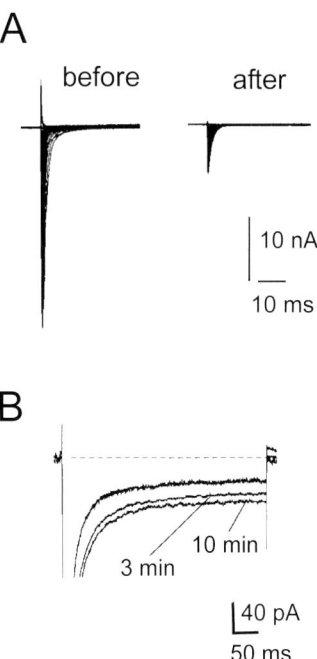

Figure 5 Nitric oxide donors alter neuronal sodium currents. (**A**) Sodium currents in C-type dorsal root ganglion neurons are shown before (*left*) and after (*right*) exposure to a nitric oxide donor. Peak sodium current amplitude is greatly reduced. (Reprinted with permission from Renganathan et al., 2002.) (**B**) Sodium currents in rat hippocampal neurons are shown before and during exposure to a nitric oxide donor. The currents are magnified to focus on the sustained or persistent component. The nitric oxide donor increased the persistent current after 3- and 10-minute exposures. (Reprinted with permission from Hammarstrom and Gage, 1999.)

(2001) reported that rat spinal cord dorsal root axons tend to undergo wallerian degeneration if they are concurrently stimulated and exposed to micromolar concentrations of nitric oxide. Prolonged exposure to nitric oxide has also been shown to damage rat isolated optic nerve (Garthwaite et al., 2002). Sodium channel blockers such as tetrodotoxin and lidocaine were able to protect optic nerve (Garthwaite et al., 2002) and dorsal root (Kapoor et al., 2003) axons from nitric oxide–induced damage. Thus, influx of sodium through voltage-gated sodium channels may contribute to nitric oxide–mediated degeneration of axons. This is somewhat surprising, given that nitric oxide can inhibit peak sodium current amplitudes (Bielefeldt et al., 1999; Li et al., 1998; Renganathan et al., 2001). However, other studies have shown that nitric oxide can also increase persistent sodium currents in muscle and neurons (Hammarstrom and Gage, 1999; Ahern et al., 2000) (Fig. 5B). Increased persistent sodium current could lead to increases in intra-axonal sodium and calcium and subsequent axonal damage. Persistent sodium currents would also be expected to depolarize cells. Depending on the degree of depolarization, this could lead to enhanced excitability or, paradoxically, prolonged depolarization could induce inactivation of normal voltage-gated sodium channels and lead to a depolarization block of impulse conduction. Indeed, prolonged depolarization induced by persistent sodium currents is thought to play a role in the reduction of muscle excitability in some of the periodic paralyses (Cannon, 1996). Nitric oxide may be able to inhibit peak sodium currents under some conditions but increase persistent sodium currents under others. Modulation of sodium currents by nitric oxide could therefore play a role in both acute and chronic impairment of impulse conduction in demyelinating disorders.

VII. Modulation of Other Ionic Currents

Factors that directly affect axonal impulse conduction could also interact with other membrane channels. For example, potassium channels play an important role in setting the resting membrane potential of neurons. Enhancing the activity of specific potassium channels can prevent the depolarization of nerve membrane needed to initiate the generation of action potentials and impulse transmission. On the other hand, reducing the activity of specific potassium channels could lead to prolonged depolarization of nerves, which, as is discussed previously, can induce inactivation of voltage-gated sodium channels, leading to a depolarization block of impulse conduction. Fatty acids can increase the activity of potassium currents (Bendahhou and Agnew, 1996) as well as inhibiting sodium currents (Hong et al., 2004; Vreugdenhil et al., 1996) and could behave as neuroelectric blocking factors. Nitric oxide has also been reported to have affects on ion channels other than sodium channels. Nitric oxide activates large-conductance calcium-activated potassium (BK) channels in pituitary nerve terminals (Ahern et al., 1999). ATP-sensitive potassium (K_{ATP}) channels are also stimulated by nitric oxide (Lin et al., 2004). An increase of BK or K_{ATP} potassium current by nitric oxide is expected to suppress nerve excitability and therefore could also contribute to decreased impulse activity. Nitric oxide may also regulate neuronal activity by modulating calcium channels (Carabelli et al., 2002; D'Ascenzo et al., 2002). Reduction of calcium channel activity by nitric oxide would be expected to reduce neuronal excitability. However, although voltage-gated calcium channels may be expressed on astrocytes and oligodendrocytes in spinal cord white matter, they do not seem to be expressed on axons (Agrawal et al., 2000); therefore it is not clear what role inhibition of these channels might play in modulating axonal conduction.

VIII. Conclusion

Although reports of neuronal blocking factors have attracted considerable attention, subsequent studies have often failed to confirm any specific relationship to demyelinating diseases or a role in their pathophysiology. Identifying the role that putative blocking factors play in MS and other inflammatory diseases is difficult because these disorders alter the intrinsic properties of axonal conduction in complex ways. The architecture and molecular makeup of demyelinated axons are distinctly different from those of normal axons; thus the sensitivity of conduction in these axons to specific factors can be difficult to predict using experimental systems. Despite decades of research into neuroelectric blocking factors, their roles, if any, in producing rapid changes in neurologic status associated with demyelinating diseases remain unclear.

Acknowledgments

Supported in part by grants from the National Multiple Sclerosis Society, the Medical Research Service and Rehabilitation Research Service, Department of Veterans Affairs, the Nancy Davis Foundation, and the Indiana Genomics Initiative. The Center for Neuroscience and Regeneration Research is a Collaboration of the Paralyzed Veterans of America and the United Spinal Association with Yale University.

References

Agrawal, S. K., Nashmi, R., and Fehlings, M. G. (2000). Role of L- and N-type calcium channels in the pathophysiology of traumatic spinal cord white matter injury. *Neuroscience* **99**, 179–188.

Ahern, G. P., Hsu, S. F., and Jackson, M. B. (1999). Direct actions of nitric oxide on rat neurohypophysial K+ channels. *J Physiol.* **520**, 165–176.

Ahern, G. P., Hsu, S. F., Klyachko, V. A., and Jackson, M. B. (2000). Induction of persistent sodium current by exogenous and endogenous nitric oxide. *J. Biol. Chem.* **275**, 28810–28815.

Arasaki, K., Kusunoki, S., Kudo, N., and Tamaki, M. (1998). The pattern of antiganglioside antibody reactivities producing myelinated nerve conduction block in vitro. *J. Neurol. Sci.* **161**,163–168.

Aulkemeyer, P., Hausner, G., Brinkmeier, H., Weber, F., Wurz, A., Heidenreich, F., and Rudel, R. (2000). The small sodium-channel blocking factor in the cerebrospinal fluid of multiple sclerosis patients is probably an oligopeptide. *J. Neurol. Sci.* **172**, 49–54.

Benatar, M., Willison, H. J., and Vincent, A. (1999). Immune-mediated peripheral neuropathies and voltage-gated sodium channels. *Muscle Nerve* **22**, 108–110.

Bendahhou, S., and Agnew, W. S. (1996). Enhancement of the Shaker B delta6-46 current by fatty acids depends on the activation of the lipoxygenase metabolic pathway. *Pflugers Arch.* **432**, 1091–1093.

Bennett, V., and Lambert, S. (1999). Physiological roles of axonal ankyrins in survival of premyelinated axons and localization of voltage-gated sodium channels. *J Neurocytol* **28**, 303–318.

Bielefeldt, K., Whiteis, C. A., Chapleau, M. W., and Abboud, F. M. (1999). Nitric oxide enhances slow inactivation of voltage-dependent sodium currents in rat nodose neurons. *Neurosci. Lett.* **271**, 159–162.

Bo, L., Dawson, T. M., Wesselingh, S., Mork, S., Choi, S., Kong, P. A., Hanley, D., and Trapp, B. D. (1994). Induction of nitric oxide synthase in demyelinating regions of multiple sclerosis brains. *Ann. Neurol.* **36**, 778–786.

Bornstein, M. B., and Crain, S. M. (1965). Functional studies of cultured brain tissues as related to "demyelinative disorders". *Science* **148**, 1242–1244.

Brinkmeier, H., Aulkemeyer, P., Wollinsky, K. H., and Rudel, R. (2000). An endogenous pentapeptide acting as a sodium channel blocker in inflammatory autoimmune disorders of the central nervous system. *Nat. Med.* **6**, 808–811.

Brinkmeier, H., Wollinsky, K. H., Seewald, M. J., Hulser, P. J., Mehrkens, H. H., Kornhuber, H. H., and Rudel, R. (1993). Factors in the cerebrospinal fluid of multiple sclerosis patients interfering with voltage-dependent sodium channels. *Neurosci. Lett.* **156**, 172–175.

Brinkmeier, H., Wollinsky, K. H., Hulser, P. J., Seewald, M. J., Mehrkens, H. H., Kornhuber, H. H., and Rudel, R. (1992b). The acute paralysis in Guillain-Barré syndrome is related to a Na+ channel blocking factor in the cerebrospinal fluid. *Pflugers Arch.* **421**, 552–557.

Brinkmeier, H., Kaspar, A., Wietholter, H., and Rudel, R. (1992a). Interleukin-2 inhibits sodium currents in human muscle cells. *Pflugers Arch.* **420**, 621–623.

Brinkmeier, H., Seewald, M. J., Wollinsky, K. H., and Rudel, R. (1996). On the nature of endogenous antiexcitatory factors in the cerebrospinal fluid of patients with demyelinating neurological disease. *Muscle Nerve* **19**, 54–62.

Buchwald, B., Toyka, K. V., Zielasek, J., Weishaupt, A., Schweiger, S., and Dudel, J. (1998). Neuromuscular blockade by IgG antibodies from patients with Guillain-Barré syndrome: A macro-patch-clamp study. *Ann. Neurol.* **44**, 913–922.

Buchwald, B., de Baets, M., Luijckx, G. J., and Toyka, K. V. (1999). Neonatal Guillain-Barré syndrome: Blocking antibodies transmitted from mother to child. *Neurology* **53**, 1246–1253.

Cannon, S. C. (1996). Sodium channel defects in myotonia and periodic paralysis. *Annu. Rev. Neurosci.* **19**, 141–164.

Cantrell, A. R., and Catterall, W. A. (2001). Neuromodulation of Na+ channels: an unexpected form of cellular plasticity. *Nat. Rev. Neurosci.* **2**, 397–407.

Carabelli, V., D'Ascenzo, M., Carbone, E., and Grassi, C. (2002). Nitric oxide inhibits neuroendocrine Ca_v1 L-channel gating via cGMP-dependent protein kinase in cell-attached patches of bovine chromaffin cells. *J. Physiol. (Lond.)* **541**, 351–366.

Coles, A. J., Wing, M. G., Molyneux, P., Paolillo, A., Davie, C. M., Hale, G., Miller, D., Waldmann, H., and Compston, A. (1999). Monoclonal antibody treatment exposes three mechanisms underlying the clinical course of multiple sclerosis. *Ann. Neurol.* **46**, 296–304.

Corbo, M., Quattrini, A., Latov, N., and Hays, A. P. (1993). Localization of GM1 and Gal(beta 1-3)GalNAc antigenic determinants in peripheral nerve. *Neurology* **43**, 809–814.

Craner, M. J., Lo, A. C., Black, J. A., and Waxman, S. G. (2003) Abnormal sodium channel distribution in optic nerve axons in a model of inflammatory demyelination. *Brain* **126**, 1552–1561.

Craner, M. J., Newcombe, J., Black, J. A., Hartle, C., Cuzner, M. L., and Waxman, S. G. (2004). Molecular changes in neurons in multiple sclerosis: altered axonal expression of Nav1.2 and Nav1.6 sodium channels and Na/Ca exchanger. *Proc. Natl. Acad. Sci. U. S. A.* **101**, 8168–8173.

Cummins, T. R., Renganathan, M., Stys, P. K., Herzog, R. I., Scarfo, K., Horn, R., Dib-Hajj, S. D., and Waxman, S. G. (2003). The pentapeptide QYNAD does not block voltage-gated sodium channels. *Neurology* **60**, 224–229.

D'Ascenzo, M., Martinotti, G., Azzena, G. B., and Grassi, C. (2002). cGMP/protein kinase G-dependent inhibition of N-type Ca2+ channels induced by nitric oxide in human neuroblastoma IMR32 cells. *J. Neurosci.* **22**, 7485–7492.

Garthwaite, G., Goodwin, D. A., Batchelor, A. M., Leeming, K., and Garthwaite, J. (2002). Nitric oxide toxicity in CNS white matter: an in vitro study using rat optic nerve. *Neuroscience* **109**, 145–155.

Giovannoni, G., Heales, S. J., Land, J. M., and Thompson, E. J. (1998). The potential role of nitric oxide in multiple sclerosis. *Multiple Sclerosis* **4**, 21221–21226.

Goldin, A. L., Barchi, R. L., Caldwell, J. H., Hofmann, F., Howe, J. R., Hunter, J. C., Kallen, R. G., Mandel, G., Meisler, M. H., Netter, Y. B., Noda, M., Tamkun, M. M., Waxman, S. G., Wood, J. N., and Catterall,

W. A. (2000). Nomenclature of voltage-gated sodium channels. *Neuron* **28**, 365–368.

Hamm, S., Rudel, R., and Brinkmeier, H. (1996). Excitatory sodium currents of NH15-CA2 neuroblastoma x glioma hybrid cells are differently affected by interleukin-2 and interleukin-1beta. *Pflugers Arch.* **433**, 160–165.

Hammarstrom, A. K., and Gage, P. W. (1999). Nitric oxide increases persistent sodium current in rat hippocampal neurons. *J. Physiol.* **520**, 451–461.

Hartung, H. P., Reiners, K., Schmidt, B., Stoll, G., and Toyka, K. V. (1991). Serum interleukin-2 concentrations in Guillain-Barré syndrome and chronic idiopathic demyelinating polyradiculoneuropathy: comparison with other neurological diseases of presumed immunopathogenesis. *Ann. Neurol.* **30**, 48–53.

Hauser, S. L., Doolittle, T. H., Lincoln, R., Brown, R. H., and Dinarello, C. A. (1990). Cytokine accumulations in CSF of multiple sclerosis patients: frequent detection of interleukin-1 and tumor necrosis factor but not interleukin-6. *Neurology* **40**, 1735–1739.

Hirota, N., Kaji, R., Bostock, H., Shindo, K., Kawasaki, T., Mizutani, K., Oka, N., Kohara, N., Saida, T., and Kimura, J. (1997). The physiological effect of anti-GM1 antibodies on saltatory conduction and transmembrane currents in single motor axons. *Brain* **120**, 2159–2169.

Hong, M. P., Kim, H. I., Shin, Y. K., Lee, C. S., Park, M., and Song, J. H. (2004). Effects of free fatty acids on sodium currents in rat dorsal root ganglion neurons. *Brain Res.* **1008**, 81–91.

Isaacs, J. D., Watts, R. A., Hazleman, B. L., Hale, G., Keogan, M. T., Cobbold, S. P., and Waldmann, H. (1992). Humanised monoclonal antibody therapy for rheumatoid arthritis. *Lancet* **340**, 748–752.

Kaplan, M. R., Cho, M. H., Ullian, E. M., Isom, L. L., Levinson, S. R., and Barres, B. A. (2001). Differential control of clustering of the sodium channels Na(v)1.2 and Na(v)1.6 at developing CNS nodes of Ranvier. *Neuron* **30**, 105–119.

Kapoor, R., Davies, M., Blaker, P. A., Hall, S. M., and Smith, K. J. (2003). Blockers of sodium and calcium entry protect axons from nitric oxide-mediated degeneration. *Ann. Neurol.* **53**, 174–180.

Kaspar, A., Brinkmeier, H., and Rudel, R. (1994). Local anaesthetic-like effect of interleukin-2 on muscular Na+ channels: no evidence for involvement of the IL-2 receptor. *Pflugers Arch.* **426**, 61–67.

Koller, H., Buchholz, J., and Siebler, M. (1996). Cerebrospinal fluid from multiple sclerosis patients inactivates neuronal Na+ current. *Brain* **119**, 457–463.

Kornberg, A. J., Pestronk, A., Bieser, K., Ho, T. W., McKhann, G. M., Wu, H. S., and Jiang, Z. (1994). The clinical correlates of high-titer IgG anti-GM1 antibodies. *Ann. Neurol.* **35**, 234–237.

Kuwabara, S., Yuki, N., Koga, M., Hattori, T., Matsuura, D., Miyake, M., and Noda, M. (1998). IgG anti-GM1 antibody is associated with reversible conduction failure and axonal degeneration in Guillain-Barre syndrome. *Ann. Neurol.* **44**, 202–208.

Li, Z., Chapleau, M. W., Bates, J. N., Bielefeldt, K., Lee, H. C., and Abboud, F. M. (1998). Nitric oxide as an autocrine regulator of sodium currents in baroreceptor neurons. *Neuron* **20**, 1039–1049.

Lin, Y. F., Raab-Graham, K., Jan, Y. N., and Jan, L. Y. (2004). NO stimulation of ATP-sensitive potassium channels: Involvement of Ras/mitogen-activated protein kinase pathway and contribution to neuroprotection. *Proc. Natl. Acad. Sci. U. S. A.* **101**, 7799–7804.

Meuth, S. G., Budde, T., Duyar, H., Landgraf, P., Broicher, T., Elbs, M., Brock, R., Weller, M., Weissert, R., and Wiendl, H. (2003). Modulation of neuronal activity by the endogenous pentapeptide QYNAD. *Eur. J. Neurosci.* **18**, 2697–2706.

Moreau, T., Coles, A., Wing, M., Isaacs, J., Hale, G., Waldmann, H., and Compston, A. (1996). Transient increase in symptoms associated with cytokine release in patients with multiple sclerosis. *Brain* **119**, 225–237.

Padmashri, R., Chakrabarti, K. S., Sahal, D., Mahalakshmi, R., Sarma, S. P., and Sikdar, S. K. (2004). Functional characterization of the pentapeptide

QYNAD on rNav1.2 channels and its NMR structure. *Pflugers Arch.* **447**, 895–907.

Parkinson, J. F., Mitrovic, B., and Merrill, J. E. (1997). The role of nitric oxide in multiple sclerosis. *J. Mol. Med.* **75**, 174–186.

Quasthoff, S., Pojer, C., Mori, A., Hofer, D., Liebmann, P., Kieseier, B. C., and Schreibmayer, W. (2003). No blocking effects of the pentapeptide QYNAD on Na+ channel subtypes expressed in Xenopus oocytes or action potential conduction in isolated rat sural nerve. *Neurosci. Lett.* **352**, 93–96.

Redford, E. J., Kapoor, R., and Smith, K. J. (1997). Nitric oxide donors reversibly block axonal conduction: Demyelinated axons are especially susceptible. *Brain* **120**, 2149–2157.

Renganathan, M., Cummins, T. R., and Waxman, S. G. (2002). Nitric oxide blocks fast, slow, and persistent Na+ channels in C-type DRG neurons by S-nitrosylation. *J. Neurophysiol.* **87**, 761–775.

Renganathan, M., Cummins, T. R., Hormuzdiar, W. N., and Waxman, S. G. (2001). Nitric oxide is an autocrine regulator of Na(+) currents in axotomized C-type DRG neurons. *J. Neurophysiol.* **83**, 2431–2442.

Sakurai, M., Mannen, T., Kanazawa, I., and Tanabe, H. (1992). Lidocaine unmasks silent demyelinative lesions in multiple sclerosis. *Neurology* **42**, 2088–2093.

Schauf, C. L., Davis, F. A., Sack, D. A., Reed, B. J., and Kesler, R. L. (1976). Neuroelectric blocking factors in human and animal sera evaluated using the isolated frog spinal cord. *J. Neurol. Neurosurg. Psychiatry* **39**, 680–685.

Schauf, C. L., Schauf, V., Davis, F. A., and Mizen, M. R. (1978). Complement-dependent serum: Neuroelectric blocking activity in multiple sclerosis. *Neurology* **28**, 426–430.

Seil, F. J., Leiman, A. L., and Kelly, J. M., 3rd. (1976). Neuroelectric blocking factors in multiple sclerosis and normal human sera. *Arch. Neurol.* **33**, 418–422.

Smith, K. J., Kapoor, R., Hall, S. M., and Davies, M. (2001). Electrically active axons degenerate when exposed to nitric oxide. *Ann. Neurol.* **49**, 470–476.

Takigawa, T., Yasuda, H., Kikkawa, R., Shigeta, Y., Saida, T., and Kitasato, H. (1995). Antibodies against GM1 ganglioside affect K+ and Na+ currents in isolated rat myelinated nerve fibers. *Ann. Neurol.* **37**, 436–442.

Vreugdenhil, M., Bruehl, C., Voskuyl, R. A., Kang, J. X., Leaf, A., and Wadman, W. J. (1996). Polyunsaturated fatty acids modulate sodium and calcium currents in CA1 neurons. *Proc. Natl. Acad. Sci. U. S. A.* **93**, 12559–12563.

Weber, F., Rudel, R., Aulkemeyer, P., and Brinkmeier, H. (2002). The endogenous pentapeptide QYNAD induces acute conduction block in the isolated rat sciatic nerve. *Neurosci. Lett.* **317**, 33–36.

Weber, F., Rudel, R., Aulkemeyer, P., and Brinkmeier, H. (2000). Anti-GM1 antibodies can block neuronal voltage-gated sodium channels. *Muscle Nerve* **23**, 1414–1420.

Weber, F., Brinkmeier, H., Aulkemeyer, P., Wollinsky, K. H., and Rudel, R. (1999). A small sodium channel blocking factor in the cerebrospinal fluid is preferentially found in Guillain-Barre syndrome: a combined cell physiological and HPLC study. *J. Neurol.* **246**, 955–960.

Wollinsky, K. H., Hulser, P. J., Brinkmeier, H., Aulkemeyer, P., Bossenecker, W., Huber-Hartmann, K. H., Rohrbach, P., Schreiber, H., Weber, F., Kron, M., Buchele, G., Mehrkens, H. H., Ludolph, A. C., and Rudel, R. (2001). CSF filtration is an effective treatment of Guillain-Barre syndrome: A randomized clinical trial. *Neurology* **57**, 774–780.

23

Evidence for Neuronal Apoptosis in Demyelinating CNS Diseases

Ricarda Diem, M.D.

Mathias Bähr, M.D.

I. Introduction

Apoptotic cell death of neurons is crucial for proper development of the nervous system. In the adult central nervous system (CNS), however, apoptosis of neuronal populations contributes to manifestation of clinical symptoms during several neurodegenerative disorders. Multiple sclerosis (MS) has been reevaluated as a disease that is associated with neuronal and axonal degeneration, in addition to inflammation and demyelination of the central nervous system (CNS). This neurodegenerative aspect of MS may have a strong impact on the development of a permanent neurological deficit in patients. Different molecular mechanisms and signal transduction pathways have been identified that are involved in developmental, as well as in lesion-induced,

apoptosis of neurons. As neuronal apoptosis and its mechanisms are difficult to investigate in human brain tissue from patients with MS, much of the present knowledge about degeneration of neurons in this disease comes from studies in experimental autoimmune encephalomyelitis (EAE), an animal model of MS. This chapter gives an overview of current data concerning features and molecular mechanisms of neuronal apoptosis in chronic inflammatory autoimmune CNS diseases. Furthermore, it describes the influence of axonal pathology, inflammation, demyelination, and neuronal function on the pathogenesis of apoptotic neuronal cell death in EAE and MS. Neuroprotective pathways and treatment approaches are critically discussed and compared with the ones in classical neurodegenerative diseases.

A. Apoptosis as a Phenomenon Involved in Developmental Processes of the CNS

Originally, the term *apoptosis* was used as a morphological description of dying vertebrate cells, which includes features such as cell shrinkage and chromatin condensation (Kerr et al., 1972). In contrast to the other main form of cell death called necrosis, apoptosis within a tissue usually occurs in a disseminated pattern without adversely affecting neighboring cells. Therefore, apoptotic cell death provides an efficient strategy for eliminating normal cells that are

327

unwanted or have lost their function at some point during development and evolution of multicellular organisms. During development of the CNS and peripheral nervous system, neuronal apoptosis appears as a phylogenetically conserved mechanism, which controls the final number of neurons. Initial overproduction and secondary elimination of neurons are thought to be an adaptive process necessary for the matching of neuronal population size to target size and for the formation of nerve cell circuits (McKay et al., 1999). The most common theory of why so many neurons become secondarily eliminated during nervous system formation involves the concept that only a proportion receives enough neurotrophic support from their target cells to survive (for review, see Raff et al., 1993). Initial evidence for the neurotrophic theory came from the experiments by Levi-Montalcini et al., which revealed that treatment of developing sympathetic and sensory neurons with nerve growth factor (NGF) prevented developmental cell death, whereas application of a neutralizing antibody to NGF largely enhanced the rate of undergoing neurons (reviewed by Levi-Montalcini et al., 1996). However, the control of neuronal apoptosis or survival during development seems to be more complex than initially proposed by the neurotrophic hypothesis: Retinal ganglion cells (RGCs), the neurons that form the axons of the optic nerve (ON), physiologically die during two cell death periods. In the early period between embryonic days 15 and 17 in the mouse, RGCs undergo developmental apoptosis induced by NGF via stimulation of the p75 receptor. In this neuronal cell type, NGF activates the same intracellular pathways as used by classical death receptor ligands such as tumor necrosis factor or Fas (for review, see Bähr, 2000). In contrast, during the later period of naturally occurring RGC death in the first postnatal week, NGF has no influence on the number of surviving RGCs. According to the multifactorial hypothesis, neuronal cell death or survival during development depend on more than one neurotrophic factor (Oppenheim, 1996). Several other neurotrophins such as brain-derived neurotrophic factor (BDNF), neurotrophin-3 (NT-3), or neurotrophin–4/5 (NT-4/5) have been shown to increase neuronal survival during nervous system formation (Hofer and Barde, 1988; Barde, 1989; Thoenen, 1991). On the other hand, at least simultaneous elimination of two of those factors, BDNF and NT-4, by the use of double knock-out mice does not lead to increased developmental neuronal apoptosis (Conover et al., 1995), which might be explained by compensatory mechanisms that are activated under these pathophysiological conditions. However, non-target-derived neurotrophic support contributes to the survival of developing neurons as well. For NT-3, it has been shown that this neurotrophin influences the survival of embryonic hippocampal pyramidal neurons before target contact via an activity-dependent autocrine loop (Boukhaddaoui et al., 2001). Electrical activity in neuronal circuits plays an important role for develop-

mental neuronal apoptosis and is closely related to neurotrophic factor signaling pathways. The balance between growth factor and neurotransmitter actions appears to be especially important for the determination of survival or death of neurons during development. As an example, the generation of hippocampal neuroarchitecture is influenced by opposing trophic and degenerative neurotransmitter-related signaling pathways such as activation of postsynaptic glutamate receptors (for review, see Mattson, 2000a).

B. Molecular Mechanisms of Developmental Neuronal Apoptosis

Studies of the nematode *Caenorhabditis elegans* first elucidated the presence of a genetically controlled suicide cascade that determines apoptotic cell death. Three apoptosis regulatory genes have been identified in this species in which 131 of 1,090 somatic cells undergo developmental apoptosis: *ced-3* and *ced-4* act in a proapoptotic way, whereas *ced-9* prevents apoptotic cell death (Horvitz, 1999). In biochemical studies, it has been shown that these three proteins function as a complex in which the antiapoptotic *ced-9* normally suppresses *ced-4* dependent activation of *ced-3*. The mammalian homologues of *ced-3, ced-4*, and *ced-9* were cloned and it became clear that these genes were core components of the mammalian apoptosis machinery as well (for review, see Bähr, 2000). The mammalian homologues of *ced-3* belong to a family of proteases called caspases, which consists of at least 14 members (Thornberry and Lazebnik, 1998). During cell death, caspases are converted from their proenzymatic forms into activated proteases in a cascade-like order and thereby mediate signaling and execution of apoptosis (Fig. 1).

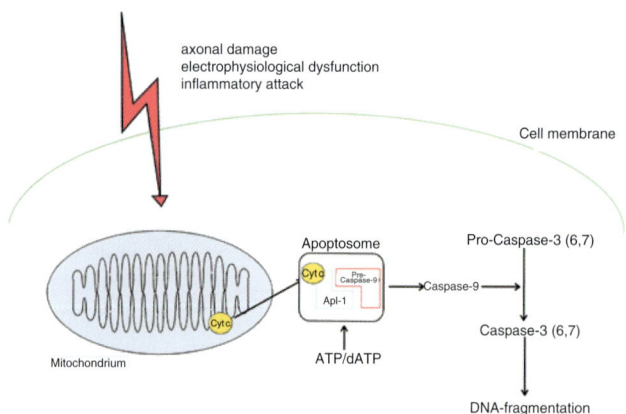

Figure 1 The mitochondrial pathway of apoptosis. Following an apoptotic trigger, cytochrome c (cyt c) is released from the mitochondrium. Cyt c liberation into the cytosol results in formation of the apoptosome (in combination with Apaf1 and pro-caspase 9), which is cleaved in the presence of ATP or dATP. This triggers the downstream caspase cascade, in which caspase-3 plays a major role in the execution of cell death. (Adapted from Bähr, 2000.)

On the basis of the peptide-sequence preference of their substrates, the caspase family can be divided into three subgroups: the Interleukin-1β-converting enzyme protease family (caspases 1, 4, 5, and 11-14), the *ced*-3 subfamily (caspases 3 and 6-10), and a third subfamily containing only caspase-2. Studies on knock-out mice revealed the individual *in vivo* relevance of each caspase. Whereas the phenotype of caspase-1-knock-out mice, for example, does not indicate any disturbances in developmental neuronal apoptosis, mice deficient in caspase-3 develop phenotypical changes characterized by an excessive number of neurons in the CNS and retina (Nicholson and Thornberry, 1997).

Ced-4 shares homology with the mammalian apoptosis regulator Apoptosis protease activated factor-1 (Apaf-1) (Zou et al., 1997), which can associate with several death proteases, including caspase-4, -8, and -9. Together with cytochrome c released from the mitochondria, complex formation of Apaf-1 and pro-caspase-9 builds the "apoptosome" as shown in Fig. 1, a trigger complex for the activation of the further downstream caspase cascade (for review, see Bähr, 2000). The phenotype of Apaf-1-knock-out mice shows similarities to caspase-3 and -9 knock-outs characterized by reduced developmental apoptosis in the CNS and consecutive brain, as well as craniofacial malformations (Cecconi et al., 1998).

Ced-9 shows sequence and structural similarities to the mammalian proto-oncogene Bcl-2 (Hengartner and Horvitz, 1994). The growing Bcl-2 family consists of at least 15 Bcl-2 homologues, which function either as antagonists (e.g., Bcl-2, Bcl-XL, or Bcl-w) or agonists (Bax, Bcl-Xs, BAD) of apoptotic cell death (for review, see Bähr, 2000). Parts of the Bcl-2 family members are located at the outer mitochondrial membrane where they can protect or disrupt membrane integrity. Whereas Bcl-2 and Bcl-XL prevent cytochrome c release from the mitochondrium, conformational changes of Bax lead to release of cytochrome c and consecutive formation of the apoptosome. This mitochondrial pathway of apoptosis is located upstream from caspase activation and triggers the further execution of cell death (Fig. 1). Studies on Bcl-2 knock-out mice revealed that this member of the Bcl-2 family is not essential for developmental neuronal cell death: At birth, the number of motoneurons, sensory, or sympathetic neurons in these mice was not significantly changed when compared to wild-type animals (Michaelidis et al., 1996). However, substantial degeneration of central and peripheral neurons occurred during the early postnatal period. In the retina, Bcl-2 knock-outs showed a loss of 29% of their RGC axons until postnatal day 15 indicating a physiological role of Bcl-2 for the maintenance of neurons soon after the period of naturally occurring cell death (Cellerino et al., 1999). In contrast, mice deficient for Bcl-XL die around embryonic day 13 because of a massive increase of developmental apoptosis in the hematopoietic and the nervous system (Motoyama et al., 1995). Knock-out mice of the death-promoting Bcl-2 family member Bax show increased numbers of motor and sympathetic neurons, as well as increased developmental survival of RGCs (Deckwerth et al., 1996; Mosinger Ogilvie et al., 1998).

II. Lesion-Induced Apoptosis: Apoptotic Neuronal Cell Death in Models of Experimental Autoimmune Encephalomyelitis

A. Apoptotic Neuronal Cell Death

In the last few years, histopathological studies of postmortem tissue of patients, as well as data from experimental animal and cell culture models, have revealed the presence of neuronal apoptosis in multiple sclerosis (MS), an autoimmune CNS disease that has long been thought to be primarily characterized by inflammation and demyelination. In human autopsy brain tissue, a limited number of apoptotic neurons could be detected in chronic active and chronic inactive lesions from patients with MS (Peterson et al., 2001). In contrast, acute active lesions did not show neurons that fulfilled the morphological or intracellular criteria of apoptotic neuronal cell death. As also known from studies of "classical" neurodegenerative diseases such as Alzheimer's disease, it is difficult to detect apoptotic neurons in human brain tissue because of the rapid time kinetics of the apoptosis-related intracellular signaling cascades (for review, see Mattson, 2000b). In addition, experiments that involve manipulation of apoptotic signaling pathways to investigate their functional relevance are not possible in patients. For these reasons, much of the present knowledge about apoptotic neuronal cell death and its mechanisms in MS comes from studies in animal models of experimental autoimmune encephalomyelitis (EAE).

By the use of different agents and modes of immunization as well as different animal strains, EAE models mimicking many aspects of the human disease have been established (Wekerle et al., 1994; Storch et al., 1998; Weissert et al., 1998; Kornek et al., 2000). EAE induced by active immunization of female brown Norway (BN) rats with the extracellular domain of recombinant rat myelin oligodendrocyte glycoprotein 1-125 (rrMOG) especially reflects the neurodegenerative aspect of MS (Meyer et al., 2001; Diem et al., 2003b). In this model, it has been demonstrated that EAE lesions often affect the ON with concomitant decrease of electrophysiological function as revealed by recordings of visual evoked potentials, the electrical cortical response to a visual stimulus. Simultaneous measurements of electroretinograms in response to pattern stimulation, which specifically correspond to RGC function, gave evidence for severe impairment of the neurons that give rise to the axons of the ON as well (Meyer et al., 2001). Immunohistochemical analysis of RGC somata showed that these neurons undergo lesion-induced apoptosis even before the onset of clinically manifest EAE (Hobom et al., 2004). RGCs positive for active caspase-3, an important member of the downstream caspase cascade, as well as those showing DNA degradation, were detected during induction and manifestation of MOG-EAE (Fig. 2 A-D). The importance of the animal's individual immunogenetic background for the kinetics and severity of neurodegeneration during EAE was emphasized by a comparative study of caspase activation in two different EAE models. Whereas neuronal caspase-3 expression in the spinal cord of Lewis rats in the interleukin-12 EAE model did not increase until the third relapse, active neuronal caspase-3 in ABH mice immunized with spinal cord homogenate was already detectable during the acute stage of the disease (Ahmed et al., 2002).

Comparing neuronal apoptosis during rrMOG-induced optic neuritis in rats with the loss of neurons in a noninflammatory, purely neurodegenerative model based on mechanical lesion of the retinocollicular fiber tract, similarities in kinetics and extent can be observed. Surgical axotomy of the ON in the rat is a frequently used model to investigate secondary neuronal cell loss in degenerative processes of the mammalian CNS because of its good surgical accessibility and well-known kinetics of cell death (Villegas-Perez et al., 1988; Bähr and Bonhoeffer, 1994; Bähr and Wizenmann, 1996; Klöcker et al., 1997, 1998; Diem et al., 2001; 2003a).

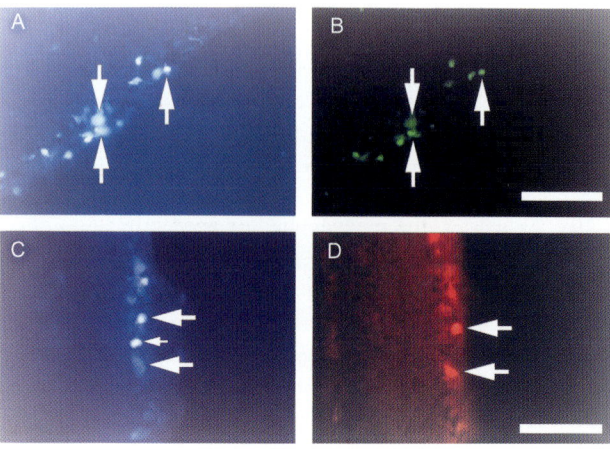

Figure 2 Cell death of retinal ganglion cells (RGCs) during autoimmune optic neuritis is accompanied by DNA-degradation and caspase-3 activation. (**A, B**) Double staining of a retinal section from a rat with optic nerve affection during experimental autoimmune encephalomyelitis induced by myelin oligodendrocyte glycoprotein. RGCs were identified by retrograde labeling with the fluorescent dye Fluorogold (FG) (**A**). FG staining colocalizes with terminal deoxynucleotidyl transferase-mediated biotinylated UTP nick end labeling indicating DNA fragmentation (**B**). (**C, D**) Detection of active caspase-3 (**D**) by immunohistochemistry in RGCs identified by FG labeling (**C**). Scale bars: (**A, B**) 100 μm; (**C, D**) 70 μm. (Reprinted from Meyer et al., 2001.)

It has been demonstrated that transection of the ON induces a delayed death of 80% to 90% of RGCs within 2 weeks, starting on or about day 4, reaching a maximum on day 7, and decreasing on or about day 14 after axotomy (Eschweiler and Bähr, 1993; Mansour-Robaey et al., 1994). In the rat model of rrMOG-induced optic neuritis, neuronal apoptosis occurred as acute and severe as after complete surgical transection of the ON: A first significant reduction of RGC density was seen at day 5 after immunization. Between day 7 after immunization and the day of disease onset, the highest rate of RGC apoptosis was observed. After this acute phase, neuronal cell death kinetics slowed down on or about day 8 of MOG-EAE (Hobom et al., 2004). At this time, rats had lost 73% of their RGCs compared to cell counts of healthy animals. Whereas these data raised the hypothesis of axonal pathology or dysfunction being responsible for the induction of apoptotic neuronal cell death in EAE as a secondary, retrograde event, the concept of primary neuronal apoptosis independent from axonal damage was suggested by *in vitro* studies on cortical neuron cultures. In this model, cerebrospinal fluid (CSF) from patients with primary progressive MS and active disease course or CSF obtained during acute relapse of relapsing-remitting MS induced apoptotic cell death of rat cortical neurons (Alcazar et al., 1998; Cid et al., 2003). Although the underlying mechanisms could not be identified, neurons were rescued from CSF-induced apoptosis by application of caspase-3 inhibitors *in vitro*.

Investigating the relationship between neuronal cell loss during EAE and neurological function, it has been shown that similar to the classical neurodegenerative disorders, a linear correlation between these two parameters could not be observed. Postmortem studies in brains from parkinsonian patients revealed that the loss of nigrostriatal dopamine neurons must be greater than 75% in order for the disease to become clinically evident (Lloyd, 1977). For amyotrophic lateral sclerosis (ALS), it has been estimated that 50% to 80% of target neurons must be degenerated before clinical disability develops (Bradley, 1987). Accordingly, in the rat optic neuritis model induced by immunization with rrMOG, visual function was not severely altered until RGC loss had reached a threshold of 50% to 60%; below that compensatory mechanisms maintained functional integrity (Meyer et al., 2001; Hobom et al., 2004). Figure 3 shows the relationship between RGC density in this model and visual acuity values determined by electroretinogram recordings. In support of these data, up to 82% of axonal loss was found in MS-like lesions from individuals with no reported neurological symptoms during their lifetime (Mews et al., 1998). After autoimmune optic neuritis, functional compensation could occur at a cortical level based on topographical changes of the primary visual cortex, as has been shown for balancing visual field defects (Safran and Landis, 1996). Local molecular mechanisms on different levels of the optic pathway that involve NMDA receptor-mediated activity (Binns and Salt,

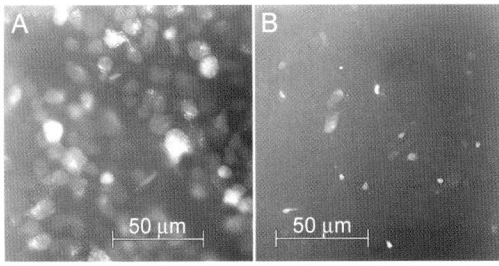

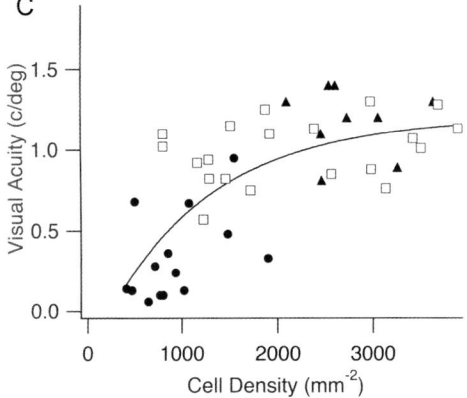

Figure 3 Correlation between retinal ganglion cell (RGC) density and visual function in rats with acute experimental autoimmune encephalomyelitis (EAE) induced by myelin oligodendrocyte glycoprotein (MOG). (**A**) Normal cell density of RGCs in a healthy control rat. (**B**) The numbers of remaining RGCs are significantly reduced in a rat with acute optic neuritis during MOG-EAE. (**C**) The decrease of RGC density in rats with optic neuritis correlates with a reduction of visual acuity determined by measurements of electroretinograms. *Filled circles* indicate visual acuities and RGC densities of rats with histopathologically proven optic neuritis, whereas *filled triangles* represent those of healthy controls. Visual acuity values and RGC counts of MOG-immunized rats without optic neuritis are given as *open squares*. Note that RGC densities in animals suffering from optic neuritis must be markedly decreased to lead to a reduction of visual acuity. (Reprinted from Meyer et al., 2001.)

1998) or substance P expression (Tu et al., 2000) may contribute to neuronal plasticity in EAE or MS. Nitric oxide (NO) has also been postulated to act as a retrograde signal that can mediate multiple aspects of synaptic plasticity in the visual system (Cogen and Cohen-Cory, 2000).

B. Molecular Mechanisms of Neuronal Apoptosis in EAE

Neurodegenerative diseases are often characterized by apoptosis of certain neuronal populations and concomitant intracellular protein depositions. In ALS, cell death of upper and lower motor neurons is associated with inclusion of proteins such as skein-like ubiquitin. In animal models of Huntington's disease, as well as in brain tissue from Huntington patients, neuronal cell death in the *striatum* related to intranuclear deposition of mutant huntingtin and ubiquitin was observed. Cell death in Parkinson's disease pre-

dominantly affects neurons of the *substantia nigra* and other subcortical nuclei that show so-called Lewy bodies in their cytoplasm (for review, see Jellinger, 2001). Distinct from those purely neurodegenerative disorders, neuronal cell death in MS or EAE does not show any clear distributional preferences. In human brain tissue, apoptotic neurons were identified in cerebral cortex lesions (Peterson et al., 2001), whereas apoptosis in different EAE models affected neuronal subpopulations such as RGCs or spinal cord neurons (Meyer et al., 2001; Diem et al., 2003b; Ahmed et al., 2002). Cytoskeleton changes or accumulation of abnormal protein during MS- or EAE-induced neuronal apoptosis are rather described for damaged axons than for the neuronal cell body itself (Kornek et al., 2000; Zhu et al., 1999). Despite these obvious differences resulting from distinct pathogenesis or pathophysiology of neurodegeneration, similar molecular mechanisms are involved because the subsequent biochemical events that execute apoptosis are highly conserved. These alterations in intracellular signal transduction occurring during early stages of neuronal apoptosis in EAE involve the Bcl-2 family of proteins. As described in context with the molecular features of developmental apoptotic neuronal cell death, this protein family includes both proapoptic and antiapoptotic members. In the rat model of rrMOG-induced EAE, a shift in the Bcl-2 family of proteins toward the proapoptotic side was observed during induction and manifestation of the disease (Hobom et al., 2004). At disease onset, RGCs showed an increase of the proapoptotic protein Bax simultaneously with a reduction of the antiapoptotic Bcl-2 protein. Figure 4 gives examples of representative retinal sections with increased protein expression of Bax in RGCs during development and manifestation of MOG-EAE.

In this model, Bcl-2 levels re-increased at day 8 of the disease when the rate of RGC death declined as shown in Fig. 5. Apoptosis of RGCs after mechanical lesion of the ON was accompanied by a reciprocal regulation of Bax and Bcl-2 as well (Isenmann et al., 1997), indicating that not only the kinetics but also the mechanisms of apoptotic RGC death are similar after autoimmune transection or surgical axotomy of the ON. From *in vitro* studies, it is known that high amounts of Bax can antagonize the antiapoptotic activity of Bcl-2 (Oltvai et al., 1993) such that the ratio of Bcl-2 to Bax determines survival or death of neurons after an apoptotic stimulus. The functional relevance of Bcl-2 for EAE-associated neurodegeneration was demonstrated in a study using transgenic mice overexpressing the Bcl-2 gene, which showed reduced axonal damage and a less severe disease course during MOG-EAE (Offen et al., 2000).

The phosphatidylinositol 3-kinase (PI3-K)/Akt pathway has originally been described as a signal transduction step involved in growth-factor-induced neuroprotection against different apoptotic stimuli *in vitro* as well as *in vivo* (Dudek et al., 1997; Kermer et al., 2000). In addition, activation of this pathway after application of pro-inflammatory

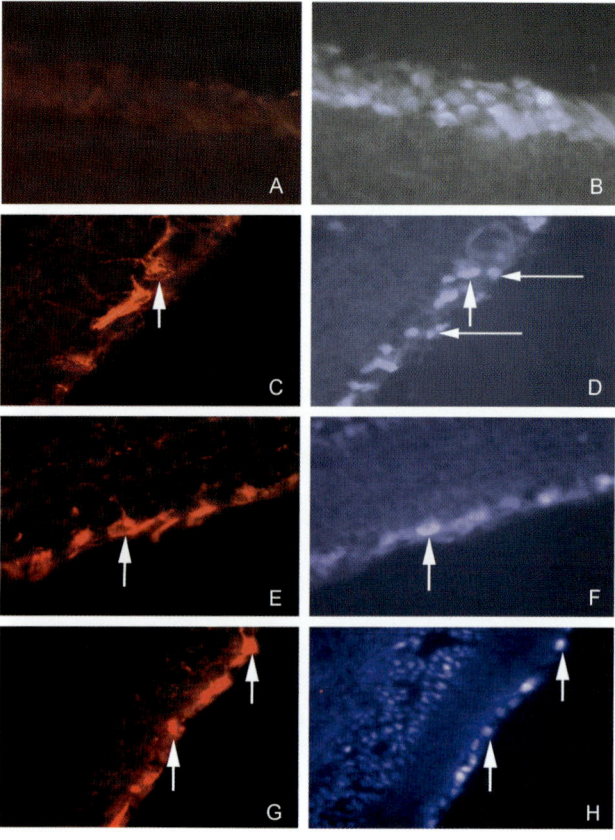

Figure 4 Increased expression of the pro-apoptotic protein Bax in retinal ganglion cells (RGCs) during development and manifestation of myelin oligodendrocyte glycoprotein (MOG)-induced experimental autoimmune encephalomyelitis (EAE) in rats. (**A, B**) Double staining of a retinal section from a healthy rat. No specific staining of Bax protein (**A**) was detected in RGCs identified by retrograde labeling with the fluorescent dye Fluorogold (FG) (**B**). (**C, D**) Retinal section from a rat at day 7 after immunization with MOG. A significant upregulation of Bax protein expression (**C**) was detected in some of the FG-positive RGCs indicated by the *vertical arrow* (**D**). *Horizontal arrows* indicate Bax-negative RGCs. (**E, F**) On day 1 of the disease, high expression levels of Bax protein in all RGCs identified by FG-labeling were discovered. (**G, H**) The amount of Bax protein in RGCs on day 8 of the disease was similar when compared to day 1 of MOG-EAE: 50μm. (Reprinted from Hobom et al., 2004.)

cytokines such as tumor necrosis factor-α or interleukin-1β led to rescue of RGCs after surgical axotomy of the ON (Diem et al., 2001; 2003a). In general, interaction of neurotrophins or cytokines with their highly specific receptors activates PI3-K, which generates various phosphorylated phosphatidylinositides. These second messengers lead to activation of protein kinase B, also called Akt (Coffer et al., 1998). Phospho-Akt, in turn, can phosphorylate and thereby inactivate the proapoptotic protein Bad (Datta et al., 1997), as well as unprocessed or active caspase-9 (Cardone et al., 1998), which leads to decreased levels of the downstream effecter caspase-3 (Li et al., 1997). In MOG-EAE, phospho-Akt levels in RGCs were decreased at day 1 of the disease as shown in Fig. 5a, which corresponds to the time point when

the most prominent RGC apoptosis occurred, as well as caspase-3 activation in RGCs peaked (Hobom et al., 2004). Simultaneously with the re-increase of Bcl-2 as described above, protein concentration of phospho-Akt normalized at day 8 of MOG-EAE, indicating a temporary breakdown of intracellular endogenous rescue mechanisms in neurons exposed to EAE-associated proapoptotic stimuli. Figure 5 compares the kinetics of phospho-Akt and Bcl-2 protein expression in RGCs during development, manifestation, and disease progression of MOG-EAE in BN rats.

Another pathway characterized in context with neurotrophin-induced neuroprotection involves phosphorylation of mitogen-activated protein kinases (MAPKs). MAPKs regulate neuronal cell growth and morphological differentiation and promote neuronal survival after neurotransmitter or neurotrophic factor stimulation (for review, see Fukunaga and Miyamoto; 1998). Multiple second messengers, such as cyclin adenosine monophosphate, protein kinase A, or calcium, control MAPK signaling via a small G protein called "Ras" (for review, see Grewal et al., 1999). MAPK phoshorylation during the time period of acute neuronal apoptosis in MOG-EAE may serve as an endogenous rescue mechanism (Diem et al., 2003b), as suggested for other neuronal cell types, which upregulate the phosphorylated, active form of MAPKs during exposure to chronic stress, brain injury, or development of neurodegenerative disorders (Ferrer et al., 2001; Dash et al., 2002; Trentani et al., 2002). In rrMOG-induced EAE in BN rats, it has been shown recently that treatment with methylprednisolone, the standard therapy of acute MS relapses, increased apoptosis of RGCs secondary to severe optic neuritis by inhibiting the phosphorylation of MAPKs (Diem et al., 2003b). This steroid effect was mimicked by treatment with a pharmacological inhibitor of MAPK kinase (MEK), which in turn phosphorylates and thereby activates MAPKs. In a study on cortical neurons under hypoxic conditions, it has been demonstrated that inhibition of MAPK phosphorylation by MEK blockade reduced the rate of surviving neurons via mechanisms such as decreasing the ability to phosphorylate and thereby inactivate the proapoptotic protein Bad (Jin et al., 2002). The negative steroid effect on RGC survival during MOG-induced EAE was further mediated by calcium influx via voltage-gated calcium channels (Diem et al., 2003b), indicating a possible involvement of transmembrane ion currents in EAE-associated neurodegeneration as well.

Increased calcium influx into neurons after activation of AMPA (α-amino-3-hydroxy-5-methyl-4-isoxazolepropionic acid)/kainate receptors may be another important mechanism for neuronal degeneration in MS and EAE. These receptors mediate toxicity induced by the excitatory neurotransmitter glutamate, which has been shown to contribute to neuronal apoptosis in neurodegenerative disorders such as Alzheimer's disease, Huntington's disease, and ALS (for review, see Mattson, 2000a). Overactivation of glutamate

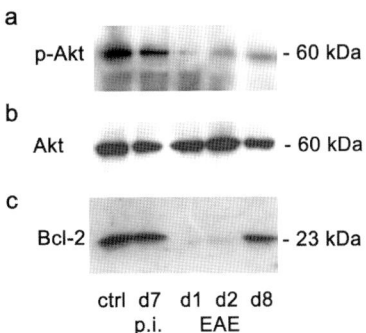

Figure 5 Western blot analysis of the anti-apoptotic proteins phospho-Akt (pAkt) (**A**) and Bcl-2 (**C**) in retinal ganglion cells during development and manifestation of myelin oligodendrocyte glycoprotein (MOG)-induced experimental autoimmune encephalomyelitis (EAE) in rats. On days 1 and 2 of MOG-EAE, phospho-Akt and Bcl-2 expression decreased to almost no detectable protein levels. The expression level of phospho-Akt and Bcl-2 re-increased on day 8 of the disease. As a control, protein concentrations of the inactive, unphosphorylated form of the Akt protein were not regulated (**B**). (Reprinted from Hobom et al., 2004.)

receptors, especially under conditions of decreased energy availability and oxidative stress, has also been proposed for pathophysiological conditions during stroke and epileptic seizures (for review, see Mody and MacDonald, 1995). In a rat model of EAE induced by immunization with myelin basic protein (MBP), it has been shown that administration of different AMPA/kainate receptor antagonists improved neurological outcome and limited apoptotic cell death of spinal cord neurons (Smith et al., 2000). Thereby it could be demonstrated that the beneficial effect of these drugs cannot be attributed to possible anti-inflammatory or immunomodulatory actions, as inflammatory histopathological changes were not influenced. The relevance of glutamate toxicity for the human disease has also been suggested by the observation of increased glutamate levels in the CSF of patients during acute MS relapse (Stover et al., 1997). Histopathological analysis of human brain and spinal cord tissue obtained at autopsy revealed a high expression of glutaminase, a marker for glutamate production, in active MS lesions. These elevated glutaminase levels were detected in macrophages and microglia in close proximity to damaged axons (Werner et al., 2001). In an adoptive transfer model in mice induced by injection of MBP-reactive T-cells, glutamine synthetase and glutamate dehydrogenase activity were downregulated in astrocytes during acute EAE, resulting in decreased ability to metabolize the excitatory neurotransmitter glutamate (Hardin-Pouzet et al., 1997). Glutamate targets not only neuronal cell types during autoimmune CNS inflammation but also oligodendrocytes that express the AMPA/kainate type of excitatory glutamate receptors are subjected to excitotoxicity. Increased oligodendrocyte survival was seen under treatment with the AMPA/kainate antagonist NBQX in adoptive transfer EAE in mice (Pitt et al., 2000), suggesting an involvement of glutamate toxicity in the pathophysiology of at least two important histopathological features of MS or EAE.

C. Role of Inflammation, Demyelination, Axonal Pathology, and Electrophysiological Dysfunction in the Pathogenesis of Neuronal Apoptosis

Currently, investigations of EAE- and MS-associated neurodegeneration devote much effort to understanding the nature of neuronal cell death in chronic inflammatory autoimmune CNS diseases. Degeneration of the axon may precede the death of the cell body and make a more important contribution to the development of chronic disability with consecutive conversion into the secondary progressive form of the disease in patients with MS. Transection and swelling of axons, changes in the axonal cytoskeleton, and impaired axonal transport have been described in acute MS (Ferguson et al., 1997; Trapp et al., 1998) and EAE lesions (Kornek et al., 2000; Meyer et al., 2001) and might induce secondary apoptotic cell death of the neuron itself. Secondary or retrograde neuronal apoptosis after surgical axotomy or crush injury of the axon is a well-characterized process in different animal models (Isenmann et al., 1997; Diem et al., 2001; Ugolini et al., 2003), which shows similarities in kinetics, extent, and mechanisms when compared with neuronal cell death in EAE (Hobom et al., 2004). Apoptotic cell death of CNS neurons in turn can lead to a reduced number of remaining projection targets for other neuronal subpopulations and thereby induce further cell death as a result of target deprivation (Theoret et al., 1997). However, apoptotic neuronal cell death during chronic inflammatory autoimmune CNS disease might have additional triggers unrelated to axonal damage.

Comparing the development of axonal injury of the ON with the time kinetics of RGC apoptosis in the rat model of MOG-induced EAE revealed that apoptosis of neurons can precede degeneration of their respective axons (Hobom et al., 2004). In this animal model, it has been demonstrated that electrophysiological dysfunction of the ON occurs simultaneously with the onset of RGC apoptosis and before histopathological abnormalities of the ON can be detected. Functional integrity can be an important survival factor for neuronal cell types as demonstrated for purified RGCs (Meyer-Franke et al., 1998), as well as for hippocampal neurons (Neumann et al., 1997). Neurons with impaired electrophysiological function might become a target for the action of cytotoxic T-cells due to cell surface expression of β_2-microglobulin and major histocompatibility complex class I molecules, whereas in electrically active neurons, expression of these proteins was suppressed (Neumann et al., 1997). Furthermore, it has been demonstrated that depolarization of purified RGCs increased cell surface levels of the neurotrophic receptor TrkB and thereby improved their trophic responsiveness and cell survival (Meyer-Franke et al., 1998; Shen et al., 1999). Depolarization was supposed to increase intracellular Ca^{2+} levels with a consecutive augmentation of intracellular cAMP concentration, which in turn promotes transport of TrkB to the cell surface. Also in the intact retina, physiological levels of electrical activity enhance the responsiveness of RGCs to peptide trophic factor stimulation (Shen et al., 1999). In MS or EAE, impairment of electrophysiological function of axons even before demyelination is detectable might be caused by elevated levels of pro-inflammatory cytokines such as tumor necrosis factor-α or interleukin-1β. For these factors, cytokine-induced alterations of voltage-gated ion channel function have been demonstrated in a rat model of ON transection (Diem et al., 2001; 2003a). For patients with MS, it has been shown that an increase of circulating pro-inflammatory cytokines in the blood after therapeutically evoked lymphopenia led to a reversible exacerbation of neurological symptoms for several hours, a time period certainly too short for demyelination and remyelination (Moreau et al., 1996). The authors suggested that this reawakening of pre-existing symptoms might be due to alterations in axonal conduction induced by direct electrophysiological effects of pro-inflammatory cytokines.

Evidence for a direct attack of autoreactive lymphocytes as the main cause for apoptotic neuronal cell death in EAE came from electron microscopy of motoneurons of the lumbar spinal cord in rats immunized with MBP (Smith et al., 2000). At the clinical peak of the disease course, motoneuron death in the ventral horn of the lumbar spine was associated with lymphocyte entry. Sequestration of lymphocytes into motoneurons led to the development of neuronal vacuoles filled with cellular debris and consecutive reduction of neuronal density in that area. Immunohistochemistry revealed that these lymphocytes entering motoneurons during the acute phase of EAE were T-lymphocytes positive for CD2, whereas an additional involvement of B- or natural killer lymphocytes, or macrophages/microglia could be

excluded. In contrast, acute RGC apoptosis in MOG-EAE in BN rats does not seem to be mediated by direct autoreactive lymphocyte action. In this model, inflammatory infiltrates in the retina consisting of T-cells or macrophages as an explanation for the degeneration of RGCs could not be detected by immunohistochemistry against T-cell receptors or as against lysosomal membrane-related antigens on macrophages and microglia (Meyer et al., 2001). Different from MOG-induced EAE, inflammatory infiltrates in the anterior segments of the eye leading to acute iridocyclitis or anterior uveitis together with optic neuritis have been described during acute MBP-EAE (Hayreh, 1981; Verhagen et al., 1994).

The concept of benign or neuroprotective effects of inflammatory infiltrates on neuronal survival as an opposite point of view has been suggested by a study using a crush injury model of the ON (Moalem et al., 1999). In this work, it has been shown that autoreactive T-lymphocytes specific for MBP reduced secondary neuronal cell death of RGCs because of a transient reduction of energy requirement caused by a decrease in nerve activity. Active immunization with encephalitogenic or nonencephalitogenic peptides of proteolipid protein or MOG can also exert neuroprotective effects on RGCs after ON crush injury (Fisher et al., 2001). In a different injury model based on avulsion of ventral roots in the rat lumbar spinal cord, it has been demonstrated that apoptotic cell death of motoneurons was reduced in rats suffering from MBP-induced EAE (Hammarberg et al., 2000). The mechanisms by which transferred T-cells or active immunization promote neuronal survival are thought to depend on the secretion of neurotrophic factors by cells of the immune system. High levels of BDNF, NT-3, and other glial cell line-derived neurotrophic factors were detected in T-cells and natural killer cells in the spinal cord from animals with MBP-EAE and simultaneous axotomy of spinal motoneurons (Hammarberg et al., 2000). Increased production of bioactive BDNF on antigen stimulation was shown in a study on T-helper (Th)1- and Th2-type CD4+ T-cell lines specific for myelin autoantigens such as MBP or MOG (Kerschensteiner et al., 1999). In this study, immune-cell-derived BDNF was demonstrated to support the survival of sensory neurons *in vitro*. BDNF immunoreactivity was also detected in inflammatory cells in lesional areas of the brain from patients with MS (Kerschensteiner et al., 1999). Although specific autoimmunity in the CNS can have a physiological neuroprotective role, the gap between benign and destructive effects of an autoreactive immune response might be small. The neuroprotective effect after immunization with immunodominant encephalitogenic epitopes, for example, could be achieved only in cases where the disease they caused was mild (Fisher et al., 2001).

Whereas the interaction between axonal and oligodendrocyte integrity is a frequently investigated phenomenon, little is known about the direct impact of demyelination on neuronal apoptosis during autoimmune CNS inflammation. In MS and EAE where axonal damage could be the consequence of demyelination, it is difficult to differentiate between the pathogenetic relevance of these two histopathological features for the induction of neuronal apoptosis. Transection of dysmyelinated ON axons in rats lacking MBP did not affect the survival rate of RGCs for time periods of up to 180 days (Phokeo and Ball, 2000), indicating that the absence of myelin did not accelerate neuronal death in this model. In a demyelinating mouse model of the human globoid cell leukodystrophy, neuronal apoptosis was reduced by lipocalin-type prostaglandin produced by perineuronal oligodendrocytes (Taniike et al., 2002), suggesting that these oligodendrocytes might be able to directly contribute to the survival of neuronal cells. At least *in vitro*, a reciprocal survival-promoting interaction between these two cell types exists, as it has been shown that purified sensory neurons can increase the survival of oligodendrocytes in culture (for review, see Raff et al., 1993).

III. Neuroprotective Pathways and Treatment Approaches

Clinically established therapeutic strategies for the treatment of MS mainly target the autoimmune response by using anti-inflammatory, immunomodulatory, and immunosuppressive agents. Although these substances have been proven to be beneficial in terms of modifying the clinical disease course, clear neuroprotective properties have been demonstrated for none of them so far. Unfortunately, the concept of achieving neuroprotective effects as a secondary phenomenon resulting from the treatment of inflammation and autoimmunity was not confirmed by many studies. In a study using magnetic resonance spectroscopy, immunomodulatory treatment with interferon-β did not prevent progression of axonal injury in patients with MS with active disease course (Parry et al., 2003). Detrimental effects of anti-inflammatory treatment on the survival of neurons have been described in a rat model of MOG-induced EAE that especially reflects the neurodegenerative aspects of the disease (Diem et al., 2003b). In this model, methylprednisolone pulse therapy, the standard treatment of acute MS exacerbations, exerted pro-apoptotic effects on RGCs by a calcium dependent inhibition of endogenous MAPK phosphorylation. In contrast, survival of RGCs in healthy rats was not affected under steroid treatment after the same protocol. From these results, it has been concluded that methylprednisolone, despite its ability to reduce inflammatory infiltration of the ON during acute optic neuritis, endangers neurons by enhancing their vulnerability to EAE-associated proapoptotic stimuli.

Current research on the neurodegenerative aspect in EAE or MS is focused on developing treatment strategies that inhibit degeneration of axons, as well as protect the neuronal cell body from apoptotic cell death by directly targeting the neuron itself. Recent data showing that the intracellular mechanisms of neuronal apoptosis in EAE closely resemble the ones in neurodegenerative disease models (Meyer et al., 2001; Diem et al., 2003b; Hobom et al, 2004) suggest that "classical" neuroprotective approaches in combination with the established disease-modifying therapies might be promising. One possible strategy would consist of the activation of intracellular antiapoptotic pathways within neurons by treatment with neurotrophic factors. Neurotrophic factors act via binding to their high-affinity tyrosine kinase receptors TrkA, TrkB, and TrkC, and the low-affinity neurotrophin receptor p75 with consecutive activation of intracellular neuroprotective pathways such as MAPKs and PI3-K/Akt (for review, see Bähr, 2000). In the last few years, treatment studies with neurotrophic factors have progressed to clinical trials in patients with neurodegenerative disorders or stroke (Borasio et al., 1998; for review, see Ay et al., 1999). However, therapeutic neuroprotective approaches involving the use of classical neurotrophic factors such as BDNF are difficult because of limitations in delivering these substances to their target cells. Similar difficulties concerning delivery or application mode occur in the context with treatment studies using the "neurocytokine" ciliary neurotrophic factor (CNTF). After binding to the α-subunit of the CNTF receptor, this cytokine activates several intracellular neuroprotective cascades such as the Janus tyrosine kinase/signal transducers and activators of transcription (JAK-STAT) pathway (for review, see Segal and Greenberg, 1996). The clinical relevance of CNTF for MS is corroborated by the observation that MS patients with homozygous CNTF null mutation have a significantly earlier onset of disease with predominant motor symptoms (Giess et al., 2002). In CNTF-deficient mice, MOG-induced EAE was more severe and recovery was poor, and an increased rate of oligodendrocyte apoptosis was found in these animals when compared with wild type mice (Linker et al., 2002). However, if administrated systemically, CNTF accumulates in the liver and does not reach the CNS in sufficient quantities, as demonstrated in a study investigating the pharmacokinetics of radioiodinated CNTF after intravenous injection in rats (Dittrich et al., 1994).

Erythropoietin (Epo), the main regulator of erythropoiesis in mammals, has been shown to exert neuroprotective effects in different animal models of brain injury (Bernaudin et al., 1999; Brines et al., 2000). Furthermore, Epo has been demonstrated to delay the onset and to reduce the severity of clinical symptoms in an EAE model induced by MBP (Brines et al., 2000). The advantage of the "atypical" neurotrophin Epo when compared with other neurotrophic agents lies in its application mode and the good clinical tolerability. In a recent study of acute ischemic stroke in humans, intravenous treatment with Epo was well tolerated and an improvement in clinical outcome as well as a reduction in infarct size was observed (Ehrenreich et al., 2002).

Additional or alternative neuroprotective approaches that have been tested in EAE models so far involve the use of AMPA/kainate receptor antagonists as already mentioned in context with the mechanisms of neuronal apoptosis during chronic inflammatory autoimmune CNS diseases. In the study done by Smith et al. (2000), two different competitive as well as two noncompetitive AMPA receptor antagonists were shown to ameliorate the clinical disease course in rats during MBP-induced EAE. The effect of AMPA receptor blockade on the density of neurons in the lumbar spinal cord was investigated after NBQX treatment that resulted in increased neuronal survival. AMPA receptor blockade in this study positively influenced neurological score and weight loss in a dose-dependent manner when the treatment was started at day 10 after immunization. At this time point, most of the animals had not yet developed severe clinical symptoms of EAE, but disease manifestation occurred within the next days. In contrast, clinical outcome was not affected when therapy was started at day 4 after immunization and was continued for 1 week, indicating that the beneficial effects of AMPA receptor blockade strongly depend on treatment during a sensitive time period around disease onset. This might differ from the treatment regimen necessary for neuroprotection induced by neurotrophin-like substances. In neurodegenerative disease models, it has been shown that treatment with neurotrophic factors was most effective when given at an early time point after inducing the lesion. As an example, the highest rate of RGC rescue after application of insulin-like growth factor-I or glial cell-line derived neurotrophic factor after ON transection in rats was achieved using a treatment protocol with the first dosage given immediately after surgery (Klöcker et al., 1997; Kermer et al., 2000). Apoptotic cell death of RGCs in this model, however, shows a delayed onset with the first reduction of cell density at day 4 after ON transection, indicating that activation of intracellular neuroprotective cascades should precede the ones necessary for the execution of neuronal apoptosis.

Another treatment approach that has been shown to exert neuroprotective effects in rodent EAE involves the use of low-molecular-weight nonenzymatic proteins called metallothioneins (MT-I+II). These proteins are characterized by a high content of zinc or copper and show an upregulated expression in microglia and reactive astrocytes during EAE (Penkowa and Hidalgo, 2000). In a rat model of MBP-induced EAE, daily systemic treatment with MT-II led to reduced axon degeneration in the brainstem and spinal cord and to a decrease in the severity of clinical symptoms. Furthermore, an increase in the number of growth cones expressing neurites in both gray and white matter of the CNS has been reported in EAE rats after

application of MT-II when treatment was started before disease onset (Penkowa and Hidalgo, 2003). The neuroprotective effect of MT-II treatment was attributed to antioxidant properties of this protein, as well as to a stimulation of the expression of neurotrophic factors and cytokines such as basic fibroblast growth factor or transforming growth factor-β.

The use of caspase inhibitors as an antiapoptotic treatment strategy to protect neurons from premature cell death during chronic inflammatory autoimmune CNS diseases has been discussed in context with an *in vitro* study on neuronal cultures (Cid et al., 2003). In this study, application of two different caspase-3 inhibitors prevented neuronal apoptosis induced by CSF obtained from patients during acute MS relapses. However, caspase activation during the process of neuronal apoptosis is generally supposed to occur late in the execution program of apoptotic cell death (for review, see Bähr, 2000). Therefore, inhibition of a single execution system located downstream of the mitochondrion might not be sufficient to protect neurons that have already been damaged on proximal levels of their cell functions. It has also been shown that certain forms of apoptotic neuronal cell death cannot be prevented by the use of caspase inhibitors (for review, see Nicotera et al., 2000). Although generally considered to be specific for the caspase family, these inhibitors can have nonspecific effects such as blocking unrelated proteases of which the activity may be necessary for cell survival (for review, see Nicotera et al., 2000). Additionally, the antiapoptotic effect of caspase-3 inhibition has been shown to be transient and resulted in a delay rather than a permanent cell rescue of RGCs after axotomy of the ON (Kermer et al., 1999).

In summary, it is evident that characterization of the molecular mechanisms, kinetics, and pathogenesis of neuronal apoptosis in chronic inflammatory autoimmune CNS diseases will have important consequences for the development of future neuroprotective therapies. In addition to axonal injury, neuronal cell death by apoptosis could reach a significant extent during the time course of MS and may thereby contribute to permanent disability in patients. New modes of delivery for growth factors or antiapoptotic agents might help to overcome current therapeutic limitations in their use in clinical studies in patients with MS. Another approach would consist of testing neuroprotective properties of substances in MS that have already been approved in the treatment of other neurological or non-neurological disorders.

Acknowledgments

Funded by the Medical Faculty of the University of Göttingen (Junior Research Group; R.D.) and the Gemeinnützige Hertie Stiftung (M.B.). The authors gratefully acknowledge the critical reading and helpful suggestions of M. Sättler.

References

Ahmed, Z., Doward, A. I., Pryce, G., Taylor, D. L., Pocock, J. M., Leonard, J. P., Baker, D., and Cuzner, M. L. (2002). A role for caspase-1 and -3 in the pathology of experimental allergic encephalomyelitis: Inflammation versus degeneration. *Am. J. Pathol.* **161**, 1577–1586.

Alcazar, A., Regidor, I., Masjuan, J., Salinas, M., and Alvarez-Cermeno, J.C. (1998). Induction of apoptosis by cerebrospinal fluid from patients with primary-progressive multiple sclerosis in cultured neurons. *Neurosci. Lett.* **255**, 75–78.

Ay, H., Ay, I., Koroshetz, W. J, and Finklestein, S. P. (1999). Potential usefulness of basic fibroblast growth factor as a treatment for stroke. *Cerebrovasc. Dis.* **9**, 131–135.

Bähr, M., and Bonhoeffer, F. (1994). Perspectives on axonal regeneration in the mammalian CNS. *Trends Neurosci.* **17**, 473–479.

Bähr, M., and Wizenmann, A. (1996). Retinal ganglion cell axons recognize specific guidance cues present in the deafferented adult rat superior colliculus. *J. Neurosci.* **16**, 5106–5116.

Bähr, M. (2000). Live or let die: Retinal ganglion cell death and survival during development and in the lesioned adult CNS. *Trends Neurosci.* **23**, 483–490.

Barde, Y. A. (1989). Trophic factors and neuronal survival. *Neuron* **2**, 1525–1534.

Bernaudin, M., Marti, H. H., Roussel, S., Divoux, D., Nouvelot, A., MacKenzie, E. T., and Petit, E. (1999). A potential role for erythropoietin in focal permanent cerebral ischemia in mice. *J. Cereb. Blood Flow Metab.* **19**, 643–651.

Binns, K. E., and Salt, T. E. (1998). Developmental changes in NMDA receptor-mediated visual activity in the rat superior colliculus, and the effect of dark rearing. *Exp. Brain Res.* **120**, 335–344.

Borasio, G. D., Robberecht, W., Leigh, P. N., Emile, J., Guiloff, R. J., Jerusalem, F., Silani, V., Vos, P. E., Wokke, J. H., and Dobbins, T. (1998). A placebo-controlled trial of insulin-like growth factor-I in amyotrophic lateral sclerosis. European ALS/IGF-I study group. *Neurology* **51**, 583–586.

Boukhaddaoui, H., Sieso, V., Scamps, F., and Valmier, J. (2001). An activity-dependent neurotrophin-3 autocrine loop regulates the phenotype of developing hippocampal pyramidal neurons before target contact. *J. Neurosci.* **21**, 8789–8797.

Bradley, W. G. (1987). Recent views on amyotrophic lateral sclerosis with emphasis on electrophysiological studies. *Muscle Nerve* **10**, 490–502.

Brines, M. L., Ghezzi, P., Keenan, S., Agnello, D., de Lanerolle, N. C., Cerami, C., and Cerami, A. (2000). Erythropoietin crosses the blood-brain barrier to protect against experimental brain injury. *Proc. Natl. Acad. Sci. U.S.A.* **97**, 10526–10531.

Cardone, M. H., Roy, N., Stennicke, H. R., Salvesen, G. S., Franke, T. F., Stanbridge, E., Frisch, S., and Reed, J. C. (1998). Regulation of cell death protease caspase-9 by phosphorylation. *Science* **282**, 1318–1321.

Cecconi, F., Alvarez-Bolado, G., Meyer B. I., Roth, K. A., and Gruss, P. (1998). Apaf1 (CED-4 homolog) regulates programmed cell death in mammalian development. *Cell* **94**, 727–737.

Cellerino, A., Michaelidis, T., Barski, J. J., Bähr, M., Thoenen, H., and Meyer, M. (1999). Retinal ganglion cell loss after the period of naturally occurring cell death in bcl-2−/− mice. *Neuroreport* **10**, 1091–1095.

Cid, C., Alvarez-Cermeno, J. C., Regidor, I., Plaza, J., Salinas, M., and Alcazar, A. (2003). Caspase inhibitors protect against neuronal apoptosis induced by cerebrospinal fluid from multiple sclerosis patients. *J. Neuroimmunol.* **136**, 119–124.

Coffer, P. J., Jin, J., and Woodgett, J. R. (1998). Protein kinase B (c-Akt): A multifunctional mediator of phosphatidylinositol 3-kinase activation. *Biochem. J.* **335**, 1–13.

Cogen, J., and Cohen-Cory, S. (2000). Nitric oxide modulates retinal ganglion cell arbor remodeling in vivo. *J. Neurobiol.* **45**, 120–133.

Conover, J. C., Erickson, J. T., Katz, D. M., Bianchi, L. M., Poueymirou, W. T., McClain, J., Pan, L., Helgren, M., Ip, N. Y., Boland, P., et al. (1995).

Neuronal deficits, not involving motor neurons, in mice lacking BDNF and/or NT4. *Nature* **375**, 235–238.

Dash, P. K., Mach, S. A., and Moore, A. N. (2002). The role of extracellular signal-regulated kinase in cognitive and motor deficits following experimental traumatic brain injury. *Neuroscience* **114**, 755–767.

Datta, S. R., Dudek, H., Tao, X., Masters, S., Fu, H., Gotoh, Y., and Greenberg, M. E. (1997). Akt phosphorylation of BAD couples survival signals to the cell-intrinsic death machinery. *Cell* **91**, 231–241.

Deckwerth, T. L., Elliott, J. L., Knudson, C. M., Johnson, E. M., Snider, W. D., and Korsmeyer, S. J. (1996). BAX is required for neuronal death after trophic factor deprivation and during development. *Neuron* **17**, 401–411.

Diem, R., Meyer, R., Weishaupt, J. H., and Bähr, M. (2001). Reduction of potassium currents and phosphatidylinositol 3-kinase-dependent Akt phosphorylation by tumor necrosis factor-α rescues axotomized retinal ganglion cells from retrograde cell death *in vivo*. *J. Neurosci.* **21**, 2058–2066.

Diem, R., Hobom, M., Grötsch, P., Kramer, B., and Bähr, M. (2003a). Interleukin-1β protects neurons via the IL-1 receptor mediated Akt pathway and by IL-1 receptor-independent decrease of transmembrane currents *in vivo*. *Mol. Cell. Neurosci.* **22**, 487–500.

Diem, R., Hobom, M., Maier, K., Weissert, R., Storch, M. K., Meyer, R., and Bähr, M. (2003b). Methylprednisolone increases neuronal apoptosis during autoimmune CNS inflammation by inhibition of an endogenous neuroprotective pathway. *J. Neurosci.* **23**, 6993–7000.

Dittrich, F., Thoenen, H., and Sendtner, M. (1994). Ciliary neurotrophic factor: pharmacokinetics and acute-phase response in rat. *Ann. Neurol.* **35**, 151–163.

Dudek, H., Datta, S. R., Franke, T. F., Birnbaum, M. J., Yao, R., Cooper, G. M., Segal, R. A., Kaplan, D. R., and Greenberg, M. E. (1997). Regulation of neuronal survival by the serine-threonine protein kinase Akt. *Science* **275**, 661–665.

Ehrenreich, H., Hasselblatt, M., Dembowski, C., Cepek, L., Lewczuk, P., Stiefel, M., Rustenbeck, H. H., Breiter, N., Jacob, S., Knerlich, F., Bohn, M., Poser, W., Rüther, E., Kochen, M., Gefeller, O., Fleiter, C., Wessel, T. C., De Ryck, M., Itri, L., Prange, H., Cerami, A., Brines, M., and Siren, A. L. (2002). Erythropoietin therapy for acute stroke is both safe and beneficial. *Mol. Med.* **8**, 495–505.

Eschweiler, G. W., and Bähr, M. (1993). Flunarizine enhances rat retinal ganglion cell survival after axotomy. *J. Neurol. Sci.* **116**, 34–40.

Ferguson, B., Matyszak, M. K., Esiri, M. M., and Perry, V. H. (1997). Axonal damage in acute multiple sclerosis lesions. *Brain* **120**, 393–399.

Ferrer, I., Blanco, R., Carmona, M., Ribera, R., Goutan, E., Puig, B., Rey, M. J., Cardozo, A., Vinals, F., and Ribalta, T. (2001). Phosphorylated map kinase (ERK1, ERK2) expression is associated with early tau deposition in neurones and glial cells, but not with increased nuclear DNA vulnerability and cell death, in Alzheimer disease, Pick's disease, progressive supranuclear palsy and corticobasal degeneration. *Brain Pathol.* **11**, 144–158.

Fisher, J., Levkovitch-Verbin, H., Schori, H., Yoles, E., Butovsky, O., Kaye, J. F., Ben-Nun, A., and Schwartz, M. (2001). Vaccination for neuroprotection in the mouse optic nerve: implications for optic neuropathies. *J. Neurosci.* **21**, 136–142.

Fukunaga, K., and Miyamoto, E. (1998). Role of MAP kinase in neurons. *Mol. Neurobiol.* **16**, 79–95.

Giess, R., Mäurer, M., Linker, R., Gold, R., Warmuth-Metz, M., Toyka, K. V., Sendtner, M., Rieckmann, P. (2002). Association of a null mutation in the CNTF gene with early onset of multiple sclerosis. *Arch. Neurol.* **59**, 407–409.

Grewal, S. S., York, R. D., and Storck, P. J. (1999). Extracellular-signal-regulated kinase signalling in neurons. *Curr. Opin. Neurobiol.* **9**, 544–553.

Hammarberg, H., Lidman, O., Lundberg, C., Eltayeb, S. Y., Gielen, A. W., Muhallab, S., Svenningsson, A., Linda, H., van Der Meide, P. H., Cullheim, S., Olsson, T., and Piehl, F. (2000). Neuroprotection by encephalomyelitis: Rescue of mechanically injured neurons and neurotrophin production by CNS-infiltrating T and natural killer cells. *J. Neurosci.* **20,** 5283–5291.

Hardin-Pouzet, H., Krakowski, M., Bourbonniere, L., Didier-Bazes, M., Tran, E., and Owens, T. (1997). Glutamate metabolism is down-regulated in astrocytes during experimental allergic encephalomyelitis. *Glia* **20,** 79–85.

Hayreh, S. S. (1981). Experimental allergic encephalomyelitis. Retinal and other ocular manifestations. *Invest. Ophthalmol. Vis. Sci.* **21,** 270–281.

Hengartner, M. O., and Horvitz, H. R. (1994). C. elegans cell survival gene ced-9 encodes a functional homolog of the mammalian proto-oncogene bcl-2. *Cell* **76,** 665–676.

Hobom, M., Storch, M. K., Weissert, R., Maier, K., Radhakrishnan, A., Kramer, B., Bähr, M., and Diem, R. (2004). Mechanisms and time course of neuronal degeneration in experimental autoimmune encephalomyelitis. *Brain Pathol.* **14,** 148–157.

Hofer, M. M., and Barde, Y. A. (1988). Brain-derived neurotrophic factor prevents neuronal death in vivo. *Nature* **331,** 261–262.

Horvitz, H. R. (1999). Genetic control of programmed cell death in the nematode *Caenorhabditis elegans. Cancer Res.* **59,** 1701–1706.

Isenmann, S., Wahl, C., Krajewski, S., Reed, J. C., and Bähr, M. (1997). Up-regulation of Bax protein in degenerating retinal ganglion cells precedes apoptotic cell death after optic nerve lesion in the rat. *Eur. J. Neurosci.* **9,** 1763–1772.

Jellinger, K. A. (2001). Cell death mechanisms in neurodegeneration. *J. Cell. Mol. Med.* **5,** 1–17.

Jin, K., Mao, X. O., Zhu, Y., and Greenberg, D. A. (2002). MEK and ERK protect hypoxic cortical neurons via phosphorylation of Bad. *J. Neurochem.* **80,** 119–125.

Kermer, P., Klöcker, N., and Bähr, M. (1999). Long-term effect of inhibition of ced 3-like caspases on the survival of axotomized retinal ganglion cells in vivo. *Exp. Neurol.* **158,** 202–205.

Kermer, P., Klöcker, N., Labes, M., and Bähr, M. (2000). Insulin-like growth factor-I protects axotomized rat retinal ganglion cells from secondary death via PI3-K-dependent Akt phosphorylation and inhibition of caspase-3 in vivo. *J. Neurosci.* **20,** 722–728.

Kerr, J. F., Wyllie, A. H., and Currie, A. R. (1972). Apoptosis: a basic biological phenomenon with wide ranging implications in tissue kinetics. *Br. J. Cancer* **26,** 239–257.

Kerschensteiner, M., Gallmeier, E., Behrens, L., Leal, V. V., Misgeld, T., Klinkert, W. E., Kolbeck, R., Hoppe, E., Oropeza-Wekerle, R. L., Bartke, I., Stadelmann, C., Lassmann, H., Wekerle, H., and Hohlfeld, R. (1999). Activated human T cells, B cells, and monocytes produce brain-derived neurotrophic factor in vitro and in inflammatory brain lesions: A neuroprotective role of inflammation? *J. Exp. Med.* **189,** 865–870.

Klöcker, N., Bräunling, F., Isenmann, S., and Bähr, M. (1997). *In vivo* neurotrophic effects of GDNF on axotomized retinal ganglion cells. *NeuroReport* **8,** 3439–3442.

Klöcker, N., Cellerino, A., and Bähr, M. (1998). Free radical scavenging and inhibition of nitric oxide synthase potentiates the neurotrophic effects of brain-derived neurotrophic factor on axotomized retinal ganglion cells *in vivo. J. Neurosci.* **18,** 1038–1046.

Kornek, B., Storch, M. K., Weissert, R., Wallstroem, E., Stefferl, A., Olsson, T., Linington, C., Schmidbauer, M., and Lassmann, H. (2000). Multiple sclerosis and chronic autoimmune encephalomyelitis: A comparative quantitative study of axonal injury in active, inactive, and remyelinated lesions. *Am. J. Pathol.* **157,** 267–276.

Levi-Montalcini, R., Skaper, S. D., Dal Toso R., Petrelli, L., and Leon, A. (1996). Nerve growth factor: from neurotrophin to neurokine. *Trends Neurosci.* **19,** 514–520.

Li, P., Nijhawan, D., Budihardjo, I., Srinivasula, S. M., Ahmad, M., Alnemri, E. S., and Wang, X. (1997). Cytochrome c and dATP-dependent formation of Apaf-1/caspase-9 complex initiates an apoptotic protease cascade. *Cell* **91,** 479–489.

Linker, R. A., Mäurer, M., Gaupp, S., Martini, R., Holtmann, B., Giess, R., Rieckmann, P., Lassmann, H., Toyka, K. V., Sendtner, M., and Gold, R.

(2002). CNTF is a major protective factor in demyelinating CNS disease: A neurotrophic cytokine as modulator in neuroinflammation. *Nat. Med.* **8,** 620–624.

Lloyd, K. G. (1977). CNS compensation to dopamine neuron loss in Parkinson's disease. *Adv. Exp. Med. Biol.* **90,** 255–266.

Mansour-Robaey, S., Clarke, D. B., Wang, Y. C., Bray, G. M., and Aguayo, A. J. (1994) Effects of ocular injury and administration of brain-derived neurotrophic factor on survival and regrowth of axotomized retinal ganglion cells. *Proc. Natl. Acad. Sci. U. S. A.* **91,** 1632–1636.

Mattson, M. P. (2000a). Apoptotic and anti-apoptotic synaptic signaling mechanisms. *Brain Pathol.* **10,** 300–312.

Mattson M. P. (2000b) Apoptosis in neurodegenerative disorders. *Nat. Rev. Mol. Cell. Biol.* **1,** 120–129.

McKay, S. E., Purcell, A. L., and Carew, T. J. (1999). Regulation of synaptic function by neurotrophic factors in vertebrates and invertebrates: Implications for development and learning. *Learn. Mem.* **6,** 193–215.

Mews, I., Bergmann, M., Bunkowski, S., Gullotta, F., and Brück, W. (1998). Oligodendrocyte and axon pathology in clinically silent multiple sclerosis lesions. *Multiple Sclerosis* **4,** 55–62.

Meyer, R., Weissert, R., Diem, R., Storch, M. K., de Graaf, K. L., Kramer, B., and Bähr, M. (2001). Acute neuronal apoptosis in a rat model of multiple sclerosis. *J. Neurosci.* **21,** 6214–6220.

Meyer-Franke, A., Wilkinson, G. A., Kruttgen, A., Hu, M., Munro, E., Hanson, M. G., Reichardt, L. F., and Barres, B. A. (1998). Depolarization and cAMP elevation rapidly recruit TrkB to the plasma membrane of CNS neurons. *Neuron* **21,** 681–693.

Michaelidis, T. M., Sendtner, M., Cooper, J. D., Airaksinen, M. S., Holtmann, B., Meyer, M., and Thoenen, H. (1996). Inactivation of bcl-2 results in progressive degeneration of motoneurons, sympathetic and sensory neurons during early postnatal development. *Neuron* **17,** 75–89.

Moalem, G., Leibowitz-Amit, R., Yoles, E., Mor, F., Cohen, I. R., and Schwartz, M. (1999). Autoimmune T cells protect neurons from secondary degeneration after central nervous system axotomy. *Nat. Med.* **5,** 49–55.

Mody, I., and MacDonald, J. F. (1995). NMDA receptor-dependent excitotoxicity: The role of intracellular Ca2+ release. *Trends Pharmacol. Sci.* **16,** 356–359.

Moreau, T., Coles, A., Wing, M., Isaacs, J., Hale, G., Waldmann, H., and Compston, A. (1996). Transient increase in symptoms associated with cytokine release in patients with multiple sclerosis. *Brain* **119,** 225–237.

Mosinger Ogilvie, J., Deckwerth, T. L., Knudson, C. M., and Korsmeyer, S. J. (1998). Suppression of developmental retinal cell death but not of photoreceptor degeneration in Bax-deficient mice. *Invest. Ophthalmol. Vis. Sci.* **39,** 1713–1720.

Motoyama, N., Wang, F., Roth, K. A., Sawa, H., Nakayama, K., Nakayama, K., Negishi, I., Senju, S., Zhang, Q., Fujii, S., et al. (1995). Massive cell death of immature hematopoietic cells and neurons in Bcl-x-deficient mice. *Science* **267,** 1506–1510.

Neumann, H., Schmidt, H., Cavalie, A., Jenne, D., and Wekerle, H. (1997). Major histocompatibility complex (MHC) class I gene expression in single neurons of the central nervous system: differential regulation by interferon (IFN)-gamma and tumor necrosis factor (TNF)-alpha. *J. Exp. Med.* **185,** 305–316.

Nicholson, D. W., and Thornberry, N. A. (1997). Caspases: killer proteases. *Trends Biochem. Sci.* **22,** 299–306.

Nicotera, P., Leist, M., Fava, E., Berliocchi, L., and Volbracht, C. (2000). Energy requirement for caspase activation and neuronal cell death. *Brain Pathol.* **10,** 276–282.

Offen, D., Kaye, J. F., Bernard, O., Merims, D., Coire, C. I., Panet, H. E., and Ben-Nun, A. (2000). Mice overexpressing Bcl-2 in their neurons are resistant to myelin oligodendrocyte glycoprotein (MOG)-induced experimental autoimmune encephalomyelitis (EAE). *J. Mol. Neurosci.* **15,** 167–175.

Oltvai, Z. N., Milliman, C. L., and Korsmeyer, S. J. (1993). Bcl-2 heterodimerizes in vivo with a conserved homolog, Bax, that accelerates programmed cell death. *Cell* **74,** 609–619.

Oppenheim, R. W. (1996). Neurotrophic survival molecules for motoneurons: an embarrassment of riches. *Neuron* **17,** 195–197.

Parry, A., Corkill, R., Blamire, A. M., Palace, J., Narayanan, S., Arnold, D., Styles, P., and Matthews, P. M. (2003). Beta-interferon treatment does not always slow the progression of axonal injury in multiple sclerosis. *J. Neurol.* **250,** 171–178.

Penkowa, M., and Hidalgo, J. (2000). Metallothionein I+II (MT-I+II) expression and their role on experimental autoimmune encephalomyelitis (EAE). *Glia* **32,** 247–263.

Penkowa, M., and Hidalgo, J. (2003). Treatment with metallothionein prevents demyelination and axonal damage and increases oligodendrocyte precursors and tissue repair during experimental autoimmune encephalomyelitis. *J. Neurosci. Res.* **72,** 574–586.

Peterson, J. W., Bö, L., Mörk, S., Chang, A., and Trapp, B. D. (2001). Transected neurites, apoptotic neurons, and reduced inflammation in cortical multiple sclerosis lesions. *Ann. Neurol.* **50,** 389–400.

Phokeo, V., and Ball, A. K. (2000). Transection of dysmyelinated optic nerve axons in adult rats lacking myelin basic protein. *Neuroreport* **11,** 3375–3379.

Pitt, D., Werner P., and Raine, C. S. (2000). Glutamate excitotoxicity in a model of multiple sclerosis. *Nat. Med.* **6,** 67–70.

Raff, M. C., Barres, B. A., Burne, J. F., Coles, H. S., Ishizaki, Y., and Jacobson, M. D. (1993). Programmed cell death and the control of cell survival: Lessons from the nervous system. *Science* **262,** 695–700.

Safran, A. B., and Landis, T. (1996). Plasticity in the adult visual cortex: Implications for the diagnosis of visual field defects and visual rehabilitation. *Curr. Opin. Ophthalmol.* **7,** 53–64.

Segal, R. A., and Greenberg, M. E. (1996). Intracellular signaling pathways activated by neurotrophic factors. *Annu. Rev. Neurosci.* **19,** 463–489.

Shen, S., Wiemelt, A. P., McMorris, F. A., and Barres, B. A. (1999). Retinal ganglion cells lose trophic responsiveness after axotomy. *Neuron* **23,** 285–295.

Smith, T., Groom, A., Zhu, B., and Turski, L. (2000). Autoimmune encephalomyelitis ameliorated by AMPA antagonists. *Nat. Med.* **6,** 62–66.

Storch, M. K., Stefferl, A., Brehm, U., Weissert, R., Wallstrom, E., Kerschensteiner, M., Olsson, T., Linington, C., and Lassmann, H. (1998). Autoimmunity to myelin oligodendrocyte glycoprotein in rats mimics the spectrum of multiple sclerosis pathology. *Brain Pathol.* **8,** 681–694.

Stover, J. F., Pleines, U. E., Morganti-Kossmann, M. C., Kossmann, T., Lowitzsch, K., and Kempski, O. S. (1997). Neurotransmitters in cerebrospinal fluid reflect pathological activity. *Eur. J. Clin. Invest.* **27,** 1038–1043.

Taniike, M., Mohri, I., Eguchi, N., Beuckmann, C. T., Suzuki, K., and Urade, Y. (2002). Perineuronal oligodendrocytes protect against neuronal apoptosis through the production of lipocalin-type prostaglandin D synthase in a genetic demyelinating model. *J. Neurosci.* **22,** 4885–4896.

Theoret, H., Herbin, M., Boire, D., and Ptito, M. (1997). Transneuronal retrograde degeneration of retinal ganglion cells following cerebral hemispherectomy in cats. *Brain Res.* **775,** 203–208.

Thoenen, H. (1991). The changing scene of neurotrophic factors. *Trends Neurosci.* **14,** 165–170.

Thornberry, N. A., and Lazebnik, Y. (1998). Caspases: Enemies within. *Science* **281,** 1312–1316.

Trapp, B. D., Peterson, J., Ransohoff, R. M., Rudick, R., Mork, S., and Bo, L. (1998). Axonal transection in multiple sclerosis lesions. *N. Engl. J. Med.* **338,** 278–285.

Trentani, A., Kuipers, S. D., Ter Horst, G. J., and Den Boer, J. A. (2002). Selective chronic stress-induced in vivo ERK1/2 hyperphosphorylation in medial prefrontocortical dendrites: Implications for stress-related cortical pathology? *Eur. J. Neurosci.* **15,** 1681–1691.

Tu, S., Butt, C. M., Pauly, J. R., and Debski, E. A. (2000). Activity-dependent regulation of substance P expression and topographic map maintenance by a cholinergic pathway. *J. Neurosci.* **20,** 5346–5357.

Ugolini, G., Raoul, C., Ferri, A., Haenggeli, C., Yamamoto, Y., Salaun, D., Henderson, C. E., Kato, A. C., Pettmann, B., and Hueber, A. O. (2003). Fas/tumor necrosis factor receptor death signaling is required for axotomy-induced death of motoneurons in vivo. *J. Neurosci.* **23,** 8526–8531.

Verhagen, C., Mor, F., and Cohen, I. R. (1994). T cell immunity to myelin basic protein induces anterior uveitis in Lewis rats. *J. Neuroimmunol.* **53,** 65–71.

Villegas-Perez, M. P., Vidal Sanz, M., Bray, G. M., and Aguayo, A. J. (1988). Influences of peripheral nerve grafts on the survival and regrowth of axotomized retinal ganglion cells in adult rats. *J. Neurosci.* **8,** 265–280.

Weissert, R., Wallstrom, E., Storch, M. K., Stefferl, A., Lorentzen, J., Lassmann, H., Linington, C., and Olsson, T. (1998). MHC haplotype-dependent regulation of MOG-induced EAE in rats. *J. Clin. Invest.* **102,** 1265–1273.

Wekerle, H., Kojima, K., Lannes-Vieira, J., Lassmann, H., and Linington, C. (1994). Animal models. *Ann. Neurol.* (Suppl.) **36,** S47–S53.

Werner, P., Pitt, D., and Raine, C. S. (2001). Multiple sclerosis: Altered glutamate homeostasis in lesions correlates with oligodendrocyte and axonal damage. *Ann. Neurol.* **50,** 169–180.

Zhu, B., Wayne Moore, G. R., Zwimpfer, T. J., Kastrukoff, L. F., Dyer, J. K., Steeves, J. D., Paty, D. W., and Cynader, M. S. (1999). Axonal cytoskeleton changes in experimental optic neurits. *Brain Res.* **824,** 204–217.

Zou, H., Henzel, W. J., Liu, X., Lutschg, A., and Wang, X. (1997). Apaf-1, a human protein homologous to *C. elegans* CED-4, participates in cytochrome c-dependent activation of caspase-3. *Cell* **90,** 389–390.

24

Mechanisms Underlying Wallerian Degeneration

Ahmet Höke, M.D., Ph.D.

John W. Griffin, M.D.

I. Introduction

When the axon of a neuron is transected, the changes that take place in the distal segment, which is separated from the cell body, are termed wallerian degeneration. In addition, there are changes that take place in the neuronal cell body and the proximal axon. The changes that occur in the neuron and in its axon are not processes that happen in isolation, but are affected by the surrounding glial cells and by the influx of immune cells. Most of what is known about wallerian degeneration comes from studies in the peripheral nervous system (PNS). However, this is changing, and understanding the mechanisms underlying wallerian degeneration in the central nervous system (CNS) is likely to shed further light onto the pathogenesis of CNS disorders such as multiple sclerosis. In this section, we review what is known about wallerian degeneration and propose new avenues of research that improve our understanding of multiple sclerosis as a neuronal disease.

II. Structural and Cellular Changes

Since the initial description by Waller (1850), structural and cellular changes and the time course of such changes that occur during wallerian degeneration have been described in increasing detail, especially in the PNS (Vial, 1958; Ohmi, 1961; Webster, 1962; Lee, 1963; Cravioto, 1969; Simon et al., 1969). For a short period after transection, most of the distal stump appears nearly normal. The segment just distal to the site of axotomy is an exception. Immediately after axotomy, there is a progressive accumulation of intra-axonal organelles at the proximal end of the disconnected nerve fibers (Zelena et al., 1968; Griffin et al., 1977) (Fig. 1). These organelles form a caplike pellet that increases in volume linearly with time until axonal breakdown supervenes (Zelena et al., 1968). This pellet results from continued retrograde transport of vesicular organelles, as well as some mitochondria, dense

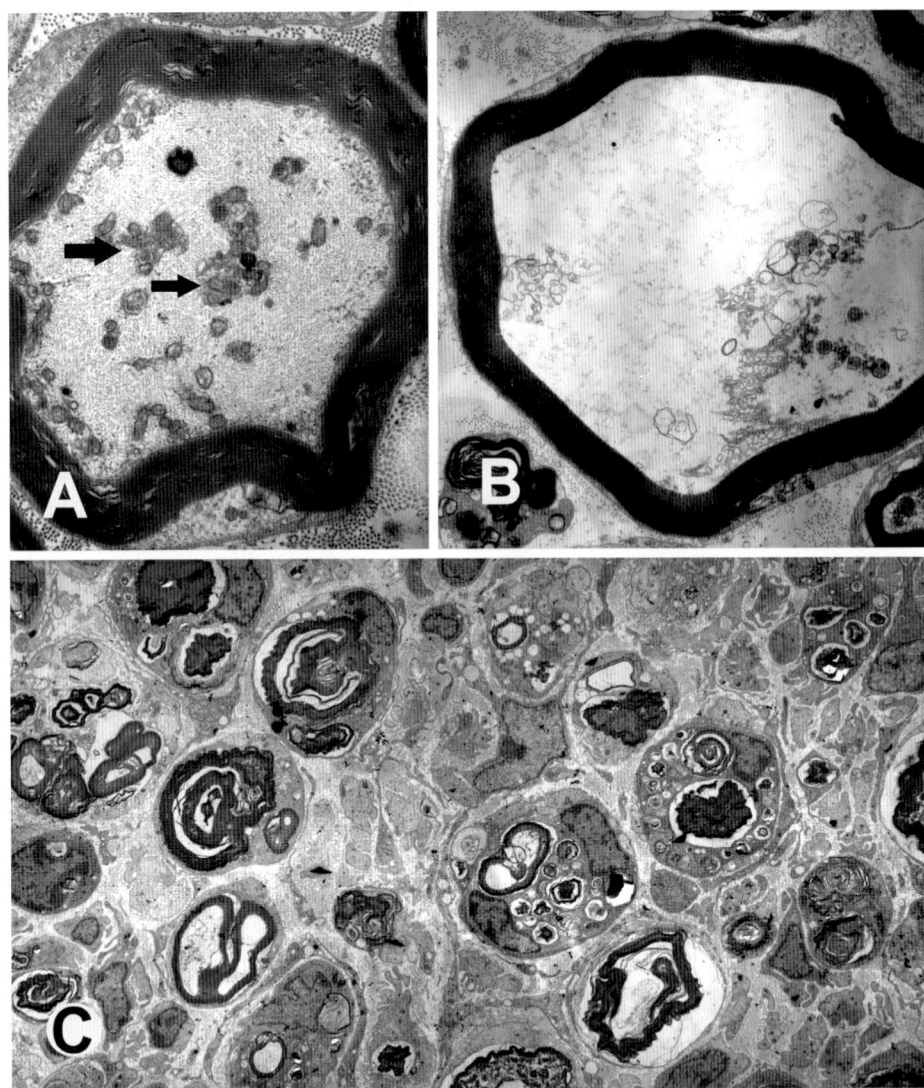

Figure 1 **Early structural changes during wwallerian degeneration** (**A**) Twelve hours after transection of the sciatic nerve of an adult rat shows one of the earliest structural changes that take place during wwallerian degeneration, accumulation or organelles, including mitochondria (*arrows*) (original magnification × 10,000.) (**B**) Within 24 hours of the transection, granular disintegration of the cytoskeleton takes place. Notice that in panel A and B, the axons are swollen as evidenced by the decrease in g-ratio (ratio of the myelin thickness to the whole fiber diameter) (original magnification × 10,000). (**C**) At 7 days after transection of the nerve, Schwann cell proliferation, macrophage infiltration, and myelin degradation are all well underway (original magnification × 2,000).

bodies, and multivesicular bodies, producing a focal accumulation at the site of axonal interruption (Zelena et al., 1968; Ranish and Ochs, 1972). During this initial stage, there are only subtle changes elsewhere along the fibers. There is a tendency for particulate organelles to accumulate beneath nodes of Ranvier and Schmidt-Lantermann incisures (Ballin and Thomas, 1969), an exaggeration of their normal enrichment in those sites and presumably indicative of some early changes in fast bidirectional transport. However, on the whole, fast transport continues at normal rates and roughly normal abundance (Ranish and Ochs, 1972; Lubinska, 1977);

even uptake of exogenous materials at the synaptic terminals persists, and electrical conduction with synaptic transmission can be elicited normally with stimulation of the distal stump (Miledi and Slater, 1970). The duration of this initial stage of wallerian degeneration varies with the species, the length of distal stump (longer with a longer stump [Miledi and Slater, 1970]), the temperature (longer in cooler distal stump [Gamble and Jha, 1958; Sea et al., 1995; Tsao et al., 1999]), and possibly with the nature of the nerve (motor vs. sensory) and the location (PNS vs. CNS) (Pesini et al., 1999) (reviewed in detail by Chaudhry and colleagues, 1992).

This brief initial stage of wallerian degeneration is followed by breakdown of the axonal cytoskeleton. Granular disintegration of the cytoskeleton describes the abrupt conversion of the axoplasm into fine particulate and amorphous debris (George and Griffin, 1994), representing cleavage products of the cytoskeleton. This change must occur in an explosive fashion at any single level of the axon, as indicated by the rarity of finding partial stages in the process. In transverse sections, each fiber either appears normal or has complete granular disintegration, suggesting a virtual "all-or-none" change without persistent intermediate stages. In the PNS, the disintegration of particulate axonal organelles and axolemma is essentially simultaneous with the breakdown of the cytoskeleton. However, in the CNS, remaining axolemma and often mitochondria frequently are found in axons that have undergone recent disintegration of their cytoskeleton (Franson and Ronnevi, 1984; George and Griffin, 1994). Although this stage appears to last only for a few hours, it serves to emphasize the early structural changes in the cytoskeleton.

The direction of spread of granular disintegration of the cytoskeleton has been a controversial issue. In the garfish olfactory nerve, the process of axonal degeneration is extremely slow, and it clearly shows a centrifugal spread (Cancalon, 1982, 1983). In mammalian axons, the axonal breakdown is much more rapid, so that the spatiotemporal sequence has been debated. Some studies suggested that degeneration is virtually synchronous all along the distal stump or that degeneration starts distally and progresses proximally with time (Lunn et al., 1990). The benchmark analysis, however, remains the rigorous quantitative study of degeneration in the rat phrenic nerve, which showed a clear centrifugal spread of early changes of wallerian degeneration (Lubinska, 1977). The phrenic nerve remains at core temperature, thereby reducing the possibility of a proximal-distal temperature gradient that might affect the results. Another system with similar advantages is the degeneration of central projections of dorsal root ganglion sensory neurons after dorsal rhizotomy close to the cell body. In this system, spread of granular disintegration of the cytoskeleton starts at the site of transection and proceeds centrifugally (away from the cell body) at a rate of about 3 mm/hr (George and Griffin, 1994).

Several cellular changes follow promptly after the breakdown of the axon, including (in the PNS) opening of the blood-nerve barrier, degranulation of mast cells, recruitment of circulating macrophages, and early changes in the Schwann cells. The sequence of vascular and glial changes and the cell–cell interactions underlying these changes are only partially understood.

One of the first changes after granular disintegration of the cytoskeleton is opening of the blood-nerve barrier in the PNS. In the transected rat sciatic nerve, this immediately follows the breakdown of the cytoskeleton, occurring 24 to 48 hours after the injury (Powell et al., 1980; Bouldin et al., 1990). Of course, at the site of the axotomy, there is a prompt breakdown (Bouldin et al., 1991), but the barrier appears to remain intact along the rest of the distal stump. Shortly after dissolution of axoplasm, there is breakdown of the blood-nerve barrier, which can be triggered by degeneration of even a small number of fibers. In the rat sciatic nerve, restoration of the blood-nerve barrier occurs only after successful regeneration of axons through the segment (Bouldin et al., 1991). However, in the frog sciatic nerve, the blood-nerve barrier is at least partially restored even in the absence of successful regeneration (Weerasuriya, 1990). The basis for breakdown of the blood-nerve barrier is unknown; the effect of degranulation of mast cells (Powell et al., 1980) and cytokines (Griffin et al., 1992) have been proposed but not directly demonstrated experimentally. The CNS responds differently. There is less breakdown of the blood-tissue-barrier along the degenerating dorsal column axonal tracts than in the PNS (George and Griffin, 1994). This cannot be due to intrinsic differences between the central and peripheral axons; the same fibers are involved in the dorsal root and dorsal column when the central branches of dorsal root ganglion neurons are transected at the dorsal root level. This is likely to be due to differences in the intrinsic differences between the glial and endothelial cells of the CNS and the PNS.

III. Wallerian Degeneration Is an Active Process

Waller's initial observation, more than 150 years ago, that the distal stumps of transected nerve fibers degenerate (Waller, 1850), and subsequent findings that most proteins in the axon are synthesized in the cell body and transported down the axons using specialized transport mechanisms led to the attractive hypothesis that degeneration of the distal stump of a transected axon occurs because of lack of necessary proteins and other materials. However, slowed wallerian degeneration observed in a strain of mice (C57Bl/Ola, now called *Wlds* for wallerian-like degeneration slow) changed that perception dramatically (Lunn et al., 1989; Perry et al., 1990; Glass and Griffin, 1991). In this spontaneously generated strain, degeneration of the transected axons is slowed significantly (Fig. 2). In a wild-type animal, transection of the sciatic nerve results in loss of electrical conductivity in the distal portion within a day or two, followed by dissolution of the axoplasm. In contrast, a transected axon in a *Wlds* mouse continues to conduct electricity for up to 2 weeks (Lunn et al., 1990; Tsao et al., 1994). This delayed process suggests that wallerian degeneration is an active process that requires the presence and activation of a cellular pathway that regulates the dissolution of the axoplasm. This cellular pathway is similar to the pathway that

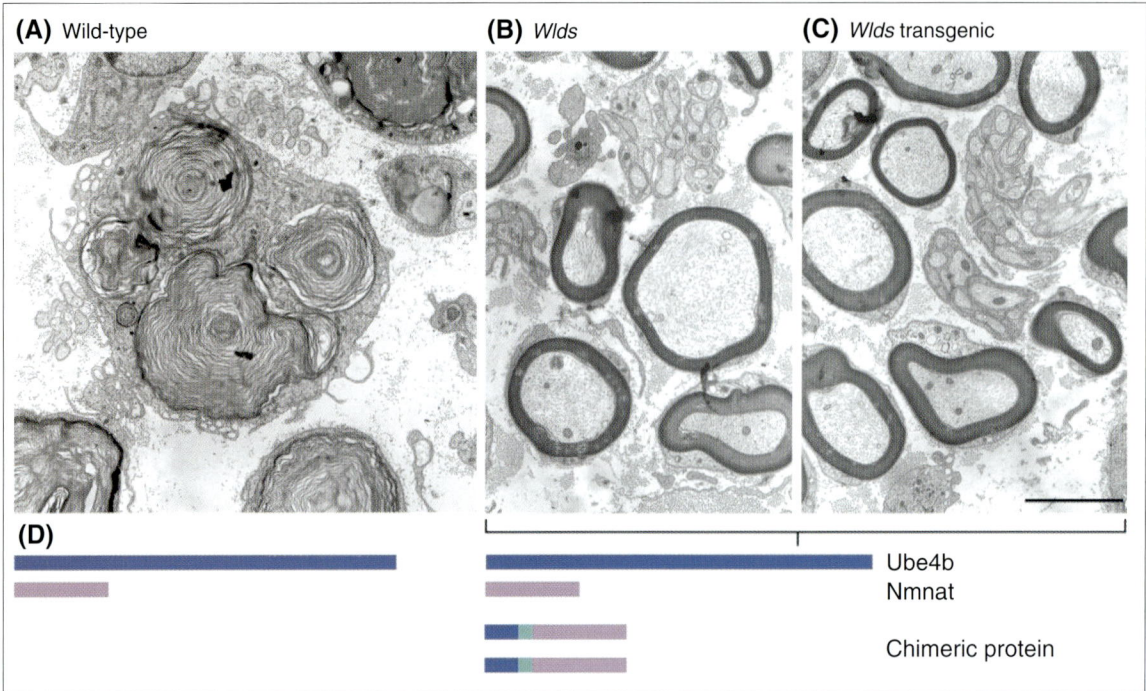

Figure 2 Axon protection in mice expressing the chimeric *Wlds* gene. Ultrathin transverse sections of (**A**) wild-type, (**B**) *Wlds,* and (**C**) transgenic *Wlds* sciatic nerve distal to a site of transection 14 days after the lesion. (**D**) *Wlds* chimeric protein and its parent proteins (drawn to scale) in these strains. The proteins below (**B**) and (**C**) are those produced in both *Wlds* and *Wlds*-transgenic mice. Two copies of the chimeric protein are shown to indicate that there are two copies of the chimeric gene per haploid genome. Abbreviations: Nmnat, nicotinamide mononucleotide adenylyltransferase; Ube4b, ubiquitination factor E4B. Scale bar, 10 μm. (With permission from Coleman and Perry, 2002.)

regulates apoptotic cell death in the sense that both are regulated active processes requiring energy, but there are significant differences as well. The molecular characters that play a role in this active self-destruct mechanism are not well understood, but are different from those involved in apoptosis (see later).

A. Role of Calcium and Calcium-Dependent Proteases

Before the observation of slow axonal degeneration in *Wlds* mice, the prevailing view was that wallerian degeneration was a passive phenomenon that involved influx of calcium in transected axons when axonal membrane integrity could not be maintained any longer due to lack of new proteins transported form the neuronal cell body (Schlaepfer, 1974b). Degeneration of axons *in vitro* was delayed when calcium was removed from the incubation media. Influx of calcium and thereby degeneration of the axon could be delayed *in vitro* if the medium was supplemented with rich energy sources and expedited if energy sources were removed from the media, again suggesting a passive process in which energy was required for maintenance of the calcium efflux mechanisms to preserve the axonal integrity

(Schlaepfer, 1974a). The potential role of calcium influx was further shown by the use of chlorpromazine, an inhibitor of calcium-binding protein calmodulin. Application of chlorpromazine inhibited the early structural changes observed during wallerian degeneration (de Medinaceli and Church, 1984).

These initial studies on the role of calcium hypothesized that once the transport of necessary materials was prevented, calcium homeostasis could not be maintained in the distal stump of a transected axon. This would lead to influx of calcium, swelling of the axon, and dissolution of the axoplasm. However, observations of slowed axonal degeneration in *Wlds* mouse challenged this hypothesis, and the researchers' attention focused on a potential role for calcium in an active process that is responsible for the degradation of axoplasm. A detailed study showed that after a lag-period, entry of extracellular calcium into the axon through an intact axolemma is both necessary and sufficient for axonal degeneration to proceed (George et al., 1995). This influx of calcium was necessary to activate calpains (calcium-dependent cysteine proteases) and result in granular degradation of the axoplasm. Blockage of entry of calcium or of activation of calpains was sufficient to delay the axonal cytoskeletal degradation. This and other similar studies

(Schlaepfer and Hasler, 1979; Badalamente et al., 1986; Mata et al., 1986) implicating a role for calcium in wallerian degeneration suggested that perhaps inhibition of calcium entry may be developed as a therapeutic tool to delay or prevent the axonal degeneration in neurodegenerative disorders. To date, however, calcium channel blockers have not been successful in preventing or slowing any neurodegenerative disorder of the PNS.

The role of calcium and calcium-dependent proteases in wallerian degeneration was further studied using the *Wlds* mouse. In the *Wlds* mouse, similar to the wild type, neurofilament degradation was dependent on the influx of calcium and activation of calpains. However, in the *Wlds* mouse, dissolution of the axoplasm required higher levels of calcium, suggesting an insensitivity of the proteases to calcium (Glass et al., 1994). To determine if there was a genetic basis for this relative insensitivity to calcium, an 80-kDa subunit of m-calpain in the *Wlds* mouse was sequenced and compared to the wild type (Glass et al., 1998). The sequence of the m-calpain subunit was similar in both the wild-type and *Wlds* mice, suggesting that either types of calpains or proteases other than calpains played a role in calcium-dependent degradation of the axonal cytoskeleton.

Another recent study on the role of calcium in pathological conditions of the axon brings attention to L-type voltage-sensitive calcium channels and intracellular calcium through ryanodine receptors (Ouardouz et al., 2003). In this study, Stys and colleagues showed that in the rat spinal cord dorsal column, ischemia results in axonal injury and an increase in intra-axonal calcium levels, even in the absence of extracellular calcium, but not when intracellular calcium stores are depleted or release of calcium from intracellular stores is blocked by ryanodine. They further show that at the initial stages of axonal degeneration, rise in intra-axonal calcium around intra-axonal endoplasmic reticulum profiles lead to dissolution of neurofilaments. Although this process is initiated by ischemia rather than axonal transection, and therefore might be different than classical wallerian degeneration, rise in intra-axonal calcium and degradation of neurofilaments is similar to what happens during granular disintegration of the axon. Further studies on different pathogenic processes in the CNS and PNS may lead to a better understanding of the role of calcium and common pathways that result in axonal pathology.

B. Role of Ubiquitin Proteasome System

One of the most important observations of the dominant mutation in the *Wlds* mouse is that there has to be an active regulator of wallerian degeneration that is present in the axon before the transection. In 1998, an 85-kb tandem triplication on the distal arm of the mouse chromosome 4 was found in the *Wlds* mouse (Coleman et al., 1998). Subsequently, within this triplication segment, exons of three genes were identified (Conforti et al., 2000) (Fig. 2D). Ubiquitin fusion degradation protein 2 (*Ufd2*) and a previously unidentified protein, *D4Cole1e* (later found to be identical to human nicotinamide mononucleotide acetyltransferase, *NMNAT*; see later) formed an in-frame fusion protein that was highly expressed in the nervous tissues. The third gene within this triplication region was a novel member of the retinoid-binding protein family, *Rbp7*. However, its expression was absent from the nervous tissues, suggesting that it did not play a role in the *Wlds* phenotype. This initial observation suggested a prominent role for the ubiquitin proteasome pathway in regulating the wallerian degeneration. It was unclear, however, how the *Ube4b/D4Cole1e* fusion protein affected the cellular mechanisms underlying wallerian degeneration. From the sequence analysis, it was not clear if either protein had any enzymatic activity (Conforti et al., 2000). A year later, the same group that identified the triplication mutation in the *Wlds* mouse recognized that the human homologue of *D4Cole1e* is *NMNAT*, a key enzyme in the synthetic pathway of NAD$^+$ (Mack et al., 2001).

To test the hypothesis that the fusion protein was responsible for the *Wlds* phenotype, the investigators generated a transgenic mouse overexpressing the *Ube4b/NMNAT* fusion protein (Mack et al., 2001). This transgenic mouse had the same phenotype as the original *Wlds* mouse with delayed wallerian degeneration of PNS axons and preservation of the neuromuscular junctions (Fig. 2). The preservation of the axons after transection was dose dependent, as the transgenic lines with low copy numbers had a phenotype that was in between the wild-type and the original *Wlds* mouse. A surprising finding was the cellular localization of the fusion protein. An antibody generated against the N-terminal of the fusion protein gave only a punctate nuclear staining in both the transgenic mouse and the original *Wlds* mouse. There was no accumulation of the fusion protein at the swollen end-bulbs of transected axons, suggesting that there was no axonal transport of the *Ube4b/NMNAT* fusion protein (Mack et al., 2001). These observations imply that the nuclear expression of the *Ube4b/NMNAT* fusion protein leads to expression and/or downregulation of other proteins that confer axonal protection. These other mediators must be transported and must be present in the axon at the time of the injury. Understanding the pathways that provide this intrinsic axonal protection may lead to novel therapies for nervous system disorders where axonal pathology is the predominant determinant of disability.

We are already seeing the benefits of this line of research as more investigators apply this tool to the study of various nervous system disorders. The *Wlds* mutation confers a period of neuroprotection against vincristine- (Wang et al., 2001a, 2001b) and paclitaxel- (Wang et al., 2002) induced neurotoxicity and neuropathy. Similarly, the *Wlds* mutation delays the loss of motor and sensory axons in a genetic model of myelin-related axonopathy in the P0-deficient mouse (Samsam et al., 2003). Moreover, in the double transgenic mouse (*Wlds* and P0-deficient), there is preservation of the motor neurons at a time when there is normally a massive loss of motor neurons in the spinal cord of the P0-deficient mouse. This suggests that preservation of the axon leads to preservation of the neuron. This observation was further confirmed in a different genetic model of axonal loss and motor neuron death. In a genetic model of spinal muscular atrophy, the progressive motor neuronopathy (*pmn/pmn*) mouse, there are deficits in axonal transport and eventual apoptosis of the spinal motor neurons. Antiapoptotic treatments, such as transgenic expression of bcl-2 gene or treatment with glial cell-derived neurotrophic factor, prevent apoptosis but do not affect the life span of the *pmn/pmn* mice (Sagot et al., 1995, 1996). However, double transgenic mice with the *Wlds* and *pmn/pmn* mutations had delayed retrograde axonal transport deficits and motor neuron death and as a result prolonged survival (Ferri et al., 2003). The observations from these studies point to the importance of preservation of axonal integrity and function in promoting therapies for diseases where there is eventual loss of the neuron. These studies are just the beginning; our understanding of the mechanisms underlying the axonal and neuronal protection provided by the *Ube4b/NMNAT* fusion is rudimentary. Many questions remain. For example, which proteins are upregulated and/or downregulated by the nuclear expression of the fusion protein? Are these proteins transported down the axon, or do they alter the characteristics of other proteins that are normally transported? Are there changes in phosphorylation states of normal constituents of the axoplasm? How is this fusion protein related to the ubiquitin-proteasome pathway?

Answers to some of these questions may come from other lines of research into the mechanisms of wallerian degeneration. As mentioned previously, the mutation in the *Wlds* mouse involves *ufd2*, one of the components of the ubiquitin-proteasome system (UPS). Polyubiquination of cellular proteins tags them for degradation by the proteasome, a multisubunit structure that acts as the cellular "garbage disposal" system (Glickman and Ciechanover, 2002). One study examined the role of UPS in early stages of axonal degeneration *in vitro* and *in vivo* (Zhai et al., 2003). He and his colleagues explanted superior cervical ganglion neurons in tissue culture and then physically severed the axons. Under normal conditions, transected axons degenerate within 8 to 10 hours. However, when they added pharmacological inhibitors of the proteasome, axonal degeneration was delayed for 16 hours or longer. This was a specific effect on the UPS pathway, as inhibitors of caspases and serine proteases did not have any effect. Similarly, systemic administration of MG132 (proteasome inhibitor) delayed the axonal degeneration after optic nerve crush *in vivo*. The effects of UPS pathway inhibition was mirrored when Zhai and colleagues used calcium chelators to remove extracellular calcium suggesting that calcium signaling is required upstream of the UPS pathway (Zhai et al., 2003).

What are the cellular targets of the UPS in wallerian degeneration? Although this is not exactly known, the work by zhai and colleagues sheds some light on this question. They demonstrated that microtubules were lost early (~4 hours) at a time when β-tubulin levels were still steady in the axoplasm, but loss of neurofilaments occurred later (~8–12 hours) and involved loss of the neurofilament subunits (Zhai et al., 2003). Both of these events were delayed by inhibition of the UPS, suggesting that cytoskeletal disintegration of the axon is downstream of the UPS. These observations suggest that depolymerization of the microtubules is the initial step of granular disintegration of the axoplasm and that it is under tight control of the UPS. It is possible that UPS controls the turnover of a variety of proteins involved in microtubule assembly and disassembly. A summary of the role of UPS in wallerian degeneration is shown in Fig. 3.

C. Caspases in Wallerian Degeneration

Before the observations that UPS was involved in the initial stages of wallerian degeneration, an attractive hypothesis was that members of the apoptotic pathway might be regulating or executing the axonal degeneration seen after injury akin to the apoptosis of injured cells. Similar to wallerian degeneration, apoptosis in the nervous system is an active process that requires energy and presence of regulatory proteins and enzymes capable of degrading cellular proteins (Yuan and Yankner, 2000). The final stages of apoptosis involve activation of caspases, the executioners of apoptosis, which then lead to degradation of cellular proteins and nuclear DNA (Hengartner, 2000). Because caspases are capable of protein degradation and their activities are tightly controlled, activated caspases could have been an ideal candidate as executers of wallerian degeneration; however, two lines of evidence argue against a strong role for caspases in wallerian degeneration. Raff and colleagues examined the role of caspase-3 in wallerian degeneration (Finn et al., 2000). At a time when caspase-3 was activated in the cell body, there were no activated caspase-3 or cleaved substrates of caspase-3 in the distal segment of a nerve after transection. Furthermore, inhibitors of the caspase pathway did not prevent wallerian degeneration, yet they prevented apoptosis of the cell body. In a second study, Raff and colleagues examined the events upstream of caspase activation (Whitmore et al., 2003). They used the optic nerve transection as a model to study the relationship between the apoptotic processes and wallerian degeneration. When the optic nerve was transected, retinal ganglion cell neurons underwent apoptotic cell death. This was prevented in double knock-out animals lacking two of the key proapoptotic proteins *Bax* and *Bak*. Yet there was no difference in the wallerian degeneration of the transected optic nerve axons in

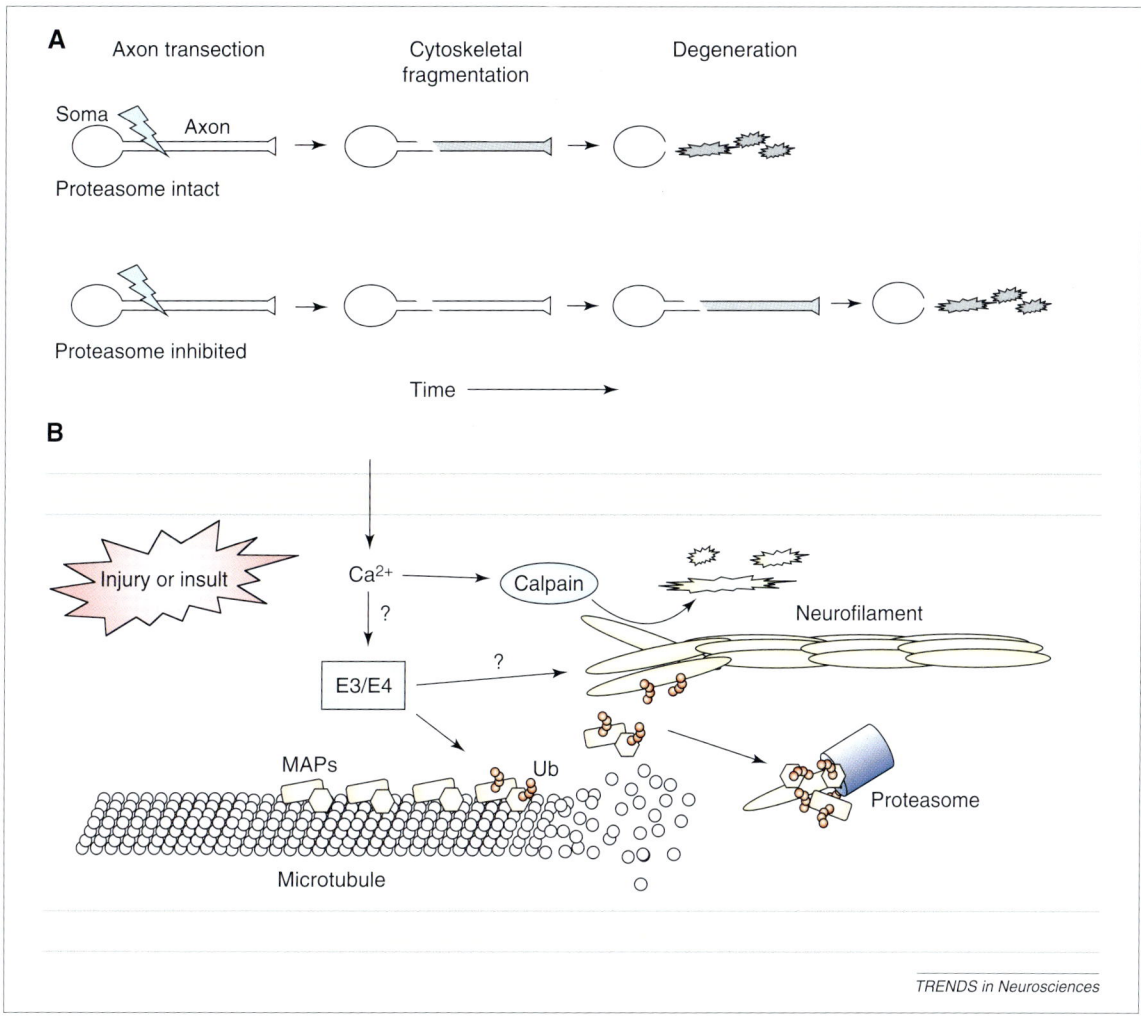

Figure 3 **Proposed role of the ubiquitin–proteasome system (UPS) in wallerian degeneration.** (**A**) Axonal injury or insult leads to fragmentation of the microtubule and neurofilament cytoskeleton followed by disintegration of the axon. Preventing polyubiquitination or proteasome-mediated degradation delays cytoskeletal fragmentation and degeneration. (**B**) Although the precise mechanisms are unknown (indicated by question marks), axonal degeneration requires Ca^{2+} influx, which leads to activation of intracellular proteases such as calpain and possibly ubiquitin (Ub)-regulatory enzymes, including E3 and E4 ubiquitin ligases. Disassembly of microtubules could proceed by ubiquitination and degradation of stabilizing microtubule-associated proteins (MAPs). Degradation of neurofilaments might be due to a combination of calpain-mediated and UPS-mediated degradation. (With permission from Ehlers, 2004.)

$Bax^{-/-}/Bak^{-/-}$ animals compared to the wild-type animals. The results were similar in the distal segment of the transected sciatic nerve. Taken together, these results argue strongly against a pivotal role for members of the apoptotic pathway in wallerian degeneration.

In another study examining the role of apoptotic machinery in wallerian degeneration, Ikegami and Koike (2003) studied the mitochondrial function in vinblastine-induced neuronal death and axonal degeneration. They found that although vinblastine caused apoptotic death of the neuron, the axonal degeneration that preceded the cell death was not mediated by the classical apoptotic machinery; there was no activated caspase-3 in the degenerating axons, and axonal degeneration was not prevented by caspase-3 inhibitors. Yet

there was a significant mitochondrial dysfunction in the axon, with loss of the mitochondrial membrane potential and loss of adenosine triphosphate synthesis before the morphological evidence of axonal degeneration. This idea that local mitochondrial dysfunction can lead to axonal degeneration is gaining momentum, although most of the evidence is indirect and circumstantial. In patients infected with the human immunodeficiency virus-1 (HIV-1), the incidence of neuropathy with distal axonal degeneration increases with the use of nucleoside reverse transcriptase inhibitors. In a detailed study of HIV-infected patients with peripheral neuropathy who are receiving nucleoside reverse transcriptase inhibitors, Dalakas and colleagues (2001) showed that there are alterations in the axonal mitochondrial morphology and accumulation of mitochondrial mutations. There is an increasing body of evidence suggesting that persistent hyperglycemia may lead to mitochondrial dysfunction and apoptotic cell death in tissue culture and animal models of diabetic neuropathy (Russell et al., 1999; Srinivasan et al., 2000; Schmeichel et al., 2003). It is likely that localized mitochondrial dysfunction may also lead to axonal degeneration before any evidence of cell death occurs. However, this remains speculative at this moment, as there is no firm experimental evidence.

IV. Dying-Back or Compartmentalized Axonal Degeneration

One of the most intriguing aspects of the axon biology is that most peripheral neuropathies, clinical or experimental, present as distal axonopathy. In most peripheral neuropathies, and many CNS disorders, distal portions of the axons degenerate, yet the neuronal cell body and the proximal axon are maintained. How does a neuron and/or an axon do this? In wallerian degeneration, the distal segment of a transected axon is separated and compartmentalized from the cell body and the proximal axon. Degeneration of the compartmentalized distal segment can ensue without any harm to the proximal axon or the cell body. However, in the case of distal axonopathies, the distal segment of the axon has to degenerate and at the same time maintain compartmentalization. The molecular mechanisms of such compartmentalization and degeneration are unknown, but may differ from the molecular mechanisms used by typical wallerian degeneration (Fig. 4). There are only a handful of experimental studies available to draw any conclusions on this matter. One experimental approach has been to use compartmentalized cell culture techniques where one can separate the neuronal cell body from the axon (Campenot, 1982). Campenot and colleagues (1994) demonstrated that local withdrawal of nerve growth factor from the chamber where the axons are located leads to degeneration of the axons only in that chamber, with no effect on the survival of the neuronal cell body (Campenot, 1994). So far, this culture technique has been used primarily to study the effects of nerve growth factor on axon biology (Riccio et al., 1997; Kuruvilla et al., 2000), but it is possible to use the same technique to study the mechanism of action of various toxic insults to the neuron and/or the axon. Furthermore, by using a co-culture paradigm in the compartmentalized culture system, one can begin to examine the interplay between various cell types in the PNS or CNS. For example, what are the roles of oligodendrocytes in neuronal survival vs. axonal survival? Are they linked to each other? Do microglia play a role in axonal survival? Are activated microglia injurious to the axon independent of their action on the neuronal cell body? These types of questions are difficult to answer using traditional co-culture systems

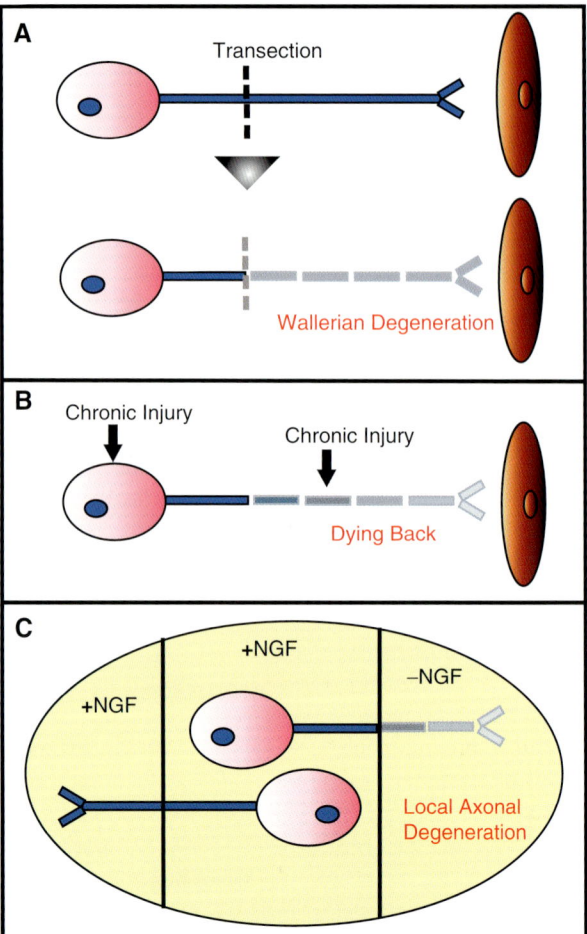

Figure 4 **Various forms of axonal degeneration.** (**A**) When an axon is cut, the isolated distal segment rapidly undergoes wallerian degeneration. When the axon of a developing neuron is cut, the cell body frequently undergoes apoptosis. (**B**) In dying-back axonal degeneration, the axonal tree of an unhealthy neuron slowly degenerates, beginning distally and progressing proximally. (**C**) When the distal part of an axon of a sympathetic neuron is locally deprived of nerve growth factor in a three-chamber culture dish, the deprived axon segment degenerates, whereas the rest of the axon and the cell survive. (With permission adapted from Raff at. al., 2002.)

because one cannot isolate the effects of the intervention on the neuronal cell body from the effects on the axons. What do we know about the role of glial cells in wallerian degeneration? This issue is discussed in the next two sections.

V. Demyelination and Wallerian Degeneration

One of the characteristic features of peripheral neuropathies with predominantly demyelinating phenotype has been that the degree of clinical severity is associated with the progressive axonal loss rather than the degree of demyelination. In recent years, as the genes underlying many of the inherited human demyelinating neuropathies have been identified, animal models of these diseases have been developed (Adlkofer et al., 1995; Anzini et al., 1997; Shy et al., 1997; Previtali et al., 2000; Wrabetz et al., 2000). In all of these animal models, the genetic abnormality is in proteins expressed primarily by the myelinating cells, oligodendrocytes and Schwann cells, and results in disturbances of proper myelination. Although there are minor differences, however, a common theme among all of these genetic disturbances has been the age-related progressive distal axonal loss (Martini et al., 1995; Muller et al., 1997).

This observation raises an important question: Does demyelination, by itself, lead to axonal loss? This important issue has specific relevance to multiple sclerosis. As discussed elsewhere in this book, in recent years, it has been recognized that axonal loss rather than demyelinating plaques are the major determinants of clinical severity in multiple sclerosis; similar to the demyelinating inherited peripheral neuropathies. This is a complex issue to answer. Although the genetic defects in these animal models of peripheral neuropathies are in different proteins, they are all components of myelin. They could easily affect axon-Schwann cell communication in such a way that Schwann cells fail to provide necessary growth factors to the axons, and this process may have nothing to do with demyelination or failed myelination.

One potential mechanism by which demyelination can lead to axonal degeneration is disruption of axonal transport through demyelinated segments (Rao et al., 1981; Guy et al., 1989; Munoz-Martinez et al., 1994; Kirkpatrick et al., 2001). This is more apparent in the optic nerve system where local injections of very small quantities of anti-Gal-C antibody can lead to focal demyelination and abnormal axonal cytoskeleton and axonal transport through the demyelinated segment (Zhu et al., 1999). Similarly, in animal models of experimental allergic neuritis, there are axonal transport deficits in the optic nerve (Rao et al., 1981; Guy et al., 1989). The issue is less clear in the PNS; demyelination in the sciatic nerve induced by focal injection of a neurotoxin from *K. humboldtiana* causes slowed fast axonal transport (Munoz-Martinez et al., 1994), but demyelination induced by intraneural injection of antigalactocerebroside does not have any effect on fast axonal transport (Armstrong et al., 1987).

The issue of axonal degeneration induced by demyelination is further complicated by the presence of inflammatory reaction in almost all of the models of inherited demyelinating peripheral neuropathies. It is possible that inflammation secondary to demyelination may result in axonal loss rather than axonal degeneration resulting from demyelination per se. In recent studies, when Martini and colleagues crossed either the P0-deficient or connexin-32-deficient mice with mice lacking mature B- and T-lymphocytes resulting from absence of recombination activating gene-1

(RAG-1), they found that the double mutants had reduced demyelination and more important, reduced axonal loss (Schmid et al., 2000; Kobsar et al., 2003). Because these animals also had reduced demyelination, it is unclear if the effect of absence of a mature immune system was on demyelination or secondary axonal loss. Further studies are needed to delineate the exact role the immune system plays in demyelination and axonal loss.

VI. Glial and Immune Cells in Wallerian Degeneration

During wallerian degeneration, most of the axonal response to transection is similar between the CNS and PNS, but there are major differences in the response of the glial and immune cells. In the PNS, within days after transection, Schwann cells of both myelinated and unmyelinated fibers sequester their myelin and divide in response to denervation (Pellegrino et al., 1986; Clemence et al., 1989; Stoll et al., 1989; Liu et al., 1995), but maintain basal lamina scaffoldings called Büngner's bands. The peak of Schwann cell proliferation occurs at 3 to 4 days, and the proliferation rate decreases to basal levels by 1 month. The mitogens for Schwann cells are unknown, but are thought to be derived from degenerating axolemma (Sobue et al., 1984). Resident as well as recruited hematogenous macrophages could also provide Schwann cell mitogens, but available data suggest that Schwann cells can divide in the absence of macrophages and degrade myelin (Fernandez-Valle et al., 1995; Kubota et al., 1998). In the denervated nerve segment, selective induction of glial growth factor subfamily of neuregulins (potent Schwann cell mitogens) occurs along with induction of neuregulin receptors (Carroll et al., 1997). However, the cellular source of these potent Schwann cell mitogens in the distal transected nerve is unknown. It is possible that these factors are produced by the Schwann cells and act in an autocrine/paracrine fashion.

Although Schwann cells can degrade myelin in the absence of macrophages, under normal circumstances, macrophages are the cell type that is responsible for the clearing of the majority of myelin debris from the peripheral nerve. Hematogenous macrophages invade the peripheral nerve starting at day 2 after transection and peak at days 4 to 7. Both resident and hematogenous macrophages contribute to the processing and removal of myelin debris (Olsson and Sjostrand, 1969; Berner et al., 1973; Stoll et al., 1989; Mueller et al., 2003) (for a thorough review of the role of macrophages in wallerian degeneration please see Friede and Bruck, 1993; Griffin et al., 1993; Bruck, 1997). The molecular mechanisms underlying Schwann cell and macrophage-mediated myelin removal are different (Hirata and Kawabuchi, 2002). Macrophage-mediated myelin removal is dependent on the activation of the complement system. Complement component C3 is present on the surface of myelin ovoids, and macrophages constitutively express the corresponding receptor, complement receptor type 3 (Bruck and Friede, 1990). Furthermore, anti-C3 antibody blocks degradation of myelin by macrophages *in vitro* (Bruck and Friede, 1990). Depletion of serum complement in rats, using cobra venom factor intravenously for 1 week, leads to reduced recruitment and activation of macrophages after sciatic nerve transection (Dailey et al., 1998). This leads to delayed clearance of myelin and delayed regeneration. In contrast, myelin removal by Schwann cells is opsonin-independent and is mediated by lectins (Reichert et al., 1994).

One of the major differences between the PNS and CNS during wallerian degeneration is the lack of rapid and effective removal of myelin debris in the CNS. As outlined previously, hematogenous macrophages play a prominent and critical role in removing the myelin debris after axonal transection in the PNS. In contrast, there is limited hematogenous macrophage recruitment in the CNS, and the myelin is not degraded rapidly (reviewed in Stoll and Jander, 1999). The mechanisms underlying these prominent differences between the CNS and the PNS are unknown. However, one potential mechanism may involve the complement system. After dorsal rhizotomy, there is active proliferation and activation of microglia (as evidenced by the presence of ED-1 immunostaining) along the degenerating dorsal column tracts (Liu et al., 1998). Despite the presence of activated microglia, there is no complement expression along the degenerating tracts. This may be due to high expression of clusterin, a potent inhibitor of the complement pathway, by astrocytes and oligodendrocytes (Liu et al., 1998). This observation may explain the lack of prompt removal of myelin debris in the CNS.

What is the significance of poor myelin removal in the CNS? Many studies in the last 10 to 20 years pointed to the presence of potent inhibitors of regeneration in myelin (reviewed in Yiu and He, 2003; Raisman, 2004; Schwab, 2004). Presence of undegraded myelin and its components may hinder the regeneration attempts of CNS axons and ultimately contribute to persistence of functional deficits after injury. These injuries need not be the mechanical type as in traumas, but could also be chemical in nature as seen in multiple sclerosis. Better understanding of the molecular mechanisms of specific activation of microglia and myelin removal after axonal injury in the CNS is likely to yield new therapeutic opportunities for the treatment of illnesses such as multiple sclerosis.

References

Adlkofer, K., Martini, R., Aguzzi, A., Zielasek, J., Toyka, K. V., and Suter, U. (1995). Hypermyelination and demyelinating peripheral neuropathy in Pmp22-deficient mice. *Nat. Genet.* **11**, 274–280.

Anzini, P., Neuberg, D. H., Schachner, M., Nelles, E., Willecke, K., Zielasek, J., Toyka, K. V., Suter, U., and Martini, R. (1997). Structural abnormalities and deficient maintenance of peripheral nerve myelin in mice lacking the gap junction protein connexin 32. *J. Neurosci.* **17**, 4545–4551.

Armstrong, R., Toews, A. D., and Morell, P. (1987). Rapid axonal transport in focally demyelinated sciatic nerve. *J. Neurosci.* **7**, 4044–4053.

Badalamente, M. A., Hurst, L. C., and Stracher, A. (1986). Calcium-induced degeneration of the cytoskeleton in monkey and human peripheral nerves. *J. Hand Surg. [Br]* **11**, 337–340.

Ballin, R. H., and Thomas, P. K. (1969). Changes at the nodes of Ranvier during wallerian degeneration: An electron microscope study. *Acta Neuropathol. (Berl.)* **14**, 237–249.

Berner, A., Torvik, A., and Stenwig, A. E. (1973). Origin of macrophages in traumatic lesions and wallerian degeneration in peripheral nerves. *Acta Neuropathol. (Berl.)* **25**, 228–236.

Bouldin, T. W., Earnhardt, T. S., and Goines, N. D. (1990). Sequential changes in the permeability of the blood-nerve barrier over the course of ricin neuronopathy in the rat. *Neurotoxicology* **11**, 23–34.

Bouldin, T. W., Earnhardt, T. S., and Goines, N. D. (1991). Restoration of blood-nerve barrier in neuropathy is associated with axonal regeneration and remyelination. *J. Neuropathol. Exp. Neurol.* **50**, 719–728.

Bruck, W. (1997). The role of macrophages in wallerian degeneration. *Brain Pathol.* **7**, 741–752.

Bruck, W., and Friede, R. L. (1990). Anti-macrophage CR3 antibody blocks myelin phagocytosis by macrophages in vitro. *Acta Neuropathol. (Berl.)* **80**, 415–418.

Campenot, R. B. (1982). Development of sympathetic neurons in compartmentalized cultures. Il Local control of neurite growth by nerve growth factor. *Dev. Biol.* **93**, 1–12.

Campenot, R. B. (1994). NGF and the local control of nerve terminal growth. *J. Neurobiol.* **25**, 599–611.

Cancalon, P. (1982). Slow flow in axons detached from their perikarya. *J. Cell Biol.* **95**, 989–992.

Cancalon, P. (1983). Proximodistal degeneration of C-fibers detached from their perikarya. *J. Cell Biol.* **97**, 6–14.

Carroll, S. L., Miller, M. L., Frohnert, P. W., Kim, S. S., and Corbett, J. A. (1997). Expression of neuregulins and their putative receptors, ErbB2 and ErbB3, is induced during wallerian degeneration. *J. Neurosci.* **17**, 1642–1659.

Chaudhry, V., Glass, J. D., and Griffin, J. W. (1992). Wallerian degeneration in peripheral nerve disease. *Neurol. Clin.* **10**, 613–627.

Clemence, A., Mirsky, R., and Jessen, K. R. (1989). Non-myelin-forming Schwann cells proliferate rapidly during wallerian degeneration in the rat sciatic nerve. *J. Neurocytol.* **18**, 185–192.

Coleman, M. P., Conforti, L., Buckmaster, E. A., Tarlton, A., Ewing, R. M., Brown, M. C., Lyon, M. F., and Perry, V. H. (1998). An 85-kb tandem triplication in the slow wallerian degeneration (Wlds) mouse. *Proc. Natl. Acad. Sci. U. S. A.* **95**, 9985–9990.

Conforti, L., Tarlton, A., Mack, T. G., Mi, W., Buckmaster, E. A., Wagner, D., Perry, V. H., and Coleman, M. P. (2000). A Ufd2/D4Cole1e chimeric protein and overexpression of Rbp7 in the slow wallerian degeneration (WldS) mouse. *Proc. Natl. Acad. Sci. U. S. A.* **97**, 11377–11382.

Cravioto, H. (1969). Wallerian degeneration: ultrastructural and histochemical studies. *Bull. Los Angeles Neurol. Soc.* **34**, 233–253.

Dailey, A. T., Avellino, A. M., Benthem, L., Silver, J., and Kliot, M. (1998). Complement depletion reduces macrophage infiltration and activation during wallerian degeneration and axonal regeneration. *J. Neurosci.* **18**, 6713–6722.

Dalakas, M. C., Semino-Mora, C., and Leon-Monzon, M. (2001). Mitochondrial alterations with mitochondrial DNA depletion in the nerves of AIDS patients with peripheral neuropathy induced by 2′3′-dideoxycytidine (ddC). *Lab. Invest.* **81**, 1537–1544.

de Medinaceli, L., and Church, A. C. (1984). Peripheral nerve reconnection: Inhibition of early degenerative processes through the use of a novel fluid medium. *Exp. Neurol.* **84**, 396–408.

Fernandez-Valle, C., Bunge, R. P., and Bunge, M. B. (1995). Schwann cells degrade myelin and proliferate in the absence of macrophages: Evidence from in vitro studies of wallerian degeneration. *J. Neurocytol.* **24,** 667–679.

Ferri, A., Sanes, J. R., Coleman, M. P., Cunningham, J. M., and Kato, A. C. (2003). Inhibiting axon degeneration and synapse loss attenuates apoptosis and disease progression in a mouse model of motoneuron disease. *Curr. Biol.* **13,** 669–673.

Finn, J. T., Weil, M., Archer, F., Siman, R., and Srinivasan, A., and Raff, M. C. (2000). Evidence that wallerian degeneration and localized axon degeneration induced by local neurotrophin deprivation do not involve caspases. *J. Neurosci.* **20,** 1333–1341.

Franson, P., and Ronnevi, L. O. (1984). Myelin breakdown and elimination in the posterior funiculus of the adult cat after dorsal rhizotomy: A light and electron microscopic qualitative and quantitative study. *J. Comp. Neurol.* **223,** 138–151.

Friede, R. L., and Bruck, W. (1993). Macrophage functional properties during myelin degradation. *Adv. Neurol.* **59,** 327–336.

Gamble, H. J., and Jha, B. D. (1958). Some effects of temperature upon the rate and progress of wallerian degeneration in mammalian nerve fibers. *J. Anat.* **92,** 171–177.

George, E. B., Glass, J. D., and Griffin, J. W. (1995). Axotomy-induced axonal degeneration is mediated by calcium influx through ion-specific channels. *J. Neurosci.* **15,** 6445–6452.

George, R., and Griffin, J. W. (1994). The proximo-distal spread of axonal degeneration in the dorsal columns of the rat. *J. Neurocytol.* **23,** 657–667.

Glass, J. D., and Griffin, J. W. (1991). Neurofilament redistribution in transected nerves: Evidence for bidirectional transport of neurofilaments. *J. Neurosci.* **11,** 3146–3154.

Glass. J. D., Schryer, B. L., and Griffin, J. W. (1994). Calcium-mediated degeneration of the axonal cytoskeleton in the Ola mouse. *J. Neurochem.* **62,** 2472–2475.

Glass, J. D., Nash, N., Dry, I., Culver, D., Levey, A. I., and Wesselingh, S. (1998). Cloning of m-calpain 80 kD subunit from the axonal degeneration-resistant WLD(S) mouse mutant. *J. Neurosci. Res.* **52,** 653–660.

Glickman, M. H., and Ciechanover, A. (2002). The ubiquitin-proteasome proteolytic pathway: Destruction for the sake of construction. *Physiol. Rev.* **82,** 373–428.

Griffin, J. W., George, R., and Ho, T. (1993). Macrophage systems in peripheral nerves. A review. *J. Neuropathol. Exp. Neurol.* **52,** 553–560.

Griffin, J. W., Price, D. L., Engel, W. K., and Drachman, D. B. (1977). The pathogenesis of reactive axonal swellings: role of axonal transport. *J. Neuropathol. Exp. Neurol.* **36,** 214–227.

Griffin, J. W., George, R., Lobato, C., Tyor, W. R., Yan, L. C., and Glass, J. D. (1992). Macrophage responses and myelin clearance during wallerian degeneration: Relevance to immune-mediated demyelination. *J. Neuroimmunol.* **40,** 153–165.

Guy, J., Ellis, E. A., Tark, E F., 3rd, Hope, G. M., and Rao, N. A. (1989). Axonal transport reductions in acute experimental allergic encephalomyelitis: Qualitative analysis of the optic nerve. *Curr. Eye Res.* **8,** 261–269.

Hengartner, M. O. (2000). The biochemistry of apoptosis. *Nature* **407,** 770–776.

Hirata, K., and Kawabuchi, M. (2002). Myelin phagocytosis by macrophages and nonmacrophages during wallerian degeneration. *Microsc. Res. Tech.* **57,** 541–547.

Ikegami, K., and Koike, T. (2003). Non-apoptotic neurite degeneration in apoptotic neuronal death: Pivotal role of mitochondrial function in neurites. *Neuroscience* **122,** 617–626.

Kirkpatrick, L. L., Witt, A. S., Payne, H. R., Shine, H. D., and Brady, S. T. (2001). Changes in microtubule stability and density in myelin-deficient shiverer mouse CNS axons. *J. Neurosci.* **21,** 2288–2297.

Kobsar, I., Berghoff, M., Samsam, M., Wessig, C., Maurer, M., Toyka, K. V., and Martini, R. (2003). Preserved myelin integrity and reduced axonopathy in connexin32-deficient mice lacking the recombination activating gene-1. *Brain* **126,** 804–813.

Kubota, A., Komiyama, A., Matsumoto, M., and Suzuki, K. (1998). Effect of macrophage suppression with silica on the proliferation of Schwann cells during wallerian degeneration. *Brain Res.* **802,** 254–258.

Kuruvilla, R., Ye, H., and Ginty, D. D. (2000). Spatially and functionally distinct roles of the PI3-K effector pathway during NGF signaling in sympathetic neurons. *Neuron* **27,** 499–512.

Lee, J. C. (1963). Electron microscopy of wallerian degeneration. *J. Comp. Neurol.* **120,** 65–79.

Liu, H. M., Yang, L. H., and Yang, Y. J. (1995). Schwann cell properties: 3. C-fos expression, bFGF production, phagocytosis and proliferation during wallerian degeneration. *J. Neuropathol. Exp. Neurol.* **54,** 487–496.

Liu, L., Persson, J. K., Svensson, M., and Aldskogius, H. (1998). Glial cell responses, complement, and clustering in the central nervous system following dorsal root transection. *Glia* **23,** 221–238.

Lubinska, L. (1977). Early course of wallerian degeneration in myelinated fibres of the rat phrenic nerve. *Brain Res.* **130,** 47–63.

Lunn, E. R., Brown, M. C., and Perry, V. H. (1990). The pattern of axonal degeneration in the peripheral nervous system varies with different types of lesion. *Neuroscience* **35,** 157–165.

Lunn, E. R., Perry, V. H., Brown, M. C., Rosen, H., and Gordon, S. (1989). Absence of wallerian degeneration does not hinder regeneration in peripheral nerve. *Eur. J. Neurosci.* **1,** 27–33.

Mack, T. G., Reiner, M., Beirowski, B., Mi, W., Emanuelli, M., Wagner, D., Thomson, D., Gillingwater, T., Court, F., Conforti, L., Fernando, F. S., Tarlton, A., Andressen, C., Addicks, K., Magni, G., Ribchester, R. R., Perry, V. H., and Coleman, M. P. (2001). Wallerian degeneration of injured axons and synapses is delayed by a Ube4b/Nmnat chimeric gene. *Nat. Neurosci.* **4,** 1199–1206.

Martini, R., Zielasek, J., Toyka, K. V., Giese, K. P., and Schachner, M. (1995). Protein zero (P0)-deficient mice show myelin degeneration in peripheral nerves characteristic of inherited human neuropathies. *Nat. Genet.* **11,** 281–286.

Mata, M., Staple, J., and Fink, D. J. (1986). Changes in intra-axonal calcium distribution following nerve crush. *J. Neurobiol.* **17,** 449–467.

Miledi, R. , and Slater, C. R. (1970). On the degeneration of rat neuromuscular junctions after nerve section. *J. Physiol.* **207,** 507–528.

Mueller, M., Leonhard, C., Wacker, K., Ringelstein, E. B., Okabe, M., Hickey, W. F., and Kiefer, R. (2003). Macrophage response to peripheral nerve injury: The quantitative contribution of resident and hematogenous macrophages. *Lab. Invest.* **83,** 175–185.

Muller, H. W., Suter, U., Van Broeckhoven, C., Hanemann, C O., Nelis, E., Timmerman, V., Sancho, S., Barrio, L., Bolhuis, P., Dermietzel, R., Frank, M., Gabreels-Festen, A., Gillen, C., Haites, N., Levi, G., Mariman, E., Martini, R., Nave, K., Rautenstrauss, B., Schachner, M., Schenone, A., Schneider, C., Schroder, M., Willecke, K., and Haneman, O. (1997). Advances in Charcot-Marie-Tooth disease research: Cellular function of CMT-related proteins, transgenic animal models, and patho-mechanisms. The European CMT Consortium. *Neurobiol. Dis.* **4,** 215–220.

Munoz-Martinez, E. J., Cuellar-Pedroza, L. H., Rubio-Franchini, C., Jauregui-Rincon, J., and Joseph-Nathan, P. (1994). Depression of fast axonal transport in axons demyelinated by intraneural injection of a neurotoxin from K. humboldtiana. *Neurochem. Res.* **19,** 1341–1348.

Ohmi, S. (1961). Electron microscopic study of wallerian degeneration of the peripheral nerve. *Z. Zellforsch. Mikrosk. Anat.* **54,** 39–67.

Olsson, Y., and Sjostrand, J. (1969). Origin of macrophages in wallerian degeneration of peripheral nerves demonstrated autoradiographically. *Exp. Neurol.* **23,** 102–112.

Ouardouz, M., Nikolaeva, M. A., Coderre, E., Zamponi, G. W., McRory, J. E., Trapp, B. D., Yin, X., Wang, W., Woulfe, J., and Stys, P. K. (2003). Depolarization-induced Ca2+ release in ischemic spinal cord white matter involves L-type Ca2+ channel activation of ryanodine receptors. *Neuron* **40,** 53–63.

Pellegrino, R. G., Politis, M J., Ritchie, J. M., and Spencer, P. S. (1986). Events in degenerating cat peripheral nerve: Induction of Schwann cell S phase and its relation to nerve fibre degeneration. *J. Neurocytol.* **15**, 17–28.

Perry, V. H., Brown, M. C., Lunn, E. R., Tree, P., and Gordon, S. (1990). Evidence that very slow wallerian degeneration in C57BL/Ola Mice is an intrinsic property of the peripheral nerve. *Eur. J. Neurosci.* **2**, 802–808.

Pesini, P., Kopp, J., Wong, H., Walsh, J. H., Grant, G., and Hokfelt, T. (1999). An immunohistochemical marker for wallerian degeneration of fibers in the central and peripheral nervous system. *Brain Res.* **828**, 41–59.

Powell, H. C., Myers, R. R., and Lampert, P. W. (1980). Edema in neurotoxic injury. *In:* "Experimental and Clinical Neurotoxicology" (P. S. Spencer and H. H. Schaumburg, eds.). pp. 118–138. Williams & Wilkins, Baltimore.

Previtali, S. C., Quattrini, A., Fasolini, M., Panzeri ,M. C., Villa, A., Filbin, M. T., Li, W., Chiu, S. Y., Messing, A., Wrabetz, L., and Feltri, M. L. (2000). Epitope-tagged P(0) glycoprotein causes Charcot-Marie-Tooth-like neuropathy in transgenic mice. *J. Cell Biol.* **151**, 1035–1046.

Raisman, G. (2004). Myelin inhibitors: Does NO mean GO? *Nat. Rev. Neurosci.* **5**, 157–161.

Ranish, N., and Ochs, S. (1972). Fast axoplasmic transport of acetylcholinesterase in mammalian nerve fibres. *J. Neurochem.* **19**, 2641–2649.

Rao, N. A., Guy, J., and Sheffield, P. S. (1981). Effects of chronic demyelination on axonal transport in experimental allergic optic neuritis. *Invest. Ophthalmol. Vis. Sci.* **21**, 606–611.

Reichert, F., Saada, A., and Rotshenker, S. (1994). Peripheral nerve injury induces Schwann cells to express two macrophage phenotypes: Phagocytosis and the galactose-specific lectin MAC-2. *J. Neurosci.* **14**, 3231–3245.

Riccio, A., Pierchala, B. A., Ciarallo, C. L., and Ginty, D. D. (1997). An NGF-TrkA-mediated retrograde signal to transcription factor CREB in sympathetic neurons. *Science* **277**, 1097–1100.

Russell, J. W., Sullivan, K. A., Windebank, A. J., Herrmann, D. N., and Feldman, E. L. (1999). Neurons undergo apoptosis in animal and cell culture models of diabetes. *Neurobiol. Dis.* **6**, 347–363.

Sagot, Y., Tan, S. A., Hammang, J. P., Aebischer, P., and Kato, A. C. (1996). GDNF slows loss of motoneurons but not axonal degeneration or premature death of pmn/pmn mice. *J. Neurosci.* **16**, 2335–2341.

Sagot, Y., Dubois-Dauphin, M., Tan, S. A., de Bilbao, F., Aebischer, P., Martinou, J. C., and Kato, A. C. (1995). Bcl-2 overexpression prevents motoneuron cell body loss but not axonal degeneration in a mouse model of a neurodegenerative disease. *J. Neurosci.* **15**, 7727–7733.

Samsam, M., Mi, W., Wessig, C., Zielasek, J., Toyka, K. V., Coleman, M. P., and Martini, R. (2003). The Wlds mutation delays robust loss of motor and sensory axons in a genetic model for myelin-related axonopathy. *J. Neurosci.* **23**, 2833–2839.

Schlaepfer, W. W. (1974a). Effects of energy deprivation on wallerian degeneration in isolated segments of rat peripheral nerve. *Brain Res.* **78**, 71–81.

Schlaepfer, W. W. (1974b). Calcium-induced degeneration of axoplasm in isolated segments of rat peripheral nerve. *Brain Res.* **69**, 203–215.

Schlaepfer, W. W., and Hasler, M. B. (1979). Characterization of the calcium-induced disruption of neurofilaments in rat peripheral nerve. *Brain Res.* **168**, 299–309.

Schmeichel, A. M., Schmelzer, J. D., and Low, P. A. (2003) Oxidative injury and apoptosis of dorsal root ganglion neurons in chronic experimental diabetic neuropathy. *Diabetes* **52**, 165–171.

Schmid, C. D., Stienekemeier, M., Oehen, S., Bootz, F., Zielasek, J., Gold, R., Toyka, K. V., Schachner, M., and Martini, R. (2000). Immune deficiency in mouse models for inherited peripheral neuropathies leads to improved myelin maintenance. *J. Neurosci.* **20**, 729–735.

Schwab, M. E. (2004). Nogo and axon regeneration. *Curr. Opin. Neurobiol.* **14**, 118–124.

Sea, T., Ballinger, M. L., and Bittner, G. D. (1995). Cooling of peripheral myelinated axons retards wallerian degeneration. *Exp. Neurol.* **133**, 85–95.

Shy, M. E., Arroyo, E., Sladky, J., Menichella, D., Jiang, H., Xu, W., Kamholz, J., and Scherer, S. S. (1997). Heterozygous P0 knockout mice develop a peripheral neuropathy that resembles chronic inflammatory demyelinating polyneuropathy (CIDP). *J. Neuropathol. Exp. Neurol.* **56**, 811–821.

Simon, R. G., Wade, R. R., DeLarco, J. E., and Baker, M. L. (1969). Wallerian degeneration: a sequential process. *J. Neurochem.* **16**, 1435–1438.

Sobue, G., Brown, M. J., Kim, S. U., and Pleasure, D. (1984). Axolemma is a mitogen for human Schwann cells. *Ann. Neurol.* **15**, 449–452.

Srinivasan, S., Stevens, M., and Wiley, J. W. (2000). Diabetic peripheral neuropathy: Evidence for apoptosis and associated mitochondrial dysfunction. *Diabetes* **49**, 1932–1938.

Stoll, G., and Jander, S. (1999). The role of microglia and macrophages in the pathophysiology of the CNS. *Prog. Neurobiol.* **58**, 233–247.

Stoll, G., Griffin, J. W., Li, C. Y., and Trapp, B. D. (1989). Wallerian degeneration in the peripheral nervous system: Participation of both Schwann cells and macrophages in myelin degradation. *J. Neurocytol.* **18**, 671–683.

Tsao, J. W., George, E. B., and Griffin, J. W. (1999). Temperature modulation reveals three distinct stages of wallerian degeneration. *J. Neurosci.* **19**, 4718–4726.

Tsao, J. W., Brown, M. C., Carden, M. J., McLean, W. G., and Perry, V. H. (1994). Loss of the compound action potential: an electrophysiological, biochemical and morphological study of early events in axonal degeneration in the C57BL/Ola mouse. *Eur. J. Neurosci.* **6**, 516–524.

Vial, J. D. (1958). The early changes in the axoplasm during wallerian degeneration. *J. Biophys. Biochem. Cytol.* 4, 551–555.

Waller, A. (1850). Experiments on the section of glossopharyngeal and hypoglossal nerves of the frog and observations of the alternatives produced thereby in the structure of their primitive fibers. *Philos. Trans. R. Soc. Lond. B Biol. Sci.* **140**, 423.

Wang, M., Wu, Y., Culver, D. G., and Glass, J. D. (2001a). The gene for slow wallerian degeneration (Wld(s)) is also protective against vincristine neuropathy. *Neurobiol. Dis.* **8**, 155–161.

Wang, M. S., Davis, A. A., Culver, D. G., and Glass, J. D. (2002). WldS mice are resistant to paclitaxel (taxol) neuropathy. *Ann. Neurol.* **52**, 442–447.

Wang, M. S., Fang, G., Culver, D. G., Davis, A. A., Rich, M. M., and Glass, J. D. (2001b). The WldS protein protects against axonal degeneration: A model of gene therapy for peripheral neuropathy. *Ann. Neurol.* **50**, 773–779.

Webster, H. D. (1962). Transient, focal accumulation of axonal mitochondria during the early stages of wallerian degeneration. *J. Cell Biol.* **12**, 361–383.

Weerasuriya, A. (1990). Patterns of change in endoneurial capillary permeability and vascular space during nerve regeneration. *Brain Res.* **510**, 135–139.

Whitmore, A. V., Lindsten, T., Raff, M. C., and Thompson, C. B. (2003). The proapoptotic proteins Bax and Bak are not involved in wallerian degeneration. *Cell Death Differ.* **10**, 260–261.

Wrabetz, L., Feltri, M. L., Quattrini, A., Imperiale, D., Previtali, S., D'Antonio, M., Martini, R., Yin, X., Trapp, B. D., Zhou, L., Chiu, S. Y., and Messing, A. (2000). P(0) glycoprotein overexpression causes congenital hypomyelination of peripheral nerves. *J. Cell Biol.* **148**, 1021–1034.

Yiu, G., and He, Z. (2003). Signaling mechanisms of the myelin inhibitors of axon regeneration. *Curr. Opin. Neurobiol.* **13**, 545–551.

Yuan, J., and Yankner, B. A. (2000). Apoptosis in the nervous system. *Nature* **407**, 802–809.

Zelena, J., Lubinska, L., and Gutmann, E. (1968). Accumulation of organelles at the ends of interrupted axons. *Z. Zellforsch. Mikrosk. Anat.* **91,** 200–219.

Zhai, Q., Wang, J., Kim, A., Liu, Q., Watts, R., Hoopfer, E., Mitchison, T., Luo, L., and He, Z. (2003). Involvement of the ubiquitin-proteasome system in the early stages of wallerian degeneration. *Neuron* **39,** 217–225.

Zhu, B., Moore, G. R., Zwimpfer, T. J., Kastrukoff, L. F., Dyer, J. K., Steeves, J. D., Paty, D. W., and Cynader, M. S. (1999) Axonal cytoskeleton changes in experimental optic neuritis. *Brain Res.* **824,** 204–217.

25

AMAN: What It Teaches Us about Mechanisms Underlying Axonal Injury

Kazim A. Sheikh, M.B.B.S.

I. Introduction

The dictum that the extent and location of neuronal and/or axonal injury in a neurological disorder correlates directly with the severity of clinical disease and inversely with extent of recovery also holds for neuropathies, that is, diseases of peripheral nerves. Autoimmunity is implicated in the pathogenesis of a small subgroup of peripheral neuropathies. Among these immune neuropathies, two acute nerve disorders, acute motor axonal neuropathy (AMAN) and Fisher syndrome (FS), both variants of Guillain-Barré syndrome (GBS), are fairly well characterized in terms of immune effectors and target antigens; and substantial evidence now exists for their autoimmune pathogenesis. In the context of multiple sclerosis (MS) and axonal injury, the AMAN variant of GBS provides instructive mechanistic insights into (1) the generation of specific immune response triggered by a preceding infection and (2) antibody-mediated axonal dysfunction and/or degeneration.

The current emphasis in research into immune-mediated neuropathies is on antibody-mediated neural injury. This is primarily driven by the characterization of pathological heterogeneity and evidence of antibody-mediated nerve injury in GBS and is in sharp contrast to the earlier work focusing on lymphocyte-orchestrated nerve injury. It is difficult to disregard parallel developments in the research area of MS, likely an autoimmune CNS disorder, where themes of pathological heterogeneity, axonal injury, and antibody- and complement-mediated injury are reemerging. Currently, the basis of neuronal and axonal injury in MS is not completely understood, but it is probable that this injury reflects a combination of factors such as specific immune attack, nonspecific injury resulting from inflammation, and short- and long-term consequences of demyelination on axonal and neuronal function. This review focuses on the theme of postinfectious molecular mimicry as a pathogenetic mechanism in AMAN. Further, the clinical and experimental evidence of anti-ganglioside antibody-mediated axonal and/or synaptic injury is reviewed to highlight issues relevant to

355

targeting of axonal antigens on myelinated nerve fibers by circulating antibodies.

II. Guillain-Barré Syndrome Variants

GBS is a prototypic autoimmune peripheral nerve disorder with acute-onset and monophasic course that is the leading cause of acute flaccid paralysis worldwide since the near eradication of polio. This syndrome of rapidly evolving flaccid paralysis and areflexia in conjunction with albuminocytologic dissociation was described by Guillain, Barré, and Strohl in 1916. Later, pathological studies on autopsy materials obtained from GBS cases showed the presence of T-cell inflammation and demyelination of peripheral nerves (Haymaker and Kernohan, 1949; Asbury et al., 1969), and the demyelinating features were confirmed by electrophysiological studies. These observations led to the concept that this disease consisted of a single pathophysiological entity characterized by inflammation and demyelination of peripheral nerves, thus explaining the synonymous use of the terms GBS and acute demyelinating polyradiculoneuropathy (AIDP). The observation that the demyelinating form of the disease (AIDP) remains by far the most common GBS variant in the developed world further supported such a notion (Arnason and Soliven, 1993; Rees et al., 1998; GBS variants in Emilia-Romagna, 1998).

In recent years it has been increasingly realized that GBS comprises a pathophysiologically heterogeneous group of disorders of peripheral nerve, and this term can no longer be equated with AIDP. The axonal forms of GBS are now widely recognized, with two patterns based on the nerve fiber type affected: AMAN, the more common form of axonal GBS, distinguished by nearly pure motor axonal injury, and the less common variant acute motor-sensory axonal neuropathy (AMSAN), characterized by degeneration of both motor and sensory axons. It has been postulated that AMAN and AMSAN represent a pathological spectrum and that AMSAN in fact represents a more severe form of AMAN. Feasby and colleagues (1986) introduced the notion of axonal GBS based on the electrophysiological and pathological description of a single case. Subsequently, American-Chinese collaborative studies and case reports originating from Japan provided initial descriptions of the AMAN pattern of GBS and reinforced the concept of axonal GBS (McKhann et al., 1991, 1993; Yuki et al., 1990). The clinical features of AMAN were largely established by studies done in northern China. The axonal forms of GBS, particularly AMAN, are much more common in China, Japan, Mexico, and other developing countries but are less frequently encountered in developed countries (McKhann et al., 1991, 1993; Ogawara et al., 2000; Ramos-Alvarez et al., 1969). Finally, Fisher (or Miller Fisher) syndrome is a minor GBS variant characterized by gait disturbance

(ataxia), areflexia, and ophthalmoplegia, initially described by C. Miller-Fisher (1956). This variant probably has a similar incidence worldwide.

These clinical observations supplemented by electrodiagnostic testing have provided a framework for classification of GBS into different variants based on (1) the predominant pathophysiological process of nerve fiber injury, namely, primary demyelination or primary axonal degeneration; (2) the nerve fiber types that are affected; and (3) regional localization of the disease process. With such a classification system, GBS can be broadly divided into primarily demyelinating and axonal types; axonal variants are further subclassified according to the fiber type affected. Minor variants of GBS are classified not on an electrophysiological basis but on the clinical constellation of symptoms implying regional distribution of pathophysiology. Based on this schema, a simple classification of GBS is proposed in Table 1.

Among the variants of GBS, significant progress has been made in our understanding of the pathogenetic sequence of AMAN and FS. The accumulated clinical and experimental evidence supports the hypothesis of postinfectious molecular mimicry as the predominant pathophysiological mechanism in AMAN and FS (Hughes et al., 1999; Yuki , 2002; Willison and Yuki, 2002). Postinfectious molecular mimicry in the peripheral nervous system (PNS) implies shared antigenic determinants between the infectious agents and nerve fibers of the PNS. This results in an immune response to the organism that initiates immune-mediated damage to nerve fibers. Arguably, post-*Campylobacter* cases of AMAN and FS provide the best available evidence to support the hypothesis of molecular mimicry as a pathogenetic mechanism underlying postinfectious autoimmune disorders.

The molecular mimicry hypothesis, besides providing a conceptual framework of pathogenesis, has also directed attention to the pathogenetic role of antibodies in the axonal variants of GBS. As a result, recent research efforts in GBS have focused on antibody-mediated nerve injury and a substantial

Table 1 Classification of GBS

Electrophysiology
Demyelinating
  AIDP
Axonal
  AMAN
  AMSAN
  AIDP with secondary axonal degeneration
Regional-Localization of symptoms
  FS
  Sensory ataxic variant
  Pharyngeal-cervical-brachial variant

AIDP, acute demyelinating polyradiculoneuropathy; AMAN, acute motor axonal neuropathy; AMSAN, acute motor-sensory axonal neuropathy; FS, Fisher syndrome.

amount of experimental work indicates that the anti-ganglioside antibodies associated with AMAN and FS have direct pathophysiological effects on nerve fibers. Although the pathophysiological or structural basis of clinical manifestations in FS are still not completely resolved, experimental studies on anti-ganglioside antibodies associated with FS have focused on dysfunction at the motor nerve terminal or neuromuscular junction (NMJ). The current discussion on AMAN also includes observations derived from experimental modeling with anti-ganglioside antibodies associated with FS.

III. Acute Motor Axonal Neuropathy

A. Clinical Features

Muscle weakness resulting from motor neuropathy is the dominant clinical feature of both the AMAN and AIDP variants of GBS. The weakness characteristically starts in the lower limbs and ascends to involve both proximal and distal muscles. Areflexia or hyporeflexia is seen in almost all patients at advanced stage of the disease. Cranial nerve involvement is common, most often affecting facial or oculomotor nerves. Patients with AMAN have minimal sensory impairment in comparison to patients with AIDP. Autonomic dysfunction can also be seen in a small proportion of patients with AMAN. The epidemiological features of AMAN are somewhat different in Chinese cases; for example, there is a strong association with preceding *Campylobacter* infection (Ho et al., 1995, 1999). Other significant epidemiological differences of GBS in northern China are a clear seasonal pattern, with peak incidence in the summer months, and an apparent predilection for rural areas and children (McKhann et al.,1991, 1993). Electrophysiology provides the most critical diagnostic evaluation, supporting clinical diagnosis and providing useful prognostic information; however, nerve conduction studies may be normal early in the disease, particularly within the first week. Typically, cases with AMAN are characterized by reduced CMAP amplitudes with normal distal latencies and motor conduction velocities and relatively normal sensory conductions (Ho et al., 1995, 1999). Both reversible and persistent loss of F-waves without other features of demyelination or remyelination are proposed to represent proximal axonal dysfunction in patients with AMAN (Kuwabara et al., 2000). These electrical features support a motor axonal pathophysiology.

B. Prognosis and Extent of Axonal Injury

The location and degree of axonal injury are the two most important variables determining the outcome after a bout of GBS. Patients with residual disability almost always have axonal degeneration. Recovery in such cases requires axon regrowth from the site of axonal transection. Because the spinal roots and proximal nerves are typically most affected and PNS axonal regeneration advances at a rate of approximately 1 inch/month, this recovery is slow and often incomplete. Despite the inherent capacity of peripheral axons to regenerate after injury, experimental evidence indicates that the following factors contribute to incomplete recovery: (1) efficiency of the axonal regeneration process decreases with time (Fu and Gordon, 1995a), (2) the denervated distal segment of peripheral nerves can optimally support axon regeneration only for a finite period (Fu and Gordon, 1995b), and (3) the efficiency of reinnervation of original pathways and targets (path finding) decreases with advanced age (Le et al., 2001). Poor recovery after axonal GBS is not always the rule; exceptions include children with electrical features of acute denervation, cases with distal axonal degeneration where regeneration is needed over only a short distance, or patients with reversible axonal conduction failure (see later). A number of clinical and electrodiagnostic predictors indicate poor recovery, including old age, ventilator dependence, preceding gastrointestinal infection, rapid progression from onset to nadir, severe motor involvement, persistent low CMAP amplitudes, inexcitable nerves, and the presence of fibrillation potentials.

C. Pathology

The pathology of axonal GBS is largely characterized by analysis of autopsied materials obtained from AMAN cases in northern China. The pathological and immunopathological changes in these cases indicate an antibody-mediated immune attack directed preferentially against motor axons causing primary axonal degeneration in the absence of prominent T-cell inflammation (Griffin et al., 1995, 1996b; Hafer-Macko et al., 1996). One important and noteworthy observation borne out by these studies is that early on there may be no axonal pathology or minimal changes, restricted to the alteration of nodal architecture at the ultrastructural level, in the presence of profound clinical weakness (Griffin et al., 1996c). This finding is of note because it would argue for a prominent contribution by axonal conduction failure as the basis of clinical weakness in AMAN. Pathological findings in AMAN are discussed further in Section IV.

D. Pathogenesis

Molecular mimicry is currently the major theme in the pathogenesis of GBS, particularly in cases that follow *Campylobacter jejuni* infection. This hypothesis is supported by the following key observations: (1) *C. jejuni* enteritis is the most commonly recognized antecedent infection in GBS; (2) different variants of GBS, particularly FS and AMAN, are strongly associated with specific anti-ganglioside antibodies; (3) the lipooligosaccharides (LOSs) of *C. jejuni* isolates from patients with GBS carry relevant ganglioside-like moieties; (4) gangliosides, the purported target antigens, are enriched in the nerve fibers; and (5) pathological and immunopathological studies in the AMAN variant of GBS indicate antibody-mediated axonal injury. The current discussion on molecular mimicry is restricted to *C. jejuni* because most of the evidence has been obtained from the post-*Campylobacter* cases, although other bacteria such as *Haemophilus influenzae* have also been reported to carry ganglioside-like moieties (Mori et al., 2001). Further, anti-ganglioside antibodies in patients with GBS can also be detected in cases preceded by viral infections (Jacobs et al., 1998). Another relatively novel feature of molecular mimicry in GBS is the nature of antigens on the infecting organism and the relevant target antigens in peripheral nerves. These purported antigens on the infectious organism and in the peripheral nerves are carbohydrates that are carried on lipid backbones. In this context, relevant pathogenetic properties/issues relating to *C. jejuni* and LOSs containing ganglioside-like moieties, anti-ganglioside antibodies, and gangliosides in peripheral nerves are discussed further.

1. Campylobacter jejuni

C. jejuni is a gram-negative non-spore-forming entero-pathogen that is one of the most common causes of bacterial gastroenteritis worldwide, especially in children (Hughes and Rees, 1997; Friedman et al., 2000; Oberhelman and Taylor, 2000). Infection with *C. jejuni* is the most frequently recognized event preceding AMAN and other variants of GBS (reviewed in Hughes and Rees, 1997). Most *Campylobacter* infections are sporadic and are associated with ingestion of improperly handled or cooked food; poultry products are a major source of human infection. In GBS cases, both stool culture and serologic methods are needed to diagnose *Campylobacter* infection, because by the time neurological symptoms develop, the yield of *C. jejuni* from stool culture is relatively low (Nachamkin, 1997). Rhodes and Tattersfield described the first case of GBS following *C. jejuni* gastroenteritis in 1982 (Rhodes and Tattersfield, 1982). Subsequent studies have confirmed this association; however, the incidence of preceding *C. jejuni* infection varies widely, ranging from 4% in North America to 74% in northern China (Hughes and Rees, 1997; Ho et al., 1999), with an overall prevalence estimated at approximately 30% (reviewed in Moran et al., 2002). Based on the known incidences of GBS and *C. jejuni* enteritis, it is estimated that 1 in 1,000 cases of *Campylobacter* infection is complicated by GBS. Because GBS is a rare complication after *C. jejuni* infection, attention has focused on host and *Campylobacter* properties that may lead to this sequela. The host properties that could confer susceptibility to GBS after *C. jejuni* infection are not well established. Although some reports indicate post-*Campylobacter* GBS cases preferentially associate with certain HLA alleles, the significance of these findings

remains unclear because of lack of confirmatory studies (Yuki et al., 1991; Rees et al., 1995c).

The issue of *Campylobacter*-related factors has been examined mainly by serotyping and characterizing the ganglioside-like mimicry in the LOS of the GBS and enteritis isolates. *C. jejuni* is genetically heterogeneous and a large number of serotypes are recognized. Penner serotyping, based on the heat-stable capsular polysaccharide antigens, is most commonly used for classification of clinical isolates, including those from patients with GBS. Numerous *C. jejuni* serotypes have been associated with GBS and of particular interest is the observation that certain GBS-associated strains are uncommon in patients with uncomplicated gastroenteritis; for example, Penner serotype HS:19 is overrepresented in GBS patients compared to diarrhea isolates in some but not all populations (Fujimoto et al., 1992; Yuki et al., 1992b; Kuroki et al., 1993; Sheikh et al., 1998; Rees et al., 1995b; Jacobs et al., 1997). Another striking example of the association of uncommon serostrains with GBS is that of serostrain HS:41 in GBS cases from Cape Town, South Africa (Goddard et al., 1997). The overrepresentation of serostrains HS:19 and HS:41 in patients with GBS has supported the notion that as yet undefined properties related to the organism are critical in determining whether or not GBS follows *C. jejuni* infection. GBS-associated isolates are not restricted to these two uncommon serotypes and other *C. jejuni* serotypes isolated from GBS include a large number of other Penner serotypes (Prendergast and Moran, 2000).

The lipopolysaccharide (LPS) of gram-negative bacteria, including *C. jejuni*, consists of three components: lipid A, the hydrophobic region inserted into the membrane; an oligosaccharide core divided into inner and outer parts; and capsular polysaccharides, also called O-chains. LOS is differentiated from LPS by lack of O-chains. In *C. jejuni* it is the oligosaccharide core region that carries ganglioside-like moieties (Fig.1A). Several studies have characterized the core regions of LPS/LOS of GBS- and diarrhea-associated *C. jejuni* strains. Yuki et al. first described the presence of a GM1-like structure in *C. jejuni* LPS isolated from a GBS patient and subsequent studies have shown the presence of GM1-, GD1a-, GalNAc-GD1a-, GM1b-, GT1a-, GD2-, GD3-, and GM2-like structures (Yuki et al., 1992a; Aspinall et al., 1993, 1994a, 1994b, 1996; Sheikh et al., 1998; Nachamkin et al., 2002). Although structural studies have failed to demonstrate a GQ1b-like structure, the purported target antigen for FS, antibody binding assays with human or murine monoclonal antibodies have shown the presence of GQ1b- and GT1a-cross-reactive moieties in *C. jejuni* LPS/LOSs (Jacobs et al., 1995, 1997; Yuki et al., 1994). Figure 1B shows the ganglioside-like moieties, as determined by mass spectrometry, in *C. jejuni* LOS implicated in AMAN and FS. It is clear that both GBS- and diarrhea-associated isolates carry ganglioside-like moieties but

A. Structure of LPS

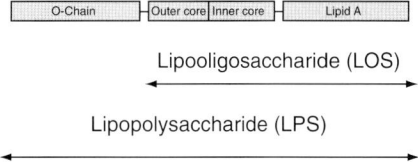

B. Structure of ganglioside-mimics in the inner core of LPS

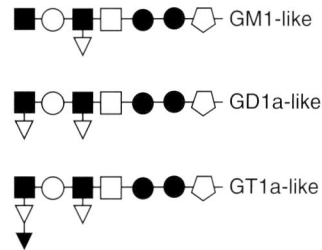

C. Structure of the gangliosides implicated as target antigens

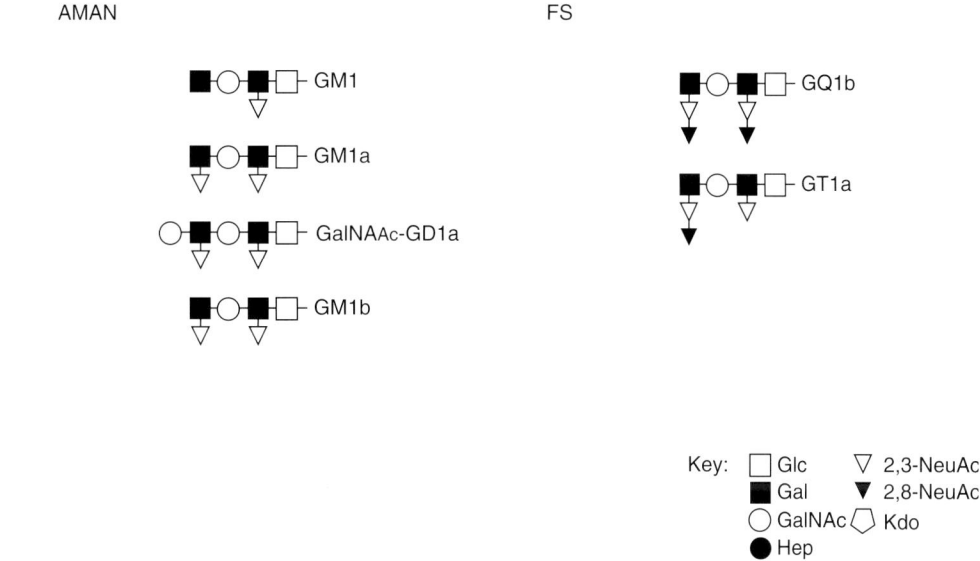

Figure 1 (**A**) Diagrammatic representation of the structure of LPS and LOS in gram-negative bacteria. (**B**) Structure of ganglioside-mimics in *C. jejuni* core oligosaccharide as determined by different mass spectroscopy studies. (**C**) Structure of gangliosides implicated as target antigens in acute motor axonal neuropathy and Fisher syndrome.

GBS-related organisms are more likely to do so (Nachamkin et al., 1999, 2002). These studies indicate that expression of ganglioside-structures in LPS by itself is not sufficient to impart GBS-inducing properties to the infecting organism.

2. Anti-Ganglioside Antibodies

The possibility that carbohydrate moieties on glycolipids could be autoantigens in neuropathic disorders was realized with the description of a case with chronic IgM parapro-teinemic neuropathy in which the paraprotein recognized a structure shared by several gangliosides (Ilyas et al., 1985). Initial descriptions of anti-ganglioside antibodies in patients with GBS were based on small case series or case reports (Ilyas et al., 1988, 1992; Yuki et al., 1990; Walsh et al., 1991). Subsequently, several large studies examined the clinicoserological correlations in GBS, leading to identifi-cation of some putative ganglioside target antigens (Rees et al., 1995a; Jacobs et al., 1996; Ho et al., 1999;

Ogawara et al., 2000). Besides identifying the target antigens, antiglycolipid serological studies tend to correlate the specificity of antibody responses with specific clinical and pathological features, such as motor vs. sensory fiber involvement or axonal vs. demyelinating injury. There are several limitations inherent to such large population-based serological studies, but despite these caveats, certain patterns/associations have emerged.

The antibody correlations for AIDP variant are not well defined. In contrast, two major gangliosides, GM1 and GD1a, and two minor gangliosides, GalNAc-GD1a and GM1b, are implicated as target antigens in AMAN (Rees et al., 1995a; Jacobs et al., 1996; Ogawara et al., 2000; Hadden et al., 1998; Ho et al., 1999; Yuki et al., 1993b; Kusunoki et al., 1994, 1996a). Antibodies against GM1 and GD1a gangliosides can be detected in up to 50% to 60% of patients with AMAN in Japanese and northern Chinese populations (Ogawara et al., 2000; Ho et al., 1999). The frequency of anti-GalNAc-GD1a and GM1b antibodies in motor-predominant syndromes is much lower, in the range of 10% to 15% (Ang et al., 1999; Yuki et al., 1999, 2000). Anti-GQ1b antibodies, frequently cross-reactive with other structurally related gangliosides containing disialosyl moieties, are present in up to 80% to 90% of patients with FS (Willison et al., 1993; Yuki et al., 1993a; Carpo et al., 1998), and this correlation provides the strongest association between antibodies to a specific ganglioside and a clinical phenotype.

In chronic neuropathies associated with anti-ganglioside reactivity, it is usually the pentameric IgM that binds to glycolipids. In contrast, the anti-ganglioside antibodies in acute neuropathic conditions such as AMAN and FS are predominantly of IgG isotype, generally complement-fixing subtypes IgG1 and IgG3 (Willison and Veitch, 1994; Ogino et al., 1995). These anti-ganglioside antibody responses in GBS are almost always polyclonal and can have a broad range of cross-reactivity with structurally related gangliosides (Koga et al., 2001). It has been proposed that differences in geography and or genetic background may affect the specificity and isotype distribution of anti-ganglioside responses in different populations (Ogawara et al., 2000; Ang et al., 2001b).

The mechanism(s) of generation of anti-ganglioside responses in GBS remain elusive. The following observations support the hypothesis of molecular mimicry in post-*Campylobacter* GBS cases. First, studies that demonstrate that either human GBS sera or purified human anti-ganglioside antibodies bind to ganglioside-like moieties contained in the core oligosaccharide region of the LPS/LOS (Wirguin et al., 1994; Oomes et al., 1995; Sheikh et al., 1998); one extension of this observation is that the cross-reactive sugar moieties in LOS triggered the production of these antibodies. Second, immunization with *C. jejuni* LPSs/LOSs can successfully induce anti-ganglioside antibodies (Wirguin et al., 1997; Goodyear et al., 1999; Ang et al., 2001a). These immune responses in experimental animals have generally

induced low-affinity, non-T-cell-dependent antibodies of IgM and IgG3 type (non-complement-fixing isotype in mice), despite the use of adjuvants to recruit T-cell help (Wirguin et al., 1997; Goodyear et al., 1999), reflecting a high level of tolerance to self-gangliosides restricting antibody responses to *C. jejuni* LPSs (Bowes et al., 2002). In contrast, serological studies in AMAN and FS indicate class switching to IgG and subclass restriction to IgG1 and IgG3 (complement-fixing isotypes in humans), both usually features of T-cell (Th1) help and atypical of the human anticarbohydrate antibody responses. The high level of tolerance to self-gangliosides in experimental animals can be reproducibly overcome, probably with successful recruitment of T-cell help and production of IgG subclasses, by immunization with gangliosides or *C. jejuni* LPSs in transgenic animals lacking complex gangliosides (Lunn et al., 2000; Bowes et al., 2002). The possibility that IgG anti-ganglioside antibody production does not require immunoglobulin class switching but reflects a primary B-cell response has not been examined in patients with GBS or experimental models.

Observations from these immunization studies raise the possibility that under some conditions, the high level of tolerance to self-gangliosides can be overcome after *C. jejuni* infection, leading to induction of T-cell-dependent IgG anti-ganglioside responses similar to those seen in human GBS cases. These experimental findings support the notion that breakdown of tolerance to self-gangliosides is critical in the pathogenesis of post-*Campylobacter* GBS. In such a model, it would not be far-fetched to propose that although generation of these antibodies reflects breakdown of strong tolerance to gangliosides, the immune system has another check to contain such an aberrant immune response, when it arises, either by turning off the anti-ganglioside antibody production by B-cells or more likely by their elimination/deletion. The existence of such a system of containment for autoreactive B-cells secreting anti-ganglioside antibodies is argued by the observations that post-*Campylobacter* GBS is monophasic, associated anti-ganglioside antibody titers reach a peak with the nadir of the disease and decay thereafter, and the extremely rare incidence of recurrence of clinical disease even in northern China, where *C. jejuni* is endemic and chances of reexposure are not trivial. An alternate explanation is that the development of these antibodies reflects thymus-independent B-cell responses, which typically do not induce long-term immunological memory. Further experimental work in this area may clarify the mechanisms involved in the generation and elimination of human anti-ganglioside antibodies after *C. jejuni* infection.

3. Peripheral Nerve Gangliosides

Gangliosides are sialic acid-containing glycosphingolipids that are widely distributed in mammalian tissues but are particularly enriched in the nervous system. Gangliosides are classified on the basis of the number and linkages of the sugar backbone and attached sialic acids. All complex gangliosides have a tetraose (four-sugar) backbone/core, consisting of galactose, *N*-acetylgalactosamine, galactose, and glucose, to which variable numbers of sialic acids are attached; the ceramide or lipid portion of the molecule is attached to the internal glucose. Although there are a large number of ganglioside species, GM1, GD1b, GD1a, and GT1b are the four most abundant complex gangliosides in the nervous system. Simpler gangliosides have a shorter core structure instead of the four-sugar backbone structure. Anti-ganglioside antibody binding to these carbohydrate moieties determines their specificities. The structures of gangliosides implicated as target antigens in AMAN and Fisher variants of GBS are depicted in Figure 1C.

One reason for defining the associations between anti-ganglioside antibody specificity and clinical variants of GBS is the simple hypothesis that differences in clinical manifestations may relate to differences in the distribution of target antigens (gangliosides) in different regions of the nervous system. A large number of biochemical studies indicate that there are no consistent differences in the ganglioside content of motor and sensory fibers to explain preferential motor nerve fiber injury, except that carbohydrate-anchoring lipids in sensory and motor nerves of gangliosides are different (Ogawa-Goto et al., 1990; Gong et al., 2002). Immunolocalization studies have examined the distribution of GM1 and GD1a in peripheral nerves. These gangliosides are localized at nodes of Ranvier and on the nodal and internodal axolemma (Fig. 2A and B) (Sheikh et al., 1999; Gong et al., 2002). GM1 is also enriched in the paranodal myelin (Fig. 2A) (Ganser et al., 1983; Sheikh et al., 1999). Most of the available data suggest that anti-ganglioside antibodies bind to the Schwann cell surface but not to compact myelin. GM1 and GD1a are also concentrated in motor nerve terminals (Fig. 2C). We have recently generated several monoclonal anti-GD1a antibodies and found that anti-GD1a monoclonal antibodies preferentially stain myelinated motor axons but not sensory myelinated axons (Fig. 3) (Gong et al., 2002), but the basis of this differential antibody binding to motor fibers remains unclear. Our finding was supported by a recent study showing the preferential staining of nodes of Ranvier in motor nerve fibers by serum with GD1a reactivity obtained from a patient with AMAN (De Angelis et al., 2002). The distribution of minor gangliosides GalNAc-GD1a and GM1b is not well characterized.

The distribution of FS targets GQ1b and related cross-reactive gangliosides in peripheral and cranial nerves have also been studied by biochemical and immunohistochemical techniques. Anti-GQ1b antibodies bind to paranodal myelin and nodes of Ranvier, and it has been shown that the extraocular cranial nerves are slightly enriched in GQ1b compared to other cranial and peripheral nerves (Chiba et al., 1993, 1997). That GQ1b is not restricted to cranial nerves is also supported by studies showing binding of disialosyl antibodies to the nodes of Ranvier in somatic nerves. Muscle spindles, motor nerve terminals in somatic and extraocular

muscles, and intrafusal muscle fibers are also labeled by antibodies cross-reactive with GQ1b (Willison et al., 1996; Goodyear et al., 1999). The observation that anti-GQ1b reactive antibodies bind to motor nerve terminals has been exploited by investigators for experimental modeling (see later) and may be relevant to FS pathogenesis.

In summary, except for GD1a localization, ganglioside distribution studies do not provide a satisfactory explanation for preferential motor fiber injury in AMAN or regional-localization of symptoms in FS. These findings suggest that it is more than likely that other factors besides ganglioside density and distribution also play important roles in anti-ganglioside antibody-mediated injury. These factors include relative differences in the blood-nerve barrier in different regions of the nerve fibers and between sensory and motor spinal roots; the motor nerve terminal provides such an example. One favored explanation for the absence of CNS involvement in AMAN despite a high level of ganglioside expression is that the blood-brain barrier is much less permeable than is the blood-nerve barrier. The existence of such differences in barrier permeability between sensory and motor roots, however, has not been reported. Further, the conduction properties of motor fibers are significantly different from those of sensory fibers, and one could speculate that these fibers are more prone to antibody-mediated conduction failure; this may be particularly relevant early in the pathogenesis of AMAN. Moreover, susceptibility to injury could also differ between motor and sensory fibers or different regions of the same nerve fiber based on the differences in expression of target gangliosides or their accessibility to anti-ganglioside antibodies. In summary, the basis of preferential motor injury in AMAN remains incompletely understood, and ongoing work is likely to provide further clues to this interesting pathogenetic issue.

The following properties of gangliosides in nerves make them suitable to serve as target antigens in nerve fibers. The ceramide portion of gangliosides anchors them into the plasma membranes, whereas oligosaccharide moieties extend into the extracelluar space from the cell surface. This membrane organization allows anti-ganglioside antibodies to bind to sugar moieties extending into the extracellular space. Immunolocalization studies have confirmed that patient-derived or experimental anti-ganglioside antibodies bind these sugars on nerve fibers, thus confirming their accessibility to immune effectors. Recent work indicates that gangliosides are focally enriched into functional domains called rafts into which protein receptors or ion channels can be actively recruited or excluded. Experimental evidence indicates that signal transduction can occur through lipid rafts, and these ganglioside-enriched microdomains can also modulate receptor function. Further, sodium and postassium channels are clustered in the ganglioside-enriched regions of myelinated nerve fibers (i.e., nodes and paranodes) (Black et al., 1990). These properties of myelinated nerve fiber gangliosides provide clues to the potential mechanisms of

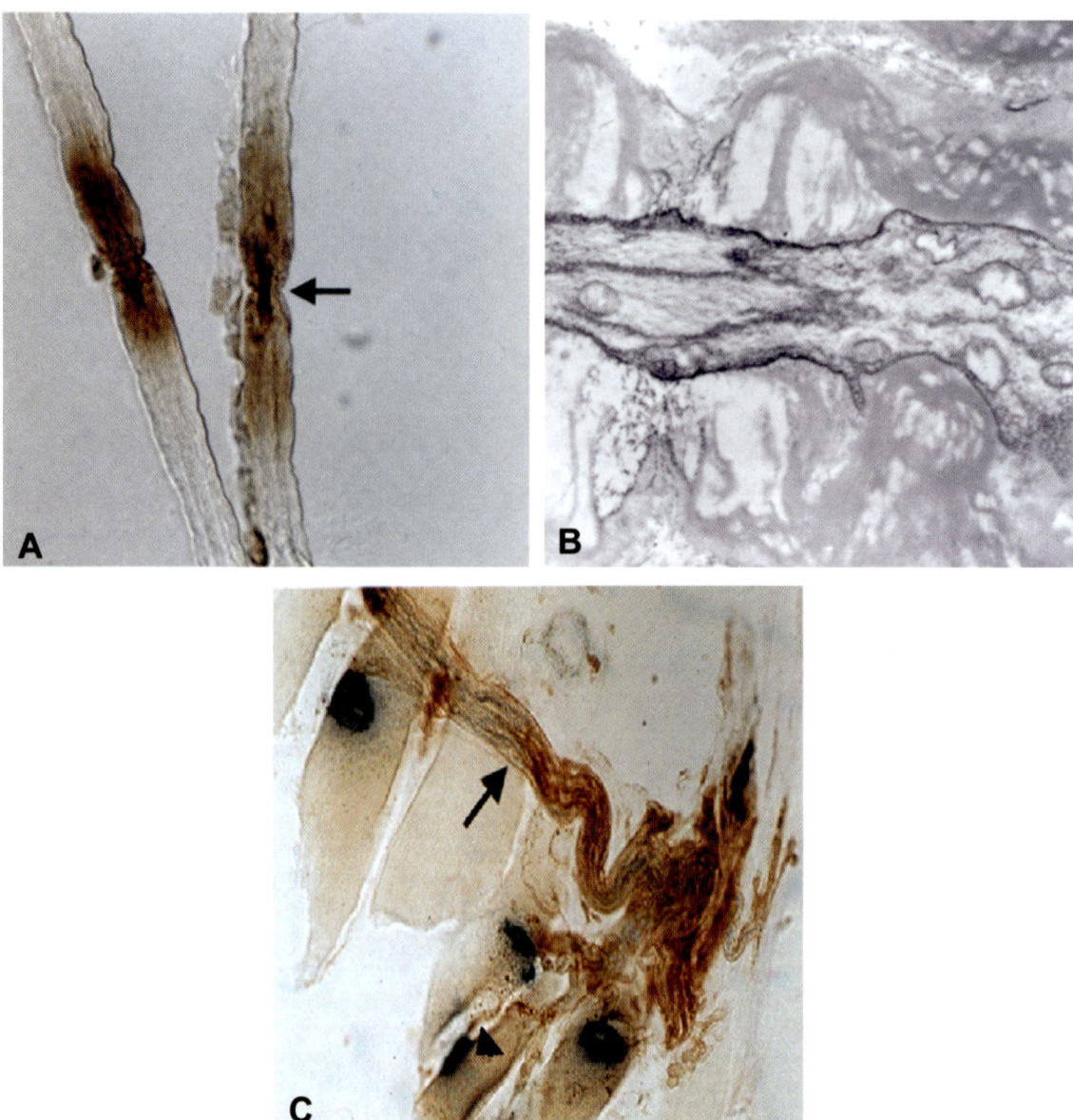

Figure 2 **Localization of GM1 ganglioside in peripheral nerves.** (**A**) Teased nerve fiber preparation showing GM1 staining at node of Ranvier (*arrow*) and paranodal Schwann cell. (**B**) Immunoelectron microscopy showing GM1 staining at the nodal axolemma and extension along paranodal axolemma. (**C**) Fresh-frozen muscle preparation showing GM1 staining (*brown*) of an intramuscular nerve (*arrow*) and a motor nerve terminal (*arrowhead*); blue staining shows motor end plates. (Adapted with permission from Sheikh et al., 1999.)

anti-ganglioside antibody-mediated nerve fiber dysfunction, as discussed in the next section.

IV. Anti-ganglioside Antibody-Mediated Axonal Injury: Possible Mechanisms

A. Pathological Effects

For last 15 years, research efforts in this area have focused on demonstrating the pathophysiological effects of anti-ganglioside antibodies, but it is only recently that the mechanism(s) of anti-ganglioside antibody-mediated axonal injury are beginning to emerge. Clinical, pathological, and experimental findings suggest that there is a spectrum of pathophysiological changes in AMAN that includes recognizable functional and structural axonal injury. Whereas the previous sections have outlined the possible mechanism(s) of generation of specific immune insult(s) directed against the axon, this section outlines evidence derived from clinical and experimental studies providing insights into the mechanisms involved in antibody-mediated axonal injury.

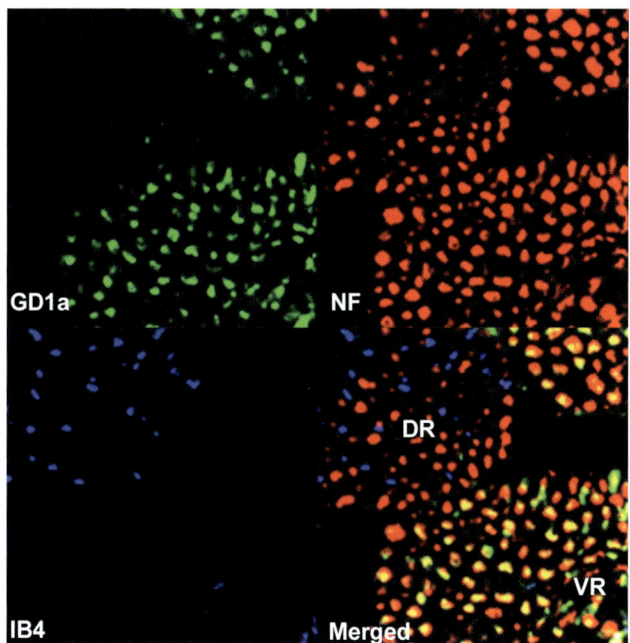

Figure 3 Fresh-frozen cross-sections of rat cauda equina (ventral and dorsal root) triple labeled with anti-ganglioside antibody GD1a-IgG1 (*green*), neurofilament (*red*), and IB-4 (*blue*). Co-localization of three labels is also shown (*merged*). Neurofilament stains all myelinated fibers, whereas IB-4 stains unmyelinated fibers in dorsal root. This figure shows that monoclonal antibody GD1a-IgG1 preferentially binds to myelinated motor axons in the ventral root but not the sensory myelinated fibers in dorsal roots. (Adapted with permission from Gong et al., 2002.)

This discussion is organized to bring out issues relevant to the means by which circulating antibody gains access to myelinated axons in nerves, keeping in view the anatomy of nerves and myelinated nerve fibers (Fig. 3).

In autoimmune diseases, accessibility of target tissues, cells, and antigens to immune effectors is critical in determining the distribution of injury. This is all the more important for the diseases of the nervous system, because the blood-tissue barriers contribute to the immune privileged status of neural tissues. For an immune effector to cause neural injury it has to cross the respective blood tissue barrier (i.e., blood-nerve-barrier for PNS and blood-brain barrier for CNS injury). Peripheral nerve fibers are organized into individual bundles or fascicles. A fibrofatty layer, the epineurium, surrounds and holds individual fascicles in nerve bundles. Each nerve fascicle is surrounded by perineurium, which consists of a variable number of layers of specialized perineurial cells attached to each other by tight junctions, with each cell layer covered by basal lamina. The thickness of perineurium varies along the course of peripheral nerves; the thickness diminishes in linear relationship to the diameter of the nerve. The perineurium plays a role in regulating the endoneurial environment, including providing a barrier to diffusion of macromolecules such as antibodies

and complement components from the epineurial space. Notably, the perineurium is open-ended near termination of the motor nerve terminal, allowing accessibility to endoneurial space and axon. The endoneurium is a space bounded by the perineurium and includes the nerve fibers, supporting glia, and extracellular matrix containing collagen. It is the endothelial cells of endoneurial blood vessels that form tight junctions with apposing cells, resulting in the formation of blood-nerve barrier. Studies with circulating tracers indicate that the permeability of the blood-nerve barrier to macromolecules, such as horseradish peroxidase, is much higher than that of the blood-brain barrier (Arvidson, 1977). This is also supported by the findings that a low level of IgG is detectable in the normal endoneurium. Further, it appears that along the course of peripheral nerve fibers the blood-nerve barrier permeability varies. This barrier is relatively more lax at the level of dorsal root ganglion and spinal roots and almost nonexistent at motor nerve terminals, making these two sites more vulnerable to attack by circulating immune effectors such as antibodies targeting peripheral nerve antigens.

We have recently examined whether circulating anti-ganglioside antibodies can access the neural tissues and cross the normal blood-nerve barrier and blood-brain barrier in mice by using tracer studies with a radiolabeled monoclonal anti-ganglioside antibody. Our results indicate a low level accumulation of this antibody in both PNS and CNS, but the accumulation in the CNS was 5- to 10-fold lower than that in the PNS. Further, there was a significant increase in the amount of antibody that accumulated in the neural tissues in the setting of experimental systemic inflammation resulting in an increase in the levels of circulating inflammatory cytokines (Sheikh et al., 2004). In addition, there is experimental evidence suggesting that sera from patients with GBS, particularly those with anti-ganglioside antibodies, perturb the permeability of an *in vitro* blood-nerve barrier model (Kanda et al., 2000, 2003). These findings suggest that in the absence of peripheral nerve antigen-specific-T-cell inflammation, anti-ganglioside antibodies can access the endoneurium and this accessibility is enhanced in the presence of circulating inflammatory cytokines, which have been reported to be elevated in patients with GBS (Sharief et al., 1993, 1997). Given these experimental findings and the absence of prominent T-cell inflammation in pathological studies of AMAN cases, it is conceivable that, in antibody-mediated neuropathies such as AMAN, T-cell-mediated breakdown of the blood-nerve barrier is not necessary for antibody accessibility to nerve.

Once the antibodies cross the blood vessels and reach the endoneurial extracellular matrix, how do they access the target antigens on nerve fibers? Does the complex endoneurial interstitium allow antibodies to diffuse through it and access the target antigens on nerve fibers, or is focal disruption of this highly organized structure required? Although uniform low-level endoneurial staining for IgG in normal nerves would favor that antibodies can diffuse through the interstitium, a definitive answer to this complex issue is not known and would require the development of sophisticated techniques to study the kinetics of macromolecules in the endoneurium.

The next step in this sequence of events is the antibody binding to axonal antigens on myelinated fibers. In myelinated fibers, there are two sites along the axon that are not covered by myelin, but only by Schwann cell basal lamina, the nodes of Ranvier, and motor nerve terminals. Therefore, these sites are relatively more accessible to immune effectors and probably more susceptible to antibody-mediated injury. The susceptibility of these two sites to antibody-mediated injury would be supported by the pathological and immunopathological findings in AMAN and experimental models demonstrating pathogenic effects of anti-ganglioside antibodies on motor nerve terminals (see later). The periaxonal space surrounding the internodal axolemma is relatively inaccessible to ions and macromolecules such as antibody and complement in endoneurial interstitial fluid, because Schwann cell terminal myelin loops attach to paranodal axolemma by gap junction-like complexes and the periaxonal space in this region only measures 3 to 5 nm compared to 12 to 14 nm in the internodal region. Factors that contribute to the differential susceptibility of different regions of a myelinated motor axon to antibody-mediated injury are summarized in Table 2.

The pathology and immunopathology of AMAN are reviewed, keeping in mind the anatomic organization of myelinated fibers as discussed previously. The pathological examination of both early and late cases has been extremely instructive and has allowed the reconstruction of pathogenetic events over the course of the disease. In AMAN the earliest pathological changes are quite subtle and involve the nodes of Ranvier of motor fibers in the ventral roots (Griffin et al., 1996c). These changes consist of lengthening of the nodal gap at times when the fibers otherwise appear normal. Macrophages are recruited to the nodes of Ranvier early on

Table 2 Properties of Different Regions of a Myelinated Motor Axon Contributing to Susceptibility to Anti-ganglioside Antibody-Mediated Injury

	Node/Paranode	Internode	Motor nerve terminal
Ganglioside antigens	++	+	++
Covered by myelin	−	+	−
Ion channels	+ (Na^+ and K^+)	−	+ (Ca^{++})
Accessibility to antibody binding	+	−/+*	+++

*When periaxonal space is breached or potentially after demyelination.

(Fig. 4A2), and these macrophages then insert into the nodal gap. The immunopathological changes correlating with motor fiber pathology in ventral roots are also initially observed at nodes of Ranvier. It is observed that early in the pathogenetic process IgG binds at nodes of Ranvier, leading to activation of complement, as suggested by C3d deposition, which causes macrophage recruitment at nodes of Ranvier through complement-derived chemoattractants (Fig. 4B and C) (Hafer-Macko et al., 1996). The currently favored pathogenetic sequence proposes that macrophages at nodes of Ranvier then open the normally impermeable periaxonal space to endoneurial constituents including antibody and complement. This sequence of events is supported by the immunocytochemical findings showing deposition of IgG and complement activation marker C3d in periaxonal space and on internodal axolemma in late cases (Fig. 4D) (Hafer-Macko et al., 1996). Subsequently macrophages are recruited to the periaxonal internodal space after the disruption of paranodal sites of attachment of the Schwann cell myelin sheath to the axon. Insertion of macrophages into the periaxonal space leads to axonal shrinkage and separation away from adaxonal Schwann cell plasmalemma. The shrunken axon surrounded by macrophage survives for some time before undergoing wallerian-like degeneration (Fig. 4E and F) (Griffin et al., 1996a). This sequence of pathological changes in early and late cases would be compatible with the distribution of gangliosides, accessibility of anti-ganglioside antibodies and complement, and anatomic organization of myelinated nerve fibers. In myelinated fibers, the motor nerve terminal is another axonal site susceptible to injury by circulating immune effectors because it is neither covered by myelin nor protected by blood-nerve barrier. A recent case report provides proof of concept for this hypothesis; this description includes a patient with AMAN who recovered rapidly after treatment with IVIg. Pathological examination of the muscle biopsy showed motor fiber degeneration largely limited to intramuscular nerves or motor nerve terminals (Ho et al., 1997a). One explanation for the rapid recovery in this instance is that regeneration over a relatively short distance can be achieved quickly.

The next critical question is this: Can anti-ganglioside antibodies with specificity similar to those in patients with AMAN cause axonal injury and reproduce the pathological and immunopathological features of AMAN in experimental animal models? Until recently there were no reproducible or reliable animal models of anti-ganglioside antibody-mediated nerve injury particularly in rodents. Recent studies indicate that repeated immunizations with a mixture of gangliosides, keyhole limpet hemocyanin, and complete Freund's adjuvant in rabbits can produce neuropathic injury. The pattern and distribution of neuropathic injury relate to the specificity of ganglioside used for immunization and the specific anti-ganglioside response. For example, studies with GD1b ganglioside led to the development of sensory ataxic

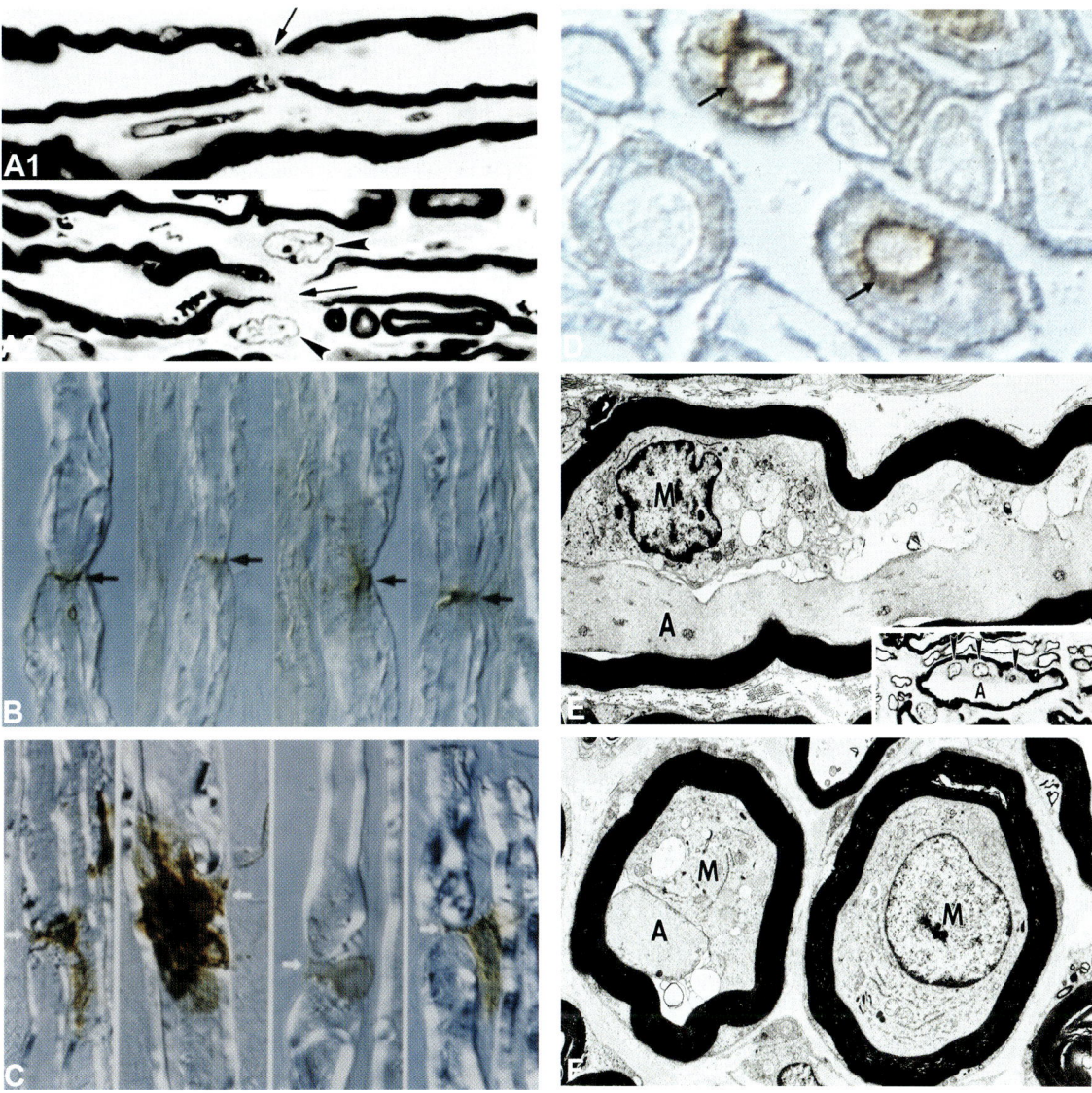

Figure 4 Representative pathology and immunopathology of early (**A–C**) and late (**D–F**) AMAN cases. (**A1**) Longitudinal section of a large myelinated fiber showing a normal node of Ranvier (*arrow*). (**A2**) Longitudinal section of a motor fiber showing lengthening of the node (*arrow*) and overlying macrophages (*arrowheads*). (**B**) Teased fiber preparations stained for C3d deposition showing deposition of this complement activation product at the nodes of Ranvier. (**C**) Teased fiber preparations stained with a macrophage marker showing macrophages overlying and inserting processes at the nodes of Ranvier. (**D**) Cross-section of a ventral root showing deposition of C3d on internodal axolemma. (**E**) Electron micrograph of a longitudinally sectioned motor nerve fiber showing a macrophage (M) entering the periaxonal space and lying adjacent to axon (A) and separating the overlying myelin sheath. (**F**) Electron micrograph of cross-sectioned motor nerve fibers at different stages of axonal degeneration; the fiber on the left shows a macrophage (M) in the periaxonal space surrounding a shrunken but intact axon (A) inside a normal appearing myelin sheath; in the fiber on the right an axon cannot be identified and macrophage (M) has occupied the position normally maintained by axon. (Adapted with permission from Griffin et al., 1995, 1996c; Hafer-Macko et al., 1996.)

neuropathy in rabbits, and pathological analysis showed degeneration of dorsal root ganglion cells and allied axonal projections (Kusunoki et al. 1996b). In contrast, use of whole bovine brain gangliosides or GM1 for immunization resulted in the development of high titer IgG anti-GM1 responses, flaccid paralysis, and degeneration of motor axons in the ventral roots (Yuki et al., 2001). The immunopathology and pathology of these animals showed deposition of IgG on motor axons and the presence of periaxonal macrophages in motor fibers, features reminiscent of human pathology (Susuki et al., 2003). Moreover, pathological analysis of some animals with severe muscle weakness and death a short time after onset of clinical weakness showed no morphological axonal changes, suggesting that in

AMAN, axonal dysfunction precedes the degeneration (Susuki et al., 2003).

With the availability of a variety of transgenic animals, we have recently taken an alternate approach to generate a mouse model of anti-ganglioside antibody-mediated neuropathy. This paradigm included the generation of monoclonal anti-ganglioside antibodies (Lunn et al., 2000) and implantation of antibody-secreting hybridoma in mice. This led to the development of axonal neuropathy when a GD1a-reactive antibody was implanted in mice (Sheikh et al., 2004). The development of neuropathy in this model was contingent on breakdown of the blood-nerve barrier by circulating cytokines generated by implantation of antibody-secreting tumor. These findings not only provide additional evidence for pathogenicity of anti-ganglioside antibodies, but also provide an example of non-T-cell-dependent breakdown of the blood-nerve barrier. Attempts of passive transfer of neuropathy in animal models with patient-derived or experimental anti-ganglioside antibodies so far have been unsuccessful.

B. Physiological Effects

Three clinicopathological observations support the hypothesis that physiological blockade of conduction at the level of the axon, in addition to motor axonal degeneration, contributes significantly to clinical weakness in AMAN. First, many patients with AMAN recover quite quickly, with or without IVIg treatment, and their time course of recovery is incompatible with nerve fiber degeneration and regeneration (Ho et al., 1997a; Kuwabara et al., 1998). Second, the pathological studies in AMAN and its animal model indicate that despite severe clinical weakness, axonal degeneration is not universal in early cases, and such degeneration affects only a proportion of motor fibers even in late cases (Griffin et al., 1996c; Susuki et al., 2003). Third, the issue of mismatch between clinical and pathological findings and axonal conduction failure was examined by serial electrophysiological studies in a set of patients with GBS. In this important study, Kuwabara and colleagues (1998) examined the electrophysiological features of a group of GBS cases with IgG anti-GM1 antibodies and classified them into axonal or demyelinating variants on the basis of initial electrodiagnostic examination. Subsequent nerve conduction studies showed that all cases classified as AIDP and some axonal cases had rapid improvement in distal compound muscle action potential amplitudes. Further, cases that were initially classified as AIDP had rapid resolution of conduction slowing and block without the appearance of slow components that indicate remyelination. These findings raise the possibility that rapid recovery of CMAP amplitudes and motor conduction slowing without features of remyelination is due to a reversible conduction failure/block at the level of axon. The recovery of CMAP amplitudes in cases initially classi-

fied as axonal could be due to dysfunction at the level of node of Ranvier or motor nerve terminal. With this in mind, experimental evidence for physiological effects of anti-ganglioside antibodies on the nodes of Raniver and motor nerve terminal is presented next.

1. Nodes of Ranvier

There are several reasons to consider the node of Ranvier as a candidate site for the pathophysiological effects of anti-ganglioside antibodies. First, most complex gangliosides are concentrated at the nodes of Ranvier. Second, in myelinated fibers axonal target antigens are particularly exposed at this site. Third, ion channels are clustered at nodes of Ranvier, and disruption of their function can lead to conduction abnormalities and finally, structural integrity of the node of Ranvier is critical for nerve fiber conduction. Therefore, experimental studies, mostly with anti-GM1 antibodies, have focused on node of Ranvier dysfunction in both animal and in vitro models. Nevertheless, discrepant findings have been reported by different investigators.

Initially, two separate studies showed that intraneural injections, in rats, of human anti-GM1 antibodies caused acute conduction block (Santoro et al., 1992; Uncini et al., 1993), but this finding was not confirmed by another group that used immunoglobulin fractions with IgG or IgM anti-GM1 reactivity purified from patients with GBS or multifocal motor neuropathy (Harvey et al., 1995). The basis for these discrepant findings has not been resolved, but it could reflect factors that were not strictly matched: (1) anti-GM1 antibody properties such as fine specificity and/or affinity, (2) whole serum versus purified immunoglobulins and anti-GM1 titers, and (3) source and activity of the exogenous complement. This issue of anti-ganglioside antibody-mediated conduction failure is rekindled by a recent report indicating that, in a rabbit model of AMAN associated with anti-GM1 antibodies, conduction abnormalities were noted in myelinated fibers in the spinal roots (Susuki et al., 2003). To explore this issue further, we have recently examined the effects of an anti-GD1a-reactive monoclonal antibody injected intraneurally in rat sciatic nerves. The serial nerve conduction studies in this model indicate development of conduction failure that reverses over time. Notably, exogenous complement was required in this model to induce conduction abnormalities (J. Spies, K. Sheikh, and colleagues, unpublished findings). Overall, these findings support the concept that anti-ganglioside antibodies with certain specificities can cause conduction failure in myelinated nerve fibers.

Different in vitro studies with anti-GM1 antibodies also report discrepant findings. The first such study examined the effects of human and rabbit sera with anti-GM1 reactivity on desheathed rat sciatic nerve preparations and found mild reduction of CMAP amplitudes (Arasaki et al., 1993). An extremely provocative finding by Takigawa and colleagues (1995) provided strong support to the concept of anti-GM1 antibody-mediated nodal ion channel dysfunction. This study, by using a voltage clamp technique on isolated single myelinated rat nerve fibers, found that rabbit sera with anti-GM1 reactivity caused increased potassium current, as elicited by step depolarization, in a complement-independent manner, whereas these antibodies in the presence of active complement caused decreased sodium currents and eventually blocked the channels irreversibly. These investigators reproduced their findings with GBS sera containing anti-GM1 antibodies (Takigawa et al., 2000). The hypothesis of sodium channel dysfunction was further supported by a report by Weber et al. (2000) showing that rabbit sera with IgG anti-GM1 reactivity caused reversible blockade of the voltage-gated sodium channels in a neural cell line. It was postulated that complexes of anti-GM1 antibodies and complement products block the ion-conducting pore of the channel directly. In contrast, two other studies *in vitro* that used human or rabbit sera with anti-GM1 reactivity did not observe acute conduction abnormalities (Hirota et al., 1997; Paparounas et al., 1999). The basis of these discrepant results is not resolved and could reflect differences in the antibody properties or methodologies used by different investigators.

One possible mechanism of sodium channel dysfunction in the Takigawa and Weber studies could be that anti-GM1 antibodies bound directly to cross-reactive oligosaccharides on highly sialylated and glycosylated sodium channels led to abnormalities in ion channel conduction. We examined this issue in the spinal roots of dystrophic mice that contained large amyelinated fibers with randomly distributed patches of sodium channels in the absence of nodes of Ranvier. This preparation allowed us to ask whether sodium channels have an obligatory co-localization with GM1-binding ligands (Sheikh et al., 1999). Our results showed that GM1-binding ligands did not co-localize with sodium channels in this situation, suggesting that anti-GM1 antibody-mediated nodal dysfunction is likely to be indirect and not due to direct targeting of sodium channels. However, this issue needs further resolution at the level of GBS-derived anti-GM1 antibodies and sodium channel isotype(s) concentrated at nodes of Ranvier in human peripheral nerves.

2. Motor Nerve Terminal

The motor nerve terminal is a susceptible site for anti-ganglioside antibody-mediated injury because it is enriched in gangliosides such as GM1, GD1a, and GQ1b, and it lacks a blood-nerve barrier. We have previously reported that this site degenerates in AMAN (Ho et al., 1997b), and an electrophysiological study suggests that this site is affected in some cases of FS (Uncini and Lugaresi, 1999). Experimental pathophysiological studies have examined both complement-dependent and complement-independent effects of anti-ganglioside antibodies on this site in phrenic nerve hemidiaphragm preparations.

a. Complement-Dependent Pathophysiological Effects
In a series of studies, Hugh Willison's group in Glasgow (Willison et al.,1996; Goodyear et al.,1999; Plomp et al., 1999) extensively investigated the effects of both human and experimental antibodies, with specificities similar to FS, on motor nerve terminal in phrenic nerve hemidiaphragm preparations both *in vitro* and *ex vivo*. They have demonstrated that anti-GQ1b reactive antibodies bind to neuromuscular junctions and induce massive quantal release of acetylcholine from nerve terminals, eventually blocking the neuromuscular transmission on a presynaptic basis. This effect is dependent on the activation of complement, probably through the alternate pathway, but neither requires activation of the classical pathway nor the formation of membrane attack complex. These anti-ganglioside antibody-mediated changes in motor nerve terminal physiology closely resemble the effects of the paralytic neurotoxin, α-latrotoxin. Subsequent studies by this group showed that in this model, there is antibody and complement deposition accompanied by morphological disruption of the nerve terminal involving the loss of major cytoskeletal components, including neurofilaments (O'Hanlon et al., 2001). Notably, both calcium depletion and calpain inhibition protected the cytoskeleton from degradation, supporting the hypothesis that calcium ingress and activation of calcium-dependent proteases, calpains, are involved in degradation of the motor nerve terminal cytoskeleton (O'Hanlon et al., 2003). It appears that α-latrotoxin like-effects at NMJ are not restricted to antibodies with GQ1b reactivity, but can also be seen with antibodies with GD1a-reactivity (H. Willison, personal communication), thus supporting the notion that motor nerve terminal is a target site for anti-ganglioside antibody-mediated injury in AMAN.

b. Complement-Independent Immunopharmacological effects of antibodies
In a parallel set of studies in a perfused macro-patch clamp electrode model, Buchwald and colleagues demonstrated blockade of evoked acetylcholine release and reduced amplitude of postsynaptic potentials, suggestive of combined presynaptic and postsynaptic blockade, after application of purified IgG from patients with GBS and FS directly to the nerve terminal and a concentration-dependent presynaptic blockade with a monoclonal antibody with GQ1b-reactivity (Buchwald et al. 1995, 1998, 2002). These effects were complement-independent and reversible, suggesting a direct immunopharmacological effect of the antibodies at the neuromuscular junction. We have examined the effects of IgG monoclonal antibodies with GD1a, GD1b, and GM1 reactivity in this model. Our results showed depressed evoked quantal release to a significant yet different extent with different mAbs, whereas the amplitude of postsynaptic currents was not significantly affected. The blockade was reversible or partially reversible after washout with these mAbs

(B. Buchwald, K. Sheikh, unpublished observations). It is possible that anti-ganglioside antibody-mediated blockade of presynaptic evoked quantal release is due to interference with presynaptic calcium channels or proteins of the vesicle release machinery. Gangliosides are expressed on the outer leaflet of the plasma membrane and anti-ganglioside antibodies could indeed form an antibody-antigen complex that alters the function of the presynaptic channel proteins. Further, these results indicate that anti-ganglioside antibodies with different specificities cause distinct pathophysiological effects, supporting the hypothesis that anti-ganglioside antibody specificity contributes to selective nerve fiber dysfunction and heterogeneity of clinical manifestations in immune neuropathies.

V. Relevance

AMAN not only provides a disease model that strongly supports the hypothesis of molecular mimicry as a pathogenetic mechanism underlying postinfectious autoimmune disorders but, more importantly, by provides an example of antibody-mediated injury of myelinated axons by targeting of specific antigens. The following observations in AMAN that might be relevant to the immunopathogenesis of axonal injury in MS are summarized as follows:

1. Autoimmune antibodies directed against axonal antigens can lead to a spectrum of pathophysiological changes, and clinical and experimental data indicate that antibody-mediated immunopharmacological axonal conduction failure and frank axonal degeneration represent two ends of this spectrum.

2. The preliminary in vitro observations, which require reconfirmation, indicate that motor nerve terminal degeneration, which is anti-ganglioside antibody-mediated and complement-dependent, involves a phase of elevated intra-axonal calcium and subsequent activation of calpains. This raises the possibility that a final common pathway of axonal degeneration is activated by multiple triggers, including immune or inflammatory insults.

3. In intact myelinated nerve fibers, nodes of Ranvier and axon terminals (at synapses) are relatively more susceptible to antibody-mediated injury. Moreover, disruption of axon-glial junctions at the nodes of Ranvier or by extension, the process of demyelination, exposes segments of axons that are normally inaccessible to immune effectors such as antibodies or complement, thereby making them prone to injury by specific or nonspecific immune insults.

The pathogenesis of MS is complex and heterogeneous, and it is likely that multiple mechanisms contribute to the axonal injury and neurological burden in this disorder. Anti-ganglioside antibodies have been proposed to be one such

pathogenetic pathway of neural injury because these antibodies are present in a proportion of MS patients (Mata et al., 1999; Sadatipour et al., 1998), raising an important but contentious question: Can anti-ganglioside antibodies contribute to ongoing neuronal and/or axonal injury in this disorder? The answer to this question remains unclear. However, the evidence of pathogenecity of anti-ganglioside antibody-mediated axonal damage in AMAN warrants further work in this area to examine this issue critically.

Acknowledgments

Supported by NIH grant NS42888. We thank Dr. Pamela Talalay for editorial assistance.

References

Ang, C. W., De Klerk, M. A., Endtz, H. P., et al. (2001a). Guillain-Barre syndrome- and Miller Fisher syndrome-associated *Campylobacter jejuni* lipopolysaccharides induce anti-GM1 and anti-GQ1b antibodies in rabbits. *Infect. Immun.* **69**, 2462–2469.

Ang, C. W., Koga, M., Jacobs, B. C., Yuki, N., van der Meche, F. G., and Van Doorn, P. A. (2001b). Differential immune response to gangliosides in Guillain-Barre syndrome patients from Japan and The Netherlands. *J. Neuroimmunol.* **121**, 83–87.

Ang, C. W., Yuki, N., Jacobs, B. C., et al. (1999). Rapidly progressive, predominantly motor Guillain-Barre syndrome with anti-GalNAc-GD1a antibodies. *Neurology* **53**, 2122–2127.

Arasaki, K., Kusunoki, S., Kudo, N., and Kanazawa, I. (1993). Acute conduction block in vitro following exposure to anti-ganglioside sera. *Muscle Nerve* **16**, 587–593.

Arnason, B. G. W., and Soliven, B. (1993). Acute inflammatory demyelinating polyradiculopathy. *In:* "Peripheral Neuropathy" (P. J. Dyck, P. K. Thomas, J. W. Griffin, P. A. Low, and J. F. Poduslo, eds.). pp. 1437–1497. W.B. Saunders, Philadelphia.

Arvidson, B. (1977). Cellular uptake of exogenous horseradish peroxidase in mouse peripheral nerve. *Acta Neuropathol.* **37**, 35–41.

Asbury, A. K., Arnason, B. G., and Adams, R. D. (1969). The inflammatory lesion in idiopathic polyneuritis. *Medicine* 48, 173–215.

Aspinall, G. O., Fujimoto, S., McDonald, A. G., et al. (1994a). Lipopolysaccharides from *Campylobacter jejuni* associated with Guillain-Barre syndrome patients mimic human gangliosides in structure. *Infect. Immunol.* **62**, 2122–2125.

Aspinall, G. O., McDonald, A. G., Pang, H., Kurjanczyk, L. A., and Penner, J. L. (1994b). Lipopolysaccharides of *Campylobacter jejuni* serotype O:19: Structures of core oligosaccharide regions from the serostrain and two bacterial isolates from patients with the Guillain-Barré syndrome. *Biochemistry* **33**, 241–249.

Aspinall, G. O., McDonald, A. G., Raju, T. S., Pang, H., and Moran, A. P. (1993). Chemical structures of the core regions of *Campylobacter jejuni* serotypes O:1, O:4, O:23, and O:36 lipopolysaccharides. *Eur. J. Biochem.* **213**, 1017–1027.

Black, J. A., Kocsis, J. D., and Waxman, S. G. (1990). Ion channel organization of the myelinated fiber. *TINS* **13**, 48–54.

Bowes, T., Wagner, E. R., Boffey, J., et al. (2002). Tolerance to self gangliosides is the major factor restricting the antibody response to lipopolysaccharide core oligosaccharides in *Campylobacter jejuni* strains associated with Guillain-Barre syndrome. *Infect. Immunol.* **70**, 5008–5018.

Buchwald, B., Ahangari, R., and Toyka, K. V. (2002). Differential blocking effects of the monoclonal anti-GQ1b IgM antibody and alpha-latrotoxin in the absence of complement at the mouse neuromuscular junction. *Neurosci. Lett.* **334**, 25–28.

Buchwald, B., Toyka, K. V., Zielasek, J., Weishaupt, A., Schweiger, S., and Dudel, J. (1998). Neuromuscular blockade by IgG antibodies from patients with Guillain-Barre syndrome: A macro-patch-clamp study. *Ann. Neurol.* **44**, 913–922.

Buchwald, B., Weishaupt, A., Toyka, K. V., and Dudel, J. (1995). Immunoglobulin G from a patient with Miller-Fisher syndrome rapidly and reversibly depresses evoked quantal release at the neuromuscular junction of mice. *Neurosci. Lett.* **201**, 163–166.

Carpo, M., Pedotti, R., Lolli, F., et al. (1998). Clinical correlate and fine specificity of anti-GQ1b antibodies in peripheral neuropathy. *J. Neurol. Sci.* **155**, 186–191.

Chiba, A., Kusunoki, S., Obata, H., Machinami, R., and Kanazawa, I. (1993). Serum anti-GQ1b IgG antibody is associated with ophthalmo-plegia in Miller Fisher syndrome and Guillain-Barre syndrome: Clinical and immunohistochemical studies. *Neurology* **43**, 1911–1917.

Chiba, A., Kusunoki, S., Obata, H., Machinami, R., and Kanazawa, I. (1997). Ganglioside composition of the human cranial nerves, with special reference to pathophysiology of Miller Fisher syndrome. *Brain Res.* **745**, 32–36.

De Angelis, M. V., Di Muzio, A., Lupo, S., Gambi, D., Uncini, A., and Lugaresi, A. (2002). Anti-GD1a antibodies from an acute motor axonal neuropathy patient selectively bind to motor nerve fiber nodes of Ranvier. *J. Neuroimmunol.* **121**, 79–82.

Feasby, T. E., Gilbert, J. J., Brown, W. F., et al. (1986). An acute axonal form of Guillain-Barre polyneuropathy. *Brain* **109**, 1115–1126.

Fisher, M. (1956). An unusual variant of acute idiopathic polyneuritis (syndrome of ophthalmoplegia ataxia and areflexia). *N. Engl. J. Med.* **255**, 57–65.

Friedman, C. R., Neimann, J., Wegener, H. C., and Tauxe, R. V. Epidemiology of *Campylobacter jejuni* infections in the United States and other industrialized nations. *In:* "Campylobacter" (I. Nachamkin and M. J. Blaser, eds.). pp. 121–138. American Society for Microbiology, Washington, D.C.

Fu, S. Y., and Gordon, T. (1995a). Contributing factors to poor functional recovery after delayed nerve repair: Prolonged axotomy. *J. Neurosci.* **15**, 3876–3885.

Fu, S. Y., and Gordon, T. (1995b). Contributing factors to poor functional recovery after delayed nerve repair: Prolonged denervation. *J. Neurosci.* **15**, 3886–3895.

Fujimoto, S., Yuki, N., Itoh, T., and Amako, K. (1992). Specific serotype of *Campylobacter jejuni* associated with Guillain-Barre syndrome. *J. Infect. Dis.* **165**, 183 (letter).

Ganser, A. L., Kirschner, D. A., and Willinger, M. (1983). Ganglioside localization on myelinated nerve fibres by cholera toxin binding. *J. Neurocytol.* **12**, 921–938.

Goddard, E. A., Lastovica, A. J., and Argent, A. C. (1997). Campylobacter 0:41 isolation in Guillain-Barre syndrome. *Arch. Dis. Child.* **76**, 526–528.

Gong, Y., Tagawa, Y., Lunn, M. P. et al. (2002). Localization of major gangliosides in the PNS: implications for immune neuropathies. *Brain* **125**, 2491–2506.

Goodyear, C. S., O'Hanlon, G. M., Plomp, J. J., et al. (1998). Monoclonal antibodies raised against Guillain-Barre syndrome variants in Emilia-Romagna, Italy, 1992–3: Incidence, clinical features, and prognosis. Emilia-Romagna Study Group on Clinical and Epidemiological Problems in Neurology. *J. Neurol. Neurosurg. Psychiatry* **65**, 218–224.

Goodyear, C. S., O'Hanlon, G. M., Plomp, J. J., et al. (1999). Monoclonal antibodies raised against Guillain-Barré syndrome–associated *Campylobacter jejuni* lipopolysaccharides react with neuronal gangliosides and paralyze muscle-nerve preparations. *J. Clin. Invest.* **104**, 697–708. Errata appears in *J. Clin. Invest.* **104**, 1771.

Griffin, J. W., Li, C. Y., Ho, T. W. et al., (1996a). Pathology of the motor-sensory axonal Guillain-Barre syndrome. *Am. Neurol. Assn.* **39**, 17–28.

Griffin, J. W., Li, C. Y., Ho, T. W. et al., (1996b). Pathology of the motor-sensory axonal Guillain-Barre syndrome. *Ann. Neurol.* **39**, 17–28.

Griffin, J. W., Li, C. Y., Ho, T. W., et al. (1995). Guillain-Barre syndrome in northern China: The spectrum of neuropathologic changes in clinically defined cases. *Brain* **118**, 577–595.

Griffin, J. W., Li, C Y., Macko, C. et al. (1996c). Early nodal changes in the acute motor axonal neuropathy pattern of the Guillain-Barre syndrome. *J. Neurocytol.* **25**, 33–51.

Hadden, R. D., Cornblath, D. R., Hughes, R. A., et al. (1998). Electrophysiological classification of Guillain-Barre syndrome: clinical associations and outcome. Plasma Exchange/Sandoglobulin Guillain-Barre Syndrome Trial Group. *Ann. Neurol.* **44**, 780–788.

Hafer-Macko, C., Hsieh, S.-T., Li, C. Y. et al. (1996). Acute motor axonal neuropathy: An antibody-mediated attack on axolemma. *Ann. Neurol.* **40**, 635–644.

Harvey, G. K., Toyka, K. V., Zielasek, J., Kiefer, R., Simonis, C., and Hartung, H.-P. (1995). Failure of anti-GM$_1$ IgG or IgM to induce conduction block following intraneural transfer. *Muscle Nerve* **18**, 388–394.

Haymaker, W., and Kernohan, J. W. (1949). The Landry-Guillain-Barre syndrome. A clinicopathologic report of fifty fatal cases and a critique of the literature. *Medicine* 28, 59–141.

Hirota, N., Kaji, R., Bostock, H., et al. (1997). The physiological effect of anti-GM1 antibodies on saltatory conduction and transmembrane currents in single motor axons. *Brain* **120**, 2159–2169.

Ho, T. W., Hsieh, S. T., Nachamkin, I. et al. (1997a). Motor nerve terminal degeneration provides a potential mechanism for rapid recovery in acute motor axonal neuropathy after *Campylobacter* infection [see comments]. *Neurology* **48**, 717–724.

Ho, T. W., Li, C. Y., Cornblath, D. R., et al. (1997b). Patterns of recovery in the Guillain-Barre syndromes [comment]. *Neurology* **48**, 695–700.

Ho, T. W., Mishu, B. , Li, C. Y. et al. (1995). Guillain-Barre syndrome in northern China: Relationship to *Campylobacter jejuni* infection and anti-glycolipid antibodies. *Brain* **118**, 597–605.

Ho, T. W., Willison, H. J., Nachamkin, I., et al. (1999). Anti-GD1a antibody is associated with axonal but not demyelinating forms of Guillain-Barre syndrome. *Ann. Neurol.* **45**, 168–173.

Hughes, R. A., Hadden, R D., Gregson, N. A., and Smith, K. J. (1999). Pathogenesis of Guillain-Barre syndrome. *J. Neuroimmunol.* **100**, 74–97.

Hughes, R. A., and Rees, J. H. (1997). Clinical and epidemiologic features of Guillain-Barre syndrome. *J. Infect. Dis.* **176 (Suppl 2)**, S92–S98.

Ilyas, A. A., Mithen, F. A., Dalakas, M. C., Chen, Z.-W., and Cook, S. D. (1992). Antibodies to acidic glycolipids in Guillain-Barré syndrome and chronic inflammatory demyelinating polyneuropathy. *J. Neurol. Sci.* **107**, 111–121.

Ilyas, A. A., Quarles, R. H., Dalakas, M. C., Fishman, P. H., and Brady, R. O. (1985). Monoclonal IgM in a patient with paraproteinemic polyneuropathy binds to gangliosides containing disialosyl groups. *Ann. Neurol.* **18**, 655–659.

Ilyas, A. A., Willison, H. J., Quarles, R. H., et al. (1988). Serum antibodies to gangliosides in Guillain-Barre syndrome. *Ann. Neurol.* **23**, 440–447.

Jacobs, B. C., Endtz, H., van der Meché, F. G. A., Hazenberg, M. P., Achtereekte, H. A., and Van Doorn, P. A. (1995). Serum anti-GQ1b IgG antibodies recognize surface epitopes on *Campylobacter jejuni* from patients with Miller Fisher syndrome. *Ann. Neurol.* **37**, 260–264.

Jacobs, B. C., Hazenberg, M. P., Van Doorn, P. A., Endtz, H. P. H., and van der Meché, F. G. A. (1997). Cross-reactive antibodies against gangliosides and *Campylobacter jejuni* lipopolysaccharides in patients with Guillain-Barré or Miller Fisher syndrome. *J. Infect. Dis.* **175**, 729–733.

Jacobs, B. C., Rothbarth, P. H., van der Meche, F. G., et al. (1998). The spectrum of antecedent infections in Guillain-Barre syndrome: A case-control study. *Neurology* **51**, 1110–1115.

Jacobs, B. C., Van Doorn, P. A., Schmitz, P. I., et al. (1996). *Campylobacter jejuni* injections and anti-GM1 antibodies in Guillain-Barré syndrome. *Ann. Neurol.* **40**, 181–187.

Kanda, T., Iwasaki, T., Yamawaki, M., Tai, T., and Mizusawa H. (2000). Anti-GM1 antibody facilitates leakage in an in vitro blood-nerve barrier model. *Neurology* **55**, 585–587.

Kanda, T., Yamawaki, M., and Mizusawa H. (2003). Sera from Guillain-Barre patients enhance leakage in blood-nerve barrier model. *Neurology* **60**, 301–306.

Koga, M., Tatsumoto, M., Yuki, N., and Hirata, K. (2001). Range of cross reactivity of anti-GM1 IgG antibody in Guillain-Barre syndrome. *J. Neurol. Neurosurg. Psychiatry* **71**, 123–124.

Kuroki, S., Saida, T., Nukina, M. et al. (1993). *Campylobacter jejuni* strains from patients with Guillain-Barre syndrome belong mostly to Penner serogroup 19 and contain beta-*N*-acetylglucosamine residues. *Ann. Neurol.* **33**, 243–247.

Kusunoki S, Chiba A, Kon K et al. *N*-acetylgalactosaminyl GD1a is a target molecule for serum antibody in Guillain-Barre syndrome. Ann. Neurol. 1994; **35**, 570–576.

Kusunoki, S., Iwamori, M., Chiba, A., et al. (1996a). GM1b is a new member of antigen for serum antibody in Guillain-Barré syndrome. *Neurology* **47**, 237–242.

Kusunoki, S., Shimizu, J., Chiba, A., Ugawa, Y., Hitoshi, S., and Kanazawa, I. (1996b). Experimental sensory neuropathy induced by sensitization with ganglioside GD1b. *Ann. Neurol.* **39**, 424–431.

Kuwabara, S., Ogawara, K., Mizobuchi, K., et al. (2000). Isolated absence of F waves and proximal axonal dysfunction in Guillain-Barre syndrome with anti-ganglioside antibodies. *J. Neurol. Neurosurg. Psychiatry* **68**, 191–195.

Kuwabara, S., Yuki, N., Koga, M., et al. (1998). IgG anti-GM1 antibody is associated with reversible conduction failure and axonal degeneration in Guillain-Barre syndrome. *Ann. Neurol.* **44**, 202–208.

Le, T. B., Aszmann, O., Chen, Y. G., Royall, R. M., and Brushart, T. M. (2001). Effects of pathway and neuronal aging on the specificity of motor axon regeneration. *Exp.Neurol.* **167**, 126–132.

Lunn, M. P., Johnson, L. A., Fromholt, S. E., et al. (2000). High-affinity anti-ganglioside IgG antibodies raised in complex ganglioside knockout mice: Reexamination of GD1a immunolocalization. *J. Neurochem.* **75**, 404–412.

Mata, S., Lolli, F., Soderstrom, M., Pinto, F., and Link, H. (1999). Multiple sclerosis is associated with enhanced B cell responses to the ganglioside GD1a. *Multiple Sclerosis* **5**, 379–388.

McKhann, G. M., Cornblath, D. R., Griffin, J. W., et al. (1993). Acute motor axonal neuropathy: A frequent cause of acute flaccid paralysis in China. *Ann. Neurol.* **33**, 333–342.

McKhann, G. M., Cornblath, D. R., Ho, T. W., et al. (1991). Clinical and electrophysiological aspects of acute paralytic disease of children and young adults in northern China. *Lancet* **338**, 593–597.

Moran, A. P., Prendergast, M. M., and Hogan, E. L. (2002). Sialosyl-galactose: A common denominator of Guillain-Barre and related disorders? *J. Neurol. Sci.* **196**, 1–7.

Mori, M., Kuwabara, S., Miyake, M., et al. (2001). *Haemophilus influenzae* infection and Guillain-Barre syndrome. *Brain* **123**, 2171–2178.

Nachamkin, I. (1997). Microbiologic approaches for studying *Campylobacter* species in patients with Guillain-Barre syndrome. *J. Infect. Dis.* **176**, S106–S114.

Nachamkin, I., Liu, J., Li, M. et al. (2002). *Campylobacter jejuni* from patients with Guillain-Barre syndrome preferentially expresses a GD(1a)-like epitope. *Infect. Immunol.* **70**, 5299–5303.

Nachamkin, I., Ung, H., Moran, A. P., et al. (1999). Ganglioside GM1 mimicry in *Campylobacter* strains from sporadic infections in the United States [published erratum appears in *J. Infect. Dis.* 1999 Jun;179(6):1593]. *J. Infect. Dis.* **179**, 1183–1189.

O'Hanlon, G. M., Humphreys, P. D., Goldman, R. S., et al. (2003). Calpain inhibitors protect against axonal degeneration in a model of anti-ganglioside antibody-mediated motor nerve terminal injury. *Brain* **126**, 2497–2509.

O'Hanlon, G. M., Plomp, J. J., Chakrabarti, M., et al. (2001). Anti-GQ1b ganglioside antibodies mediate complement-dependent destruction of the motor nerve terminal. *Brain* **124**, 893–906.

Oberhelman, R. A., and Taylor, D. N. (2000). *Campylobacter* infections in developing countries. *In:* "Camplyobacter" (I. Nachamkin and M. J. Blaser, eds.). pp. 139–153. American Society for Microbiology, Washington, D.C.

Ogawa-Goto, K., Funamoto, N., Abe, T., and Nagashima, K. (1990). Different ceramide compositions of gangliosides between human motor and sensory nerves. *J. Neurochem.* **55**, 1486–1493.

Ogawara, K., Kuwabara, S., Mori, M., Hattori, T., Koga, M., and Yuki, N. (2000). Axonal Guillain-Barre syndrome: Relation to anti-ganglioside antibodies and *Campylobacter jejuni* infection in Japan. *Ann. Neurol.* **48**, 624–631.

Ogino, M., Orazio, N., and Latov, N. (1995). IgG anti-GM1 antibodies from patients with acute motor neuropathy are predominantly of the IgG1 and IgG3 subclasses. *J. Neuroimmunol.* **58**, 77–80.

Oomes, P. G., Jacobs, B. C., Hazenberg, M. P. H., and Banffer, J. R. J., and van der Meché, F. G. A.. Anti-GM1 IgG antibodies and *Campylobacter jejuni* bacteria in Guillain-Barre syndrome: Evidence of molecular mimicry. *Ann. Neurol.* **38**, 170–175.

Paparounas, K., O'Hanlon, G. M., O'Leary, C. P., Rowan, E. G., and Willison, H. J. (1999). Anti-ganglioside antibodies can bind peripheral nerve nodes of Ranvier and activate the complement cascade without inducing acute conduction block in vitro [see comments]. *Brain* **122**, 807–816.

Plomp, J. J., Molenaar, P. C., O'Hanlon, G M., et al. (1999). Miller Fisher anti-GQ1b antibodies: Alpha-latrotoxin-like effects on motor end plates [published erratum appears in *Ann. Neurol.* 1999 Jun;45(6):823]. *Ann. Neurol.* **45**, 189–199.

Prendergast, M. M., and Moran, A. P. (2000). Lipopolysaccharides in the development of the Guillain-Barre syndrome and Miller Fisher syndrome forms of acute inflammatory peripheral neuropathies. *J. Endotoxin. Res.* **6**, 341–359.

Ramos-Alvarez, M., Bessudo, L., and Sabin, A. (1969). Paralytic syndromes associated with noninflammatory cytoplasmic or nuclear neuronopathy: acute paralytic disease in Mexican children, neuropathologically distinguishable from Landry-Guillain-Barre syndrome. *JAMA* **207**, 1481–1492.

Rees, J. H., Gregson, N. A., and Hughes, R. A. C. (1995a). Anti-ganglioside GM1 antibodies in Guillain-Barre syndrome and their relationship to *Campylobacter jejuni* infection. *Ann. Neurol.* **38**, 809–816.

Rees, J. H., Soudain, S. E., Gregson, N. A., and Hughes, R. A. (1995b). *Campylobacter jejuni* infection and Guillain-Barré syndrome. *N. Engl. J. Med.* **333**, 1374–1379.

Rees, J. H., Thompson, R. D., Smeeton, N. C., and Hughes, R. A. (1998). Epidemiological study of Guillain-Barre syndrome in south east England. *J. Neurol. Neurosurg.Psychiatry* **64**, 74–77.

Rees, J. H., Vaughan, R. W., Kondeatis, E., and Hughes, R. A. C. (1995c). HLA-class II alleles in Guillain-Barre syndrome and Miller Fisher syndrome and their association with preceding *Campylobacter jejuni* infection. *J. Neuroimmunol.* **62**, 53–57.

Rhodes, K. M., and Tattersfield, A. E. (1982). Guillain-Barre syndrome associated with *Campylobacter* infection. *Br. Med. J.(Clin. Res. Ed)* **285**, 173–174.

Sadatipour, B. T., Greer, J. M., and Pender, M. P. (1998). Increased circulating anti-ganglioside antibodies in primary and secondary progressive multiple sclerosis. *Ann. Neurol.* **44**, 980–983.

Santoro, M., Uncini, A., Corbo, M., et al. (1992). Experimental conduction block induced by serum from a patient with anti-GM1 antibodies. *Ann. Neurol.* **31**, 385–390.

Sharief, M. K., Ingram, D. A., and Swash, M. (1997). Circulating tumor necrosis factor-alpha correlates with electrodiagnostic abnormalities in Guillain-Barre syndrome. *Ann. Neurol.* **42**, 68–73.

Sharief, M. K., McLean, B., and Thompson, E. J. (1993). Elevated serum levels of tumor necrosis factor-alpha in Guillain-Barre syndrome. *Ann. Neurol.* **33**, 591–596.

Sheikh, K. A., Deerinck, T. J., Ellisman, M. H., and Griffin, J. W. (1999). The distribution of ganglioside-like moieties in peripheral nerves. *Brain* **122**, 449–460.

Sheikh, K. A., Nachamkin, I., Ho, T. W., et al. (1998). *Campylobacter jejuni* lipopolysaccharides in Guillain-Barre syndrome: Molecular mimicry and host susceptibility. *Neurology* **51**, 371–378.

Sheikh, K. A., Zhang, G., Gong, Y., Schnaar, R. L., and Griffin, J. W. (2004). An anti-ganglioside antibody-secreting hybridoma induces neuropathy in mice. *Ann. Neurol.* **56**, 228–239.

Susuki, K., Nishimoto, Y., Yamada, M., et al. (2003). Acute motor axonal neuropathy rabbit model: Immune attack on nerve root axons. *Ann. Neurol.* **54**, 383–388.

Takigawa, T., Yasuda, H., Kikkawa, R., Shigeta, Y., Saida, T., and Kitasato, H. (1995). Antibodies against GM1 ganglioside affect K$^+$ and Na$^+$ currents in isolated rat myelinated nerve fibers. *Ann. Neurol.* **37**, 436–442.

Takigawa, T., Yasuda, H., Terada, M., et al. (2000). The sera from GM1 ganglioside antibody positive patients with Guillain-Barre syndrome or chronic inflammatory demyelinating polyneuropathy blocks Na+ currents in rat single myelinated nerve fibers. *Intern. Med.* **39**, 123–127.

Uncini, A., and Lugaresi, A. (1999). Fisher syndrome with tetraparesis and antibody to GQ1b: Evidence for motor nerve terminal block. *Muscle Nerve* **22**, 640–644.

Uncini, A., Santoro, M., Corbo, M., Lugaresi, A., and Latov, N. (1993). Conduction abnormalities induced by sera of patients with multifocal motor neuropathy and anti-GM1 antibodies. *Muscle Nerve* **16**, 610–615.

Walsh, F. S., Cronin, M., Koblar, S., et al. (1991). Association between glycoconjugate antibodies and *Campylobacter* infection in patients with Guillain-Barre syndrome. *J. Neuroimmunol.* **34**, 43–51.

Weber, F., Rudel, R., Aulkemeyer, P., and Brinkmeier, H. (2000). Anti-GM1 antibodies can block neuronal voltage-gated sodium channels. *Muscle Nerve* **23**, 1414–1420.

Willison, H. J., O'Hanlon, G. M., Paterson, G., et al. (1996). A somatically mutated human anti-ganglioside IgM antibody that induces experimental neuropathy in mice is encoded by the variable region heavy chain gene, V1-18. *J. Clin. Invest.* **97**, 1155–1164.

Willison, H. J., and Veitch, J. (1994). Immunoglobulin subclass distribution and binding characteristics of anti-GQ1b antibodies in Miller Fisher syndrome. *J. Neuroimmunol.* **50**, 159–165.

Willison, H. J., Veitch, J., Patterson, G., Kennedy, P. G. E. (1993). Miller Fisher syndrome is associated with serum antibodies to GQ1b ganglioside. *J. Neurol. Neurosurg. Psychiatry* **56**, 204–206, 1993.

Willison, H. J., and Yuki, N. (2002). Peripheral neuropathies and anti-glycolipid antibodies. *Brain* **125**, 2591–2625.

Wirguin, I., Briani, C., Suturkova-Milosevic, L., et al. (1997). Induction of anti-GM1 ganglioside antibodies by *Campylobacter jejuni* lipopolysaccharides. *J. Neuroimmunol.* **78**, 138–142.

Wirguin, I., Suturkova-Milosevic, L. J., Della-Latta, P., Fisher, T., Brown, R. H., Jr., and Latov, N. (1994). Monoclonal IgM antibodies to GM1 and asialo-GM1 in chronic neuropathies cross-react with *Campylobacter jejuni* lipopolysaccharides. *Ann. Neurol.* **35**, 698–703.

Yuki, N. (2002). Current cases in which epitope mimicry is considered a component cause of autoimmune disease: Guillain-Barre syndrome. *Cell Mol. Life Sci.* **57(4)**, 527–533.

Yuki, N., Ang, C. W., Koga, M., et al. (2000). Clinical features and response to treatment in Guillain-Barre syndrome associated with antibodies to GM1b ganglioside [In Process Citation]. *Ann. Neurol.* **47**, 314–321.

Yuki, N., Handa, S., Taki, T., Kasama, T., Takahashi, M., and Saito, K. (1992a). Cross-reactive antigen between nervous tissue and a bacterium elicits Guillain-Barre syndrome: Molecular mimicry between ganglioside GM1 and lipopolysaccharide from Penner's serotype 19 of *Campylobacter jejuni*. *Biomed. Res.* **13**, 451–453.

Yuki, N., Ho, T. W., Tagawa, Y., et al. (1999). Autoantibodies to GM1b and GalNAc-GD1a: Relationship to *Campylobacter jejuni* infection and acute motor axonal neuropathy in China. *J. Neurol. Sci.* **164**, 134–138.

Yuki, N., Sato, S., Fujimoto, S., Yamada, Y., Kinoshita, A., and Itoh, T. (1992b). Serotype of *Campylobacter jejuni*, HLA, and the Guillain-Barre syndrome. *Muscle Nerve* **16**, 968–969.

Yuki, N., Sato, S., Itoh, T., and Miyatake, T. (1991). HLA-B35 and acute axonal polyneuropathy following *Campylobacter jejuni* infection. *Neurology* **41**, 1561–1563.

Yuki, N., Sato, S., Tsuji, S., Ohsawa, T., and Miyatake, T. (1993a). Frequent presence of anti-GQ1b antibody in Fisher's syndrome. *Neurology* **43**, 414–417.

Yuki, N., Taki, T., and Handa, S. (1996). Antibody to GalNAc-GD1a and GalNAc-GM1b in Guillain-Barre syndrome subsequent to *Campylobacter jejuni* enteritis. *J. Neuroimmunol.* **71**, 155–161.

Yuki, N., Taki, T., Takahashi, M., et al. (1994). Molecular mimicry between GQ$_{1b}$ ganglioside and lipopolysaccharides of *Campylobacter jejuni* isolated from patients with Fisher's syndrome. *Ann. Neurol.* **36**, 791–793.

Yuki, N., Yamada, M., Koga, M., et al. (2001). Animal model of axonal Guillain-Barre syndrome induced by sensitization with GM1 ganglioside. *Ann. Neurol.* **49**, 712–20.

Yuki, N., Yamada, M., Sato, S., et al. (1993b). Association of IgG anti-GD1a antibody with severe Guillain-Barre syndrome. *Muscle Nerve* **16**, 642–647.

Yuki, N., Yoshino, H., Sato, S., and Miyatake, T. (1990). Acute axonal polyneuropathy associated with anti-GM1 antibodies following *Campylobacter* enteritis. *Neurology* **40**, 1900–1902.

26

Axonal Degeneration as a Predictor of Outcome in Neurological Disorders

Isabelle M. Medana, Ph. D.

Gabriele C. DeLuca, D.Phil.

Margaret M. Esiri, D.M.

I. Introduction

The significance of axons in pathological processes that affect the central nervous system (CNS) has been relatively underappreciated until recently. In neurodegenerative conditions, neuron cell bodies, dendrites, and synapses have generally gained the lion's share of attention, whereas in white matter diseases, the myelin sheath has traditionally been the main focus of interest. It has, of course, long been recognized that axons degenerate when the cell bodies of neurons die, but this was considered a secondary event of only subsidiary interest when the aim was to understand the cause of the primary neuronal death. Similarly, in white matter diseases, the death of axons was recognized to occur, but its significance for functional disability was hardly appreciated until recently. Three developments have come together to change this situation. First, surrogates of axonal loss, such as *N*-acetyl aspartate in magnetic resonance spectroscopy (Davie et al., 1995; de Stefano et al., 1998), and cerebral atrophy in magnetic resonance imaging studies (Chard et al., 2003; Filippi et al., 1995; Losseff et al., 1996) became recognized and allowed axon loss to be appreciated and measured for the first time in living subjects, paving the way for better correlative clinical studies. Second, more systematic quantitative studies of axons started to be performed in neuropathological material (Ganter et al., 1999; Lovas et al., 2000). Third, techniques were developed that allowed axonal damage to be readily detected in the same material. (Sherriff et al., 1994a, b) These developments have allowed axon degeneration to be viewed in a new light, as a final common pathway in many different diseases and one that can be evaluated as a guide to the severity of a disease process and a predictor of its outcome. There is still much work to be done, but a start has been made to explore the potential of this guide, as reviewed in this chapter, which provides a broad perspective by reviewing the role of axon degeneration as a predictor of clinical outcome in a spectrum of neurological disorders.

Some of the work on the significance of axonal degeneration for the outcome of neurological disorders has been performed in the context of long-standing diseases such as multiple sclerosis (MS). The value of surrogate markers in predicting outcome in MS is covered in other chapters in this book. However, there are more acute disorders where measures of axonal degeneration are also being shown to have a bearing on outcome. These conditions are as varied as head trauma and cerebral malaria. Studies in experimental models of human disorders are also finding that axonal degeneration relates closely to outcome, as reviewed here.

II. Assessing Damaged Axons

A. Amyloid Precursor Protein Immunocytochemistry

The traditional stains for visualizing axons—the single, slender processes that emerge from neurons at the axon hillocks and extend with a relatively uniform caliber to the terminals up to a meter or more away—are silver stains that bind to the neurofilaments. With such stains damaged axons appear swollen because of the interruption in their fast transport system and the proximal accumulation of organelles and fluid.

Immunocytochemical staining for β-amyloid precursor protein (APP) more sensitively detects axons that have impaired fast axonal transport (Fig. 1). In normally functioning axons, the protein is transported in this way and never builds up to a concentration that allows its detection in tissue sections. However, axons that have this transport system disrupted rapidly accumulate APP proximal to the disrupted segment. This occurs before the development of conventional morphological evidence of axonal damage (e.g., in the form of axonal end-bulbs), so the immunocytochemical method for detecting APP is more sensitive than routine histological methods for detecting axon damage. Other proteins transported by fast axonal transport also accumulate, but antibodies to APP have been shown to be the most sensitive for detecting this type of damage (Grady et al., 1993; Gultekin and Smith, 1994; Li et al., 1995; Ng et al., 1994; Pesini et al., 1999; Sherriff et al., 1994a). Experimental animal studies of brain trauma have shown that some axonal damage is reversible, but it is not known if axonal damage severe enough to be detected with APP immunoreactivity in humans is ever reversible; in general this has been thought unlikely. With regard to timing of dam-

age detectable in this way, the immunoreaction in damaged axons for APP becomes positive in head trauma 1 to 3 hours after the insult (McKenzie et al., 1996; Oehmichen et al., 1998; Sherriff et al., 1994b) and remains positive for up to 1 month (Geddes et al., 2000). The distal parts of irreversibly damaged axons will undergo wallerian degeneration, which can be detected by such traditional methods as the Marchi technique on tissue sections and in living subjects by neuroimaging with (Banati et al., 2000) or without (Simon et al., 2000) novel ligands. An estimate of the scale of long-previous irreversible axonal damage can be obtained by performing estimates of axon numbers, a relatively straightforward task using modern computerized image analysis facilities.

B. Cerebrospinal Fluid "Surrogates"

The immunocytochemical method for detecting APP is one of the most sensitive methods for detecting axonal damage; however, this method is confined only to fatal cases. Therefore, the question arises: How can we examine axonal injury during life and in patients who eventually recover from their disease? Electrophysiological and neuropsychological tests and brain imaging can help identify parenchymal abnormalities, although imaging often underestimates the abnormalities later seen at pathologic examination (Patankar et al., 2002) and is not cell-type specific.

One method that is gaining popularity is the measurement by enzyme-linked immunosorbent assays (ELISA) of markers of axonal damage released into the cerebrospinal fluid (CSF) or blood of patients with various neurological disorders. A marker that is often used is τ, a phosphorylated microtubule-associated protein, considered to be important for maintaining the stability of axonal microtubules involved in the mediation of fast axonal transport of synaptic constituents (Green et al., 2000; Jimenez-Jimenez et al., 2002). Another surrogate marker for degenerated axons that can be measured in CSF is the light subunit of the neurofilament protein (NFL) (Hagberg et al., 2000).

Although immunocytochemistry for APP and ELISA for τ or NFL give a measure of axonal damage the results do not provide completely analogous information (Table 1). For example, the CSF markers only give an indication of acute, irreversible, axonal degeneration, as the cytoskeletal components must be released into the extracellular fluid and gain access to the CSF, which has a turnover time of approximately 6 hours. Serial CSF measurements can be made during the course of patients' disease but performing multiple lumbar punctures on ill patients may not be clinically or ethically appropriate. In comparison, APP immunohistochemistry allows the detection of a spectrum of axonal injury ranging from mild, reversible damage to irreversible degeneration. Immunoreaction in damaged axons for APP

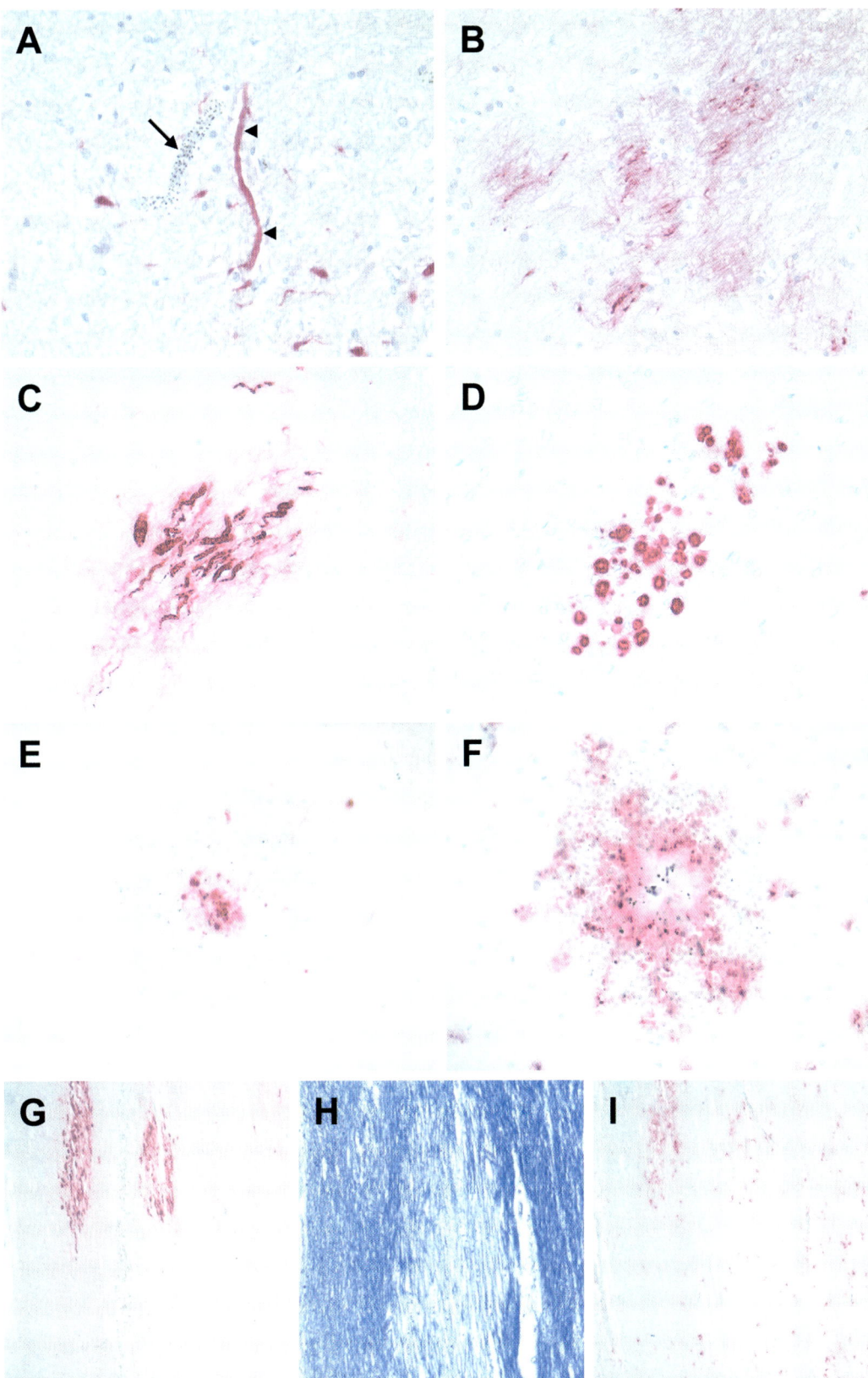

Figure 1 Brain sections from severe malaria patients stained for the β-amyloid precursor protein (β-APP). (A–D) Different staining patterns of β-APP: single axons (*arrow heads*) in close association with a vessel containing parasitized erythrocytes (*arrow*) (**A**) Linear arrays with lesion boundary not well defined. (**B**) Focal area containing swollen and club-shaped axons. (**C**) Axonal bulbs. (**D**). (**E–I**) Serial sections stained for either β-APP to visualize areas of axonal damage (**E, G**) or CD68 to identify microglia (**F, I**) or Luxol Fast Blue Cresyl Violet to identify demyelination (**H**). (**E–F**) Axonal damage (**E**) and microglial response (**F**) to a ring hemorrhage. (**G–I**) Two focal areas of axonal damage (**G**). The right foci of axonal damage is associated with a larger area of demyelination (**H**) and the left focus of axonal damage is associated with a stronger microglial response (**I**).

Table 1

	Immunocytochemistry on brain tissue	Biochemical analysis of CSF
Markers	β-APP	τ, neurofilament
Patient	Fatal cases only	Fatal cases and survivors
Time course measurements	No	Yes
Spatial information	Yes	No
Type of axonal injury	Spectrum—mild reversible to irreversible degeneration	Acute, axonal degeneration only
Window of marker detection	Months	Hours

β-amyloid precursor protein (APP), β-APP.

becomes positive within hours after the insult and may remain positive for at least a month (see previous discussion). β-APP immunohistochemistry gives spatial information, whereas the CSF measurements provide a crude measure of the total extent and degree of axonal damage during life and may reflect preferentially those axons closest to the subarachnoid space. This last point must be emphasized as lesion location is probably more relevant to functional impairment than the total amount of damaged axons.

Imaging surrogates of axonal damage and loss are discussed in other chapters of this book (see Chapters 13, 14, and 15).

III. Head Trauma

Even before the development of any new techniques, the significance of axonal damage in head injury for outcome, in terms of both mortality and morbidity, was well recognized. Injury to axons, particularly diffuse axonal injury, is one of the most important of several components of a complex and variable pathological picture (reviewed by Graham et al., 2002). According to a grading system defined originally using a model of head trauma in primates (Gennarelli et al., 1982), diffuse axonal injury is now classified into three grades of severity. In the first and mildest grade, there is no macroscopic change, but widespread microscopic injury to axons is visible in the corpus callosum, intracerebral white matter, particularly in the parasagittal regions, and the brainstem. Such microscopic axonal injury is now best demonstrated using an antibody to the APP, but in earlier studies it was demonstrated, albeit with less sensitivity, with silver impregnation or with hematoxylin and eosin to demonstrate axonal spheroids. The focal microglial reaction at the site of axonal injury was also a sensitive means of detection in early studies (Oppenheimer, 1968) and had the merit of persisting for months or years (Adams et al., 2001). In the second, intermediate grade of axonal injury, there are small macroscopically visible abnormalities in the corpus callosum associated with small hemorrhages. In the third, most severe grade, there are superadded focal tears in the upper brain stem. Very mild degrees of diffuse axonal injury are seen in survivors of trauma who die subsequently not of their head injury but of other injury or disease up to 99 days later (Blumbergs et al., 1994; Gennarelli, 1993; Oppenheimer, 1968). In such cases there may be loss of consciousness as short as 60 seconds. In contrast, grades 2 and 3 diffuse axonal injury is seen in those with short or more prolonged unconscious survival or in those who regain consciousness but are quite severely disabled until death.

Only 1% to 2% of patients admitted to the hospital after traumatic brain injury will die of their injuries. Of the remainder, a sizeable minority will be left with significant sequelae chiefly in the form of cognitive and behavioral problems. In one study of young people, this applied to a similar proportion of those with a head injury originally assessed as mild and to those whose original head injury was assessed as moderate or severe (Thornhill et al., 2000). Diffuse axonal injury is thought to play a major role in the damage responsible for this very substantial morbidity. However, this is not the only type of pathology found in moderately or severely disabled survivors of head injury. For example, in two studies of such cases that survived for at least a month, grade 2 or 3 diffuse axonal injury was seen in half, and in the other half severe focal brain damage or ischemic injury was the main form of pathology (Adams et al., 2000, 2001; Jennett et al., 2001). Other factors that are known to be significant in predicting a poor outcome after head injury are age greater than 50 years, long duration of posttraumatic amnesia (Capruso and Levin, 2000), and possession of the *APOE ε4* gene allele (Teasdale et al., 1997).

Boxers subject themselves to repeated episodes of relatively mild head trauma. A "punch drunk" state or *dementia pugilistica* develops in some of them, although it is much less commonly seen now than previously. In a study of 224 randomly selected boxers examined by Roberts (1969), 17% had clinically demonstrable prominent CNS lesions including ataxia, dysarthria, pyramidal tract signs or symptoms, rigidity, and tremor. A few had intellectual deficits, particularly memory impairment. These features were significantly more common in those who had fought many professional bouts and had had a long boxer's career. Neuropathological studies identified damage to the cerebellar cortex, septum, midbrain, and cerebral hemispheres in professional boxers (Adams and Bruton, 1989; Corsellis et al., 1973). The damage reported in the cerebral hemispheres took the form of neurofibrillary tangles to a greater extent than axonal injury in white matter so that, in contrast to other forms of head injury, diffuse axonal injury appears to contribute less to clinical impairment in boxers. Instead boxers seem to manifest a form of pathology to which other head injury victims are also susceptible—a heightened risk of Alzheimer-type changes (Smith et al., 2004).

IV. Vascular Disease

In acute strokes, substantial amounts of cerebral white matter can be rendered ischemic in addition to gray matter. However, there has been little investigation of how the extent of white matter damage and loss correlates with clinical severity of a stroke. The nature and severity of the clinical deficit will, of course, depend on the localization of the infarct, as well as on its volume. It might be of interest to investigate the significance of white matter damage not only for the resulting clinical deficit but also for its recovery. In animal models of acute ischemia, APP immunocytochemistry has been used as a marker of damage in white matter in studies that explored the ability of protective interventions to reduce such damage (Imai et al., 2001; Schabitz et al., 2000).

Some studies have reported on more chronic forms of vascular disease, particularly subcortical small vessel disease. This type of disease commonly underlies vascular cognitive impairment (Esiri et al., 1997). Because vascular dementia can be difficult to distinguish clinically from Alzheimer's disease (AD), and because the treatment of the two conditions may differ, there has been interest in searching for ways in which to distinguish them. Neuroimaging frequently demonstrates degrees of leukoaraiosis in both, but leukoaraiosis correlates poorly with cognitive deficits; however, callosal atrophy was correlated with cognitive deficits in subcortical vascular disease (Yamauchi et al., 1994). Attention has been directed to an alternative marker of significant white matter vascular pathology in the form of measures of proteins in CSF. The pathology of vascular dementia on the basis of subcortical small vessel disease consists principally of damage to myelin and axons, although there is frequently coexisting hippocampal sclerosis, which may contribute to the clinical deficits (Kril et al., 2002). CSF levels of myelin basic protein (Ohta et al., 2002) sulphatide (Tullberg et al., 2000) and neurofilament proteins (Sjogren et al., 2001) have been shown to reflect this type of damage quite reliably. In contrast, Alzheimer's disease as a form of τ-opathy results in elevated levels of CSF tau and soluble APP with elevations also in neurofilament protein (Sjogren et al., 2001; Skoog et al., 1995; Wallin et al., 1999). The latter presumably results from wallerian degeneration of axons secondary to neuron loss in AD. As yet there is still considerable overlap between the different clinical categories and neuropathological confirmation of the diagnosis is still lacking but the approach of using CSF markers of axon degeneration and pathological markers looks promising.

An interesting example of a specific form of vascular dementia is provided by the inherited condition of CADASIL (cerebral autosomal dominant arteriopathy with subcortical infarcts and leukoencephalopathy). In this condition it has been possible to monitor development of dementia in those carrying mutations in the relevant gene on chromosome 19 and compare this with imaged white matter lesions. The lesions begin as small periventricular hyperintensities, which then progress through a multifocal nodular stage to full confluence of lesions throughout the cerebral hemispheres (Chabriat et al., 1998). Total lesion volume correlated significantly with disability in terms of reduced executive function (Dichgans et al., 1999). Diminished frontal lobe function is the chief cognitive manifestation of the disease. The pathology consists of multiple small lacunar-infarcts in white matter and deep gray matter. The relative abundance of axonal vs. myelin damage does not seem to have been specifically investigated. Likewise, in hereditary cerebral hemorrhage with amyloidosis-Dutch type, another inherited condition with dementia in some cases, the presence of dementia correlated with the number of focal lesions on computed tomography scan, though not with white matter hypodensity (Haan et al., 1990).

V. Infections

A. Malaria

Impairment of consciousness and other signs of cerebral dysfunction are important clinical features of severe falciparum malaria. The majority of neurological complications are transient, but a significant minority of patients develop sequelae. The mechanism by which malaria infection induces severe but potentially reversible neurological dysfunction remains elusive. The malaria parasite invades and develops within erythrocytes, which sequester in the cerebral microvasculature by adhesion to specific endothelial receptors. However, it is not known how malaria parasites, which remain within the vascular space and do not infect brain cells, influence parenchymal brain function to induce coma and possibly death.

Cerebral white matter lesions have been strongly associated with neurological complications in malaria infection (Davis et al., 1992; Dugbartey et al., 1998; Kochar and Makkar, 1994; Lewallen et al., 1999; Medana et al., 2002). In our studies of cerebral malaria (CM) in Vietnamese adults (Medana et al., 2002), we have identified impairment of transport within axons as a pathological correlate and possible cause of reversible neurological complications. APP immunocytochemistry was performed on brain sections from 54 adult Vietnamese cases with falciparum malaria to determine whether defects in axonal transport would reflect cerebral impairment in this group. The extent and distribution of axonal damage were found to distinguish the groups of patients infected with *P. falciparum* with and without cerebral complications during life. This is the only finding of positive quantitative associations with clinical manifestations of CM with the exception of parasite sequestration. There were significant associations between axonal damage and important clinical and biochemical parameters, including lactate, CSF protein, and Glasgow coma score. APP staining also was found in patients with pure cerebral malaria without other organ complications.

More recently, we found biochemical evidence of axonal damage in the CSF of adult Vietnamese patients with severe malaria during their illness (Medana et al., unpublished data). These experiments complement the neuropathological study described above (Medana et al., 2002) by giving an indication of axonal damage in patients who eventually recover from the disease. The mean concentration of τ proteins in the CSF was significantly raised in patients with severe malaria compared with controls. This confirms that axonal damage is evident in patients on admission to the hospital, most of whom survive, and is not an agonal event. This study also highlights that not all of the axonal injury observed in postmortem brain sections would have been reversible had the patient survived, as CSF τ levels reflect acute irreversible axonal degeneration. Systemic complications of severe malaria including renal and hepatic dysfunction were correlated with CSF τ levels, indicating a role in irreversible axonal injury. These findings suggest that axons are vulnerable to a broad range of cerebral insults that occur during falciparum malaria infection. Disruption in axonal transport may represent a final common pathway leading to neurological dysfunction in CM.

The APP immunocytochemical findings are also consistent with other studies of patients with CM. Impairment of somatosensory discrimination and conduction has been found in patients with a history of CM (Dugbartey et al., 1998; Kochar and Makkar, 1994). Also, cotton wool spots have been found in retinae of patients with CM (Davis et al., 1992; Lewallen et al., 1999). In both cases the findings are likely to be manifestations of axonal disruption or obstruction of axonal flow (McLeod et al., 1977).

Kochar and Makkar (1994) recorded somatosensory evoked potentials by median nerve stimulation in 10 adult patients from India with CM. They observed abnormalities in 80% of patients, of which the most common problem was prolongation of central conduction time. It was not possible for the authors to elucidate the exact pathogenetic mechanisms responsible for the electrophysiological changes. However, they suggested that a phase exists in CM that causes delay in the conduction of traveling impulses in the brain as a result of damage in the white matter and changes in volume conduction at the partition of geometric boundaries.

Dugbartey and colleagues (1998) also have investigated, using neuropsychological tests, neuropathological changes in

pediatric patients with a history of CM. They pointed out that the corpus callosum is the largest neocortical fiber tract in the brain that facilitates efficient communication between the cerebral hemispheres. They reasoned that if CM shows a predilection for cerebral white matter, interhemispheric transfer inefficiencies should be demonstrable. Bimanual tactile roughness discrimination was found to be significantly impaired in the CM group. In contrast, intrahemispheric processing of tactile information was intact. This group suggested that inefficiency in the integrity of the callosal fibers could account for these findings, although damage to alternative subcortical pathways involved in transfer across the cerebral hemispheres could not be ruled out entirely.

Cotton wool spots have been found in retinae of patients with CM (Davis et al., 1992; Lewallen et al., 1999). The intense retinal whiteness of small cotton wool spots represents gross localized axonal distensions secondary to the cessation of axoplasmic flow (McLeod et al., 1977). Davis and colleagues found that cotton wool spots were observed much more frequently than retinal hemorrhages in adult Thai patients with severe malaria. Further, all but one of the patients with cotton wool spots at presentation had an impairment of consciousness. In these cases the cotton wool spots were found in association with capillary nonperfusion. However, two comatose patients had neither cotton wool spots nor nonperfusion. The lack of cotton wool spots in these patients probably reflects the marked variability in the sequestered parasite biomass among patients with severe malaria, as well as the variations within individuals and tissues. Cotton wool spots are less common in African children, occurring in 5% of those with CM (Lewallen et al., 1999).

B. HIV

Neurological disease is a common occurrence in patients with acquired immunodeficiency syndrome (AIDS), causing clinical symptoms ranging from cognitive impairments, motor disturbances, behavioral changes, headache, and peripheral neuropathy (reviewed by Lawrence and Major, 2002). It has been estimated that 10% of patients with AIDS will have a CNS lesion as the first clinical manifestation, 40% will have some type of neurological complication during the course of the disease, and more than 70% of AIDS autopsies will demonstrate neuropathological findings (reviewed by Gonzalez et al., 1998). A proportion of neurological disease will be associated with opportunistic infections as a result of immunodeficiency. However, in the absence of these infections 20% to 30% of patients will develop neurocognitive defects—HIV-1-associated cognitive motor complex also termed HIV dementia (HIVD). At autopsy, the brains of patients with HIVD show numerous disseminated foci composed of microglia, macrophages, and multinucleated giant cells (Gray et al., 1998), termed HIV encephalitis (Masliah et al., 1992). The presence of subclinical decline in cognitive performances in HIV patients before development of significant immunodeficiency is controversial. However, it has been shown that HIV is present in CSF and brain during early asymptomatic phases of HIV infection (An et al., 1997).

Although the neuropathological correlates of the clinical manifestations remain unclear, several candidates have been proposed including viral load (Ellis et al., 2002), myelin pallor, and neuronal loss. In line with CM, an intriguing problem is that neurons are not the target of infection. In addition, some evidence supports the reversibility of neurological complications. An example highlighted by Lawrence and Major (2002) is that some patients may improve after treatment, and further deterioration may be delayed suggesting that irreversible nerve cell loss is unlikely to be involved.

With the introduction of APP immunohistochemistry, widespread axonal damage in white matter of patients with AIDS, and to a lesser degree in those with pre-AIDS, has been revealed (Adle-Biasette et al., 1999; An et al., 1997; Giometto et al., 1997; Gray et al., 1998; Raja et al., 1997). APP+ axons have been found predominantly in the subcortical white matter, basal ganglia (Adle-Biasette et al., 1999; An et al., 1997; Giometto et al., 1997; Gray et al., 1998; Raja et al., 1997), and the brainstem, including pontocerebellar fibers (Adle-Biasette et al., 1999; Gray et al., 1998). APP+ axons are commonly found in association with microglia/macrophages and multinucleated giant cells. These results have led some authors to hypothesize that areas of disturbed axons in clinically active regions of the brain may contribute to the appearance of neuropsychological symptoms (Giometto et al., 1997).

Associations between axonal damage and other neuropathological findings have been made to try to define the possible mechanisms of axonal damage in HIV infection. Diffuse myelin pallor is a common autopsy finding in HIV infection and is more frequent in those who show features of encephalopathy (reviewed in Raja et al., 1997). In the majority of reports, there is a parallel between APP+ axons and myelin pallor. However, axonal damage is also present in the absence of pallor. This led Raja and colleagues (1997) to suggest that APP staining is a more sensitive marker of some forms of white matter damage in HIV infection. The link between myelin pallor and axonal damage is less clear in some reports of HIV+ individuals without AIDS (An et al., 1997) and is clearly not involved in a featured case of AIDS with a relapsing course with neurological signs (Gray et al., 1998). In the former study of 29 HIV-1+ asymptomatic patients, pallor was minimal in three cases and absent in the others. Axonal damage in the absence of myelin pathology also has been described in a patient who died after a relapsing course of neurological signs. In this case, axonal damage was an extremely frequent finding without other neuropathological changes or evidence of productive HIV infection of the brain (Gray et al., 1998). Further, in a monkey model of

HIV using simian immunodeficiency virus-infected macaques, significant increases in APP were found in white matter in the absence of myelin pallor (Mankowski et al., 2002). From these results it is clear that axonal damage can be a primary manifestation of HIV infection in the brain.

On the other hand, the association between myelin pathological changes and axonal dysfunction has been demonstrated in vacuolar myelopathy (Rottnek et al., 2002), which is the most common AIDS-related spinal cord disease. Clinical features of the disease include lower extremity spasticity and weakness, paraparesis, urinary frequency, urgency, incontinence, and erectile dysfunction. Rottnek and colleagues (2002) have shown a time course of changes starting with significant infiltration by activated macrophages, and then, as myelin disease progresses, abnormalities in axons such as spheroids. During the initial stage of the disease, clinical signs and symptoms are infrequent, but the authors suggest that symptomatic vacuolar myelopathy may arise only when a threshold of axonal injury is reached.

The association of axonal damage with vessels has also been a topic of interest with variable findings. In the report by Raja and colleagues (1997), APP+ foci showed an approximately perivascular distribution. Similar results were found in the case report of Gray and colleagues (1998). In both cases the authors emphasized the potential role of systemic vascular-related factors in the pathogenesis of the axonal damage. In contrast, the study of HIV individuals without AIDS showed that the majority of APP did not colocalize with vessels (An et al., 1997). Similar findings were made in another study by the same group (Giometto et al., 1997). In this study the authors made a distinction between APP positive structures, ballooned structures representing chronic axonal damage, and bundles of parallel formations representing acute axonal damage. They reported that, with few exceptions, acute axonal damage was not related to blood vessels.

Several groups have now assessed CSF levels of markers of axonal degeneration in HIV-1 infection. One study found elevated levels of tau only in association with complications that caused cerebral necrosis (Green et al., 2000). In a study of 52 patients with HIV-1 however, a higher mean concentration was found in patients with AIDS dementia complex (ADC) compared with patients with asymptomatic HIV-1 infection and HIV-negative controls (Andersson et al., 1999). However, CSF τ levels could not discriminate between patients with ADC and patients with AIDS with other neurological complications. Similar findings were made by Hagberg and colleagues (2000). This group analyzed CSF levels of the light subunit of the NF protein (NFL) as a marker for degenerated axons. In patients with AIDS, the CSF NFL levels were high compared with patients who were HIV seropositive but without AIDS. They also found that CSF levels of NFL were higher in cytomegalovirus encephalitis compared with other neurological disease of infectious origin.

Both groups also found that immune activation rather than HIV viral load was associated with neurochemical signs of axonal destruction in the CNS. These results led the authors to suggest that immune activation is a pathogenic mechanism for neural injury, and a high CNS viral load is not a direct prerequisite for axonal degeneration (Andersson et al., 1999; Hagberg et al., 2000).

Human T-Lymphotropic Virus Type I (HTLV-1)

HIV is not the only viral disease that indirectly leads to axonal injury in the CNS. Another example is HTLV-I, which is associated with adult T-cell leukemia and chronic progressive disease of the spinal cord termed HTLV-I-associated myelopathy (HAM)/tropical spastic paraparesis (TSP) (Umehara et al., 2000). Signs and symptoms are referable to the corticospinal tract and the posterior columns, although the former dominate clinically and include weakness, hyperreflexia, and extensor plantar responses. Neurophysiological testing has demonstrated a delay in central motor and sensory conduction times (reviewed in Jernigan et al., 2003). Neuropathological changes correlate with the clinical presentation of HAM/TSP and include infiltration of T-lymphocytes and macrophages and increased expression of cytokines. However, demyelination and axonal loss have been described as the histological hallmarks of inflamed lesions of HAM/TSP and the pathological correlates of persistent disability that characterizes spastic paraparesis and urinary disturbance.

How the CNS damage develops is unclear, but, like HIV, it is unlikely to be the result of direct infection with virus (Levin et al., 2002); however, systemic viral expression was higher in HAM/TSP than in asymptomatic HTLV-I carriers (Yamano et al., 2002). Other findings in line with HIV are the association with myelin pallor and degeneration, although axonal damage can be found in the absence of myelin pathology. Further, APP+ axons tend to be located in relation to blood vessels, particularly veins, with or without inflammatory cell infiltrates. Again, these findings led to the conclusion that alteration in the blood-brain barrier, and seepage of neurotoxins into the CNS might relate to the primary axonal changes in HAM/TSP (Umehara et al., 2000). Unlike HIV, the neurotoxic mechanisms are more clear, with evidence pointing toward an autoimmune etiology (Levin et al., 2002) involving autoantibodies and cytotoxic T-cells. Jernigan and colleagues (2003) showed that antibodies to neurons and axons are likely to play a role in this disease. Specifically, the antibody is thought to bind to the heterogeneous nuclear ribonucleoprotein A1, a CNS autoantigen associated with molecular mimicry in HTLV-1-associated neurological disease. IgG was found to be deposited on these elements within areas that clinically, neurophysiologically, and pathologically show severe damage. These areas include the corticospinal tract and posterior column-medial lemniscal system (Jernigan et al., 2003).

VI. Multiple Sclerosis

Clinical descriptions have often failed to point out that the predilection for myelin damage in MS is only relative or have left unmentioned the development of axonal damage and loss even though this has been a consistent theme in most careful pathological descriptions (Charcot, 1868; Dawson, 1916; Ganter et al., 1999; Bjartmar et al., 2000; Evangelou et al., 2000; Lovas et al., 2000; Lassmann, 2003). Despite the fact that axonal changes in MS have been documented for more than a century, the substantial extent of axonal damage and its contribution to functional disability have only been emphasised in recent years (Davie et al., 1995; Lossef et al., 1996; Wujek et al., 2002).

Pathological studies validate the existence of axonal damage and build on the significance of axonal pathology in MS by revealing not only that axonal damage is an early feature of the disease, but that axonal loss is substantial (Ganter et al., 1999; Lovas et al., 2000; DeLuca et al., 2004). Through the use of β-APP immunohistochemistry, it has been demonstrated that the bulk of acute axonal injury occurs during early lesion formation and is most pronounced in actively demyelinating regions of both active and chronic active plaques (Ferguson et al., 1997; Kornek et al., 2000; Kuhlmann 2002). Although it is not known to what extent such axonal damage is reversible, there is evidence that some acutely injured axons become transected resulting in axonal degeneration distal to the site of injury (Trapp et al., 1998). Recent postmortem studies confirm such axonal degeneration by quantifying the amount of axonal loss in normal-appearing white matter (NAWM). In one study examining the distribution and extent of axonal loss of the functionally important long tracts (i.e., the corticospinal and sensory tracts), it was observed that axonal loss in MS was widespread, and its extent was tract-specific (Table 1) (DeLuca et al., 2004a). In the corticospinal tracts, axonal loss occurred throughout the length of the spinal cord, with maximal axonal loss in the NAWM of approximately 41%. The sensory tracts, in contrast, only showed a reduction in total axon number in the upper regions of the spinal cord, with a maximal axonal loss of approximately 24%. In both tracts, the nerve fiber loss appeared to be size selective, in that only fibers of small diameter (i.e., $<3~\mu m^2$) were affected, with large fibers remaining relatively preserved (Fig. 2, top right). The axonal loss observed in these tracts did not correlate with duration of disease, validating the idea that axonal loss begins at an early stage of the disease, at least in some patients.

Although axonal damage and loss may be an early feature of MS pathology, most patients acquire irreversible functional disability only after they have entered the progressive

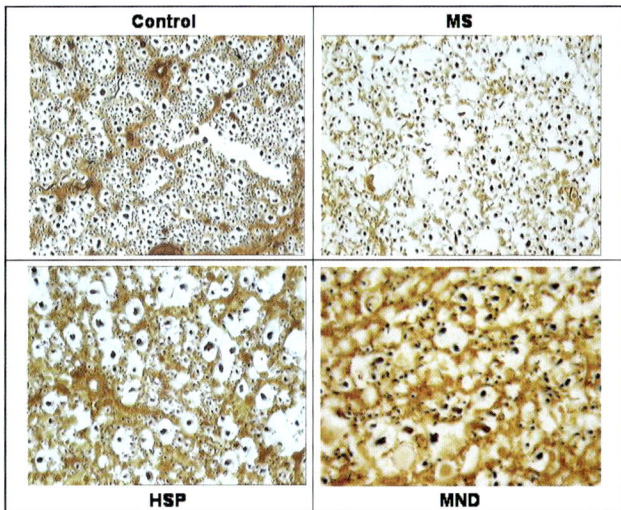

Figure 2 Palmgren-stained transverse sections of corticospinal tract axons in the spinal cord in a control case, a multiple sclerosis case, a case of hereditary spastic paraplegia, and amyotrophic lateral sclerosis (× 400). There is a reduction in the density of axonal fibres in the corticospinal tract in each condition.

phase of the disease. Pathological studies examining the extent of axonal loss in secondary progressive MS (SP-MS) have reported reductions in axonal density of approximately 57% to 61% in spinal cord lesions. (Bjartmar et al., 2000; Lovas et al., 2000). In a prospective postmortem analysis, axonal loss in both lesions and NAWM was found to be significantly correlated with a decrease in *N*-acetyl aspartate (NAA) as measured by high-performance liquid chromatography. Therefore, the observations that (1) axonal loss is significant in SP-MS, (2) axonal loss correlates with reductions in NAA in postmortem tissue, (3) magnetic resonance spectroscopy (MRS) measures of NAA *in vivo* decrease in MS brains over time, and (4) MRS NAA reduction correlates with permanent neurological disability all support the claim that axonal loss in excess of a certain threshold contributes to the acquisition of permanent neurological disability (Bjartmar et al., 2000). Experimental evidence relating the loss of axons to clinical disability in a chronic relapsing-remitting mouse model of MS (EAE) directly supports the hypothesis that cumulative axonal loss determines disability in patients with MS (Wujek et al., 2002).

There is no doubt that pathological studies have provided valuable insight into the distribution and extent of axonal loss in MS; however, they have not been overwhelmingly successful at directly relating changes in axonal populations to functional disability. Studies performed using autopsy material often lack detailed retrospective clinical information, making it difficult to relate pathological findings to various clinical parameters, such as the Expanded Disability Status Scale. In addition, autopsy material is necessarily biased toward including patients with increased disability

and longer duration of disease than might be ideal in understanding the dynamics of axonal loss. Although there is evidence that patients with short duration of disease have extensive axonal loss, it must be acknowledged that patients with disease of short duration coming to autopsy will have been selected for more aggressive disease. These limitations of human autopsy material in studying the clinical effects of axonal loss underline the importance of using surrogates for this feature in living human patients and animal models of MS described elsewhere in this chapter.

VII. Neurodegenerative Disorders

Amyotrophic lateral sclerosis (ALS) and hereditary spastic paraplegia (HSP), unlike MS, are classic neurodegenerative diseases, each with distinct clinical and pathological features. A unifying element of these disorders, however, is the presence of significant nerve fiber loss in various tracts (Fig. 2).

A. ALS

ALS is a form of motor neuron disease characterized by progressive weakness and paralysis of skeletal muscle resulting from the selective degeneration of motor neurons in the brain and spinal cord. With a typical age of onset in the sixth and seventh decade of life, the clinical course is relentlessly progressive, with death usually resulting within 1 to 5 years (Nguyen et al., 2000). Approximately 90% of ALS cases are sporadic, and 10% are familial, with up to 20% of the familial cases having a missense mutation in the gene for Cu/Zn superoxide dismutase 1 (SOD1).

The motor system is the cardinal target of the pathological insult with both upper and lower motor neurons being affected; however, cases of ALS usually demonstrate either predominantly upper or lower motor neuron involvement. The degeneration of motor neurons appears to be size selective, with motor neurons of large axonal diameter (α-motor neurons) primarily affected with relative preservation of the motor neurons of small axonal caliber (Nguyen et al., 2000). Acute neuronal injury, as visualized by APP immunohistochemistry, has been shown to occur in the perikarya of anterior horn neurons and proximal axonal swellings in cases with mild lesions and shorter disease duration and not in areas of more severe pathology or of longer duration (Sasaki and Iwata, 1999). APP expression has also been described in the corticospinal tracts, anterior columns, and anterior roots (Murakami et al., 1995). The temporally acute nature of APP expression suggests that neuronal injury is an early event in ALS that may precede the progressive neurodegenerative processes characteristic of the disease.

It has been shown that neuronal and axonal loss occurs in ALS. Severe neuronal loss associated with fibrillary gliosis is known to affect the anterior horn cells at all levels of the spinal cord and in Clarke's column at the thoracic segments. Axonal loss has been described in the corpus callosum, posterior limb of the internal capsule, middle third of the crus cerebri, centrum semiovale, and the lateral column of all spinal cord segments (Takahashi et al., 1997). The abundant presence of ubiquinated dystrophic neurites at the end of the corticospinal tracts compared to the motor cortex indicate a "dying-back" process may be operative in the corticospinal axonal degeneration observed in the disease (Schiffer et al., 1994). Unfortunately, clinicopathological studies relating the distribution and extent of such axonal loss to functional disability in ALS are notably sparse and warrant attention in future studies (Fig. 3).

B. HSP

HSP encompasses a heterogeneous group of rare, genetic neurodegenerative disorders unified by the presence of progressive weakness and spasticity predominantly affecting the lower limbs. Conventionally, the disease is categorized into pure and complicated forms, the latter defined by the presence of additional neurological and non-neurological manifestations such as optic atrophy, retinopathy, cognitive decline, epilepsy, cerebellar ataxia, extrapyramidal disease, amyotrophy, and muscle atrophy (Crosby and Proukakis, 2002; Okuda et al., 2002). The mode of inheritance in HSP is varied, with autosomal dominant, autosomal recessive, and X-linked forms having been described in both pure and complicated subtypes (reviewed in Reid et al., 2003).

Pathological studies have classified the pattern of damage seen in HSP as that of a "dying back" process in which the long ascending (sensory) and long descending (corticospinal) tracts in the spinal cord degenerate progressively from their distal ends. Diffuse axonal swellings are not a prominent feature (Schwarz and Liu, 1956; Behan and Maia, 1974). A study investigating the distribution and extent of

axonal loss of the long tracts found that axonal loss in HSP was widespread and tract-specific. In the corticospinal tracts, axonal loss occurred throughout the spinal cord, with an average axonal loss of 62%. In contrast, axonal loss in the sensory tracts was restricted to the cervical and upper thoracic regions of the spinal cord, with an average axonal loss of 29%. Unlike in MS, the axonal loss observed in HSP appears to affect both the small- (≤ 3 μm^2) and large- (>3 μm^2) diameter nerve fiber populations. The lack of correlations between axonal loss and disease duration in HSP suggest that axonal loss occurs at an early, subclinical stage with symptoms visible only once a threshold of axonal loss has been surpassed (DeLuca et al., 2004b).

VIII. Acute Encephalopathies

Although much of the damage inflicted by acute metabolic insults, such as hypoxia, hypoglycemia, and carbon monoxide poisoning, is on gray matter, secondary wallerian degeneration may correlate with clinical deficits. Thus, in an MR study of verbal memory deficits after carbon monoxide poisoning, these deficits were correlated with fornix atrophy at 6 months (Kesler et al., 2001). Considerable damage to white matter has been demonstrated pathologically in carbon monoxide poisoning (Dolinak et al., 2000a). In hypoxia occurring after cardiac arrest, diffuse axonal injury has also been described (Kaur et al., 1999; Lambri et al., 2001), and this can be distinguished from that resulting from trauma based on its distribution and the appearance of the damaged axons on APP immunostaining (Lambri et al., 2001; Dolinak et al., 2000a, 2000b). Severe hypoglycemia can also be associated with axonal injury, although in this condition, as well as in hypoxia, raised intracranial pressure can contribute to the damage that is produced (Dolinak et al., 2000b).

IX. Leukodystrophies

The relative rarity of these conditions of white matter makes it difficult for large groups of cases to be studied clinicopathologically. Although the damage to myelin predominates, damage to axons, with progressive loss of axons as the disease progresses, is also characteristic (Schaumburg et al., 1975). Brainstem and spinal cord descending tracts show consequent wallerian degeneration, but this has not been assessed in quantitative terms and related to clinical severity.

X. Experimental Models of Neurological Disorders

Animal models are essential tools in axonal injury research. There are several ways that animal models can help

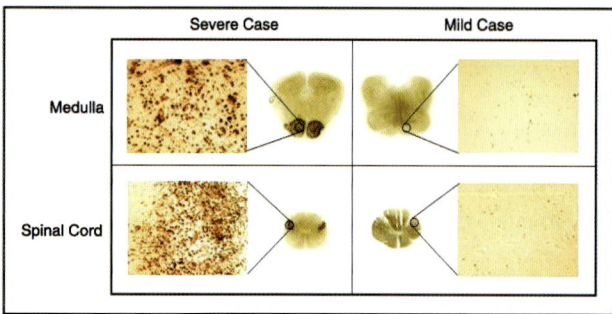

Figure 3 Marchi-stained transverse sections of the medulla (*upper panel*) and spinal cord (*lower panel*) taken from mild (*right*) and severe (*left*) cases of amyotrophic lateral sclerosis. Note the degree of Marchi-positivity in the corticospinal tracts of severe cases of amyotrophic lateral sclerosis. Positive Marchi-staining represents axonal degeneration. Magnified images (× 100) are taken from the corticospinal tracts in the medullary pyramids and lateral columns of the spinal cord.

overcome the hurdles that arise during neuropathological studies in humans. Time course analyses can be performed, which are critical for examining mechanisms of disease. In most human studies, brain pathology investigations are limited to the end stage, because the tissue is inaccessible to direct observation. Second, the neurological diseases can take several years to develop and involve complex interactions between resident brain cells, limiting the ability of researchers to model these mechanisms in culture. Furthermore, transgenic and knock-out mice can be used to directly determine factors that contribute to pathology and neurological deficits in various models of disease. Finally, animal models allow the researcher to assess therapeutic interventions.

Axonal injury has been observed in various animal models of trauma, ischemia autoimmune diseases, viral infections, toxic injury, and neurodegenerative disorders, and many of these studies have been mentioned in the various sections of this chapter. However, research using animal models of two neurological diseases, ALS and MS, merit special attention.

A. ALS

Transgenic mice with alterations in either the SOD1 or neurofilament (NF) genes display motor neuron pathology and deficits in motor function and are the most commonly used animal models to study the mechanisms of ALS neurodegeneration. Studies using these models have shown that damage to axons, in particular axonal transport defects, are one of the earliest known abnormalities, occurring months before clinical changes can be detected. Additional support for the view that axonal transport defects may play a critical role in the pathogenesis of ALS came from inhibition of axonal transport machinery in mice. Transgenic mice overexpressing dynamitin develop a late-onset and progressive motor neuron disease resembling ALS, with neurofilamentous swellings in motor axons. Transgenic mice overexpressing the shortest tau isoform exhibit axonal degeneration of spinal neurons and motor weakness (reviewed in Robertson et al., 2002).

1. SOD Transgenic Mouse Models

Approximately 15% to 20% of autosomal dominant familial ALS cases (FALS; ~ 2% of all cases) have mutations in the SOD1 gene. However, the mechanisms of how these ubiquitously expressed mutant proteins lead to selective vulnerability of motor neurons are not understood. Several lines of transgenic mouse models that express several of the mutant forms of the SOD1 gene have been established. These transgenic mice develop phenotypes similar to human FALS and show motor dysfunction at 3 to 9 months of age (Warita et al., 1999).

Defects in axonal transport in these mice have become a focus for several groups. Axonal transport can be divided into two rate components: fast (100- to 400-mm/day) and slow (0.1–3-mm/day). Warita and colleagues (1999) have investigated whether fast axonal components are modified in ligated sciatic nerves of SOD1 transgenic mice and how they are altered developmentally from an early preclinical stage. Defects in fast anterograde transport machinery (decreased accumulation of the microtubule activated ATPase kinesin after ligation of the sciatic nerve) were observed, and led the authors to hypothesize that this impairment may contribute to selective motor neuron death.

Other groups have also shown that slowing of axonal transport is an early event in the toxicity of the ALS-linked SOD1 mutants to motor neurons (Williamson and Cleveland, 1999); however, this group showed some selectivity toward the slow component of axonal transport. They used transgenic mice expressing the human SOD1^{G37R} and SOD1^{G85R} mutants. [^{35}S]Methionine was injected into the spinal cord of SOD1 mice and labeled proteins were quantified in consecutive segments from the spinal cord. Retardation of slow axonal transport was an early event in these transgenic mice. Tubulin transport was found to slow more dramatically at earlier stages, whereas the transport of neurofilaments and other cargoes was affected later. The authors interpreted these findings as an indication of a worsening defect, reflecting a decline in neuronal health and function with time; they highlighted that this is consistent with the slow accumulation of damage over a long period, ultimately culminating in late-onset disease in both mice and humans. Unlike the Warita study, no changes were detected in fast axonal transport, suggesting some selectivity toward slow transport. Results from this study provided evidence of a unifying mechanism of SOD1 mutant action that occurs long before the onset of clinical symptoms. Thus, compromised transport of selected cargoes may contribute to motor neuron vulnerability through chronic reduction in these key axonal components (Williamson and Cleveland, 1999).

2. Neurofilament Models of ALS

ALS is characterized by depositions of neurofilament proteins in the perikarya and proximal axons. To investigate how disorganized NFs might cause neurodegeneration, Collard and colleagues (1995) examined axonal transport of newly synthesized proteins in mice that overexpress the human NF heavy-subunit gene. These mice show muscle weakness, a fine tremor, and a disturbance of gait and pathology similar to ALS; but these mice do not become fully paralyzed, and the spinal cords do not show significant motor neuron loss. This group observed dramatic defects of axonal transport of the neurofilament proteins, as well as other proteins such as tubulin and actin. Ultrastructural analysis revealed a dramatic lack of cytoskeletal elements, smooth endoplasmic reticulum, and mitochondria of the degenerating axons. They proposed that the neurofilament accumulations observed in these mice cause axonal degeneration and subsequent weakness by impeding the transport of important cellular components required for axonal maintenance.

B. Multiple Sclerosis

Numerous animal models have been developed that reproduce some aspect of MS. However, it is experimental autoimmune encephalomyelitis (EAE) in rats (Kornek et al., 2000) and mice (Lo et al., 2003; Wujek et al., 2002) and Theiler's murine encephalomyelitis virus (TMEV) in mice (McGavern et al., 1999) that most closely mimic, and are most often used to investigate, the disability-related axonal loss seen in MS.

Kornek and colleagues (2000) performed a quantitative analysis of axonal injury in rats with myelin-oligodendrocyte glycoprotein-induced chronic EAE. The use of APP immunostaining allowed a better comparison with MS lesions than was previously possible. The patterns of axonal pathology in chronic EAE were qualitatively and quantitatively similar to those found in MS. More specifically the acute phase of axonal destruction in actively demyelinating lesions was most closely reflected in this model. Axonal loss within the spinal cord has been well described in rodent models of EAE (Raine and Cross, 1989; White et al., 1992), and there is a general consensus that axonal damage and loss are a reliable correlate of permanent clinical disability (Kornek et al., 2001).

More recently, efforts have been made to quantify axonal loss and relate it to clinical disability. Reminiscent of the findings in animal models of trauma, axonal loss in spinal cord above a threshold was found to determine the extent of neurological disability. Wujek and colleagues (2002), using a chronic relapsing-remitting EAE mouse model, found a causal relationship between the number of inflammatory attacks, axonal loss and permanent neurological disability. Lo and colleagues (2003) treated mice with EAE with phenytoin, a drug originally developed as an antiepileptic. Phenytoin was shown to reduce the degeneration of spinal cord axons in this model, and this was paralleled by preservation of axonal conduction within the spinal cord and amelioration of clinical deficits.

TMEV infection of susceptible mice is another popular model for studying axonal injury in MS. McGavern and colleagues (1999) have used Daniels' strain of the virus, which in susceptible mice results in a biphasic disease characterized by an acute neuronal infection, followed by chronic immune-mediated demyelination. They analyzed the temporal profile of demyelination and axonal loss to determine the independent contributions to clinical and electrophysiological abnormalities. They demonstrated a preferential loss of medium to large myelinated axons; this was accompanied by electrophysiological abnormalities and strongly correlated with reduced motor coordination and spinal atrophy.

McGavern and colleagues (2000) went on to focus specifically on hind-limb gait during the late, chronic stage of TMEV-induced demyelinating disease and addressed whether or not this functional abnormality is an indicator of the severity of spinal cord axonal loss observed at this time. In the first instance, reductions in hind-limb width coincided temporally with loss of medium and large normally myelinated fibers in the same mice rather than demyelination. To confirm that the heterogeneity in hind-limb width changes was related to axonal loss, the authors went on to correlate the relationship between the percentage of medium and large fiber loss and the change in hind-limb width from baseline. A near-perfect correlation was obtained between the percentage of medium and large normally myelinated fiber loss and the change in hind-limb width from baseline. From the linear relationship, a threshold of axonal loss was established. A reduction in medium and large normally myelinated axons greater than 33% resulted in a decrease in hind-limb stride width. A functional measurement changed only when a threshold of axonal loss was reached. Therefore, this study elegantly showed that axonal loss can follow primary, immune-mediated demyelination in the CNS and that the severity of axonal loss correlates almost perfectly with the degree of spinal cord atrophy and neurological deficits (McGavern et al., 2000).

XI. Conclusions

In the last few years, axonal degeneration and loss, together with their surrogate markers, have emerged as important measures of the extent of damage to the CNS. This is reflected in studies of conditions as diverse as head trauma, cerebral malaria, MS, viral infections, metabolic disease, and ischemic damage. This chapter reviewed the progress made in examining these measures not only in human diseases but also in animal models of disease, where a degree of precision in correlative studies can be reached that is as yet unmatched in human pathology. A common theme emerges: Axon damage and loss result in clinical deficits only after a certain threshold is crossed; but after that threshold is crossed axon deficits and functional deficits closely mirror each other. This understanding opens the way to develop better prognostic measures of human disease outcome for the assessment of interventions that can potentially improve outcome. It also allows for new therapeutic approaches to be developed that are based on the foundation of nurturing and preserving axons, whatever the nature of the disease that is damaging them.

References

Adams, C. W., and Bruton, C. J. (1989). The cerebral vasculature in dementia pugilistica. *J. Neurol. Neurosurg. Psychiatry* **52,** 600–604.

Adams, J. H., Graham, D. I., and Jennett, B. (2000). The neuropathology of the vegetative state after an acute brain insult. *Brain* **123**, 1327–1338.

Adams, J. H., Graham, D. I., and Jennett, B. (2001). The structural basis of moderate disability after traumatic brain damage. *J. Neurol. Neurosurg. Psychiatry* **71**, 521–524.

Adle-Biassette, H., Chretien, F., Wingertsmann, L., Hery, C., Ereau, T., Scaravilli, F., Tardieu, M., and Gray, F. (1999). Neuronal apoptosis does not correlate with dementia in HIV infection but is related to microglial activation and axonal damage. *Neuropathol. Appl. Neurobiol.* **25**, 123–133.

An, S. F., Giometto, B., Groves, M., Miller, R. F., Beckett, A. A., Gray, F., Tavolato, B., and Scaravilli, F. (1997). Axonal damage revealed by accumulation of beta-APP in HIV-positive individuals without AIDS. *J. Neuropathol. Exp. Neurol.* **56**, 1262–1268.

Andersson, L., Blennow, K., Fuchs, D., Svennerholm, B., and Gisslen, M. (1999). Increased cerebrospinal fluid protein tau concentration in neuro-AIDS. *J. Neurol. Sci.* **171**, 92–96.

Banati, R. B., Newcombe, J., Gunn, R. N., Cagnin, A., Turkheimer, F., Heppner, F., Price, G., Wegner, F., Giovannoni, G., Miller, D. H., Perkin, G. D., Smith, T., Hewson, A. K., Bydder, G., Kreutzberg, G. W., Jones, T., Cuzner, M. L., and Myers, R. (2000). The peripheral benzodiazepine binding site in the brain in multiple sclerosis: Quantitative in vivo imaging of microglia as a measure of disease activity. *Brain* **123**, 2321–2337.

Barkhof, F. (2004). Assessing treatment effects on axonal loss-evidence from MRI monitored clinical trials. *J Neurol* **251 Suppl 4, IV**, 6–12.

Behan, W. M., and Maia, M. (1974). Strumpell's familial spastic paraplegia: Genetics and neuropathology. *J. Neurol. Neurosurg. Psychiatry* **37**, 8–20.

Bjartmar, C., Kidd, G., Mork, S., Rudick, R., and Trapp, B. D. (2000). Neurological disability correlates with spinal cord axonal loss and reduced N-acetyl aspartate in chronic multiple sclerosis patients. *Ann. Neurol.* **48**, 893–901.

Blumbergs, P. C., Scott, G., Manavis, J., Wainwright, H., Simpson, D. A., and McLean, A. J. (1994). Staining of amyloid precursor protein to study axonal damage in mild head injury. *Lancet* **344**, 1055–1056.

Capruso, D. X., and Levin, H. S. (2000). Neurobehavioural sequelae of head injury. *In:* "Head Injury" (P. R. Cooper, ed.). pp. 525–553. McGraw-Hill, New York.

Chabriat, H., Levy, C., Taillia, H., Iba-Zizen, M. T., Vahedi, K., Joutel, A., Tournier-Lasserve, E., and Bousser, M. G. (1998). Patterns of MRI lesions in CADASIL. *Neurology* **51**, 452–457.

Charcot, M. (1868). Histologie de le sclerose en plaques. *Gaz. Hop.* **141**, 554–558.

Chard, D. T., Griffin, C. M., Parker, G. J., Kapoor, R., Thompson, A. J., Miller, D. H. (2002). Brain atrophy in clinically early relapsing remitting multiple sclerosis. *Brain* **125**, 327–337.

Collard, J. F., Cote, F., and Julien, J. P. (1995). Defective axonal transport in a transgenic mouse model of amyotrophic lateral sclerosis. *Nature* **375**, 61–64.

Corsellis, J. A., Bruton, C. J., and Freeman-Browne, D. (1973). The aftermath of boxing. *Psychol. Med.* **3**, 270–303.

Crosby, A. H., and Proukakis, C. (2002). Is the transportation highway the right road for hereditary spastic paraplegia? *Am. J. Hum. Genet.* **71**, 1009–1016.

Davie, C. A., Barker, G. J., Webb, S., Tofts, P. S., Thompson, A. J., Harding, A. E., McDonald, W. I., and Miller, D. H. (1995). Persistent functional deficit in multiple sclerosis and autosomal dominant cerebellar ataxia is associated with axon loss. *Brain* **118**, 1583–1592.

Davis, T. M., Suputtamongkol, Y., Spencer, J. L., Ford, S., Chienkul, N., Schulenburg, W. E., and White, N. J. (1992). Measures of capillary permeability in acute falciparum malaria: Relation to severity of infection and treatment. *Clin. Infect. Dis.* **15**, 256–266.

Dawson, J. W. (1916). The histology of disseminated sclerosis. *Trans. Roy. Soc.* **1**, 517–740.

DeLuca, G. C., Ebers, G. C., and Esiri, M. M. (2004). Axonal loss in multiple sclerosis: a pathological survey of the corticospinal and sensory tracts. *Brain* **127**, 1009–1018.

DeLuca, G. C., Ebers, G. C., and Esiri, M. M. (2004). The extent of axonal loss in hereditary spastic paraplegia. Submitted.

de Stefano, N., Gruidi, L., Stromillo, M. L., Bartolozzi, M. L., Federico, A. (2003). Imaging neuronal and axonal degeneration in multiple sclerosis *Neurol. Sci.* **24 Suppl 5**, S283–286.

De Stefano, N., Matthews, P. M., Fu, L., Narayanan, S., Stanley, J., Francis, G. S., Antel, J. P., and Arnold, D. L. (1998). Axonal damage correlates with disability in patients with relapsing-remitting multiple sclerosis. Results of a longitudinal magnetic resonance spectroscopy study. *Brain* **121**, 1469–1477.

Dichgans, M., Filippi, M., Bruning, R., Iannucci, G., Berchtenbreiter, C., Minicucci, L., Uttner, I., Crispin, A., Ludwig, H., Gasser, T., and Yousry, T. A. (1999). Quantitative MRI in CADASIL: correlation with disability and cognitive performance. *Neurology* **52**, 1361–1367.

Dolinak, D., Smith, C., and Graham, D. I. (2000a). Global hypoxia per se is an unusual cause of axonal injury. *Acta. Neuropathol. (Berl.)* **100**, 553–560.

Dolinak, D., Smith, C., and Graham, D. I. (2000b). Hypoglycaemia is a cause of axonal injury. *Neuropathol. Appl. Neurobiol.* **26**, 448–453.

Dugbartey, A. T., Spellacy, F. J., and Dugbartey, M. T. (1998). Somatosensory discrimination deficits following pediatric cerebral malaria. *Am. J. Trop. Med. Hyg.* **59**, 393–396.

Ellis, R. J., Moore, D. J., Childers, M. E., Letendre, S., McCutchan, J. A., Wolfson, T., Spector, S. A., Hsia, K., Heaton, R. K., and Grant, I. (2002). Progression to neuropsychological impairment in human immunodeficiency virus infection predicted by elevated cerebrospinal fluid levels of human immunodeficiency virus RNA. *Arch. Neurol.* **59**, 923–928.

Esiri, M. M., Wilcock, G. K., and Morris, J. H. (1997). Neuropathological assessment of the lesions of significance in vascular dementia. *J. Neurol. Neurosurg. Psychiatry* **63**, 749–753.

Evangelou, N., Esiri, M. M., Smith, S., Palace, J., and Matthews, P. M. (2000). Quantitative pathological evidence for axonal loss in normal appearing white matter in multiple sclerosis. *Ann. Neurol.* **47**, 391–395.

Ferguson, B., Matyszak, M. K., Esiri, M. M., and Perry, V. H. (1997). Axonal damage in acute multiple sclerosis lesions. *Brain* **120**, 393–399.

Ganter, P., Prince, C., and Esiri, M. M. (1999). Spinal cord axonal loss in multiple sclerosis: A post-mortem study. *Neuropathol. Appl. Neurobiol.* **25**, 459–467.

Ge, Y., Gonen, O., Inglese, M., Babb, J. S., Markowitz, C. E., Grossman, R. I. (2004). Neuronal injury precedes brain atrophy in multiple sclerosis. *Neurology* **62**, 624–627.

Geddes, J. F., Whitwell, H. L., and Graham, D. I. (2000). Traumatic or diffuse axonal injury? Author's response. *Neuropathol. Appl. Neurobiol.* **26**, 491.

Gennarelli, T. A. (1993). Cerebral concussion and brain injuries. *In:* "Head Injury" (P. R. Cooper, ed.). pp. 137–158. Williams and Wilkins, Baltimore.

Gennarelli, T. A., Thibault, L. E., Adams, J. H., Graham, D. I., Thompson, C. J., and Marcincin, R. P. (1982). Diffuse axonal injury and traumatic coma in the primate. *Ann. Neurol.* **12**, 564–574.

Giometto, B., An, S. F., Groves, M., Scaravilli, T., Geddes, J. F., Miller, R., Tavolato, B., Beckett, A. A., and Scaravilli, F. (1997). Accumulation of beta-amyloid precursor protein in HIV encephalitis: Relationship with neuropsychological abnormalities. *Ann. Neurol.* **42**, 34–40.

Gonzalez, R. G., Ruiz, A., Tracey, I., and McConnell, J. (1998). Structural, functional and molecular neuroimaging in AIDS. *In:* "The Neurology of AIDS" (H. Gendelman, S. A. Lipton, L. Epstein, and S. Swindells, eds.). pp. 333–353. Chapman and Hall, New York.

Grady, M. S., McLaughlin, M. R., Christman, C. W., Valadka, A. B., Fligner, C. L., and Povlishock, J. T. (1993). The use of antibodies targeted against the neurofilament subunits for the detection of diffuse axonal injury in humans. *J. Neuropathol. Exp. Neurol.* **52**, 143–152.

Graham, D. I., Genarelli, T. A., and McIntosh, T. K. (2002). Trauma. In: "Greenfield's Neuropathology" (D. I. Graham, P. L. Lantos, Eds.). Vol. 1. pp. 823–898. Arnold, London.

Gray, F., Belec, L., Chretien, F., Dubreuil-Lemaire, M. L., Ricolfi, F., Wingertsmann, L., Poron, F., and Gherardi, R. (1998). Acute, relapsing brain oedema with diffuse blood-brain barrier alteration and axonal damage in the acquired immunodeficiency syndrome. Neuropathol. Appl. Neurobiol. 24, 209–216.

Green, A. J., Giovannoni, G., Hall-Craggs, M. A., Thompson, E. J., and Miller, R. F. (2000). Cerebrospinal fluid tau concentrations in HIV infected patients with suspected neurological disease. Sex Transm. Infect. 76, 443–446.

Gultekin, S. H., and Smith, T. W. (1994). Diffuse axonal injury in craniocerebral trauma. A comparative histologic and immunohistochemical study. Arch. Pathol. Lab. Med. 118, 168–171.

Haan, J., Lanser, J. B., Zijderveld, I., van der Does, I. G., and Roos, R. A. (1990). Dementia in hereditary cerebral hemorrhage with amyloidosis-Dutch type. Arch. Neurol. 47, 965–967.

Hagberg, L., Fuchs, D., Rosengren, L., and Gisslen, M. (2000). Intrathecal immune activation is associated with cerebrospinal fluid markers of neuronal destruction in AIDS patients. J. Neuroimmunol. 102, 51–55.

Imai, H., Masayasu, H., Dewar, D., Graham, D. I., and Macrae, I. M. (2001). Ebselen protects both gray and white matter in a rodent model of focal cerebral ischemia. Stroke 32, 2149–2154.

Jennett, B., Adams, J. H., Murray, L. S., and Graham, D. I. (2001). Neuropathology in vegetative and severely disabled patients after head injury. Neurology 56, 486–490.

Jernigan, M., Morcos, Y., Lee, S. M., Dohan, F. C., Jr., Raine, C., and Levin, M. C. (2003). IgG in brain correlates with clinicopathological damage in HTLV-1 associated neurologic disease. Neurology 60, 1320–1327.

Jimenez-Jimenez, F. J., Zurdo, J. M., Hernanz, A., Medina-Acebron, S., de Bustos, F., Barcenilla, B., Sayed, Y., and Ayuso-Peralta, L. (2002). Tau protein concentrations in cerebrospinal fluid of patients with multiple sclerosis. Acta Neurol. Scand. 106, 351–354.

Kaur, B., Rutty, G. N., and Timperley, W. R. (1999). The possible role of hypoxia in the formation of axonal bulbs. J. Clin. Pathol. 52, 203–209.

Kesler, S. R., Hopkins, R. O., Blatter, D. D., Edge-Booth, H., and Bigler, E. D. (2001). Verbal memory deficits associated with fornix atrophy in carbon monoxide poisoning. J. Int. Neuropsychol. Soc. 7, 640–646.

Kochar, D. K., Makkar, R. K. (1994). Somatosensory evoked potentials in cerebral malaria. A preliminary study. Electromyogr. Clin. Neurophysiol. 34, 301–307.

Kornek, B., Storch, M. K., Bauer, J., Djamshidian, A., Weissert, R., Wallstroem, E., Stefferl, A., Zimprich, F., Olsson, T., Linington, C., Schmidbauer, M., Lassmann, H. (2001). Distribution of a calcium channel subunit in dystrophic axons in multiple sclerosis and experimental autoimmune encephalomyelitis. Brain 124, 1114–1124.

Kornek, B., Storch, M. K., Weissert, R., Wallstroem, E., Stefferl, A., Olsson, T., Linington, C., Schmidbauer, M., and Lassmann, H. (2000). Multiple sclerosis and chronic autoimmune encephalomyelitis: A comparative quantitative study of axonal injury in active, inactive, and remyelinated lesions. Am. J. Pathol. 157, 267–276.

Kril, J. J., Patel, S., Harding, A. J., and Halliday, G. M. (2002). Patients with vascular dementia due to microvascular pathology have significant hippocampal neuronal loss. J. Neurol. Neurosurg. Psychiatry 72, 747–751.

Kuhlmann, T., Lingfeld, G., Bitsch, A., Schuchardt, J., and Bruck, W. (2002). Acute axonal damage in multiple sclerosis is most extensive in early disease stages and decreases over time. Brain 125, 2202–2212.

Lambri, M., Djurovic, V., Kibble, M., Cairns, N., and Al-Sarraj, S. (2001). Specificity and sensitivity of beta APP in head injury. Clin. Neuropathol. 20, 263–271.

Lassmann, H. (2003). Axonal injury in multiple sclerosis. J. Neurol. Neurosurg. Psychiatry 74, 695–697.

Lawrence, D. M., Major, E. O. (2002). HIV-1 and the brain: Connections between HIV-1-associated dementia, neuropathology and neuroimmunology. Microbes Infect. 4, 301–308.

Levin, M. C., Lee, S. M., Kalume, F., Morcos, Y., Dohan, F. C., Jr., Hasty, K. A., Callaway, J. C., Zunt, J., Desiderio, D., and Stuart, J. M. (2002). Autoimmunity due to molecular mimicry as a cause of neurological disease. Nat. Med. 8, 509–513.

Lewallen, S., Harding, S. P., Ajewole, J., Schulenburg, W. E., Molyneux, M. E., Marsh, K., Usen, S., White, N. J., and Taylor, T. E. (1999). A review of the spectrum of clinical ocular fundus findings in P. falciparum malaria in African children with a proposed classification and grading system. Trans. R. Soc. Trop. Med. Hyg. 93, 619–622.

Li, G. L., Farooque, M., Holtz, A., and Olsson, Y. (1995). Changes of beta-amyloid precursor protein after compression trauma to the spinal cord: An experimental study in the rat using immunohistochemistry. J. Neurotrauma. 12, 269–277.

Lin, X., Blumhardt, L. D., Constantinesan, C. S. (2003). The relationship of brain and cervical cord volume to disability in clinical subtypes of multiple sclerosis: a three-dimensional MRI study. Acta Neurol. Scand. 108, 401–406.

Lo, A. C., Saab, C. Y., Black, J. A., and Waxman, S. G. (2003). Phenytoin protects spinal cord axons and preserves axonal conduction and neurological function in a model of neuroinflammation in vivo. J. Neurophysiol. 90, 3566–3571.

Losseff, N. A., Webb, S. L., O'Riordan, J. I., Page, R., Wang, L., Barker, G. J., Tofts, P. S., McDonald, W. I., Miller, D. H., and Thompson, A. J. (1996). Spinal cord atrophy and disability in multiple sclerosis. A new reproducible and sensitive MRI method with potential to monitor disease progression. Brain 119, 701–708.

Lovas, G., Szilagyi, N., Majtenyi, K., Palkovits, M., and Komoly, S. (2000). Axonal changes in chronic demyelinated cervical spinal cord plaques. Brain 123, 308–317.

Mankowski, J. L., Queen, S. E., Tarwater, P. M., Fox, K. J., and Perry, V. H. (2002). Accumulation of beta-amyloid precursor protein in axons correlates with CNS expression of SIV gp41. J. Neuropathol. Exp. Neurol. 61, 85–90.

Masliah, E., Achim, C. L., Ge, N., DeTeresa, R., Terry, R. D., and Wiley, C. A. (1992). Spectrum of human immunodeficiency virus-associated neocortical damage. Ann. Neurol. 32, 321–329.

McGavern, D. B., Zoecklein, L., Drescher, K. M., and Rodriguez, M. (1999). Quantitative assessment of neurologic deficits in a chronic progressive murine model of CNS demyelination. Exp. Neurol. 158, 171–181.

McGavern, D. B., Zoecklein, L., Sathornsumetee, S., and Rodriguez, M. (2000). Assessment of hindlimb gait as a powerful indicator of axonal loss in a murine model of progressive CNS demyelination. Brain Res. 877, 396–400.

McKenzie, K. J., McLellan, D. R., Gentleman, S. M., Maxwell, W. L., Gennarelli, T. A., and Graham, D. I. (1996). Is beta-APP a marker of axonal damage in short-surviving head injury? Acta Neuropathol. (Berl.) 92, 608–613.

McLeod, D., Marshall, J., Kohner, E. M., and Bird, A. C. (1977). The role of axoplasmic transport in the pathogenesis of retinal cotton-wool spots. Br. J. Ophthalmol. 61, 177–191.

Medana, I. M., Day, N. P., Hien, T. T., Mai, N. T., Bethell, D., Phu, N. H., Farrar, J., Esiri, M. M., White, N. J., and Turner, G. D. (2002). Axonal injury in cerebral malaria. Am. J. Pathol. 160, 655–666.

Murakami, S., Sheriff, F. E., and Morris, J. H. (1995). APP immunoreactivity in axonal lesions in motor neuron disease in comparison with cerebral infarction patients [abstract]. Neuropathology 15, 289.

Ng, H. K., Mahaliyana, R. D., and Poon, W. S. (1994). The pathological spectrum of diffuse axonal injury in blunt head trauma: Assessment with axon and myelin strains. Clin. Neurol. Neurosurg. 96, 24–31.

Nguyen, M. D., Lariviere, R. C., and Julien, J. P. (2000). Reduction of axonal caliber does not alleviate motor neuron disease caused by mutant superoxide dismutase 1. Proc. Natl. Acad. Sci. U. S. A. 97, 12306–12311.

Oehmichen, M., Meissner, C., Schmidt, V., Pedal, I., Konig, H. G., and Saternus, K. S. (1998). Axonal injury: A diagnostic tool in forensic neuropathology? A review. Forensic Sci. Int. 95, 67–83.

Ohta, M., Ohta, K., Nishimura, M., and Saida, T. (2002). Detection of myelin basic protein in cerebrospinal fluid and serum from patients with HTLV-1-associated myelopathy/tropical spastic paraparesis. *Ann. Clin. Biochem.* **39**, 603–605.

Okuda, B., Iwamoto, Y., and Tachibana, H. (2002). Hereditary spastic paraplegia with thin corpus callosum and cataract: a clinical description of two siblings. *Acta Neurol. Scand.* **106**, 222–224.

Oppenheimer, D. R. (1968). Microscopic lesions in the brain following head injury. *J. Neurol. Neurosurg. Psychiatry* **31**, 299–306.

Patankar, T. F., Karnad, D. R., Shetty, P. G., Desai, A. P., and Prasad, S. R. (2002). Adult cerebral malaria: prognostic importance of imaging findings and correlation with postmortem findings. *Radiology* **224**, 811–816.

Pesini, P., Kopp, J., Wong, H., Walsh, J. H., Grant, G., and Hokfelt, T. (1999). An immunohistochemical marker for Wallerian degeneration of fibers in the central and peripheral nervous system. *Brain Res.* **828**, 41–59.

Raine, C. S., and Cross, A. H. (1989). Axonal dystrophy as a consequence of long-term demyelination. *Lab. Invest.* **60**, 714–725.

Raja, F., Sherriff, F. E., Morris, C. S., Bridges, L. R., and Esiri, M. M. (1997). Cerebral white matter damage in HIV infection demonstrated using beta-amyloid precursor protein immunoreactivity. *Acta Neuropathol. (Berl.)* **93**, 184–189.

Reid, E. (2003). Science in motion: Common molecular pathological themes emerge in the hereditary spastic paraplegias. *J. Med. Genet.* **40**, 81–86.

Roberts, A. H. (1969). "Brain damage in boxers. A study of prevalence of traumatic encephalopathy among ex-professional boxers." Pitman, London.

Robertson, J., Kriz, J., Nguyen, M. D., and Julien, J. P. (2002). Pathways to motor neuron degeneration in transgenic mouse models. *Biochimie* **84**, 1151–1160.

Rottnek, M., Di Rocco, A., Laudier, D., and Morgello, S. (2002). Axonal damage is a late component of vacuolar myelopathy. *Neurology* **58**, 479–481.

Sasaki, S., and Iwata, M. (1999). Immunoreactivity of beta-amyloid precursor protein in amyotrophic lateral sclerosis. *Acta Neuropathol. (Berl.)* **97**, 463–468.

Sastre-Garriga, J., Ingle, G. T., Chard, D. T., Ramio-Torrenta, L, Miller, D. H., Thompson, A. J. (2004). Grey and white matter atrophy in early clinical stages of primary progressive multiple sclerosis *Neuroimage* **22**, 353–359.

Schabitz, W. R., Li, F., and Fisher, M. (2000). The *N*-methyl-D-aspartate antagonist CNS 1102 protects cerebral gray and white matter from ischemic injury following temporary focal ischemia in rats. *Stroke* **31**, 1709–1714.

Schaumburg, H. H., Powers, J. M., Raine, C. S., Suzuki, K., and Richardson, E. P., Jr. (1975). Adrenoleukodystrophy. A clinical and pathological study of 17 cases. *Arch. Neurol.* **32**, 577–591.

Schiffer, D., Attanasio, A., Chio, A., Migheli, A., and Pezzulo, T. (1994). Ubiquitinated dystrophic neurites suggest corticospinal derangement in patients with amyotrophic lateral sclerosis. *Neurosci. Lett.* **180**, 21–24.

Schwarz, G. A., and Liu, C. N. (1956). Hereditary (familial) spastic paraplegia; further clinical and pathologic observations. *AMA Arch. Neurol. Psychiatry* **75**, 144–162.

Sherriff, F. E., Bridges, L. R., Gentleman, S. M., Sivaloganathan, S., and Wilson, S. (1994a). Markers of axonal injury in post mortem human brain. *Acta Neuropathol. (Berl.)* **88**, 433–439.

Sherriff, F. E., Bridges, L. R., and Sivaloganathan, S. (1994b). Early detection of axonal injury after human head trauma using immunocytochemistry for beta-amyloid precursor protein. *Acta Neuropathol. (Berl.)* **87**, 55–62.

Sjogren, M., Blomberg, M., Jonsson, M., Wahlund, L. O., Edman, A., Lind, K., Rosengren, L., Blennow, K., and Wallin, A. (2001). Neurofilament protein in cerebrospinal fluid: a marker of white matter changes. *J. Neurosci. Res.* **66**, 510–516.

Skoog, I., Vanmechelen, E., Andreasson, L. A., Palmertz, B., Davidsson, P., Hesse, C., and Blennow, K. (1995). A population-based study of tau protein and ubiquitin in cerebrospinal fluid in 85-year-olds: Relation to severity of dementia and cerebral atrophy, but not to the apolipoprotein E4 allele. *Neurodegeneration* **4**, 433–442.

Simon, J. H., Kinkel, R. P., Jacobs, L., Bub, L., and Simonian, N. (2000). A Wallerian degeneration pattern in patients at risk for MS. *Neurology* **54**, 1155–1160.

Smith, C., Nicoll, J. A., and Graham, D. I. (2004). Head injury and dementia. *In:* "The Neuropathology of Dementia" (M. M. Esiri, V. M.-Y. Lee, and J. Q. Trojanowski, eds.). pp. 455–469. Cambridge University Press, Cambridge.

Takahashi, T., Yagishita, S., Amano, N., Yamaoka, K., and Kamei, T. (1997). Amyotrophic lateral sclerosis with numerous axonal spheroids in the corticospinal tract and massive degeneration of the cortex. *Acta Neuropathol. (Berl.)* **94**, 294–299.

Teasdale, G. M., Nicoll, J. A., Murray, G., and Fiddes, M. (1997). Association of apolipoprotein E polymorphism with outcome after head injury. *Lancet* **350**, 1069–1071.

Thornhill, S., Teasdale, G. M., Murray, G. D., McEwen, J., Roy, C. W., and Penny, K. I. (2000). Disability in young people and adults one year after head injury: prospective cohort study. *BMJ* **320**, 1631–1635.

Traboulsee, A., Dehmeshki, J., Peters, K. R., Griffin, C. M., Bres, P. A., Silver, N., Ciccarrelli, O., Chard, D. T., Barkar, G. J., Thompson A. J., Miller, D. H. (2003) Disability in multiple sclerosis is related to normal appearing brain tissue MTR histogram. *Mult Scler* **9**, 566–73

Trapp, B. D., Peterson, J., Ransohoff, R. M., Rudick, R., Mork, S., and Bo, L. (1998). Axonal transection in the lesions of multiple sclerosis. *N. Engl. J. Med.* **338**, 278–285.

Tullberg, M., Mansson, J. E., Fredman, P., Lekman, A., Blennow, K., Ekman, R., Rosengren, L. E., Tisell, M., and Wikkelso, C. (2000). CSF sulfatide distinguishes between normal pressure hydrocephalus and subcortical arteriosclerotic encephalopathy. *J. Neurol. Neurosurg. Psychiatry* **69**, 74–81.

Ukkonen, M., Dastidov, P., Heinonen, T., Laasonen, E., Elovaara, I. (2003). Volumetric quantitation by MRI in primary progressive multiple sclerosis: volume of plaques and atrophy correlated with neurological disability. *Eur. J. Neurol* **10**, 663–669.

Umehara, F., Abe, M., Koreeda, Y., Izumo, S., and Osame, M. (2000). Axonal damage revealed by accumulation of beta-amyloid precursor protein in HTLV-I-associated myelopathy. *J. Neurol. Sci.* **176**, 95–101.

Wallin, A., Blennow, K., and Rosengren, L. (1999). Cerebrospinal fluid markers of pathogenetic processes in vascular dementia, with special reference to the subcortical subtype. *Alzheimer Dis. Assoc. Disord.* **13 Suppl 3**, S102–105.

Warita, H., Itoyama, Y., and Abe, K. (1999). Selective impairment of fast anterograde axonal transport in the peripheral nerves of asymptomatic transgenic mice with a G93A mutant SOD1 gene. *Brain Res.* **819**, 120–131.

White, S. R., Black, P. C., Samathanam, G. K., and Paros, K. C. (1992). Prazosin suppresses development of axonal damage in rats inoculated for experimental allergic encephalomyelitis. *J. Neuroimmunol.* **39**, 211–218.

Williamson, T. L., and Cleveland, D. W. (1999). Slowing of axonal transport is a very early event in the toxicity of ALS-linked SOD1 mutants to motor neurons. *Nat. Neurosci.* **2**, 50–56.

Wujek, J. R., Bjartmar, C., Richer, E., Ransohoff, R. M., Yu, M., Tuohy, V. K., and Trapp, B. D. (2002). Axon loss in the spinal cord determines permanent neurological disability in an animal model of multiple sclerosis. *J. Neuropathol. Exp. Neurol.* **61**, 23–32.

Yamauchi, H., Fukuyama, H., Ogawa, M., Ouchi, Y., and Kimura, J. (1994). Callosal atrophy in patients with lacunar infarction and extensive leukoaraiosis. An indicator of cognitive impairment. *Stroke* **25**, 1788–1793.

Yamano, Y., Nagai, M., Brennan, M., Mora, C. A., Soldan, S. S., Tomaru, U., Takenouchi, N., Izumo, S., Osame, M., and Jacobson, S. (2002). Correlation of human T-cell lymphotropic virus type 1 (HTLV-1) mRNA with proviral DNA load, virus-specific CD8(+) T cells, and disease severity in HTLV-1-associated myelopathy (HAM/TSP). *Blood* **99**, 88–94.

27

Remyelination as Neuroprotection

Charles L. Howe, Ph.D.
Moses Rodriguez, M.D.

I. Introduction

A major area of investigation in the neurosciences is directed at understanding the factors that participate in neurological deficits. In demyelinating diseases of the central nervous system (CNS), it has been assumed that demyelination by itself contributes to functional deficits. Previous physiological studies demonstrated that demyelination in the CNS can result in conduction slowing and conduction block (McDonald and Sears, 1969). Such observations appeared sufficient to explain the majority of deficits in demyelinating human diseases such as multiple sclerosis (MS). However, clinical and basic science observations have begun to challenge this hypothesis.

II. Multiple Sclerosis

MS is one of the most frequent neurological diseases of early adulthood, affecting as many as 400,000 patients in the United States, 85% of whom are between the ages of 20 and 50 years old (Mayr et al., 2003). Clinically, this disease is most often marked by a relapsing and remitting pattern of neurological dysfunction, frequently leading over time to a secondary progressive disease pattern marked by accumulative loss of neurological function (Noseworthy et al., 2000). The relapsing-remitting phase is characterized by clinical symptoms such as loss of visual acuity, weakness, ataxia, fatigue, and clumsiness that develop over a period of several days, stabilize, and then resolve over the course of several weeks (Noseworthy et al., 2000). At least early in the disease, corticosteroid treatment accelerates recovery from clinical deficit. Frequently, some dysfunction may persist after relapse, and an accumulation of such persistant clinical deficit ultimately results in a progressive impairment termed secondary progressive MS (Noseworthy et al., 2000).

Although clinically characterized by pathological and functional hallmarks such as focally demyelinated lesions and gadolinium enhancement, as detected by magnetic resonance imaging (MRI), the cellular and molecular locus of MS is distinctly heterogeneous (Lucchinetti et al., 2000). Although all lesions contain an inflammatory infiltration of T-cells and macrophages, further analysis suggests that four distinct patterns of pathology are present in active lesions. The first two patterns are marked by well-delineated perivascular demyelination and simultaneous loss of immunoreactivity for all myelin proteins within the lesion, but relative sparing of oligodendrocytes and active repopulation of demyelinated lesions with oligodendrocytes during remyelination (Lucchinetti et al., 2000) (Fig. 1). This is consistent with previous reports show-

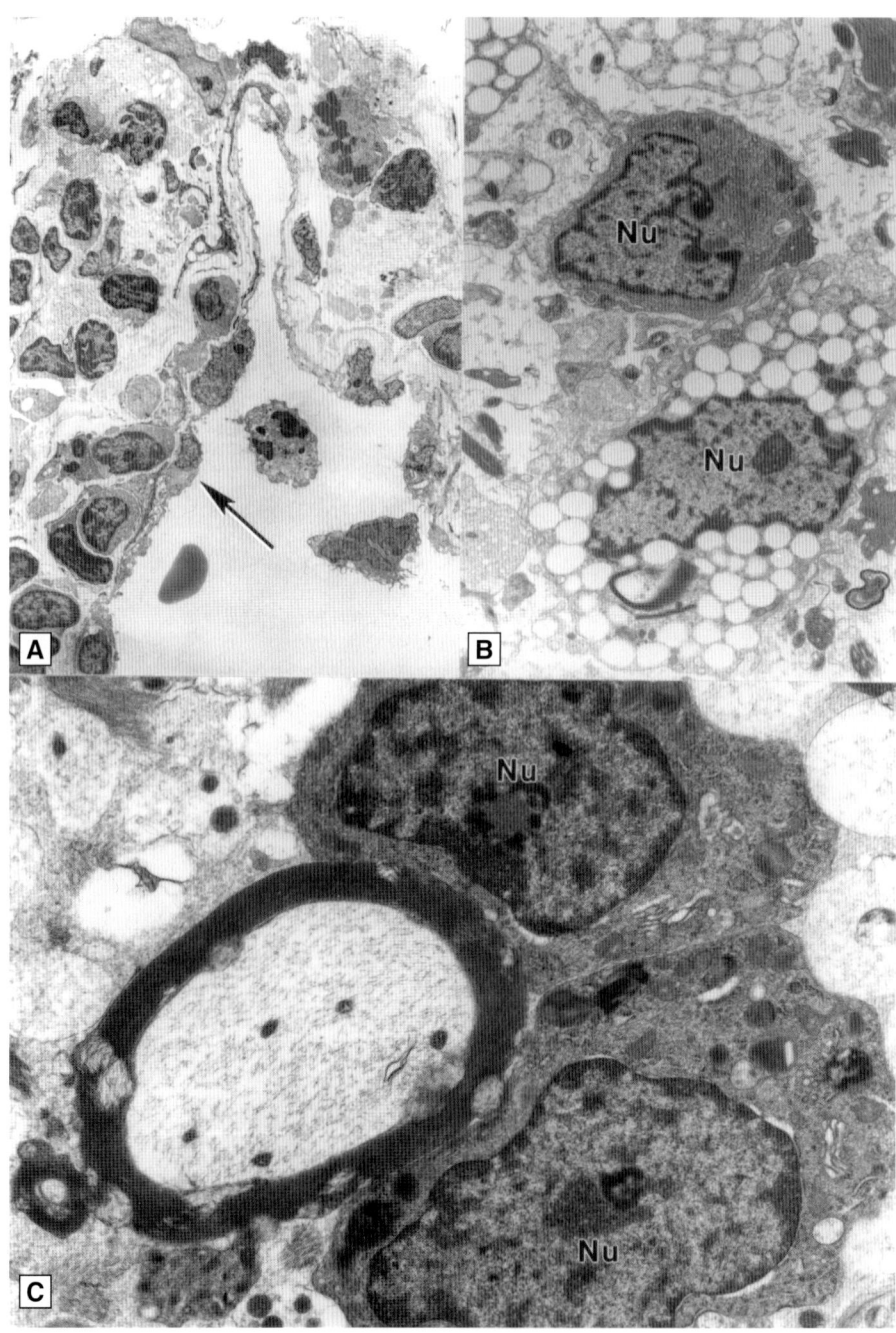

Figure 1 **Examples of immune cell infiltration in a mouse model of MS.** (**A**) Evidence of perivascular immune cells near a demyelinated lesion. (**B**) Macrophage with lipid inclusions associated with a demyelinated lesion. (**C**) Two immune effector cells in direct contact with the myelin sheath of an axon. Immune cell infiltration is strongly associated with Pattern I and Pattern II MS pathology.

ing abortive attempts at remyelination in MS lesions (Prineas and Connell, 1979; Prineas et al., 1989) (Fig. 2). The second pattern is unique in that actively degenerating myelin is associated with pronounced immunoglobulin and complement reactivity (Lucchinetti et al., 2000). The third and fourth patterns do not exhibit perivascular localization, and the borders of active lesions are only poorly defined. Oligodendrocytes are not spared and repopulation of lesions is not observed. Finally, the third pattern is uniquely associated with greater loss of myelin-associated glycoprotein immunoreactivity than other myelin proteins (Lucchinetti et al., 2000). This pattern is consistent with the concept of "dying-back oligodendrogliopathy," in which the primary injury is to the oligodendrocyte. The earliest morphological manifestation of this pattern is degeneration of the inner myelin sheath and oligodendroglial loops, the most distal extensions of the oligodendrocyte (Rodriguez, 2003) (Fig. 3). Of importance, heterogeneity is found among patients but not within individuals. All lesions of any given patient are of the same phenotype, suggesting a single pathogenic mechanism within a patient but multiple mechanisms across the population.

The heterogeneity observed in patients with MS is also reflected in animal models of MS. The two best studied models of human MS are immune-mediated encephalo-myelitis induced by immunization with CNS antigens and viral-induced demyelination. Lesions commonly found in patients with the first and second pattern of MS pathology are similar to those observed in T-cell-mediated and antibody-mediated autoimmune demyelination. Likewise, lesions observed in the third and fourth patterns of human MS are typical of the oligodendrogliopathy and demyelination induced by viral infection (Lucchinetti et al., 2000; Paz Soldan and Rodriguez, 2002; Rodriguez, 1985).

The functional correlate of any of the patterns described previously is generally considered to be loss of axon conduction resulting from demyelination. During the relapsing-remitting phase of MS, the regression of symptoms is likely due to resolution of inflammation and remyelination, resulting in a return of axon function. However, as the disease progresses and as each round of repair accumulates demyelination that is not resolved, axonal function deteriorates (Noseworthy et al., 2000) (Fig. 4). This is marked by redistribution of sodium channels along demyelinated axon segments, and eventually by loss of the axon altogether (Rivera-Quinones et al., 1998) (see Chapters 7 and 8). Because axons are the absolute locus of neuronal function and transmission, it is likely that understanding and reversing axon failure and loss will be required for any rational therapeutic program.

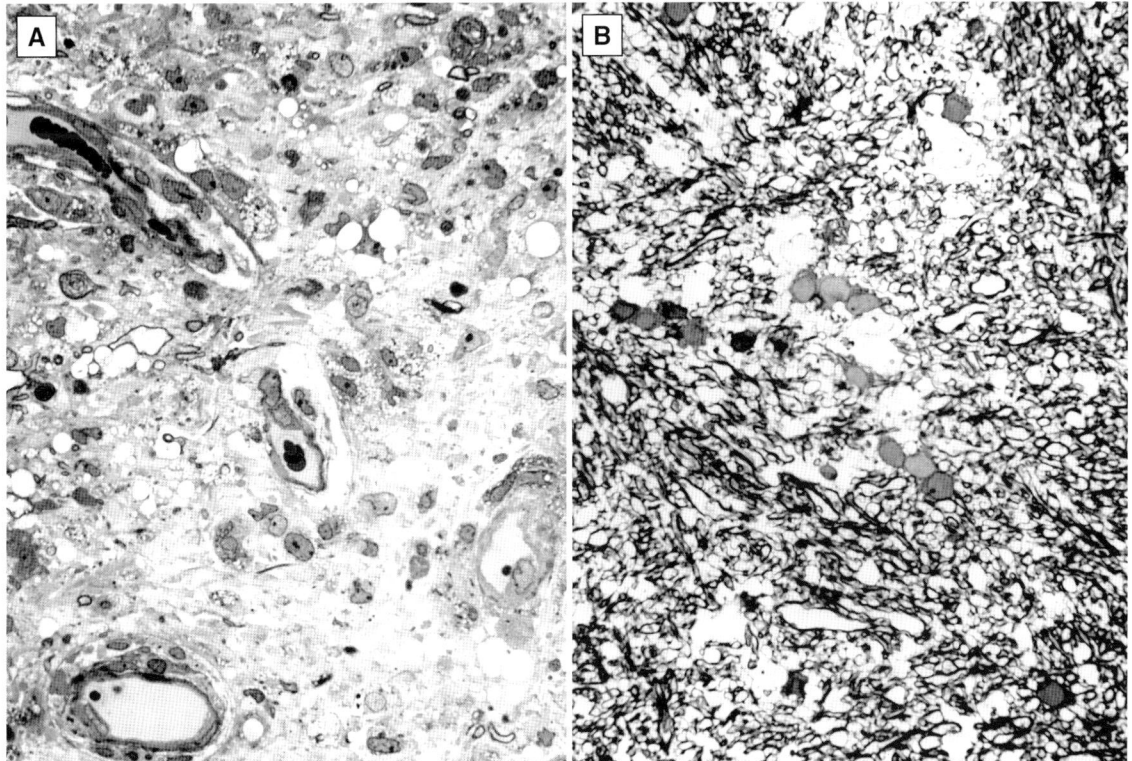

Figure 2 (**A**) Demyelination in the brain of a patient with MS. (**B**) Evidence of spontaneous remyelination in the brain of a patient with MS. Spontaneous remyelination occurs in Patterns I and II lesions, but fails to occur in Pattern III MS lesions.

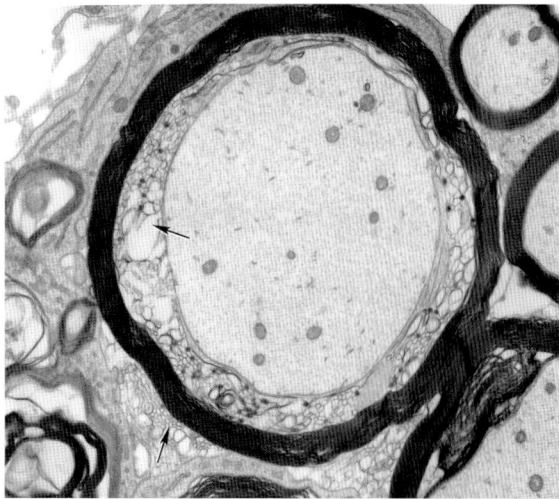

Figure 3 Evidence of "dying-back" oligodendrogliopathy. Note the degeneration of the inner myelin sheath, presenting an "inside-out" type of myelin damage. This type of pathology is present in Pattern III MS lesions in which the attack is primarily directed against the oligodendrocyte. The most distal extension of the oligodendrocyte is the inner myelin lamellae. Therefore, injury to the inner sheath with relative preservation of the other myelin lamellae is indicative of primary injury to the myelin-producing cell.

III. Evidence of Axon Loss in MS

Magnetic resonance imaging (MRI) studies in patients with MS have demonstrated only a weak correlation between lesion load and clinical deficits (Stevens et al., 1986). Moreover, pathological studies have demonstrated that some lesions observed by MRI are indeed demyelinated and frequently involve areas of CNS that should have resulted in neurological deficits, but do not (Bruck et al., 1997). Likewise, autopsy analysis has demonstrated that demyelination, sufficient to make the pathological diagnosis of MS, can be observed in individuals who during life remained normal in neurological function (Mews et al., 1998). These observations have suggested that demyelination may be required but not sufficient for the development of permanent neurological deficits.

Further challenge to the demyelination hypothesis is provided by studies that use magnetic resonance spectroscopy to sensitively and quantitatively measure axon-specific metabolites such as *N*-acetyl aspartate (NAA). These studies found that active lesions are significantly reduced in NAA, and that as the disease progresses from the relapsing-remitting phase to the chronic-progressive phase, a reduction in NAA can be measured even in normal-appearing white matter (Matthews et al., 1996). This finding suggests that a reduction in NAA may reflect both acute, but potentially reversible, axonal dysfunction associated with temporary demyelination, as well as chronic, irreversible loss of axons as a result of degeneration beyond the scope of any given demyelinated lesion. The

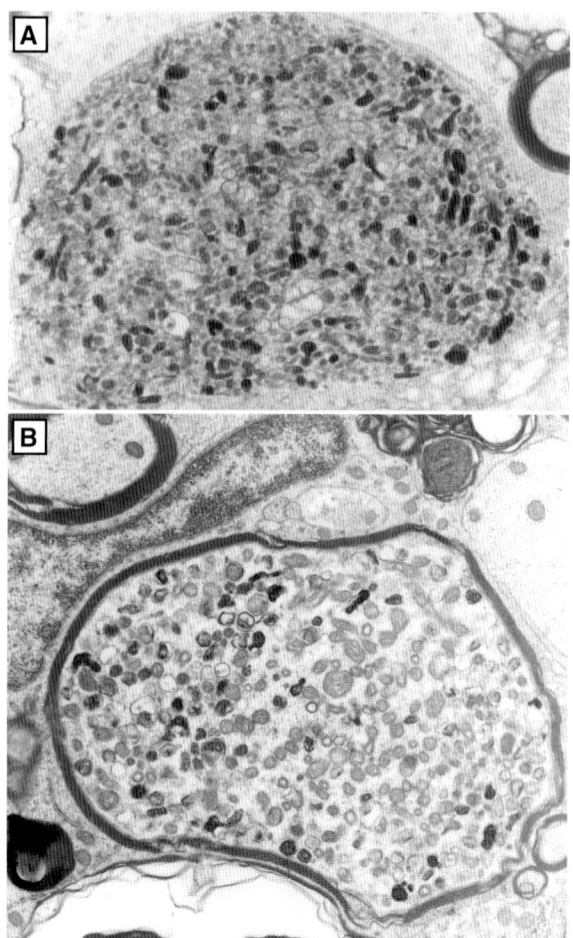

Figure 4 Two examples of degenerating axons. (**A**) Human MS patient. (**B**) Mouse with demyelination after infection with Theiler's virus. Note the accumulation of electron dense organelles characteristic of dying axons.

mechanisms by which demyelination induces axon dysfunction and axon degeneration remain unclear (Trapp et al., 1998), but a number of recent studies suggest that multiple factors may be involved, ranging from increased accessibility of inflammatory mediators and immune effector cells, to a loss of trophic support. For example, CD8+ cytotoxic T-cells have been observed in contact with demyelinated axons in active MS lesions (Neumann et al., 2002), and the terminal swellings of transected axons have been found to be engulfed by macrophages and microglia (Trapp et al., 1998). Likewise, myelination is known to provide trophic and maintenance cues to axons, controlling axon caliber, and neurofilament phosphorylation and spacing (Sanchez et al., 1996; Windebank et al., 1985). Finally, changes in NAA associated with MS may reflect defects or dysregulation of axonal energy-storage mechanisms, as NAA-derived metabolic products such as acetyl coenzyme A may function to meet the high energy demands of axonal electrochemical conduction (Mehta and Namboodiri, 1995). This idea is particularly intriguing in light of evidence that both lesion load and Expanded Disability Status Score (EDSS) are negatively correlated with levels of NAA found in normal-appearing white matter of patients with MS (Sarchielli et al., 1999), suggesting that axonal loss, axonal metabolic dysfunction, or both, are primarily responsible for neurological deficit in MS.

IV. Evidence of Axon Loss in Animal Models of MS

A. Theiler's Virus

Animal experiments have also questioned the hypothesis that demyelination alone is sufficient to explain permanent deficits in demyelinating diseases. Theiler's murine encephalomyelitis virus (TMEV) was isolated and identified by Theiler nearly 70 years ago as a picornavirus responsible for ubiquitous enteric infection and infrequent paralysis in mice (Theiler, 1937). Although initially used as a mouse model of polio, later work identified a strain of TMEV (the DA or Daniels' strain) that induced a chronic-progressive demyelinating disease in susceptible mice (Daniels et al., 1952). Further work in the 1970s suggested that Theiler's

virus-induced demyelinating disease resembled human MS (Lipton, 1975; Lipton and Dal Canto, 1976a; 1976b; 1979), and numerous investigators have extended our understanding of MS using a variety of TMEV strains (Brahic 2002; Monteyne et al., 1997). After intracerebral injection of Theiler's virus, and during the first 10 to 12 days of infection, the virus replicates primarily in neurons of the hippocampus (Fig. 5), striatum, cortex, and anterior horn of the spinal cord, and then is rapidly cleared from the brain (Drescher et al., 1999). Oligodendrocytes and macrophages are also infected early (Njenga et al., 1997a).

In mice of resistant major histocompatibility complex (MHC) haplotypes (H-2^{b,d,k}), no demyelination or viral persistence develops. However, in animals of susceptible MHC haplotypes (H-2^{s,q,r,v,f,p}), the virus is cleared from neurons in the brain but persists in glial cells (Brahic et al., 1981; Rodriguez et al., 1983) and macrophages (Dal Canto and Lipton, 1982; Levy et al., 1992; Rossi et al., 1997) of the spinal cord white matter and brainstem (Fig. 6). This viral persistence is associated with chronic demyelination and stereotypical neurological impairment and paralysis due to the loss of axons (Drescher et al., 1997; Lipton 1975; Rodriguez and Miller, 1994) (Fig. 7). Demyelination in this model is in part mediated by a "dying-back" oligoden-

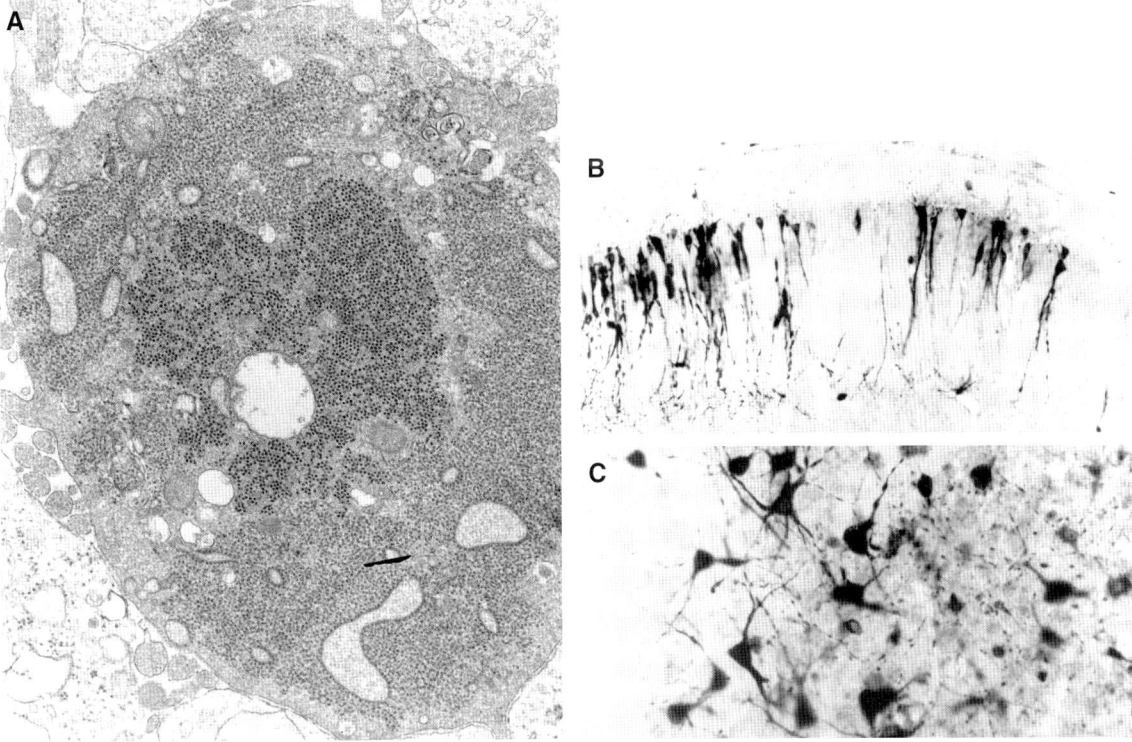

Figure 5 (**A**) High magnification view of a cell infected with Theiler's virus. Note the high density of dark, regularly shaped virions filling the cell. (**B, C**) Theiler's virus-infected neurons in the hippocampus (**B**) and spinal cord (**C**), as marked by immunostaining for viral antigens. Note the presence of viral antigen in the axons of these cells.

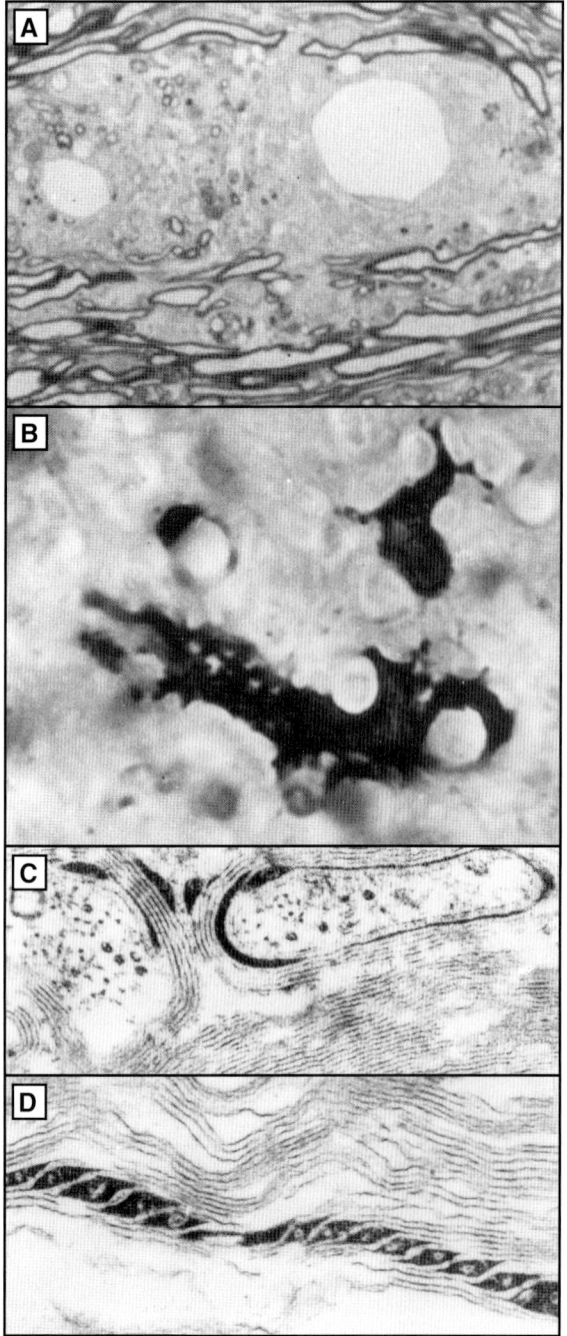

Figure 6 **Immuno-electron micrograph evidence of Theiler's virus persistence in oligodendrocytes and myelin.** (**A**) An area of demyelination in a longitudinal section, showing myelin injury and inflammatory cells. (**B**) Vibratome section of the region shown in (**A**) stained for viral antigen, demonstrating an infected oligodendrocyte ensheathing an axon. (**C**) Electron micrograph of cells shown in (**B**). Note the presence of viral antigen (electron-dense immunoperoxidase reaction product) in the inner and outer glial loops. The location of the viral antigen is consistent with the concept of "dying-back" oligodendrogliopathy. (**D**) Viral antigen present in the Schmidt-Lanterman clefts. The presence of labeled Schmidt-Lanterman incisures in Theiler's infected oligodendrocytes may represent an early response to virus-mediated injury.

drogliopathy (Ludwin and Johnson, 1981) manifested by injury to the most distal extensions of the oligodendrocyte (Rodriguez, 1985).

Of the H-2 genes, it is the D locus that is of major importance for resistance vs. susceptibility. Resistance is a dominant trait that maps to H-2D, and genetic deletion or mutation of the D locus results in viral persistance and chronic demyelinating disease (Rodriguez et al., 1986). Specific introduction of H-2D^b or H-2D^d genes into normally susceptible mice results in the acquisition of resistance to viral persistence (Rodriguez and David, 1995). This resistance is associated with a robust antiviral cytotoxic T-cell response that develops in the gray matter of infected C57BL6 mice (Pena Rossi et al., 1991), and immunological depletion of CD8$^+$ T-cells or the genetic deletion of CD8$^+$ T cells observed in β2-microglobulin knock-out mice results in viral persistence within otherwise resistant genetic backgrounds. Consistent with the genetics of resistance discussed previously, the cytotoxic T-cell response observed during the acute phase of Theiler's virus infection is restricted to the D^b molecule (Lin et al., 1997). Moreover, after Theiler's virus infection of resistant mice of the H-2^b haplotype, we have identified an immunodominant cytotoxic T-cell population within the CNS that is specific for the VP2$_{121-130}$ viral capsid peptide presented within the context of D^b (Johnson et al., 1999). We have also previously demonstrated that cytotoxic T-cells appear to play a critical role in the injury of neurons and axons in both the acute (Howe and Rodriguez, unpublished observations) and chronic phases of Theiler's virus infection (Rivera-Quinones et al., 1998; Ure and Rodriguez, 2000; 2002).

B. Experimental Allergic Encephalomyelitis

Experimental allergic (or autoimmune) encephalomyelitis (EAE) has been a central model of inflammatory demyelinating disease since Rivers and Schwentker induced myelin destruction in monkeys immunized with brain tissue in 1935 (Rivers and Schwentker, 1935). Since that time, it has become clear that EAE can be induced in essentially all mammals, from rodents to humans (Lassmann and Wekerle, 1998; Raine and Bornstein, 1970) (Fig. 8). CNS protein-reactive T-cells are required for induction of EAE, and adoptive transfer of T-cells from immunized animals into naïve animals can elicit autoimmune-mediated inflammation. In contrast to Theiler's virus-mediated demyelination, EAE-related encephalitogenic T-cells are almost entirely CD4$^+$, recognizing CNS antigens only within the context of MHC class II (Swanborg, 2001). While some evidence suggests that CD8$^+$ and γδ-T cells may play a regulatory role in EAE (Segal, 2003), CD4$^+$ T-cells are considered to be the primary mediators of autoimmune-mediated demyelination. This is an important distinction, as well as an important difference between human MS and EAE in animals.

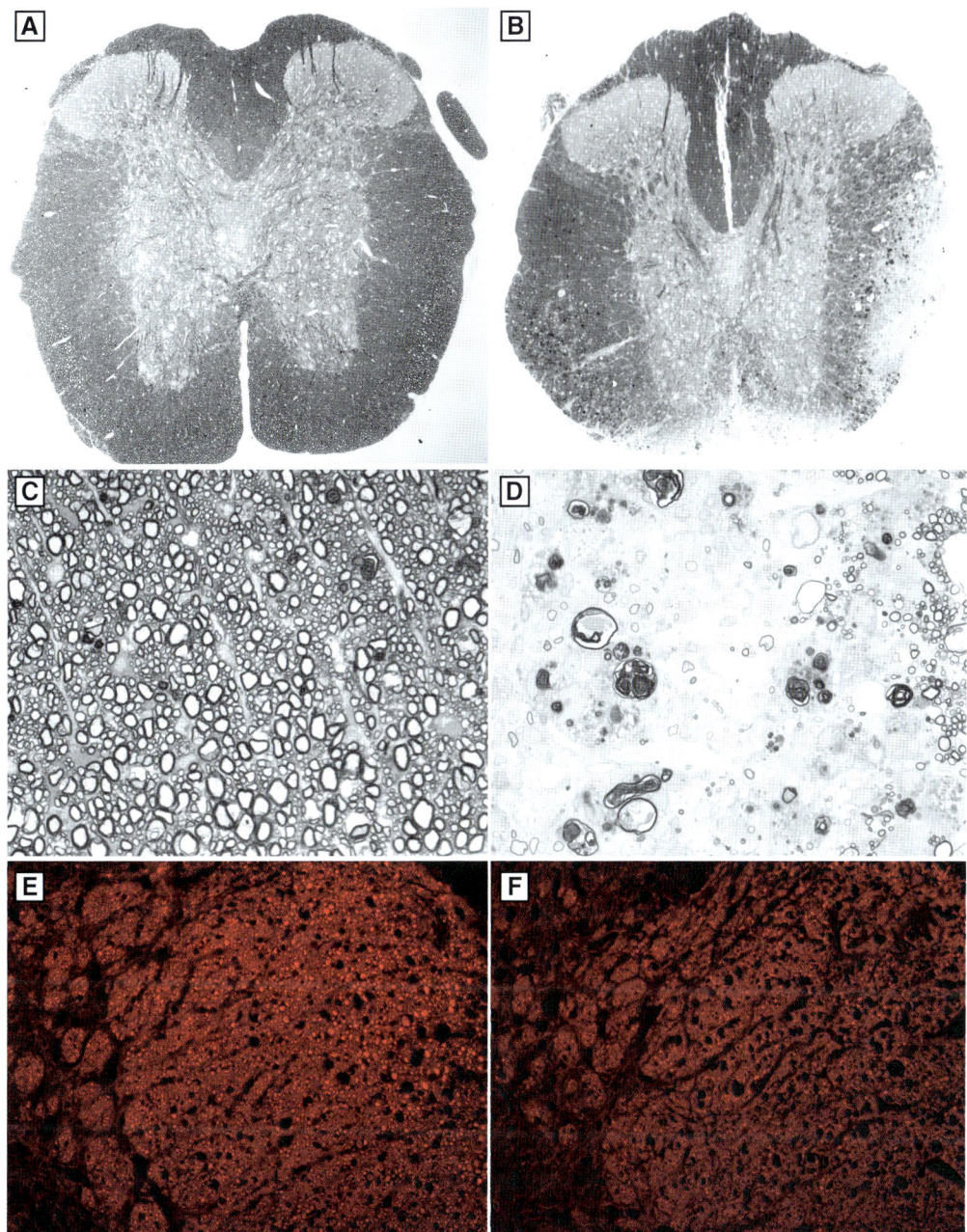

Figure 7 **Evidence of demyelination and axon loss in the Theiler's virus model of MS.** (**A**) Appearance of normal white matter in an uninfected SJL/J mouse. Ultrathin sections of araldite-embedded spinal cord were stained with 4% paraphenylenediamine to visualize myelin. (**B**) Extensive demyelination evident in the spinal cord of an SJL/J mouse infected for 180 days with Theiler's virus. (**C**) Higher magnification of white matter from a normal, uninfected mouse. Note the thick myelin sheaths. (**D**) Higher magnification view of a demyelinated lesion in (**B**). Note the almost complete loss of myelinated profiles, the thinness of the myelin sheaths that are present, and the presence of a large number of dark debris inclusions. (**E**) Immunostaining for the neurofilament heavy chain in an area of normal white matter in an uninfected mouse. Note the intensely stained axon profiles seen in cross-section. (**F**) A comparable region in a mouse chronically infected with Theiler's virus. This demyelinated region shows substantial loss of neurofilament staining.

(Continues)

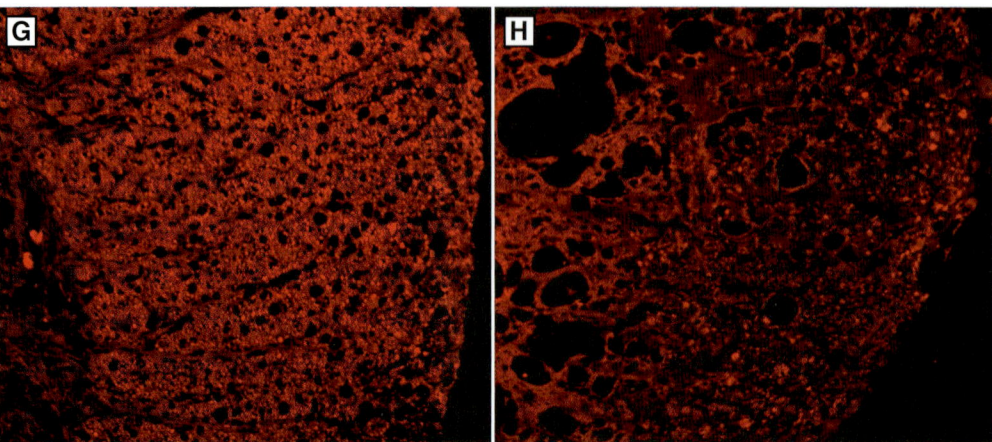

Figure 7—cont'd (**G**) Another example of neurofilament staining in a normally myelinated area of the spinal cord of an uninfected mouse. (**H**) The same location as in (**G**) within the demyelinated lesion of a chronically infected mouse. (**F**) and (**G**) suggest that severe axon loss is associated with demyelination in the Theiler's virus model of MS.

Axon damage is also associated with EAE (Ahmed et al., 2002; Bjartmar and Trapp, 2003; Bjartmar et al., 2003; Kornek et al., 2000, 2001; Linker et al., 2002; Madrid and

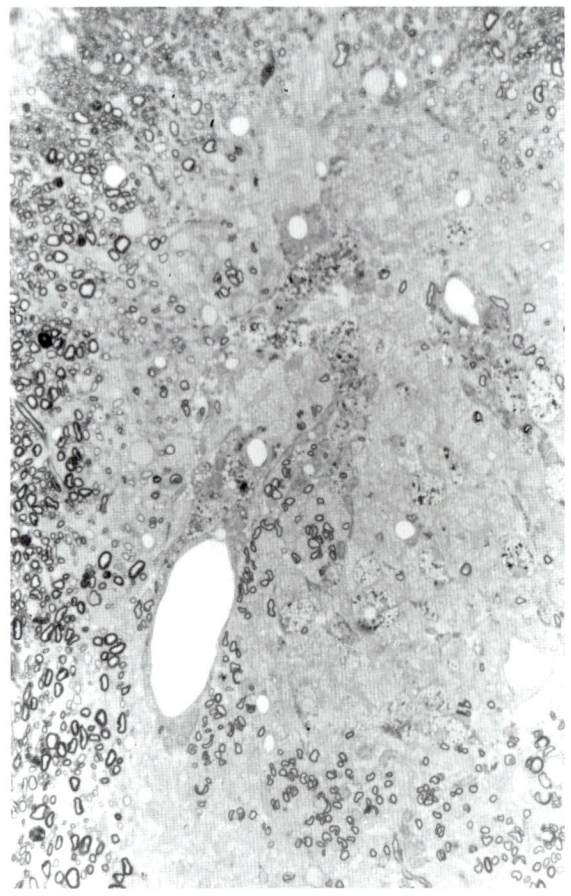

Figure 8 An example of demyelination in the spinal cord associated with EAE. Note the focal nature of the lesion, surrounded by relatively normal appearing white matter.

Wisniewski, 1977; Mancardi et al., 2001; Mead et al., 2002; Penkowa et al., 2003; Penkowa and Hidalgo, 2003; Petzold et al., 2003; Pluchino et al., 2003; Raine and Cross, 1989; Raine et al., 1984; Storch et al., 2002). Both acute axonal damage within actively demyelinating lesions, and chronic axonal injury within inactive lesions and normal-appearing white matter are observed in EAE (Kornek et al., 2000). However, the mechanisms responsible for this axon damage are unclear, and, in contrast to the Theiler's virus model of MS, no study to date has identified a specific effector cell or process that is indispensable for axon injury but dispensable for demyelination.

C. Chemically Induced Demyelination

A variety of toxins, when injected into the spinal cord, rapidly induce demyelinating lesions without significant impact on cells other than oligodendrocytes (Matsushima and Morell, 2001; van Engelen et al., 1997). These include lysolecithin (lysophosphatidylcholine), an activator of phospholipase A_2, and cuprizone, a copper chelator. Although a significant amount of evidence supports the role of the immune system in mediating and repairing the myelin damage induced by these two toxins, very little evidence is available regarding the extent of axon damage associated with these models. That said, Redford et al. (1997) showed that lysolecithin-induced demyelination sensitizes axons to conduction blockade induced by nitric oxide donors, suggesting that naked axons are more susceptible to soluble effector molecules released by immune cells. Likewise, Jean et al. (2002) have described a dramatic reduction in neurofilament staining of axons within lysolecithin-damaged areas, and have shown that acceleration of remyelination with platelet-derived growth factor ameliorates this loss of axon immuno-labeling. Finally, a subtantial reduction in axon caliber was associated with chronic demyelination induced by cuprizone treatment, with axon diameter being reduced to 60% of normal after 16 weeks of demyelination (Mason et al., 2001).

Thus, every major animal model of demyelinating disease is associated with axon damage. Because the methods used to induce demyelination in these models are extremely disparate, and because the cellular effectors of demyelination are variable across each of these models, it seems that axon failure, rather than mechanism of demyelination, is the critical feature of MS and animal models of MS. Therefore, from the perspective of controlling and reversing the neurological dysfunction associated with MS, it is important to understand the cellular mechanisms and the cellular effectors involved in axon damage and axon dropout. Experiments carried out by our group suggest that at least one important cellular effector of axon damage is the CD8+ T-cell.

V. The CD8+ T-Cell Hypothesis

Using the Theiler's virus model of MS, we have investigated the role of MHC class I and class II in the progression of demyelination and the development of functional neurological deficits. We found that C57BL/6 × 129/J mice (H-2^b haplotype) were resistant to demyelination induced by Theiler's virus and never developed clinical disease. In contrast, mice of the identical haplotype that were deficient in expression of MHC class I (C57BL/6 × 129/J β_2-microglobulin$^{-/-}$) developed extensive demyelination (Fig. 9). These animals failed to develop significant clinical signs of functional deficit as measured by hind-limb motor-evoked potentials, spontaneous vertical and horizontal movement assessment, rotarod performance, and activity wheel behavior (Fiette et al., 1993; Pullen et al., 1993; Rivera-Quinones et al., 1998; Rodriguez et al., 1993; Ure and Rodriguez, 2002). On the other hand, mice of the same haplotype that were deficient in expression of MHC class II (C57BL/6 × 129/J Ab^0) developed not only extensive demyelination but also severe neurological impairment, and were, in fact, frequently moribund by 120 days postinfection (Njenga et al., 1996; Rivera-Quinones et al., 1998). Our findings indicate that physiological function was likely preserved secondary to the upregulation and redistribution of sodium channels along demyelinated axons. In fact, whereas chronically infected mice of a susceptible haplotype (SJL/J mice) showed a severe loss of sodium channel density and intensity along axons, chronically infected β_2-microglobulin$^{-/-}$ mice showed a dramatic upregulation and redistribution of axonal sodium channels, even though overall levels of myelin loss and distribution of demyelinated lesions were similiar between the two strains (Rivera-Quinones et al., 1998) (Fig. 10). Furthermore, axons, as marked by either Bielschowski staining or antineurofilament staining, were preserved in chronically infected β_2-microglobulin$^{-/-}$ mice, even in regions of significant cellular infiltrate and demyelination (Fig. 11). In contrast, there was significant disruption and degeneration of axons in chronically infected SJL/J mice (Rivera-Quinones et al., 1998). These findings indicate

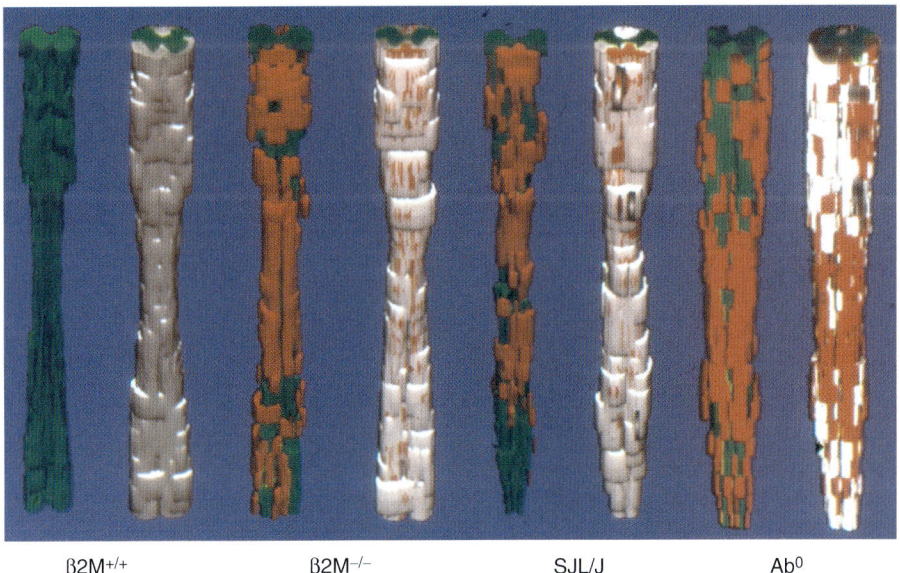

β2M$^{+/+}$ β2M$^{-/-}$ SJL/J   Ab^0

Figure 9 Three-dimensional reconstruction of demyelinated lesions in chronically infected mice. Infected β2m$^{+/+}$ mice do not exhibit demyelination, whereas the extent and distribution of demyelinated lesions is qualitatively similar in class I-deficient mice (β2m$^{-/-}$), SJL/J mice, and class II-deficient mice (Ab^0). For each pair of reconstructions, the left profile shows gray matter (*green*) with an overlay of demyelinated areas (*red*); the right profile shows normal white matter (*white*) and demyelinated lesions (*red*).

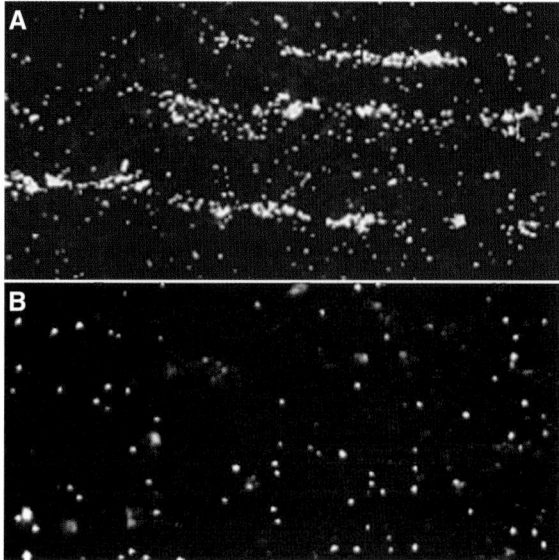

Figure 10 Saxitoxin binding associated with voltage-dependent sodium channels in mouse spinal cord. Normal axons have a distribution of sodium channels corresponding to the spacing of the nodes of Ranvier, and this distribution is integral to the normal saltatory conduction of the axon potential along myelinated axons. After demyelination, sodium channels are redistributed to a more uniform pattern, while axon loss results in loss of sodium channel labeling. (**A**) Spinal cord from infected class I-deficient mice ($\beta2m^{-/-}$) showing evidence of sodium channel redistribution but intense channel labeling. (**B**) In contrast, spinal cord sections from chronically infected SJL/J mice show substantial loss of sodium channel labeling, consistent with a loss of axons.

that MHC class I-restricted CD8⁺ T-cells are likely to be critical mediators of axon damage associated with demyelination in susceptible strains of mice (Fig. 12).

Further evidence in support of this CD8⁺ T-cell hypothesis is provided by our recent studies assessing axon transport in chronically infected mice. Using retrograde labeling of spinal axon tracts, we have demonstrated a failure of retrograde axon transport in mice with demyelination and functional deficits (Ure and Rodriguez, 2000) (Fig. 13). However, we found that retrograde axonal transport was preserved in demyelinated mice with deletion of MHC class I (Ure and Rodriguez, 2002), suggesting that the lack of CD8⁺ cytotoxic T-cells protected axonal integrity while not affecting demyelinated lesion load (Ure and Rodriguez, 2002). A specific CD8+ T-cell-mediated response is further supported by our experiments showing that depletion of antigen-specific cytotoxic T-cells restricted to a viral peptide (VP2$_{121-130}$) resulted in preservation of neurological function, as measured by rotarod performance (Johnson et al., 2001). Therefore, specific presentation of a Theiler's viral epitope within the context of H-2D^b is necessary for at least a component of the neurological dysfunction associated with infection, although VP2 peptide depletion has no effect on the extent of viral infection or the level of demyelination

induced by infection (Johnson et al., 2001). Finally, ongoing experiments in our laboratory indicate that VP2 peptide depletion of the MHC class I cytotoxic T-cell response to Theiler's virus infection preserves spinal axons, as measured by neurofilament staining, axon counting, and retrograde labeling. Thus, antiviral CD8⁺ cytotoxic T-cells are clearly important for the loss of axons and development of neurological dysfunction associated with chronic demyelination in the Theiler's virus model of MS.

The hypothesis that CD8⁺ T-cells are critical in the pathogenesis of Theiler's virus infection is relevant specifically to mice of the H-2^b haplotype. Observations regarding the role of MHC class I in resistance vs. susceptibility to viral persistance and demyelination were made in recombinant inbred strains of the C57BL background (Rodriguez and David, 1985; Rodriguez et al., 1986), and the immunodominant VP2$_{121-130}$ peptide response was observed only in H-2^b mice (Fig. 14). The hypothesis probably does not explain the mechanism of demyelination and neurological deficit in susceptible strains such as SJL/J mice (H-2^s haplotype). For example, disruption of MHC class I function by deletion of β_2-microglobulin in SJL/J mice results in more demyelination and increased neurological deficit (Begolka et al., 2001), and in the SJL/J strain it has been suggested that MHC class II-restricted T-cell response (Miller et al., 1987), and epitope-spreading to myelin antigens may be the mechanism of demyelination and neurological deficit (Croxford et al., 2002; Miller et al., 1997). However, CD8⁺ MHC class I-restricted cytotoxic T-cells have definitely been implicated in human MS, and it is likely that demyelination and neurological dysfunction in humans are a combination of both CD8⁺- and CD4⁺-mediated mechanisms (Neumann, 2003). Recent pathological studies have shown that CD8⁺ T-cells may be the most common subset of T-cells in the MS brain and appear to be clonally expanded in MS lesions (Babbe et al., 2000). Recent experiments in collaboration with Hans Lassmann have demonstrated intense expression of MHC class I in oligodendrocytes, neurons, axons, and astrocytes in the MS lesion (Hoftberger et al., 2003), and autopsy studies have demonstrated that CD8⁺ T-cells are statistically associated with axonal injury in MS (Bitsch et al., 2000). In addition, CD8⁺ T-cells have been shown to injure neurons and transect axons *in vitro* (Medana et al., 2000, 2001), and imaging studies have indicated that axonal loss in MS is a direct correlate for disability (Narayanan et al., 1997; Truyen et al., 1996; van Waesberghe et al., 1999). These studies suggest that CD8⁺ T-cells may be the primary effectors for axonal injury and neurological deficits in MS.

VI. Effector Molecules

Cytotoxic T-cell-induced cytotoxicity is mediated predominantly by two independent pathways. The first is a

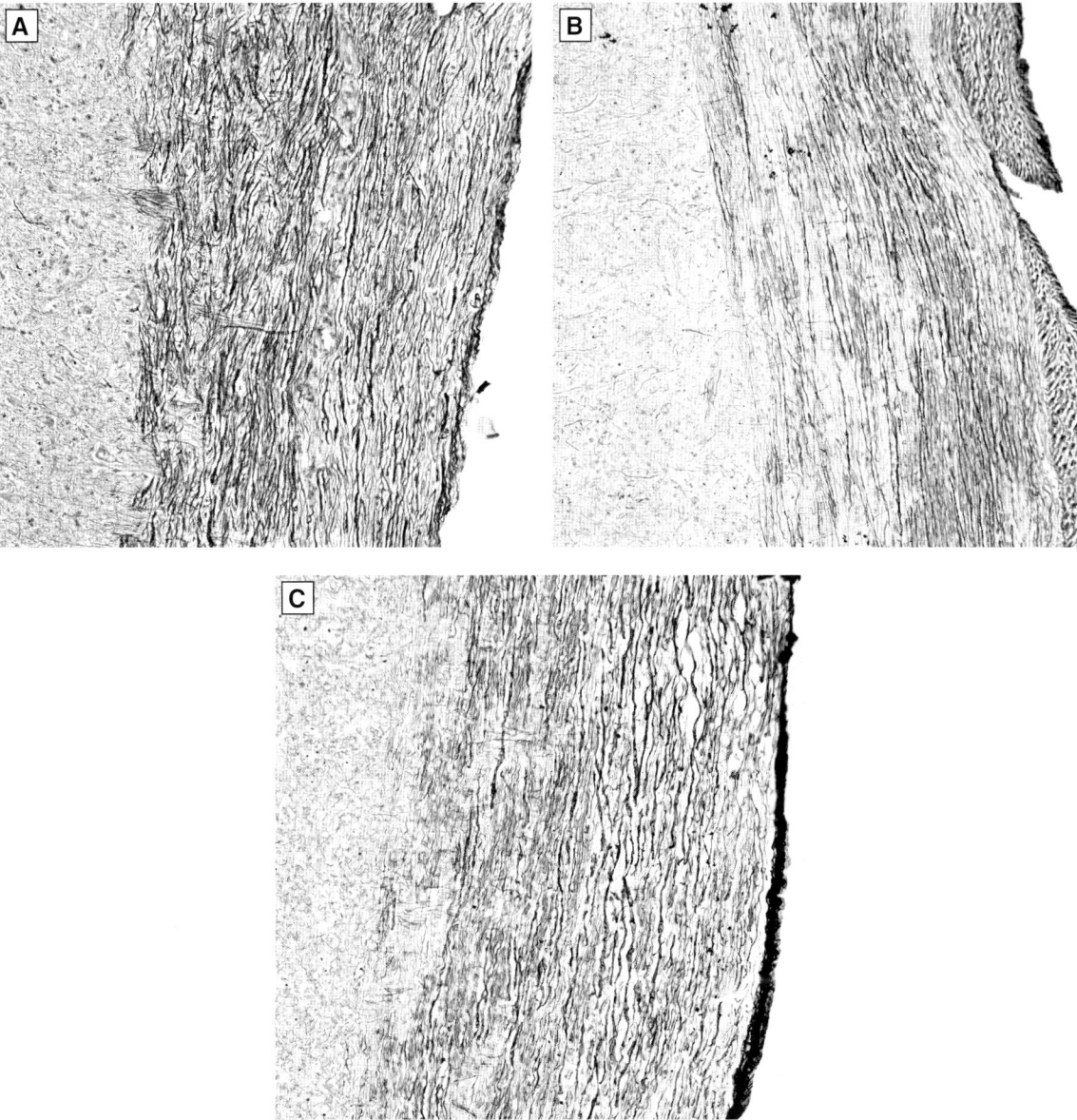

Figure 11 Bielschowski staining of spinal cord sections reveals axon preservation in infected class I-deficient mice ($\beta2m^{-/-}$) and significant axon loss in infected SJL/J mice. (**A**) Normal Bielschowski staining in an uninfected SJL/J mouse. (**B**) Severe loss of axon staining within a demyelinated lesion of an infected SJL/J mouse. (**C**) Preservation of axon staining in a demyelinated lesion of a chronically infected $\beta2m^{-/-}$ mouse.

granule-mediated process involving the pore-forming molecule perforin and granzymes. The second is a receptor ligand interaction that induces apoptosis through Fas (CD95/Apo-1) on the target and Fas ligand (FasL/CD95L/Apo-1ligand) on the effector cell. Both mechanisms are implicated in neurological injury, and both require contact between the target cell and the cytotoxic T-cell. At least one means of such physical contact is the generation of an "immune synapse," formed when the T-cell receptor complex of a cytotoxic T-cell encounters and binds to an MHC class I molecule presenting an appropriate peptide epitope on the surface of a target cell. It was assumed previously that neurons escape immune surveillance through their inability to express MHC class I on the cell surface. However, it has been shown *in vivo* that during pathological processes, the expression of MHC class I on the surface of neurons is rapidly upregulated. For example, after Theiler's virus infection, MHC class I is rapidly upregulated in most CNS cells, including neurons (Altintas et al., 1993; Lindsley et al., 1991). Therefore, after viral infection, axons and neurons become suitable targets for cytotoxic T-cells that are specific for CD8[+]-restricted viral epitopes. In addition, soluble

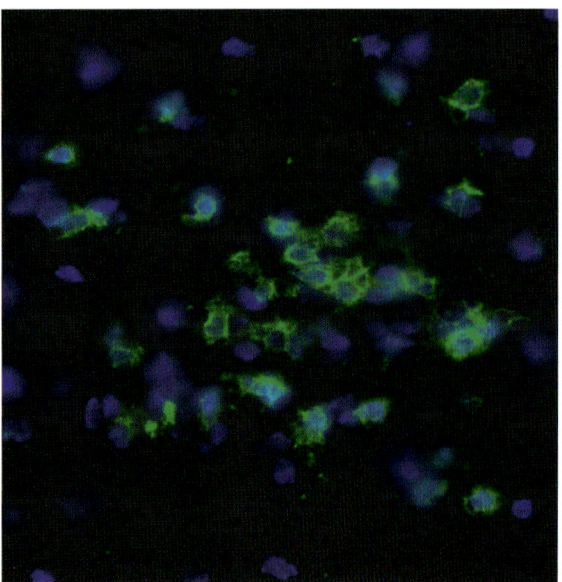

Figure 12 Immunostaining reveals the presence of substantial numbers of CD8[+] T-cells within demyelinated lesions of the spinal cord. Green represents anti-CD8 staining; blue shows DAPI-labeled nuclei.

factors such as interferon-α/β (IFN-α/β), released as a result of infection, appear to be involved in the induction of MHC class I on CNS cells (Njenga et al., 1997b). Of interest, electrically silent neurons upregulate MHC class I molecules on their surface (Neumann et al., 1995), thus predisposing them to cytotoxic attack. This suggests that pathological processes such as demyelination that lead to conduction block may cause axons to become particularly vulnerable to cytotoxic T-cell-mediated killing.

A. Perforin

The dominant mechanism for cytotoxic CD8[+] T-cell-mediated viral clearance and killing of virally infected cells is the release of cytolytic granules containing the pore-forming protein perforin, the proteoglycan serglycin, and a family of serine proteases known as the granzymes. Granzymes A and B are the most abundant granzymes in cytolytic granules, and granzyme B is a mediator of caspase-dependent apoptosis. Granzymes appear to be packaged within the cytolytic granule in complex with serglycin. Approximately 30 to 50 granzyme molecules bind to each molecule of serglycin, forming a large granzyme particle that ranges in size from 40 to 200 nm in diameter. After T-cell receptor recognition of the appropriate peptide/MHC class I complex on target cells and the formation of the immune synapse, the granzyme/serglycin complex and perforin are exocytosed by the cytotoxic T-cell (Lieberman, 2003). Some confusion currently exists regarding the role of perforin in the steps subsequent to cytolytic granule exocytosis, but the current

model suggests that granzymes, either free or in complex with serglycin, bind to the surface of the target cell and are endocytosed. This event appears to occur in the absence of perforin (Froelich et al., 1996; Pinkoski et al., 1998; Shi et al., 1997). Once endocytosed, however, perforin may function to facilitate the transfer of granzymes from target cell endosomes to the cytosol via endosomolysis, apparently without plasma membrane pore formation (Browne et al., 1999; Froelich et al., 1996; Metkar et al., 2002). Regardless of the precise mechanism of action, perforin is clearly required for the full killing function of cytotoxic T-cells, and it was therefore logical to assess the role of perforin in T-cell-mediated axon killing.

Our laboratory has demonstrated, using Theiler's virus infection of C57BL/6 H-2[b] mice, that perforin may be a critical component in the induction of neurological deficits once demyelination is established (Murray et al., 1998). We found that perforin deficiency broke viral resistance, resulting in viral persistence and consequent demyelination (Fig. 15). Despite significant demyelination throughout the spinal cord, however, perforin-deficient C57BL/6 H-2[b] mice failed to develop the significant functional deficits associated with demyelination in susceptible strains of mice. Perforin-deficient mice did not acquire hind-limb paralysis, did not show a decrease in spontaneous activity, and did not develop significant changes in hind-limb stride, suggesting that neurological deficits associated with demyelination are dependent on perforin, and, by extension, on functional cytotoxic T-cells (Murray et al., 1998). Furthermore, we have recently observed that the number of large axons in the spinal cord does not differ between infected wild-type C57BL/6 mice and perforin-deficient C57BL/6 mice, strengthening the argument that neurological function in these animals is preserved as a result of axon preservation. Likewise, perforin contributes to neurological deficit and axon dropout in susceptible B10.Q H-2[q] mice. In these experiments, we found that wild-type B10.Q mice developed significant demyelination, a dramatic decrease in the frequency of large axons in the spinal cord, and significant neurological dysfunction, as measured by rotarod performance, but that large axon frequency and neurological function were relatively preserved in perforin-deficient B10.Q mice, despite marked demyelination.

B. Fas/FasL

Fas is a member of the tumor necrosis factor (TNF) receptor superfamily that is expressed on target cells as a receptor for the Fas ligand (FasL) present on the surface of cytotoxic T-cells. The intracellular domain of Fas contains a death domain (DD) region necessary for induction of apoptosis. Upon binding of FasL to Fas on a target cell, the DD is induced to recruit an adaptor protein called Fas-associated death domain (FADD). FADD bears both a death domain, via which it binds to Fas, and a death effector domain,

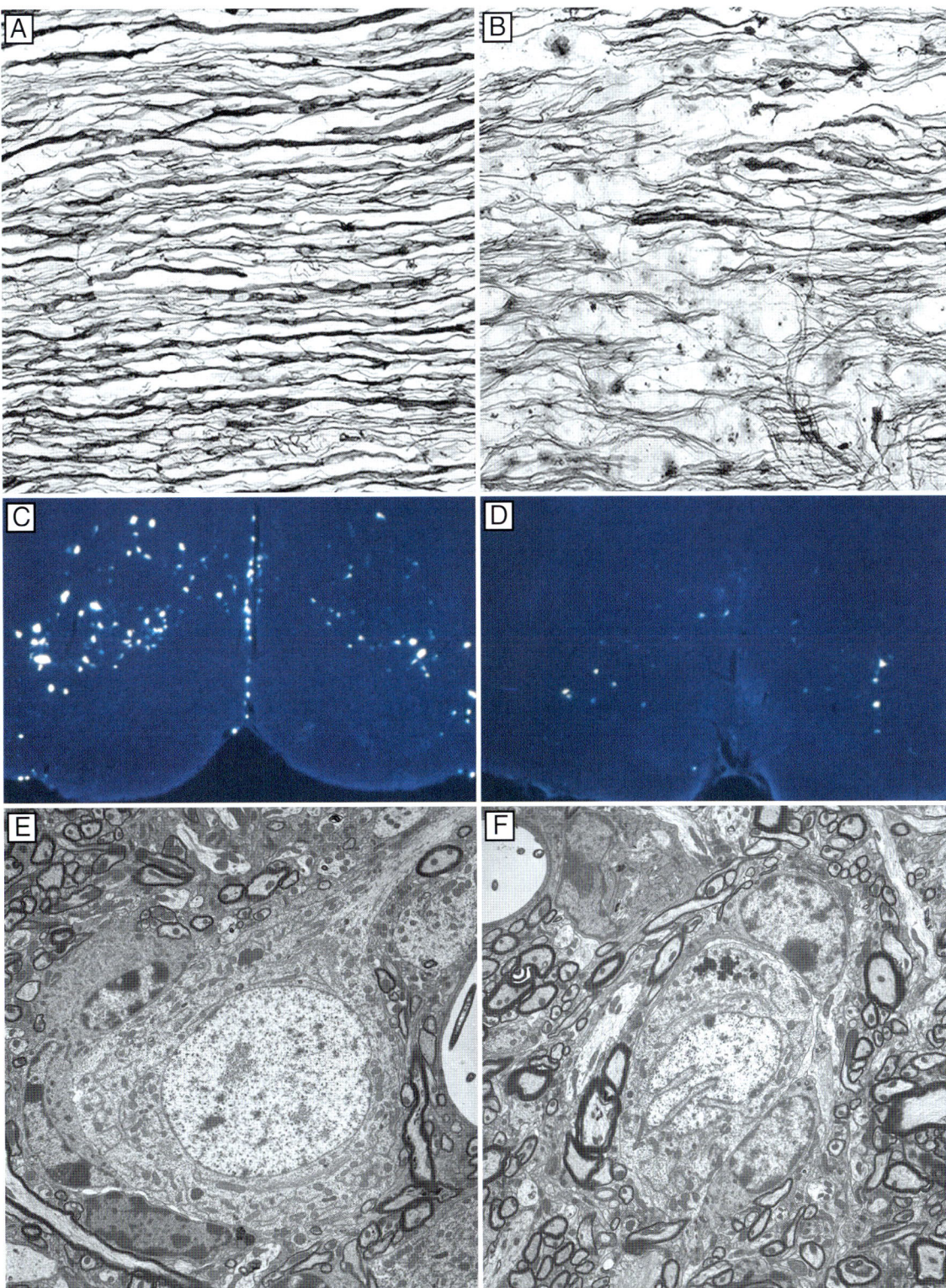

Figure 13 **Chronically infected SJL/J mice exhibit profound loss of axons in the spinal cord.** (**A**) Bielschowski-stained axons in uninfected, aged SJL/J mouse spinal cord. (**B**) Bielschowski-stained axons in the spinal cord of a chronically infected (180 days) SJL/J mouse. Note the loss of stained axons and the relative disarray of the axons that are present. (**C**) Brainstem neurons in an uninfected SJL/J mouse labeled in a retrograde fashion. Fluorogold was applied to the surface of a hemisectioned spinal cord. After recovery and adequate time for retrograde axonal transport of the fluorogold, brainstem and spinal cord were sectioned and analyzed for the presence of fluorogold within neurons of the brainstem. Uninfected animals exhibit reproducible and robust retrograde transport of the dye. (**D**) However, chronically infected SJL/J mice exhibit a profound defect in retrograde transport of fluorogold, suggesting that the descending axons of brainstem neurons are completely lost or dysfunctional. (**E**) Electron micrograph of a normal rubrospinal neuron in an uninfected SJL/J mouse. (**F**) Example of a degenerating rubrospinal neuron in a chronically infected SJL/J mouse. No such degenerating profiles were observed in the uninfected mouse. This finding suggests that the loss of retrograde transport and normal axon staining is correlated with loss of brainstem neurons. This may be the cellular substrate of the neurological deficits observed in these animals.

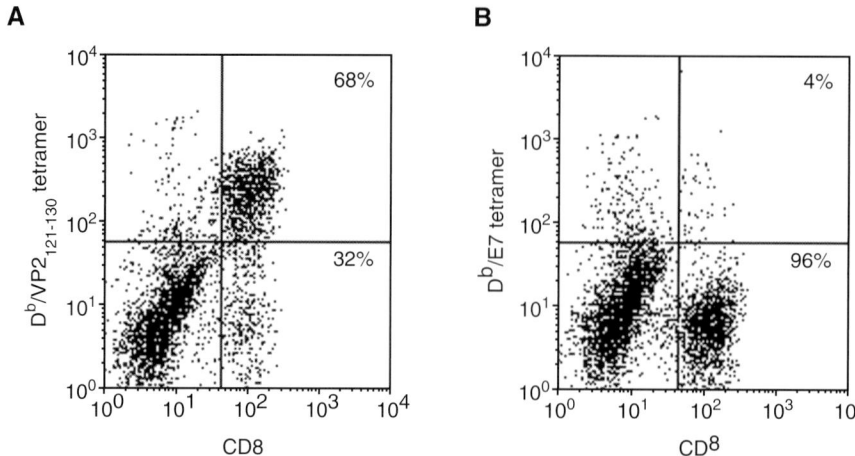

Figure 14 Brain-infiltrating lymphocytes were isolated from mice that were infected for 7 days with Theiler's virus. These cells were stained with fluorescently labeled tetramers that presented either the Theiler's virus immunodominant VP2$_{121-130}$ peptide within the context of H-2D^b or the irrelevant E7 peptide in the context of H-2D^b. Using flow cytometry for analysis of cells positive for tetramer and CD8, we observed that 68% of CD8$^+$ brain infiltrating lymphocytes were specific for the VP2$_{121-130}$ peptide, but only 4% of such cells labeled with the irrelevant tetramer.

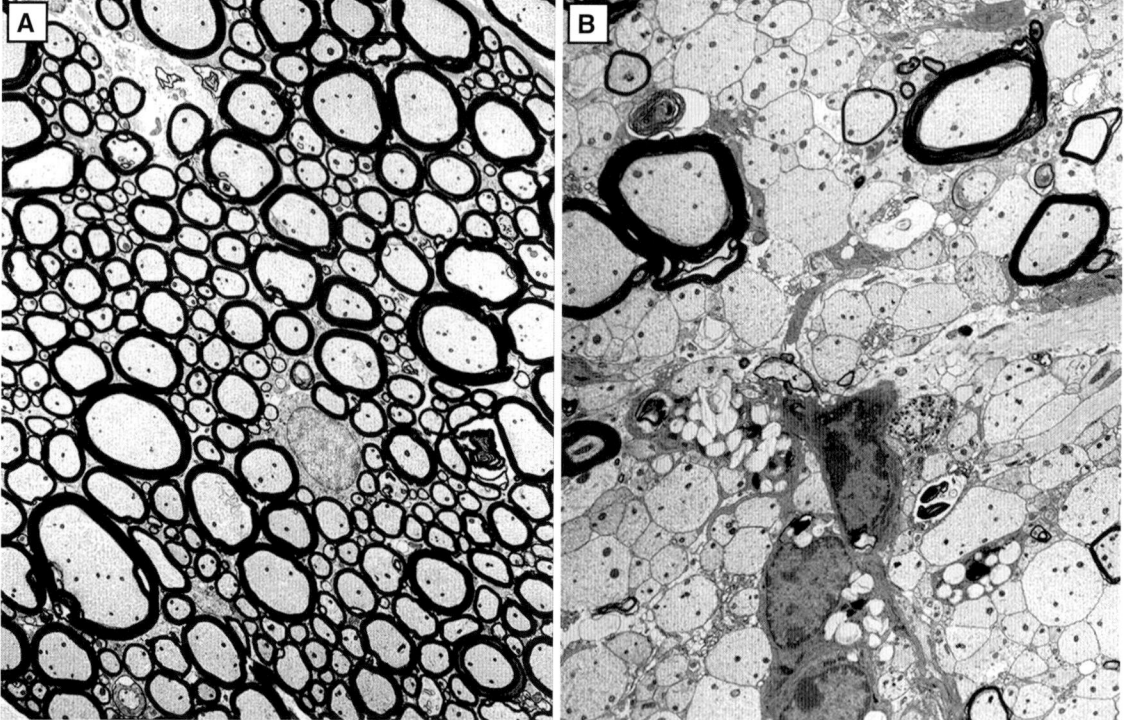

Figure 15 (**A**) Normally myelinated axons in the white matter of an infected C57BL/6 H-2^b mouse. (**B**) Theiler's virus infection of perforin-deficient C57BL/6 H-2^b mice results in extensive demyelination. Despite such widespread demyelination, however, these animals do not exhibit significant functional impairment. This finding suggests that perforin-mediated killing by CD8$^+$ T-cells is required for axon loss and functional deficits, but not for demyelination.

through which it associates with pro-caspase-8. Thus, a death-inducing complex, called the death-inducing signaling complex (DISC), is formed at the Fas receptor. Pro-caspase-8 recruitment to the DISC results in autocleavage and activation of caspase-8, which then goes on to activate effector caspases such as caspase-3, resulting in apoptosis (Thorburn, 2004).

The Fas/FasL pathway is active in essentially all cytotoxic cells, but is apparently most important for CD4[+] cells of the T_H1 phenotype (Ju et al., 1994). Although cultured CD4[+] and CD8[+] T-cells can engage both the perforin and the Fas/FasL pathways, *in vivo* experiments suggest that MHC class I-dependent killing is dominated by the perforin pathway, whereas MHC class II-dependent elimination is almost entirely mediated by Fas/FasL interactions (Graubert et al., 1997; Schulz et al., 1995). Thus, a comparison between the relative role of perforin and Fas/FasL in demyelination and neurological deficit associated with Theiler's virus infection is a reasonable approach to address the CD8[+] hypothesis.

Indeed, in support of the CD8[+] hypothesis, and in contrast to the findings for perforin, the Fas/FasL system appears to play a minimal role in determining resistance to Theiler's virus infection. Neither the *lpr* mutant, deficient in Fas, nor the *gld* mutant, defective in FasL binding, developed demyelination or neurological deficit in response to Theiler's virus infection (Murray et al., 1998). Moreover, Rensing-Ehl and colleagues have reported that neurons express only low levels of Fas, even after cytokine stimulation, and are resistant to FasL-mediated killing (Rensing-Ehl et al., 1996). In contrast, other investigators have suggested that in certain situations, MHC class I-restricted killing of neurons by virus-specific CD8[+] T-lymphocytes is mediated through the Fas/FasL pathway, but not the perforin pathway (Medana et al., 2000). Likewise, the role of Fas/FasL in human MS is less clear than in the Theiler's virus model. Although one report indicates that Fas is irrelevant to oligodendrocyte loss in MS lesions (Bonetti and Raine, 1997), another provides evidence, at least *in vitro*, that Fas-mediated signaling contributes to a nonapoptotic injury of oligodendrocytes. Of particular interest, FasL has been shown to protect neurons against perforin-mediated cytotoxicity (Medana et al., 2001), raising the possibility that both these mechanisms of neuronal killing may interact with one another in as yet uncharacterized, and potentially extremely complicated, ways.

C. Interferon γ

Interferon γ (IFNγ) is another important molecule involved in the effector functions of cytotoxic T-cells. IFNγ is a T_H1 antiviral and immunomodulatory cytokine that is critically involved in host resistance to multiple pathogens. IFNγ induces a wide range of effects on CNS cells, including macrophage activation, enhancement of leukocyte adhe-

sion, release of TNF-α and other cytokines, and upregulation of MHC expression on microglia and macrophages (Munoz-Fernandez and Fresno, 1998). We evaluated the role of IFNγ in protecting neurons from virus-induced injury after infection with Theiler's virus. During viral infections, IFNγ is produced by natural killer (NK) cells, CD4[+], and CD8[+] T-cells; however, the proportion of lymphocyte subsets responding to virus infection influences the contributions to IFNγ-mediated protection. To determine the lymphocyte subsets that produce IFNγ to maintain resistance, we used adoptive transfer strategies to generate mice with lymphocyte-specific deficiencies in IFNγ production. We demonstrated that IFNγ production by both CD4[+] and CD8[+] T-cell subsets is critical for resistance to Theiler's virus-induced demyelination and neurological disease, and that CD4[+] T-cells make a greater contribution to IFNγ-mediated protection. To determine the cellular targets of IFNγ-mediated responses, we used adoptive transfer studies and bone marrow chimerism to generate mice in which either hematopoietic or somatic cells lacked the ability to express IFNγ receptor. We demonstrated that IFNγ receptor must be present on CNS glia, but not bone marrow-derived lymphocytes, in order to maintain resistance to Theiler's virus-induced demyelination (Murray et al., 2002). In addition, we found that both IFNγ[−/−] and IFNγ[+/+] mice of resistant MHC H-2[b] haplotype cleared Theiler's virus infection from spinal motor neurons, but whereas IFNγ[+/+] H-2[b] mice eventually cleared virus from the spinal cord white matter, IFNγ[−/−] H-2[b] mice developed viral persistence in glial cells of the white matter and consequent spinal cord demyelination. Moreover, infection of susceptible H-2[q] haplotype IFNγ[−/−] mice resulted in frequent deaths and severe neurological deficits within 11 to 16 days of infection as compared to infected IFNγ[+/−] H-2[q] littermate controls and parental IFNγ[+/+] H-2[q] B10.Q controls (Fig. 16). Morphological analysis demonstrated severe injury to spinal cord neurons of IFNγ[−/−] H-2[q] mice during early infection, with less than 20% of mice surviving 45 days after infection. More viral RNA was detected in the brain and spinal cord of IFNγ[−/−] H-2[q] mice as compared to IFNγ[+/−] H-2[q] or IFNγ[+/+] H-2[q] mice at 14 and 21 days after TMEV infection, and virus antigen was localized predominantly to spinal motor neurons in infected IFNγ[−/−] H-2[q] mice. Virus antigen persisted in neurons in these mice for as long as 45 days after infection. IFNγ deletion did not affect the humoral response directed against the virus; however, there was less expression of CD4, CD8, MHC class I, and MHC class II in the CNS of IFNγ[−/−] H-2[q] mice as compared to IFNγ[+/+] H-2[q] mice. Finally, *in vitro* analysis of virus-induced death of NSC-34 spinal motor neurons and primary spinal motor neurons showed that IFNγ exerted a neuroprotective effect in the absence of other aspects of the immune response (Rodriguez et al., 2003) (Fig. 16). These findings suggest that IFNγ plays a critical role in protecting spinal cord neurons from persistent infection and death, and that

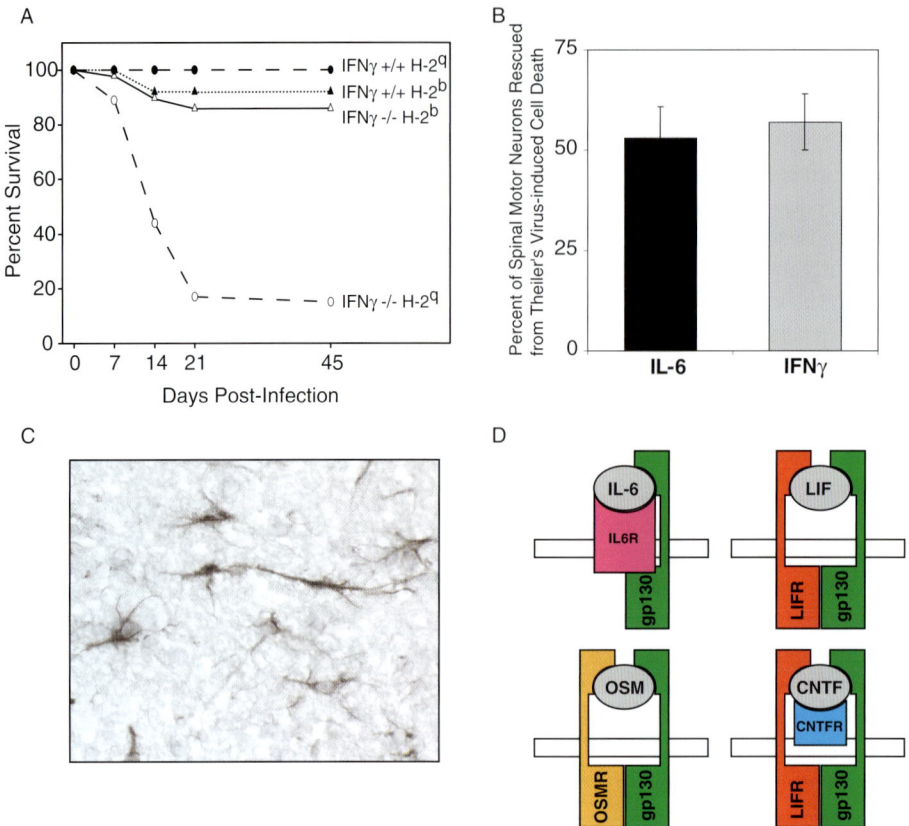

Figure 16 Interferon-γ and IL-6 function as neuroprotective factors during Theiler's virus infection. (**A**) Susceptible IFNγ$^{-/-}$ mice on an H-2^q background exhibit dramatically reduced survival and significant neurological impairment after infection with Theiler's virus as compared to IFNγ$^{+/+}$ H-2^q mice and H-2^b mice. (**B**) Spinal motor neurons infected *in vitro* with Theiler's virus exhibit profound apoptotic death. Treatment of these cells with IFNγ or IL-6 rescued approximately half of the cells in culture without affecting the extent of infection. This suggests that IFNγ and IL-6 directly stimulated the survival of spinal motor neurons. (**C**) After Theiler's virus infection astrocytes dramatically upregulate expression of IL-6, suggesting that they may be the local source of this factor necessary for protection of neurons. (**D**) IL-6, leukemia inhibitory factor (LIF), oncostatin M (OSM), and ciliary neurotrophic factor (CNTF) all share the gp130 receptor subunit, suggesting that the neuroprotective signaling effects of all of these molecules may be mediated in common by gp130.

the cells responsible for production of this protective IFNγ appear to be cytotoxic T-cells. Thus, a model in which CD8$^+$ T-cells attack and kill axons and neurons via perforin must also include CD8$^+$ and CD4$^+$ T-cells that release potentially neuroprotective cytokines that accelerate viral clearance while sparing irreplacable neurons.

D. Other Cytokines

In addition to IFNγ, other cytokines also display unexpected neuroprotective effects. For example, we have shown that interleukin-6 (IL-6) protects anterior horn neurons from death induced by Theiler's virus without altering the development of the normal antiviral humoral response or the development of normal viral titer (Pavelko et al., 2003).

Instead, we found that IL-6 protects anterior horn neurons, as well as NSC-34 motor neurons (Cashman et al., 1992), from death induced by viral infection via a direct neuroprotective mechanism (Pavelko et al., 2003) (Fig. 16). This finding is in agreement with other reports that IL-6 promotes neurite outgrowth and survival of cultured enteric neurons (Schafer et al., 1999), and that IL-6 delays the progression of motor neuron disease in wobbler mice (Ikeda et al., 1996). Infection with a neurotropic coronavirus activated astrocytes to produce IL-6 (Sun et al., 1995), and we observed a similar upregulation in astrocytic expression of IL-6 after Theiler's virus infection (Pavelko et al., 2003) (Fig. 16). Therefore, we suggest that IL-6, normally considered to be an immune modulator during inflammation, signals to protect motor neurons from death, potentially in a manner analogous to ciliary neurotrophic factor (CNTF), a neurotrophic factor that also uses the gp130 signal transduction module (Pavelko et al., 2003; Ransohoff et al., 2002) (Fig. 16). The relevance of IL-6-mediated neuroprotection to MS remains to be delineated, but the concentrations of IL-6 receptor components are altered in the cerebrospinal fluid and serum of patients with MS (Padberg et al., 1999), suggesting that IL-6 signaling may be important to protect neurons during a demyelinating insult (Ransohoff et al., 2002).

A variety of other cytokines are also implicated in MS and animal models of MS, including TNFα (Arnett et al., 2001, 2003; Paya et al., 1990), CNTF (Linker et al., 2002), leukemia inhibitory factor (Butzkueven et al., 2002), oncostatin M (Repovic et al., 2003), IL-10 (Petereit et al., 2003), and IL-4 (Hulshof et al., 2002), and a number of these cytokines use the common gp130 signal transduction module described previously. However, the exact mechanism(s) via which these factors function in MS, and the role each may play in protection of axons and neurons from damage or death associated with demyelination, remains to be discovered. Likewise, numerous neurotrophic factors and cytokines are known to support the survival of neurons and axons, including nerve growth factor, brain-derived neurotrophic factor, neurotrophin-3, neurotrophin-4/5, glial cell line-derived neurotrophic factor, CNTF (Ransohoff et al., 2002; Sofroniew et al., 2001), insulin-like growth factor-1 (Kaspar et al., 2003), vascular endothelial growth factor (Lambrechts et al., 2003), hepatocyte growth factor (Sun et al., 2002), cardiotrophin-like cytokine/cytokine-like factor 1 (Forger et al., 2003; Ransohoff et al., 2002), and other immune cell-derived factors (Yin et al., 2003). The role of each of these factors in limiting neurological dysfunction in MS is unknown, but is likely to be important, both for understanding the pathophysiology of the disease and for designing appropriate therapeutic interventions (Ransohoff et al., 2002). Moreover, the complexity of interactions possible between these factors and between elements of the immune system is certainly a critical consideration (Bonini et al., 2003). Obviously, the most efficacious therapy will be one that displays exquisite sensitivity and specificity. We have proposed the use of growth factor-like natural autoantibodies to rapidly promote remyelination, and thereby protect axons from the deleterious effects of exposure to immune effectors.

VII. Protection of Axons via Facilitation of Remyelination

The existence of pathogenic autoantibodies is well established for several peripheral neurological syndromes including myasthenia gravis, Lambert-Eaton syndrome, Guillain-Barré syndrome, and acquired neuromyotonia (Vincent et al., 1999). Involvement of pathogenic autoantibodies in a particular disease has been defined by several lines of experimental and clinical evidence. For example, antibodies to a defined target should be present in the majority of patients that present with the disease. The presence of these antibodies is often demonstrated by using the purified antibodies to immunostain tissues that express the target antigen. Moreover, immunization with the target antigen, passive transfer of antibodies against the antigen, or transfer of antibodies from patients with the disease to naïve animals should induce disease. Finally, reduction of serum antibody levels, by plasma exchange or by immunosuppression, generally leads to clinical improvement in patients, whereas an increase in antibody levels induces a return of clinical symptoms. Autoantibodies may also play a role in MS. When antibodies to myelin oligodendrocyte glycoprotein (MOG) are injected after the induction of EAE, the severity of the disease is dramatically increased and large demyelinating lesions develop (Genain et al., 1995; Linington et al., 1992; Schluesener et al., 1987). In addition, antibodies to MOG have been detected in association with disintegrating myelin in both human MS patients and in a marmoset model of EAE (Genain et al., 1999). Likewise, EAE-like Type II MS lesions, responsible for 30% to 50% of lesions in patients, are characterized by the deposition of immunoglobulin and complement (Lucchinetti et al., 1998, 2000). Finally, we have shown that plasma exchange is effective in approximately 40% of cases with fulminant MS exacerbations, suggesting the presence of pathogenic autoantibodies in these patients (Weinshenker et al., 1999).

In a novel application of many of the same criteria used to define pathogenic antibodies, we have tried to define autoantibodies that promote tissue repair. A direct demonstration that autoreactive antibodies can enhance endogenous myelin repair came from our studies using Theiler's virus to induce chronic demyelinating disease in mice (Rodriguez et al., 1987a). As described previously, intracerebral infection of susceptible mice with Theiler's virus results in a disease course characterized by acute encephalitis that is resolved in 14 to 21 days, followed by chronic viral persistence in spinal cord white matter. Persistent Theiler's virus infection eventually leads to chronic demyelination and progressive loss of motor function, a clinical pattern similar to that observed for progressive MS in humans. Myelin pathology in Theiler's virus infected mice is immune-mediated, with chronically infected animals demonstrating a wide range of disease phenotypes depending on their specific genetic background. In the SJL strain, demyelination is evident within 30 days after infection and by 1 to 3 months the animals develop neurological deficits including spasticity and gait abnormalities, weakness of the lower extremities, and bladder incontinence. Paralysis eventually occurs by 6 to 9 months after infection. Spontaneous remyelination is common in many mouse strains, but is limited in the SJL strain; often less than 10% of the total demyelinated lesion area is repaired. The low background of spontaneous repair in these animals makes them an excellent model for the study of strategies to promote endogenous remyelination (Rodriguez et al., 1987b).

Our initial observation of a beneficial humoral immune response occurred when significant remyelination was demonstrated in SJL mice that were chronically infected with Theiler's virus and immunized with spinal cord homogenate (SCH) prepared in incomplete Freund's adjuvant. Histological examination of spinal cord lesions from immunized animals revealed substantial remyelination compared to control animals. Passive transfer of antiserum (Rodriguez et al., 1987a) or purified immunoglobulin (Rodriguez and Lennon, 1990) from uninfected animals that had been immunized with SCH also enhanced remyelination in infected SJL mice, directly demonstrating for the first time a beneficial role of the humoral immune response in promoting myelin repair. This enhancement of remyelination was associated with

proliferation or preservation of mature oligodendrocytes (Ludwin and Bakker, 1988; Prayoonwiwat and Rodriguez, 1993).

To further explore the nature of this beneficial immune response, hybridomas were generated from SJL mice after SCH immunization, in an attempt to identify monoclonal antibodies that promote remyelination. Two mouse monoclonal antibodies that enhance remyelination were identified and designated SCH94.03 and SCH79.08 (Miller et al., 1994) (Fig. 17). Both of these monoclonal antibodies are polyreactive IgMs that bind to antigens on the surface of oligodendrocytes, suggesting that the activity of these monoclonal antibodies may involve direct stimulation of the myelin-producing cells (Asakura et al., 1996). Four additional oligodendrocyte-specific mouse IgMs (O4, O1, A2B5, and HNK1) were also shown to promote CNS remyelination (Asakura et al., 1998), suggesting that this phenomenon was a general principle rather than an isolated immunological aberration.

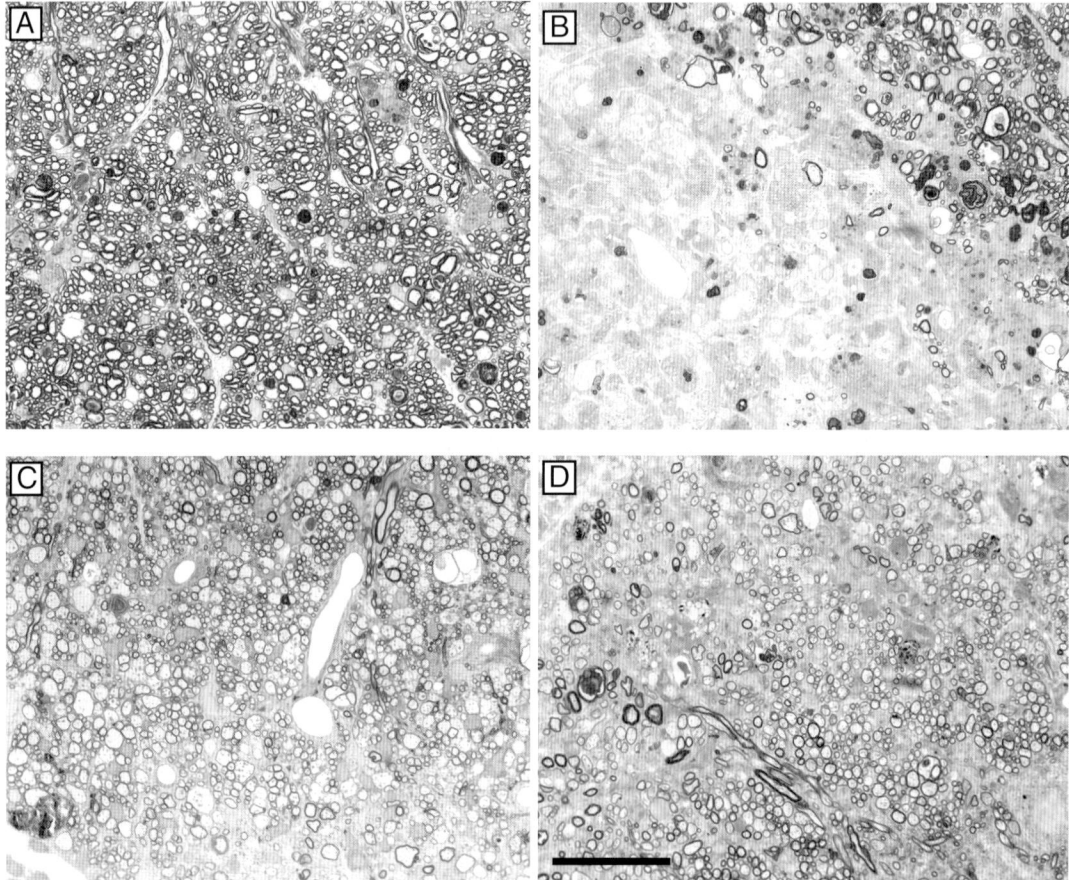

Figure 17 **Antibody-mediated remyelination.** (**A**) Normal myelin in an uninfected SJL/J mouse. (**B**) Severe demyelination is observed in a chronically infected SJL/J mouse. (**C**) Five weeks after a single treatment with the mouse IgM 94.03 there is significant remyelination within demyelinated lesions of a chronically infected SJL/J mouse. (**D**) Likewise, 5 weeks after a single treatment with the human antibody rHIgM22 there is a dramatic increase in remyelinated axons within demyelinated lesions. Scale bar in (**D**) is 50 μm and refers to all panels.

Using oligodendrocyte binding as a screening assay, we identified candidate human monoclonal antibodies that might also promote remyelination (Warrington et al., 2000). Human monoclonal antibodies were isolated from patients with monoclonal gammopathy, a relatively common condition characterized by high concentrations of monoclonal serum antibody. A total of 52 serum-derived human monoclonal IgMs (sHIgMs) were screened, and six were found to bind to the surface of morphologically mature rat oligodendrocytes in culture. In contrast, none of the 50 serum-derived human monoclonal IgGs (sHIgG) bound to oligodendrocytes. The six oligodendrocyte-binding sHIgMs were tested *in vivo*, and two, designated sHIgM22 and sHIgM46, were found to promote substantial remyelination (Warrington et al., 2000) (Fig. 17). More recently, we have engineered a recombinant form of sHIgM22, designated rHIgM22, that exhibits the same pattern of oligodendrocyte binding (Fig. 18) and induces the same level of remyelination as sHIgM22 (Mitsunaga et al., 2002) (Fig. 17). Generation of this recombinant monoclonal human IgM marked an important step forward in the production of a potential therapeutic agent aimed at ameliorating demyelination in patients with MS, as this antibody is available in essentially unlimited quantities and will not induce cross-species reactivity if administered to humans.

As outlined previously, there are several properties used to define autoantibodies as pathogenic agents. Similar criteria can be applied to autoreactive antibodies involved in tissue repair. For example, recognition of appropriate tissues or molecules is an important defining characteristic. All of the antibodies that promote remyelination bind to antigens on the surface of oligodendrocytes, suggesting that these antibodies function through direct stimulation of the myelin-producing cells. It is important to note that these antibodies are polyreactive, recognizing a variety of chemical haptens and proteins as measured by enzyme-linked immunosorbent assay, and also robustly recognizing intracellular proteins in permeablized cells. Despite this antigenic promiscuity, however, remyelination-promoting antibodies bind only to a limited number of antigens on the surface of live oligodendrocytes. The surface antigens bound by several of these monoclonal antibodies have been characterized and are generally lipid or carbohydrate in nature (Asakura et al., 1998; Sommer and Schachner, 1981).

Remyelination-promoting antibodies appear to be naturally occurring autoantibodies. Antibodies of this type are present in the serum of normal individuals and are often polyreactive IgMs capable of binding to a variety of structurally unrelated, self and non-self antigens (Lacroix-Desmazes et al., 1998). Such antibodies may represent a primordial form of the immune system that evolved to perform largely physiological functions rather than classical immune functions (Bouvet and Dighiero, 1998; Stewart, 1992). One of these nonimmunological functions may be to promote tissue repair, serving effectively as trophic factors for specific cell types (Bieber et al., 2001).

The concept of an endogenous antibody-mediated repair system is consistent with our initial observation of enhanced remyelination after SCH or myelin antigen immunization (Rodriguez et al., 1987a). Immunization may mimic immune system exposure to CNS antigens that occurs after injury, resulting in an increased titer of anti-CNS antibodies. Human IgMs from patients with macroglobulinemia were found to bind at high frequency to myelin antigens, suggesting that anti-CNS antibodies are common in the serum of individuals with no history of neurological damage (Warrington et al., 2000). Therefore, increasing the serum concentration of specific anti-CNS monoclonal antibodies may be a novel therapeutic treatment for human neurological injury and disease.

Because all of the remyelination-promoting monoclonal antibodies that we have identified so far bind to oligodendrocytes or myelin, it seems reasonable to suggest a direct effect on the recognized cells. Other laboratories have demonstrated that oligodendrocyte-specific antibodies can induce biochemical and morphological changes in glial cells. For example, Dyer and colleagues showed that antibodies directed against oligodendrocyte surface epitopes, including antibodies to galactocerebroside, sulfatide, and myelin/oligodendrocyte-specific protein, can induce changes in the organization of oligodendrocyte plasma membrane and can alter cytoskeletal structure (Dyer and Benjamins, 1988; 1989; Dyer and Matthieu, 1994). These changes in cellular structure were preceded by antibody-induced calcium influx (Dyer, 1993; Dyer and Benjamins, 1990; 1991), suggesting that the gating of calcium may play an important role in the regulation of oligodendrocyte structure and function, and may play a role in antibody-induced remyelination. In support of this hypothesis, we recently reported similar changes in intracellular calcium concentration in oligodendrocytes after treatment with remyelination-promoting monoclonal antibodies (Howe et al., 2004; Paz Soldan et al., 2003). We assessed the direct effect of mouse and human monoclonal IgMs on CNS glial cells by using ratiometric fluorescent monitoring of intracellular calcium concentration ($[Ca^{2+}]_i$). A change in $[Ca^{2+}]_i$ was used as a marker for physiological activation. We found that remyelination-promoting antibodies stimulated a transient elevation of $[Ca^{2+}]_i$ in both astrocytes and oligodendrocytes. Of importance, all remyelination-promoting antibodies tested evoked Ca^{2+} transients in mixed glial cultures; isotype- and species-matched control antibodies did not (Paz Soldan et al., 2003) (Fig. 19).

We observed calcium responses of two types: a rapid transient calcium increase that occurred immediately upon exposure to antibody, and a slower transient calcium increase that was slightly delayed after antibody exposure. Morphological examination of the responding cells revealed

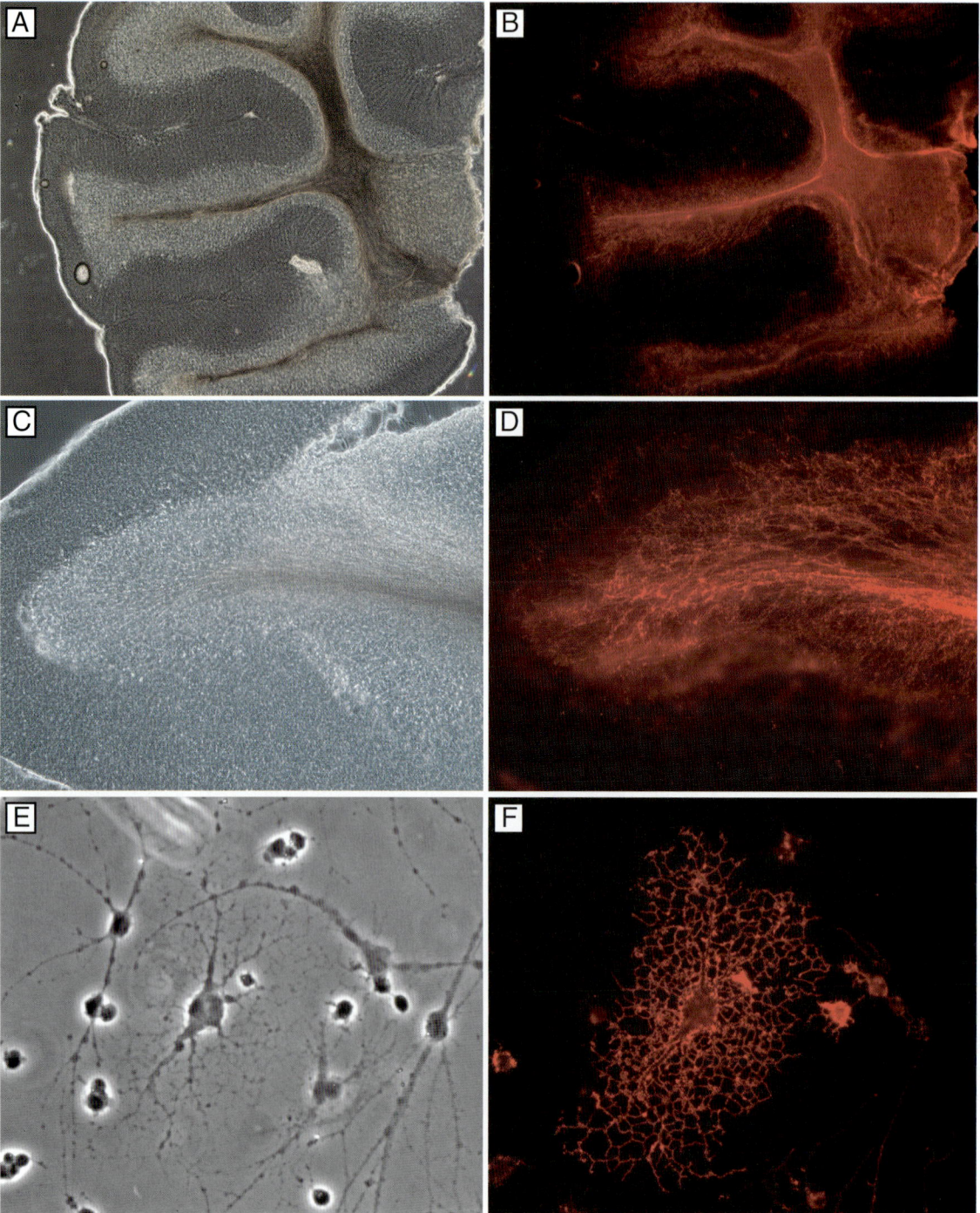

Figure 18 **rHIgM22 stains white matter and human oligodendrocytes.** (**A**) Phase contrast image of a slice of mouse cerebellum. The phase dark material is white matter. (**B**) rHIgM22 specifically stains the white matter tracts of the same cerebellar section shown in (**A**). (**C**) Higher magnification phase contrast view of a white matter tract in the cerebellum. (**D**) rHIgM22 staining in the same section shown in (**C**). Note the finely stained myelinated axons. (**E**) Phase contrast image of human glial cells, with a mature, highly branched oligodendrocyte present in the center of the field. (**F**) rHIgM22 only labels the oligodendrocyte. Note the extensive labeling of the elaborate myelin branches.

that the immediate type response occurred in astrocytes, whereas the delayed type response occurred in oligodendrocytes (Paz Soldan et al., 2003). We also investigated the state of differentiation in oligodendrocytes that showed the delayed calcium response, and found that approximately 60% of delayed response cells showed surface immunoreac-

A

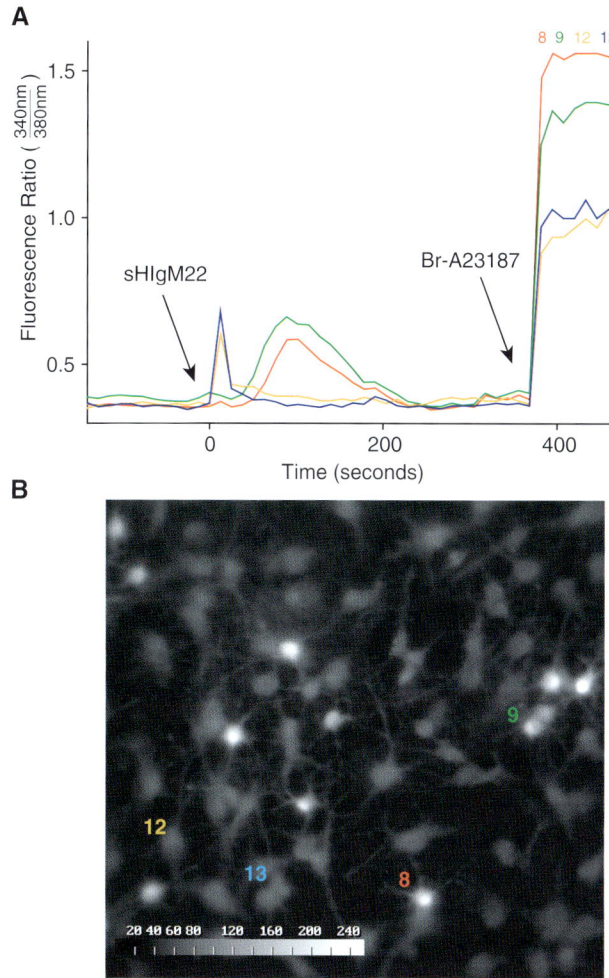

B

Figure 19 sHIgM22 induces transient calcium influx in mixed glial cells in culture as detected by ratiometric imaging using Fura-2. (**A**) Immediately after treatment with sHIgM22, there is a brief influx of calcium in astrocytes, followed by a slower but transient influx of calcium in oligodendrocytes. Ionophore (Bromo-A23187) induces maximal calcium influx in all cells. (**B**) Fluorescent image of two cells (8, 9) fluxing calcium in response to sHIgM22 treatment. It is important to note that after treatment with antibody, calcium levels return to baseline, suggesting that the calcium influx is not toxic but is rather an element in a specific signal transduction cascade elicited by the antibody.

tivity to A2B5, a marker for preoligodendrocytes. The remaining 40% of cells exhibiting the delayed type response showed surface immunoreactivity to O4, an antisulfatide antibody that serves as a marker for more mature oligodendrocytes (Paz Soldan et al., 2003).

Further characterization showed that the immediate astrocyte and delayed oligodendrocyte responses use distinct Ca^{2+} entry pathways. We found that the immediate Ca^{2+} response occurred in either the presence or absence of extracellular calcium, but that thapsigargin-induced depletion of endoplasmic reticulum calcium stores abrogated this response. In contrast, the delayed type response was pre-

vented by removal and chelation of extracellular Ca^{2+} (Paz Soldan et al., 2003). Moreover, although the number of cells exhibiting an immediate response to treatment with the O4 monoclonal IgM was not affected by blocking several classes of plasma membrane Ca^{2+} channels, pharmacologically blocking the activity of phospholipase C (PLC) significantly decreased the percentage of astrocytes that exhibited elevated intracellular Ca^{2+}. In contrast, the delayed Ca^{2+} response in oligodendrocytes was not dependent on intracellular stores, but was sensitive to pharmacological inhibition of Ca^{2+} flux through α-amino-3-hydroxy-5-methyl-4-isoxazolepropionic acid (AMPA)-sensitive glutamate channels (Paz Soldan et al., 2003). These data support the conclusion that the delayed response in oligodendrocytes is dependent on Ca^{2+} entry through AMPA receptor Ca^{2+} channels, whereas the immediate response in astrocytes is dependent on Ca^{2+} release from endoplasmic reticulum stores, likely through PLC-mediated generation of IP_3 and gating of IP_3-sensitive calcium channels.

We also determined that the antigen-binding domain of remyelination-promoting antibodies is required for Ca^{2+} signaling in glial cells. As described previously, Theiler's virus-infected mice treated with mouse monoclonal IgM antibody 94.03 exhibit enhanced remyelination. In contrast, mice treated with species- and isotype-matched control monoclonal antibody CH12 exhibit fourfold to sixfold less myelin repair, similar to saline treatment; 94.03 and CH12 have greater than 99% amino acid identity, differing only in the third complementarity determining region (CDR3) by five amino acids (Asakura et al., 1998). The CDR3 is critical in the formation of the antigen-binding domain, and the difference in remyelination potential engendered by the sequence difference between 94.03 and CH12 suggests that antigen specificity, rather than some other component of antibody structure, is required for remyelination. Finally, mixed primary glial cultures exposed to SCH 94.03 exhibited a transient rise in $[Ca^{2+}]_i$, while similar cultures exposed to CH12 showed no calcium changes. Therefore, remyelination-promoting antibody-induced Ca^{2+} signaling in glial cells depends on antigen specificity defined by the CDR3 region of the antibody.

Of primary importance, antibody-mediated Ca^{2+} signaling *in vitro* correlated statistically with remyelination promotion *in vivo*. To establish a relationship between the ability of an antibody to elicit a Ca^{2+} response and its ability to promote remyelination, we studied several remyelination-promoting and control antibodies. Mouse remyelination-promoting antibodies SCH 94.03, SCH 79.08, and O4 all mediated Ca^{2+} responses in astrocytes and oligodendrocytes. The control mouse antibody CH12, which did not promote remyelination, also did not evoke Ca^{2+} responses. Likewise, human remyelination-promoting antibodies sHIgM22, sHIgM46, and CB2BG8 all mediated Ca^{2+} responses in astrocytes and oligodendrocytes, whereas the control human antibodies sHIgM12, sHIgM14, sHIgM47, and AKJR4, which did not promote remyelination, did not evoke Ca²⁺ responses (Paz Soldan et al., 2003). Thus, there appears to be a high degree of correlation between the ability of monoclonal IgM antibodies to promote remyelination and the stimulation of calcium influx, suggesting a potential signaling connection between these two phenomena.

Further evidence in support of a causal link between calcium signaling and remyelination is provided by experiments showing that rHIgM22 elicits a transient elevation in intracellular calcium in CG4 cells, a model of premyelinating oligodendrocytes (Howe et al., 2004). As with primary oligodendrocytes, we found that this calcium signal was dependent on the influx of extracellular calcium through AMPA receptor calcium channels. More importantly, we showed that rHIgM22 was able to rescue CG4 cells from death induced by either hydrogen peroxide or TNFα, and that this rescue was dependent on calcium flux through CNQX-sensitive calcium channels (Howe et al., 2004). Biochemically, rHIgM22 appears to block cell death by preventing c-jun N-terminal kinase (JNK) signaling and caspase-3 activation. In support of this model for rHIgM22 survival signaling, we also found that antibody treatment of SJL mice chronically infected with Theiler's virus led to a significant decrease in caspase family gene expression and caspase-3 activity within demyelinated lesions of the cervical spinal cord (Howe et al., 2004). As rHIgM22 induced substantial remyelination in these animals, we concluded that rHIgM22-induced calcium signaling blocked caspase-3 activation in premyelinating oligodendrocytes and thereby promoted their survival and consequent differentiation into myelin-producing oligodendrocytes (Howe et al., 2004).

Another important clue as to the mechanism of remyelination-promoting antibody action was provided by experiments showing that the ability of rHIgM22 to induce calcium influx and rescue CG4 cells from death was dependent on the integrity of lipid rafts in the plasma membrane of these cells (Howe et al., 2004). Treatment with β-methylcyclodextrin, a cholesterol-chelating compound that effectively destroys lipid raft structure, prevented rHIgM22-induced survival signaling, suggesting that perhaps redistribution or aggregation of lipid raft domains is necessary for antibody-mediated signal transduction (Howe et al., 2004) (Fig. 20). This hypothesis is further supported by evidence that monovalent forms of sHIgM22 are unable to elicit remyelination or calcium signaling (Ciric et al., 2003), suggesting that multivalency, and therefore oligomerization of cognate antigen, is necessary for the function of remyelination-promoting antibodies. In fact, on the basis of the evidence at hand regarding antibody-induced signaling, we hypothesize that remyelination-promoting antibodies function as soluble initiators of the type of clustering and consequent signaling described for integrins and proteoglycans involved in cell–cell adhesion and contact-mediated signaling (Fig. 21).

Integrins and cell surface proteoglycans are associated with plasma membrane lipid raft microdomains and with the oligomeric scaffolding protein caveolin (Baron et al., 2003). Therefore, lipid rafts, enriched in a number of receptor and nonreceptor kinases, serve as a locus of integrin- and proteoglycan-related signaling. As a result of clustering induced by binding to extracellular matrix elements, integrin-associated structural and signaling molecules are also clustered within lipid raft domains, and the resulting increase in density and proximity of these molecules results in the initiation of several important signals (Harder et al., 1998; Harder and Simons, 1997). The reorganization of actin filaments into stress fibers occurs at the focal point of this clustering activity, and results in a positive feedback loop that encourages further integrin and proteoglycan clustering and signaling. These focal adhesions are highly enriched in signaling molecules such as FAK (focal adhesion kinase) and members of the Src-family of nonreceptor tyrosine kinase (Hanks et al., 2003). FAK is recruited to integrin clusters either through direct interaction with the integrin β subunit or via interaction with reorganized actin fibers. Activated FAK in turn activates phosphoinositide-3 kinase (PI3-K), Src, and elements of the mitogen-activated protein kinase (MAPK) cascades (Bernfield et al., 1999; Bokoch, 2003; Juliano, 2002). Likewise, lipid raft clustering leads to signaling through the myristoylated and palmitoylated Src-family kinases Src, Fyn, Yes, and Lck (Hoessli et al., 2000). These nonreceptor tyrosine kinases are activated by clustering, and they initiate signaling cascades that result in activation of the MAPK Erk1/2. Erk1/2 signaling results in phosphorylation of elements of the ternary complex factor, and thus promotes transcription of the immediate early gene c-fos (Sofroniew et al., 2001). In parallel, lipid raft clustering of integrins and proteoglycans engages the MAPK JNK, leading to phosphorylation of the transcription factor c-jun, and association of c-jun with c-fos to form the AP-1 transcription factor complex. This complex is a critical regulator of genes involved in cell proliferation (Lin, 2003). Likewise, clustering-induced activation of FAK and PI3-K leads to signaling through Akt, a protein kinase that promotes survival by phosphorylating and inactivating the proapoptotic proteins Bad and caspase-9 (Sofroniew et al., 2001). Finally, lipid raft clustering of integrins in response to extracellular matrix binding results in the activation of the Rho family of small guanine nucleotide-binding proteins. These molecules include Rac, Cdc42, and RhoA, which are involved in induction of filopodia and formation of focal adhesions (Kaibuchi et al., 1999).

An additional signaling mechanism invoked by clustering of integrins within lipid rafts involves the concomitant aggregation of growth factor receptors and ion channels. Aggregation of growth factor receptors results in partial activation via proximity-dependent transphosphorylation (Ferguson, 2003). This partial activation brings the growth

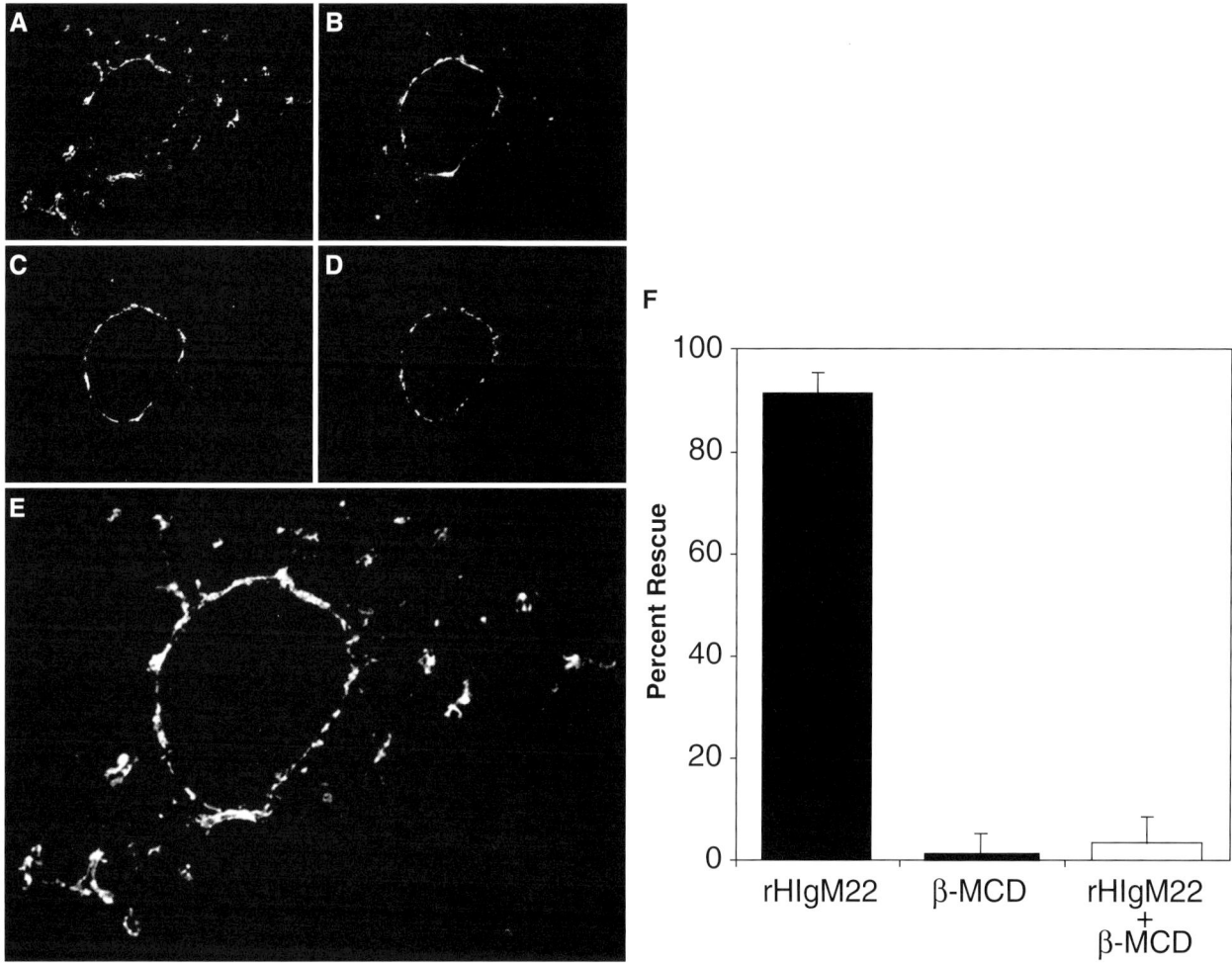

Figure 20 **Evidence of lipid raft involvement in rHIgM22 signaling.** (**A-E**) rHIgM22 immunostains patches of plasma membrane, as observed in serial z-sections throughout the cell (**A–D**). Stacking of the individual images shows the relative "patchiness" of the rHIgM22 staining pattern, suggesting that rHIgM22 antigen is localized to a specific plasma membrane microdomain. (**F**) rHIgM22 rescues premyelinating oligodendrocytes from death induced by treatment with hydrogen peroxide for 30 minutes. Cholesterol chelation with methyl-β-cyclodextrin (β-MCD) completely abrogates the protective effect of rHIgM22, suggesting that signaling from lipid rafts is critical for the ability of rHIgM22 to rescue oligodendrocytes from oxidative stress-induced apoptosis.

factor receptors closer to a threshold for full activation induced by substantially less extracellular growth factor. For example, PDGFα receptors (PDGFR) are sequestered in lipid rafts of oligodendrocytes committed to terminal differentiation, and PDGFR signaling from these rafts is required for survival of oligodendrocytes (Frost et al., 2003; Park et al., 2001). Likewise, axonal laminin-2 provides a target-dependent survival signal for differentiating oligodendrocytes via signaling through the lipid raft localized α6β1 integrin. Laminin-induced clustering of integrin within lipid rafts leads to substantial amplification of PI3-K and Akt signaling downstream from the PDGFR (Baron et al., 2003). Therefore, lipid raft microdomain-localized clustering of integrins and subsequent amplification of growth factor receptor signaling is an important signaling mechanism within oligodendrocytes. Similarly, integrin clustering within lipid rafts leads to a signaling cascade that uses Src

and calcium calmodulin-dependent protein kinase II (CaMKII) activation to phosphorylate AMPA receptors, resulting in a slow-building potentiation of calcium flux through the AMPA receptor calcium channel (Kramar et al., 2003).

Clustering of oligodendrocyte cell surface proteoglycans within lipid raft microdomains initiates many of the same signaling events as integrin clustering (Simons and Horowitz, 2001). For example, syndecan-4 is a transmembrane heparan sulfate proteoglycan that is recruited to focal adhesions in response to extracellular matrix-dependent clustering or antibody-induced clustering (Lim et al., 2003; Tkachenko and Simons 2002). Syndecan-4 signals through protein kinase Cα (PKCα) by potentiating its response to phosphatidylinositol 4,5-bisphosphate (PIP_2). This potentiation is accomplished by a clustering-dependent increase in the association of syndecan-4 with both PIP_2 and PKCα,

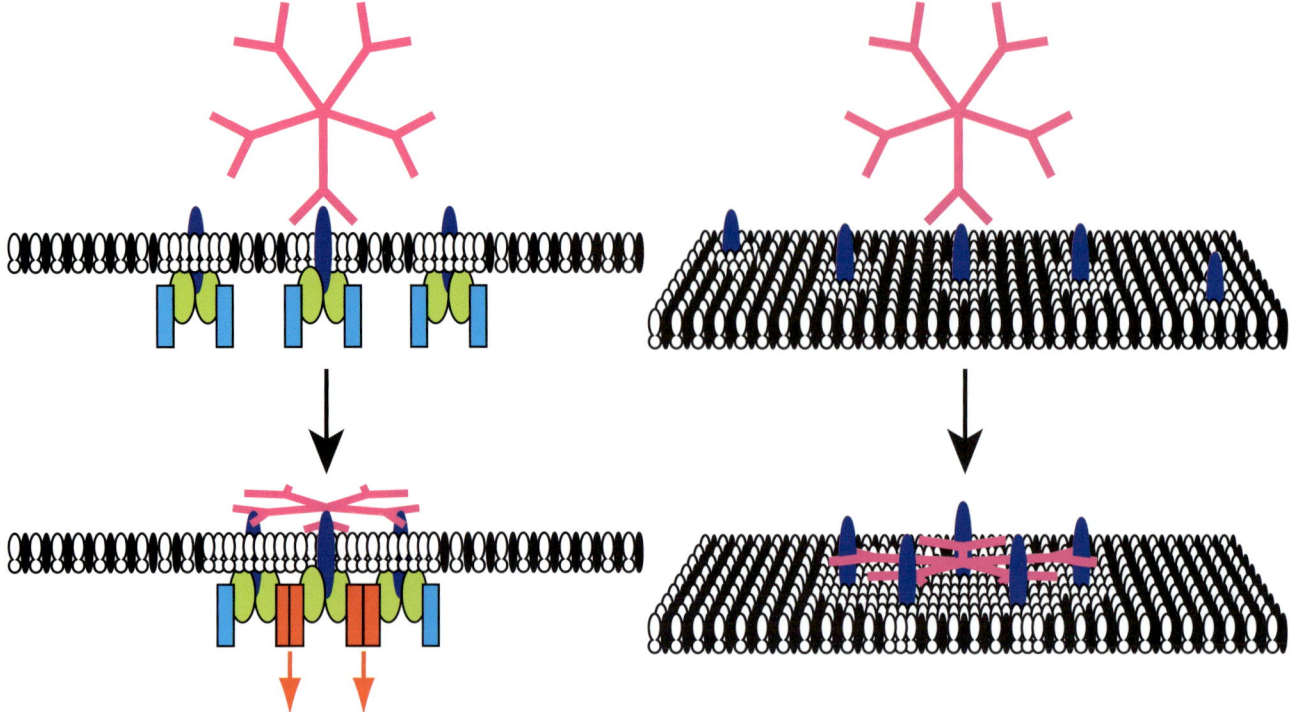

Figure 21 A model of rHIgM22 and remyelination-promoting antibody signal induction. Pentameric rHIgM22 may bind to a surface antigen that is associated intracellularly with signal transduction elements that are activated by clustering. rHIgM22-mediated aggregation of cell surface epitopes translates into lipid raft clustering and concomitant induction of intracellular signals.

resulting in the formation of a multimeric ternary complex of these three molecules (Bass and Humphries, 2002; Lim et al., 2003). Syndecan-4 clustering also induces the activation of Rho family GTPases and FAK, leading to substantial reorganization of the actin cytoskeleton downstream from syndecan-4 multimerization (Yoneda and Couchman, 2003).

Proteoglycan clustering within lipid raft microdomains also results in substantial modification of calcium channel activity. NG2 is a transmembrane proteoglycan that is enriched on the surface of oligodendrocyte progenitors (Dawson et al., 2000). This proteoglycan associates with the glutamate receptor interaction protein (GRIP1) via a PDZ domain-mediated interaction (Stegmuller et al., 2003). As a result of this molecular linkage, NG2 is indirectly associated with the AMPA receptor within lipid rafts of oligodendrocyte progenitors (Hering et al., 2003; Stegmuller et al., 2003). Immature oligodendrocyte AMPA channels are involved in regulation of proliferation and differentiation (Yuan et al., 1998), and the association of AMPA channels with NG2 suggests that adhesion-mediated clustering of NG2 may modify glial calcium signaling and thereby control maturation of oligodendrocytes. It is interesting to note that AMPA channel function is substantially modified by lectin binding, and concanavalin A binding leads to desensitization of the AMPA channel and a consequent increase in calcium permeability in the absence of changes in glutamate

binding (Thalhammer et al., 2002). Moreover, sialidase treatment modulates AMPA function by alleviating desensitization, and this effect is indirect, as sialic acid residues are not found on the AMPA receptor (Hoffman et al., 1997). Because NG2 does bear sialic acid residues, it is reasonable to speculate that the effect of deglycosylation or lectin binding is mediated by an alteration in NG2 association with the AMPA receptor. Therefore, as with integrins, multimerization of proteoglycans is an important modulator of oligodendrocyte signaling, survival, proliferation, and differentiation.

The pentameric structure of the IgM antibodies we have identified as remyelination-promoting antibodies immediately suggests that clustering and multimerization of cell surface antigens is an important element in the signal transduction elicited downstream from antibody binding (Asakura et al., 1996, 1998; Bieber et al., 2001; Miller et al., 1994; Rodriguez and Lennon 1990; Sommer and Schachner 1981; Warrington et al., 2000). Therefore, we propose that our remyelination-promoting antibodies function as soluble initiators of the type of clustering described previously for integrins and proteoglycans. It is important to note that several of the antibodies we have shown to promote remyelination are reactive with sialic acid residues (A2B5), other carbohydrate domains (HNK-1), and lipid raft-localized molecules (O1, O4) (Asakura et al., 1998; Warrington et al.,

2000). Moreover, several of these antibodies have been shown to alter oligodendrocyte morphology, initiate calcium signals, and induce differentiation (Dyer 1993; Dyer and Benjamins, 1989; 1990; 1991), and the general lack of similar effects induced by IgG antibodies reactive with similar epitopes suggests that multimerization is an important element in the transduction of these effects. It is also important to note, however, that cellular context is a critical factor in the signaling initiated by remyelination-promoting antibodies, as many of these antibodies recognize rather broad classes of molecules but only initiate signals in a limited manner. Thus we hypothesize that remyelination-promoting antibodies recognize oligodendrocyte surface molecules that are presented within specific contexts, and that this recognition event leads to the clustering of signal transducers within plasma membrane lipid raft microdomains.

Myelin reactive autoantibodies may also enhance repair through more indirect mechanisms. Antibodies binding to damaged oligodendrocytes and myelin may stimulate repair by enhancing the opsonization and clearance of myelin debris by macrophages (DeJong and Smith, 1997). Large numbers of macrophages are often observed in demyelinated lesions, and phagocytosis of myelin debris may be an important prerequisite to efficient remyelination. However, our most recent data indicate definitively that the Fc portion of the antibodies is not required for remyelination induced by sHIgM22 (Ciric et al., 2003), and this critical piece of information has focused our attention on the direct hypothesis.

Expanding the concept of antibody-mediated CNS repair from remyelination to axon regeneration, McKerracher and colleagues immunized animals with SCH before spinal cord hemisection or optic nerve crush (Ellezam et al., 2003; Huang et al., 1999). An identical preimmunization strategy was used, and therefore the antibody response is likely to be the same as in our earlier studies using the Theiler's virus-mediated model of demyelination. Preimmunization with SCH resulted in significant axonal regrowth in both spinal cord and optic nerve lesion models and resulted in a functional recovery in the spinal cord lesion model. Sera from animals demonstrating axon regrowth contained increased titers of myelin-reactive antibodies, which, when used *in vitro*, allowed the outgrowth of neurites on normally inhibitory CNS myelin. It was hypothesized that anti-SCH antibodies promoted axon regeneration by blocking *in vivo* myelin-associated inhibitors of axon outgrowth (Ellezam et al., 2003; Huang et al., 1999). However, the SCH antisera did not contain elevated titers of antibodies to known myelin inhibitors (Nogo, myelin associated glycoprotein, chondroitin sulfate proteoglycan). Therefore, myelin reactive antibodies might be useful not only to promote myelin repair after demyelinating disease but also for the treatment of axonal damage after spinal cord injury. Such antibodies may be administered exogenously or generated *in vivo* via appropriate immunization strategies. Recent work with the IN-1

antibody, also an oligodendrocyte reactive IgM, has led to very similar conclusions (Bregman et al., 1995; Chen et al., 2000; GrandPre et al., 2000).

There are currently few effective therapies to promote tissue repair or to prevent or reverse neurological deficits after CNS injury or disease; therefore, the characterization of endogenous immune-mediated repair mechanisms is important. An understanding of these mechanisms should open up significant new areas for the development of antibody-based therapeutics and perhaps small molecule-based therapeutics and vaccines for induction of the reparative response. Remyelination is an important therapeutic goal for the treatment of neurological disease and is likely to protect axons from further injury. Human monoclonal antibodies that promote remyelination represent a new class of therapeutics for diseases such as MS, spinal cord injury, neurodegeneration, and stroke.

VIII. Conclusions

The loss of oligodendrocytes and myelin normally associated with demyelinating diseases such as MS is, of course, devastating. However, rational therapeutic approaches that may be within reach, including treatment with remyelination-promoting antibodies or transplantation of oligodendrocyte progenitors, will likely repair and reverse myelin-related damage and dysfunction. In contrast, the loss of neurons, axons, and synaptic connections that may result after repeated bouts of demyelination is likely to be a far more complex and intractable problem to solve. Axons and synapses are the final physical manifestation of the neural connectivity and plasticity that develops over the lifetime of an individual; replacing these structures once lost may simply prove to be impossible. Therefore, it is critical that strategies be developed for protecting and maintaining axons during demyelinating episodes associated with MS. Obviously, the ultimate goal is to prevent MS altogether, but in the short term, a reasonable goal is to rapidly promote remyelination and thereby protect neurons and axons from damage and death inflicted by exposure to immune mediators. We propose that treatment with remyelination-promoting growth factor-like human IgM natural autoantibodies may be an efficacious method for quickly repairing demyelinated lesions and maintaining axonal connectivity. Likewise, another important goal of our group is to better understand the immune effector cells involved in damaging axons and neurons. There is substantial evidence that CD8[+] T-cells are a key mediator of axon killing in patients with MS, and we will continue to study the role of these cells in a number of animal models of MS, including the Theiler's virus model.

There is strong evidence to support the role of MHC class I in the pathogenesis of Theiler's virus-induced disease. The data to support this hypothesis can be summarized as follows. First, susceptibility vs. resistance to viral persistance and demyelination maps to the D region molecule of the class I gene (Rodriguez et al., 1986). Second, class I genes are upregulated in neurons, astrocytes, and oligodendrocytes immediately after infection (Redwine et al., 2001). Third, the upregulation of class I MHC is differentially regulated such that both K and D region molecules are upregulated during the acute phase of the infection, but only D region molecules are upregulated during the chronic demyelinating disease (Altintas et al., 1993). Fourth, cytotoxic T-cell-mediated killing can be demonstrated for T-cells isolated directly from the infected CNS without *in vitro* stimulation (Lin et al., 1995). Fifth, cytotoxic T-cell-mediated killing is directed against the viral capsid proteins of Theiler's virus, primarily VP2, and to a lesser extent VP1 (Lin et al., 1995). Sixth, in mice of the H-2^b haplotype, VP2$_{121-130}$ is the immunodominant peptide recognized specifically within the context of the H-2D^b molecule (Borson et al., 1997). Seventh, FACS using fluorescently labeled tetramers of VP2$_{121-130}$/D^b demonstrate that 60% to 80% of all CD8$^+$ T-cells in the CNS of infected mice are directed against this one immunodominant peptide (Johnson et al., 1999). Eighth, we have shown that mice with a dysfunctional MHC class I induced by genetic deletion of β2-microglobulin exhibit profound demyelination of the spinal cord despite normal neurological function (Rivera-Quinones et al., 1998). Preservation of physiological function was likely due to preservation of axons, and, in fact, we showed that axons upregulated and redistributed sodium channels along demyelinated segments. Ninth, retrograde labeling of descending axon tracts demonstrated a failure in retrograde axonal transport in mice with demyelination and functional deficits (Ure and Rodriguez, 2000). However, axonal transport was preserved in demyelinated mice with deletion of β2-microglobulin (Ure and Rodriguez, 2002). Tenth, we recently showed that depletion of antigen-specific cytotoxic T-cells restricted to VP2$_{121-130}$ resulted in preservation of neurological function (Johnson et al., 2001). These results suggest that axonal injury mediates neurological impairment during the chronic phase of Theiler's virus infection that is separable from virus-induced demyelination, and also suggest that CD8$^+$ cytotoxic T-lymphocytes directed against a specific viral peptide presented by MHC class I on axons and neurons may play an important role in this process.

We favor the hypothesis that demyelination is necessary but not sufficient for development of permanent deficits in primary demyelinating disorders of humans and animals. Demyelination predisposes axons to subsequent secondary injury. A major function of myelin is to protect axons against subsequent injury or loss. This secondary injury to the axon may be the result of either (1) T-cell cytotoxicity or (2) failure of neurotrophic support from death of myelinating oligodendrocytes. It is not known how long an axon can remain demyelinated in the CNS before death or remyelination takes place; however, strategies to prevent cytotoxic T-cell-mediated injury to axons and strategies to maintain axons may ultimately prove to be the most efficacious means of preventing long-term disability after demyelination. Rapid remyelination of these preserved axons, induced perhaps by treatment with growth factor-like human monoclonal IgM antibodies directed against myelin antigens, may protect them from further injury and thereby preserve neurological function.

References

Ahmed, Z., Doward, A. I., Pryce, G., Taylor, D. L., Pocock, J. M., Leonard, J. P., Baker, D., and Cuzner, M. L. (2002). A role for caspase-1 and -3 in the pathology of experimental allergic encephalomyelitis: Inflammation versus degeneration. *Am. J. Pathol.* **161,** 1577–1586.

Altintas, A., Cai, Z., Pease, L. R., and Rodriguez, M. (1993). Differential expression of H-2K and H-2D in the central nervous system of mice infected with Theiler's virus. *J. Immunol.* **151,** 2803–2812.

Arnett, H. A., Mason, J., Marino, M., Suzuki, K., Matsushima, G. K., and Ting, J. P. (2001). TNF alpha promotes proliferation of oligodendrocyte progenitors and remyelination. *Nat. Neurosci.* **4,** 1116–1122.

Arnett, H. A., Wang, Y., Matsushima, G. K., Suzuki, K., and Ting, J. P. (2003). Functional genomic analysis of remyelination reveals importance of inflammation in oligodendrocyte regeneration. *J. Neurosci.* **23,** 9824–9832.

Asakura, K., Miller, D. J., Murray, K., Bansal, R., Pfeiffer, S. E., and Rodriguez, M. (1996). Monoclonal autoantibody SCH94.03, which promotes central nervous system remyelination, recognizes an antigen on the surface of oligodendrocytes. *J. Neurosci. Res.* **43,** 273–281.

Asakura, K., Miller, D. J., Pease, L. R., and Rodriguez, M. (1998). Targeting of IgMkappa antibodies to oligodendrocytes promotes CNS remyelination. *J. Neurosci.* **18,** 7700–7708.

Babbe, H., Roers, A., Waisman, A., Lassmann, H., Goebels, N., Hohlfeld, R., Friese, M., Schroder, R., Deckert, M., Schmidt, S., Ravid, R., and Rajewsky, K. (2000). Clonal expansions of CD8(+) T cells dominate the T cell infiltrate in active multiple sclerosis lesions as shown by micromanipulation and single cell polymerase chain reaction. *J. Exp. Med.* **192,** 393–404.

Baron, W., Decker, L., Colognato, H., and ffrench-Constant, C. (2003). Regulation of integrin growth factor interactions in oligodendrocytes by lipid raft microdomains. *Curr. Biol.* **13,** 151–155.

Bass, M. D., and Humphries, M. J. (2002). Cytoplasmic interactions of syndecan-4 orchestrate adhesion receptor and growth factor receptor signalling. *Biochem. J.* **368,** 1–15.

Begolka, W. S., Haynes, L. M., Olson, J. K., Padilla, J., Neville, K. L., Dal Canto, M., Palma, J., Kim, B. S. and Miller, S. D. (2001). CD8-deficient SJL mice display enhanced susceptibility to Theiler's virus infection and increased demyelinating pathology. *J. Neurovirol.* **7,** 409–420.

Bernfield, M., Gotte, M., Park, P. W., Reizes, O., Fitzgerald, M. L., Lincecum, J., and Zako, M. (1999). Functions of cell surface heparan sulfate proteoglycans. *Annu. Rev. Biochem.* **68,** 729–777.

Bieber, A. J., Warrington, A., Pease, L. R., and Rodriguez, M. (2001). Humoral autoimmunity as a mediator of CNS repair. *Trends Neurosci.* **24,** S39–44.

Bitsch, A., Schuchardt, J., Bunkowski, S., Kuhlmann, T., and Bruck, W. (2000). Acute axonal injury in multiple sclerosis. Correlation with demyelination and inflammation. *Brain* **123,** 1174–1183.

Bjartmar, C., and Trapp, B. D. (2003). Axonal degeneration and progressive neurologic disability in multiple sclerosis. *Neurotox. Res.* **5,** 157–164.

Bjartmar, C., Wujek, J. R., and Trapp, B. D. (2003). Axonal loss in the pathology of MS: consequences for understanding the progressive phase of the disease. *J. Neurol. Sci.* **206,** 165–171.

Bokoch, G. M. (2003). Biology of the p21-Activated Kinases. *Annu. Rev. Biochem.* **72,** 743–781.

Bonetti, B., and Raine, C. S. (1997). Multiple sclerosis: oligodendrocytes display cell death-related molecules in situ but do not undergo apoptosis. *Ann. Neurol.* **42,** 74–84.

Bonini, S., Rasi, G., Bracci-Laudiero, M. L., Procoli, A., and Aloe, L. (2003). Nerve growth factor: neurotrophin or cytokine? *Int. Arch. Allergy Immunol.* **131,** 80–84.

Borson, N. D., Paul, C., Lin, X., Nevala, W. K., Strausbauch, M. A., Rodriguez, M., and Wettstein, P. J. (1997). Brain-infiltrating cytolytic T lymphocytes specific for Theiler's virus recognize H2Db molecules complexed with a viral VP2 peptide lacking a consensus anchor residue. *J. Virol.* **71,** 5244–5250.

Bouvet, J. P., and Dighiero, G. (1998). From natural polyreactive autoantibodies to a la carte monoreactive antibodies to infectious agents: Is it a small world after all? *Infect. Immunol.* **66,** 1–4.

Brahic, M. (2002). Theiler's virus infection of the mouse, or of the importance of studying animal models. *Virology* **301,** 1–5.

Brahic, M., Stroop, W. G., and Baringer, J. R. (1981). Theiler's virus persists in glial cells during demyelinating disease. *Cell* **26,** 123–128.

Bregman, B. S., Kunkel-Bagden, E., Schnell, L., Dai, H. N., Gao, D., and Schwab, M. E. (1995). Recovery from spinal cord injury mediated by antibodies to neurite growth inhibitors. *Nature* **378,** 498–501.

Browne, K. A., Blink, E., Sutton, V. R., Froelich, C. J., Jans, D. A., and Trapani, J. A. (1999). Cytosolic delivery of granzyme B by bacterial toxins: evidence that endosomal disruption, in addition to transmembrane pore formation, is an important function of perforin. *Mol. Cell Biol.* **19,** 8604–8615.

Bruck, W., Bitsch, A., Kolenda, H., Bruck, Y., Stiefel, M., and Lassmann, H. (1997). Inflammatory central nervous system demyelination: Correlation of magnetic resonance imaging findings with lesion pathology. *Ann. Neurol.* **42,** 783–793.

Butzkueven, H., Zhang, J. G., Soilu-Hanninen, M., Hochrein, H., Chionh, F., Shipham, K. A., Emery, B., Turnley, A. M., Petratos, S., Ernst, M., Bartlett, P. F., and Kilpatrick, T. J. (2002). LIF receptor signaling limits immune-mediated demyelination by enhancing oligodendrocyte survival. *Nat. Med.* **8,** 613–619.

Cashman, N. R., Durham, H. D., Blusztajn, J. K., Oda, K., Tabira, T., Shaw, I. T., Dahrouge, S., and Antel, J. P. (1992). Neuroblastoma x spinal cord (NSC) hybrid cell lines resemble developing motor neurons. *Dev. Dyn.* **194,** 209–221.

Chen, M. S., Huber, A. B., van der Haar, M. E., Frank, M., Schnell, L., Spillmann, A. A., Christ, F., and Schwab, M. E. (2000). Nogo-A is a myelin-associated neurite outgrowth inhibitor and an antigen for monoclonal antibody IN-1. *Nature* **403,** 434–439.

Ciric, B., Howe, C. L., Paz Soldan, M., Warrington, A. E., Bieber, A. J., Van Keulen, V., Rodriguez, M., and Pease, L. R. (2003). Human monoclonal IgM antibody promotes CNS myelin repair independent of Fc function. *Brain Pathol.* **13,** 608–616.

Croxford, J. L., Olson, J. K., and Miller, S. D. (2002). Epitope spreading and molecular mimicry as triggers of autoimmunity in the Theiler's virus-induced demyelinating disease model of multiple sclerosis. *Autoimmun. Rev.* **1,** 251–260.

Dal Canto, M. C., and Lipton, H. L. (1982). Ultrastructural immunohistochemical localization of virus in acute and chronic demyelinating Theiler's virus infection. *Am. J. Pathol.* **106,** 20–29.

Daniels, J. B., Pappenheimer, A. M., and Richardson, S. (1952). Observations on encephalomyelitis of mice (DA strain). *J. Exp. Med.* **96,** 517–530.

Dawson, M. R., Levine, J. M., and Reynolds, R. (2000). NG2-expressing cells in the central nervous system: Are they oligodendroglial progenitors? *J. Neurosci. Res.* **61,** 471–479.

DeJong, B. A., and Smith, M. E. (1997). A role for complement in phagocytosis of myelin. *Neurochem. Res.* **22,** 491–498.

Drescher, K. M., Murray, P. D., David, C. S., Pease, L. R., and Rodriguez, M. (1999). CNS cell populations are protected from virus-induced pathology by distinct arms of the immune system. *Brain Pathol.* **9,** 21–31.

Drescher, K. M., Pease, L. R., and Rodriguez, M. (1997). Antiviral immune responses modulate the nature of central nervous system (CNS) disease in a murine model of multiple sclerosis. *Immunol. Rev.* **159,** 177–193.

Dyer, C. A., (1993). Novel oligodendrocyte transmembrane signaling systems. Investigations utilizing antibodies as ligands. *Mol. Neurobiol.* **7,** 1–22.

Dyer, C. A., and Benjamins, J. A. (1988). Antibody to galactocerebroside alters organization of oligodendroglial membrane sheets in culture. *J. Neurosci.* **8,** 4307–4318.

Dyer, C. A., and Benjamins, J. A. (1989). Organization of oligodendroglial membrane sheets: II. Galctocerebroside:antibody interactions signal changes in cytoskeleton and myelin basic protein. *J. Neurosci. Res.* **24,** 212–221.

Dyer, C. A., and Benjamins, J. A. (1990). Glycolipids and transmembrane signaling: Antibodies to galactocerebroside cause an influx of calcium in oligodendrocytes. *J. Cell Biol.* **111,** 625–633.

Dyer, C. A., and Benjamins, J. A. (1991). Galactocerebroside and sulfatide independently mediate Ca2+ responses in oligodendrocytes. *J. Neurosci. Res.* **30,** 699–711.

Dyer, C. A., and Matthieu, J. M. (1994). Antibodies to myelin/oligodendrocyte-specific protein and myelin/oligodendrocyte glycoprotein signal distinct changes in the organization of cultured oligodendroglial membrane sheets. *J. Neurochem.* **62,** 777–787.

Ellezam, B., Bertrand, J., Dergham, P., and McKerracher, L. (2003). Vaccination stimulates retinal ganglion cell regeneration in the adult optic nerve. *Neurobiol. Dis.* **12,** 1–10.

Ferguson, S. S. (2003). Receptor tyrosine kinase transactivation: Fine-tuning synaptic transmission. *Trends Neurosci.* **26,** 119–122.

Fiette, L., Aubert, C., Brahic, M., and Rossi, C. P. (1993). Theiler's virus infection of beta 2-microglobulin-deficient mice. *J. Virol.* **67,** 589–592.

Forger, N. G., Prevette, D., deLapeyriere, O., de Bovis, B., Wang, S., Bartlett, P., and Oppenheim, R. W. (2003). Cardiotrophin-like cytokine/cytokine-like factor 1 is an essential trophic factor for lumbar and facial motoneurons in vivo. *J. Neurosci.* **23,** 8854–8858.

Froelich, C. J., Orth, K., Turbov, J., Seth, P., Gottlieb, R., Babior, B., Shah, G. M., Bleackley, R. C., Dixit, V. M., and Hanna, W. (1996). New paradigm for lymphocyte granule-mediated cytotoxicity. Target cells bind and internalize granzyme B, but an endosomolytic agent is necessary for cytosolic delivery and subsequent apoptosis. *J. Biol. Chem.* **271,** 29073–29079.

Frost, E. E., Nielsen, J. A., Le, T. Q., and Armstrong, R. C. (2003). PDGF and FGF2 regulate oligodendrocyte progenitor responses to demyelination. *J. Neurobiol.* **54,** 457–472.

Genain, C. P., Cannella, B., Hauser, S. L., and Raine, C. S. (1999). Identification of autoantibodies associated with myelin damage in multiple sclerosis. *Nat. Med.* **5,** 170–175.

Genain, C. P., Nguyen, M. H., Letvin, N. L., Pearl, R., Davis, R. L., Adelman, M., Lees, M. B., Linington, C., and Hauser, S. L. (1995). Antibody facilitation of multiple sclerosis-like lesions in a nonhuman primate. *J. Clin. Invest.* **96,** 2966–2974.

GrandPre, T., Nakamura, F., Vartanian, T., and Strittmatter, S. M. (2000). Identification of the Nogo inhibitor of axon regeneration as a Reticulon protein. *Nature* **403,** 439–444.

Graubert, T. A., DiPersio, J. F., Russell, J. H., and Ley, T. J. (1997). Perforin/granzyme-dependent and independent mechanisms are both important for the development of graft-versus-host disease after murine bone marrow transplantation. *J. Clin. Invest.* **100,** 904–911.

Hanks, S. K., Ryzhova, L., Shin, N. Y., and Brabek, J. (2003). Focal adhesion kinase signaling activities and their implications in the control of cell survival and motility. *Front. Biosci.* **8,** D982–996.

Harder, T., Scheiffele, P., Verkade, P., and Simons, K. (1998). Lipid domain structure of the plasma membrane revealed by patching of membrane components. *J. Cell Biol.* **141,** 929–942.

Harder, T. and Simons, K. (1997). Caveolae, DIGs, and the dynamics of sphingolipid-cholesterol microdomains. *Curr. Opin. Cell Biol.* **9,** 534–542.

Hering, H., Lin, C. C., and Sheng, M. (2003). Lipid rafts in the maintenance of synapses, dendritic spines, and surface AMPA receptor stability. *J. Neurosci.* **23,** 3262–3271.

Hoessli, D. C., Ilangumaran, S., Soltermann, A., Robinson, P. J., Borisch, B., and Nasir Ud, D. (2000). Signaling through sphingolipid microdomains of the plasma membrane: The concept of signaling platform. *Glycoconj. J.* **17,** 191–197.

Hoffman, K. B., Kessler, M., and Lynch, G. (1997). Sialic acid residues indirectly modulate the binding properties of AMPA-type glutamate receptors. *Brain Res.* **753,** 309–314.

Hoftberger, R., Aboul-Enein, F., Brueck, W., Lucchinetti, C., Rodriguez, M., Schmidbauer, M., Jellinger, K., and Lassmann, H. (2004). Expression of major histocompatibility complex class I molecules on the different cell types in multiple sclerosis lesions. *Brain Pathol.* **14,** 43–50.

Howe, C. L., Bieber, A. J., Warrington, A. E., Pease, L. R., and Rodriguez, M. (2004). Antiapoptotic signaling by a remyelination-promoting human antimyelin antibody. *Neurobiol. Dis.* **15,** 120–131.

Huang, D. W., McKerracher, L., Braun, P. E., and David, S. (1999). A therapeutic vaccine approach to stimulate axon regeneration in the adult mammalian spinal cord. *Neuron* **24,** 639–647.

Hulshof, S., Montagne, L., De Groot, C. J., and Van Der Valk, P. (2002). Cellular localization and expression patterns of interleukin-10, interleukin-4, and their receptors in multiple sclerosis lesions. *Glia* **38,** 24–35.

Ikeda, K., Kinoshita, M., Tagaya, N., Shiojima, T., Taga, T., Yasukawa, K., Suzuki, H., and Okano, A. (1996). Coadministration of interleukin-6 (IL-6) and soluble IL-6 receptor delays progression of wobbler mouse motor neuron disease. *Brain Res.* **726,** 91–97.

Jean, I., Allamargot, C., Barthelaix-Pouplard, A., and Fressinaud, C. (2002). Axonal lesions and PDGF-enhanced remyelination in the rat corpus callosum after lysolecithin demyelination. *Neuroreport* **13,** 627–631.

Johnson, A. J., Njenga, M. K., Hansen, M. J., Kuhns, S. T., Chen, L., Rodriguez, M., and Pease, L. R. (1999). Prevalent class I-restricted T-cell response to the Theiler's virus epitope Db:VP2121-130 in the absence of endogenous CD4 help, tumor necrosis factor alpha, gamma interferon, perforin, or costimulation through CD28. *J. Virol.* **73,** 3702–3708.

Johnson, A. J., Upshaw, J., Pavelko, K. D., Rodriguez, M., and Pease, L. R. (2001). Preservation of motor function by inhibition of CD8+ virus peptide-specific T cells in Theiler's virus infection. *FASEB J.* **15,** 2760–2762.

Ju, S. T., Cui, H., Panka, D. J., Ettinger, R., and Marshak-Rothstein, A. (1994). Participation of target Fas protein in apoptosis pathway induced by CD4+ Th1 and CD8+ cytotoxic T cells. *Proc. Natl. Acad. Sci. U. S. A.* **91,** 4185–4189.

Juliano, R. L. (2002). Signal transduction by cell adhesion receptors and the cytoskeleton: Functions of integrins, cadherins, selectins, and immunoglobulin-superfamily members. *Annu. Rev. Pharmacol. Toxicol.* **42,** 283–323.

Kaibuchi, K., Kuroda, S., and Amano, M. (1999). Regulation of the cytoskeleton and cell adhesion by the Rho family GTPases in mammalian cells. *Annu. Rev. Biochem.* **68,** 459–486.

Kaspar, B. K., Llado, J., Sherkat, N., Rothstein, J. D., and Gage, F. H. (2003). Retrograde viral delivery of IGF-1 prolongs survival in a mouse ALS model. *Science* **301,** 839–842.

Kornek, B., Storch, M. K., Bauer, J., Djamshidian, A., Weissert, R., Wallstroem, E., Stefferl, A., Zimprich, F., Olsson, T., Linington, C., Schmidbauer, M., and Lassmann, H. (2001). Distribution of a calcium channel subunit in dystrophic axons in multiple sclerosis and experimental autoimmune encephalomyelitis. *Brain* **124,** 1114–1124.

Kornek, B., Storch, M. K., Weissert, R., Wallstroem, E., Stefferl, A., Olsson, T., Linington, C., Schmidbauer, M., and Lassmann, H. (2000). Multiple sclerosis and chronic autoimmune encephalomyelitis: A comparative quantitative study of axonal injury in active, inactive, and remyelinated lesions. *Am. J. Pathol.* **157,** 267–276.

Kramar, E. A., Bernard, J. A., Gall, C. M., and Lynch, G. (2003). Integrins modulate fast excitatory transmission at hippocampal synapses. *J. Biol. Chem.* **278,** 10722–10730.

Lacroix-Desmazes, S., Kaveri, S. V., Mouthon, L., Ayouba, A., Malanchere, E., Coutinho, A., and Kazatchkine, M. D. (1998). Self-reactive antibodies (natural autoantibodies) in healthy individuals. *J. Immunol. Methods* **216,** 117–137.

Lambrechts, D., Storkebaum, E., Morimoto, M., Del-Favero, J., Desmet, F., Marklund, S. L., Wyns, S., Thijs, V., Andersson, J., van Marion, I., Al-Chalabi, A., Bornes, S., Musson, R., Hansen, V., Beckman, K., Adolfsson, R., Pall, H. S., Prats, H., Vermeire, S., Rutgeerts, P., Katayama, S., Awata, T., Leigh, N., Lang-Lazdunski, L., Dewerchin, M., Shaw, C., Moons, L., Vlietinck, R., Morrison, K. E., Robberecht, W., Van Broeckhoven, C., Collen, D., Andersen, P. M., and Carmeliet, P. (2003). VEGF is a modifier of amyotrophic lateral sclerosis in mice and humans and protects motoneurons against ischemic death. *Nat. Genet.* **34,** 383–394.

Lassmann, H., and Wekerle, H. (1998). Experimental models of multiple sclerosis. *In:* "McAlpine's Multiple Sclerosis" (A. Compston, G. Ebers, H. Lassmann, I. McDonald, B. Matthews, and H. Wekerle, Eds.). pp. 409–433. Churchill Livingstone, London.

Levy, M., Aubert, C., and Brahic, M. (1992). Theiler's virus replication in brain macrophages cultured in vitro. *J. Virol.* **66,** 3188–3193.

Lieberman, J. (2003). The ABCs of granule-mediated cytotoxicity: New weapons in the arsenal. *Nat. Rev. Immunol.* **3,** 361–370.

Lim, S. T., Longley, R. L., Couchman, J. R., and Woods, A. (2003). Direct binding of syndecan-4 cytoplasmic domain to the catalytic domain of protein kinase C alpha (PKC alpha) increases focal adhesion localization of PKC alpha. *J. Biol. Chem.* **278,** 13795–13802.

Lin, A. (2003). Activation of the JNK signaling pathway: breaking the brake on apoptosis. *Bioessays* **25,** 17–24.

Lin, X., Pease, L. R., and Rodriguez, M. (1997). Differential generation of class I H-2D-versus H-2K-restricted cytotoxicity against a demyelinating virus following central nervous system infection. *Eur. J. Immunol.* **27,** 963–970.

Lin, X., Thiemann, N. R., Pease, L. R., and Rodriguez, M. (1995). VP1 and VP2 capsid proteins of Theiler's virus are targets of H-2D-restricted cytotoxic lymphocytes in the central nervous system of B10 mice. *Virology* **214,** 91–99.

Lindsley, M. D., Thiemann, R., and Rodriguez, M. (1991). Cytotoxic T cells isolated from the central nervous systems of mice infected with Theiler's virus. *J. Virol.* **65,** 6612–6620.

Linington, C., Engelhardt, B., Kapocs, G., and Lassman, H. (1992). Induction of persistently demyelinated lesions in the rat following the repeated adoptive transfer of encephalitogenic T cells and demyelinating antibody. *J. Neuroimmunol.* **40,** 219–224.

Linker, R. A., Maurer, M., Gaupp, S., Martini, R., Holtmann, B., Giess, R., Rieckmann, P., Lassmann, H., Toyka, K. V., Sendtner, M., and Gold, R. (2002). CNTF is a major protective factor in demyelinating CNS disease: A neurotrophic cytokine as modulator in neuroinflammation. *Nat. Med.* **8,** 620–624.

Lipton, H. L., (1975). Theiler's virus infection in mice: an unusual biphasic disease process leading to demyelination. *Infect. Immunol.* **11,** 1147–1155.

Lipton, H. L., and Dal Canto, M. C. (1976a). Chronic neurologic disease in Theiler's virus infection of SJL/J mice. *J. Neurol. Sci.* **30,** 201–207.

Lipton, H. L., and Dal Canto, M. C. (1976b). Theiler's virus-induced demyelination: Prevention by immunosuppression. *Science* **192,** 62–64.

Lipton, H. L., and Dal Canto, M. C. (1979). Susceptibility of inbred mice to chronic central nervous system infection by Theiler's murine encephalomyelitis virus. *Infect. Immunol.* **26,** 369–374.

Lucchinetti, C., Bruck, W., Parisi, J., Scheithauer, B., Rodriguez, M., and Lassmann, H. (2000). Heterogeneity of multiple sclerosis lesions: implications for the pathogenesis of demyelination. *Ann. Neurol.* **47,** 707–717.

Lucchinetti, C. F., Brueck, W., Rodriguez, M., and Lassmann, H. (1998). Multiple sclerosis: Lessons from neuropathology. *Semin. Neurol.* **18,** 337–349.

Ludwin, S. K., and Bakker, D. A. (1988). Can oligodendrocytes attached to myelin proliferate? *J. Neurosci.* **8,** 1239–1244.

Ludwin, S. K., and Johnson, E. S. (1981). Evidence for a "dying-back" gliopathy in demyelinating disease. *Ann. Neurol.* **9,** 301–305.

Madrid, R. E., and Wisniewski, H. M. (1977). Axonal degeneration in demyelinating disorders. *J. Neurocytol.* **6,** 103–117.

Mancardi, G., Hart, B., Roccatagliata, L., Brok, H., Giunti, D., Bontrop, R., Massacesi, L., Capello, E., and Uccelli, A. (2001). Demyelination and axonal damage in a non-human primate model of multiple sclerosis. *J. Neurol. Sci.* **184,** 41–49.

Mason, J. L., Langaman, C., Morell, P., Suzuki, K., and Matsushima, G. K. (2001). Episodic demyelination and subsequent remyelination within the murine central nervous system: Changes in axonal calibre. *Neuropathol. Appl. Neurobiol.* **27,** 50–58.

Matsushima, G. K., and Morell, P. (2001). The neurotoxicant, cuprizone, as a model to study demyelination and remyelination in the central nervous system. *Brain Pathol.* **11,** 107–116.

Matthews, P. M., Pioro, E., Narayanan, S., De Stefano, N., Fu, L., Francis, G., Antel, J., Wolfson, C., and Arnold, D. L. (1996). Assessment of lesion pathology in multiple sclerosis using quantitative MRI morphometry and magnetic resonance spectroscopy. *Brain* **119,** 715–722.

Mayr, W. T., Pittock, S. J., McClelland, R. L., Jorgensen, Nw, Noseworthy, J. H., and Rodriguez, M. (2003). Incidence and prevalence of multiple sclerosis in Olmsted County, Minnesota, 1985-2000. *Neurology* **61,** 1373–1377.

McDonald, W. I., and Sears, T. A. (1969). Effect of demyelination on conduction in the central nervous system. *Nature* **221,** 182–183.

Mead, R. J., Singhrao, S. K., Neal, J. W., Lassmann, H., and Morgan, B. P. (2002). The membrane attack complex of complement causes severe demyelination associated with acute axonal injury. *J. Immunol.* **168,** 458–465.

Medana, I., Martinic, M. A., Wekerle, H., and Neumann, H. (2001). Transection of major histocompatibility complex class I-induced neurites by cytotoxic T lymphocytes. *Am. J. Pathol.* **159,** 809–815.

Medana, I. M., Gallimore, A., Oxenius, A., Martinic, M. M., Wekerle, H., and Neumann, H. (2000). MHC class I-restricted killing of neurons by virus-specific CD8+ T lymphocytes is effected through the Fas/FasL, but not the perforin pathway. *Eur. J. Immunol.* **30,** 3623–3633.

Mehta, V., and Namboodiri, M. A. (1995). N-acetylaspartate as an acetyl source in the nervous system. *Brain Res. Mol. Brain Res.* **31,** 151–157.

Metkar, S. S., Wang, B., Aguilar-Santelises, M., Raja, S. M., Uhlin-Hansen, L., Podack, E., Trapani, J. A., and Froelich, C. J. (2002). Cytotoxic cell granule-mediated apoptosis: Perforin delivers granzyme B-serglycin complexes into target cells without plasma membrane pore formation. *Immunity* **16,** 417–428.

Mews, I., Bergmann, M., Bunkowski, S., Gullotta, F., and Bruck, W. (1998). Oligodendrocyte and axon pathology in clinically silent multiple sclerosis lesions. *Multiple Sclerosis* **4,** 55–62.

Miller, D. J., Sanborn, K. S., Katzmann, J. A., and Rodriguez, M. (1994). Monoclonal autoantibodies promote central nervous system repair in an animal model of multiple sclerosis. *J. Neurosci.* **14,** 6230–6238.

Miller, S. D., Clatch, R. J., Pevear, D. C., Trotter, J. L., and Lipton, H. L. (1987). Class II-restricted T cell responses in Theiler's murine encephalomyelitis virus (TMEV)-induced demyelinating disease. I.

Cross-specificity among TMEV substrains and related picornaviruses, but not myelin proteins. *J. Immunol.* **138,** 3776–3784.

Miller, S. D., Vanderlugt, C. L., Begolka, W. S., Pao, W., Neville, K. L., Yauch, R. L., and Kim, B. S. (1997). Epitope spreading leads to myelin-specific autoimmune responses in SJL mice chronically infected with Theiler's virus. *J. Neurovirology.* **3,** S62–S65.

Mitsunaga, Y., Ciric, B., Van Keulen, V., Warrington, A. E., Paz Soldan, M., Bieber, A. J., Rodriguez, M., and Pease, L. R. (2002). Direct evidence that a human antibody derived from patient serum can promote myelin repair in a mouse model of chronic-progressive demyelinating disease. *FASEB J.* **16,** 1325–1327.

Monteyne, P., Bureau, J. F., and Brahic, M. (1997). The infection of mouse by Theiler's virus: from genetics to immunology. *Immunol. Rev.* **159,** 163–176.

Munoz-Fernandez, M. A., and Fresno, M. (1998). The role of tumour necrosis factor, interleukin 6, interferon-gamma and inducible nitric oxide synthase in the development and pathology of the nervous system. *Prog. Neurobiol.* **56,** 307–340.

Murray, P. D., McGavern, D. B., Lin, X., Njenga, M. K., Leibowitz, J., Pease, L. R., and Rodriguez, M. (1998). Perforin-dependent neurologic injury in a viral model of multiple sclerosis. *J. Neurosci.* **18,** 7306–7314.

Murray, P. D., McGavern, D. B., Pease, L. R., and Rodriguez, M. (2002). Cellular sources and targets of IFN-gamma-mediated protection against viral demyelination and neurological deficits. *Eur. J. Immunol.* **32,** 606–615.

Narayanan, S., Fu, L., Pioro, E., De Stefano, N., Collins, D. L., Francis, G. S., Antel, J. P., Matthews, P. M., and Arnold, D. L. (1997). Imaging of axonal damage in multiple sclerosis: Spatial distribution of magnetic resonance imaging lesions. *Ann. Neurol.* **41,** 385–391.

Neumann, H. (2003). Molecular mechanisms of axonal damage in inflammatory central nervous system diseases. *Curr. Opin. Neurol.* **16,** 267–273.

Neumann, H., Cavalie, A., Jenne, D. E., and Wekerle, H. (1995). Induction of MHC class I genes in neurons. *Science* **269,** 549–552.

Neumann, H., Medana, I. M., Bauer, J., and Lassmann, H. (2002). Cytotoxic T lymphocytes in autoimmune and degenerative CNS diseases. *Trends Neurosci.* **25,** 313–319.

Njenga, M. K., Asakura, K., Hunter, S. F., Wettstein, P., Pease, L. R., and Rodriguez, M. (1997a). The immune system preferentially clears Theiler's virus from the gray matter of the central nervous system. *J. Virol.* **71,** 8592–8601.

Njenga, M. K., Pavelko, K. D., Baisch, J., Lin, X., David, C., Leibowitz, J., and Rodriguez, M. (1996). Theiler's virus persistence and demyelination in major histocompatibility complex class II-deficient mice. *J. Virol.* **70,** 1729–1737.

Njenga, M. K., Pease, L. P., Wettstein, P., Mak, T., and Rodriguez, M. (1997b). Interferon a/b mediates early virus-induced expresson of H-2D and H-2K in the central nervous system. *Lab. Invest.* **77,** 71–84.

Noseworthy, J. H., Lucchinetti, C., Rodriguez, M., and Weinshenker, B. G. (2000). Multiple sclerosis. *N. Engl. J. Med.* **343,** 938–952.

Padberg, F., Feneberg, W., Schmidt, S., Schwarz, M. J., Korschenhausen, D., Greenberg, B. D., Nolde, T., Muller, N., Trapmann, H., Konig, N., Moller, H. J., and Hampel, H. (1999). CSF and serum levels of soluble interleukin-6 receptors (sIL-6R and sgp130), but not of interleukin-6 are altered in multiple sclerosis. *J. Neuroimmunol.* **99,** 218–223.

Park, S. K., Solomon, D., and Vartanian, T. (2001). Growth factor control of CNS myelination. *Dev. Neurosci.* **23,** 327–337.

Pavelko, K. D., Howe, C. L., Drescher, K. M., Gamez, J. D., Johnson, A. J., Wei, T., Ransohoff, R. M., and Rodriguez, M. (2003). Interleukin-6 protects anterior horn neurons from lethal virus-induced injury. *J. Neurosci.* **23,** 481–492.

Paya, C. V., Leibson, P. J., Patick, A. K., and Rodriguez, M. (1990). Inhibition of Theiler's virus-induced demyelination in vivo by tumor necrosis factor alpha. *Int. Immunol.* **2,** 909–913.

Paz Soldan, M. M. and Rodriguez, M. (2002). Heterogeneity of pathogenesis in multiple sclerosis: Implications for promotion of remyelination. *J. Infect. Dis.* **186**, S248–253.

Paz Soldan, M. M., Warrington, A. E., Bieber, A. J., Ciric, B., Van Keulen, V., Pease, L. R., and Rodriguez, M. (2003). Remyelination-promoting antibodies activate distinct Ca2+ influx pathways in astrocytes and oligodendrocytes: relationship to the mechanism of myelin repair. *Mol. Cell Neurosci.* **22**, 14–24.

Pena Rossi, C., McAllister, A., Fiette, L., and Brahic, M. (1991). Theiler's virus infection induces a specific cytotoxic T lymphocyte response. *Cell Immunol.* **138**, 341–348.

Penkowa, M., Espejo, C., Martinez-Caceres, E. M., Montalban, X., and Hidalgo, J. (2003). Increased demyelination and axonal damage in metallothionein I+II-deficient mice during experimental autoimmune encephalomyelitis. *Cell Mol. Life Sci.* **60**, 185–197.

Penkowa, M. and Hidalgo, J. (2003). Treatment with metallothionein prevents demyelination and axonal damage and increases oligodendrocyte precursors and tissue repair during experimental autoimmune encephalomyelitis. *J. Neurosci. Res.* **72**, 574–586.

Petereit, H. F., Pukrop, R., Fazekas, F., Bamborschke, S. U., Ropele, S., Kolmel, H. W., Merkelbach, S., Japp, G., Jongen, P. J., Hartung, H. P., and Hommes, O. R. (2003). Low interleukin-10 production is associated with higher disability and MRI lesion load in secondary progressive multiple sclerosis. *J. Neurol. Sci.* **206**, 209–214.

Petzold, A., Baker, D., Pryce, G., Keir, G., Thompson, E. J., and Giovannoni, G. (2003). Quantification of neurodegeneration by measurement of brain-specific proteins. *J. Neuroimmunol.* **138**, 45–48.

Pinkoski, M. J., Hobman, M., Heibein, J. A., Tomaselli, K., Li, F., Seth, P., Froelich, C. J., and Bleackley, R. C. (1998). Entry and trafficking of granzyme B in target cells during granzyme B-perforin-mediated apoptosis. *Blood* **92**, 1044–1054.

Pluchino, S., Quattrini, A., Brambilla, E., Gritti, A., Salani, G., Dina, G., Galli, R., Del Carro, U., Amadio, S., Bergami, A., Furlan, R., Comi, G., Vescovi, A. L., and Martino, G. (2003). Injection of adult neurospheres induces recovery in a chronic model of multiple sclerosis. *Nature* **422**, 688–-694.

Prayoonwiwat, N. and Rodriguez, M. (1993). The potential for oligodendrocyte proliferation during demyelinating disease. *J. Neuropathol. Exp. Neurol.* **52**, 55–63.

Prineas, J. W. and Connell, F. (1979). Remyelination in multiple sclerosis. *Ann. Neurol.* **5**, 22–31.

Prineas, J. W., Kwon, E. E., Goldenberg, P. Z., Ilyas, A. A., Quarles, R. H., Benjamins, J. A., and Sprinkle, T. J. (1989). Multiple sclerosis. Oligodendrocyte proliferation and differentiation in fresh lesions. *Lab. Invest.* **61**, 489–503.

Pullen, L. C., Miller, S. D., Dal Canto, M. C., and Kim, B. S. (1993). Class I-deficient resistant mice intracerebrally inoculated with Theiler's virus show an increased T cell response to viral antigens and susceptibility to demyelination. *Eur. J. Immunol.* **23**, 2287–2293.

Raine, C. S. and Bornstein, M. B. (1970). Experimental allergic encephalomyelitis: A light and electron microscope study of remyelination and "sclerosis" in vitro. *J. Neuropathol. Exp. Neurol.* **29**, 552–574.

Raine, C. S. and Cross, A. H. (1989). Axonal dystrophy as a consequence of long-term demyelination. *Lab. Invest.* **60**, 714–725.

Raine, C. S., Mokhtarian, F., and McFarlin, D. E. (1984). Adoptively transferred chronic relapsing experimental autoimmune encephalomyelitis in the mouse. Neuropathologic analysis. *Lab. Invest.* **51**, 534–546.

Ransohoff, R. M., Howe, C. L., and Rodriguez, M. (2002). Growth factor treatment of demyelinating disease: at last, a leap into the light. *Trends Immunol.* **23**, 512–516.

Redford, E. J., Kapoor, R., and Smith, K. J. (1997). Nitric oxide donors reversibly block axonal conduction: Demyelinated axons are especially susceptible. *Brain* **120**, 2149–2157.

Redwine, J. M., Buchmeier, M. J., and Evans, C. F. (2001). In vivo expression of major histocompatibility complex molecules on oligodendrocytes and neurons during viral infection. *Am. J. Pathol.* **159**, 1219–1224.

Rensing-Ehl, A., Malipiero, U., Irmler, M., Tschopp, J., Constam, D., and Fontana, A. (1996). Neurons induced to express major histocompatibility complex class I antigen are killed via the perforin and not the Fas (APO-1/CD95) pathway. *Eur. J. Immunol.* **26**, 2271–2274.

Repovic, P., Mi, K., and Benveniste, E. N. (2003). Oncostatin M enhances the expression of prostaglandin E2 and cyclooxygenase-2 in astrocytes: Synergy with interleukin-1beta, tumor necrosis factor-alpha, and bacterial lipopolysaccharide. *Glia* **42**, 433–446.

Rivera-Quinones, C., McGavern, D., Schmelzer, J. D., Hunter, S. F., Low, P. A., and Rodriguez, M. (1998). Absence of neurological deficits following extensive demyelination in a class I-deficient murine model of multiple sclerosis. *Nat. Med.* **4**, 187–193.

Rivers, T. M. and Schwentker, F. F. (1935). Encephalomyelitis accompanied by myelin destruction experimentally produced in monkeys. *J. Exp. Med.* **61**, 689–702.

Rodriguez, M. (1985). Virus-induced demyelination in mice: "dying back" of oligodendrocytes. *Mayo Clin. Proc.* **60**, 433–438.

Rodriguez, M. (2003). A function of myelin is to protect axons from subsequent injury: Implications for deficits in multiple sclerosis. *Brain* **126**, 751–752.

Rodriguez, M. and David, C. S. (1985). Demyelination induced by Theiler's virus: Influence of the H-2 haplotype. *J. Immunol.* **135**, 2145–2148.

Rodriguez, M. and David, C. S. (1995). H-2 Dd transgene suppresses Theiler's virus-induced demyelination in susceptible strains of mice. *J. Neurovirol.* **1**, 111–117.

Rodriguez, M., Dunkel, A. J., Thiemann, R. L., Leibowitz, J., Zijlstra, M., and Jaenisch, R. (1993). Abrogation of resistance to Theiler's virus-induced demyelination in H-2b mice deficient in beta 2-microglobulin. *J. Immunol.* **151**, 266–276.

Rodriguez, M., Leibowitz, J., and David, C. S. (1986). Susceptibility to Theiler's virus-induced demyelination. Mapping of the gene within the H-2D region. *J. Exp. Med.* **163**, 620–631.

Rodriguez, M., Leibowitz, J. L., and Lampert, P. W. (1983). Persistent infection of oligodendrocytes in Theiler's virus-induced encephalomyelitis. *Ann. Neurol.* **13**, 426–433.

Rodriguez, M. and Lennon, V. A. (1990). Immunoglobulins promote remyelination in the central nervous system. *Ann. Neurol.* **27**, 12–17.

Rodriguez, M., Lennon, V. A., Benveniste, E. N., and Merrill, J. E. (1987a). Remyelination by oligodendrocytes stimulated by antiserum to spinal cord. *J. Neuropathol. Exp. Neurol.* **46**, 84–95.

Rodriguez, M. and Miller, D. J. (1994). Immune promotion of central nervous system remyelination. *Prog. Brain Res.* **103**, 343–355.

Rodriguez, M., Oleszak, E., and Leibowitz, J. (1987b). Theiler's murine encephalomyelitis: A model of demyelination and persistence of virus. *Crit. Rev. Immunol.* **7**, 325–365.

Rodriguez, M., Zoecklein, L. J., Howe, C. L., Pavelko, K. D., Gamez, J. D., Nakane, S., and Papke, L. M. (2003). Gamma interferon is critical for neuronal viral clearance and protection in a susceptible mouse strain following early intracranial Theiler's murine encephalomyelitis virus infection. *J. Virol.* **77**, 12252–12265.

Rossi, C. P., Delcroix, M., Huitinga, I., McAllister, A., van, R. N., Claassen, E., and Brahic, M. (1997). Role of macrophages during Theiler's virus infection. *J. Virol.* **71**, 3336–3340.

Sanchez, I., Hassinger, L., Paskevich, P. A., Shine, H. D., and Nixon, R. A. (1996). Oligodendroglia regulate the regional expansion of axon caliber and local accumulation of neurofilaments during development independently of myelin formation. *J. Neurosci.* **16**, 5095–5105.

Sarchielli, P., Presciutti, O., Pelliccioli, G. P., Tarducci, R., Gobbi, G., Chiarini, P., Alberti, A., Vicinanza, F., and Gallai, V. (1999). Absolute quantification of brain metabolites by proton magnetic resonance spectroscopy in normal-appearing white matter of multiple sclerosis patients. *Brain* **122**, 513–521.

Schafer, K. H., Mestres, P., Marz, P., and Rose-John, S. (1999). The IL-6/sIL-6R fusion protein hyper-IL-6 promotes neurite outgrowth and neuron survival in cultured enteric neurons. *J. Interferon Cytokine Res.* **19**, 527–532.

Schluesener, H. J., Sobel, R. A., Linington, C., and Weiner, H. L. (1987). A monoclonal antibody against a myelin oligodendrocyte glycoprotein induces relapses and demyelination in central nervous system autoimmune disease. *J. Immunol.* **139**, 4016–4021.

Schulz, M., Schuurman, H. J., Joergensen, J., Steiner, C., Meerloo, T., Kagi, D., Hengartner, H., Zinkernagel, R. M., Schreier, M. H., Burki, K. et al. (1995). Acute rejection of vascular heart allografts by perforin-deficient mice. *Eur. J. Immunol.* **25**, 474–480.

Segal, B. M. (2003). Experimental autoimmune encephalomyelitis: Cytokines, effector T cells, and antigen-presenting cells in a prototypical Th1-mediated autoimmune disease. *Curr. Allergy Asthma Rep.* **3**, 86–93.

Shi, L., Mai, S., Israels, S., Browne, K., Trapani, J. A., and Greenberg, A. H. (1997). Granzyme B (GraB) autonomously crosses the cell membrane and perforin initiates apoptosis and GraB nuclear localization. *J. Exp. Med.* **185**, 855–866.

Simons, M., and Horowitz, A. (2001). Syndecan-4-mediated signalling. *Cell Signal* **13**, 855–862.

Sofroniew, M. V., Howe, C. L., and Mobley, W. C. (2001). Nerve growth factor signaling, neuroprotection, and neural repair. *Annu. Rev. Neurosci.* **24**, 1217–1281.

Sommer, I., and Schachner, M. (1981). Monoclonal antibodies (O1 to O4) to oligodendrocyte cell surfaces: An immunocytological study in the central nervous system. *Dev. Biol.* **83**, 311–327.

Stegmuller, J., Werner, H., Nave, K. A., and Trotter, J. (2003). The proteoglycan NG2 is complexed with alpha-amino-3-hydroxy-5-methyl-4-isoxazolepropionic acid (AMPA) receptors by the PDZ glutamate receptor interaction protein (GRIP) in glial progenitor cells. Implications for glial-neuronal signaling. *J. Biol. Chem.* **278**, 3590–3598.

Stevens, J. C., Farlow, M. R., Edwards, M. K., and Yu, P. L. (1986). Magnetic resonance imaging. Clinical correlation in 64 patients with multiple sclerosis. *Arch. Neurol.* **43**, 1145–1148.

Stewart, J. (1992). Immunoglobulins did not arise in evolution to fight infection. *Immunol. Today* **13**, 396–399; discussion 399–400.

Storch, M. K., Weissert, R., Steffer, A., Birnbacher, R., Wallstrom, E., Dahlman, I., Ostensson, C. G., Linington, C., Olsson, T., and Lassmann, H. (2002). MHC gene related effects on microglia and macrophages in experimental autoimmune encephalomyelitis determine the extent of axonal injury. *Brain Pathol.* **12**, 287–299.

Sun, N., Grzybicki, D., Castro, R. F., Murphy, S., and Perlman, S. (1995). Activation of astrocytes in the spinal cord of mice chronically infected with a neurotropic coronavirus. *Virology* **213**, 482–493.

Sun, W., Funakoshi, H., and Nakamura, T. (2002). Overexpression of HGF retards disease progression and prolongs life span in a transgenic mouse model of ALS. *J. Neurosci.* **22**, 6537–6548.

Swanborg, R. H. (2001). Experimental autoimmune encephalomyelitis in the rat: lessons in T-cell immunology and autoreactivity. *Immunol. Rev.* **184**, 129–135.

Thalhammer, A., Everts, I., and Hollmann, M. (2002). Inhibition by lectins of glutamate receptor desensitization is determined by the lectin's sugar specificity at kainate but not AMPA receptors. *Mol. Cell Neurosci.* **21**, 521–533.

Theiler, M. (1937). Spontaneous encephalomyelitis of mice, a new virus disease. *J. Exp. Med.* **65**, 705–719.

Thorburn, A. (2004). Death receptor-induced cell killing. *Cell Signal* **16**, 139–144.

Tkachenko, E., and Simons, M. (2002). Clustering induces redistribution of syndecan-4 core protein into raft membrane domains. *J. Biol. Chem.* **277**, 19946–19951.

Trapp, B. D., Peterson, J., Ransohoff, R. M., Rudick, R., Mork, S., and Bo, L. (1998). Axonal transection in the lesions of multiple sclerosis. *N. Engl. J. Med.* **338**, 278–285.

Truyen, L., van Waesberghe, J. H., van Walderveen, M. A., van Oosten, B. W., Polman, C. H., Hommes, O. R., Ader, H. J., and Barkhof, F. (1996). Accumulation of hypointense lesions ("black holes") on T1 spin-echo MRI correlates with disease progression in multiple sclerosis. *Neurology* **47**, 1469–1476.

Ure, D., and Rodriguez, M. (2000). Extensive injury of descending neurons demonstrated by retrograde labeling in a virus-induced murine model of chronic inflammatory demyelination. *J. Neuropathol. Exp. Neurol.* **59**, 664–678.

Ure, D. R., and Rodriguez, M. (2002). Preservation of neurologic function during inflammatory demyelination correlates with axon sparing in a mouse model of multiple sclerosis. *Neuroscience* **111**, 399–411.

van Engelen, B. G., Pavelko, K. D., and Rodriguez, M. (1997). Enhancement of central nervous system remyelination in immune and non-immune experimental models of demyelination. *Multiple Sclerosis* **3**, 76–79.

van Waesberghe, J. H., Kamphorst, W., De Groot, C. J., van Walderveen, M. A., Castelijns, J. A., Ravid, R., Lycklama a Nijeholt, G. J., van der Valk, P., Polman, C. H., Thompson, A. J., and Barkhof, F. (1999). Axonal loss in multiple sclerosis lesions: Magnetic resonance imaging insights into substrates of disability. *Ann. Neurol.* **46**, 747–754.

Vincent, A., Lily, O., and Palace, J. (1999). Pathogenic autoantibodies to neuronal proteins in neurological disorders. *J. Neuroimmunol.* **100**, 169–180.

Warrington, A. E., Asakura, K., Bieber, A. J., Ciric, B., Van Keulen, V., Kaveri, S. V., Kyle, R. A., Pease, L. R., and Rodriguez, M. (2000). Human monoclonal antibodies reactive to oligodendrocytes promote remyelination in a model of multiple sclerosis. *Proc. Natl. Acad. Sci. U. S. A.* **97**, 6820–6825.

Weinshenker, B. G., O'Brien, P. C., Petterson, T. M., Noseworthy, J. H., Lucchinetti, C. F., Dodick, D. W., Pineda, A. A., Stevens, L. N., and Rodriguez, M. (1999). A randomized trial of plasma exchange in acute central nervous system inflammatory demyelinating disease. *Ann. Neurol.* **46**, 878–886.

Windebank, A. J., Wood, P., Bunge, R. P., and Dyck, P. J. (1985). Myelination determines the caliber of dorsal root ganglion neurons in culture. *J. Neurosci.* **5**, 1563–1569.

Yin, Y., Cui, Q., Li, Y., Irwin, N., Fischer, D., Harvey, A. R., and Benowitz, L. I. (2003). Macrophage-derived factors stimulate optic nerve regeneration. *J. Neurosci.* **23**, 2284–2293.

Yoneda, A., and Couchman, J. R. (2003). Regulation of cytoskeletal organization by syndecan transmembrane proteoglycans. *Matrix Biol.* **22**, 25–33.

Yuan, X., Eisen, A. M., McBain, C. J., and Gallo, V. (1998). A role for glutamate and its receptors in the regulation of oligodendrocyte development in cerebellar tissue slices. *Development* **125**, 2901–2914.

28

Transplantation of Peripheral-Myelin-Forming Cells to Repair Demyelinated Axons

Jeffery D. Kocsis, Ph.D.

Masanori Sasaki, M.D., Ph.D.

I. Introduction

Multiple sclerosis (MS) is associated with variable degrees of axonal demyelination and transection in the brain and spinal cord (Trapp et al., 1998). Although very limited in the normal injured mammalian central nervous system (CNS), substantial endogenous axonal regeneration and remyelination can occur in peripheral nerve under certain conditions. Part of this regenerative capacity of peripheral nerve has been linked to several unique properties of

Schwann cells (SCs) including their production of extracellular matrix and trophic factors and their lack of growth inhibitory proteins that are present on oligodendrocytes (see Ide, 1996 for overview). Ramon y Cajal (1928) demonstrated that CNS axons can invade peripheral nerve engrafted into the CNS and that the regenerated axons become myelinated by SCs in the nerve grafts. Blakemore (1977) made the important observation that, when segments of peripheral nerve were placed over demyelinated spinal cord, the demyelinated CNS axons became myelinated by SCs. Moreover, transplantation of SCs into demyelinated spinal cord white matter results in significant improvement in conduction velocity (Honmou et al., 1996).

Another cell type that has attracted much attention over the past decade as a cell candidate to both encourage axonal regeneration and remyelination is the olfactory ensheathing cell (OEC). OECs, which are located in olfactory nerves and the outer nerve layer of the olfactory bulb, normally do not form myelin, but can do so when transplanted into the CNS (Franklin et al., 1996; Imaizumi et al. 1998). OECs are an unusual population of glial cells in that they share characteristics with both astrocytes in the CNS and SCs in the peripheral nervous system (PNS) (Ramon-Cueto and Valverde, 1995), and are the only glial cells known to cross the PNS-CNS transitional zone, accompanying the axons that they ensheath (Doucette, 1991). An interesting observation with both SCs and OECs is that in addition to remyelinating CNS axons, they can enhance axonal regeneration in the spinal cord when transplanted into axonal transection lesion sites (Li et al., 1997; Ramon-Cueto et al., 1998; Imaizumi et al., 2000a, 2000b). In this chapter we discuss cell transplantation as a strategy for protection and repair of the CNS in disorders such as MS. Because these cells are especially well understood, we discuss SCs and OECs as potential cellular tools to remyelinate and to enhance axonal regeneration in the injured spinal cord, and the prospect of using subpopulations of bone marrow cells to remyelinate CNS axons.

II. Schwann Cell Transplantation to Remyelinate the Spinal Cord

Transplantation of SCs into the demyelinated rodent spinal cord results in remyelination with a characteristic peripheral pattern (Blakemore and Crang, 1985; Baron-von Evercooren et al., 1992; Honmou et al., 1996). Moreover, when anatomical repair is achieved subsequent to SC transplantation, near-normal conduction velocity of the remyelinated axons is achieved (Honmou et al., 1996). Endogenous remyelination of demyelinated CNS axons by oligodendrocytes (Gledhill et al., 1973) or SCs (Blight and Young, 1989; Felts and Smith 1992) results in the reestablishment of relatively normal impulse conduction in animal models of demyelination. However, endogenous remyelination is very limited in human demyelinating diseases such as MS (Prineas and Connell, 1979). Given the success of cell transplantation to form functional myelin in animal models, myelin-forming cell transplantation has been suggested as a potential repair strategy for demyelinated CNS axons.

Transplantation of human SCs derived from human sural nerve can remyelinate spinal cord axons in the immunosuppressed rat (Kohama et al., 2001). In these experiments a focal demyelinated lesion was created in the dorsal column of the spinal cord of 12-week-old rats by X-irradiation and ethidium bromide injection (X-EB) (see Kohama et al., 2001, for technical details). This lesion presents as a persistent area of demyelination that lacks astrocytes. An example of a remyelinated axon region of the spinal cord 3 weeks after focal injection of reconstituted cryopreserved human SCs is shown in Fig. 1. Note the relatively large number of myelinated axons with typical SC morphology (i.e., large cytoplasmic and nuclear regions). Electron micrographs (not shown) reveal the presence of a basement membrane and extracellular collagen deposition. The conduction velocity of the axons remyelinated by the human SCs was improved (Fig. 2), indicating that electrophysiological function of the remyelinated axons was improved.

Autologous tissue represents one possible source of SCs for transplantation into patients with demyelinating disease.

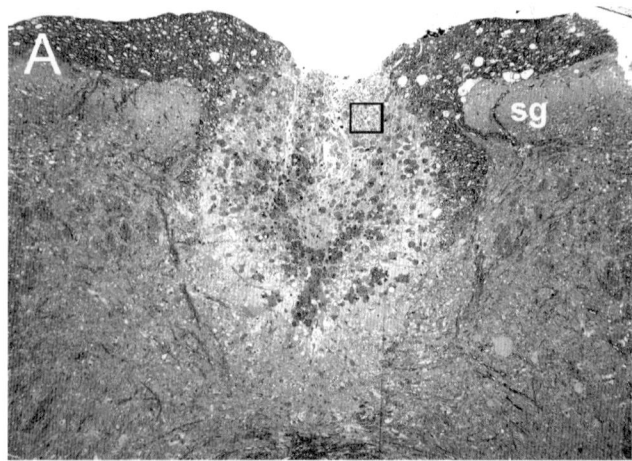

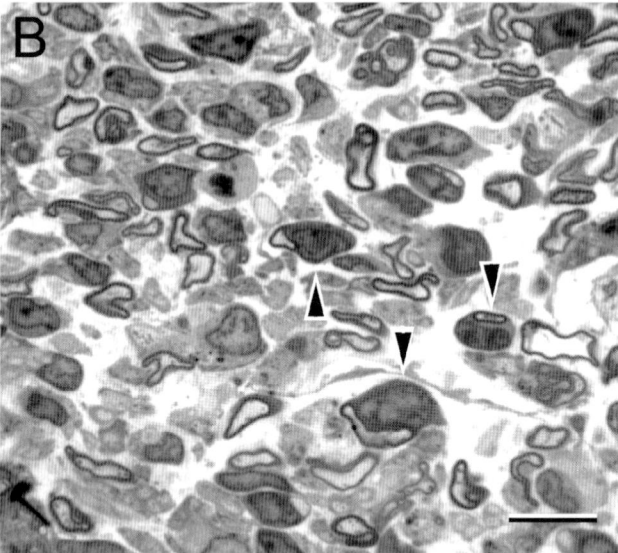

Figure 1 Remyelinated axons after human Schwann cell transplantation showing a peripheral pattern of myelination. Photomicrograhs were obtained from spinal cords placed in fixative after *in vitro* electrophysiological recordings. (**A**) Lesion area of dorsal columns 3 weeks after induction of the X-EB lesion. Sg refers to substantia gelatinosa of in the dorsal horn. (**B**) Higher power micrograph from the boxed region of the lesion showing remyelinated axons. Arrows in **B** indicate examples of axons myelinated by cells with large nuclear and cytoplasmic domains characteristic of peripheral myelin. Calibration in **B** corresponds to 100 μm in **A** and 10 μm in **B**. (Modified from Kohama et al., 2002.)

Presumably, SCs are not antigenically predisposed to the immunological attack seen in MS as are oligodendrocytes. The demonstration of anatomical and electrophysiological repair of demyelinated axons by adult human SCs is an important prerequisite for future consideration of these cells as candidates for autologous transplantation studies in humans. One potential problem with the use of SCs to remyelinate lesions in patients with MS is the presence of a glial scar in MS lesion sites that could limit cell migration and remyelination potential. In the X-EB lesion in the rat where relatively extensive remyelination is observed, it is

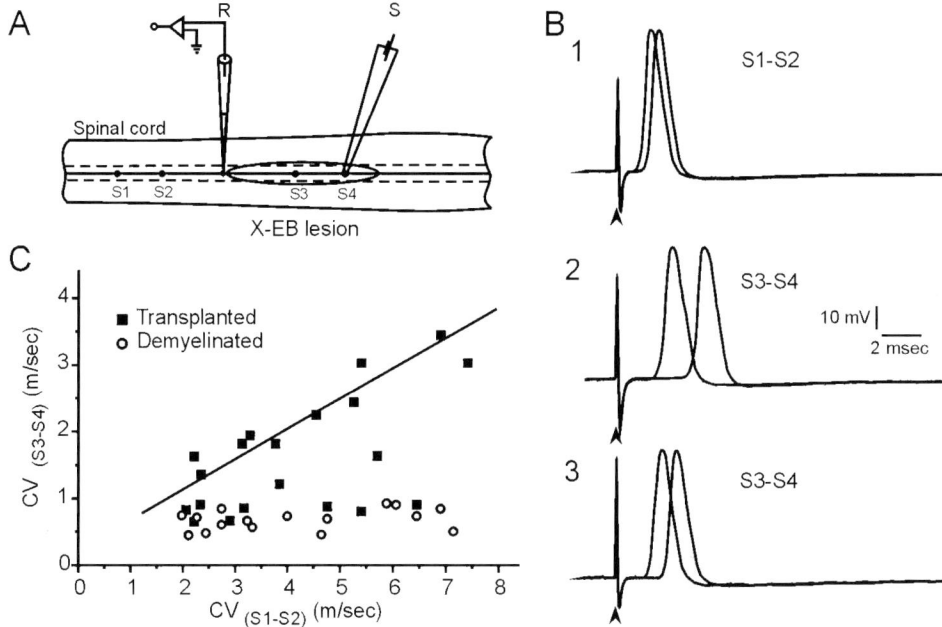

Figure 2 Intra-axonal recordings from demyelinated and remyelinated dorsal column axons. (**A**) Schematic showing arrangement of intra-axonal recording and stimulation sites. Intra-axonal recordings were obtained from dorsal column axons outside of the lesion where the axons were normally myelinated. Stimulating electrodes were positioned outside (S1-S2) and within (S3-S4) the X-EB lesion zone to assess single axon conduction velocity over both the demyelinated or remyelinated axon segment and the normally myelinated axon segment of the same axon. (**B**) Pairs of action potentials recorded from S1-S2 stimulation (1), S3-S4 in the demyelinated dorsal columns (2), and S3-S4 following cell transplantation (3). Recordings were obtained at comparable conduction distances. (**C**) Plot of the conduction velocity of axon segments within the lesion (S3-S4) versus conduction velocity of the axon segment outside of the lesion (S1-S2) for X-EB lesioned spinal cord without (*open circles*) and with (*closed squares*) transplantation. (Modified from Kohama et al., 2002.)

important to note that the lesion is agliotic, and thus the potential impediment of gliosis is not an issue. However, SCs transplanted into a contusion injury model in the spinal cord where gliosis does occur lead to increased myelination, axon sparing/regeneration, and improved functional outcome in rodents (Takami et al., 2002).

Experimental *in vitro* studies have shown that astrocytes inhibit both SC proliferation and SC myelination potential (Guénard et al., 1994). When SCs are transplanted into the demyelinated spinal cord (Blakemore et al., 1986), they remyelinate axons throughout the area from which astrocytes are absent but not beyond. On the basis of this type of observation, it has been suggested that SCs and astrocytes are mutually exclusive. In contrast, OECs coexist with astrocytes within the olfactory bulb, are associated with olfactory receptor neurons from their peripheral origin to their central projection in the outer nerve layer of the olfactory bulb, and share in the formation of the glia limitans (Doucette, 1984, 1991). One assumption favoring the use of OECs in CNS repair studies, therefore, was that the use of OECs instead of SCs might prevent the astrocytic response to nerve injury (Franklin and Barnett, 1997, 2000), which is thought to block the regeneration response. Studies including the co-culture of either SCs or OECs with astrocytes have shown

that OECs, in contrast to SCs, intermingle with astrocytes (Lakatos et al., 2000). Moreover, contact with SCs, but not with OECs, induced apoptosis of astrocytes (Lakatos et al., 2000). After induction of an electrolytic lesion of the rat corticospinal tract, injection of OECs induced axonal elongation across and beyond the lesion, and a reduced upregulation of GFAP expression in the adjacent astrocytic processes compared with nontransplanted lesions (Li et al., 1997; 1998). The assumption emerging from these studies that OECs in contrast to SCs might reduce astrocytosis *in vivo* was recently tested by application of OECs into the photochemically lesioned spinal cord (Verdu et al., 2001). It was found that OECs reduced the number of hypertrophic astrocytes as well as the maximal area and volume of the cystic cavity (Verdu et al., 2001) compared to nontransplanted controls.

III. Transplantation of Olfactory Ensheathing Cells (OECs) to Remyelinate the Spinal Cord

Adult olfactory receptor neurons continually undergo turnover from an endogenous progenitor pool, and their nascent axons grow through the olfactory nerves and cross the PNS-CNS interface where they form new synaptic connections in the olfactory bulb (Graziadei et al., 1978). This apparent support role of OECs in axonal growth in the adult CNS has spawned extensive research aimed at studying the potential of OEC transplants to encourage axonal regeneration and functional recovery in spinal cord injury models (Li et al., 1997, 1998; Ramon-Cueto et al., 1998, 2000; Imaizumi et al., 2000a, 2000b). In the normal nervous system, OECs surround or ensheath bundles of nonmyelinated axons in the olfactory nerve and do not form myelin. OECs share with SCs the ability to support axonal ensheathment and regrowth, but they do not share the same developmental origin or some immunocytochemical and morphological features of SCs (Ramon-Cueto and Valverde, 1995). The SC-like morphology of OECs includes p75 and S100 expression, as well as a spindle-shaped morphology in culture (Pixley, 1992).

A large body of work supports the proposal that transplantation of OECs into various spinal cord injury and demyelination models can promote axonal regeneration, remyelination, and functional recovery (Franklin et al., 1996; Li et al., 1997, 1998; Ramon-Cueto et al., 1998, 2000; Imaizumi et al., 2000a, 2000b; Lu et al., 2002; Keyvan-Fouladi et al., 2003; Plant et al., 2003). Yet, there is an important controversy as to whether the transplanted OECs associate with axons and form peripheral myelin, as opposed to recruiting endogenous SCs that form myelin (Takami et al., 2002; Boyd et al., 2004). OECs can express a number of trophic factors, transcription factors, and extracellular matrix molecules (Ramon-Cueto and Avila, 1998; Chuah and West, 2002; Au and Roskams, 2003; Ramer et al., 2004), which could facilitate endogenous SC cell invasion, angiogenesis, and activation of progenitor cells to facilitate repair.

A recent study failed to observe myelination *in vitro* in a co-culture experiment with dorsal root ganglion neurons and immunoselected (p75) OECs under culture conditions permissive for myelination by SCs (Plant et al., 2002). These investigators raise the important question as to whether transplanted OECs might induce or enhance the migration of endogenous SCs into the transplantation site (Brook et al., 1998). Moreover, although numerous reports suggest that OECs can form myelin when transplanted into the demyelinated (Franklin et al., 1996; Imaizumi et al., 1998; Barnett et al., 2000; Kato et al., 2000; Akiyama et al., 2004; Radtke et al., 2004) or injured spinal cord (Li et al., 1997, 1998; Imaizumi et al., 2000a, 2000b), one study was unable to find evidence of OEC myelination in the compressed spinal cord, suggesting that OEC (derived from embryos) transplantation may facilitate endogenous SC invasion into the lesion site (Boyd et al., 2004). To address this issue, we prepared cell suspensions of OECs from the olfactory bulb of alkaline phosphatase expressing adult transgenic rats (Kisseberth et al., 1999). The marker gene, human placental alkaline phosphatase

(hPAP), is linked to the ubiquitous active R26 gene promoter, and its stable expression has been demonstrated by neural precursor cells in culture and after transplantation into the CNS (Mujtaba et al., 2002; Han et al., 2002). Transplantation of cell suspensions enriched in adult OECs (>95% p75+ and S100+) derived from hPAP transgenic rats can be readily identified *in vivo* and are associated with myelin formation (Fig. 3) (Akiyama et al., 2004). The extensive degree of remyelination by identified SCs and OECs indicates that both cell types under appropriate *in vivo* conditions are capable of forming myelin in the spinal cord.

In rodents, considerable endogenous remyelination can occur after development of a chemically-induced demyelinating lesion (Akiyama et al., 2004). A large number of myelinated profiles are present by 3 weeks after induction of focal demyelinating lesions in the rat spinal cord (Akiyama et al., 2004). Figure 4 shows a progressive increase in conduction velocity from 1 to 6 weeks after a focal injection of ethidium bromide (EB) into the rat spinal cord. When the spinal cord is X-irradiated 3 days before EB injection to block mitosis of progenitor cells and endogenous repair, a persistent region of demyelination is observed even at 6 weeks postinjury. The conduction velocity of the persistently demyelinated axons remains low (about 1.0 m/sec) throughout this period. However, when SCs or OECs are transplanted into the X-EB lesion, one can see that, for both cell types, conduction velocity is improved at both 3 and 6 weeks posttransplantation. In this lesion model system, improvement in conduction velocity was comparable after transplantation of SCs and OECs.

Most of the experimental work showing axonal repair using OECs was done on the rodent system, and the OEC preparations were of varying purity and cellular composition. The robust capability of rodents in terms of endogenous myelin repair may differ in primates. Unlike what occurs in the rodent, very little endogenous repair was observed after EB lesions in the nonhuman primate spinal cord at 4 weeks postinjection (Radtke et al., 2004). However, after grafting of OECs derived from a transgenic pig model expressing H-transferase to alter carbohydrate structure of the cells to mimic that of the human Type O blood group, considerable peripheral-like myelin was observed in the primate spinal cord (Fig. 5). These results suggest that although endogenous repair of myelin may be less robust in primates than in rodents, transplantation of peripheral-myelin forming cells are capable of remyelinating primate spinal cord axons.

IV. Cell Transplantation and Axonal Regeneration of Spinal Cord Axons

Although several studies suggest that transplantation of OECs into various spinal cord injury and demyelination

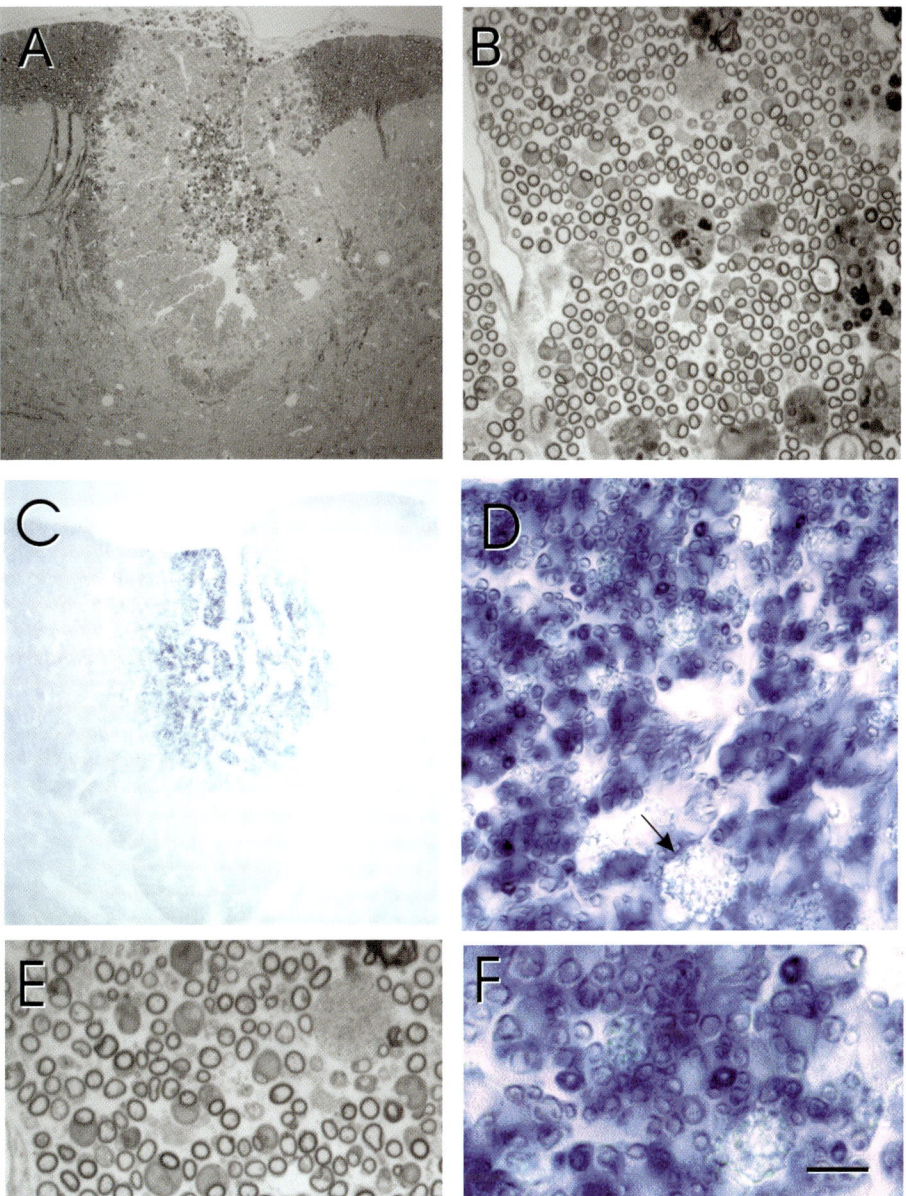

Figure 3 Remyelination after transplantation of hPAP OECs into the X-EB dorsal funiculus lesion. (**A**) Low power plastic embedded section of the dorsal spinal cord 3 weeks after hPAP OEC transplantation. (**B**) A higher power micrograph shows extensive myelinated profiles throughout the transplantation site. In adjacent frozen sections reacted for ALP, blue reaction product can be observed in the transplantation site (**C**). Higher power of this area shows numerous blue profiles characteristic of myelinated axons similar to that observed for SC transplantation in Fig. 2 (**D**). (**E**) Higher power images of plastic embedded sections shows myelinated axons many of which are associated with large cytoplasmic and nuclear surrounds characteristic of peripheral myelination. (**F**) These profiles are associated with hPAP reaction product (**F**). Scale bar in **D**; 200 μm in **A, C**; 25 μm in B, D; 7 μm in **E, F.** (Modified from Akiyama et al., 2004.)

models can promote axonal regeneration, remyelination, and functional recovery (Franklin et al., 1996; Li et al., 1997, 1998; Ramon-Cueto et al., 1998, 2000; Imaizumi et al., 2000a, 2000b; Lu et al., 2002; Keyvan-Fouladi et al., 2003; Plant et al., 2003), Takami et al. (2002) reported that transplantation of SCs, but not OEC transplantation, results in improved hind-limb locomotor function in contusive spinal

cord injury. Transplantation of OECs into spinal cord injury models mediates some degree of axonal regeneration and functional improvement even when transplantation is delayed (Lu et al., 2002; Keyvan-Fouladi et al., 2003). Myelinated axons spanning the lesion site have a characteristic peripheral pattern of myelination similar to that of SC myelination (Li et al., 1997, 1998; Imaizumi et al., 1998,

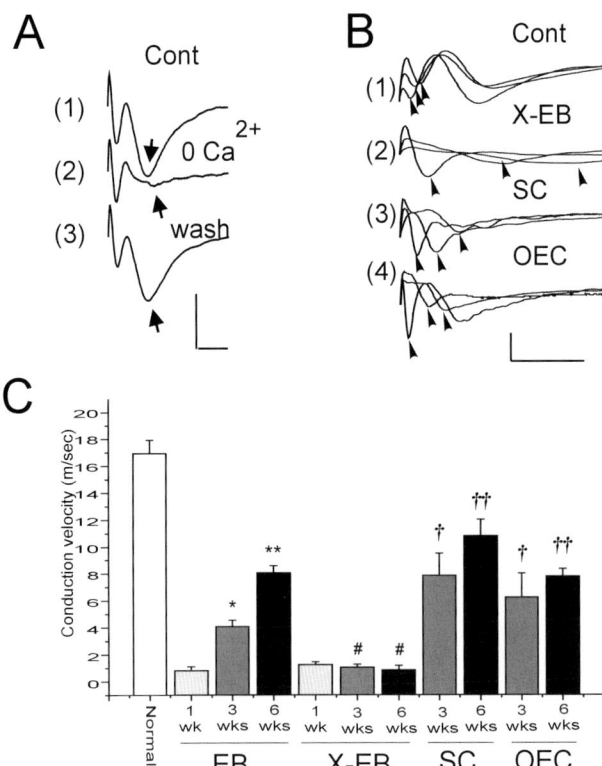

Figure 4 Conduction velocity measurements of demyelinated axons and after remyelination by Schwann cells or OECs. (**A**) Compound action potentials recorded from the dorsal columns (near midline and within 100 μm of the surface) with a glass microelectrode *in vivo* after stimulation of the dorsal column surface near the midline. Note an early and late negativity. When the surface of the spinal cord was washed with a 0 calcium and high (6 mM) magnesium Krebs' solution (2), the second negativity was eliminated indicating its synaptic nature. Thus the first negativity corresponds to conducting dorsal column axons. (**B**) Superimposed compound action potentials recorded at 1.0-mm increments longitudinally along the dorsal columns in normal (cont; 1), X-EB lesion (2), and 3 weeks after SC (3) and OEC (4) transplantation. (**C**) Histograms of conduction velocity (error bars indicate SEM) of dorsal column axons obtained from normal, 1, 3, and 6 weeks after EB injection without prior X-irradiation, after X-EB lesion induction, and 3 and 6 weeks after SC and OEC transplantation into the X-EB lesion. $^*P < 0.1$, $^{**}P < 0.01$, $†P < 0.05$, $††P < 0.05$, and # not statistically significant. (Modified from Akiyama et al., 2004.)

2000a). Spinal cord injuries without OEC transplants can show limited SC-like myelination, presumably from invasion of the injury site from endogenous SCs (Brook et al., 1998; Imaizumi et al., 2000a, 2000b; Namiki et al., 2000; Takami et al., 2002) or possibly from precursor cells.

A unique feature associated with axonal regeneration after OEC transplantation is the occurrence of groups of axons within the transection lesion site with a peripheral pattern of myelination surrounded by a fibroblast-like cell that forms a "tunnel" around small clusters of myelinated axons (Li et al., 1997). An example of groupings of myelinated fibers surrounded by fibroblast-like cells is shown in Fig. 6. This section was taken from the center of the tran-

section zone indicating that the axons were regenerated. These tunnels have not been reported after SC transplantation into transection lesions (Imaizumi et al., 2000a, 2000b) or SC transplantation into demyelinating lesions (Lankford et al., 2002), suggesting that they are unique to OEC preparations. Li et al. (1998) referred to the surrounding fibroblast-like cells as "A" cells and the myelin-forming cells as "S" cells and suggest that both can be derived from the donor OECs. Although transplanted SCs can myelinate spinal cord axons (Blakemore and Crang, 1985; Baron-Van Evercooren et al., 1992; Honmou et al., 1996) and are associated with improved functional outcome (Takami et al., 2002), the "A" and "S" cell organization appears to be unique to OEC transplantation (Li et al., 1997, 1998; Imaizumi et al., 2000a, 2000b). However, Boyd et al. (2004) did not find LacZ-expressing "S" cells after transplantation of E18-derived OECs into a spinal cord compression injury model, but only LacZ-expressing fibroblast-like cells. They conclude that only the fibroblast-like cell ("A" cells) is derived from the OEC transplantation and that the "S" cells are exclusively derived from invading SCs.

We used an anti-GFP antibody in conjunction with immunoperoxidase staining on the electron microscopic level to identify the fate of donor GFP-expressing OECs transplanted in dorsal sectioned spinal cords of rat. We found evidence of GFP immunoreactivity on an ultrastrutual level in the cytoplasm of cells within the lesion site that were forming peripheral-like myelin (Sasaki et al., 2004). These data indicate that transplantation of adult OECs prepared at relatively high purity (>95% p75+) and not maintained in culture for extensive periods are able to form peripheral-like myelin around axons spanning a dorsal funiculus transection.

A difficulty in comparing results from OEC transplantation studies from various laboratories is that differences are present in the age of the animals used for cell harvesting, purification procedures, and lesion models into which the cells were transplanted. OECs used in our studies were prepared relatively acutely from the outer nerve layer of the adult olfactory bulb, an area rich in OECs *in vivo* (Devon and Doucette, 1992). The degree of cell purity (>95%) in our cell suspension as assessed using p75/S100 immunostaining was about the same as in other studies where immunopanning techniques were used (Takami et al., 2002; Lakatos et al., 2003) or where OECs were prepared from embryonic tissue (Devon and Doucette, 1992). Mitotic inhibitors and stimulators of cell proliferation and differentiation were used in those studies. In our cell preparation method from adult tissue, we did not use mitotic inhibitors, nor did we stimulate proliferation and differentiation *in vivo*. Contamination by SCs, which are also p75/S100 positive, in our cultures would be problematic in the interpretation that adult OECs are able to form peripheral-like myelin. However, one would expect at best a very minor contamina-

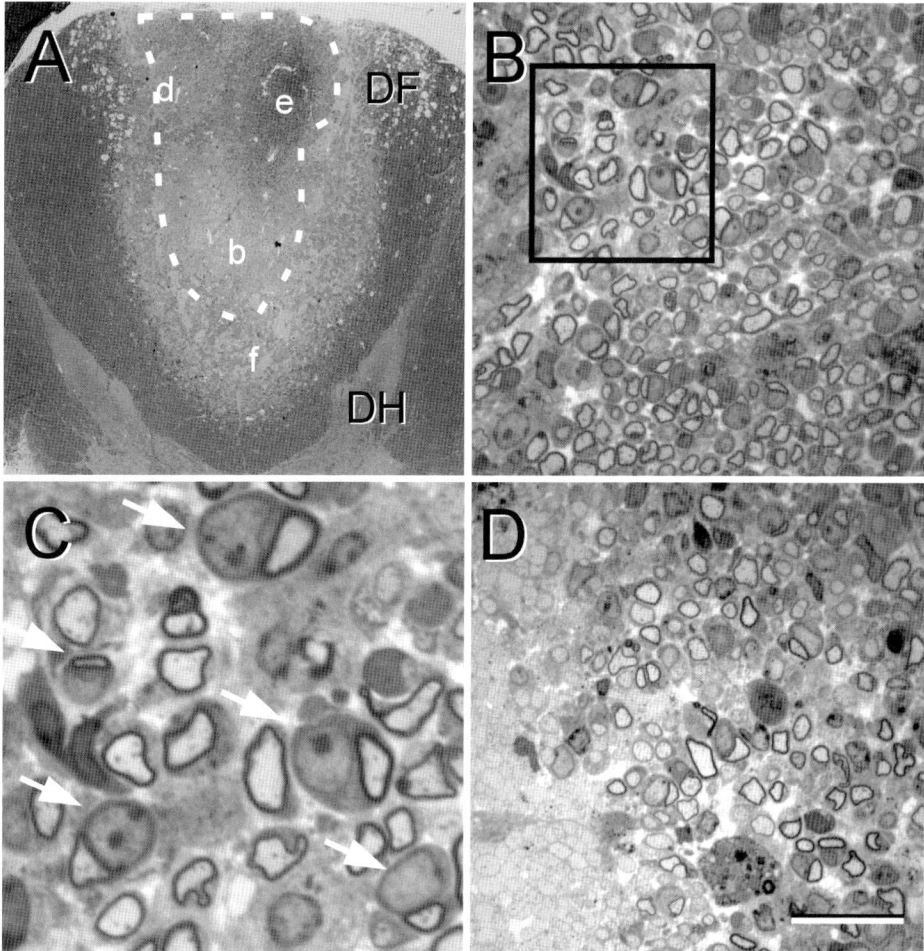

Figure 5 Transplantation of transgenic pig OECs into the demyelinated monkey spinal cord. (**A**) Low-power micrograph of lesion after cell transplantation in the dorsal funiculus (DF). Remyelination was observed within the white dashed lines and most of the dorsal funicular region outside of the dashed lines remained demyelination. (**B**) The central core of the lesion was densely remyelinated. (**C**) The boxed area in (**B**), showing myelinated axon profiles exhibiting a peripheral pattern of remyelination. (**D**) The edge of the densely remyelinated zone a transition from demyelinated (*left*) to remyelinated axons can be seen. Scale bar, (a) = 1.25 mm, (c) = 50 μm, (b, d) = 125 μm. (Modified from Radtke et al., 2004.)

tion of SCs, possibly associated with blood vessel innervation (Takami et al., 2002). Such minor contamination could not account for the vast majority (>95%) of our cells displaying a p75/S100 phenotype. Yet, the issue of cell contamination with SCs or meningeal cells (Lakatos et al., 2003) is important and clearly should be addressed in future studies.

The mechanisms for the functional improvement observed after OEC transplantation into spinal cord injury models are not clear and have been suggested to include long-tract regeneration (Li et al., 1997; Ramon-Cueto et al., 2000), axonal sparing and neuroprotection (Plant et al., 2003), sprouting and plasticity associated with novel polysynaptic pathways (Keyvan-Fouladi et al., 2003), recruitment of endogenous SCs (Takami et al., 2002; Boyd et al.,

2004), and remyelination (Franklin et al., 1996; Imaizumi et al., 2000a, 2000b). OECs secrete a number of trophic factors such as nerve growth factor, glial-derived neurotrophic factor, brain-derived neurotrophic factor, and ciliary neurotrophic factor that could contribute to these events (Woodhall et al., 2001). It is possible that more than one of these mechanisms is operative.

OECs have emerged as an important cell candidate for cell transplantation strategies to improve functional outcome in adult spinal cord injury. Clinical investigations in spinal cord injury using OEC engraftment are in progress (Senior, 2002; Huang et al., 2003). Although it is generally agreed that, under appropriate cell preparation and transplantation conditions, functional outcome can be enhanced by OEC transplantation, questions still remain with regard to the

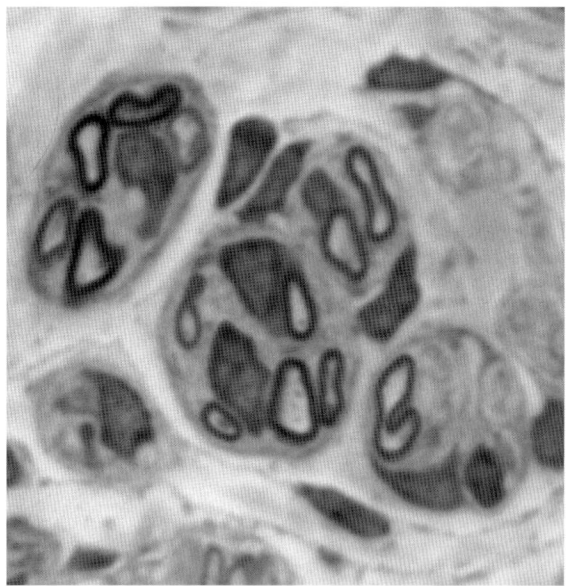

Figure 6 Semithin plastic sections stained with methylene blue/Azure II through the transection site 5 weeks after transplantation of OECs. Note the clustering of myelinated axons surrounded by a cellular element. These surrounding cells are not observed after transplantation of SCs and appear to be unique to OEC transplantation. Scale bar = 8 μm.

in vivo fate of transplanted OECs. Determination of the relative contribution of cellular repair such as remyelination vs. trophic support for endogenous recruitment of cells, neuroprotection, and synaptic plasticity by OECs will be important for a comprehensive evaluation of the potential therapeutic efficacy of OECs as a cell therapy in spinal cord injury. As our understanding of potential trophic influences of OECs is expanded, this could suggest novel pharmacological approaches to the treatment of spinal cord injury.

Another aspect of spinal cord injury is the reduction in cyclic adenosine monophosphate (cAMP) in injured neurons (Pearse et al., 2004). Increased cAMP levels in growth cones has been shown to enable neurons to extent neurites across inhibitory substrates such as myelin (Cai et al., 2001). One study demonstrated the combined transplantation of SCs with inhibition of cAMP hydrolysis (Rolipram treatment) and db-cAMP treatment promoted axonal growth and functional recovery after spinal cord injury (Pearse et al., 2004). This study emphasizes that a combination of cell therapy and pharmacological approaches may maximize functional recovery in spinal cord injury.

V. Bone Marrow–Derived Stem Cells as a Potential Cell Source for Neural Repair

Bone marrow cell transplantation into demyelinated (Sasaki et al., 2001; Akiyama et al., 2002a, 2002b; Inoue

et al., 2003) or contused spinal cord (Hofstetter et al., 2002) has demonstrated remyelination and improved functional recovery, respectively. Moreover, transplantation of bone marrow cells into cerebral ischemia models has demonstrated reduced lesion size and improved functional outcome (Li et al., 2002; Iihoshi et al., 2004). The precise cell population in bone marrow responsible for these putative therapeutic effects is uncertain. However, bone marrow-derived stromal cells (MSCs) have been suggested to differentiate into bone, cartilage, cardiac myocytes, and neurons and glia both *in vitro* and *in vivo*. MSCs are thought to represent a very small proportion of cells in the mononuclear population of bone marrow, and a method to isolate and expand them in culture would provide a valuable tool to study their potential therapeutic efficacy *in vivo*.

Bone marrow cells can be enriched in MSCs by selecting for plastic-adherent cells. These stromal cells will grow to confluency in appropriate culture conditions as flattened fibroblast-like cells (Friedenstein, 1976). MSCs may be present in different proportions in the stromal cell fraction of various species. MSCs have a distinct cell surface antigen pattern including SH2[+], SH3[+], and CD34[−] (Majumdar et al., 1998). Methodologies have been established to culture human MSCs in very high purity. However, these cells had reduced mitogenic activity after about five cell doublings over the course of about 6 weeks. To generate larger numbers of human MSCs, they have been transfected with the human telomerase gene for immortalization (Kobune et al, 2003).

Autologous bone marrow cells isolated by density gradient (mononuclear layer) can remyelinate demyelinated spinal cord axons (X-EB lesion model) after either direct (Sasaki et al., 2001; Akiyama et al., 2002b) or intravenous (Akiyama et al., 2002a; Inoue et al. 2003) administration or direct microinjection into the lesion. Figure 7 shows myelinated profiles in the X-EB demyelinated spinal cord after intravenous delivery of mononuclear cells isolated from bone marrow. Many of the myelin profiles were SC-like. Several lines of evidence indicate that the remyelination following bone marrow cell transplantation was from the transplanted bone marrow cells and not from endogenous host cells. Our studies were carried out within 3 weeks after X-EB lesion induction, which is well within the time at which persistent demyelination is confirmed in a large number of control studies (Akiyama et al., 2002a, 2002b, 2004; Blakemore and Crang, 1985; Franklin et al., 1996; Honmou et al., 1996, Kato et al., 2000; Kohama et al., 2001; Sasaki et al., 2001). However, the possible recruitment of cells outside of the lesion zone by the injection procedure cannot be completely ruled out. We used acutely prepared autologous bone marrow mononuclear cells prepared on density gradient that were not expanded in culture and were therefore not able to incorporate reporter genes into the cells for more definitive assessment of the fate of the injected cells. However, sham injections of medium alone did not result in remyelination.

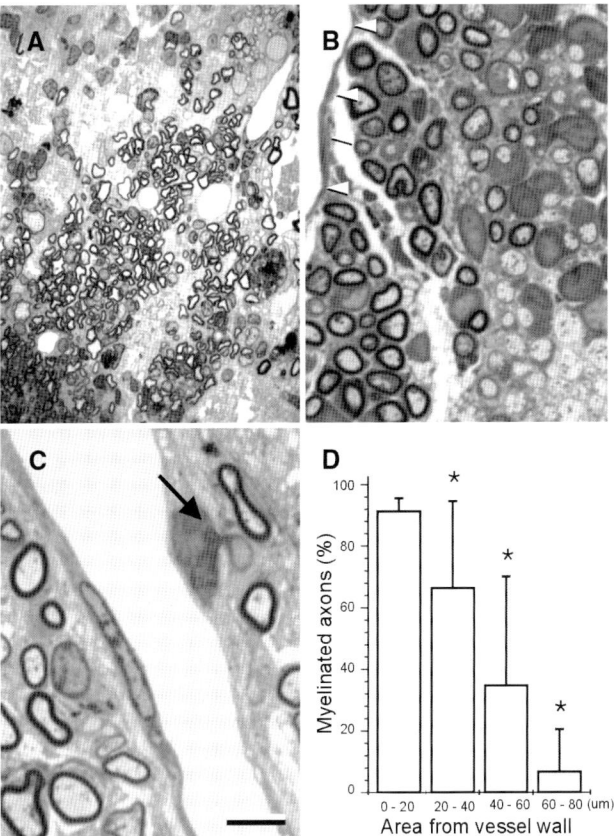

Figure 7 **Remyelination in perivascular regions after intravenous injections of bone marrow.** (**A**) A relatively large number of axons are remyelinated near a bed of capillaries. (**B**) A higher power micrograph shows endothelium of a capillary (*arrowheads*) and myelinated axon profiles near the capillary. Axons away from this capillary are not remyelinated (*right*). However, note that cells with dark nuclei are present in this non-myelinated zone and some appear to be associated with axons, possibly in the process of remyelinating. (**C**) Longitudinal section through a capillary showing myelinated axons near the vessel, and a dark cell close to the capillary wall. (**D**) Histograms showing percentage of myelinated axons at various distances from vessel walls. Scale bar in **C** corresponds to 20 μm in **A**, 8 μm in **B**, and 5 μm in **C**. *$P < 0.01$ Analysis of variation (ANOVA). (Modified from Akiyama et al., 2002a.)

Moreover, the "dose-response" relationship of myelination with the number of injected cells further suggests that the donor cells were responsible for the remyelination (Inoue et al., 2003). Future studies with high-efficiency reporter gene incorporation into the endogenous cells will be critical to definitively distinguish between facilitation of endogenous repair vs. homing of injected cells into the lesion.

Intravenously delivered cells are unlikely to migrate across the blood-brain barrier (BBB) into normal spinal cord tissue, because the BBB would prevent cell access to the parenchyma. Indeed, we did not observe cells entering the nonlesion zone after intravenous delivery. Intravenously transplanted bone marrow cells appear to be recruited through the vascular system (Ferrari et al., 1998) and might

be allowed to enter the spinal cord lesions because of the partial disruption of BBB in the X-EB lesions. In addition there may be active targeting mechanisms in the pathological environment of the lesion. Expression of chemotactic factors such as monocyte chemoattractant protein-1 is increased in damaged CNS tissues (Kim, 1996), and injured tissue extract selectively induces chemotaxis of mesenchymal progenitors *in vitro* (Chen et al., 2001). Adhesion molecules such as intercellular adhesion molecule (Zhang et al., 1995), vascular adhesion molecule-1, and E-selectin are also highly expressed on the endothelial cells in the damaged lesions (Blann et al., 1999; Haraldsen et al., 1996; Quesenberry and Becker, 1998; Zhang et al., 1995). Other unknown molecules may also promote migration of transplanted bone marrow cells into the demyelinated lesions. In addition, migration of bone marrow cells from the hematopoietic environment to the other nonhematopoietic tissues is associated with genetic transformation, in part through changes in expression of cell surface adhesion molecules such as intercellular adhesion molecule-1, vascular cell adhesion molecule-1, and neural cell adhesion molecules (Haraldson et al., 1996; Quesenberry and Becker, 1998; Vermeulen et al., 1998). Thus, the interaction of these molecules may promote the transplanted bone marrow cells to target the spinal cord lesions.

The autologous bone marrow cells injected into the X-EB model rats were acutely prepared from the same demyelinated rats, with cells isolated by centrifugation through a density gradient (mononuclear cell layer) to remove erythrocytes, platelets, and debris. The recovered mononuclear cell layer consisted of stromal cells, mesenchymal stem cells, hematopoietic and nonhematopoietic stem and precursor cells, and lymphocytes (Azizi et al., 1998). It remains unclear as to which type of cell within the bone marrow cell fraction is responsible for the *in vivo* differentiation of myelin-forming cells. Local injection of CD34+ cells (referred to as hematopoietic stem cells) did not result in remyelination in our demyelinated model system (Sasaki, et al., 2001), suggesting that hematopoietic stem cells are not a candidate cell for remyelination. MSCs have been reported to differentiate into neurons, astrocytes, and myelin-forming cells (Akiyama et al., 2002b; Woodbury et al., 2000), suggesting that cells within this fraction may be responsible for the myelin repair.

A large number of transplanted bone marrow cells into demyelinated lesions differentiated *in vivo* into myelin-forming cells (Inoue et al., 2003), although bone marrow cells predominantly differentiated into astrocytic and neuronal cell types in normal or ischemic brain (Eglitis et al., 1999). It is well established that stem cells from one region will, when placed in ectopic CNS sites, differentiate with a terminal phenotype appropriate for that ectopic site (e.g., Akiyama et al., 2001; Brustle et al., 1999; Gage et al., 1995; Hammang et al., 1997; Snyder et al., 1997). The extracellular environment into which transplanted stem cells are delivered has an important influence on their fate *in vivo* (Akiyama et al., 2001; Brustle et al., 1999; Hammang et al., 1997; Snyder et al., 1997). Pathological CNS tissue is a different environment than intact CNS tissue and markedly alters the terminal differentiated phenotype of transplanted cells (Gage et al., 1995). The lesion into which the cells were placed in our model was enriched in axons because virtually all glia including astrocytes and oligodendrocytes were killed by the lesion protocol (Honmou et al., 1996). This abundance of axon membrane may be an important local environmental signal for bone marrow cell differentiation into myelin-forming cells. In the current demyelinated model, transplanted bone marrow cells retained the capacity to respond to local epigenetic signals in the demyelinated lesions, as they can differentiate into myelin-forming cell phenotypes.

VI. Conclusions

Experimental studies of demyelination and axonal transection of the spinal cord indicate the feasibility of cell transplantation as an approach that may elicit at least some degree of functional recovery, raising the possibility that this approach might be useful in the treatment of disorders such as MS. One of the primary challenges to develop such therapies will be selecting the appropriate cell type and delivery method for the appropriate neurological condition. Although oligodendrocytes normally form myelin in the CNS, the prospect of using SCs, OECs, or bone marrow-derived cells to remyelinate CNS lesions in patients with MS is intriguing because they can be harvested autologously, and they may not have antigens present on oligodendrocytes that may be immunogenic. Yet, there are limitations with the use of these cells. One is that these peripheral-myelinating cells do not precisely recapitulate the pattern of remyelination by oligodendroctyes. The density of axonal spacing is less with SC and OEC myelination, and one must ask what potential negative effects this could have on the system. Indeed, it has speculated that a selective force for the evolution of oligodendrocytes was to provide for maximum conduction velocity conferred by myelin deposition, with the most economic utilization of space. The advantage this organization achieves with oligodendrocyte myelination is a relatively compact CNS, but a disadvantage is that pathology to a single oligodendrocyte will affect a number of myelin segments. In spite of this limitation, however, it seems reasonable to suggest that restoration of myelin and conduction in even a limited subset of axons might potentially result in significant functional recovery.

Another important concern with regard to cell transplantation therapies is the harvesting of sufficient numbers of cells for transplantation. Although a number of cell types can be expanded in culture with trophic factors and mito-

gens, it is not clear if such expansion will alter the physiology of the cells in a way that impairs their ability to form functional myelin. Further studies to examine the myelinogenic potential of expanded cells is required. Another concern with expanded cells is the potential risk of tumor formation. It will be essential to determine whether experimental *in vivo* transplantation of expanded cells not only retains their ability to carry out neural repair, but does not form tumors.

Transplanted cells may provide neurotrophic support for endogenous cell survival, but additionally may contribute to neural repair by, for example, remyelination. An advantage of MSCs is that they can be easily and safety obtained in large numbers from autologous bone marrow aspirates, and they display a higher efficiency to migrate from the vascular system into the CNS. Although controversial (Castro et al., 2002; Alvarez-Dolado et al., 2003) because of the potential for cell fusion of bone marrow cells with resident cells, transdifferentiation of bone marrow cells into astrocytes, neurons, and into myelin-forming cells may occur in the CNS after direct or intravenous delivery. Irrespective of whether transdifferentiation, cell fusion, or a combination occurs, it is important to note that functional improvement has been reported after bone marrow cell transplantation in spinal cord injury and stroke models. The prospect that intravenous delivery of these cells could lead to a global neuroprotection, with subsequent repair such as remyelination, is intriguing and should be further explored. Future research to study the repair potential of systemic bone marrow cell delivery in other lesion models and research to study more restricted cell types within the mononuclear layer will provide important information on the potential of these cells as candidates for clinical studies in human neurological diseases such as MS.

Acknowledgments

Supported in part by Rehabilitation Research and Development Service of the Department of Veterans Affairs, the NIH, and the National Multiple Sclerosis Society.

References

Akiyama, Y., Radtke, C., Honmou, O., and Kocsis, J. D. (2002a). Remyelination of the spinal cord following intravenous delivery of bone marrow cells. *Glia* **39**, 229–236.

Akiyama, Y., Radtke, C., and Kocsis, J. D. (2002b). Remyelination of the rat spinal cord by transplantation of identified bone marrow stromal cells. *J. Neurosci.* **22**, 6623–6630.

Akiyama, Y., Lankford, K. L., Radtke, C., Greer, C. A., and Kocsis, J. D. (2004). Remyelination of spinal cord axons by olfactory ensheathing cells and Schwann cells derived from a transgenic rat expressing alkaline phosphatase marker gene. *Neuron Glia Biol.* **1**, 1–9.

Alvarez-Dolado, M., Pardal, R., Garcia-Verdugo, J. M., Fike, J. R., Lee, H. O., Pfeffer, K., Lois, C., Morrison, S. J., and Alvarez-Buylla, A. (2003). Fusion of bone-marrow-derived cells with Purkinje neurons, cardiomyocytes and hepatocytes. *Nature* **425**, 968–973.

Au, E., and Roskams, A. J. (2003). Olfactory ensheathing cells of the lamina propria in vivo and in vitro. *Glia* **41**, 224–236.

Azizi, S. A., Stokes, D., Augelli, B. J., DiGirolamo, C., and Prockop, D. J. (1998). Engraftment and migration of human bone marrow stromal cells implanted in the brains of albino rats: Similarities to astrocyte grafts. *Proc. Natl. Acad. Sci. U. S. A.* **95**, 3908–3913

Barnett, S. C., Alexander, C. L., Iwashita, Y., Gilson, J. M., Crowther, J., Clark, L., Dunn, L. T., Papanastassiou, V., Kennedy, P. G., and Franklin, R. J. (2000). Identification of a human olfactory ensheathing cell that can effect transplant-mediated remyelination of demyelinated CNS axons. *Brain* **123**, 1581–1588.

Baron-Van Evercooren, A., Gansmuller, A., Duhamel, E., Pascal, F., and Gumpel, M. (1992). Repair of a myelin lesion by Schwann cells transplanted in the adult mouse spinal cord. *J. Neuroimmunol.* **40**, 235–242.

Blakemore, W. F. (1977). Remyelination of CNS axons by Schwann cells transplanted from the sciatic nerve. *Nature* **266**, 88–69.

Blakemore, W. F., and Crang, A. J. (1985). The use of cultured autologous Schwann cells to remyelinate areas of persistent demyelination in the central nervous system. *J. Neurol. Sci.* **70**, 207–223.

Blakemore, W. F., Crang, A. J., et al. (1986). The interaction of Schwann cells with CNS axons in regions containing normal astrocytes. *Acta Neuropathol.* **71(3-4)**, 295–300.

Blann, A., Kumar, P., Krupinski, J., McCollum, C., Beevers, D. G., and Lip, G. Y. (1999). Soluble intercelluar adhesion molecule-1, E-selectin, vascular cell adhesion molecule-1 and von Willebrand factor in stroke. *Blood Coagul. Fibrinolysis* **10**, 277–284.

Blight, A. R., and Young, W. (1989). Central axons in injured cat spinal cord recover electrophysiological function following remyelination by Schwann cells. *J. Neurol. Sci.* **91**, 15–34.

Boyd, J. G., Lee, J., Skihar, V., Doucette, R., and Kawaja, M. D. (2004). LacZ-expressing olfactory ensheathing cells do not associate with myelinated axons after implantation into the compressed spinal cord. *Proc. Natl. Acad. Sci. U. S. A.* **101**, 2162–2166.

Brook, G. A., Plate, D., Franzen, R., Martin, D., Moonen, G., Schoenen, J., Schmitt, A. B., Noth, J., and Nacimiento, W. (1998). Spontaneous longitudinally orientated axonal regeneration is associated with the Schwann cell framework within the lesion site following spinal cord compression injury of the rat. *J. Neurosci. Res.* **53**, 51–65.

Brustle, O., Jones, K. N., Learish, R. D., Karram, K., Choudhary, K., Wiestler, O. D., Duncan, I. D., and McKay, R. D. (1999). Embryonic stem cell-derived glial precursors: A source of myelinating transplants. *Science* **285**, 754–756.

Cai, D., Qiu, J., Cao, Z., McAtee, M., Bregman, B. S., and Filbin, M. T. (2001) Neuronal cyclic AMP controls the developmental loss in ability of axons to regenerate. *J. Neurosci.* **21**, 4731–4739.

Cajal, S. R. Y. (1928). "Degeneration and Regeneration in the Nervous System." Oxford University Press, London.

Castro, R. F., Jackson, K. A., Goodell, M. A., Robertson, C. S., Liu, H., and Shine, H. D. (2002). Failure of bone marrow cells to transdifferentiate into neural cells in vivo. *Science* **297**, 1299.

Chen, J., Sanberg, P. R., Li, Y., Wang, L., Lu, M., Willing, A. E., Sanchez-Ramos, J., and Chopp, M. (2001). Intravenous administration of human umbilical cord blood reduces behavioral deficits after stroke in rats. *Stroke* **32**, 2682–2688.

Chuah, M. I., and West, A. K. (2002). Cellular and molecular biology of ensheathing cells. *Microsc. Res. Tech.* **58**, 216–227.

Devon, R., and Doucette, R. (1992). Olfactory ensheathing cells myelinate dorsal root ganglion neurites. *Brain Res.* **589**, 175–179.

Doucette, R. (1984). The glial cells in the nerve fiber layer of the rat olfactory bulb. *Anat. Rec.* **210(2)**, 385–391.

Doucette, R. (1991). PNS-CNS transitional zone of the first cranial nerve. *J. Comp. Neurol.* **312**, 451–466.

Eglitis, M. A., Dawson, D., Park, K. W., and Mouradian, M. M. (1999). Targeting of marrow-derived astrocytes to the ischemic brain. *Neuroreport* **10**, 1289–1292.

Felts, P. A., and Smith, K. J. (1992). Conduction properties of central nerve fibers remyelinated by Schwann cells. *Brain Res.* **574**, 178–192.

Ferrari, G., Cusella-De Angelis, G., Coletta, M., Paolucci, E., Stornaiuolo, A., Cossu, G., and Mavilio, F. (1998). Muscle regeneration by bone marrow-derived myogenic progenitors. *Science* **279**, 1528–1530.

Franklin, R. J., Gilson, J. M., Franceschini, I. A., and Barnett, S. C. (1996). Schwann cell-like myelination following transplantation of an olfactory bulb-ensheathing cell line into areas of demyelination in the adult CNS. *Glia* **17**, 217–224.

Franklin, R. J., and Barnett, S. C. (1997). Do olfactory glia have advantages over Schwann cells for CNS repair? *J. Neurosci. Res.* **50(5)**, 665–672.

Franklin, R. J., and Barnett, S. C. (2000). Olfactory ensheathing cells and CNS regeneration: The sweet smell of success? *Neuron* **28(1)**, 15–18.

Friedenstein, A. J. (1976). Precursor cells of mechanocytes. *Int. Rev. Cytol.* **47**, 327–359.

Gage, F. H., Ray, J., and Fisher, L. J. (1995). Isolation, characterization, and use of stem cells from the CNS. *Annu. Rev. Neurosci.* **18**, 159–192

Gledhill, R. F., Harrison, B. M., and McDonald, W. I. (1973). Pattern of remyelination in the CNS. *Nature* **244**, 443–444.

Graziadei, P. P., Levine, R. R., and Graziadei, G. A. (1978). Regeneration of olfactory axons and synapse formation in the forebrain after bulbectomy in neonatal mice. *Proc. Natl. Acad. Sci. U. S. A.* **75**, 5230–5234.

Guénard, V., Gwynn, L. A., et al. (1994). Astrocytes inhibit Schwann cell proliferation and myelination of dorsal root ganglion neurons in vitro. *J. Neurosci.* **14(5 Pt 2)**, 2980–2992.

Hammang, J. P., Archer, D. R., and Duncan, I. D. (1997). Myelination following transplantation of EGF-responsive neural stem cells into a myelin-deficient environment. *Exp. Neurol.* **147**, 84–95.

Han, S. S., Kang, D. Y., Mujtaba, T., Rao, M. S., and Fischer, I. (2002). Grafted lineage-restricted precursors differentiate exclusively into neurons in the adult spinal cord. *Exp. Neurol,* **177**, 360–375.

Haraldsen, G., Kvale, D., Lien, B., Farstad, I. N., and Brandtzaeg, P. (1996). Cytokine-regulated expression of E-selectin, intercellular adhesion molecule-1 (ICAM-1), and vascular cell adhesion molecule-1 (VCAM-1) in human microvascular endothelial cells. *J. Immunol.* **156**, 2558–2565.

Hofstetter, C. P., Schwarz, E. J., Hess, D., Widenfalk, J., El Manira, A., Prockop, D. J., and Olson, L. (2002). Marrow stromal cells form guiding strands in the injured spinal cord and promote recovery. *Proc. Natl. Acad. Sci. U. S. A.* **99**, 2199–2204.

Honmou, O., Felts, P. A., Waxman, S. G., and Kocsis, J. D. (1996). Restoration of normal conduction properties in demyelinated spinal cord axons in the adult rat by transplantation of exogenous Schwann cells. *J. Neurosci.* **16**, 3199–3208.

Huang, H., Chen, L., Wang, H., Xiu, B., Wang, R., Zhang, J., Zhang, F., Gu, Z., Li, Y., Song, Y., Hao, W., Pang, S., and Sun. J. (2003). Influence of patients' age on functional recovery after transplantation of olfactory ensheathing cells into injured spinal cord injury. *Chin. Med. J. (Engl.)* **116**, 1488–1491.

Ide, C. (1996) Peripheral nerve regeneration. *Neurosci. Res.* **25**, 101–121.

Iihoshi, S., Honmou, O., Houkin, K., Kazuo, H., and Kocsis, J. D. (2004). A therapeutic window for an intravenous administration of autologous bone marrow after cerebral ischemia in adult rats. *Brain Res.* **1007**, 1–9.

Imaizumi, T., Lankford, K. L., Waxman, S. G., Greer, C. A., and Kocsis, J. D. (1998). Transplanted olfactory ensheathing cells remyelinate and enhance axonal conduction in the demyelinated dorsal columns of the rat spinal cord. *J. Neurosci.* **18**, 6176–6185.

Imaizumi, T., Lankford, K. L., and Kocsis, J. D. (2000a). Transplantation of olfactory ensheathing cells or Schwann cells restores rapid and secure conduction across the transected spinal cord. *Brain Res.* **854**, 70–78.

Imaizumi, T., Lankford, K. L., Burton, W. V., Fodor, W. L., and Kocsis, J. D. (2000b). Xenotransplantation of transgenic pig olfactory ensheathing cells promotes axonal regeneration in rat spinal cord. Nat Biotechnol **18**, 949-953.

Inoue M, Honmou O, Oka S, Houkin K, Hashi K, Kocsis JD. (2003) Comparative analysis of remyelinating potential of focal and intravenous administration of autologous bone marrow cells into the rat demyelinated spinal cord. *Glia* **44**, 111–118.

Kato, T., Honmou, O., Uede, T., Hashi, K., and Kocsis, J. D. (2000). Transplantation of human olfactory ensheathing cells elicits remyelination of demyelinated rat spinal cord. *Glia* **30**, 209–218.

Keyvan-Fouladi, N., Raisman, G., and Li, Y. (2003). Functional repair of the corticospinal tract by delayed transplantation of olfactory ensheathing cells in adult rats. *J. Neurosci.* **23**, 9428–9434.

Kim, J. S. (1996). Cytokines and adhesion molecules in stroke and related diseases. *J. Neurol. Sci.* **137**, 69–78.

Kisseberth, W. C., Brettingen, N. T., Lohse, J. K., and Sandgren, E. P. (1999). Ubiquitous expression of marker transgenes in mice and rats. *Dev. Biol.* **214**, 128–138.

Kobune, M., Kawano, Y., Ito, Y., Chiba, H., Nakamura, K., Tsuda, H., Sasaki, K., Dehari, H., Uchida, H., Honmou, O., Takahashi, S., Bizen, A., Takimoto, R., Matsunaga, T., Kato, J., Kato, K., Houkin, K., Niitsu, Y., and Hamada, H. (2003). Telomerized human multipotent mesenchymal cells can differentiate into hematopoietic and cobblestone area-supporting cells. *Exp. Hematol.* **31(8)**, 715–722.

Kohama, I., Lankford, K. L., Preiningerova, J., White, F. A., Vollmer, T. L., and Kocsis, J. D. (2001). Transplantation of cryopreserved adult human Schwann cells enhances axonal conduction in demyelinated spinal cord. *J. Neurosci.* **21**, 944–950.

Lakatos, A., Franklin, R. J., et al. (2000). Olfactory ensheathing cells and Schwann cells differ in their in vitro interactions with astrocytes. *Glia* **32(3)**, 214–225.

Lakatos, A., Smith, P. M., Barnett, S. C., and Franklin, R. J. (2003). Meningeal cells enhance limited CNS remyelination by transplanted olfactory ensheathing cells. *Brain* **126**, 598–609.

Lankford, K. L., Imaizumi, T., Honmou, O., and Kocsis, J. D. (2002). A quantitative morphometric analysis of rat spinal cord remyelination following transplantation of allogenic Schwann cells. *J. Comp. Neurol.* **443**, 259–274.

Li, Y., Field, P. M., and Raisman, G. (1997). Repair of adult rat corticospinal tract by transplants of olfactory ensheathing cells. *Science* **277**, 2000–2002.

Li, Y., Field, P. M., and Raisman, G. (1998). Regeneration of adult rat corticospinal axons induced by transplanted olfactory ensheathing cells. *J. Neurosci.* **18**, 10514–10524.

Li, Y., Chen, J., Chen, X. G., Wang, L., Gautam, S. C., Xu, Y. X., Katakowski, M., Zhang, L. J., Lu, M., Janakiraman, N., and Chopp, M. (2002). Human marrow stromal cell therapy for stroke in rat: Neurotrophins and functional recovery. *Neurology* **59**, 514–523

Lu, J., Feron, F., Mackay-Sim, A., and Waite, P. M. (2002). Olfactory ensheathing cells promote locomotor recovery after delayed transplantation into transected spinal cord. *Brain* **125**, 14–21.

Majumdar, M. K., Thiede, M. A., Mosca, J. D., Moorman, M., and Gerson, S. L. (1998). Phenotypic and functional comparison of cultures of marrow-derived mesenchymal stem cells (MSCs) and stromal cells. *J. Cell Physiol.* **176**, 57–66.

Mujtaba, T., Han, S. S., Fischer, I., Sandgren, E., and Rao, M. S. (2002). Stable expression of the alkaline phosphatase marker gene by neural cells in culture and after transplantation into the CNS using cells derived from a transgenic rat. *Exp. Neurol.* **174**, 48–57.

Namiki, J., Kojima, A., and Tator, C. H. (2000). Effect of brain-derived neurotrophic factor, nerve growth factor, and neurotrophin-3 on functional recovery and regeneration after spinal cord injury in adult rats. *J. Neurotrauma* **17**, 1219–1231.

Pearse, D. D., Pereira, F. C., Marcillo, A. E., Bates, M. L., Berrocal, Y. A., Filbin, M. T., and Bunge, M. B. (2004). cAMP and Schwann cells promote axonal growth and functional recovery after spinal cord injury. *Nat. Med.* **10**, 610–616.

Pixley, S. K. (1992). The olfactory nerve contains two populations of glia, identified both in vivo and in vitro. *Glia* **5**, 269–284.

Plant, G. W., Currier, P. F., Cuervo, E. P., Bates, M. L., Pressman, Y., Bunge, M. B., and Wood, P. M. (2002). Purified adult ensheathing glia fail to myelinate axons under culture conditions that enable Schwann cells to form myelin. *J. Neurosci.* **22**, 6083–6091.

Plant, G. W., Christensen, C. L., Oudega, M., and Bunge, M. B. (2003). Delayed transplantation of olfactory ensheathing glia promotes sparing/regeneration of supraspinal axons in the contused adult rat spinal cord. *J. Neurotrauma* **20**, 1–16.

Prineas, J. W., and Connell, F. (1979). Remyelination in multiple sclerosis. *Ann. Neurol.* **5**, 22–31.

Quesenberry, P. J., and Becker, P. S. (1998). Stem cell homing: Rolling, crawling, and nesting. *Proc. Natl. Acad. Sci. U. S. A.* **95**, 15155–15157.

Radtke, C., Akiyama, Y., Brokaw, J., Lankford, K. L., Wewetzer, K., Fodor, W. L., and Kocsis, J. D. (2004). Remyelination of the nonhuman primate spinal cord by transplantation of H-transferase transgenic adult pig olfactory ensheathing cells. *FASEB J.* **18**, 335–337. Full text: FASEB Journal Express Article 10.1096/fj.03-021 fje 2003.

Ramer, L. M., Au, E., Richter, M. W., Liu, J., Tetzlaff, W., and Roskams, A. J. (2004) Peripheral olfactory ensheathing cells reduce scar and cavity formation and promote regeneration after spinal cord injury. *J. Comp. Neurol.* **473**, 1–15.

Ramon-Cueto, A., and Avila, J. (1998). Olfactory ensheathing glia: properties and function. *Brain Res. Bull.* **46**, 175–187.

Ramon-Cueto, A., Plant, G. W., Avila, J., and Bunge, M. B. (1998). Long-distance axonal regeneration in the transected adult rat spinal cord is promoted by olfactory ensheathing glia transplants. *J. Neurosci.* **18**, 3803–3815.

Ramon-Cueto, A., Cordero, M. I., Santos-Benito, F. F., and Avila, J. (2000). Functional recovery of paraplegic rats and motor axon regeneration in their spinal cords by olfactory ensheathing glia. *Neuron* **25**, 425–435.

Ramon-Cueto, A., and Valverde, F. (1995). Olfactory bulb ensheathing glia: A unique cell type with axonal growth-promoting properties. *Glia* **14(3)**, 163–173.

Sasaki, M., Honmou, O., Akiyama, Y., Uede, T., Hashi, K., and Kocsis, J. D. (2001). Transplantation of an acutely isolated bone marrow fraction repairs demyelinated adult rat spinal cord axons. *Glia* **35**, 26–34.

Sasaki, M., Lankford, K. L., Zemedkun, M., and Kocsis, J. D. (2004). Olfactory ensheathing cells transplanted into the transected dorsal funiculus bridge the lesion and form myelin. *J. Neurosci.* **24**, 8485–8493.

Senior, K. (2002). Olfactory ensheathing cells to be used in spinal-cord repair trial. *Lancet Neurology* **1**, 269.

Snyder, E. Y., Yoon, C., Flax, J. D., and Macklis, J. D. (1997). Multipotent neural precursors can differentiate toward replacement of neurons undergoing targeted apoptotic degeneration in adult mouse neocortex. *Proc. Natl. Acad. Sci. U. S. A.* **94**, 11663–11668.

Takami, T., Oudega, M., Bates, M. L., Wood, P. M., Kleitman, N., and Bunge, M. B. (2002). Schwann cell but not olfactory ensheathing glia transplants improve hindlimb locomotor performance in the moderately contused adult rat thoracic spinal cord. *J. Neurosci.* **22**, 6670–6681.

Trapp, B. D., Peterson, J., Ransohoff, R. M., Rudick, R., Mort, S., and B., L. (1998). Axonal transection in the lesions of multiple sclerosis. *N. Engl. J. Med.* **338**, 278–285.

Verdu, E., Garcia-Alias, G., et al. (2001). Effects of ensheathing cells transplanted into photochemically damaged spinal cord. *Neuroreport* **12(11)**, 2303–2309.

Vermeulen, M., Le Pesteur, F., Gagnerault, M. C., Mary, J. Y., Sainteny, F., and Lepault, F. (1998). Role of adhesion molecules in the homing and mobilization of murine hematopoietic stem and progenitor cells. *Blood* **92,** 894–900.

Woodbury, D., Schwarz, E. J., Prockop, D. J., and Black, I. B. (2000). Adult rat and human bone marrow stromal cells differentiate into neurons. *J. Neurosci. Res.* **61,** 364–370.

Woodhall, E., West, A. K., and Chuah, M. I. (2001). Cultured olfactory ensheathing cells express nerve growth factor, brain-derived neu-

rotrophic factor, glia cell line-derived neurotrophic factor and their receptors. *Brain Res. Mol. Brain Res.* **88,** 203–213.

Zhang, R. L., Chopp, M., Zaloga, C., Zhang, Z. G., Jiang, N., Gautam, S. C., Tang, W. X., Tsang, W., Anderson, D. C., and Manning, A. M. (1995). The temporal profiles of ICAM-1 protein and mRNA expression after transient MCA occlusion in the rat. *Brain Res.* **682,** 182–188.

29

Blocking the Axonal Injury Cascade: Neuroprotection in Multiple Sclerosis and Its Models

Stephen G. Waxman, M.D., Ph.D.
Albert C. Lo, M.D., Ph. D.

I. Introduction

It is becoming increasingly appreciated that multiple sclerosis (MS), besides being an inflammatory demyelinating disorder, is also a neurodegenerative disease with significant loss of axons and neurons, even at early stages of the disease (Ferguson et al., 1997; Trapp et al., 1998; Filippi et al., 2003). Evidence from human studies shows that the loss of axons and neurons, as a result of neurodegeneration, contributes substantially to nonremitting neurological deficits (Davie et al., 1999; Lee et al., 2000). It might be expected, therefore, that protective approaches that prevent axonal and neuronal degeneration should also slow or halt the progression of disability in MS.

The currently available MS disease modifying agents have been developed to suppress or control the inflammatory-immune component of MS pathology. Since 1993, several disease-modifying medications (primarily based in β-interferon or glatiramer acetate) have been introduced into clinical practice (Goodin et al., 2002). Because of the importance of preventing neurodegeneration to maintain neurological function, however, there is now increased interest from the clinical community and patients in the identification and clinical development of new therapeutic agents that provide *neuroprotection*. In this chapter, we use the term *neuroprotection* to refer to protection of neurons and axons, so that they do not degenerate as a result of the targeting of neuronal molecules (Table 1). In using this operational definition, we do not mean to neglect immunomodulatory interventions that also can prevent neuronal injury. On the contrary, we focus on neuroprotective approaches that act directly on neurons not only because of their protective action but also because, as a result of their actions on different molecular or cellular targets, they may

Table 1 Neuroprotection in MS and Its Models: Agents Targeting Neurons and Axons

I. Sodium Channel Blockers
    a. Tetrodotoxin and Saxitoxin
    b. Tertiary anesthetics (lidocaine, procaine)
    c. Quanternary anesthetics (QX-314, QX-222)
    d. Anticonvulsant drugs (phenytoin, carbamazepine, lamotrigine)
    e. Antiarrhythmic drugs (e.g., bupivacaine, flecainide)

II. Calcium Channel Blockers
    a. L-type blockade (dilitaizen, nifedipine, verapamil)
    b. N-type blockage (SNX-124, synthetic conotoxin)

III. Blockade of Na^+/Ca^{++} Exchanger
    a. Bepridil
    b. Amiloride derivatives: Benzamil and dichlorobenzamil

IV. Adenosine and GABA
    a. Exogenous
    b. Endogenous autoprotection

V. Other Mechanisms and Agents
    a. Blockage of α-adrenergic receptors (prazocin).
    b. Na-K-ATPase, Na/H exchanger
    c. Riluzole
    d. Sipatrigine
    e. Non-glucocorticoid steroids (tirilazad mesylate)

VI. Temperature
    a. Hypothermia

ultimately be used in combination with immunomodulatory interventions.

The majority of data on neuroprotection in white matter are derived from studies that are still in preclinical stages, using either *in vitro* or *in vivo* systems to model aspects of MS pathobiology. Given the uncertainty that remains about the pathogenesis of MS, and in view of its clinical heterogeneity, no animal model is able to perfectly mimic the human disease, but each model system attempts to replicate specific pathological or pathophysiological characteristics of the MS white matter injury process. Experimental studies have reflected the heterogeneity of MS and have used models that involve a spectrum of disease triggers including hypoxic, nitric oxide-induced, and central nervous system (CNS) inflammatory insults. The studies reviewed in this chapter range accordingly from investigations on anoxia-induced white matter injury of isolated optic nerves studied *in vitro*, to experiments using *in vivo* preparations of spinal cord and spinal nerves, to studies in whole-organism level models such as experimental autoimmune encephalomyelitis (EAE). Some of these studies use anoxia or nitric oxide (NO) as triggers of axonal injury, with a basis in findings derived from human MS lesions. Pathological evidence indicates that some patterns of MS pathology bear close similarities to white matter hypoxic injury (Lassmann, 2003), and physiological studies raise the possibility that energy depletion is a contributor to axonal injury in MS (e.g., Smith et al., 2001). Although *in vitro* studies cannot reproduce all the conditions that occur *in vivo*, the anoxic optic nerve preparation has provided a highly tractable, pure white matter model tract where physiologically relevant parameters can be tightly controlled and precise biophysical measurements can be made, which has helped to provide insight into the molecular mechanisms of white matter axonal injury and neuroprotection. In a similar manner, NO is found in MS plaques and has been hypothesized to cause conduction block, axonopathy, and axonal degeneration. Other studies reviewed in this chapter have used models developed to mimic the immunopathologies of MS, such as EAE, which is a well-established, immunologically induced model that is known to reproduce many of the behavioral and histopathological features of MS.

II. Persistent Na^+ Channels and the Na^+/Ca^{2+} Exchanger

A number of *in vitro* experiments have shown that intra-axonal influx of calcium via the Na^+/Ca^{2+} exchanger can produce irreversible physiological failure and subsequent degeneration of the white matter axon (Stys et al., 1992a; see also Chapter 19). Stys et al. (1990) performed a series of experiments that have delineated the cascading interaction of persistently activated Na^+ channels, the Na^+/Ca^{2+} exchanger (which can import calcium when operating in its "reverse" mode in response to high levels of intracellular Na^+ and/or depolarization), and the resultant inflow of calcium into the axon. In these studies, the isolated optic nerve was used as a model and was subjected to a standardized insult consisting of 60 minutes of anoxia. After the anoxic challenge, quantitative analysis of compound action potential (CAP) recovery is used as a functional outcome measure of axonal integrity. When measured after 60 minutes of anoxia, the area of the postanoxic CAP is substantially depressed and remains at only about 30% of preanoxia levels with no additional recovery, indicating that only 30% of the axons are capable of conducting action potentials (Stys et al. 1990, 1991a, 1991b). At the ultrastructural level, the development of permanent structural damage parallels the reduced functional capacity. Anoxia produces injury to the axonal membrane and mitochondria, and severe disruption of cytoskeletal structures, similar to calcium-mediated injury of the cytoskeleton within axons (Waxman et al., 1993).

Notably, even though excitotoxicity is not the trigger for neuronal damage in this model of white matter injury (Ransom et al., 1990), the presence of extracellular Ca^{2+} is necessary for anoxia-induced axonal degeneration to occur. Removing Ca^{2+} from the perfusate, and then subjecting optic nerves to the same duration (60 minutes) of anoxia results in complete (100%) recovery of CAP to preanoxia levels (Stys et al., 1990). Ultrastructural examination of anoxia-exposed axons in Ca^{2+}-free conditions reveals the retention of normal axonal cytoarchitecture (Waxman et al., 1993).

In this form of axonal injury, calcium enters the axon via reverse operation of the Na^+/Ca^{2+} exchanger (Fig. 1.) (Stys et al., 1991a; 1992a; see also Chapter 19). In its normal mode, this exchanger functions as an antiporter—extruding one Ca^{2+}

EXTRACELLULAR

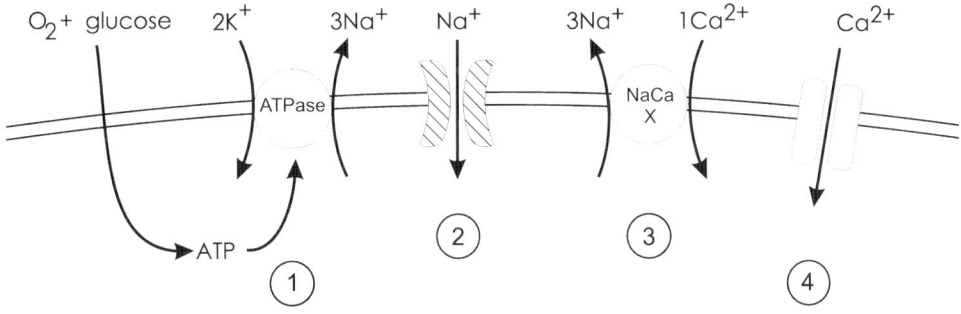

INTRACELLULAR

Figure 1 Cellular pathophysiological events leading to terminal intracellular influx of calcium. Anoxia leads to ATP depletion with resultant failure of ATPase activity and depolarization (1). Persistent Na^+ channels (2) provide a route for Na^+ influx. Collapse of the Na^+ gradient forces the Na^+/Ca^{2+} exchanger (3) to operate in reverse causing influx of Ca^{2+} into the axon. Voltage Ca^{2+} channels (4) provide a route for Ca^{2+}. (Modified from Stys et al., 1992a.)

ion in exchange for three Na^+ ions—as Na^+ ions run down their gradient from the extracellular compartment to the intracellular compartment. However, in situations where the normal Na^+ transmembrane gradient has collapsed or has even been reversed because of the intracellular rise of Na^+, or when there is membrane depolarization, the Na^+/Ca^{2+} exchanger can be forced to operate backward, now driving Ca^{2+} ion into the axon (Baker et al., 1969; Cervetto et al., 1989). Anoxia appears to trigger an elevation of intra-axonal Na^+ via ATPase run-down because of energy failure and activation of Na^+ channels resulting from depolarization (Stys et al., 1992a). High concentrations of intra-axonal Na^+ have been correlated with reverse action of the Na^+/Ca^{2+} exchanger; using electron probe microanalysis during membrane depolarization or anoxia of optic nerve, levels of intracellular Na^+ are observed to rise concomitant with parallel increases in Ca^{2+}, consistent with reverse function of the exchanger (LoPachin and Stys. 1995).

Of importance, the time-course of sodium influx in the anoxic optic nerve indicates that the increase in intra-axonal Na^+ levels is the result of persistent Na^+ influx via a noninactivating Na^+ conductance (Stys et al., 1992a). Although the presence of this standing Na^+ conductance was not directly demonstrated in the studies of anoxic injury, sucrose gap studies on the normal optic nerve have shown the presence of a noninactivating tetrodotoxin (TTX)-sensitive Na^+ conductance in optic nerve axons (Stys et al., 1993). Although the channel(s) responsible for the persistent Na^+ influx in injured axons has not been definitively identified, several studies suggest that Nav1.6 sodium channels, which are present in high density in the axonal membrane at the nodes of Ranvier (Caldwell et al., 2000), contribute a significant fraction (if not all) of the noninactivating Na^+ conductance. Biophysical studies have demonstrated that the Nav1.6 sodium channel produces a sizable persistent current (Smith et al., 1998;

Burbidge et al., 2002; Herzog et al., 2003). Furthermore, immunochemical studies demonstrate the co-localization of Nav1.6 sodium channels and the Na^+/Ca^{2+} exchanger within degenerating axons in EAE (Craner et al., 2004a) and in MS (Craner et al., 2004b), as described in Chapter 7.

III. Voltage-Gated Ca^{2+} Channels

Although a major route for calcium influx into the axon involves persistent Na^+ channel opening and the eventual reversal of the Na^+/Ca^{2+} exchanger, N-type and L-type voltage-gated calcium channels (VGCC) may also play a role in calcium-mediated axonal degeneration in MS (Fern et al., 1995b; Kornek et al., 2001). There is some evidence for the presence of VGCC in normal axons (see Chapter 5). Moreover, it has been reported that α1B subunits of N-type calcium channels accumulate within dystrophic (presumably degenerating) axons in EAE and MS (Kornek et al., 2001). Although it is not known whether these channels are inserted into the axon membrane and the functional role of these abnormally distributed VGCC along dystrophic axons is not clear, results from *in vitro* studies on white matter tract experiments indicate that VGCC can contribute to axonal dysfunction. Fern et al. (1995a) have shown that block of L-type Ca^{2+} channels before anoxic insult can provide significant physiological axonal neuroprotection; furthermore, by simultaneously blocking both L-type and N-type Ca^{2+} channels, even greater protection of axon conduction can be achieved (Fern et al., 1995b).

IV. Nitric Oxide

There is evolving data linking nitric oxide (NO) to axonal degeneration in neuroinflammatory disease (see Chapter

18). It is known that NO is present at increased concentrations in EAE (Staykova et al., 2002) and within MS plaques (Bo et al., 1994; Brosnan et al., 1994; Cross et al., 1998). Exposing CNS white matter directly to NO, at concentrations consistent with what would be found pathologically in human inflammatory CNS lesions, causes axonal conduction block (Redford et al., 1997; Shrager et al., 1998), and it has been shown that demyelinated axons are particularly vulnerable (Redford et al., 1997). Impulse activity appears to lower the threshold for NO-induced injury, and exposure of electrically active axons to NO can induce degeneration (Smith et al., 2001).

Physiological evidence suggests that NO induces physiological dysfunction and structural degeneration by producing energy depletion within axons (Smith et al., 2001). There is evidence indicating that NO can impair mitochondrial function within neurons (Brown et al., 1995; Bolanos et al., 1997). Inadequate mitochondrial respiration would be expected, like anoxia, to result in run-down of Na/K-ATPase, which would be predicted to produce axonal depolarization and Na$^+$ influx via sodium channels, in turn evoking reverse Na$^+$/Ca^{2+} exchange that injures axons (Fig. 2). Impulse activity, particularly at high frequencies, would be expected to increase the demand for energy (or ATP) depletion. Consistent with this hypothesis, axons can be protected from NO-induced degeneration with blockers of the Na$^+$/Ca^{2+} exchanger and with the sodium channel blocker flecainide (Kapoor et al., 2003), as discussed by Smith (see Chapter 18) and reviewed later in this chapter.

V. Pharmacological Manipulation of the Axonal Injury Cascade

This section reviews the effect of drugs and other interventions that can modulate or interfere with the axonal calcium influx cascade.

A. Sodium Channel Blockers

1. Tetrodotoxin and Saxitoxin

From the molecular cascade depicted in Fig. 1, block of Na$^+$ channels with tetrodotoxin (TTX) or saxitoxin (STX) would be predicted to confer protection of axons in various models of axon degeneration. Experimental studies using the *in vitro* anoxic optic nerve injury and spinal cord injury models support this prediction (Stys et al., 1992a; Agrawal and Fehlings, 1996; Imaizumi et al., 1997; Teng and Wrathall, 1997). In the optic nerve anoxic-injury model, for example, 1μM TTX provides greater than 80% of preanoxic recovery of CAP after 60 minutes of anoxic insult; 1μM of STX also preserves CAP function after anoxic injury, although not to as great an extent (58%) (Stys et al., 1992a).

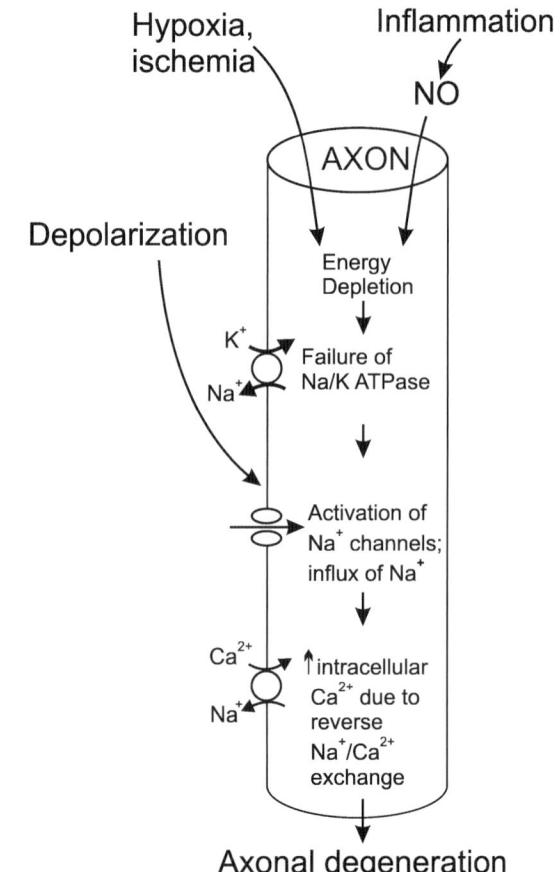

Figure 2 Molecular cascade leading to elevations of intracellular Ca^{2+}, which can result in axonal degeneration. Depolarization, anoxia, and nitric oxide (NO) can each trigger downstream events causing the intra-axonal influx of Na$^+$ and the reverse function of the Na$^+$/Ca^{2+} exchanger, leading to axonal degeneration.

TTX also prevents against the morphological axonopathy caused by exposure of isolated optic nerve to NO (Garthwaite et al., 2002).

Further support for neuroprotection of white matter axons by TTX has been reported in an *in vivo* spinal cord injury model. TTX has a protective effect on spinal cord axons after contusive dorsal column injury (Teng and Wrathall, 1997; Rosenberg et al., 1999), suggesting that sodium channels may be generally involved in a final common injury cascade that produces degeneration of spinal cord axons after a variety of insults. Phenytoin also has a neuroprotective effect in experimental spinal cord contusive injury (Hains et al., 2004).

2. Tertiary Anesthetics

Tertiary anesthetics are known to reversibly block sodium channels (Narahashi et al., 1967; Strichartz, 1973; Cahalan, 1978). Administration of lidocaine or procaine (1μM) *in vitro* significantly enhances CAP recovery in the anoxic optic nerve (88% to 94%, compared to 34% recovery of nontreated, optic nerve [Stys et al., 1992c]). Lower concentrations (0.1 μM) of lidocaine and procaine that were neuroprotective in the anoxic optic nerve (with CAP recovery of 72% to 74%) did not markedly block normoxic conduction, suggesting that it is possible to use some sodium channel blocking agents to protect axons at concentrations that do not compromise axonal function. Procaine treatment has also been reported to provide some improvement of recovery of spinal cord dorsal column white matter CAP (83% vs. 72% for untreated control) after *in vitro* dorsal column compression injury (Agrawal and Fehlings, 1996).

Lidocaine also protects isolated ventral and dorsal roots from NO-induced injury. Using an *in vivo* spinal cord preparation to examine NO-induced axonal pathology, Kapoor et al. (2003) have shown that in spinal cord perfused in medium containing lidocaine, 83% of spinal roots exposed to NO regained "good" impulse conduction (defined as >50% CAP amplitude) compared to only 43% of spinal roots that regained conduction after NO exposure without treatment (Kapoor et al., 2003). Lidocaine treatment was also reported to prevent structural injury of axons in this study.

3. Quaternary Anesthetics

Some quaternary anesthetic analogs, such as QX-314 and QX-222, offer state-specific Na$^+$ channel block, where the agents preferentially bind open Na$^+$ channels (Wang et al., 1987; Khodorov, 1991). This characteristic is therapeutically advantageous because doses that achieve neuroprotection potentially may have little or no effect in terms of impeding normal action potential (Stys et al., 1992c). In the anoxic optic nerve model of white matter injury, QX-314 and QX-222 used at neuroprotective concentrations caused only minimal reduction in the CAP under normoxic conditions (5% of CAP for QX-314 and no reduction for QX-222). Nonetheless, the neuroprotective effects of these quaternary agents were substantial, with dramatic treatment recovery of the CAP after 60 minutes of anoxic injury (CAP recovery = 99.6% for QX-314 and 81.4% for QX-222) (Stys et al., 1992c).

Investigations of neuroprotection by QX-314 have been extended to an *in vivo* model of spinal cord compression injury (Agrawal and Fehlings, 1997). In these studies, after T1 spinal cord injury, animals were randomized to placebo or to receive 2 to −10 nM QX-314, delivered by microinjection to the injury site 15 minutes postinjury, as a one-time dose. Six weeks later, QX-314-treated animals demonstrated significantly increased functional integrity of spinal cord long tract axons, recognized through retrograde fluorogold labeling of supraspinal nuclei, with ~50% more fluorogold-positive neurons in the QX-314 animals compared to control animals. However, there was no clear difference in injury-site morphometrics or in final hind-limb behavioral testing

between treated and untreated animals (Agrawal and Fehlings 1997).

4. Anticonvulsant Drugs

Phenytoin and carbamazepine are two clinically available and widely used anticonvulsant agents known to inhibit persistent neuronal sodium channels (Schwarz and Grigat, 1989; Ragsdale et al., 1996; Ragsdale and Avoli, 1998). These agents were demonstrated to be effective as neuroprotective agents in the optic nerve anoxia model of white matter injury (Fern et al., 1993). Both agents promoted significant recovery of postanoxic CAP in a dose-dependent manner, where maximal neuroprotection plateaued below the clinical reference range, and at concentrations that had no suppressing effect on conduction under normoxic conditions (Fig. 3). At these concentrations, phenytoin produced 69% recovery and carbamazepine produced 53% recovery of the CAP, compared to 34% recovery for untreated anoxic axons (Fern et al., 1993).

Lamotrigine, a newer anticonvulsant agent, is also known to block sodium channels (Kuo, 1998) and has been shown to be structurally neuroprotective of optic nerve axons subjected to oxygen-glucose deprivation injury *in vitro* (Garthwaite et al., 1999). Lamotrigine-treated optic nerves showed greater than 50% preservation of axons after oxygen-glucose deprivation in this study, compared to 100% axonopathy of oxygen-deprived axons. Lamotrigine at the concentration used for neuroprotection had only a small inhibitory effect on the normal optic nerve CAP. A clinically relevant note is that even the lowest neuroprotective concentration of lamotrigine used in this study (100 μM) was still significantly in excess of levels seen in the cerebrospinal fluid of epileptic patients taking lamotrigine (Garthwaite et al., 1999).

Lo et al. (2002, 2003) carried out a series of studies to test whether oral administration of sodium channel-blocking anticonvulsant drugs in an animal model of MS would have neuroprotective properties similar to those seen within the isolated optic nerve model. Because phenytoin was more efficacious at neuroprotection than carbamazepine in the *in vitro* optic nerve anoxia experiments (Fern et al., 1993), phenytoin was tested as an neuroprotective agent in an *in vivo* animal model of MS, oligodendrocyte glycoprotein (MOG)-induced EAE.

The first study (Lo et al., 2002) extrapolated from the earlier *in vitro* demonstration (Fern et al., 1993) of a neuroprotection effect in the optic nerve, and examined optic nerve axon loss in EAE to assess the possible protective effects of phenytoin. In this study, mice with EAE were treated with oral phenytoin, beginning 10 days after immunological induction with MOG peptide, at doses that were titrated to achieve serum phenytoin levels within the human therapeutic range. At 28 days post-MOG injection, the number of axons in treated and untreated optic nerves

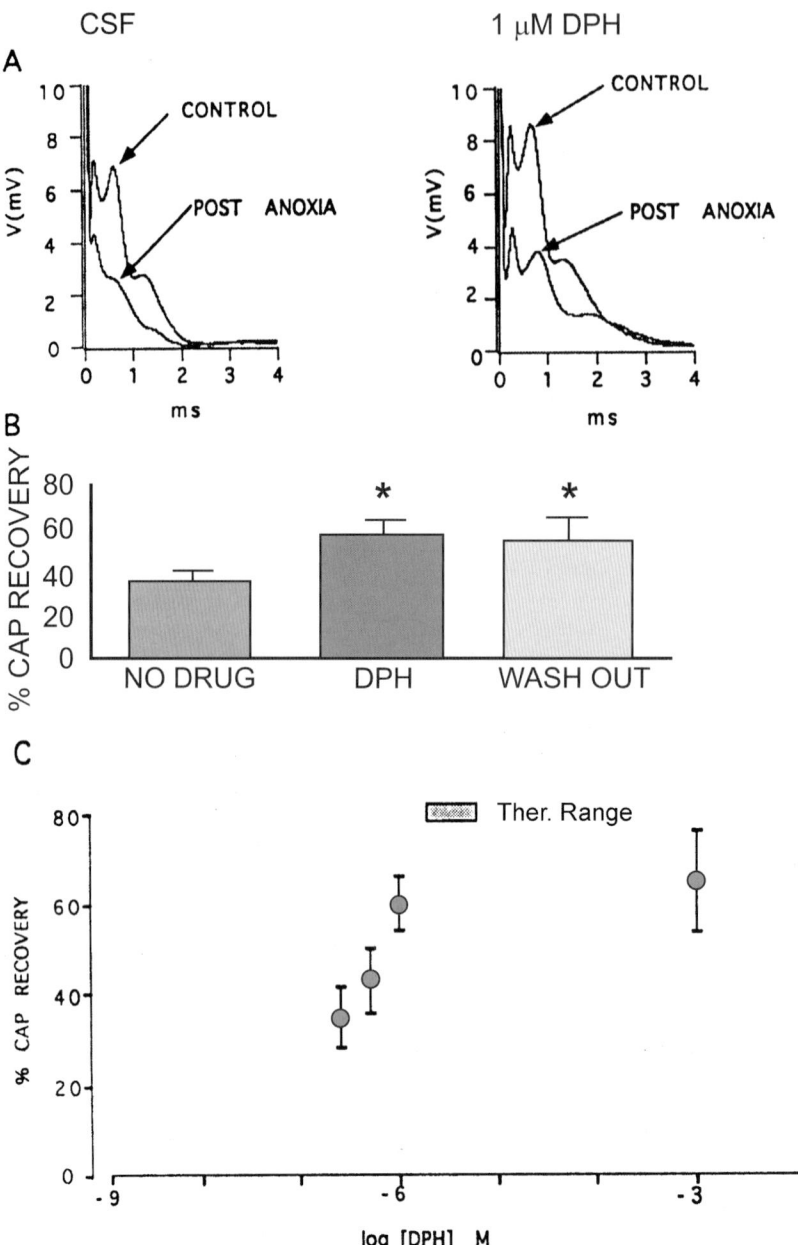

Figure 3 *In vitro* administration of phenytoin prevents irreversible optic nerve dysfunction. (**A**) One hour of anoxia substantially reduces the compound action potential (CAP) of an isolated rodent optic nerve, whereas treatment with 1 μM of phenytoin significantly restores postanoxic CAP recovery. (**B**) The presence of 1 μM phenytoin increases CAP recovery from 35% to 58% and a wash-out after the initial 60 minutes of reoxygenation has no additional effect. (**C**) Significant effects on CAP recovery occurs at concentrations below the clinically defined therapeutic range for phenytoin. (From Fern et al., 1993.)

were compared after immunolabeling with antineurofilament antibodies. To identify all axons within these fields, nerve fibers were labeled using a combination of antibodies directed against both phosphorylated (SMI-31) and nonphosphorylated (SMI-32) neurofilaments (Lovas et al., 2000; Lo et al., 2002; Wujek et al., 2002). Axon counts of untreated EAE revealed 49% loss of optic nerve axons. EAE treated with oral phenytoin showed robust neuroprotection,

with only 12% loss of optic nerve axons (Fig. 4). Clinical scores were significantly better, indicating less functional impairment, in phenytoin-treated mice.

Given the neuroprotective effects seen of phenytoin treatment in optic nerve, and in view of the substantial contribution of spinal cord atrophy to disability in MS, the effect of phenytoin was examined in a second study (Lo et al., 2003) on spinal cord white matter axons in EAE. In this study cer-

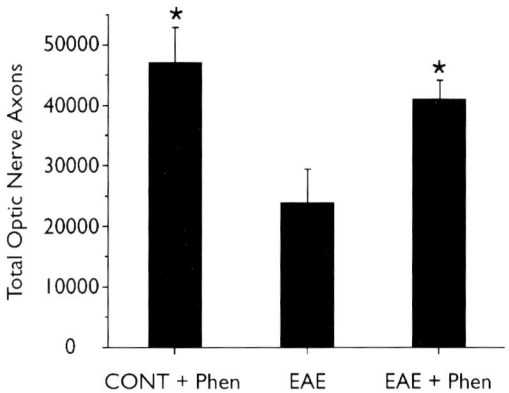

Figure 4 Oral administration of phenytoin *in vivo* to EAE mice results in significant axonal neuroprotection in the optic nerve. In EAE, there is a considerable loss of optic nerve axons as is quantified by neurofilament counts. Phenytoin administration in EAE results in a significant increase in optic nerve axon numbers. (Modified from Lo et al., 2002.)

vical spinal cord axons were counted within standardized 500 μm^2 fields located at predetermined sites in the corticospinal tract, dorsal, lateral, and ventral columns. (This lesion-independent method of axon counting permitted the same white matter tract regions to be compared in different animals, and avoided selection bias due to lesion variability.) Mice with untreated EAE displayed a significant loss of axons within the corticospinal tracts and dorsal columns compared to control animals (non-EAE) (Fig. 5A,B). The density of axons labeled with neurofilament antibodies after 27 to 28 days of untreated EAE decreased substantially, with a 63% dropout of axons in the corticospinal tract and a 43% loss of axons in the dorsal columns (cuneate fasciculus). Treatment with phenytoin beginning at day 10 reduced the loss of corticospinal axons from 63% to 28% and reduced

the loss of cuneate fasciculus axons from 43% to 17% (Lo et al., 2003).

Protection of axons by phenytoin was reflected functionally both in the electrophysiological recordings of the spinal cord CAP, which measures function in dorsal column axons, and in clinical behavioral testing (Figs. 6 and 7). The CAP in the untreated EAE group was significantly smaller or even unrecordable compared to the phenytoin-treated control group (Fig. 6B). In contrast, robust CAPs with a normal positive-negative configuration were observed in phenytoin-treated EAE, with a threshold similar to that in controls, and the average CAP amplitude in the phenytoin-treated EAE group was not significantly different than in the phenytoin-treated control group. (Fig. 6C). Thus in addition to protecting the structural integrity of spinal cord axons in EAE, phenytoin maintains their ability to conduct action potentials.

Clinical scores were assessed in this study using a standard EAE rating scale. Untreated EAE mice manifested progressive clinical impairment, with an average clinical score of 3.8 ± 0.18 (representing complete hind-limb paralysis) at days 27 and 28. Phenytoin-treated EAE mice at day 27 and 28 exhibited a less severe clinical course, with an average clinical score of 1.5 ± 0.26, which represents a limp tail and minor righting reflex abnormalities (Fig. 7) (Lo et al., 2003).

More recently, the effects of carbamazepine in EAE have been assessed in EAE (Lo and Waxman, unpublished), and protective effects similar to those of phenytoin have been observed.

4. Sodium Channel Blocking Antiarrhythmic Drugs

Of the four established classes of antiarrhythmic drugs, class I agents function by acting on sodium channels, a mechanism of action that predicts this class of agent to be reason-

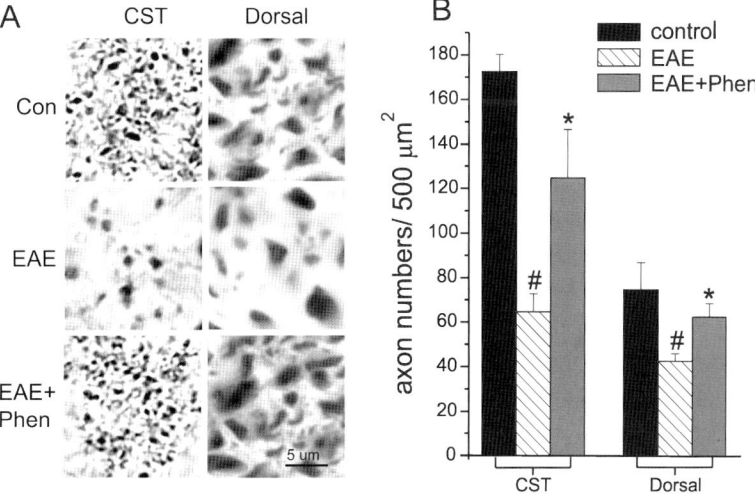

Figure 5 (**A**) Cervical spinal cord axons in the corticospinal tract (CST) and dorsal column are lost in untreated EAE. (**B**) Quantification of neurofilaments in the CST and dorsal columns of untreated EAE compared to phenytoin-treated EAE demonstrates reduction of both CST and dorsal column axon counts in untreated EAE ($\#P < 0.05$) and a significant increase in axons in phenytoin-treated EAE ($^*P < 0.05$). (Modified from Lo et al., 2003.)

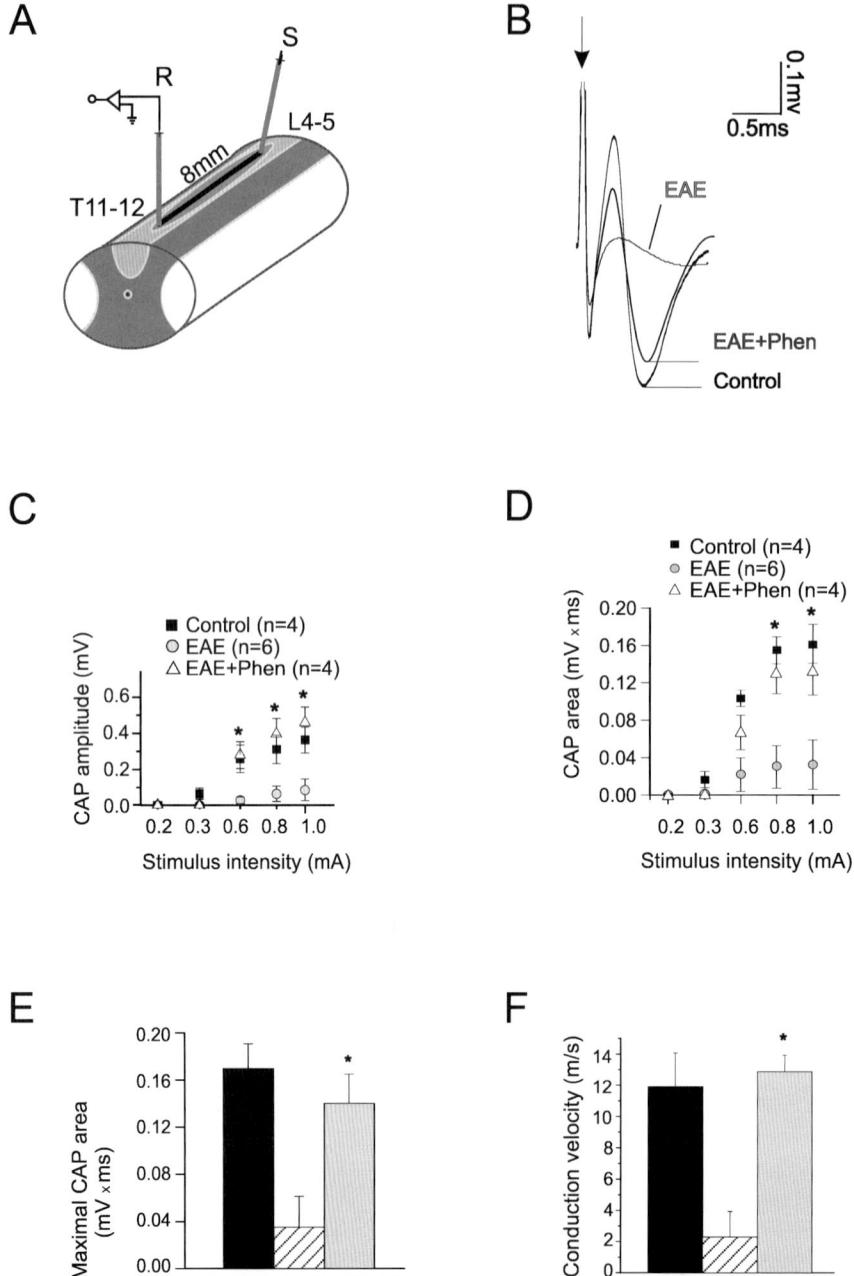

Figure 6 Neurophysiological spinal cord compound action potential (CAP) recordings of untreated and phenytoin-treated EAE. (**A**) Stimulating "S" and recording "R" electrodes are placed 8 mm apart at L4–5 and T11–T12, respectively. (**B**) The biphasic CAP wave seen in controls is highly attenuated in untreated EAE, and is restored in phenytoin-treated EAE (arrow indicates stimulus artifact). (**C**) Average CAP amplitudes (± SEM, mV) in phenytoin-treated controls, untreated EAE, and phenytoin-treated EAE at different stimulating current intensities ($^*P < 0.01$, phenytoin-treated EAE compared to untreated EAE). (**D**) Average CAP area (± SEM, mV × ms) at different stimulus intensities in phenytoin-treated control, untreated EAE, and phenytoin-treated EAE ($^*P < 0.05$, phenytoin-treated EAE compared to untreated EAE). (**E**) Average supramaximal CAP area (± SEM, mV × ms) in phenytoin-treated control, untreated EAE, and phenytoin-treated EAE ($^*P < 0.05$ phenytoin-treated EAE compared to untreated EAE). (**F**) Average conduction velocity (±SEM, m/s) in phenytoin-treated control, untreated EAE, and phenytoin-treated EAE ($^*P < 0.05$, phenytoin-treated EAE compared to untreated EAE). (From Lo et al., 2003.)

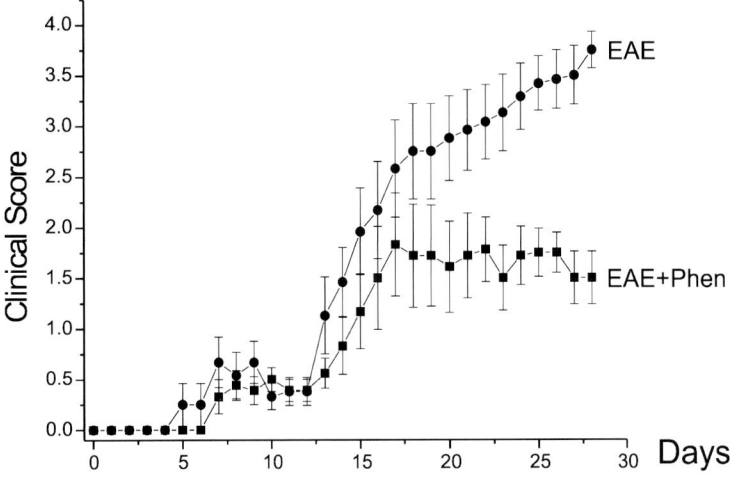

Figure 7 Phenytoin treatment ameliorates EAE clinical dysfunction. Clinical scores (mean ± SEM) are shown for untreated-EAE (*filled circles*) and phenytoin-treated EAE (*filled boxes*). Oral administration of phenytoin was started on day 10, as indicated by the horizontal bar. (From Lo et al., 2003.)

able candidates with neuroprotective properties in disorders of white matter. Various antiarrhythmic agents, some of which are used in clinical practice, have been tested in the rat optic nerve anoxia model (Stys, 1995) as well as in NO-mediated axonal degeneration models (Kapoor et al., 2003) and EAE (Bechtold et al., 2004). In the *in vitro* anoxia optic nerve model, the most effective agent tested (as assessed by postanoxic CAP restoration) was prajmaline, with 82% CAP recovery. Tocainide provided 79% recovery and ajmaline provided 79% recovery (untreated controls had 32% recovery in postanoxia electrophysiological testing). Disopyramide and bupivacaine were slightly less effective and resulted in CAP recovery in the range of 72% to 75%, and procainamide was ineffective. However, an important consideration for any of these agents for potential clinical use is their "efficacy index," which depends on the dose required for neuroprotection and any effect of that dose on normal conduction, which is undesirable. Prajmaline and tocainide at neuroprotective doses suppressed the preanoxic CAP by only 10%, whereas ajmaline (which provided almost the same magnitude of CAP protection as prajmaline) significantly depressed normal conduction by about 21%. Disopyramide, bupivacaine, and verapamil produced a 12% to 15% reduction in preanoxia CAP.

Stys and Lesiuk (1996) demonstrated that mexiletine provides neuroprotection of both in the *in vitro* anoxic optic nerve model and in an *in situ* ischemia-induced optic nerve injury model. Within the concentration range tested (10 μM to 1 mM) for mexiletine, the peak postanoxic recovery was seen at 100 μM (53% recovery of postanoxic CAP vs. 21% for untreated anoxic optic nerves). The magnitude of recovery above and below 100 μM was reduced. At this maximum

neuroprotective concentration, the preanoxic CAP was suppressed slightly by 15%. In another set of *in vivo* experiments using ischemic conditions, the optic nerve electrophysiological responses to ischemia with and without mexiletine were examined *in situ*. The postischemic (60 minutes) CAP of untreated optic nerves in these experiments was dramatically reduced to 21% of control levels. Treatment with mexiletine (80 mg/kg) resulted in modestly improved recovery of the CAP, to 31% of preischemic control (Stys and Lesiuk, 1996).

Another Na^+ channel-blocking antiarrhythmic agent, flecainide, was studied using a model of the NO-mediated injury of spinal roots (Kapoor et al., 2003; see also Chapter 18). Flecainide, at concentrations that allow normal impulse propagation, was perfused over spinal dorsal roots, resulting in a significant increase in the number of spinal roots which regained conduction following NO exposure. Whereas only 27% of spinal roots (3 of 11 roots assessed) recovered "good" conduction (defined as >50% CAP amplitude) after exposure to NO, 88% of flecainide-treated spinal roots (22 of 25 roots) showed good CAP recovery after NO exposure (Kapoor et al., 2003). Furthermore morphological analysis demonstrated that treatment with flecainide maintained the axonal structural integrity of axons, whereas exposure to NO alone caused dispersion of the axolemma and dissolution of organelles within the axoplasma, consistent with wallerian degeneration (Kapoor et al., 2003).

Bechtold et al. (2004) (see also Chapter 18) recently reported that flecainide (delivered subcutaneously) has a protective effect in EAE induced by inoculation of dark agouti rats with syngeneic spinal cord homogenate, reducing axon loss in the spinal cord from 48% to 3% to 17% depending on the dose schedule. As with phenytoin, treatment with flecainide protected axonal conduction and improved clinical outcome. Thus two sodium-channel blocking drugs, phenytoin and flecainide, have been demonstrated to protect against loss of spinal cord axons in EAE.

B. Calcium Channel Blockers

The ability of calcium channel antagonists to provide neuroprotection has been studied using the anoxic optic nerve model (Fern et al., 1995b). L-type Ca^{2+} channel blockers, verapamil, diltiazem, and nifedipine all provide partial but significant protection of CAP recovery (51% to 66% postanoxic CAP recovery) after anoxic exposure to optic nerves. These agents were used at concentration ranges corresponding to doses known to block Ca^{2+} channels. Within this concentration range, diltiazem offered the greatest magnitude of recovery. For both diltiazem and verapamil, the degree of neuroprotection was dose-dependent. Blocking both L-type and N-type Ca^{2+} channels by co-administration of diltiazem and SNX-124 (synthetic w-conotoxin) resulted in even greater protection (74% postanoxic CAP) than diltiazem or SNX-124 alone (no significant protection when used alone), perhaps suggesting that Ca^{2+} influx through N-type channels becomes important in anoxic injury only when L-type channels are blocked.

Studies also suggest that activation of calcium channels may trigger release of calcium from intracellular stores within axons. Ouardouz et al. (2003) have demonstrated, in dorsal column axons, that ischemia can trigger a rise in intracellular calcium via ryanodine-sensitive intracellular calcium release channels that is triggered by L-type calcium channels. These results suggest a previously unsuspected role for Ca^{2+} channels in axons and implicate Ca^{2+} release from intracellular stores in axons.

C. Blockade of Na^+/Ca^{2+} Exchanger

As might be predicted from the mechanism illustrated in Fig. 1, blocking of the Na/Ca exchanger also results in neuroprotection of white matter. Bepridil, as well as benzamil and dichlorobenzamil (both derivatives of amiloride, a clinically used K+ sparing diuretic) (Kleyman and Cragoe, 1988) all exhibit neuroprotective properties in the anoxic optic nerve model, attenuating the loss of the CAP after anoxic challenge. Benzamil neuroprotection exhibited a dose-dependent response curve, with a maximal protective effect of 71% postanoxic CAP recovery at a concentration of 500 μm. Bepridil provided 69% postanoxic CAP recovery at 50 μM (Stys et al., 1992a).

Bepridil also has been reported to protect myelinated spinal roots axons from axonal degeneration (with axonal damage scores at about a third of the severity of nontreated axons) in the NO-mediated axonal injury model studied *in vitro* (Kapoor et al., 2003).

D. Adenosine and γ-Aminobutyric Acid (GABA) Autoprotection

Neuroprotective effects of neurotransmitters and neuromodulators such as adenosine and GABA have been demonstrated in the anoxic optic nerve model (Fern et al., 1994, 1995a). Protection from anoxia was found regardless of whether these molecules were delivered from exogenous sources or released from endogenous stores.

Adenosine provided significant neuroprotection in a dose-responsive manner with a maximal recovery of postanoxic CAP at 2.5 μM (51% recovery vs. 29% for controls). Confirmation that adenosine acts through the adenosine receptor was provided by the demonstration that theophylline, an adenosine receptor antagonist, completely abolished adenosine's neuroprotective activity. Administration of exogenous GABA (1 μM) also significantly increased recovery of the postanoxic optic nerve CAP (56% compared to 36% for nontreated optic nerves) (Fern et al., 1995a).

Fern et al. (1994, 1995a) have suggested that the axon possess an autoprotective compensatory mechanism involving the release of endogenous GABA and adenosine to maintain axon integrity in response to pathological insults. They proposed that the white matter autoprotective system responds to energy depletion anoxia by releasing endogenous stores of GABA and adenosine, which act synergistically on GABA-B and adenosine receptors, in turn triggering activation of protein kinase C and G protein.

Agonists of GABA receptors such as diazepam provide significant protection of postanoxic optic nerves (69% recovery of CAP) (Fern et al., 1993). However, these neuroprotective concentrations (1–10 μM) are significantly greater than clinically used doses (20-40 nM).

E. Other Mechanisms and Agents

Although the mechanism of action is not clear, antagonists of α-adrenergic receptors have been reported to reduce spinal cord axonal degeneration in EAE (White et al., 1992). Prazosin, an α-adrenergic receptor antagonist, was delivered twice daily to mice with EAE, starting 1 week after the immunoinduction of EAE. This study assessed inflammation and axonal damage by focusing on lesions found within the ventral and lateral funiculi of the cervical and lumbar enlargements of the spinal cord. Within these regions, the densities of inflammatory loci were measured and compared between groups; damage to monoaminergic axons was also evaluated by identifying serotonin (5HT-) or tyrosine hydroxylase (TH) immunostained axons. The results of this study were interpreted as showing significant axonal protection (more so for 5HT labeled axons [>50%] than for TH axons). Behavioral examination showed less severe neurological deficits in prazosin-treated animals compared to saline-treated control animals.

The Na^+-K^+-ATPase pump and the Na^+-H^+ exchanger may also participate in the response of the axon to injury and are also potential targets for neuroprotection, as both have been implicated in alternative pathways for modulating intracellular Na^+ loading during pathological conditions (Murphy et al., 1991). Metabolic collapse, as might be expected during axonal injury, halts sodium extrusion via the Na^+-K^+-ATPase pump, and intracellular Na^+ will slowly rise, which, as described previously through reversal of the Na^+/Ca^{2+} exchanger, would be predicted to produce an exacerbation of axonal injury. Experimental inhibition of the Na^+-K^+-ATPase pump reduces extrusion of Na^+ through the pump and, in fact, further worsened postinjury CAP measures. Agrawal and Fehlings (1996) used ouabain to inhibit the Na^+-K^+-ATPase pump, and observed a worsening of the postcompression dorsal column CAP after experimental spinal cord injury by an additional ~15%. As opposed to worsening of axon injury through blocking of the Na^+-K^+-ATPase pump, antagonism of the Na^+-H^+ exchanger has been reported to confer partial neuroprotection. Blocking the Na^+-H^+ exchanger with either harmaline or amiloride, both of which are selective Na^+-H^+ exchanger blockers (Hartley and Dubinsky, 1993), was reported to improve postinjury spinal cord function (Agrawal and Fehlings, 1996). In these experiments, the isolated spinal cord *in vitro* was bathed in media that contained either harmaline or amiloride before dorsal column compression injury. After postcompression cord injury, harmaline or amiloride-treated dorsal columns displayed improved CAP outcomes, but only modestly, with 86% to 90% recovery with Na^+-H^+ blockers compared to 71% to 72% for untreated controls.

Riluzole is an agent with mixed pharmacological actions, including block of sodium and glutamatergic channels, which is approved for clinical use in motor neuron disease. Recent studies have examined riluzole's effect in an animal model of MS and in MS. The action of riluzole as a neuroprotective agent was studied in MOG-induced EAE, where it was delivered intraperitoneally twice a day. A number of paradigms for treatment onset were studied, and irrespective of whether riluzole was delivered immediately at the time of EAE induction or delayed, the clinical severity of EAE behavior was attenuated (Gilgun-Sherki et al., 2003). The authors reported axonal neuroprotection in the spinal cord of riluzole-treated EAE compared to non-treated EAE, but did not report axon counts. There was also a reduction of non-phosphorylated neurofilament immunolabel in riluzole-treated animals, which the authors interpreted as suggesting reduced demyelination in animals treated with riluzole (Gilgun-Sherki et al., 2003).

Riluzole was also studied clinically in a small open-label pilot clinical study in Europe in which nine patients with primary-progressive MS were treated (riluzole, 50 mg twice a day) (Kalkers et al., 2002). Patients were monitored with magnetic resonance imaging of spinal cord atrophy every 6 months for 1 year. Imaging data after patients received riluzole for 1 year was compared to scans taken at 12 months and 6 months before the start of treatment. During the year before treatment with riluzole, spinal cord area atrophied by 2%. After initiation of riluzole, spinal cord area essentially did not change significantly over the subsequent year (0.2% decrease). Unfortunately, although the data might be viewed as suggesting a beneficial effect that reduced the rate of spinal cord atrophy, interpretation of the results is compromised by omission of data from two patients who dropped out of the study as a results of side effects and because of the small sample size and lack of statistical analysis.

Sipatrigin, a derivative of lamotrigine, has mixed ion channel blocking actions. It provides state-dependent block of sodium channels, but it is also reported to block calcium channels (Graham et al., 1994; Calabresi et al., 2000). In the *in vitro* NO-mediated optic nerve axonopathy model, treatment with 100 μM of sipatrigine has been reported to prevent axon loss as assessed by morphological quantitation (Garthwaite et al., 2002).

Lessons may also be learned from other agents that have been studied in models of peripheral axon degeneration. One example is a study of tirilazad mesylate in experimental allergic neuritis (EAN) (Feasby et al., 1994). As opposed to glucocorticoid agents such as methylprednisolone, which is thought to suppress EAN through anti-inflammatory actions, tirilazad mesylate is a no-glucocorticoid, 21-amino steroid, with evidence to suggest that it acts by inhibiting oxygen free-radical induced lipid peroxidation of axonal membranes (Koc et al., 1999). The rationale for use of this agent is based on suppression of axonal lipid peroxidation. Semiquantitative analysis revealed that axonal degeneration was significantly inhibited by tirilazad mesylate, whereas assessment scores for demyelination and inflammation were similar to untreated EAN controls. Clinical examination showed that although peak clinical disability for tirilazad mesylate-treated animals was slightly less severe, the final clinical outcomes for treated and untreated animals were not significantly different (Feasby et al., 1994). Nevertheless these data provide some suggestion of an action of tirilazad in preventing axon degeneration without influencing inflammatory or demyelination responses.

VI. Temperature

Small reductions in temperature during anoxia-induced white matter injury can strongly and favorably influence nerve functional outcome. Using the *in vitro* optic nerve anoxia model to evaluate the effect of temperature (through a 10°C range, 32–42°C) on postanoxic CAP, Stys et al. (1992b) observed that there were protective effects of lower temperature and worsened outcomes from increased temperature. Lowering temperature by only 2.5°C during anoxic exposure resulted in near doubling of CAP recovery during the postanoxic period (65% recovery at 34.5°C vs. 35% at 37°C). Reducing temperature further, by a total of 5°C (37–32°C), resulted in complete recovery of post-anoxic CAP. The converse relationship, of worsened functional recovery at higher temperature, was also seen.

The neuroprotective mechanism of action of hypothermia is not entirely clear. It may be due to reduced metabolic requirements of hypothermic tissue including white matter, since it is known that oxygen consumption is reduced on the order of 6% to 8% per degree C from 37°C (Nishizaki et al., 1988), which extrapolates to a 15% to 20% total reduction of oxygen consumption for a 2.5°C drop. However the Q_{10}s of other events in the axonal injury cascade may also contribute to the protective effect of hypothermia. As discussed above, the reversal of the Na^+/Ca^{2+} exchanger is a critical step in the final influx on calcium into axons, and it is known that the rate of Ca^{2+} movement through this exchanger is highly temperature-dependent, with lower temperatures causing slower exchange (Russell and Blaustein, 1974).

VII. Limitations of Studies *in vitro* and in Animal Models

Although studies *in vitro* and in animal models, as outlined in this chapter, have clear operational and ethical advantages compared to human studies, they also have limitations and must be interpreted appropriately.

The question "How well does it represent the *in vivo* situation?" can be posed about any *in vitro* study. This is especially so for a disorder as heterogeneous and incompletely understood as MS, where pathogenesis remains only partially explored and may vary between various subgroups of patients and at different times during the course of the disease. Mechanisms indicated by *in vitro* studies and agents shown to be promising *in vitro* must clearly be tested *in vivo*.

A similar question "How well does it apply to humans?" can be posed with respect to all animal models. In this regard, EAE has a number of relatively unique limitations. There are many models of EAE, ranging from monophasic to progressive to chronic-relapsing. The histopathology varies between models, and there is no consensus as to which model will be most predictive of neuroprotective efficacy in humans. Although primate models of EAE are available, most EAE studies are carried out in rodents, and their limited life spans,

as well as expense, has limited the duration of most rodent studies. Thus an effect that appears to have prevented axonal degeneration in short- or medium-term studies may turn out, in long-term studies, to be due to a delay in axonal degeneration, rather than a truly protective effect.

In this latter context it is also important to recall that some of the molecules targeted by putative neuroprotective agents are also present on immune cells. Ion channels, for example, are present in a variety of immune cells. In parallel with *neuroprotective* effects, these agents may thus modulate immunopathogenesis. If this turns out to be the case, it should not dampen enthusiasm for investigating these drugs, but it does underscore the need for multidisciplinary studies that examine immunobiological, as well as neurobiological, actions.

VIII. Conclusions and Future Prospects

The last 10 years have seen an important step forward in the effort to find effective treatments for MS: the successful development of the first generation of clinically effective disease modifying agents (e.g., interferons and glatiramer acetate). These agents were developed as immunomodulatory drugs, and they are effective at reducing inflammation and relapse rate (which is a clinical manifestation of acute inflammation). They have not been as successful in preventing the development of nonremitting disability (Kappos et al., 2001; Cohen et al., 2002).

Axonal degeneration appears to be a major contributor to disability in MS, and with renewed interest in neuronal/axonal destruction, there exists a therapeutic opportunity and urgent clinical need for the development of neuroprotective agents for MS. Although only some of the molecules reviewed in this chapter have the high clinical index needed for translation into the clinical realm, most of them contribute to proof-of-principle, and a number of agents in this chapter are being considered for clinical trial evaluation. The development of neuroprotective agents, which may complement immunomodulatory drugs, is a promising multipronged strategy that may provide clinicians and patients with new therapeutic tools that will slow or prevent progressive neurological impairment in MS.

Acknowledgments

Supported, in part, by grants from the National Multiple Sclerosis Society (RG-1912) and the Medical Research Service and Rehabilitation Research Service, Department of Veterans Affairs. We thank the Nancy Davis Foundation, and Destination Cure for support. The Center for Neuroscience and Regeneration Research is a collaboration of the Paralyzed Veterans of America and the United Spinal Association with Yale University. A.C.L. was supported by VA Rehabilitation Research and Development Award #B3230V.

References

Agrawal, S. K., and Fehlings, M. G. (1996). Mechanisms of secondary injury to spinal cord axons in vitro: Role of Na^+, Na^+-K^+-ATPase, the Na^+-H^+ exchanger, and the Na^+-Ca^{2+} exchanger. *J. Neurosci.* **16**, 545–552.

Agrawal, S. K., and Fehlings, M. G. (1997). The effect of the sodium channel blocker QX-314 on recovery after acute spinal cord injury. *J. Neurotrauma* **14**, 81–88.

Baker, P. F., Blaustein, M. P., Keynes, R. D., Manil, J., Shaw, T. I., and Steinhardt, R. A. (1969). The ouabain-sensitive fluxes of sodium and potassium in squid giant axons. *J. Physiol. (Lond).* **200**, 459–496.

Bechtold, D. A., Kapoor, R., and Smith, K. J. (2004). Axonal protection using flecainide in experimental autoimmune encephalomyelitis. *Ann. Neurol.* **55**, 607–616.

Bo, L., Dawson, T. M., Wesselingh, S., Mork, S., Choi, S., Kong, P. A., Hanley, D., and Trapp, B. D. (1994). Induction of nitric oxide synthase in demyelinating regions of multiple sclerosis brains. *Ann. Neurol.* **36**, 778–786.

Bolanos, J. P., Almeida, A., Stewart, V., Peuchen, S., Land, J. M., Clark, J. B., and Heales, S. J. (1997). Nitric oxide-mediated mitochondrial damage in the brain: Mechanisms and implications for neurodegenerative diseases. *J. Neurochem.* **68**, 2227–2240.

Brosnan, C. F., Battistini, L., Raine, C. S., Dickson, D. W., Casadevall, A., and Lee, S. C. (1994). Reactive nitrogen intermediates in human neuropathology: An overview. *Dev. Neurosci.* **16**, 152–161.

Brown, G. C., Bolanos, J. P., Heales, S. J., and Clark, J. B. (1995). Nitric oxide produced by activated astrocytes rapidly and reversibly inhibits cellular respiration. *Neurosci. Lett.* **193**, 201–204.

Burbidge, S. A., Dale, T. J., Powell, A. J., Whitaker, W. R., Xie, X. M., Romanos, M. A., and Clare, J. J. (2002). Molecular cloning, distribution and functional analysis of the NA(V)1.6. Voltage-gated sodium channel from human brain. *Brain Res. Mol. Brain Res.* **103**, 80–90.

Cahalan, M. D. (1978). Local anesthetic block of sodium channels in normal and pronase-treated squid giant axons. *Biophys. J.* **23**, 285–311.

Calabresi, P., Stefani, A., Marfia, G. A., Hainsworth, A. H., Centonze, D., Saulle, E., Spadoni, F., Leach, M. J., Giacomini, P., and Bernardi, G. (2000). Electrophysiology of sipatrigine: A lamotrigine derivative exhibiting neuroprotective effects. *Exp. Neurol.* **162**, 171–179.

Caldwell, J. H., Schaller, K. L., Lasher, R. S., Peles, E., and Levinson, S. R. (2000). Sodium channel Na(v)1.6 is localized at nodes of Ranvier, dendrites, and synapses. *Proc. Natl. Acad. Sci. U. S. A.* **97**, 5616–5620.

Cervetto, L., Lagnado, L., Perry, R. J., Robinson, D. W., and McNaughton, P. A. (1989). Extrusion of calcium from rod outer segments is driven by both sodium and potassium gradients. *Nature* **337**, 740–743.

Cohen, J. A., Cutter, G. R., Fischer, J. S., Goodman, A. D., Heidenreich, F. R., Kooijmans, M. F., Sandrock, A. W., Rudick, R. A., Simon, J. H., Simonian, N. A., Tsao, E. C., Whitaker, J. N., and Investigators I. (2002). Benefit of interferon beta-1a on MSFC progression in secondary progressive MS. *Neurology* **59**, 679–687.

Craner, M. J., Hains, B. C., Lo, A. C., Black, J. A., and Waxman, S. G. (2004a). Co-localization of sodium channel Nav 1.6 and the sodium-calcium exchanger at sites of axonal injury in the spinal cord in EAE. *Brain* **127**, 294–303.

Craner, M. J., Newcombe, J., Black, J. A., Hartle, C., Cuzner, M. L., and Waxman, S. G. (2004b). Molecular changes in neurons in MS: altered axonal expression of Na_v1.2 and Na_v1.6 sodium channels and Na^+/Ca^{2+} exchanger. *Proc. Natl. Acad. Sci.* **101**, 8168–8173.

Cross, A. H., Manning, P. T., Keeling, R. M., Schmidt, R. E., and Misko T. P. (1998). Peroxynitrite formation within the central nervous system in active multiple sclerosis. *J. Neuroimmunol.* **88**, 45–56.

Davie, C. A., Silver, N. C., Barker, G. J., Tofts, P. S., Thompson, A. J., McDonald, W. I., and Miller, D. H. (1999). Does the extent of axonal loss and demyelination from chronic lesions in multiple sclerosis correlate with the clinical subgroup? *J. Neurol. Neurosurg. Psychiatry* **67**, 710–715.

Feasby, T. E., Hahn, A. F., Lovgren, D., and Wilkie, L. (1994). Lewis rat EAN is suppressed by the 21-aminosteroid tirilazad mesylate (U-74006F). *Neuropathol. Appl. Neurobiol.* **20**, 384–391.

Ferguson, B., Matyszak, M. K., Esiri, M. M., and Perry, V. H. (1997). Axonal damage in acute multiple sclerosis lesions. *Brain* **120**, 393–399.

Fern, R., Waxman, S. G., and Ransom, B. R. (1994). Modulation of anoxic injury in CNS white matter by adenosine and interaction between adenosine and GABA. *J. Neurophysiol.* **72**, 2609–2616.

Fern, R., Waxman, S. G., and Ransom, B. R. (1995a). Endogenous GABA attenuates CNS white matter dysfunction following anoxia. *J. Neurosci.* **15**, 699–708.

Fern, R., Ransom, B. R., and Waxman, S. G. (1995b). Voltage-gated calcium channels in CNS white matter: Role in anoxic injury. *J. Neurophysiol.* **74**, 369–377.

Fern, R., Ransom, B. R., Stys, P. K., and Waxman, S. G. (1993). Pharmacological protection of CNS white matter during anoxia: actions of phenytoin, carbamazepine and diazepam. *J. Pharmacol. Exp. Ther.* **266**, 1549–1555.

Filippi, M., Bozzali, M., Rovaris, M., Gonen, O., Kesavadas, C., Ghezzi, A., Martinelli, V., Grossman, R. I., Scotti, G., and Comi, G., et al. (2003). Evidence for widespread axonal damage at the earliest clinical stage of multiple sclerosis. *Brain* **126**, 433–437.

Garthwaite, G., Brown, G., Batchelor, A. M., Goodwin, D. A., and Garthwaite, J. (1999) Mechanisms of ischaemic damage to central white matter axons: a quantitative histological analysis using rat optic nerve. *Neuroscience* 94, 1219–1230.

Garthwaite, G., Goodwin, D. A., Batchelor, A. M., Leeming, K., and Garthwaite, J. (2002). Nitric oxide toxicity in CNS white matter: an in vitro study using rat optic nerve. *Neuroscience* 109, 145–155.

Gilgun-Sherki, Y., Panet, H., Melamed, E., and Offen, D. (2003). Riluzole suppresses experimental autoimmune encephalomyelitis: Implications for the treatment of multiple sclerosis. *Brain Res.* **989**, 196–204.

Goodin, D. S., Frohman, E. M., Garmany, G. P. Jr., Halper, J., Likosky, W. H., Lublin, F. D., Silberberg, D. H., Stuart, W. H., van den Noort, S., and Therapeutics Technology Assessment Subcommittee of the American Academy of N. and the M. S. C. f. C. P. G. (2002). Disease modifying therapies in multiple sclerosis: report of the Therapeutics and Technology Assessment Subcommittee of the American Academy of Neurology and the MS Council for Clinical Practice Guidelines. *Neurology* **58**, 169–178.

Graham, S. H., Chen, J., Lan, J., Leach, M. J., and Simon, R. P. (1994). Neuroprotective effects of a use-dependent blocker of voltage-dependent sodium channels, BW619C89, in rat middle cerebral artery occlusion. *J. Pharmacol. Exp. Ther.* **269**, 854–859.

Hains, B. C., Saab, C. Y., Lo, A. C., Black, J. A., and Waxman, S. G. (2004). Stabilization of sodium influx with phenytoin enhances outcome recovery following contusion (SCI). *Exp. Neurol.* **188**, 365–377.

Hartley, Z., and Dubinsky, J. M. (1993). Changes in intracellular pH associated with glutamate excitotoxicity. *J. Neurosci.* **13**, 4690–4699.

Herzog, R. I., Cummins, T. R., Ghassemi, F., Dib-Hajj, S. D., and Waxman, S. G. (2003). Distinct repriming and closed-state inactivation kinetics of Nav1.6 and Nav1.7 sodium channels in mouse spinal sensory neurons. *J. Physiol.* **551**, 741–750.

Imaizumi, T., Kocsis, J. D., and Waxman, S. G. (1997). Anoxic injury in the rat spinal cord: pharmacological evidence for multiple steps in Ca^{2+}-dependent injury of the dorsal columns. *J. Neurotrauma* **14**, 299–311.

Kalkers, N. F., Barkhof, F., Bergers, E., van Schijndel, R., and Polman, C. H. (2002). The effect of the neuroprotective agent riluzole on MRI parameters in primary progressive multiple sclerosis: a pilot study. *Multiple Sclerosis* **8**, 532–533.

Kapoor, R., Davies, M., Blaker, P. A., Hall, S. M., and Smith, K. J. (2003). Blockers of sodium and calcium entry protect axons from nitric oxide-mediated degeneration. *Ann. Neurol.* **53**, 174–180.

Kappos, L., Polman, C., Pozzilli, C., Thompson, A., Beckmann, K., Dahlke, F., and European Study Group in Interferon beta-1b in Secondary-Progressive M. S. (2001). Final analysis of the European multicenter trial on IFNbeta-1b in secondary-progressive MS. *Neurology* **57**, 1969–1975.

Khodorov, B. I. (1991). Role of inactivation in local anesthetic action. *Ann. N. Y. Acad. Sci.* **625**, 224–248.

Kleyman, T. R., and Cragoe, E. J. Jr. (1988). Amiloride and its analogs as tools in the study of ion transport. *J. Membr. Biol.* **105**, 1–21.

Koc, R. K., Akdemir, H., Karakucuk, E. I., Oktem, I. S., and Menku, A. (1999). Effect of methylprednisolone, tirilazad mesylate and vitamin E on lipid peroxidation after experimental spinal cord injury. *Spinal Cord* **37**, 29–32.

Kornek, B., Storch, M. K., Bauer, J., Djamshidian, A., Weissert, R., Wallstroem, E., Stefferl, A., Zimprich, F., Olsson, T., Linington, C., Schmidbauer, M., and Lassmann, H. (2001). Distribution of a calcium channel subunit in dystrophic axons in multiple sclerosis and experimental autoimmune encephalomyelitis. *Brain* **124**, 1114–1124.

Kuo, C. C. (1998). A common anticonvulsant binding site for phenytoin, carbamazepine, and lamotrigine in neuronal Na$^+$ channels. *Mol. Pharmacol.* **54**, 712–721.

Lassmann, H. (2003). Hypoxia-like tissue injury as a component of multiple sclerosis lesions. *J. Neurol. Sci.* **206**, 187–191.

Lee, M. A., Blamire, A. M., Pendlebury, S., Ho, K. H., Mills, K. R., Styles, P., Palace, J., and Matthews, P. M. (2000). Axonal injury or loss in the internal capsule and motor impairment in multiple sclerosis. *Arch. Neurol.* **57**, 65–70.

Lo, A. C., Black, J. A., and Waxman, S. G. (2002). Neuroprotection of axons with phenytoin in experimental allergic encephalomyelitis. *NeuroReport* **13**, 1909–1912.

Lo, A. C., Saab, C. Y., Black, J. A., and Waxman, S. G. (2003). Phenytoin protects spinal cord axons and preserves axonal conduction and neurological function in a model of neuroinflammation in vivo. *J. Neurophysiol.* **90**, 3566–3571.

LoPachin, R. M, Jr., and Stys, P. K. (1995). Elemental composition and water content of rat optic nerve myelinated axons and glial cells: effects of in vitro anoxia and reoxygenation. *J. Neurosci.* **15**, 6735–6746.

Lovas, G., Szilagyi, N., Majtenyi, K., Palkovits, M., and Komoly, S. (2000). Axonal changes in chronic demyelinated cervical spinal cord plaques. *Brain* **123**, 308–317.

Murphy, E., Perlman, M., London, R. E., and Steenbergen, C. (1991). Amiloride delays the ischemia-induced rise in cytosolic free calcium. *Circ. Res.* **68**, 1250–1258.

Narahashi, T., Anderson, N. C., and Moore, J. W. (1967). Comparison of tetrodotoxin and procaine in internally perfused squid giant axons. *J. Gen. Physiol.* **50**, 1413–1428.

Nishizaki, T., Yamauchi, R., Tanimoto, M., and Okada, Y. (1988). Effects of temperature on the oxygen consumption in thin slices from different brain regions. *Neurosci. Lett.* **86**, 301–305.

Ouardouz, M., Nikolaeva, M. A., Coderre, E., Zamponi, G. W., McRory, J. E., Trapp, B. D., Yin, X., Wang, W., Woulfe, J., and Stys, P. K. (2003). Depolarization-induced Ca^{2+} release in ischemic spinal cord white matter involves L-type Ca^{2+} channel activation of ryanodine receptors. *Neuron* **40**, 53–63.

Ragsdale, D. S., and Avoli, M. (1998). Sodium channels as molecular targets for antiepileptic drugs. *Brain Res. Brain Res. Rev.* **26**, 16–28.

Ragsdale, D. S., McPhee, J. C., Scheuer, T. and Catterall, W. A. (1996). Common molecular determinants of local anesthetic, antiarrhythmic, and anticonvulsant block of voltage-gated Na$^+$ channels. *Proc. Natl. Acad. Sci. U. S. Am.* **93**, 9270–9275.

Ransom, B. R., Waxman, S. G., and Davis, P. K. (1990). Anoxic injury of CNS white matter: Protective effect of ketamine. *Neurology* **40**, 1399–1403.

Ransom, B. R., Walz, W., Davis, P. K., and Carlini, W. G. (1992). Anoxia-induced changes in extracellular K$^+$ and pH in mammalian central white matter. *J. Cereb. Blood Flow Metab.* **12**, 593–602.

Redford, E. J., Kapoor, R., and Smith, K. J. (1997). Nitric oxide donors reversibly block axonal conduction: Demyelinated axons are especially susceptible. *Brain* **120**, 2149–2157.

Rosenberg, L. J., Teng, Y. D., and Wrathall, J. R. (1999). Effects of the sodium channel blocker tetrodotoxin on acute white matter pathology after experimental contusive spinal cord injury. *J. Neurosci.* **19**, 6122–6133.

Russell, J. M., and Blaustein, M. P. (1974). Calcium efflux from barnacle muscle fibers. Dependence on external cations. *J. Gen. Physiol.* **63**, 144–167.

Schwarz, J. R., and Grigat, G. (1989). Phenytoin and carbamazepine: potential- and frequency-dependent block of Na currents in mammalian myelinated nerve fibers. *Epilepsia* **30**, 286–294.

Shrager, P., Custer, A. W., Kazarinova, K., Rasband, M. N., and Mattson, D. (1998). Nerve conduction block by nitric oxide that is mediated by the axonal environment. *J. Neurophysiol.* **79**, 529–536.

Smith, K. J., Kapoor, R., Hall, S. M., and Davies, M. (2001). Electrically active axons degenerate when exposed to nitric oxide. *Ann. Neurol.* **49**, 470–476.

Smith, M. R., Smith, R. D., Plummer, N. W., Meisler, M. H., and Goldin, A. L. (1998). Functional analysis of the mouse Scn8a sodium channel. *J. Neurosci.* **18**, 6093–6102.

Staykova, M. A., Cowden, W., and Willenborg, D. O. (2002). Macrophages and nitric oxide as the possible cellular and molecular basis for strain and gender differences in susceptibility to autoimmune central nervous system inflammation. *Immunol. Cell Biol.* **80**, 188–197.

Strichartz, G. R. (1973). The inhibition of sodium currents in myelinated nerve by quaternary derivatives of lidocaine. *J. Gen. Physiol.* **62**, 37–57.

Stys, P. K. (1995). Protective effects of antiarrhythmic agents against anoxic injury in CNS white matter. *J. Cereb. Blood Flow Metab.* **15**, 425–432.

Stys, P. K., and Lesiuk, H. (1996). Correlation between electrophysiological effects of mexiletine and ischemic protection in central nervous system white matter. *Neuroscience* **71**, 27–36.

Stys, P. K., Waxman, S. G., and Ransom, B. R. (1991a). Reverse operation of the Na$^+$-Ca^{2+} exchanger mediates Ca^{2+} influx during anoxia in mammalian CNS white matter. *Ann. N. Y. Acad. Sci.* **639**, 328–332.

Stys, P. K., Ransom, B. R., and Waxman, S. G. (1991b). Compound action potential of nerve recorded by suction electrode: a theoretical and experimental analysis. *Brain Res.* **546**, 18–32.

Stys, P. K., Waxman, S. G., and Ransom, B. R. (1992a). Ionic mechanisms of anoxic injury in mammalian CNS white matter: role of Na$^+$ channels and Na$^+$-Ca^{2+} exchanger. *J. Neurosci.* **12**, 430–439.

Stys, P. K., Waxman, S. G., and Ransom B. R. (1992b). Effects of temperature on evoked electrical activity and anoxic injury in CNS white matter. *J. Cereb. Blood Flow Metab.* **12**, 977–986.

Stys, P. K., Ransom, B. R., and Waxman, S. G. (1992c). Tertiary and quaternary local anesthetics protect CNS white matter from anoxic injury at concentrations that do not block excitability. *J. Neurophysiol.* **67**, 236–240.

Stys, P. K., Ransom, B. R., Waxman, S. G., and Davis, P. K. (1990). Role of extracellular calcium in anoxic injury of mammalian central white matter. *Proc. Natl. Acad. Sci. U. S. A.* **87**, 4212–4216.

Stys, P. K., Sontheimer, H., Ransom, B. R., and Waxman, S. G. (1993). Noninactivating, tetrodotoxin-sensitive Na$^+$ conductance in rat optic nerve axons. *Proc. Natl. Acad. Sci. U. S. A.* **90**, 6976–6980.

Teng, Y. D., and Wrathall, J. R. (1997). Local blockade of sodium channels by tetrodotoxin ameliorates tissue loss and long-term functional deficits resulting from experimental spinal cord injury. *J. Neurosci.* **17**, 4359–4366.

Trapp, B. D., Peterson, J., Ransohoff, R. M., Rudick, R., Mork, S., and Bo, L. (1998). Axonal transection in the lesions of multiple sclerosis. *N. Engl. J. Med.* **338**, 278–285.

Wang, G. K., Brodwick, M. S., Eaton, D. C., and Strichartz, G. R. (1987). Inhibition of sodium currents by local anesthetics in chloramine-T-treated squid axons. The role of channel activation. *J. Gen. Physiol.* **89,** 645–667.

Waxman, S. G., Black, J. A., Ransom, B. R., and Stys, P. K. (1993). Protection of the axonal cytoskeleton in anoxic optic nerve by decreased extracellular calcium. *Brain Res.* **614,** 137–145.

White, S. R., Black, P. C., Samathanam, G. K., and Paros, K. C. (1992). Prazosin suppresses development of axonal damage in rats inoculated for experimental allergic encephalomyelitis. *J. Neuroimmunol.* **39,** 211–218.

Wujek, J. R., Bjartmar, C., Richer, E., Ransohoff, R. M., Yu, M., Tuohy, V. K., and Trapp, B. D. (2002). Axon loss in the spinal cord determines permanent neurological disability in an animal model of multiple sclerosis. *J. Neuropathol. Exp. Neurol.* **61,** 23–32.

30

Functional Brain Reorganization and Recovery after Injury to White Matter

P. M. Matthews, M.D., D.Phil.

I. Introduction

II. New Tools for Studying Brain Functional Organization in Health and Disease

III. Motor Learning by the Healthy Brain Provides a Basis for Understanding Adaptive Functional Reorganization of the Brain After Injury

IV. Direct Observations on Patients After Brain Injury: Common Brain Mechanisms Contribute to Adaptive Changes After Corticospinal Tract Injury

V. Potentially Adaptive Functional Changes Are Widely Distributed in Brains of Patients with MS

VI. Distinguishing Functional Changes Related to Altered Patterns of Use

VII. Limitations to Adaptive Plasticity in MS

VIII. Studying Brain Recovery and Rehabilitation Using Approaches from Cognitive Neuroscience: Recognizing the Importance of "Context"

IX. Conclusion and Practical Implications

I. Introduction

Although demyelination is still the most characteristic histopathological feature of multiple sclerosis (MS), more recently a central role for axonal loss has been recognized in determining chronic disability (Matthews et al., 1998). Axonal loss has been recognized even since the days of Charcot, but it was not until the last decade, with the advent of magnetic resonance spectroscopic imaging applications in MS, that the magnitude of axonal loss in the disease was appreciated (Arnold et al., 1990). The notion that axonal injury and loss are linked closely with inflammation and demyelination has gained wide acceptance since the publication of two elegant histopathological studies (Trapp et al., 1998; Ferguson et al., 1997). Axonal loss also is found in and around lesions of the spinal cord. Substantial axonal loss even occurs in so-called "normal appearing" white matter. There is some evidence that there may be some selectivity, with smaller axons being more likely to be injured (Evangelou et al., 2000; Ganter et al., 1999).

More recent work has made clear that there is substantial neuronal loss even early in the disease. Evidence for cortical injury in MS is not new, although focus on it has been a more recent development. Microscopic features of gray matter damage have been recognized, including neuronal apoptosis and inflammatory infiltrates of a different character than those in the white matter (Peterson et al., 2001; Cifelli et al., 2002; Wylezinska et al., 2003).

Direct magnetic resonance imaging (MRI) definition of cortical inflammatory lesions in MS is highly insensitive because the cortex is thin relative to the size of imaging voxels, and contrast changes between lesions and adjacent tissue are not so great as in white matter. However, there is clear evidence for cortical and deep gray matter atrophy, with clinical progression of MS related to gray matter injury (Fox et al., 2000; De Stefano et al., 2003; Chard et al., 2002). In addition, as described later, there is now further indirect evidence for neuronal evolvement with the identification of widespread neuronal functional changes in the brain.

MS can thus be considered a disease in which the primary (i.e., clinically most important) pathology involves progressive injury to neurons and axons. In this way (and others), it shares important features with most forms of brain injury. Similar to the situation highlighted long ago with stroke (Luria, 2000), the problem of understanding the progression of disability in MS becomes one of understanding not the roles of the specific functional regions that are injured and *dysfunctional,* but how the remaining *functional* brain responds as a whole.

The increasingly widespread availability of newer methods of functional brain imaging allow us to make observations characterizing these global brain functional responses. Observations made at a *systems* level with functional imaging techniques can then be linked conceptually to phenomena on a *molecular* or *cellular* level to develop hypotheses regarding potential new pharmacological (e.g., paroxetine) (Pariente et al., 2001; Loubinoux et al., 2002), electrophysiological (e.g., repetitive transcranial magnetic stimulation [TMS]) (Siebner and Rothwell, 2003), or other therapies (e.g., constraint-induced neurorehabilitation) (Taub et al., 1993, 2002, 2003).

The application of functional MRI (fMRI) and related techniques to understanding brain recovery in MS is still in its early stages. The primary focus of this review is on understanding motor recovery, because it has been in this area that most effort has been directed thus far. However, extensions of the strategy to other areas (e.g., cognitive rehabilitation) have already begun and these are discussed briefly (Penner et al. 2003; Parry et al. 2003).

The brain has a limited repertoire of responses to brain injury (whatever the cause). Three general mechanisms for recovery can be defined:

1. *Repair* refers to restoration of the damaged system itself after an injury. For example, oligodendroglial cell death after white matter ischemia leads to local demyelination and conduction block. Repair can occur with generation of new oligodendroglial cells from progenitors and remyelination, restoring normal conduction and glial trophic support for axons (Halfpenny et al., 2002). Redistribution and changes in membrane sodium channel expression profile may also contribute, particularly if remyelination is incomplete (Craner et al., 2003).

2. *Compensation* involves development of an altered strategy for completing a task. For example, there may be increased use of truncal movements to point accurately with a hemiparetic limb (Cirstea and Levin 2000; Friel and Nudo, 1998).

3. *Adaptation* is the major focus of this review. Brain adaptation involves recruitment of new systems that can activate the same final output pathway (in the case of movement, this may mean the same motor units) as used before the injury. Recruitment of uninjured, parallel pathways for controlling the normal set of antagonist muscles in pointing with a limb made paretic by a stroke is one example. Functional adaptive change involves several distinct mechanisms (Seil, 1997) including the unmasking of existing latent corticocortical connections (Jacobs and Donoghue, 1991), synaptic rearrangement, and axonal growth coupled with new synapse formation (Donoghue et al., 1990). These occur with different time courses, ranging from seconds (or less) for "unmasking" to days and weeks for new axonal growth.

The relative contributions of these different mechanisms to recovery change with the nature of the pathology and its context. For example, in the early stages of MS, remyelination may be robust (Halfpenny et al., 2002). In other situations, with irreversible loss of neurons and axons, the relative contributions of compensation and adaptation must vary with the extent and localization of the lesions. In well-controlled correlations between surgical brain lesions and behavior in monkeys, Friel and Nudo (1998) demonstrated that monkeys with larger lesions of motor cortex needed to develop compensatory movement strategies, while those with smaller lesions were able to recover prelesional movement behaviors fully (Friel and Nudo, 1998). Presumably, this reflects a limited capacity of the brain to adaptively recruit any specific output pathway. The relative contributions of different mechanisms thus provides another putative phenotype for expression of genetic factors (e.g., the apoE4 haplotype) (Enzinger et al., 2004), which is implicated in lipid homeostasis and neuronal repair, or neurotrophic factor polymorphisms that may help to determine the potential for synaptic reorganization (Egan et al., 2003; Stoop and Poo, 1996; Linker et al., 2002). Local synaptic reorganization is substantial (Trachtenberg et al., 2002), although it may decline with age (Gan et al., 2003).

II. New Tools for Studying Brain Functional Organization in Health and Disease

Two basic classes of "functional brain mapping" techniques have evolved over the last several decades: (1) those techniques that directly map electrical activity of the brain and (2) those that map local physiological or metabolic consequences of this altered brain electrical activity. Among the former are the noninvasive neural electromagnetic techniques of electroencephalography and magnetoencephalography. TMS can be used to assess physiological characteristics of the cortex, such as excitability, and to map its organization by assessing behavioral responses to cortical stimulations at different locations (Boniface and Ziemann, 2003). These methods allow exquisite temporal resolution of neural processing (typically on a 10- to 100-ms time scale), but suffer from relatively poor spatial resolution (between one and several centimeters).

fMRI methods are in the second category (see Jezzard et al., 2001, for a complete review) along with positron emission tomography (PET). They can be used to detect changes in regional blood perfusion, blood volume, or blood oxygenation that accompany neuronal activity. PET demands injection of radioactive tracers and highly specialized equipment, limiting the number of scans that can be made with any single subject and the availability of the technique. Blood oxygenation level dependent (BOLD) fMRI has become the overwhelmingly most important of these methods because it has a similar spatial (on the order of a few mm) to PET and a better temporal resolution (seconds, limited by the hemodynamic response itself). Moreover, the technique can be implemented on any modern high-field MRI system, making it widely available at a reasonable cost.

A. Principles of BOLD fMRI

BOLD fMRI relies on detecting consequences of the locally increased blood flow (and blood volume) associated with increased neuronal activity (Fig. 1) (Kim et al. 1993; Ogawa et al. 1990, 1992, 1993). Because the increase in local blood flow is in excess of the increased metabolic demands, there is reduced oxygen extraction and a higher ratio of oxy- to deoxyhemoglobin ("redder blood") in the region of neuronal activation. Greater blood oxygenation

leads to greater signal on an appropriately (T_2^*) sensitized MRI scan. The BOLD fMRI arises from the different magnetic properties of oxygenated (oxyHb) and deoxygenated hemoglobin (deoxyHb): deoxyHb is paramagnetic (and distorts an applied magnetic field for imaging), whereas oxyHb is diamagnetic (and does not perturb the applied magnetic field significantly).

Arterioles carrying oxygenated arterial blood thus cause little distortion to the magnetic field, whereas capillaries and veins containing blood that is partially deoxygenated distort the magnetic field locally. The (microscopic) magnetic field inhomogeneities associated with distortions from deoxyHb leads to destructive interference of signal within the tissue voxel, which shortens the so-called T2* "relaxation time." A shorter T2* leads to lower signal from a voxel (and thus a darker image pixel). Alternatively, the increased oxy-/deoxy-hemoglobin ratio associated with activation leads to a longer T_2^*, more signal from the voxel, and a relatively brighter pixel on the gradient echo image.

In the fMRI experiment, a large (typically hundreds) series of images are acquired rapidly (using a fast imaging technique, such as echo planar imaging) while the subject performs a task in which brain activity alternates between two or more well-defined states (e.g., rest vs. movement of the hand) (Matthews and Jezzard, 2003). By correlating the signal time course from each voxel with the known time course of the task, it is possible to identify those voxels in the brain that show task-associated signal changes corresponding to "activation." Although PET provides an absolute measure of tissue metabolism, BOLD fMRI can at present be used only for determining *relative* signal intensity changes between different cognitive states studied within a single imaging session. Also, the magnitude of the signal intensity changes being measured with fMRI is only on the order of 0.5% to 5.0%. As this is much smaller than the intrinsic local tissue contrast (e.g., between gray matter and CSF), one of the most significant practical confounds in fMRI is an extreme sensitivity to *motion,* which can mix signals from

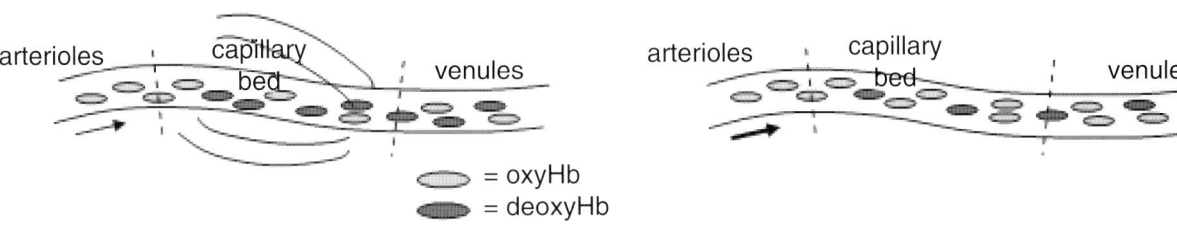

Basal state: higher deoxy/oxy
Hb ratio, *lower* relative signal

Activated state: lower deoxy/oxy
Hb ratio, *higher* relative signal

Figure 1 Hemodynamic parameters that change during neuronal activity. In the basal state deoxyhemoglobin in the capillaries and venules causes microscopic field gradients to be established around the blood vessels. This in turn leads to a decreased signal in a gradient-echo MRI sequence. In the activated state, there is a significant increase in flow, but only a modest increase in oxygen consumption. This results in a lower concentration of deoxyhemoglobin in the capillaries and venules, and hence to a reduction in the microscopic field gradients and to an increase in the signal intensity. (Figure modified from material provided by Prof. P. Jezzard.)

neighboring voxels over an extended series of images. If movement occurs synchronously with the task, movement-associated signal changes will be found along with those associated specifically with any brain functional changes.

B. The Genesis of the BOLD Signal

Although neuronal activity is accompanied by increased energy utilization, it is not the increased energy use itself that directly triggers the associated increase in blood flow. Instead, the increased blood flow is a direct consequence of presynaptic neurotransmitter action (Attwell and Iadecola, 2002) and thus reflects local neuronal *signaling*. Increases in the BOLD signal are correlated electrophysiologically most strongly with the local field potential rather than the neuronal firing rate (Logothetis et al., 2001). The volume over which blood flow increases associated with neuronal activity is determined by the perfusion territory of local arterioles.

There may be multiple mediators of the arteriolar response, but nitric oxide (NO) and eicosanoids clearly are important under normal circumstances (Buerk et al., 2003; St. Lawrence et al., 2003). Binding of glutamate to receptors on astrocytes triggers NO release. Neuronal-hemodynamic coupling thus may change with disease (D'Esposito et al., 2003). For example, early after ischemic infarction, regional cerebral blood flow (rCBF) may be uncoupled (lack of response) from regional cerebral metabolic rate for glucose consumption (rCMRglu) (persistent response) as a consequence of ischemia-induced inhibition of nitric oxide syn-

thetase (NOS). Even chronically there may be changes in brain neuronal-hemodynamic coupling related to this or other mechanisms (Pineiro et al., 2002).

In MS there is widespread upregulation of NOS (Smith and Lassmann, 2002). We have made an initial assessment of potential changes in hemodynamic coupling in patients with relapsing-remitting MS (Saini et al., 2004). Hemodynamic responses to motor activation reassuringly appear well preserved, suggesting that there are no major confounds to inferring functional localization on the basis of fMRI in studies of MS (Fig. 2).

III. Motor Learning by the Healthy Brain Provides a Basis for Understanding Adaptive Functional Reorganization of the Brain after Injury

The brain arguably has not evolved so much to adapt to injury as to adapt its responses to changing external or internal environments. It is attractive to hypothesize that the broad range of examples of functional reorganization of the brain in response to altered external stimuli or internal state rely on common mechanisms. Studies in animal models have shown that similar functional changes in sensorimotor cortical areas are associated with peripheral nerve injury (Seil, 1997), amputation (Florence et al., 1998), or repeated direct cortical stimulation (Nudo et al., 1990), for example. Peripheral

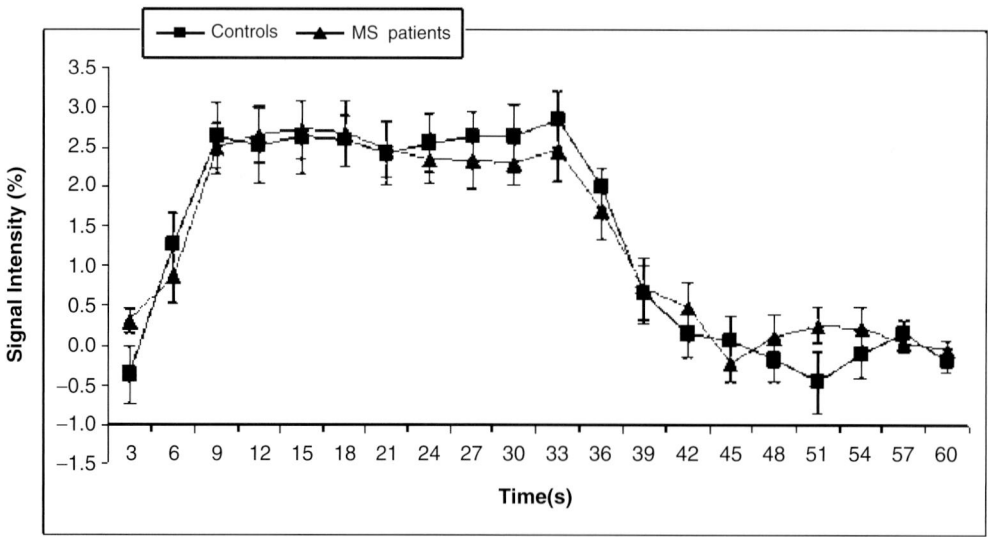

Figure 2 Group mean hemodynamic responses are shown for the single most highly activated voxel in the primary sensorimotor cortex of healthy controls and patients with clinically stable relapsing-remitting multiple sclerosis during a repetitive writing task performed with the right hand (see Saini et al., 2004). No significant differences in the rate of signal intensity rise or maximum increase in blood oxygenation level dependent (BOLD) signal are between control and patient groups. These results suggest that the relationship between neuronal activity and the BOLD response is not altered in these patients with MS.

deafferentation in monkeys leads to a reduction of the area of cortical responsiveness for the deafferented limb (Merzenich et al., 1983; Garraghty and Kaas, 1991) that mirrors enlargements of cortical responsiveness with motor-skill learning (Kleim et al., 1998) or repetitive intracortical microstimulation (Nudo et al., 1990). Changes in functional organization of the cortex related to altered afferent or efferent activity must share at least some common mechanisms, whatever the specific cause of the altered activity; however, the most common manifestation of this type of change is for learning. Most generally formulated learning involves changing the brain representations for the relationship between a stimulus and its consequences. Studies of learning therefore may provide important lessons to help understand responses of the brain to injury.

Motor learning can occur over both the short and long term. Different patterns of behavioral and brain functional activity changes are associated with the two time frames for learning. With short-term learning, there is a rapid improvement in performance associated with a decrease in the specific attentional demands of the task (Floyer-Lea and Matthews, 2003). This is associated with decreasing activity in prefrontal cortex and a progressive "focusing" of activity in the primary motor cortex contralateral to the limb moved (Fig. 3) (see for example, Ramnani et al., 2000; Toni et al., 2001a; Grafton et al., 1992; Karni et al., 1995, 1998) as performance becomes more automatic with increasing practice. It is intriguing to note the substantial similarities between the dynamic change in activation patterns illustrated in Fig. 3 and the dynamic changes in brain activity with recovery after acute stroke (see for example, Ward et al., 2003).

The acquisition of motor skills of many types appears to be associated with altered primary motor cortex representations;

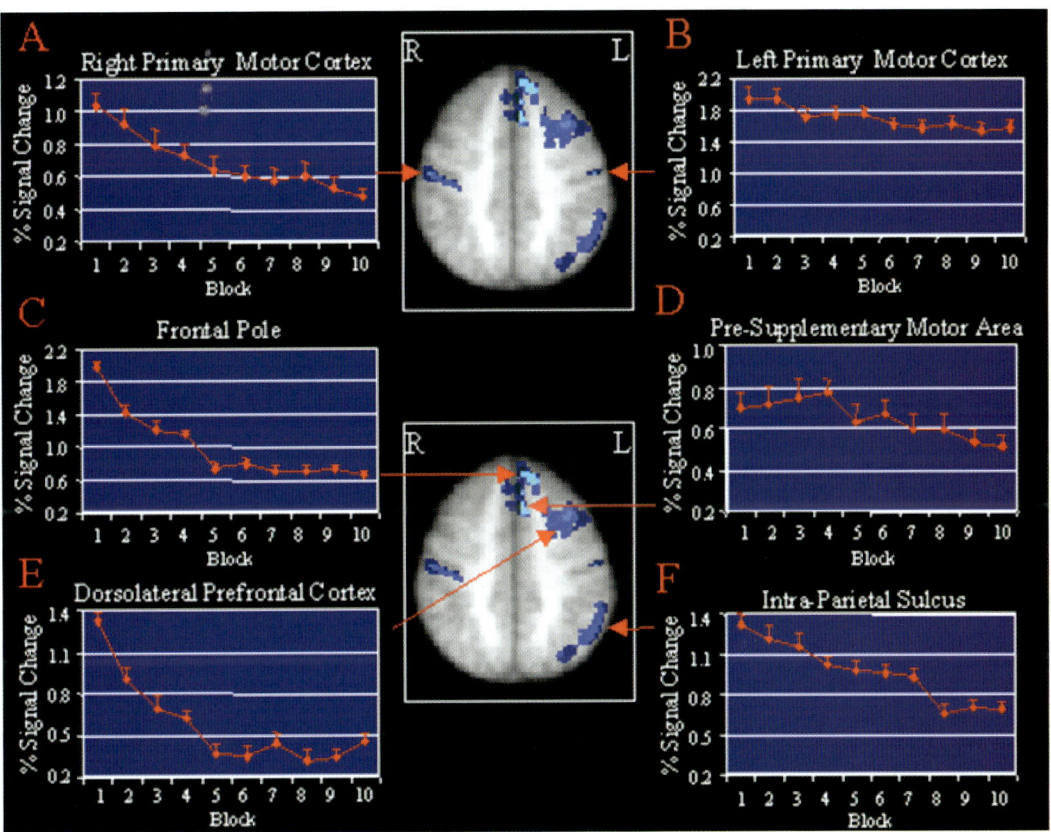

Figure 3 Brain activation correlated with improvement in performance for a group of healthy subjects when learning to exert finger flexion pressure with the (dominant) right hand according to a visually-presented pattern, together with their time courses (group random effects image, z < 2.3, P < 0.01, corrected). Areas that showed an increase in activation are shown in red; those areas that showed a decrease in activation are shown in blue. At the start of the experiment the level of activation is similar in the right (**A**) and left (**B**) motor cortex. Although both sides show a decrease in activation over the course of the experiment, the right hemisphere shows a more significant decrease than the left hemisphere, so that by the end of the experiment, the activation is almost completely left-lateralized. The dorsolateral prefrontal cortex (DLPFC) and the presupplementary motor area (pre-SMA) show contrasting time courses. The DLPFC (**E**) shows initially high activation that drops off sharply, reaching baseline levels before the early learning phase is complete. The pre-SMA (**D**) shows an initial increase in activation before decreasing, reaching a peak at the time when activation in the DLPFC has declined. The frontal pole (**C**) has a time course closer to that of the behavioral learning itself, whereas the intraparietal sulcus (IPS) (**F**) shows a more sustained decrease that continues into the postlearning phase.

for example, qualitatively similar phenomena are found after learning an isometric tracking task (Floyer-Lea et al., unpublished) or after development of skills in a sport such as badminton (Pearce et al., 2000). Analogous changes have been described in the nonhuman primate primary motor cortex based on invasive cortical mapping. For example, as monkeys learn to draw peanuts from smaller wells, there is reorganization of motor representations for limb movement in the primary motor cortex (Nudo et al., 1996a). It is important to note, however, that both human and primate studies have emphasized that these changes in patterns of brain activity associated with learning are task specific (Floyer-Lea and Matthews, 2003; Karni et al., 1995; Kleim et al., 1998). Even two similar (but distinct) finger movement sequences do not use precisely the same representation (Karni et al., 1995).

This suggests that the substrate for *general* skill learning (e.g., being able to play the piano, as opposed to being able to play any specific piece on the piano) is not simply a change in motor representation in the primary motor cortex. One may speculate that this form of learning, which possibly is central to understanding recovery, is mediated by changes that are much more widely distributed. A potentially important part of such a network for change involves frontoparietal circuits. Activity in the dorsolateral prefrontal cortex is associated with problem solving and shows performance-related increases in activity (Duncan et al., 2000). Parietal activity is involved in evaluating the potential significance of stimuli (Driver and Mattingley, 1998; Mort et al., 2003). The posterior parietal cortex is also concerned with aspects of visual and spatial stimulus selection (Fink et al., 1996). Consistent with this, the preparation to move is associated with frontoparietal activation.

It has been more difficult to study subcortical activity, but subcortical regions clearly also contribute substantially to the brain circuits involved in learning. Subcortical circuits appear to be involved particularly for learning implicit tasks (Doyon et al., 2002; Laforce, Jr. and Doyon, 2001) or when tasks become more automatic (when performance is less affected by distracters) (Floyer-Lea and Matthews, 2003).

Although lessons can be drawn from learning in the healthy brain, however, it is unlikely that motor recovery after brain injury simply represents learning *redux*. A number of special mechanisms may alter the potential for functional reorganization in the context of brain injury (Witte, 1998). Ischemic brain injury triggers complex changes in cortical excitability (Witte et al., 2000): local to the infarct, excitability is decreased (Neumann-Haefelin and Witte, 2000), but more distantly, excitability is increased. The latter occurs in association with downregulation of inhibitory γ-aminobutyric acid (GABA) receptor levels (Redecker et al., 2002). Studies in the healthy brain suggest that functional reorganization in motor cortex could be strongly affected by GABAergic activity (Butefisch et al., 2000), as well as the excitatory glutaminergic system acting through N-methy-

D-aspartate (NMDA) receptors (Hess et al., 1994). Deafferentation induces at least transiently increased excitability in the contralateral hemisphere (Werhahn et al., 2002, 2003). Loss of sensory afferents alone reduce local GABA concentrations, potentially helping to drive short-term functional reorganization. These factors may even contribute to the structural and functional changes that occur in the brain many months after the injury, when primary repair has slowed or stopped (Taub et al., 2002, 2003). Although similar phenomena are much less well characterized in MS, TMS data, for example, suggest that such changes may be important (Ho et al., 1999).

Another distinction between simple motor learning and recovery after brain injury is that the latter represents *relearning* to perform tasks in different ways. Either compensatory strategies must be developed or new pathways must be recruited adaptively. In general, this must involve some systems distinct from those engaged for naïve motor learning. Exciting work has begun to explore the more general mechanisms by which feedback relevant to the action plan is processed that emphasizes these differences. Ramnani et al. used a simple visuomotor association learning task and distinguished between activity time-locked to positive, negative, and neutral (control) feedback (Ramnani and Matthews, 2003). Specific brain regions (including the dorsal prefrontal cortex, cingulate cortex, anterior temporal cortex, ventral striatum/pallidum, thalamus, and the amygdala) showed increased activity with meaningful feedback. When the contingencies between stimuli and actions were changed to create a *relearning* trial, meaningful feedback activated the supramarginal gyrus (left-lateralized for negative feedback, right-lateralized for positive feedback) to a significantly greater degree than with the initial learning. Two conclusions relevant to the current discussion can be drawn from this. First, specific mechanisms are responsible for responding to the feedback necessary to modify behavior. Second, the specific pathways engaged with performance feedback are determined in part by the context in which they are engaged.

IV. Direct Observations on Patients After Brain Injury: Common Brain Mechanisms Contribute to Adaptive Changes After Corticospinal Tract Injury

A. Cortical Plasticity

Adaptive functional reorganization is an example of the more general phenomenon of "plasticity." Donaghue defines this as "any enduring change in cortical properties, either morphological or functional" (Sanes and Donoghue, 2000). Such changes can be defined by fMRI (or related methods) as an expansion of brain regions local to the usual functions, recruitment of additional cortical areas, or as local shifts in centers of activity associated with specific behaviors. Direct electrophysiological studies (still perhaps the gold standard) have shown empirically that there must be a dual focus in defining postinjury plasticity; both local and anatomically more distant functional changes can be found. For example, reorganization after injury to the corticospinal tract involves both a local expansion (or shift) in motor representations and new recruitment of motor cortex in the undamaged hemisphere (Nudo et al., 1996b, 2001). These observations (and related work) suggest that postinjury reorganization depends to a significant extent on modifications to existing pathways rather than the development of entirely new circuits (e.g., recruitment of existing motor pathways in the hemisphere ipsilateral to the hand moved) (Cole and Glees, 1952) that may be used to only a minor extent by the healthy brain (Kim et al., 1993) or only under different conditions (e.g., with more complex tasks) (Rao et al., 1993).

B. Evidence for Cortical Plasticity with MS

MS may be a particularly appropriate disease for the study of brain plasticity (see Cifelli and Matthews, 2002), as most patients show good recovery from clinical expression of new lesions (relapses) in the earlier stages of the illness, despite evidence for axonal injury with each attack (Fu et al., 1998; Evangelou et al., 2000). Some aspects of axonal injury may be partially reversible (de Stefano et al., 1995), which must contribute to the potential for clinical recovery. However, irreversible axonal injury can be substantial (Evangelou et al., 2000; Trapp et al., 1998), suggesting that other factors, such as adaptive functional reorganization, also must be important (Cifelli et al., 2002).

Yousry et al. (1998) first provided fMRI-based evidence suggesting that patients with MS who have motor weakness show potentially adaptive increased activation of ipsilateral and accessory motor areas, reminiscent of earlier findings with subcortical ischemic stroke (Weiller et al., 1993). Later studies have refined these observations and related patterns of functional change directly to measures of injury or disability (see, for example, Filippi et al., 2003; Rocca et al., 2002; Lee et al., 2000; Reddy et al. 2000c, 2000d; Pantano et al., 2002).

To interpret these changes in brain functional organization as evidence for adaptive plasticity related to disease, at least three conditions need to be fulfilled:

1. The extent of the functional reorganization must be related to the burden of disease (and thus evolve dynamically through the course of the disease).
2. Evidence for functional reorganization must be found even in the absence of disease-associated behavioral impairment (consistent with the notion that adaptive plasticity *limits* clinical expression of the disease).

3. Altered patterns of functional activation in patients must be independent of conscious patterns of recruitment (as the latter are associated with development of strategies for compensation).

Ideally, it may also be possible to demonstrate that ascribing a relevant, adaptive functional role to the new pattern of brain activation is physiologically reasonable. Not all functional brain changes are either directly relevant to the task or desirable. Brain functional changes simply may be epiphenomena (e.g., a result of sensory stimulation by an ambulatory aid while a hemiparetic patient walks) rather than a direct manifestation of altered central programs for motor control. Functional changes can be incidental (e.g., the perceived need to attend more closely to cues if movement is impaired). Brain functional changes also can be *maladaptive*. For example, the intense training used by professional musicians may lead to focal hand dystonia, in which representations for digit movements become linked, leading to awkward or frankly uncomfortable finger postures (Pujol et al., 2000).

1. Functional Brain Changes in Patients with MS Are Related to Disease Burden

Functional reorganization defined by fMRI in patients with MS is related to the burden of disease. Using a simple hand movement task, Lee et al. (2000) first reported that brain T2 lesion load was correlated with a decreasing relative activation in motor cortex ipsilateral to the hand moved (Fig. 4). For a more specific test, the need to use measures of pathology in the corticospinal tracts (CSTs) is suggested by previous work with focal ischemic brain injury, which established direct correlations between motor functional impairment and damage to the CST (Feydy et al., 2002; Binkofski et al., 1996; Fukui et al., 1994). Reddy et al. (2000c) demonstrated a correlation between NAA decreases (a measure of axonal injury) in the corticospinal tract and changes in patterns of functional activity with hand movement in patients who did not have clinical deficits affecting the limb tested. Pantano et al. (2002) showed a similar correlation between changes in the pattern of brain activation and lesion load pathology in the CST of patients with MS after a first episode of hemiparesis. They confirmed that, with increasing time after clinical presentation (during which disease burden may be expected to rise), there was an increasingly abnormal pattern of brain activity with hand movement. Similar, more intensive correlations with pathology have been reported by the Filippi group in patients with relapsing-remitting (Filippi et al., 2003) and primary-progressive MS (Rocca et al., 2002), although this approach has been more sensitive to changes elsewhere than in the ipsilateral motor cortex.

Aspects of this phenomenon can be generalized to other systems. Staffen et al. (2002) studied patients with MS and healthy controls performing a sustained attention task. Although performance was equivalent between the two

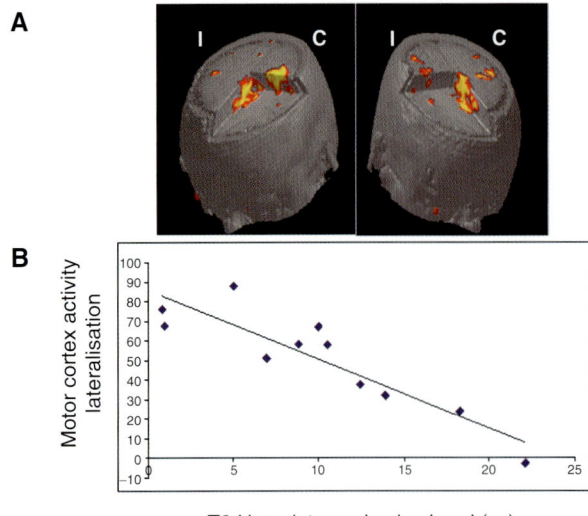

Figure 4 (**A**) With simple finger flexion, the major regions of brain activation in healthy subjects are the sensorimotor cortex contralateral (*C*) to the hand moved and the midline supplementary motor area. Patients with multiple sclerosis and corticospinal tract injury show increased relative ipsilateral (*I*) sensorimotor cortex activation. (**B**) This difference is highlighted by an activation hemispheric lateralization index (*LI*), defined as the ratio of sensorimotor cortex activation contralateral to that ipsilateral to the hand moved. The LI decreases (i.e., activation becomes more bihemispheric) as disease burden rises, consistent with the notion that ipsilateral sensorimotor cortex recruitment represents cortical adaptive plasticity (see Johansen-Berg et al., 2002b; figure from Lee et al., 2000.)

groups, patients with MS showed activation in right frontal and left parietal cortex not found in healthy controls, suggesting adaptive recruitment of additional, multimodal control regions. Werring et al. (2000) examined patients with MS who had recovered from optic neuritis using visual stimulation with fMRI. Although the patients showed decreased activation of the visual cortex receiving projections from the affected optic nerve, there were additional extensive task-associated *decreases* in activation in the claustrum, the lateral temporal and posterior parietal cortices, and the thalamus. All of these brain regions are involved in higher order visual processing or object recognition. The extent to which activity in these additional regions was suppressed was related to the severity of optic nerve pathology as assessed from visual-evoked potentials. A speculative explanation for this observation is that suppression of activity in these areas is a manifestation of adaptively increased attentional mechanisms, which may enhance information processing specifically in primary visual cortex immediately after presentation of the visual stimulus.

2. Functional Brain Changes in Patients with MS Are Dynamic

As predicted from evidence that brain activity patterns change with disease burden, functional reorganization observed by fMRI is dynamic, changing as lesions evolve

pathologically. In an early report by Reddy et al. (2000d), a patient with a new large demyelinating lesion affecting the corticospinal tract was monitored with serial MRI, MRS, and fMRI studies after the onset of hemiparesis. Clinical recovery *preceded* normalization of NAA concentrations (an index of structural repair after the lesion) and was associated with relative increases in premotor area and supplementary motor area activation in the hemisphere ipsilateral to the hand moved (an index of functional adaptation). The observation that clinical recovery occurred faster than the structural repair, and was associated with changing patterns of brain activation, is consistent with a functional role for the latter. The general correlation between changes in fMRI responses and magnetic resonance spectroscopy (MRS) measures suggests a progressive normalization of patterns of functional organization in motor cortex in response to the repair of axonal injury associated with the lesion. Qualitatively similar dynamic changes occur after focal ischemic stroke as recovery progresses (Marshall et al., 2000; Ward et al., 2003), Results are consistent with prior cross-sectional studies demonstrating that the magnitude of activation changes was greater with poorer functional recovery (Calautti and Baron, 2003; Johansen-Berg et al., 2002a; Jang et al., 2003).

A key point is that brain functional changes associated with movement are (at least to a large degree) independent of the specific cause of neuroaxonal damage in the CST. The pattern of change discussed previously for MS is similar to that found with serial fMRI studies of motor activation in patients with stroke. These studies have shown a similar initial bilateral activation with lesions of the contralateral motor cortex that reverts toward a more lateralized activation pattern with progression of recovery (Ward et al., 2003; Marshall et al., 2000; Feydy et al., 2002). Altered patterns of recruitment may help to maintain functions (e.g., via adaptive recruitment of additional descending motor pathways) despite persistent injury to the corticospinal tract.

Aspects of these potentially adaptive functional changes may occur rapidly, suggesting that some aspects may rely on unmasking preexisting pathways. Parry and colleagues (2003) studied brain responses to the Stroop paradigm, a test of attention and prepotent inhibition. Patients with MS and healthy controls were studied using a fMRI counting Stroop task. The two subject groups had comparable performances, but patients showed a deficit of activation in a right frontal region (including Brodman's area 45 and the basal ganglia) implicated by modeling studies in key aspects of the task (Cohen et al., 1996). The patients also showed relatively increased activation in a predominantly left medial prefrontal region previously implicated in supramodal monitoring and related tasks. A direct relationship between these activation measures and relative brain atrophy was consistent with the notion that left prefrontal activation represented a functional adaptation to the deficits. Parry et al.

(2003) tested the effects of acute administration of rivastigmine, a central cholinesterase inhibitor, on the patterns of brain activation. It was hypothesized that this drug might be able to partially correct functional impairment in the dysfunctional right hemisphere circuit. Within 90 minutes of oral drug administration, there was a relative normalization of the abnormal, Stroop-associated brain activation in all of the patients with MS (with no change in the patterns of brain activation in any of the healthy controls).

The potential time-frame for adaptive functional changes after injury has been reduced further by studies in the healthy brain. For example, Bütefisch demonstrated that changes in movement representation for the thumb can occur over training periods as short as minutes (Butefisch et al., 2000). Strens et al. (2002) demonstrated that TMS delivered to the motor cortex to locally disrupt activity is associated with increased excitability in the motor cortex of the opposite hemisphere. Similarly, Lee et al. (2003) used TMS to interfere with activity in the primary motor cortex while monitoring the metabolic response of the entire motor system using PET. Although the TMS parameters used (30 minutes of slow 1-Hz stimulation) should have decreased excitability of the left motor cortex, no behavioral consequences of the disruption were observed with a simple motor task, suggesting that unaffected regions of the motor network were able to compensate for the effects of disruption in the primary motor cortex. A candidate adaptive change was identified in PET scans acquired after the stimulation showing that, after repetitive TMS interference to the left primary motor cortex, increased activation of the opposite premotor cortex was seen with right hand movement. This recalls the interhemispheric functional reorganization that occurs in the premotor cortex after corticospinal tract damage (see previously).

3. Functional Brain Changes with MS Are Found in Patients Without Clinical Deficits Limiting Performance

The second criterion for adaptive functional reorganization—that it can be found even without behavioral changes—has also been demonstrated. Changes in cortical activation occur early in the course of MS and in patients without symptoms in the affected functional system. Patients with MS without motor or sensory impairment of the upper limbs were investigated with fMRI and MRS using a hand-tapping paradigm (Reddy et al., 2000c). LI was abnormally low in the patients and decreased progressively, with decreases in relative brain NAA concentrations. Because these results were obtained from patients who had normal hand function, the potential confound that arises from performance differences in comparison with healthy controls was absent. Patients with optic neuritis as their only clinical manifestation of MS also show brain functional changes with movement compared to healthy controls, suggesting that even low levels of injury in the motor system are

associated with adaptive functional changes (Pantano et al., 2002). Again, emphasizing that the changes are not determined solely by the pathology, qualitatively similar changes were noted in the well-recovered patients with capsular infarcts studied by PET more than a decade ago (Weiller et al., 1993).

4. Functional Brain Changes with MS Occur Independent of Conscious Control

The third criterion for adaptive brain plasticity—that brain functional changes are independent of volitional activity—can also be confirmed in some patients. Because fMRI assesses predominantly presynaptic activity (see previously) and there is strong afferent sensory input into motor cortical regions, parts of the cortical network for limb movement (including primary sensorimotor and premotor cortex) should be defined by patterns of brain activity with passive movement of a limb (Sahyoun et al., 2003; Reddy et al., 2001; Weiller et al. 1996). A passive movement task, therefore, can be used to test for abnormal patterns of brain activity in patients relative to healthy controls. Although only some components of the network for motor control can be defined, the use of a passive task has the advantage of being free from potential confounds arising from differences in movement preparation and planning (Reddy et al., 2001; Sahyoun et al., 2003). Reddy et al. (2002) tested a group of patients with MS using both an active and a passive hand movement task, verifying with surface electromyography that the passive task was not associated with motor unit activation. A strong, quantitative correlation was found between indices of relative activation with the active and passive tasks. Separate studies confirmed that the activation was independent of movement imagery, and that it is absent in patients with pure sensory neuropathies who lack hand perception or somatic sensation. The recruitment of ipsilateral motor cortex during movement in MS pathology, therefore, is not dependent on factors related to volition.

5. Demonstrating a Functional Role for the Brain reorganization

In general, behaviorally relevant roles for functional changes such as those found in patients with MS have not been directly established. The observation of clinical recovery in the absence of resolution of structural changes in a functional system provides *indirect* evidence that functional reorganization is adaptive. More commonly, the rationale is one of physiological reasonableness. For example, increased sensory cortical activity may be expected as an adaptation to the need to alter motor representation with corticospinal tract injury affecting the hand (Rocca et al., 2002). More evidence is available regarding the potential role of increased activity in motor cortex ipsilateral to the hand moved after injury to the CST. Clinical observations have suggested that sensorimotor cortex opposite to a focal lesion affecting motor control may support important new functions. For example, Fisher (1992) described two patients whose functional deficits deteriorated after partial recovery from a second stroke in the other hemisphere and Ago et al. (2003) reported a patient with a right hemisphere stroke and left hemiparesis who sustained deterioration of residual function after a new lacunar infarct in the left corona radiata. Transient cortical "lesioning" using TMS also supports this notion. Johansen-Berg et al. (2002b) described measurable functional impairments in cued finger movements after TMS pulse delivery to the dorsal premotor cortex contralateral to a focal ischemic lesion. The extent of this impairment after TMS was correlated with relative activity in the ipsilateral motor cortex measured using fMRI.

C. Functional Changes in MS Are Similar to Those Found in Other Forms of Brain Injury

MS has been a useful model disease with which to study functional reorganization because of the slow progression of the pathology and the availability of well-validated MRI indices of pathological progression and clinical indices of disability. There is compelling evidence that fundamental principles regarding functional reorganization in the motor system are generalizable. As noted previously, functional cortical changes have been demonstrated in patients with other brain pathology, for example, after strokes (e.g., Weiller et al., 1993; Cramer et al., 1997) or with the growth of tumors (Seitz et al., 1995). Reddy et al. (2002) tested the notion of generalizability more directly using a vascular disease "analog" of MS. They studied patients with diffuse ischemic changes in white matter from cerebral autosomal dominant arteriopathy with subcortical infarcts and leukoencephalopathy (CADASIL) using both MRS and fMRI. The relationship between axonal injury, disability, and cortical functional organization were evaluated. Just as was found with patients with MS, for a simple motor task, increases in ipsilateral motor cortical activation correlated with severity of the disease in the patients with CADASIL.

V. Potentially Adaptive Functional Changes Are Widely Distributed in Brains of Patients with MS

A. Functional Changes Occur Throughout the Motor Control Network

Motor control in the brain is highly distributed. Although it may be viewed as hierarchical, the preceding arguments make clear that there is substantial parallel processing and interaction within the network. Altered function at a single "node" in the network, therefore, would be expected to have

widespread effects, as other "nodes" adjust their output in response.

Sensorimotor cortex function is altered locally as well as in the opposite hemisphere. Lee et al. (2000) demonstrated a net posterior shift in activity in a group of patients with MS. Relative posterior shifts have been found in patients with recovery after stroke (Pineiro et al., 2001; Calautti and Baron, 2003), similar to previous reports from observations of patients with brain tumors (Seitz et al., 1995); however, the specific relative shift may depend on the extent and localization of the pathology. It is possible that it is more apparent in the postcentral gyrus than in the precentral gyrus because of differences in relative somatotopy. The somatosensory cortex shows clear somatotopy (Sutherling et al., 1992), whereas representations are overlapping to a much greater extent in the primary motor cortex of the relatively precentral gyrus (Sanes et al., 1995).

Studies of patients with MS also have consistently identified increased activation in the premotor cortex and in the midline cortex, including supplementary motor and cingulate motor areas with hand movement (Lee et al., 2000; Pantano et al., 2002; Rocca et al., 2002). These may represent unmasking of areas with "parallel" motor projections to anterior brain cells. However, the lack of evidence for fine finger movement representation outside of the contralateral CST, the (previously cited) strong evidence for the importance of the CST in determining the outcome after stroke, and prominent involvement of similar areas in healthy controls during motor learning suggest that increased activity in these regions may provide mechanisms for flexible optimization of output.

B. The Importance of Sensory-Motor Integration

As noted previously, there is a close relationship between sensory and motor functions in movement. For example, monkeys show a transient motor deficit after selective lesioning of the primary sensory motor cortex (Asanuma and Arissian, 1984). Deafferented patients learn new movement patterns poorly (Xerri et al., 1998). There are strong reciprocal anatomical connections between primary sensorimotor cortex. Thus, it is not surprising that, as well as changes in the motor network, patients with MS may show altered patterns of activation in secondary somatosensory cortex and in multimodal sensory integration regions.

Recent fMRI studies have shown that patients with MS have enhanced sensory cortical activation (e.g., in the secondary somatosensory area in addition to changes directly in the motor cortex) (Rocca et al., 2002). In some cases, a specific rationale for these changes is apparent, as in the substitution of visuomotor for somatosensory information (Seitz et al., 1999). For example, Altschueller et al. (1999) found that when hemiparetic patients performed bilateral movements for rehabilitation, viewing the normal arm through a mirror positioned between the two arms enhanced functional gains. Patients with MS may also show functional changes in regions of the brain involved in multimodal sensory integration such as the claustrum and insula (Werring et al., 2000; Pantano et al., 2002; Filippi et al., 2003). As described previously, in some cases, there may be suppression of activity in brain regions responsible for sensory integration, a possible adaptation for enhancement of responses in the primary sensory cortex being tested (Werring et al., 2000).

Increased parietal lobe activation is also a relatively consistent finding in patients with MS, but specific interpretation is limited by the complexity of functions of this brain region. Parietal activity seems to be involved in evaluating the potential significance of stimuli (Driver and Mattingley, 1998; Mort et al., 2003). The posterior parietal cortex is concerned with aspects of visual and spatial stimulus selection (Fink et al., 1996). The intraparietal sulcus projects to the premotor cortex (Cavada and Goldman-Rakic, 1989). Consistent with this, the anticipation of a movement or preparation to move is associated with frontoparietal activation in the healthy brain (Sahyoun et al., 2003; Toni et al., 2001b). Increased parietal activation can also be found in this region in patients with MS performing hand movements (Pantano et al., 2002). Activity in the intraparietal sulcus appears important for transformations of actions from an external to internal reference frame and must change with brain injury. Increased parietal activity is seen in the healthy brain with novel, complex finger movement tasks (Sakai et al., 1998). A strong correlation was found between activation in this region in a group of patients with relapsing-remitting MS and multiple measures of their brain pathology (Rocca et al., 2002).

C. The Cerebellum and Motor Recovery

A potentially important brain region mediating recovery is the cerebellum. Contralesional cerebellar activity shows increased or sustained activity after an acute ischemic lesion associated with hemiparesis (Feydy et al., 2002; Fraser et al., 2002; Calautti and Baron, 2003). Increased cerebellar activity may distinguish patients with a more favorable outcome after stroke (Small et al., 2002). Cerebellar pathways have been implicated in circuitry mediating recovery and could be particularly important for adaptive responses to injury because of their high intrinsic synaptic plasticity (Voogd and Glickstein, 1998). The cerebellum has a well-described and key role in functional plasticity of the motor system during skill learning by the healthy brain, for example (Doyon et al., 2002; Lafleur et al., 2002; Ungerleider et al., 2002). Cerebellar activation may be critical for sensory processing (Ito, 1993), specifically in monitoring and optimizing movements based on proprioceptive feedback. This role could link these changes to those in secondary somatosensory areas, recalling the specifically *disability*-associated activations reported by Reddy et al. (2002) (Fig. 5).

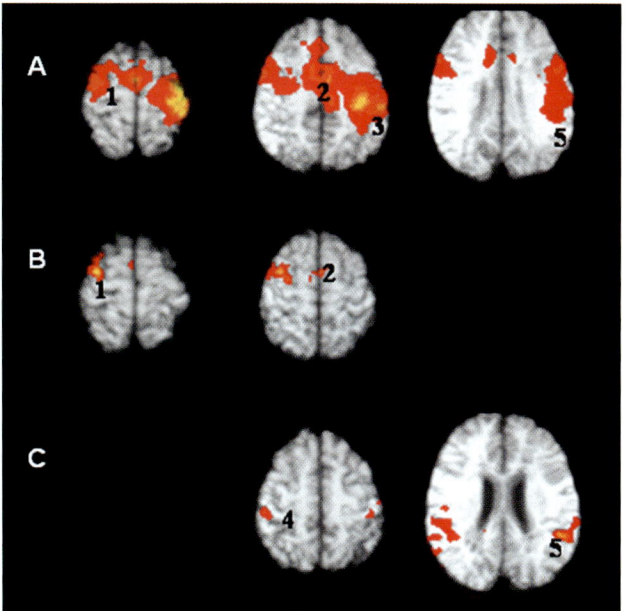

Figure 5 To test whether behavioral changes associated with increased disability and greater disease burden make independent contributions to altered patterns of brain activity in patients with multiple sclerosis, patients were matched for either disability or burden of disease, and fMRI was performed with a finger flexion task. (**A**) For all subjects, the task was associated with activation in a distributed motor control network, including the primary sensorimotor and premotor cortex and the supplementary motor area. (**B**) Patients with greater corticospinal tract injury who were matched for disability showed relatively increased activation in the dorsal premotor cortex and supplementary motor area. (**C**) In contrast, patients matched for corticospinal tract injury, but with greater disability, showed relatively increased activation in secondary somatosensory and parietal cortex. 1 = ipsilateral dorsal premotor cortex; 2 = supplementary motor cortex; 3 = contralateral sensorimotor cortex; 4 = primary somatosensory cortex; 5 = secondary somatosensory cortex.

A recent study explored the potential role of cerebellar-cortical interactions in patients with MS through a measure of functional connectivity that was defined as the strength of the correlation between regional time courses for brain BOLD responses (Saini et al., 2004). Predominantly patients with early relapsing-remitting MS were studied, along with age-matched, healthy controls. The control group showed the expected strong "crossed" correlation between activation changes in the left primary motor cortex and right cerebellar dentate nuclei (DiPiero et al., 1990; Meyer et al., 1994). This was not found in patients with MS. In contrast, increased connectivity was found between the left premotor cortex (contralateral to the hand moved) and the cerebellar cortex (the input region for the cortico-ponto-cerebellar projection system) on the same side. Increases in activity in the cerebellar hemisphere contralateral to the hand moved are also found with motor learning in healthy subjects (Doyon et al., 2002). This may reflect recruitment of uncrossed pontocerebellar projections. In studies of the cat, although the majority of pontocerebellar projections are crossed, almost a quarter were found to project to the same side (Brodal, 1983). One possible role for activity in the cerebellum contralateral to the hand moved would be changing excitability of premotor cortex *ipsilateral* to the hand moved via crossed dentate-thalamo-cortical projections. A subcortical pathway linking activity in motor cortices of the two hemispheres is suggested by observations such as that showing motor cortex activation ipsilateral to the hand moved does not require an intact corpus callosum (Reddy et al., 2000a, 2000b).

VI. Distinguishing Functional Changes Related to Altered Patterns of Use

The integration of specific functional systems (e.g., those responsible for cognition, perception, and action) in distributed networks controlling task performance suggests that adaptive functional changes need not be confined to the primary effector system for the task. For example, as described previously, abnormal activation in patients with MS performing a simple motor task may be found not only in primary motor control regions but also in sensory and association cortex including the insula and temporal, parietal, and occipital areas (Filippi et al., 2003; Rocca et al., 2002). However, some of the additional activation in patients may be a consequence of the changes in patterns of use (e.g., associated with disability) that accompany injury in patients rather than adaptive functional responses to injury itself. Altered patterns of somatosensory feedback and use certainly lead to changes in the functional organization of the brain in other contexts (Jenkins et al., 1990; Plautz et al., 2000). One fMRI study directly tested whether the effects of injury and disability could be distinguished (Reddy et al., 2002) (Fig. 5). Patients with greater brain injury but no functional impairment showed larger ipsilateral premotor and bilateral supplementary motor area activations. A separate fMRI testing the effects of greater disability alone, and controlling for the extent of injury, showed greater activation in bilateral primary and secondary somatosensory cortex.

VII. Limitations to Adaptive Plasticity in MS

The observation that functional impairments inevitably progress in most patients leads immediately to the conclusion that adaptive plasticity in MS is limited. What limits this adaptive plasticity? That the brain cannot maintain normal behaviors with even isolated focal lesions, if they are large enough, suggests an intrinsic limitation based on local specializations for processing and connectivity. In the evolution of the brain, a compromise has been achieved between parallelism of structure and functional specializa-

tions. Thus, there is a limited scope for recovery of function after major damage to a critical functional system.

In a diffuse disease such as MS, other factors also play a role. Principal among these factors must be diffuse cortical injury and neurodegeneration (Peterson et al., 2001; Cifelli et al., 2002; Wylezinska et al., 2003). Several studies have demonstrated that cortical function is impaired in patients with MS. PET measures of resting cerebral blood flow and metabolism have shown decreases of cortical metabolism associated with clinical progression in MS (Blinkenberg et al., 1999). Sun et al. (1998) reported a correlation between decreased oxidative metabolism and increasing disability Flexible connectivity and adaptive functional reorganization demand widely distributed, intact connectivity. As connectivity is progressively impaired or limited by pathology, the potential for recruitment of parallel pathways decreases.

VIII. Studying Brain Recovery and Rehabilitation Using Approaches from Cognitive Neuroscience: Recognizing the Importance of "Context"

Functional imaging has allowed increasingly informative study of motor control and related cognition in the healthy brain. This has provided a framework for understanding functional brain changes associated with injury and recovery in MS. This work has emphasized that there are widespread changes in response to even focal brain injury, consistent with expectations for adaptive changes that may limit clinical expression of the pathology.

These functional observations also provide insights by emphasizing that behavior and function interact in molding brain responses in disease. The use dependence of functional reorganization implies that brain activity itself helps to determine brain functional outcomes in concert with pathology. The "context" of tasks is also important. For example, Ramnani and Matthews (2003) noted distinct differences in the way in which the brain processes meaningful feedback regarding behavior for initial learning and for relearning. Thus, although studies of motor learning offer useful insights into potential mechanisms of neurorehabilitation, it also must be appreciated that neurorehabilitation (a *recovery* of movement) is more accurately a specialized form of *relearning*.

The importance of context has been emphasized in a different way by a study showing that the manner by which the motor cortex becomes activated is important in determining associated functional reorganization: Lotze and Cohen showed that motor learning depends on more than just movement even when alertness and kinematic aspects of training are well controlled (Lotze et al., 2003). Although both active and passive movements led to activation of the same general area within the primary motor cortex, active training led to more prominent increases in the extent of activation in the primary motor cortex over time, as well as changes in TMS recruitment curves, reflecting the relative degree of intracortical facilitation.

The pathological context of the injury is also important. It has long been recognized that the heterogeneity of localization, size, and severity of lesions, for example, has an effect on disability (Riahi et al., 1998). With appreciation of the interacting cognitive systems for perception, movement planning sensorimotor transformation, and execution of a movement and its control by feedback, new approaches to characterizing motor impairment in terms of deficits in specific brain functional systems become possible. This promises the potential for better targeted therapies, moving away from the notion that one therapeutic approach will be optimally suited to all patients.

IX. Conclusions and Practical Implications

fMRI and related methods provide powerful new ways of exploring systems-level responses of the brain after injury from MS. Cognitive neuroscience provides a useful framework for interpreting these observations and for generating new hypotheses. This offers opportunities for neurobiologically based therapeutic regimens. For example, the Taub constraint-induced therapy procedure is based on the concept of reversing "learned non-use," that is, explicitly enhancing sensorimotor representations of a paretic limb by repetitive movements (Taub et al., 1993, 2002). Muelbacher and colleagues have demonstrated a complementary approach in which the paretic limb representation is transiently increased by reducing that for an adjacent territory (Muellbacher et al., 2002). They anesthetized the upper arm region of the paretic limb so that somatosensory afferents and motor efferents were blocked (Muellbacher et al., 2002). With this regional anesthesia, the paretic hand gained immediately in pinch strength—gains that were maintained for as long as 2 weeks. Even simply increasing sensory input to a brain region may help to increase representation of the relevant body part and drive functional changes. For example, augmenting pharyngeal sensory stimulation can induce changes in its cortical motor representation and improve swallowing (Fraser et al., 2002; Hamdy and Rothwell, 1998). This offers a clear theoretical justification for rehabilitation in MS, as well as the opportunity to develop specific new, neurobiologically based strategies.

An understanding of brain activity at the systems level provides an opportunity for making inferences about the neurotransmitter changes underlying these activities. This knowledge can be used to develop strategies by which pharmacological neuromodulators may be used to enhance recovery. Measures of outcome can also be made more specific in therapeutic trials.

Particularly exciting is that appreciation of MS as a neuronal disease emphasizes that major problems of brain injury and recovery are shared between MS, acute injuries such as stroke, and neurodegenerative conditions. This allows harnessing of a broad range of research to the task of developing a new generation of treatment for MS.

Acknowledgments

PMM is grateful to the MRC (UK) for personal support and for core support of the FMRIB center. Important contributions to this review have come from discussion and joint writings with Prof. P. Jezzard, Dr H. Reddy, H. Johansen-Berg, N. Ramnani, and S. Saini.

References

Ago, T., Kitazono, T., Ooboshi, H., et al. (2003). Deterioration of pre-existing hemiparesis brought about by subsequent ipsilateral lacunar infarction. *J. Neurol. Neurosurg. Psychiatry* **74,** 1152–1153.

Altschuler, E. L., Wisdom, S. B., Stone, L., et al. (1999). Rehabilitation of hemiparesis after stroke with a mirror. *Lancet* **353,** 2035–2036.

Arnold, D. L., Matthews, P. M., Francis, G., and Antel, J. (1990). Proton magnetic resonance spectroscopy of human brain in vivo in the evaluation of multiple sclerosis: Assessment of the load of disease. *Magn. Reson. Med.* **14,** 154–159.

Asanuma, H., and Arissian, K. (1984). Experiments on functional role of peripheral input to motor cortex during voluntary movements in the monkey. *J. Neurophysiol.* **52,** 212–227.

Attwell, D., and Iadecola, C. (2002). The neural basis of functional brain imaging signals. *Trends Neurosci.* **25,** 621–625.

Binkofski, F., Seitz, R. J., Arnold, S., Classen, J., Benecke, R., and Freund, H. J. (1996). Thalamic metabolism and corticospinal tract integrity determine motor recovery in stroke. *Ann. Neurol.* **39,** 460–470.

Blinkenberg, M., Jensen, C. V., Holm, S., Paulson, O. B., and Sorensen, P. S. (1999). A longitudinal study of cerebral glucose metabolism, MRI, and disability in patients with MS. *Neurology* **53,** 149–153.

Boniface, S., and Ziemann, U. (2003). "Plasticity in the Human Nervous System: Investigations with Transcranial Magnetic Stimulation." Cambridge University Press, Cambridge.

Brodal, P. (1983). Principles of organization of the corticopontocerebellar projection to crus II in the cat with particular reference to the parietal cortical areas. *Neuroscience* **10,** 621–638.

Buerk, D. G., Ances, B. M., Greenberg, J. H., and Detre, J. A. (2003). Temporal dynamics of brain tissue nitric oxide during functional forepaw stimulation in rats. *Neuroimage* **18,** 1–9.

Butefisch, C. M., Davis, B. C., Wise, S. P., et al., (2000). Mechanisms of use-dependent plasticity in the human motor cortex. *Proc. Natl. Acad. Sci. U. S. A.* **97,** 3661–3665.

Calautti, C., and Baron, J. C. (2003). Functional neuroimaging studies of motor recovery after stroke in adults: A review. *Stroke* **34,** 1553–1566.

Cavada, C., and Goldman-Rakic, P. S. (1989). Posterior parietal cortex in rhesus monkey. I. Parcellation of areas based on distinctive limbic and sensory corticocortical connections. *J. Comp. Neurol.* **287,** 393–421.

Chard, D. T., Griffin, C. M., Parker, G. J., Kapoor, R., Thompson, A. J., and Miller, D. H. (2002). Brain atrophy in clinically early relapsing-remitting multiple sclerosis. *Brain* **125,** 327–337.

Cifelli, A., Arridge, M., Jezzard, P., Esiri, M. M., Palace, J., and Matthews, P. M. (2002). Thalamic neurodegeneration in multiple sclerosis. *Ann. Neurol.* **52,** 650–653.

Cifelli, A., and Matthews, P. M. (2002). Cerebral plasticity in multiple sclerosis: Insights from fMRI. *Multiple Sclerosis* **8**, 193–199.

Cirstea, M. C., and Levin, M. F. (2000). Compensatory strategies for reaching in stroke. *Brain* **123 (Pt 5)**, 940–953.

Cohen, J. D., Braver, T. S., and O'Reilly, R. C. (1996). A computational approach to prefrontal cortex, cognitive control and schizophrenia: recent developments and current challenges. *Philos. Trans. R. Soc. Lond. B Biol. Sci.* **351**, 1515–1527.

Cole, J., and Glees, P. (1952). Ipsilateral impairment following area 4 lesions in monkeys. *J. Physiol.* **117**, 54P.

Cramer, S. C., Nelles, G., Benson, R. R., et al. (1997). A functional MRI study of subjects recovered from hemiparetic stroke. *Stroke* **28**, 2518–2527.

Craner, M. J., Lo, A. C., Black, J. A., and Waxman, S. G. (2003). Abnormal sodium channel distribution in optic nerve axons in a model of inflammatory demyelination. *Brain* **126**, 1552–1561.

D'Esposito, M., Deouell, L. Y., and Gazzaley, A. (2003). Alterations in the BOLD fMRI signal with ageing and disease: a challenge for neuroimaging. *Nat. Rev. Neurosci.* **4**, 863–872.

de Stefano, N., Matthews, P. M., and Arnold, D. L. (1995). Reversible decreases in *N*-acetylaspartate after acute brain injury. *Magn, Reson, Med.* **34**, 721–727.

de Stefano, N., Matthews, P. M., Filippi, M., et al. (2003). Evidence of early cortical atrophy in MS: Relevance to white matter changes and disability. *Neurology* **60**, 1157–1162.

DiPiero, V., Chollet, F., Dolan, R. J., Thomas, D. J., and Frackowiak, R. (1990). The functional nature of cerebellar diaschisis. *Stroke* **21**, 1365–1369.

Donoghue, J. P., Suner, S., and Sanes, J. N. (1990). Dynamic organization of primary motor cortex output to target muscles in adult rats. II. Rapid reorganization following motor nerve lesions. *Exp. Brain Res.* **79**, 492–503.

Doyon, J., Song, A. W., Karni, A., Lalonde, F., Adams, M. M., and Ungerleider, L. G. (2002). Experience-dependent changes in cerebellar contributions to motor sequence learning. *Proc. Natl. Acad. Sci. U. S. A* **99**, 1017–1022.

Driver, J., and Mattingley, J. B. (1998). Parietal neglect and visual awareness. *Nat. Neurosci.* **1**, 17–22.

Duncan, J., Seitz, R. J., Kolodny, J., et al. (2000). A neural basis for general intelligence. *Science* **289**, 457–460.

Egan, M. F., Kojima, M., Callicott, J. H. et al. (2003). The BDNF val66met polymorphism affects activity-dependent secretion of BDNF and human memory and hippocampal function. *Cell* **112**, 257–269.

Enzinger, C., Ropele, S., Smith, S., et al. (2004). Accelerated evolution of brain atrophy and "black holes" in MS patients with *APOE*4. *Ann. Neurol.* **55**, 563–569.

Evangelou, N., Esiri, M. M., Smith, S., Palace, J., and Matthews, P. M. (2000). Quantitative pathological evidence for axonal loss in normal appearing white matter in multiple sclerosis. *Ann. Neurol.* **47**, 391–395.

Ferguson, B., Matyszak, M. K., Esiri, M. M., and Perry, V. H. (1997). Axonal damage in acute multiple sclerosis lesions. *Brain* **120**, 393–399.

Feydy, A., Carlier, R., Roby-Brami, A., et al. (2002). Longitudinal study of motor recovery after stroke: Recruitment and focusing of brain activation. *Stroke* **33**, 1610–1617.

Filippi, M., Rocca, M. A., Falini, A., et al. (2003). Correlations between structural CNS damage and functional MRI changes in primary progressive MS. *Neuroimage* **15**, 537–546.

Fink, G. R., Halligan, P. W., Marshall, J. C., Frith, C. D., Frackowiak, R. S., and Dolan, R. J. (1996). Where in the brain does visual attention select the forest and the trees? *Nature* **382**, 626–628.

Fisher, C. M. (1992). Concerning the mechanism of recovery in stroke hemiplegia. *Can. J. Neurol. Sci.* **19**, 57–63.

Florence, S. L., Taub, H. B., and Kaas, J. H. (1998). Large-scale sprouting of cortical connections after peripheral injury in adult macaque monkeys. *Science* **282**, 1117–1121.

Floyer-Lea, A., and Matthews, P. M. (2003). Transition of activity from prefrontal cortex to pre-SMA during early motor learning. *Neuroimage* **19 (Part 2)**, 156.

Fox, N. C., Jenkins, R., Leary, S. M., et al. (2000). Progressive cerebral atrophy in MS: a serial study using registered, volumetric MRI. *Neurology* **54**, 807–812.

Fraser, C., Power, M., Hamdy, S., et al. (2002). Driving plasticity in human adult motor cortex is associated with improved motor function after brain injury. *Neuron* **34**, 831–840.

Friel, K. M., and Nudo, R. J. (1998). Recovery of motor function after focal cortical injury in primates: Compensatory movement patterns used during rehabilitative training. *Somatosens. Mot. Res.* **15**, 173–189.

Fu, L., Matthews, P. M., De Stefano, N., et al. (1998). Imaging axonal damage of normal-appearing white matter in multiple sclerosis. *Brain* **121**, 103–113.

Fukui, K., Iguchi, I., Kito, A., Watanabe, Y., and Sugita, K. (1994). Extent of pontine pyramidal tract Wallerian degeneration and outcome after supratentorial hemorrhagic stroke. *Stroke* **25**, 1207–1210.

Gan, W. B., Kwon, E., Feng, G., Sanes, J. R., and Lichtman, J. W. (2003). Synaptic dynamism measured over minutes to months: Age-dependent decline in an autonomic ganglion. *Nat. Neurosci.* **6**, 956–960.

Ganter, P., Prince, C., and Esiri, M. M. (1999). Spinal cord axonal loss in multiple sclerosis: A post-mortem study. *Neuropathol. Appl. Neurobiol.* **25**, 459–467.

Garraghty, P. E., and Kaas, J. H. (1991). Large-scale functional reorganization in adult monkey cortex after peripheral nerve injury. *Proc. Natl. Acad. Sci. U. S. A* **88**, 6976–6980.

Grafton, S. T., Mazziotta, J. C., Presty, S., Friston, K. J., Frackowiak, R. S., and Phelps, M. E. (1992). Functional anatomy of human procedural learning determined with regional cerebral blood flow and PET. *J. Neurosci.* **12**, 2542–2548.

Halfpenny, C., Benn, T., and Scolding, N. (2002). Cell transplantation, myelin repair, and multiple sclerosis. *Lancet Neurol.* **1**, 31–40.

Hamdy, S., and Rothwell, J. C. (1998). Gut feelings about recovery after stroke: The organization and reorganization of human swallowing motor cortex. *Trends Neurosci.* **21**, 278–282.

Hess, G., Jacobs, K. M., and Donoghue, J. P. (1994). *N*-methyl-D-aspartate receptor mediated component of field potentials evoked in horizontal pathways of rat motor cortex. *Neuroscience* **61**, 225–235.

Ho, K. H., Lee, M., Nithi, K., Palace, J., and Mills, K. (1999). Changes in motor evoked potentials to short-interval paired transcranial magnetic stimuli in multiple sclerosis. *Clin. Neurophysiol.* **110**, 712–719.

Ito, M. (1993). Synaptic plasticity in the cerebellar cortex and its role in motor learning. *Can. J. Neurol. Sci.* **20 Suppl 3:S70-4.**, S70–S74.

Jacobs, K. M., and Donoghue, J. P. (1991). Reshaping the cortical motor map by unmasking latent intracortical connections. *Science* **251**, 944–947.

Jang, S. H., Kim, Y. H., Cho, S. H., Chang, Y., Lee, Z. I., and Ha, J. S. (2003). Cortical reorganization associated with motor recovery in hemiparetic stroke patients. *Neuroreport* **14**, 1305–1310.

Jenkins, W. M., Merzenich, M. M., Ochs, M. T., Allard, T., and Guic-Robles, E. (1990). Functional reorganization of primary somatosensory cortex in adult owl monkeys after behaviorally controlled tactile stimulation. *J. Neurophysiol.* **63**, 82–104.

Jezzard, P., Matthews, P. M., and Smith, S. M. (2001). "Functional MRI: An Introduction to Methods." Oxford University Press, Oxford.

Johansen-Berg, H., Dawes, H., Guy, C., Smith, S. M., Wade, D. T., and Matthews, P. M. (2002a). Correlation between motor improvements and altered fMRI activity after rehabilitative therapy. *Brain* **125**, 2731–2742.

Johansen-Berg, H., Rushworth, M. F., Bogdanovic, M. D., Kischka, U., Wimalaratna, S., and Matthews, P. M. (2002b). The role of ipsilateral premotor cortex in hand movement after stroke. *Proc. Natl. Acad. Sci. U. S. A.* **99**, 14518–14523.

Karni, A., Meyer, G., Jezzard, P., Adams, M. M., Turner, R., and Ungerleider, L. G. (1995). Functional MRI evidence for adult motor cortex plasticity during motor skill learning. *Nature* **377**, 155–158.

Karni, A., Meyer, G., Rey-Hipolito, C., et al. (1998). The acquisition of skilled motor performance: Fast and slow experience-driven changes in primary motor cortex. *Proc. Natl. Acad. Sci. U. S. A.* **95**, 861–868.

Kim, S. G., Ashe, J., Georgopoulos, A. P., et al. (1993). Functional imaging of human motor cortex at high magnetic field. *J. Neurophysiol.* **69**, 297–302.

Kleim, J. A., Barbay, S., and Nudo, R. J. (1998). Functional reorganization of the rat motor cortex following motor skill learning. *J. Neurophysiol.* **80**, 3321–3325.

Lafleur, M. F., Jackson, P. L., Malouin, F., Richards, C. L., Evans, A. C., and Doyon, J. (2002). Motor learning produces parallel dynamic functional changes during the execution and imagination of sequential foot movements. *Neuroimage* **16**, 142–157.

Laforce, R, Jr., and Doyon, J. (2001). Distinct contribution of the striatum and cerebellum to motor learning. *Brain Cogn.* **45**, 189–211.

Lee, L., Siebner, H. R., Rowe, J. B., et al. (2003). Acute remapping within the motor system induced by low-frequency repetitive transcranial magnetic stimulation. *J. Neurosci.* **23**, 5308–5318.

Lee, M., Reddy, H., Johansen-Berg, H., et al. (2000). The motor cortex shows adaptive functional changes to brain injury from multiple sclerosis. *Ann. Neurol.* **47**, 606–613.

Linker, R. A., Maurer, M., Gaupp, S., et al. (2002). CNTF is a major protective factor in demyelinating CNS disease: A neurotrophic cytokine as modulator in neuroinflammation. *Nat. Med.* **8**, 620–624.

Logothetis, N. K., Pauls, J., Augath, M., Trinath, T., and Oeltermann, A. (2001). Neurophysiological investigation of the basis of the fMRI signal. *Nature* **412**, 150–157.

Lotze, M., Braun, C., Birbaumer, N., Anders, S., and Cohen, L. G. (2003). Motor learning elicited by voluntary drive. *Brain* **126**, 866–872.

Loubinoux, I., Pariente, J., Rascol, O., Celsis, P., and Chollet, F. (2002). Selective serotonin reuptake inhibitor paroxetine modulates motor behavior through practice. A double-blind, placebo-controlled, multi-dose study in healthy subjects. *Neuropsychologia* **40**, 1815–1821.

Luria, A. R. (2000) "The Man with a Shattered World." Harvard Press, Cambridge.

Marshall, R. S., Perera, G. M., Lazar, R. M., Krakauer, J. W., Constantine, R. C., and DeLaPaz, R. L. (2000). Evolution of cortical activation during recovery from corticospinal tract infarction. *Stroke* **31**, 656–661.

Matthews, P. M., De Stefano, N., Narayanan, S., et al. (1998). Putting magnetic resonance spectroscopy studies in context: Axonal damage and disability in multiple sclerosis. *Semin. Neurol.* **18**, 327–336.

Matthews, P. M., and Jezzard, P. (2003). Functional magnetic resonance imaging. *J. Neurol Neurosurg. Psychiatry.* **75**, 6–12.

Merzenich, M. M., Kaas, J. H., Wall, J., Nelson, R. J., Sur, M., and Felleman, D. (1983). Topographic reorganization of somatosensory cortical areas 3b and 1 in adult monkeys following restricted deafferentation. *Neuroscience* **8**, 33–55.

Meyer, B. U., Roricht, S., and Machetanz, J. (1994). Reduction of corticospinal excitability by magnetic stimulation over the cerebellum in patients with large defects of one cerebellar hemisphere. *Electroencephalogr. Clin. Neurophysiol.* **93**, 372–379.

Mort, D. J., Malhotra, P., Mannan, S. K., et al. (2003). The anatomy of visual neglect. *Brain* **126**, 1986–1997.

Muellbacher, W., Richards, C., Ziemann, U., et al. (2002). Improving hand function in chronic stroke. *Arch. Neurol.* **59**, 1278–1282.

Neumann-Haefelin, T., and Witte, O. W. (2000). Periinfarct and remote excitability changes after transient middle cerebral artery occlusion. *J. Cereb. Blood Flow Metab.* **20**, 45–52.

Nudo, R. J., Jenkins, W. M., and Merzenich, M. M. (1990). Repetitive microstimulation alters the cortical representation of movements in adult rats. *Somatosens. Mot. Res.* **7**, 463–483.

Nudo, R. J., Milliken, G. W., Jenkins, W. M., and Merzenich, M. M. (1996a) Use-dependent alterations of movement representations in primary motor cortex of adult squirrel monkeys. *J. Neurosci.* **16**, 785–807.

Nudo, R. J., Plautz, E. J., and Frost, S. B. (2001). Role of adaptive plasticity in recovery of function after damage to motor cortex. *Muscle Nerve* **24**, 1000–1019.

Nudo, R. J., Wise, B. M., SiFuentes, F., and Milliken, G. W. (1996b). Neural substrates for the effects of rehabilitative training on motor recovery after ischemic infarct. *Science* **272**, 1791–1794.

Ogawa, S., Lee, T. M., Nayak, A. S., and Glynn, P. (1990). Oxygenation-sensitive contrast in magnetic resonance image of rodent brain at high magnetic fields. *Magn. Reson. Med.* **14**, 68–78.

Ogawa, S., Menon, R. S., Tank, D. W., et al. (1993). Functional brain mapping by blood oxygenation level-dependent contrast magnetic resonance imaging. A comparison of signal characteristics with a biophysical model. *Biophys. J.* **64**, 803–812.

Ogawa, S., Tank, D. W., Menon, R., et al. (1992). Intrinsic signal changes accompanying sensory stimulation: functional brain mapping with magnetic resonance imaging. *Proc. Natl. Acad. Sci. U. S. A.* **89**, 5951–5955.

Pantano, P., Iannetti, G. D., Caramia, F., et al. (2002). Cortical motor reorganization after a single clinical attack of multiple sclerosis. *Brain* **125**, 1607–1615.

Pariente, J., Loubinoux, I., Carel, C., et al. (2001). Fluoxetine modulates motor performance and cerebral activation of patients recovering from stroke. *Ann. Neurol.* **50**, 718–729.

Parry, A. M., Scott, R. B., Palace, J., Smith, S., and Matthews, P. M. (2003). Potentially adaptive functional changes in cognitive processing for patients with multiple sclerosis and their acute modulation by rivastigmine. *Brain* **126**, 2750–2760.

Pearce, A. J., Thickbroom, G. W., Byrnes, M. L., and Mastaglia, F. L. (2000). Functional reorganisation of the corticomotor projection to the hand in skilled racquet players. *Exp. Brain Res.* **130**, 238–243.

Penner, I. K., Rausch, M., Kappos, L., Opwis, K., and Radu, E. W. (2003). Analysis of impairment related functional architecture in MS patients during performance of different attention tasks. *J. Neurol.* **250**, 461–472.

Peterson, J. W., Bo, L., Mork, S., Chang, A., Trapp, B. D. (2001). Transected neurites, apoptotic neurons, and reduced inflammation in cortical multiple sclerosis lesions. *Ann. Neurol.* **50**, 389–400.

Pineiro, R., Pendlebury, S., Johansen-Berg, H., and Matthews, P. M. (2001). Functional MRI detects posterior shifts in primary sensorimotor cortex activation after stroke: evidence of local adaptive reorganization? *Stroke* **32**, 1134–1139.

Pineiro, R., Pendlebury, S., Johansen-Berg, H., and Matthews, P. M. (2002). Altered hemodynamic responses in patients after subcortical stroke measured by functional MRI. *Stroke* **33**, 103–109.

Plautz, E. J., Milliken, G. W., and Nudo, R. J. (2000). Effects of repetitive motor training on movement representations in adult squirrel monkeys: Role of use versus learning. *Neurobiol. Learn. Mem.* **74**, 27–55.

Pujol, J., Roset-Llobet, J., Rosines-Cubells, D., et al. (2000). Brain cortical activation during guitar-induced hand dystonia studied by functional MRI. *Neuroimage* **12**, 257–267.

Ramnani, N., and Matthews, P. M. (2003). Initial learning and subsequent remapping of arbitrary visuomotor associations: an fMRI study of feedback-specific activity during conditional motor learning. *Proc. Organ. Hum. Brain Mapp. http://11208.164.121.55//hbm2003,* 207. 2003.

Ramnani, N., Toni, I., Josephs, O., Ashburner, J., and Passingham, R. E. (2000). Learning- and expectation-related changes in the human brain during motor learning. *J. Neurophysiol.* **84**, 3026–3035.

Rao, S. M., Binder, J. R., Bandettini, P. A., et al. (1993). Functional magnetic resonance imaging of complex human movements. *Neurology* **43**, 2311–2318.

Reddy, H., Floyer, A., Donaghy, M., and Matthews, P. M. (2001). Altered cortical activation with finger movement after peripheral denervation: comparison of active and passive tasks. *Exp. Brain Res.* **138**, 484–491.

Reddy, H., Lassonde, M., Bemasconi, N., et al. (2000a). An fMRI study of the lateralization of motor cortex activation in acallosal patients. *Neuroreport* **11**, 2409–2413.

Reddy, H., Matthews, P. M., and Lassonde, M. (2000b). Functional MRI cerebral activation and deactivation during finger movement. *Neurology* **55**, 1244.

Reddy, H., Narayanan, S., Arnoutelis, R., et al. (2000c). Evidence for adaptive functional changes in the cerebral cortex with axonal injury from multiple sclerosis. *Brain* **123 (Pt 11)**, 2314–2320.

Reddy, H., Narayanan, S., Matthews, P. M., et al. (2000d). Relating axonal injury to functional recovery in MS. *Neurology* **54**, 236–239.

Reddy, H., Narayanan, S., Woolrich, M., et al. (2002). Functional brain reorganization for hand movement in patients with multiple sclerosis: Defining distinct effects of injury and disability. *Brain* **125**, 2646–2657.

Redecker, C., Wang, W., Fritschy, J. M., and Witte, O. W. (2002). Widespread and long-lasting alterations in GABA(A)-receptor subtypes after focal cortical infarcts in rats: Mediation by NMDA-dependent processes. *J. Cereb. Blood Flow Metab.* **22**, 1463–1475.

Riahi, F., Zijdenbos, A., Narayanan, S., et al. (1998). Improved correlation between scores on the expanded disability status scale and cerebral lesion load in relapsing-remitting multiple sclerosis. Results of the application of new imaging methods. *Brain* **121**, 1305–1312.

Rocca, M. A., Matthews, P. M., Caputo, D., et al. (2002). Evidence for widespread movement-associated functional MRI changes in patients with PPMS. *Neurology* **58**, 866–872.

Sahyoun, C., Floyer, A., Johansen-Berg, H., and Matthews, P. M. (2003). Towards an understanding of gait control: Brain activation during the anticipation, preparation and execution of foot movements. *Neuroimage.* **21**, 568–575.

Saini, S., de Stefano, N., Smith, S., et al. (2004). Altered cerebellar functional connectivity mediates potential adaptive plasticity in patients with MS. *J. Neurol. Neurosurg. Psychiatry.* **75**, 840–846.

Sakai, H., Hikosaka, O., Miyauchi, S., Takino, R., Sasaki, Y., Putz, B. (1998). Transition of brain activation from frontal to parietal areas in visuomotor sequence learning. *J. Neurosci.* **18**, 1827–1840.

Sanes, J. N., and Donoghue, J. P. (2000). Plasticity and primary motor cortex. *Annu. Rev. Neurosci.* **23**, 393–415.

Sanes, J. N., Donoghue, J. P., Thangaraj, V., Edelman, R. R., and Warach, S. (1995). Shared neural substrates controlling hand movements in human motor cortex. *Science* **268**, 1775–1777.

Seil, F. J. (1997). Recovery and repair issues after stroke from the scientific perspective. *Curr. Opin. Neurol.* **10**, 49–51.

Seitz, R. J., Huang, Y., Knorr, U., Tellmann, L., Herzog, H., and Freund, H. J. (1995). Large-scale plasticity of the human motor cortex. *Neuroreport* **6**, 742–744.

Seitz, R. J., Knorr, U., Azari, N. P., Herzog, H., and Freund, H. J. (1999). Visual network activation in recovery from sensorimotor stroke. *Restor. Neurol Neurosci.* **14**, 25–33.

Siebner, H. R., and Rothwell, J. (2003). Transcranial magnetic stimulation: new insights into representational cortical plasticity. *Exp. Brain Res.* **148**, 1–16.

Small, S. L., Hlustik, P., Noll, D. C., Genovese, C., and Solodkin, A. (2002). Cerebellar hemispheric activation ipsilateral to the paretic hand correlates with functional recovery after stroke. *Brain* **125**, 1544–1557.

Smith, K. J., and Lassmann, H. (2002). The role of nitric oxide in multiple sclerosis. *Lancet Neurol.* **1**, 232–241.

St. Lawrence, K. S., Ye, F. Q., Lewis, B. K., Frank, J. A., and McLaughlin, A. C. (2003). Measuring the effects of indomethacin on changes in cerebral oxidative metabolism and cerebral blood flow during sensorimotor activation. *Magn. Reson. Med.* **50**, 99–106.

Staffen, W., Mair, A., Zauner, H., et al. (2002). Cognitive function and fMRI in patients with multiple sclerosis: Evidence for compensatory cortical activation during an attention task. *Brain* **125**, 1275–1282.

Stoop, R., and Poo, M. M. (1996). Synaptic modulation by neurotrophic factors: Differential and synergistic effects of brain-derived neurotrophic factor and ciliary neurotrophic factor. *J. Neurosci.* **16**, 3256–3264.

Strens, L. H., Oliviero, A., Bloem, B. R., Gerschlager, W., Rothwell, J. C., and Brown, P. (2002). The effects of subthreshold 1 Hz repetitive TMS on cortico-cortical and interhemispheric coherence. *Clin. Neurophysiol.* **113**, 1279–1285.

Sun, X., Tanaka, M., Kondo, S., Okamoto, K., and Hirai, S. (1998). Clinical significance of reduced cerebral metabolism in multiple sclerosis: A combined PET and MRI study. *Ann. Nucl. Med.* **12**, 89–94.

Sutherling, W. W., Levesque, M. F., and Baumgartner, C. (1992). Cortical sensory representation of the human hand: Size of finger regions and nonoverlapping digit somatotopy. *Neurology* **42**, 1020–1028.

Taub, E., Miller, N. E., Novack, T. A., et al. (1993). Technique to improve chronic motor deficit after stroke. *Arch. Phys. Med. Rehabil.* **74**, 347–354.

Taub, E., Uswatte, G., and Elbert, T. (2002). New treatments in neurorehabilitation founded on basic research. *Nat. Rev. Neurosci.* **3**, 228–236.

Taub, E., Uswatte, G., and Morris, D. M. (2003). Improved motor recovery after stroke and massive cortical reorganization following constraint-induced movement therapy. *Phys. Med. Rehabil. Clin. North Am.* **14**, S77–91, ix.

Toni, I., Ramnani, N., Josephs, O., Ashburner, J., and Passingham, R. E. (2001a). Learning arbitrary visuomotor associations: Temporal dynamic of brain activity. *Neuroimage* **14**, 1048–1057.

Toni, I., Thoenissen, D., and Zilles, K. (2001b). Movement preparation and motor intention. *Neuroimage* **14**, S110–S117.

Trachtenberg, J. T., Chen, B. E., Knott, G. W., et al. (2002). Long-term in vivo imaging of experience-dependent synaptic plasticity in adult cortex. *Nature* **420**, 788–794.

Trapp, B. D., Peterson, J., Ransohoff, R. M., Rudick, R., Mork, S., and Bo, L. (1998). Axonal transection in the lesions of multiple sclerosis. *N. Engl. J Med.* **338**, 278–285.

Ungerleider, L. G., Doyon, J., and Karni, A. (2002). Imaging brain plasticity during motor skill learning. *Neurobiol. Learn. Mem.* **78**, 553–564.

Voogd, J., and Glickstein, M. (1998). The anatomy of the cerebellum. *Trends Neurosci.* **21**, 370–375.

Ward, N. S., Brown, M. M., Thompson, A. J., and Frackowiak, R. S. (2003). Neural correlates of motor recovery after stroke: A longitudinal fMRI study. *Brain* **126**, 2476–2496.

Weiller, C., Juptner, M., Fellows, S., et al. (1996). Brain representation of active and passive movements. *Neuroimage* **4**, 105–110.

Weiller, C., Ramsay, S. C., Wise, R. J, Friston, K. J., Frackowiak, R. S. (1993). Individual patterns of functional reorganization in the human cerebral cortex after capsular infarction. *Ann. Neurol.* **33**, 181–189.

Werhahn, K. J., Conforto, A. B., Kadom, N., Hallett, M., and Cohen, L. G. (2003). Contribution of the ipsilateral motor cortex to recovery after chronic stroke. *Ann. Neurol.* **54**, 464–472.

Werhahn, K. J., Mortensen, J., Kaelin-Lang, A., Boroojerdi, B., and Cohen, L. G. (2002). Cortical excitability changes induced by deafferentation of the contralateral hemisphere. *Brain* **125**, 1402–1413.

Werring, D. J., Bullmore, E. T., Toosy, A. T., et al (2000). Recovery from optic neuritis is associated with a change in the distribution of cerebral response to visual stimulation: A functional magnetic resonance imaging study. *J. Neurol. Neurosurg. Psychiatry* **68**, 441–449.

Witte, O. W. (1998). Lesion-induced plasticity as a potential mechanism for recovery and rehabilitative training. *Curr. Opin. Neurol.* **11**, 655–662.

Witte, O. W., Bidmon, H. J., Schiene, K., Redecker, C., and Hagemann, G. (2000). Functional differentiation of multiple perilesional zones after focal cerebral ischemia. *J. Cereb. Blood Flow Metab.* **20**, 1149–1165.

Wylezinska, M., Cifelli, A., Jezzard, P., Palace, J., Alecci, M., and Matthews, P. M. (2003). Thalamic neurodegeneration in relapsing-remitting multiple sclerosis. *Neurology* **60**, 1949–1954.

Xerri, C., Merzenich, M. M., Peterson, B. E., and Jenkins, W. (1998). Plasticity of primary somatosensory cortex paralleling sensorimotor skill recovery from stroke in adult monkeys. *J. Neurophysiol.* **79**, 2119–2148.

Yousry, T. A., Berry, I., and Filippi, M. (1998). Functional magnetic resonance imaging in multiple sclerosis. *J. Neurol. Neurosurg. Psychiatry* **64 Suppl 1**, S85–S87.

Index

Note: Page numbers followed by "f" denote figures; "t" tables.